AF327517

A. M. De Schepper (Editor)

Imaging of Soft Tissue Tumors

A. M. De Schepper (Editor)

F. Vanhoenacker
P. M. Parizel   J. Gielen (Coeditors)

Imaging of
Soft Tissue Tumors

Third Edition
with 411 Figures in 1158 Separate Illustrations
and 38 Tables

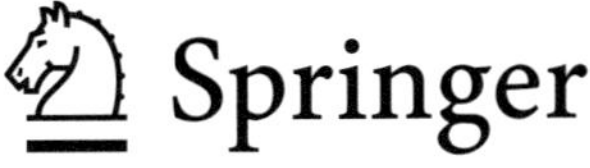 Springer

Arthur M. De Schepper, MD, PhD – Professor emeritus, University of Antwerp* –
Consultant-Professor, Leiden University Medical Center, The Netherlands
Filip Vanhoenacker, MD, PhD – Consultant-Radiologist, University Hospital, Antwerp*
Jan Gielen, MD, PhD – Staff Radiologist, University Hospital, Antwerp*
Paul M.Parizel, MD, PhD – Professor and Chairman, University Hospital, Antwerp*

* Department of Radiology, University Hospital of Antwerp
  Wilrijkstraat 10, 2650 Edegem, Belgium

ISBN-10 3-540-24809-0 Springer Berlin Heidelberg New York
ISBN-13 978-3-540-24809-5 Springer Berlin Heidelberg New York

ISBN-10 3-540-41405-3 Second Editon Springer-Verlag Berlin Heidelberg New York

Library of Congress Control Number: 2005930319

Springer-Verlag is a part of Springer Science+Business Media
springeronline.com
© Springer-Verlag Berlin Heidelberg 1997, 2001, 2006
Printed in Germany

Editor: Dr. Ute Heilmann, Heidelberg
Desk Editor: Wilma McHugh, Heidelberg
Cover design: Frido Steinen-Broo, EStudio Calamar, Spain
Reproduction and Typesetting: AM-productions GmbH, Wiesloch
Production: LE-TEX Jelonek, Schmidt & Vöckler GbR, Leipzig

Printed on acid-free paper   21/2152/YL   5 4 3 2 1 0

Preface of the Third Edition

The Belgian Soft Tissue Neoplasm Registry (BSTNR) is a multiinstitutional database project involving the cooperation of nearly all magnetic resonance imaging (MRI) centers in Belgium. This initiative, which was started in 2001, had two main goals. First, the BSTNR provided a second opinion report (within 48 h) as a professional courtesy toward all cooperating radiologists. Second, the BSTNR served as a scientific data bank of soft tissue tumors, which are rare lesions in daily radiological practice. All cooperating radiologists had access to the data of the register for use in clinical scientific studies. The scientific value of the BSTNR increased with the installation of a peer-review group of pathologists, all of whom shared a large amount of experience in soft tissue tumor pathology. They reviewed the pathological findings of all malignant tumors, all exceptional tumors, and all tumors in which there was a discordance between MRI and histopathological findings. They guarantee that the pathological standard remains "gold."

Until now we have included more than 1,500 histologically proven soft tissue tumors. This exceptional material constitutes the foundation of this third edition. We are grateful to all the coinvestigators of the BSTNR for their long-term contribution. We asked all coauthors to update their chapters with pertinent new data and images. We also asked them to respect the new World Health Organization classification of soft tissue tumors, which changed considerably in 2002, taking into account the usefulness of the classification for the radiologist. This implies that tumors have moved from one chapter to another according to their tissue of origin and their malignancy grade, e.g., the formerly named malignant fibrous histiocytoma, the synovial cell sarcoma, the hemangiopericytoma, and the solitary fibrous tumor. We also asked our coauthors to include at the end of their chapters a shortlist of striking features and a concise message to take home. The content of many chapters has changed substantially, e.g., the chapter on tumors of connective tissue, on pseudotumors, on biopsy of soft tissue tumors, and on posttreatment follow-up. The chapter on imaging strategy is tuned according to evolution of the MR technique and sequences. In the chapter on MRI, we omit the general principles of the method and focus on the sequences that are currently used in the study of soft tissue tumors. The index at the end of the book is better organized and more comprehensive. Finally we have added two new chapters, one on pathology and a second on molecular biology and genetics. We asked both authors to focus on those features that are most important to radiologists, who will be the main readers of this book. We are grateful to Springer-Verlag for giving us the opportunity to produce a third edition of a book on a radiological subject, which is a rather exceptional event.

Antwerp, March 2005   **Arthur M. De Schepper**

Preface of the Second Edition

At the time of writing, our group has had more than 10 years' experience in the imaging of soft tissue tumors. We are now, – more than ever, – convinced that a multidisciplinary dialogue between orthopedic surgeons, oncologists, pathologists and radiologists is imperative for the medical management of these lesions. The common goals of all specialists dealing with soft tissue tumors should be: early detection, minimally invasive staging and grading procedures, specific diagnosis (or suitably ordered differential diagnosis), guided percutaneous biopsies, and the most suitable therapy. This approach will guarantee the patient the optimal chances of survival with the best possible quality of life. To help us achieve these goals, we have established a Commission for Bone and Soft Tissue Tumors at the University Hospital in Antwerp, which convenes every 2 weeks. This multidisciplinary group formulates opinions and recommendations on diagnosis, prognosis, treatment and follow-up, and is highly valued by referring physicians. In addition, we are organizing a Belgian Registry of Soft Tissue Tumors with the cooperation of all Belgian centers in which MRI equipment is available and intend to invite students and investigators from all over the world to share our scientific interest in this fascinating field of medical imaging.

The main objective of this second edition of *"Imaging of Soft Tissue Tumors"* is to provide radiologists with an updated and easy-to-read reference work. This second edition includes new literature references and illustrations. Older illustrations have been replaced with higher quality images, generated by newer equipment and/or MRI pulse sequences. New tables organizing information into summaries have been included and the subject index has been updated. Most importantly, the text contains newer insights (for instance about fibrohistiocytic tumors), and reflects our own experience of increasing understanding of soft tissue tumors and their imaging. The chapter about magnetic resonance imaging has been shortened, and now focuses mainly on principles, pulse sequences and applications that are directly related to the examination of soft tissues and soft tissue tumors. We have included new chapters on "Soft Tissue Tumors in Pediatric Patients" and "Soft Tissue Lymphoma", and also a chapter on the controversial subject of (percutaneous) biopsy.

The readers and the reviewers of our book will judge whether we have succeeded in our objectives.

Finally, we would like to thank our editor and Mrs. Mennecke-Bühler at Springer-Verlag for sharing in the challenge of editing a second edition of this book on a rare pathology.

Antwerp, July 2001   **Arthur M. De Schepper**

Preface of the First Edition

Although the soft tissues constitute a large part of the human body, soft tissue tumors are rare, accounting for less than 1% of all neoplasms. The annual incidence of benign soft tissue tumors in a hospital population is 300 per 100000. Moreover, benign lesions outnumber their malignant counterparts by about 100 to 1. The clinical and biochemical findings of soft tissue tumors are frequently nonspecific. The first sign is usually a soft tissue swelling or a palpable mass with or without pain or tenderness. Laboratory results are frequently normal or show minimal nonspecific changes.

Until a few decades ago, detection of soft tissue tumors usually did not take place until late in the course of disease. This resulted from their low incidence and nonspecific clinical findings and from the poor sensitivity of conventional radiography, which was the only imaging technique available. Soft tissue tumors and soft tissue disorders in general were practically unknown to radiologists until the introduction of ultrasound and computed tomography (CT). Unfortunately, these methods suffered from inherent drawbacks, such as the poor specificity of ultrasound and the poor contrast resolution of CT.

Many of these problems were solved by the introduction of magnetic resonance imaging (MRI). Thanks to its high contrast tissue resolution and its multiplanar imaging capability, new horizons were opened for imaging soft tissues. Today, a correct assessment of disorders of bones, joints, or soft tissues is unimaginable without MRI.

In view of recent developments in surgery, radiation therapy, systemic chemotherapy, and regional perfusion techniques, the imaging of soft tissue tumors is gaining in importance. Correct diagnosis includes the detection, characterization, and staging of the lesions. The inadequate diagnosis and therapy of soft tissue sarcomas frequently results in tumor recurrence, necessitating major therapeutic "aggression." MRI is the optimal imaging technique for avoiding inadequate assessment.

Despite the interest of many groups of radiologists in the subject and despite the considerable number of overview articles that have been published in the radiologic literature, soft tissue tumors receive only minimal attention in modern state-of-the-art books on musculoskeletal imaging. Nevertheless, since all radiologists involved in the fascinating field of MRI are now confronted with tumoral pathology of soft tissues, there is a need for an illustrated radiologic guide on the subject.

From the beginning of our experience using MRI, back in 1985, we have been interested in soft tissue tumors. Our initial findings were discussed at an international congress in 1992. Conflicting findings in the literature concerning the sensitivity and specificity of MRI, which were mainly caused by the limited number of patients in published series, prompted us to start a multicenter European study. At the European Congress of Radiology 1993 in Vienna, 29 co-investigators from all over Europe agreed to participate (see the list 'Investigators of Multicentric European Study on Magnetic Resonance Imaging of Soft Tissue Tumors'). More than 1000 cases were collected, which constitute the basis of the radiologic work we prepared.

It was not our intention to write the 'all you ever wanted to know' book on soft tissue tumors. This objective has already been achieved for the pathology of soft tissue tumors by Enzinger and Weiss. Although their famous textbook contains a brief discussion of modern medical imaging, you will find it rarely on the office desk of radiologists. This present book is intended to serve as a reference guide for practising radiologists and clinicians seeking the optimal imaging approach for their patients with a soft tissue tumor.

The book is divided into four sections. In the first section we discuss the different imaging modalities and their respective contribution to the diagnosis of oft tissue tumors. As MRI is generally accepted to be the method of choice, there is a detailed theoretical description of this technique combined with a short discussion of imaging sequences. We also included a chapter on scintigraphy of soft tissue tumors, in which the current literature on the subject is summarized because scintigraphy was hardly used in our own patient material.

The second part deals with staging and characterization of soft tissue tumors and is concluded by a chapter on general imaging strategy. Tumor-specific imaging strategy is, where needed, added at the end of the tumor-specific chapters, which are collected in Part III. These chapters include a short description of epidemiology, clinical and pathological presentation, and a detailed discussion of imaging findings. For this Part, we used the classification of E.B.Chung (Current classification of soft tissue tumors. In: Fletcher CD, McKee PH (eds) Pathobiology of soft tissue tumors, 1st edn. Churchill Livingstone, Edinburgh, 1990, pp 43–81), which is an updated version of the most comprehensive system of classification, that of the World Health Organization. Because the illustrations originate from different institutions using different MR systems and pulse sequences, the figure legends only mention the plane of imaging (sagittal, axial, coronal), the kind of sequence (SE, TSE, GRE, ...), and the weighting (T1, T2).

The fourth part consists of only one chapter dealing with post-treatment imaging findings.

I would like to thank my co-editors Dr. Paul Parizel, Dr. Frank Ramon, Dr. Luc De Beuckeleer, and Dr. Jan Vandevenne, and all the coauthors for the tremendous job they have done. From this work I learned that writing a good book requires a sabaticcal leave, which good fortune I did not have.

As previously mentioned, it has been possible to include many of the illustrations shown in the book only because of the cooperation of the 29 European investigators, to whom I owe my gratitude. We gratefully acknowledge the support of Prof. Eric Van Marck, pathologist at our institution, for reviewing the manuscript, and of Ingrid Van der Heyden (secretary) for her aid in preparing so many chapters.

Finally, I wish to express my gratitude to Springer-Verlag and to Dr. Ute Heilmann for sharing the challenge of preparing this book with us.

Antwerp, June 1996   **Arthur M. De Schepper**

Contents

List of Contributors

J. Alexiou, MD
Department of Radiology, Institut Bordet
Rue Héger-Bordet 1, 1000 Brussels, Belgium

P.P. Blockx, MD
Department of Nuclear Medicine
Universitair Ziekenhuis Antwerpen
University of Antwerp
Wilrijkstraat 10, 2650 Edegem, Belgium

Johan L. Bloem, MD, PhD
Department of Diagnostic Radiology
and Nuclear Medicine
Leids Universitair Medisch Centrum (LUMC)
PB 9600, 2300 RC Leiden, The Netherlands

H. Bosmans, MD, PhD
Department of Radiology
Universitaire ziekenhuizen Leuven
Katholieke Universiteit Leuven
Herestraat 49, 3000 Leuven, Belgium

P. Bracke, MD
Department of Radiology, KLINA, Brasschaat
Augustijnslei 100, 2930 Brasschaat, Belgium

P. Brys, MD
Department of Radiology
Universitaire Ziekenhuizen Leuven
Katholieke Universiteit Leuven
Herestraat 49, 3000 Leuven, Belgium

L. Carp, MD
Department of Nuclear Medicine
Universitair Ziekenhuis Antwerpen
University of Antwerp
Wilrijkstraat 10, 2650 Edegem, Belgium

Ruth Ceulemans, MD
Department of Radiology
Northwestern Medical Faculty Foundation
676 North St. Clair Street South 800
Chicago, IL 60611, USA

A.M. Davies, MD
MRI Centre, Royal Orthopaedic Hospital
The Woodlands, Bristol Road South
Birmingham, B31 2AP, UK

L.H.L. De Beuckeleer, MD
Department of Radiology
Sint Augustinus Ziekenhuis
Wilrijk, Oosterveldlaan 24, 2610 Wilrijk, Belgium

H.R. Degryse, MD
Department of Radiology
KLINA, Brasschaat, Augustijnslei 100
2930 Brasschaat, Belgium

A. De Schepper, MD, PhD
Department of Radiology
Universitair Ziekenhuis Antwerpen
University of Antwerp
Wilrijkstraat 10, 2650 Edegem, Belgium

H. Garcia, MD
Department of Pathology
Hospitais da Universidade de Coimbra
Prac. Prof. Mota Pinto, 3000 Coimbra, Portugal

Jan Gielen, PhD
Department of Radiology
Universitair Ziekenhuis Antwerpen
University of Antwerp
Wilrijkstraat 10, 2650 Edegem, Belgium

K. Geniets, MD
Department of Radiology
Universitair Ziekenhuis Antwerpen
University of Antwerp
Wilrijkstraat 10, 2650 Edegem, Belgium

Timothy J. Hough, MD
Department of Diagnostic Imaging
Rhode Island Hospital
Brown University School of Medicine
593 Eddy Street, Providence, RI 02093, USA

S. Khan, MD
Department of Radiology
East Lancashire NHS Trust
Blackburn Royal Infirmary
Bolton Road, Blackburn
Lancashire, BB2 3LR, UK

Scott M. Levine, MD
Department of Diagnostic Imaging
Rhode Island Hospital
Brown University School of Medicine
593 Eddy Street, Providence, RI 02093, USA

M. Cristina Marques, MD
Department of Radiology
Hospitais da Universidade de Coimbra
Prac. Prof. Mota Pinto
3049 Coimbra, Portugal

L.L. Mortelmans, MD
Department of Diagnostic Radiology
Algemeen Ziekenhuis Middelheim
Lindendreef 1, 2020 Antwerp, Belgium

Parizel P.M., MD, PhD
Department of Radiology
Universitair Ziekenhuis Antwerpen
University of Antwerp
Wilrijkstraat 10, 2650 Edegem, Belgium

Ramon F., MD
Department of Radiology
Algemeen Ziekenhuis Maria Middelares
Hospitaalstraat 17, 9100 St.-Niklaas, Belgium

Roberto Salgado, MD
Department of Pathology
Universitair Ziekenhuis Antwerpen
University of Antwerp
Wilrijkstraat 10, 2650 Edegem, Belgium

Rodrigo Salgado, MD
Department of Radiology
Universitair Ziekenhuis Antwerpen
University of Antwerp
Wilrijkstraat 10, 2650 Edegem, Belgium

Avery A. Sandberg, MD, DSc
Department of DNA Diagnostics
St. Joseph's Hospital and Medical Center
350 West Thomas Road
Phoenix, AZ 85013, USA

P.C. Seynaeve, MD
Department of Diagnostic Radiology
MR Unit CAZK Groeninghe
Loofstraat 43, 8500 Kortrijk, Belgium

M. Shahabpour, MD
Department of Diagnostic Radiology
Academisch Ziekenhuis Vrije Universiteit Brussel
Laarbeeklaan 101, 1090 Brussels, Belgium

Richard M. Terek, MD
Department of Orthopedic Surgery
Rhode Island Hospital
Brown University School of Medicine
593 Eddy Street, Providence, RI 02093, USA

Glenn A. Tung, MD
Department of Diagnostic Imaging
Rhode Island Hospital
Brown University School of Medicine
593 Eddy Street, Providence, RI 02093, USA

L. van den Hauwe, MD
Department of Radiology, KLINA, Brasschaat
Augustijnslei 100, 2930 Brasschaat, Belgium

H.J. van der Woude, MD
Department of Radiology, O.L.V. Gasthuis Amsterdam,
Postbus 95500, 1090 HM Amsterdam

J.E. Vandevenne, MD
Department of Radiology
ZOL. St.-Jan
Schiepse Bos 6
3600 Genk, Belgium

P. Van Dyck, MD
Department of Radiology
Universitair Ziekenhuis Antwerpen
University of Antwerp
Wilrijkstraat 10, 2650 Edegem, Belgium

J.W.M. Van Goethem, MD, PhD
Department of Radiology
Universitair Ziekenhuis Antwerpen
University of Antwerp
Wilrijkstraat 10, 2650 Edegem, Belgium

F.M. Vanhoenacker, MD, PhD
Department of Radiology
University Hospital Antwerp
Wilrijkstraat, 10, B-2650 Edegem, Belgium

Marnix Van Holsbeeck, MD
Department of Diagnostic Radiology
Section Musculoskeletal Radiology
and Emergency Radiology, Henry Ford Hospital
2799 West Grand Boulevard, Detroit, MI 48202, USA

E. Van Marck, MD, PhD
Department of Anatomopathology
Universitair Ziekenhuis Antwerpen
University of Antwerp
Wilrijkstraat 10, 2650 Edegem, Belgium

C. Van Rijswijk, MD
Department of Diagnostic Radiology
and Nuclear Medicine
Leids Universitair Centrum (LUMC)
PB 9600, 2300 RC Leiden, The Netherlands

Koenraad L. Verstraete, MD, PhD
Department of Magnetic Resonance
MR, -1K 12 I.B., Ghent University Hospital
De Pintelaan 185, 9000 Gent, Belgium

Part 1
Diagnostic Modalities

Ultrasound of Soft Tissue Tumors

1

J. Gielen, R. Ceulemans, M. van Holsbeeck

Contents

1.1 Introduction

This chapter illustrates how ultrasound is currently used in imaging soft tissue tumors and also details the advantages and drawbacks of this modality.

In daily practice ultrasound is a powerful tool for differentiating a lot of benign tumors (neurogenic tumors, superficial lipoma) and tumor-like lesions (cysts, ganglia, scars, synovial chondromatosis, lipoma arborescens, etc.) from real tumors. Greyscale imaging, as well as (power) Doppler vascular imaging and dynamic interpretation plays an important role in the recognition of potentially malignant lesions. By differentiating benign from potentially malignant lesions, further diag-nostic and therapeutic work up may be reorientated in the majority of cases. Dynamic on-line interpretation of the examination is self-evident. Diagnosis on the basis of hard copies alone is erroneous. The use of ultrasound-guided aspiration (FNAB) or core biopsy (CNB) is emphasized and new applications described that are being developed in the field of dermatology. Specificity of ultrasound characterization of benign cases is higher than malignant cases. Thus the appearance of the most common, benign soft tissue tumors on ultrasound images is briefly discussed and documented.

1.2 General Principles

In the case of a peripheral, small to moderate-sized soft tissue mass, high-resolution (5–10 MHz) ultrasound can document the size and extent, intra- or extra-articular localization, and relationship to surrounding anatomical structures as well as magnetic resonance imaging (MRI). This holds true for the skin and hypodermis, neck, all peripheral joints, and especially for the wrist, hand, and fingers [31, 32, 71, 73]. Despite new developments with extended field of view (panoramic ultrasound), ultrasound has no role, however, in the staging of large, primary soft tissue sarcomas and bone tumors with soft tissue extension. In this setting magnetic resonance is the imaging modality of choice.

For the purpose of grading, ultrasound-guided biopsy can provide samples for histological and immunohistochemical diagnosis [30, 83]. This applies to soft tissue tumors, as well as to bone tumors with marked extraosseous tumor extension.

Malignant soft tissue tumors are rare; the majority of presenting soft tissue swellings are benign in character [43]. Even if this benign character is already clinically suspected, ultrasound can be used to reassure the patient and the referring physician that this is indeed the case, and thereby obviate the need for further (imaging) workup. If malignancy is suspected, on the other hand, ultrasound can be used to guide an 18- up to 14-gauge (automated gun or Tru-Cut) core biopsy (CNB). Since tissue sampling can be guided by ultrasound to avoid areas of hemorrhage and tumor necrosis, a high-yield solid component is possible [37, 82, 83]. The constant real-time visualization of the needle-tip position that is available on ultrasound images may shorten the procedure time considerably, in contrast to computed tomography (CT) and MRI [17].

The advantages of ultrasound over MRI are its low cost and availability at short notice: an ultrasound examination can often be performed the same day or within a few days of the outpatient's initial visit. One advantage over CT is the lack of radiation exposure.

The drawback of ultrasound is its poor specificity in defining the tumor's histological nature. Most benign tumors, sarcomas, lymphomas, nerve tumors, and benign and malignant skin lesions are hypoechoic, solid soft-tissue masses [17, 31, 37, 62, 79]. Additionally, the appearance of a given soft tissue tumor may vary on ultrasound images, e.g., cystic hygroma, skeletal muscle hemangioma, lipoma, melanoma [31, 32, 72].

Ultrasound criteria that suggest malignancy are nonhomogeneous echotexture and architectural distortion due to infiltration of adjacent structures (Fig. 1.1). Benign tumors are more likely to posses a homogeneous echotexture and regular delineation and to displace rather than to invade adjacent structures [37, 79]. In reality, there is considerable overlap between these two groups. Benign tumors such as skeletal muscle hemangioma, neurofibroma, and schwannoma can present with features of poor delineation and nonhomogeneous echotexture, while sarcomas on the other hand often demonstrate sharply defined margins due to pseudocapsule formation [18]. If these sarcomas are small in size at the time of detection, the tumor necrosis that would result in nonhomogeneity on ultrasound images may not yet have occurred. Some lesions are, however, also characterized by their location, e.g., subungual glomus tumor and branchial cyst [32]. Color Doppler imaging and spectral Doppler analysis of soft tissue tumors is of limited value when differentiating benign from malignant tumors. If an organized vascular pattern is present, the tumor is more likely to be benign. Flow characteristics are not specific enough to be applicable in clinical practice [35] Resistive indices cannot be used to distinguish benign from malignant musculoskeletal soft tissue masses [47].

The best practical approach is to select lesions ultrasonographically that are confidently diagnosed as benign. To prevent delay in diagnosis, all other lesions are potentially malignant and have to be subject of further diagnostic workup by MRI and imaging-guided CNB in that order [10]. Benign lesions confidently diagnosed from ultrasound images are homogeneous cystic lesions with strong back-wall enhancement and sharp margins that do not show any vascular signal with power Doppler (at highest sensitivity). Careful ultrasound examination combined with clinical correlation may

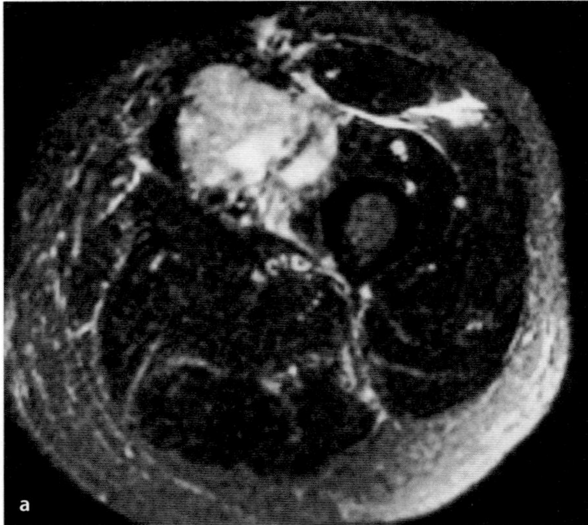
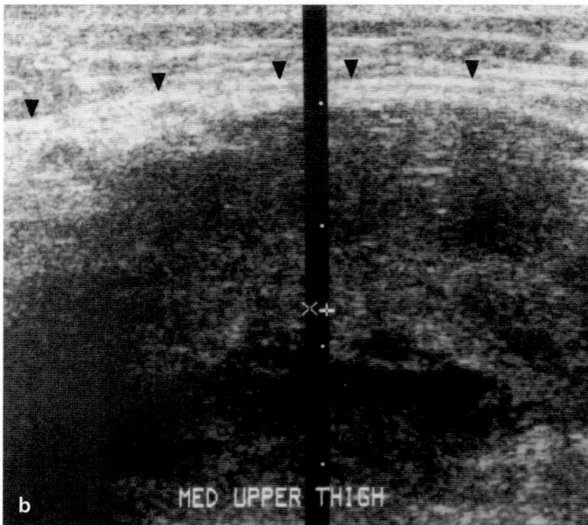

Fig. 1.1 a, b. Recurrence of myxofibrosarcoma in the proximal, medial aspect of the left thigh. **a** Axial, fat-suppressed, fast spin-echo T2-weighted MR image. **b** Longitudinal ultrasound image. Status after resection of vastus medialis muscle. Tumor recurrence in situ, invading the sartorius muscle and vastus intermedius muscles. Loss of fat plane delineation between predominantly intermediate signal intensity mass on fast spin-echo T2-weighted MR image and the superficial femoral neurovascular bundle (**a**). Ill-defined, nodular, solid soft tissue mass causing bulging of fascia lata (*arrowheads*). Inhomogeneous echotexture with deep anechoic component (**b**). Fine-needle aspiration and Tru-Cut biopsy confirmed tumor recurrence

suggest a specific diagnosis in the case of a sebaceous cyst (Fig. 1.2), a lipoma, or, in the presence of a phlebolith, a skeletal muscle hemangioma [71, 79]. Also, in patients with an initial diagnosis of hematoma or muscle tear, it is important that an accurate history is taken. A hematoma does not arise spontaneously, except in patients with a coagulation disorder or who are on anticoagulation medication. Hematomas do not keep on growing, and they are caused by trauma, usually quite severe trauma.

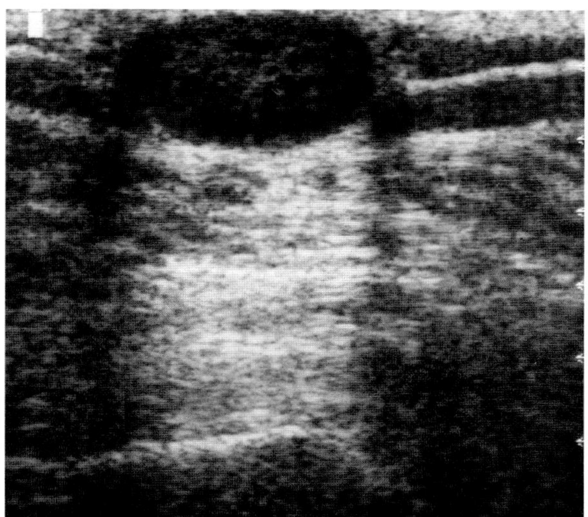

Fig. 1.2. Sebaceous cyst. Transverse ultrasound image. The subcutaneous localization, marked posterior acoustic enhancement, and edge shadowing are highly specific for sebaceous cysts

The trade-off for high-frequency, linear, musculoskeletal transducers is their limited depth of penetration and the small, static scan field. This is a disadvantage if the soft tissue swelling is large, if it is localized deep in the flexor compartment of the calf, the proximal thigh, buttocks, or trunk, or if the patient is heavily built. Extended field-of-view sonography (EFOVS) overcomes the disadvantage of a limited, standard field of view. By generating a panoramic image, it better displays size and anatomical spatial relationships of a soft tissue mass. It is beneficial in communication of imaging findings to the referring clinician. The reproducibility of the examination also improves. This allows for better evaluation of change in progress studies [3, 53, 80]. If EFOVS is unavailable, ultrasound is not the preferred imaging modality due to its lack of overview and penetration, and MRI should be used for the first examination [6]. These characteristics of high-frequency transducers turn into benefits, however, when it comes to diagnosing very small lesions in the wrist, hand and foot, and lesions of skin and peripheral neural origin. The scanning plane can be easily adjusted to the complicated local anatomy in the hand, wrist, and foot. Magnetic resonance coils of different shapes and sizes are not necessary.

More recent applications of ultrasound in soft tissue tumor imaging are ultrasound-guided interventional procedures, staging, and grading of dermatological lesions. Diagnostic procedures and therapeutic interventions that are guided by ultrasound are gaining in popularity in the musculoskeletal subdiscipline, following the already more established use of this technique in mammography and the abdominal-genitourinary field.

Percutaneous interventions range from ganglion aspiration (18–22 gauge), fine-needle aspiration biopsy (FNAB), in suspected local recurrence of a soft tissue sarcoma, core needle biopsy (CNB) of extra- and intra-articular solid soft tissue masses, preoperative needle-wire localization of nonpalpable, and solid soft tissue and vascular tumors to aspiration and culture sampling of a fluid collection, percutaneous catheter drainage of subperiostal abscess and muscle biopsy in neuromuscular disease [8,9,13,17,39,54,69,70,83,]. The procedures can be performed after ultrasound selection of the approach (site, depth, and needle angulation) and subsequent skin marking or, better, under real-time ultrasound guidance (Figs. 1.3, 1.4) [17, 83].

In screening for nonpalpable subcutaneous metastases of melanoma and cancers of the lung, breast, colorectum, stomach, or ovary and for melanoma recurrences, 7.5-MHz linear array transducers can dynamically screen a wide area of the body [1, 25]. CT has been reported to underestimate the number of lesions [63]. Ultrahigh-resolution ultrasound (20 MHz) is being used in imaging of nodular and infiltrative epidermal and dermal lesions. The width of the field of view is 1.2 cm and the depth of penetration only 2 cm.

Although epidermal lesions are visible, accurate clinical assessment of their depth of extension is not possible. Dermal lesions are not always visible. Ultrahigh-frequency ultrasound is a sensitive tool in lesion detection and delineation of its deep margin. In the majority of lesions, it cannot differentiate malignant from benign lesions and will not obviate the need for biopsy [31]. Even with these ultrahigh-frequency transducers, the normal epidermis cannot be visualized. Exceptions are the sole of the foot and the hypothenar area. Hypodermis can be visualized as a hyperechoic layer.

In the detection of local recurrences of soft tissue sarcoma, MRI and ultrasound appear to be equally sensitive. Ultrasound is the most cost-effective method in the detection of early local recurrences of soft tissue sarcomas and should therefore be used for initial routine follow-up and guided biopsies [2]. The presence of a nonelongated, hypoechoic mass is considered ultrasound evidence of local recurrence [15].

Ultrasound may be inconclusive in the early postoperative period (3–6 months postoperatively), as inhomogeneous, hypoechoic masses may also represent hematoma, abscess, or granulation tissue. Ultrasound follow-up with comparison to a baseline study on MRI, both performed 4–6 weeks after surgery, can help differentiate in such cases. Ultrasound-guided FNAB and/or CNB represents a possible alternative. MRI diagnosis of a soft tissue tumor recurrence in the immediate postoperative period or after irradiation can be extremely difficult due to the diffuse, high signal intensity background in (fast) spin-echo T2-weighted images or postcontrast (fat-suppressed) spin-echo T1-weighted

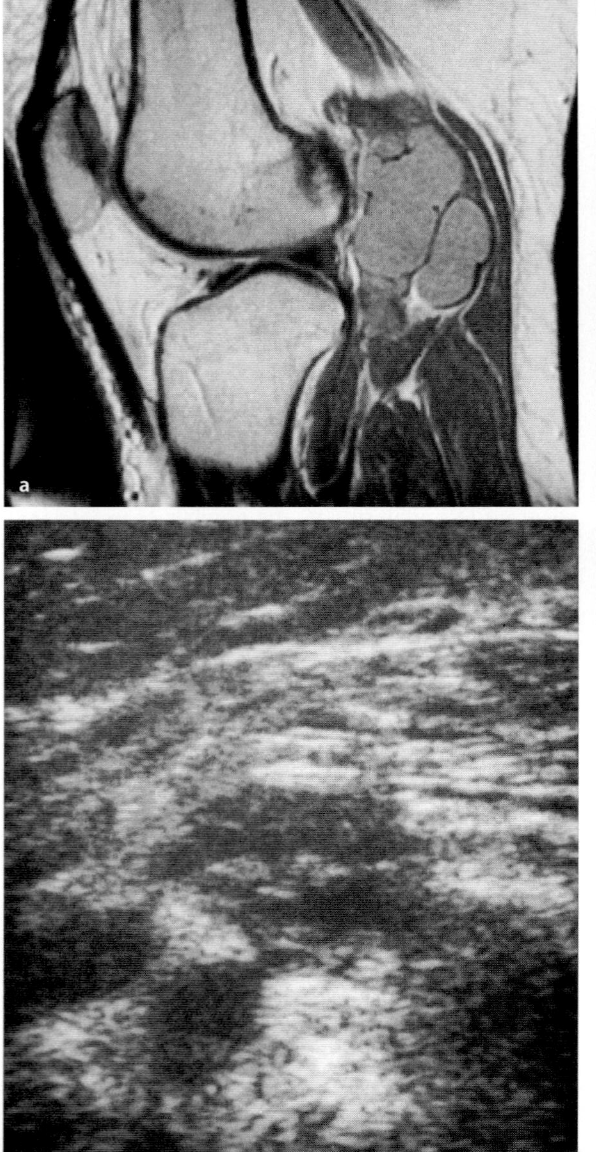

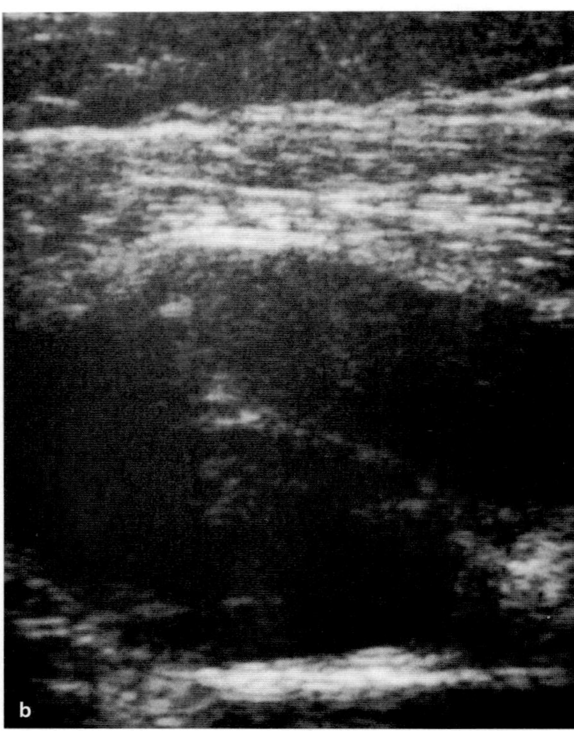

Fig. 1.3 a–c. Ganglion. **a** Sagittal fast spin-echo proton density-weighted MR image of left knee, immediately lateral to popliteal neurovascular bundle. **b** Longitudinal ultrasound image. **c** Longitudinal ultrasound image, following ultrasound-guided ganglion aspiration. A large ganglion (**a, b**), localized midline through lateral in the popliteal fossa, causes compression and displacement of the popliteal artery and vein. Two consecutive punctures (one lateral, one midline superficial) drained 16 ml of pale yellow, viscous ganglion content and resulted in near-total collapse and vascular decompression (**c**)

sequences. If the tumor recurs in poorly vascularized postoperative scar tissue, intravenous gadolinium contrast administration may have little effect in terms of tumor enhancement and thereby increased conspicuousness [15]. If scar tissue and recurrence cannot be differentiated, ultrasound-guided percutaneous biopsy should be considered [6, 15]. Under those circumstances the examination has prime prognostic and therapeutic value [83].

Obtaining a CT or an MRI time slot will be a practical problem in most institutions if the imaging-guided biopsy has to be performed at short notice. In an ultrasound-guided procedure, there will be no such problem. The technical crew to be mobilized may consist only of the ultrasound operator.

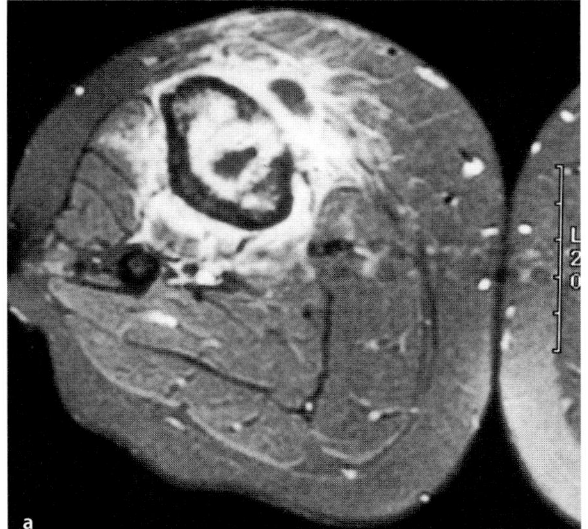

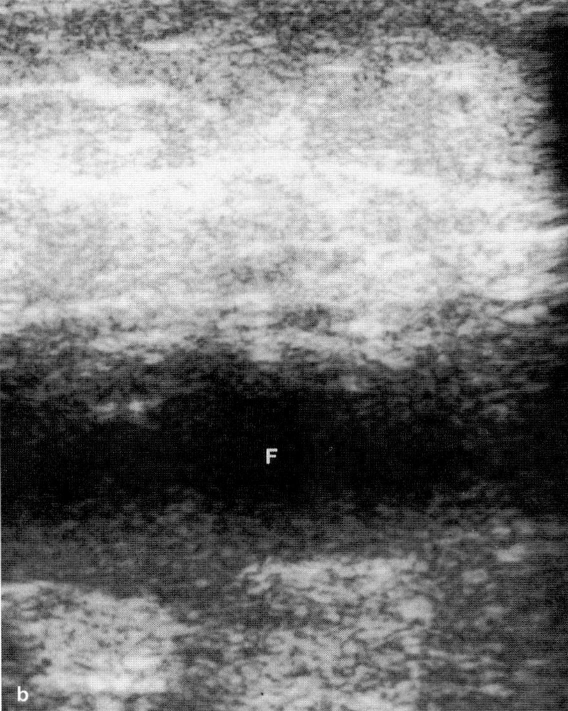

Fig. 1.4 a, b. Chronic osteomyelitis of right tibia with acute exacerbation. **a** Axial, fat-suppressed, spin-echo T1-weighted MR image after gadolinium contrast injection. **b** Transverse ultrasound image of subcutaneous abscess. The intraosseous and superficial soft tissue abscess can be identified as nonenhancing hypointense soft tissue structures (**a**). Ultrasound-guided fluid pocket (*F*) aspiration was performed (**b**). Culture yielded *Staphylococcus aureus*. Bacterial growth and culture sensitivity are crucial for adequate antibiotic therapy

1.3 Ultrasound Findings in Specific Soft Tissue Tumors of the Extremities

1.3.1 Synovial Soft Tissue Tumors

1.3.1.1 Synovial Osteochondromatosis or Synovial Chondromatosis

The condition known as synovial osteochondromatosis or synovial chondromatosis is a metaplastic transformation of synovial cells into cartilage. These cartilaginous nodules often calcify and/or ossify as nodules of equal size. Ultrasound is the imaging modality of choice when the disease is suggested by clinical examination or radiographs [61]. Both the purely cartilaginous and calcified nodules can be identified by ultrasound (Figs. 1.5, 1.6). Due to its dynamic scanning ability, ultrasound can also differentiate freely moving bodies from nodules embedded in synovium. Nodules may form an acoustic shadow front if calcified [58, 61, 67]. Synovial osteochondromatosis or chondromatosis is usually a monoarticular disease. Rarely bursae and tendon sheaths undergo synovial metaplasia.

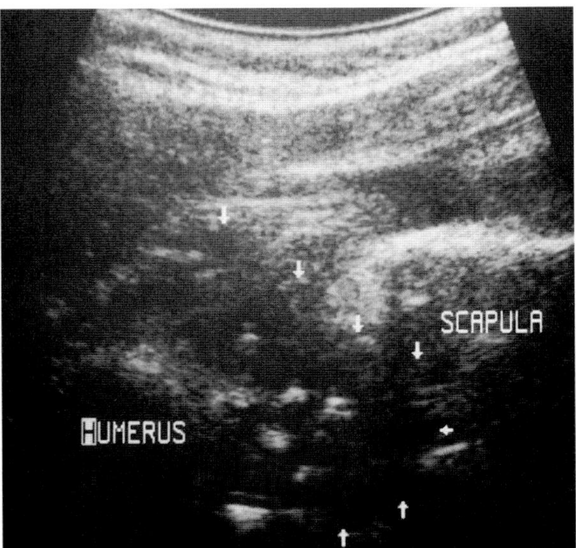

Fig. 1.5. Synovial osteochondromatosis of left shoulder joint in a 20-year-old woman. Transverse ultrasound image of the posterior, caudad aspect of the left shoulder (5-MHz curvilinear transducer). Marked distention of axillary recess (outlined by *small arrows*), filled with synovial proliferation. Embedded are multiple, equalsized cartilaginous bodies. Synovial proliferation was also noted in the infraspinatus recess and biceps tendon sheath (not shown). The biceps tendon sheath contained multiple, partially calcified, metaplastic nodules. The patient was treated by synovectomy

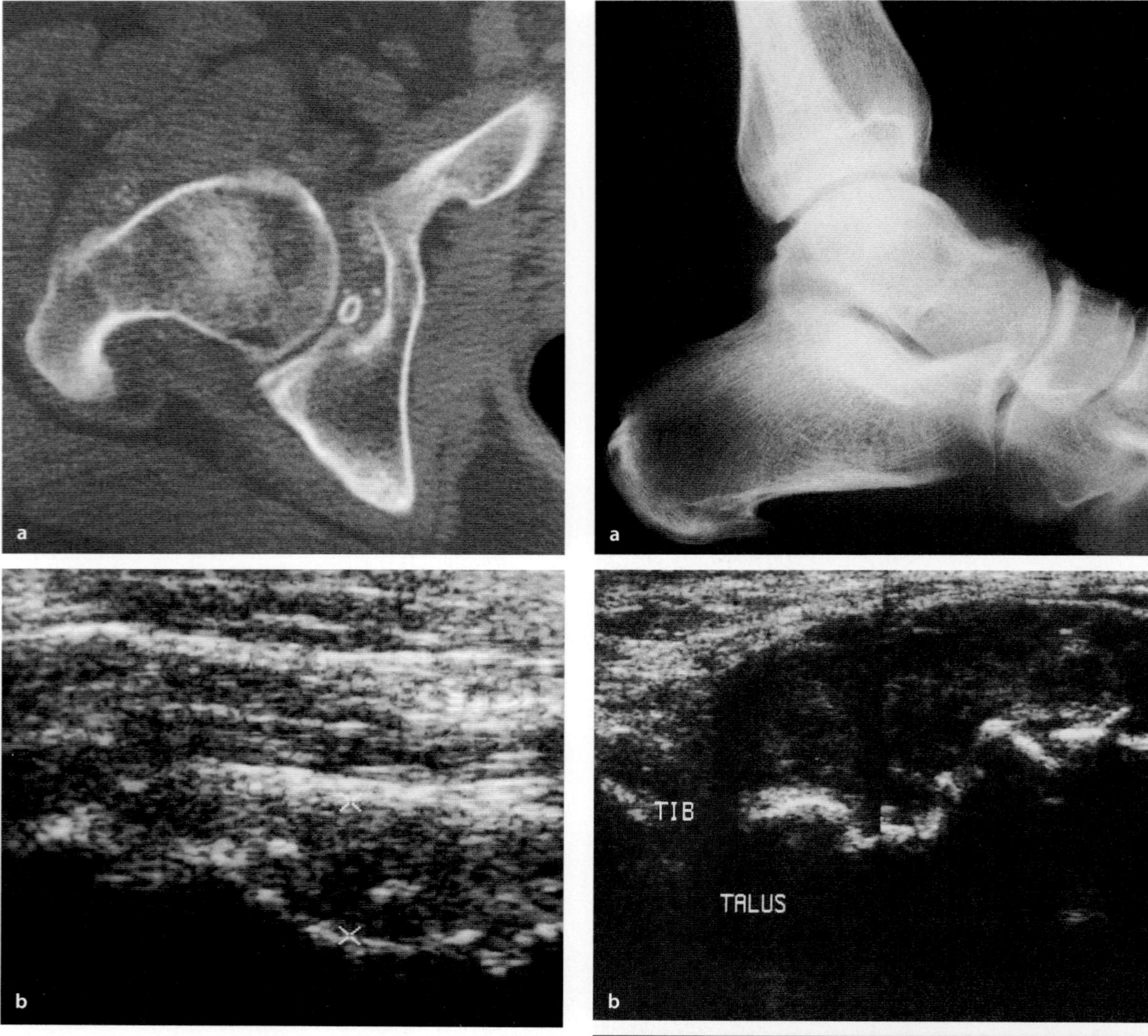

Fig. 1.6 a, b. Synovial osteochondromatosis of right hip joint in a 40-year-old white man with a 2-year history of right hip pain. **a** Axial CT scan section at tip of greater trochanter; bone window setting. **b** Longitudinal, anterior ultrasound image. One larger, peripherally calcified nodule and numerous small, faintly calcified nodules can be identified, predominantly in the medial and anterior joint space (**a**). Marked distention of the anterior hip joint space (**b**) (between calipers). Intra-articular synovial proliferation; two embedded metaplastic nodules. The most proximal, calcified nodule demonstrates posterior acoustic shadowing

Fig. 1.7 a–c. Pigmented villonodular synovitis (PVNS) involving the left talocalcaneonavicular joint in 47-year-old man. **a** Lateral radiograph. **b** Longitudinal ultrasound image of dorsum of hind foot. **c** Sagittal gradient echo T2-weighted MR image. Radiograph shows dense soft tissue mass along the dorsal aspect of talus and navicular, which contains a single calcification (**a**). Well-defined, inhomogeneous, but predominantly hypoechoic solid soft tissue mass. Minute anechoic foci and small hyperechoic areas are also present (**b**). Note secondary pressure erosion of the talar neck. The low-signal intensity, hemosiderin-laden soft tissue mass involves the talonavicular and communicating anterior and middle subtalar joint (**c**)

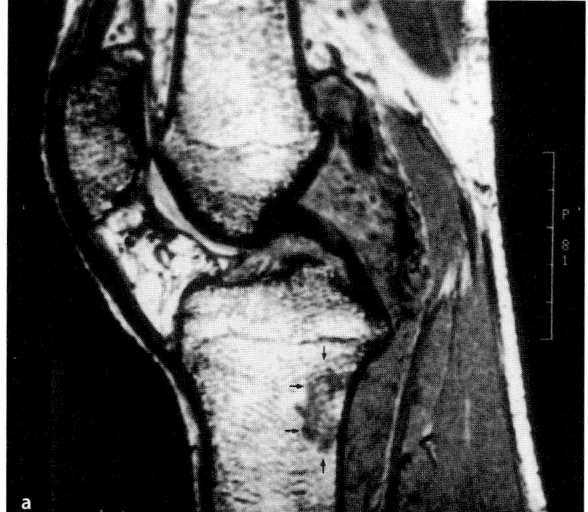

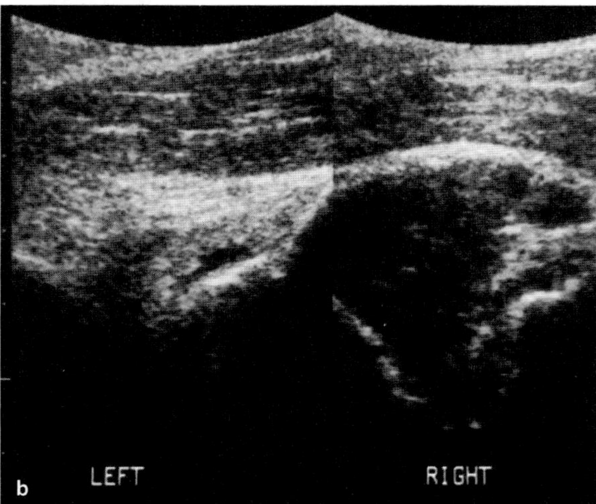

Fig. 1.8 a, b. Bifocal pigmented villonodular synovitis of right knee. **a** Sagittal gradient echo MR image. **b** Longitudinal ultrasound image; split-screen comparison view of dorsal femorotibial joint space. Marked distention of posterior femorotibial joint space, filled with soft tissue mass of intermediate signal intensity (**a**). Multiple foci of low signal intensity are present both in the deep and superficial dorsal aspect of the mass. Intraosseous tumor extension in the dorsolateral aspect of the tibial proximal metaphysis (**a**, *arrows*) is also noted. The symptomatic right side (**b**) shows a slightly inhomogeneous, predominantly hypoechoic synovial soft tissue mass, enveloping the posterior cruciate ligament insertion. The mass displaces the posterior capsule. A second tumor focus was localized in the medial aspect of the suprapatellar pouch and was biopsied

1.3.1.2 Pigmented Villonodular Synovitis

Pigmented villonodular synovitis (PVNS), also known as giant cell tumor when it affects the tendon sheath, is a benign inflammatory disorder resulting in diffuse or localized synovial hypertrophy.

In articular PVNS, ultrasound depicts hypoechoic synovial proliferation of variable thickness, affecting the entire synovial cavity or only a limited portion (Figs. 1.7, 1.8). Lobulated soft tissue nodules may pro-

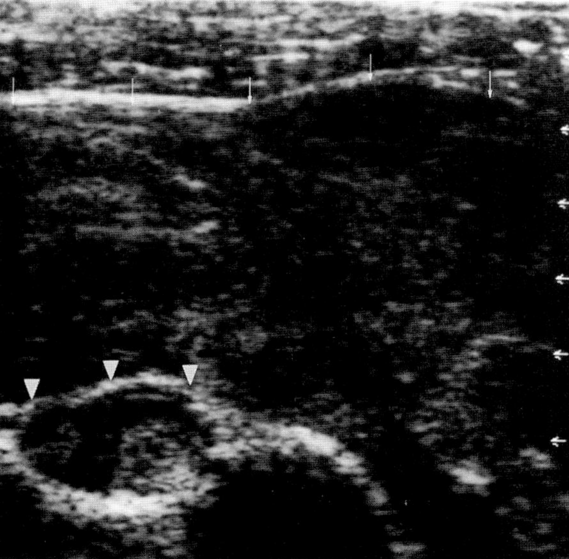

Fig. 1.9. Symmetrical amyloid shoulder arthropathy in multiple myeloma patient. Transverse ultrasound image of the anterior aspect of the shoulder. Marked distention of the subacromial-subdeltoid bursa (*arrows*) and the synovial tendon sheath of the long head of the biceps, causing anterior displacement of the transverse ligament (*arrowheads*). Mixture of predominantly hypoechoic and faintly hyperechoic synovial amyloid deposits

ject from the synovium into a hypoechoic or anechoic joint effusion, as a result of debris or hemorrhage. Loculations of joint fluid may be created by the synovial infolding [46].

Rheumatoid arthritis, seronegative inflammatory arthritis, hemophiliac arthropathy, and gout arthritis should be considered in the differential diagnosis of diffuse synovial hypertrophy on ultrasound images [46].

PVNS of the tendon sheath is a common tumor of the hand. Ultrasound depicts it as a well-defined, occasionally slightly nonhomogeneous or lobular, hypoechoic, solid soft tissue mass, abutting or eccentrically enveloping the tendon [28, 29, 41].

1.3.1.3 Amyloidosis

β_2-Amyloid arthropathy occurs in patients undergoing long-standing hemodialysis (more than 5 years) with cuprophane membranes and in patients with multiple myeloma.

The ultrasound parameters of shoulder amyloid arthropathy are enlargement of the rotator cuff tendons (supraspinatus tendon larger than 8 mm in thickness, its normal range being 4–8 mm), focal intratendinous areas of increased echogenicity, distention of the glenohumeral joint space, the synovial tendon sheath of the long head of the biceps and the subacromial-subdeltoid bursa, irregularity of the humeral head, and abnormal fluid collections around the joint [48] (Fig. 1.9).

The capsular and articular or bursal synovial amyloid deposits have a slightly heterogeneous hypoechoic echotexture.

The ultrasound findings of a maximal rotator cuff thickness greater than 8 mm or the presence of hypoechoic pads between the muscle layers of the rotator cuff has a 72–79% sensitivity and 97–100% specificity for amyloidosis, in the setting of longstanding hemodialysis [12, 48, 56].

1.3.2 Peripheral Neurogenic Tumors

Large peripheral nerves of the extremities such as the sciatic, popliteal, ulnar and median nerves can be routinely identified by high- and ultrahigh-resolution real-time ultrasound [23, 33, 41, 74]. In a high-frequency ultrasound examination, also smaller superficial peripheral normal nerves can be identified as a hyperechoic, fascicular soft tissue structure in its course between muscle bellies [16]. The configuration is concentric in transverse section and oval or tubular on longitudinal view. Occasionally, an internal punctate architecture can be seen on transverse section. Ultrahigh-frequency transducers show an alternating pattern of hypo- and hyperechogenicity. The parallel-oriented, but discontinuous, linear hypoechoic areas represent coalescing bundles of neuronal fascicles, embedded in a hyperechoic background of connective tissue, called epineurium. Ultrasound underestimates the number of neuronal fascicles, when compared with histological sections. Presumed explanations are the undulating neural course and its resultant obliquity and lateral deformation. With the use of lower ultrasound frequencies, the hypoechoic areas within the nerve become less defined and less numerous as a result of degradation in image resolution [74]. The nerve remains immobile in comparison with its surrounding musculotendinous structures during (passive or active) dynamic examination. This is best visualized using longitudinal view. Of key importance in the diagnosis of a peripheral neurogenic tumor is recognition of the location along the peripheral nerve course.

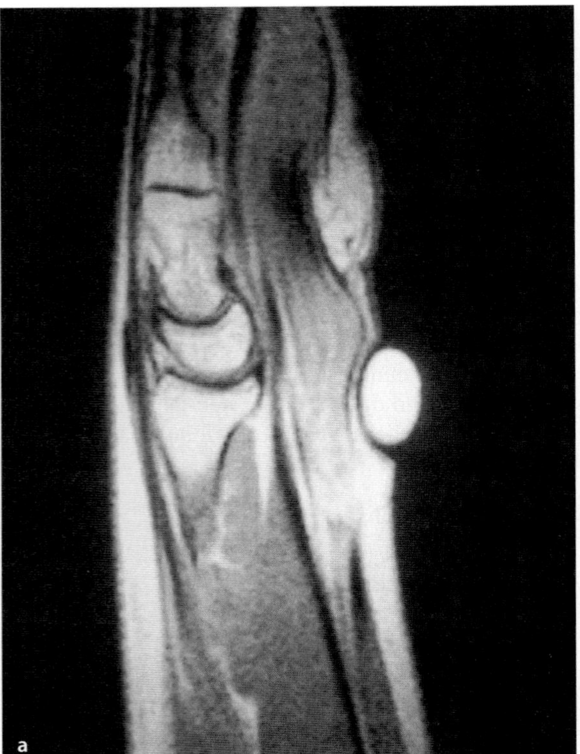

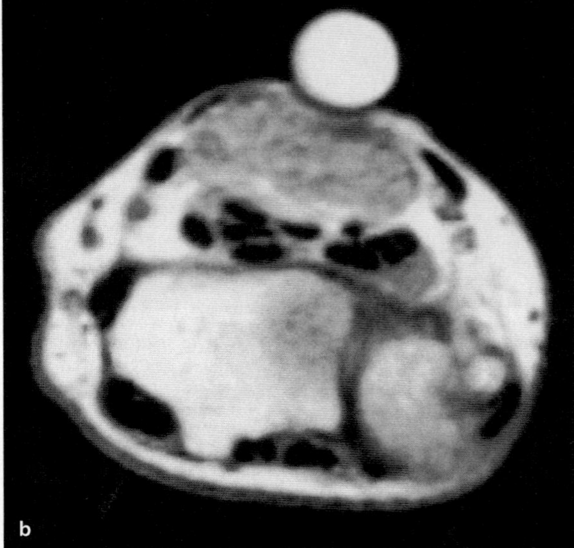

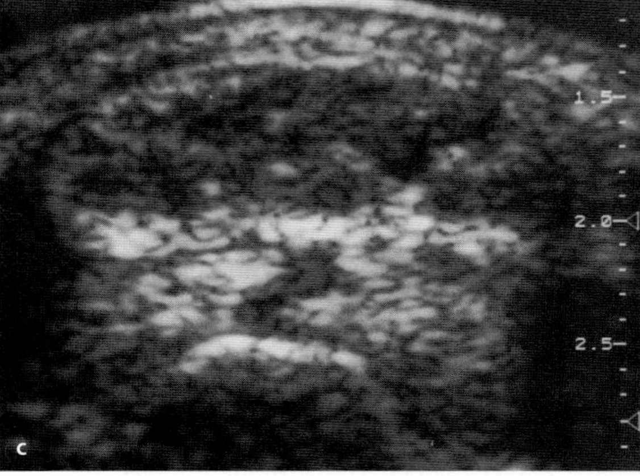

Fig. 1.10 a–c. Longstanding fibrolipohamartoma of median nerve in a 54-year-old woman. **a** Sagittal spin-echo T1-weighted MR image of the wrist. **b** Axial spin-echo T1-weighted MR image proximal to the carpal tunnel. **c** Transverse ultrasound image of carpal tunnel. Enlargement of the median nerve in the distal forearm (**b**), carpal tunnel (**c**), and metacarpus (**a**). The enlarged median nerve contains dot-like, thickened neuronal fascicles and some fatty tissue, especially in its deep aspect (**b, c**). The thickened bundles of neuronal fascicles are of intermediate signal intensity in (**a, b**) and hypoechoic in (**c**)

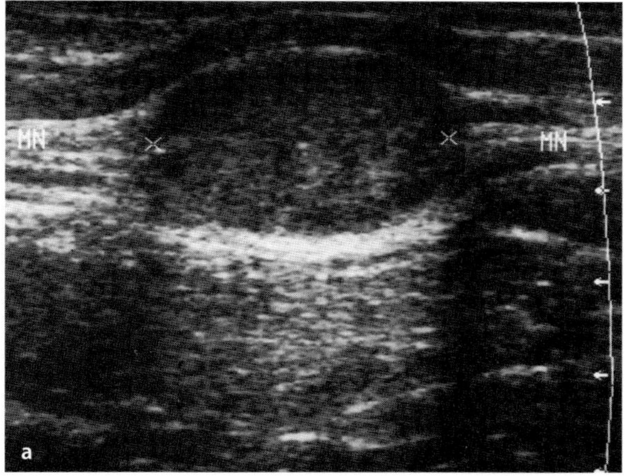

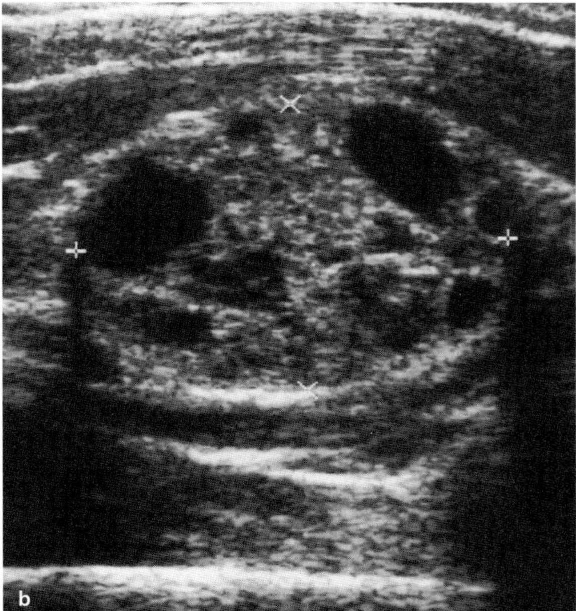

Fig. 1.11a, b. Schwannoma of median nerve in forearm. **a** Longitudinal, linear 5-MHz ultrasound image. **b**. Longitudinal, linear 7.5-MHz ultrasound image. The median nerve (MN) courses in and out of the well-defined hypoechoic nerve sheath tumor (**a**). The internal echotexture of the tumor drastically changes when the 7.5-MHz transducer is applied (**b**)

1.3.2.1 Nerve and Nerve Sheath Tumors

Tumors of peripheral nerves are rare, usually benign, and located subcutaneously. Ultrasound reports have documented schwannoma, neurofibroma, neural fibrolipoma (fibrolipohamartoma), and intraneural ganglion [4, 14, 19, 29, 40, 42, 50, 51] (Fig. 1.10). With the exception of intraneural ganglion and neural fibrolipoma, all these nerve-related tumors and tumor-like lesions were hypoechoic masses [14, 19, 22, 23, 40, 41, 42, 50, 51]. A plexiform neurofibroma was reported as an almost echofree mass with poor back-wall enhancement [66]. The majority of reported schwannomas and two neurofibro-

mas, both of them in von Recklinghausen's disease, showed posterior acoustic enhancement [14, 23, 42] (Fig. 1.11). A tarsal malignant peripheral nerve sheath tumor, arising at the site of multiple, postsurgical in situ recurrences of an initial schwannoma, showed poor delineation, homogeneous hypoechogenicity, and some dorsal acoustic enhancement.

Schwannomas and neurofibromas may show poorly defined contours [29, 40]. Some schwannomas and neurofibromas show intratumoral nonhomogeneity [59] (Fig. 1.11). The majority of reported schwannomas are well-defined, the majority of neurofibromas poorly defined.

Intraneural ganglion is a cystic, glue-like mass containing fluid and lined with collagen within the epineurium that may cause pain and motor dysfunction due to compression [50, 51]. Histological examination shows nerve fibers dispersed within the mucinous substance of the cyst. Most frequently the peroneal nerve is involved, with drop foot at presentation. Ultrasound shows a spindle-shaped anechoic soft tissue structure within or abutting the nerve course [50, 51].

These ganglia are common along the course of the suprascapular nerve in the shoulder [38, 76, 77, 78]. They invariably cause infraspinatus weakness and in some cases supraspinatus weakness as well. In the last 4,000 shoulder ultrasound studies we conducted, we recognized this entity in five patients. Two of them were cured by repetitive aspiration under ultrasound guidance.

1.3.2.2 Nerve-Related Tumor-like Lesions

In a reported tuberculoid leprosy of the external popliteal nerve [22], the well-defined hypoechoic mass proved surgically to be a caseous pouch. Within it, the thickened sheath of the enlarged lateral popliteal nerve could be identified as two parallel linear hyperreflectivities on longitudinal view.

Traumatic neuromas occur in postsurgical, postamputation, or posttraumatic patients [23, 29]. Traumatic friction or irritation of a nondisrupted nerve trunk as well as partial or complete transection of the nerve may induce this failed repair mechanism [75]. A traumatic neuroma is usually an ill-defined, hypoechoic mass.

Morton's neuroma represents focal perineural fibrosis involving a plantar digital nerve [52, 64, 65]. It occurs between the metatarsal heads and is quite common. Most commonly affected is the digital nerve of the third web space, followed, in decreasing order of frequency, by web spaces two, one, and four. Neuroma can be solitary or can simultaneously involve multiple web spaces. Bilateral lesions may also occur.

The neuroma is at least 5 mm in size in the majority of cases (95%). If greater than 20 mm in length, the interdigital mass should suggest an abnormality other than neuroma, such as a ganglion cyst, a synovial cyst, or a Giant cell tumor from an adjacent tendon sheath [64].

Middle-aged women are most commonly affected, and they typically complain of pain and numbness in the forefoot, elicited by ambulation and mediolateral compression of the forefoot, when narrow-toed shoes are worn. The normal plantar nerve is not sonographically detectable. However, in the presence of a neuroma, ultrasound can identify on longitudinal views the presumed plantar digital nerve coursing into the pseudotumoral mass. The abnormal, possibly edematous nerve is linear, 2–3 mm thick, and hypoechoic; its demonstration in continuity with the interdigital mass improves diagnostic confidence. Morton's neuroma is a predominantly well-defined but occasionally poorly defined soft tissue structure. The majority are hypoechoic masses, a minority demonstrate a mixed echo pattern or anechogenicity. They are shown poorly or are not seen to be vascularized on power color Doppler. A plantar transducer approach is preferred with imaging in both the longitudinal and the transverse plane. The correct transverse section should visualize the hypoechoic rim of cartilage covering the corresponding metatarsal heads.

Extreme flexion of the toes in the direction opposite the transducer or the Mulder maneuver (mediolateral compression of the forefoot and manual digital plantar displacement of the soft tissues in the examined web space, with the transducer applied to the sole of the foot), help in rendering the neuroma more superficial and allow it to be better appreciated [52, 64].

1.3.3 Vascular Tumors

1.3.3.1 Glomus Tumor

Glomus tumors originate from the neuromyoarterial glomus bodies and have a homogeneous, markedly hypoechoic or even sonolucent echotexture (Fig. 1.12). The most common site is the finger tip, although the tumor may occur everywhere. In the distal finger, the subungual space is more affected than the pulpar soft tissues [28].

Average lesion size is 6 mm, and lesions as small as 2 mm can be detected. Therefore, ultrasound investigation with at least a linear-array 10-MHz transducer is recommended. Although exquisitely tender to palpation, most lesions are not palpable as such.

Glomus tumor may have a flattened configuration when subungually localized and in that case may present as a less conspicuous, thickened hypoechoic subungual space. The normal subungual space is only 1–2 mm thick. If localized lateral to the nail bed or in

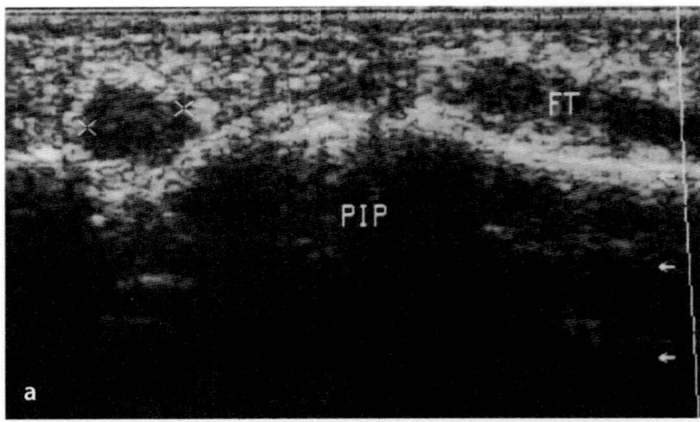

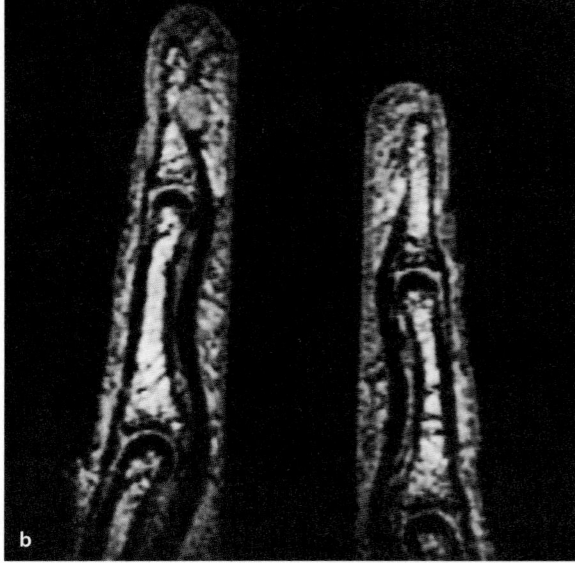

Fig. 1.12a, b. Glomus tumor of the distal phalanx of digit 3. **a** Longitudinal ultrasound image. **b** Sagittal gradient-echo MR image. Ultrasound identifies the 5-mm hypoechoic nodule (**a**, between calipers) along the palmar aspect of the tuft (FT). MRI depicts intermediate signal intensity tumor (**b**) causing pressure erosion of the underlying cortex

the palmar digital soft tissues, it assumes an ellipsoid or concentric shape [26]. These lesions show a marked (power) Doppler vascular signal, which equals the vascular signal of the normal nail bed. Differential diagnosis of a thickened hypoechoic subungual space should include angioma and mucoid cyst. Mucoid cysts can also present as small, concentric, hypoechoic solid soft tissue mass underlying the nail matrix [28].

1.3.3.2 Hemangioma, Angioma, and Vascular malformations

■ **Subcutaneous Hemangioma.** Subcutaneous hemangiomas usually present as hypoechoic soft tissue masses. Fornage has, however, reported two hyperechoic angiomas [26].

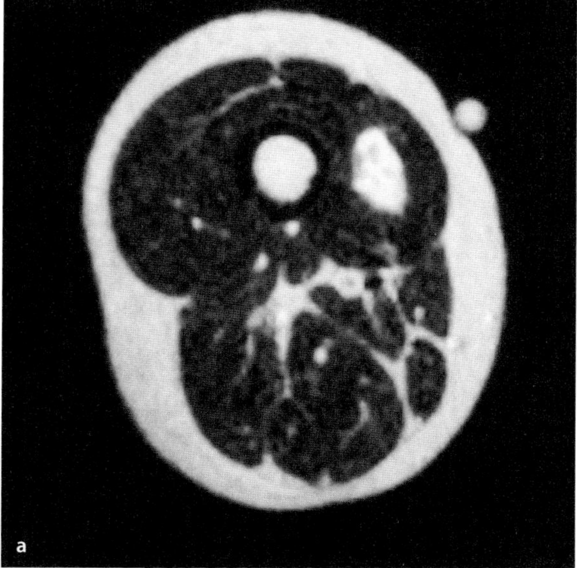

Fig. 1.13 a–c. Skeletal muscle hemangioma of vastus medialis muscle in young woman, who complained of swelling and vague pain. **a** Axial fast spin-echo T2-weighted MR image. **b, c** Transverse ultrasound images. Well-defined, inhomogeneous, high signal-intensity soft tissue structure in the medial vastus (**a**). A small amount of intratumoral fatty tissue was visualized on coronal, spin-echo T1-weighted image (not shown). Intramuscular, inhomogeneous, mixed hypo- and hyperechoic, partially ill-defined soft tissue mass (*arrows*) (**b**). The presence of a single phlebolith (*arrow*) within the mass confirms the diagnosis (**c**)

■ **Hemangioma of Skeletal Muscle.** Skeletal muscle hemangiomas are relatively common congenital vascular hamartomas and represent less than 1% of all hemangiomas. Patients are usually children, teenagers, or young adults, presenting with either a palpable, painful soft tissue mass or ill-defined muscular pain. The predilection site of skeletal muscle hemangiomas is the lower extremity [57].

An ultrasound examination readily detects the intramuscular soft tissue mass, which is well-defined in the majority of cases but may have an ominous ill-defined and irregular margin. There is no specific echo pattern; the majority of the reported muscle hemangiomas appear as homogeneous hyperechoic masses. However, both homogeneous hypoechoic lesions and mixed masses (Fig. 1.13) have been reported.

Ultrasound should not be the modality of choice to identify intratumoral phleboliths, but can readily appreciate them if they are large enough [21, 34] (Fig. 1.13). Intratumoral phleboliths are only present in 25% of cases.

Pressure erosion of underlying cortical bone can be visualized. One reported skeletal muscle arteriovenous hemangioma exhibited increased color flow and low-resistance arterial Doppler signal [34]. Venous, cavernous, capillary, and mixed hemangioma usually do not show any color or duplex Doppler signal due to the slow blood flow within the lesion.

Early experience with sonographically guided percutaneous injection of 1% polidocanol for sclerosis of peripheral vascular lesions shows that it is simple, effective, and safe. This technique is especially effective in cases of soft tissue venous malformation and lymphangioma [45].

1.3.3.3 Lymphangioma (Cystic Hygroma)

Lymphangiomas (cystic hygromas) are developmental benign tumors that are rare and result from a regional block in lymphatic drainage. Predilection site is the neck, although they can occur everywhere. Fifty percent of them are present at birth, and the majority are discovered by 2 years of age. Usually they are slow-growing, painless soft tissue masses; in other instances rapid

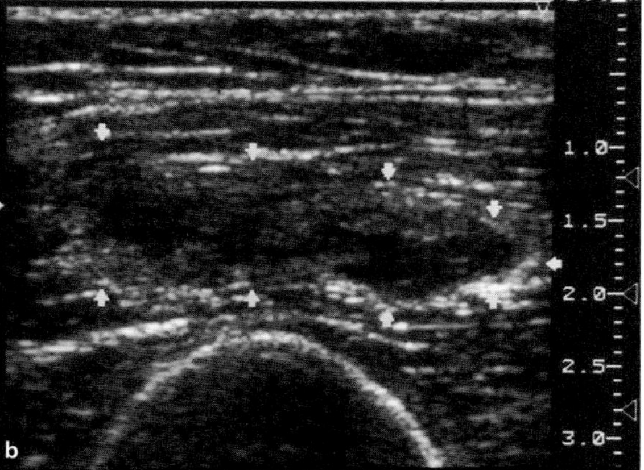

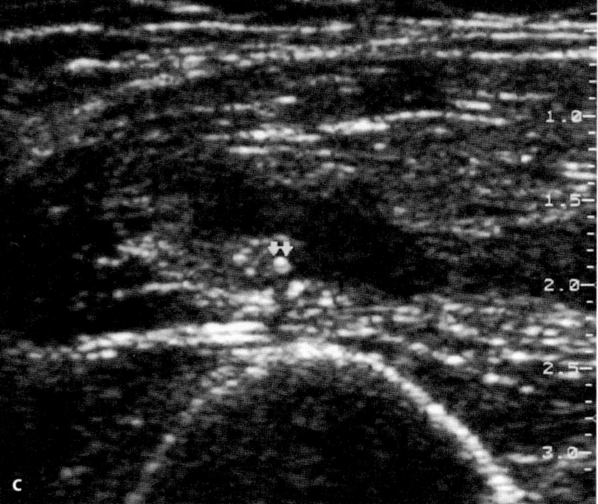

growth may occur due to intralesional hemorrhage or infection. These tumors are usually isolated findings, but can also be part of a syndrome.

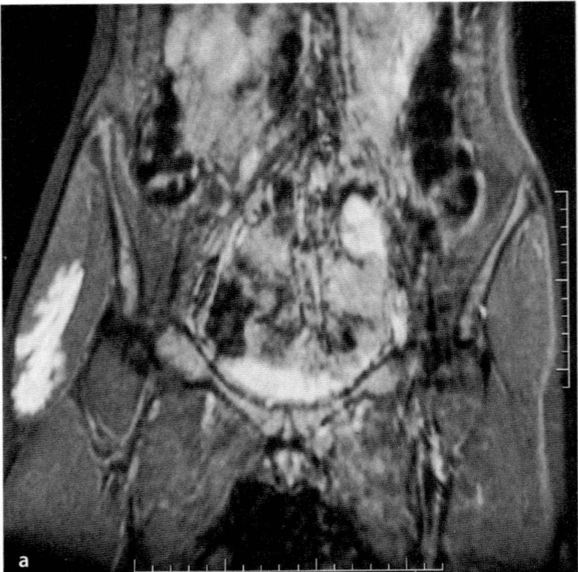

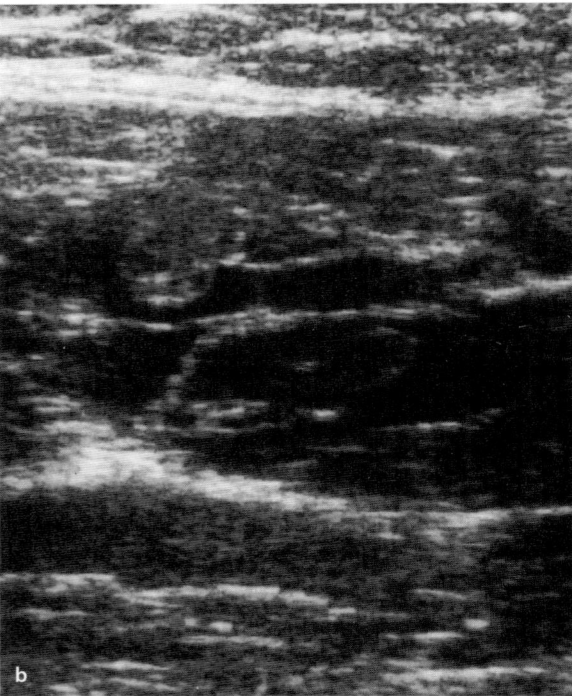

Fig. 1.14a,b. Lymphangioma of right gluteus maximus. The patient complained of swelling of right buttock and thigh when seated. **a** Coronal gradient-echo MR image. **b** Longitudinal ultrasound image. Intramuscular, tubular, hyperintense soft tissue structure (**a**). Septate, cystic, anechoic soft tissue mass (**b**)

Cystic hygroma is one of the three histological subtypes of lymphangioma, capillary or simple lymphangioma and cavernous lymphangioma being the other two. The three subtypes will often coexist within the same lesion. Cystic hygroma has a variable appearance on ultrasound images [49, 72]. It may present as a multiloculated, predominantly anechoic mass with through transmission and internal linear septations, which can

vary in thickness (Fig. 1.14). Cystic hygromas may also contain solid components arising from the cyst wall or septa, which pathologically correspond to abnormal lymphatic channels that are too small to be resolved. Less commonly, a complex, hypoechoic mass with a few internal, small cystic areas is visualized [49]. Occasionally, an organizing or calcified thrombus will be present in the mass. Larger lesions tend to be poorly defined. The cysts form along tissue planes and render complete resection difficult.

1.3.4 Lipoma

Lipomas have an elongated shape and most are oriented parallel to the skin surface [5, 27, 36, 62]. The echo pattern varies according to the number of internal interfaces between fat and connective elements [27]. In a series of 35 superficial lipomas studied by ultrasound, 29% were homogeneously hypoechoic, 29% were homogeneously hyperechoic, 22% were isoechoic, and 20% showed a mixed pattern (Fig. 1.15). The mixed pattern consisted either of intratumoral linear hyperechoic strands parallel to the skin surface or focal areas of hyperechogenicity.

Sixty-six percent of superficial lipomas are well-marginated, the remainder poorly defined [27, 62]. Occasionally a distinct echogenic capsule can be identified. Transverse diameter and shape of subcutaneous lipomas is variable with external compression; they are invariably avascular on power Doppler images. Intramuscular lipoma has a high postsurgical recurrence rate that results from incomplete resection due to lipomatous infiltration between muscle fibers, which is not fully appreciated when investigated by ultrasound. An elongated iso- or hyperechoic mass should suggest a lipoma, whereas a hypoechoic mass is associated with a broader differential diagnosis, including malignant tumor. Malignant masses, however, rarely have an elongated or flattened shape [27]. Superficially located lesions that are easily compressable, avascular, and with iso- or hyperreflective ultrasound texture compared with normal subcutaneous tissue are confidently characterized as lipomas on ultrasound examination. Diagnosis on the basis of hard copies alone is erroneous and may lead to underscoring of ultrasound as a diagnostic tool. This is demonstrated in a retrospective study by Inampudi et al. with sensitivies of only 40–52% and accuracies from 49 to 64% to differentiate lipomas from nonlipomas [44]. The major differential at the subcutaneous compartment is synovial sarcoma that, if bleeding components are present, may be compressed but is nonhomogeneous and hypervascular on power Doppler images. Also in lipomatous tumors, location is an important diagnostic criterion. Deep-seated lesions always need further diagnostic workup by MRI.

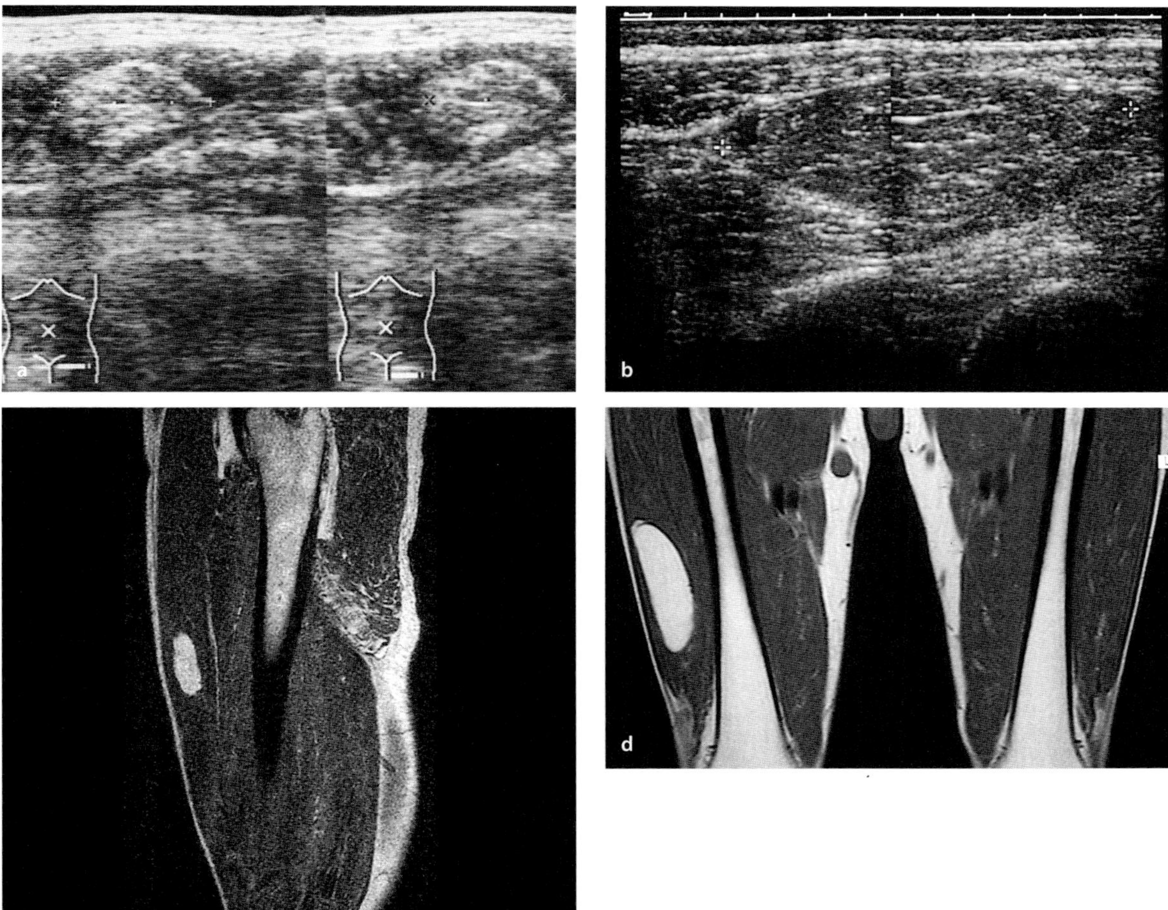

Fig. 1.15 a–d. Two cases of intramuscular lipoma of the thigh in a 57-year-old man (**a, b**) and in a 66-year-old man (**c, d**). **a** Ultrasound of the thigh. **b** Sagittal spin-echo, T1-weighted MR image. **c** Ultrasound of the thigh. **d** Coronal spin-echo T1-weighted MR image. Two examples of intramuscular lipoma showing a charac-teristic elongated shape and orientation parallel to the skin but with nonspecific reflectivity. One lesion is hyperreflective (**a**), while the other is hypo- to isoreflective (**c**) compared with muscle. On MRI both lesions show the same signal intensity as fat on all pulse sequences (**b, d**)

1.3.5 Ganglion Cyst

A ganglion is a well-defined, anechoic soft tissue structure with posterior acoustic enhancement which arises from a joint or is closely related to a tendon [7, 8, 60]. It may be loculated and contain internal septations. Anechogenicity, posterior acoustic enhancement, and sharp delineation cannot always be demonstrated in a small cyst [20]. The ganglion cyst wall is composed of compressed collagen fibers with flattened cells without evidence of an epithelial or synovial lining. The wall is usually thin and regular. In recurrent or long-standing lesions, a thicker wall and intraluminal echoes, thought to be caused by some degree of organization of the cystic fluid or particulate cholesterol crystals, can be visualized [76, 81].

In a minority of wrist ganglion cysts (27–30%), the communicating stalk with the joint of origin may go un-detected [11, 20]. No communicating duct has been documented so far in digital ganglion cysts [7, 68]. Ultrasound is equally as sensitive as MRI in the detection of occult dorsal wrist ganglion cysts, but it offers a slight advantage in differentiating between a small, compressible joint effusion and a small ganglion cyst which does not collapse under compression [11]. A frequent location is the dorsal and volar aspect of the wrist [29, 79], the finger, and the peroneal compartment [8, 11]. Dorsal wrist ganglion cysts predominantly arise from the scapholunate joint, with average size ranging between 3 mm and 3.5 cm. Volar ganglia usually extend superficially between the radial artery and flexor carpi radialis tendon and may arise from the radioscaphoid, scapholunate, scaphotrapezoid, or second carpometacarpal joint, in that order of decreasing frequency [8]. Aspiration followed by a short immobilization period is one method of conservative treatment [8, 20, 68].

1.3.6 Epidermoid Cyst

Epidermoid inclusion cysts are hypoechoic, relatively regular soft tissue tumors. They may contain small intralesional hyperreflectivities, presumably representing keratin clusters [29].

1.3.7 Sarcoma

1.3.7.1 Synovial Sarcoma

Synovial sarcoma is a misnomer. This lesion has no relation to joint or synovium. It is a rare, malignant mesenchymal tumor of unknown differentiation. Bleeding components are often present. The ultrasound appearance of this tumor is aspecific, as all malignant soft tissue sarcomas are, and may be easily confused with benign cystic lesions such as acute bursitis or organizing hematoma [55].

1.4 Conclusion

Ultrasound is an important imaging technique in the initial assessment of a soft tissue swelling. In the majority of cases, it will establish that the swelling is benign in character (e.g., in wrist ganglions, meniscal cysts, or tenosynovitis) and obviate unnecessary further imaging workup.

In soft tissue tumors in the wrist, hand, fingers, and skin and in peripheral nerve tumors, ultrasound imaging is superior to MRI by virtue of its small field of view and excellent anatomical depiction. The drawback of ultrasound is its nonspecificity in the setting of a hypoechoic solid soft tissue mass. In institutions without a biopsy-dedicated CT or MRI suite, ultrasound is the most accessible and least time-consuming modality for imaging-guided aspiration and biopsy.

> **Things to remember:**
> 1. Ultrasound is an important imaging technique in the initial assessment of a soft tissue swelling.
> 2. In the majority of cases, ultrasound will establish that the soft tissue swelling is benign (cystic) in character and obviate unnecessary further imaging workup.
> 3. The drawback of ultrasound is its nonspecificity in the setting of a hypoechoic, solid soft tissue mass.
> 4. Ultrasound is the most accessible and least time-consuming modality for imaging-guided aspiration and biopsy for superficially located lesions.

References

1. Alexander AA, Nazarian LN, Feld RI (1997) Superficial soft tissue masses suggestive of recurrent malignancy : sonographic localization and biopsy. Am J Roentgenol 169:1449–1451
2. Arya S, Nagarkatti DG, Dudhat SB, Nadkarni KS, Joshi MS, Shinde SR (2000) Soft tissue sarcomas: ultrasonographic evaluation of local recurrences. Clin Radiol 55(3):193–197
3. Barberie JE, Wong AD, Cooperberg PL, Caron BW (1998) Extended field of view sonography in musculoskeletal disorders. Am J Roentgenol 171:751–757
4. Beggs I (1997) Pictorial review: imaging of peripheral nerve tumors. Clin Radiol 52:8–17
5. Behan M, Kazam E (1978) The echographic characteristics of fatty tissues and tumors. Radiology 129:143
6. Bernardino ME, Jing BS, Thomas JL, Lindell MM, Zornoza J (1981) The extremity soft-tissue lesion: a comparative study of ultrasound, computed tomography and xerography. Radiology 139:53–59
7. Bianchi S, Abdelwahab IF, Zwass A, Calogera R, Banderali A, Brovero P, Votano P (1993) Sonographic findings in examination of digital ganglia: retrospective study. Clin Radiol 48:45–47
8. Bianchi S, Abdelwahab IF, Zwass A, Giacomello P (1994) Ultrasonographic evaluation of wrist ganglia. Skeletal Radiol 23:201–203
9. Braunstein EM, Silver TM, Martel W, Jaffe M (1981) Ultrasonographic diagnosis of extremity masses. Skeletal Radiol 6:157–163
10. Brouns F, Stas M, De Wever I (2003) Delay in diagnosis of soft tissue sarcomas. Eur J Surg Oncol 29(5):440–445
11. Cardinal E, Buckwalter KA, Braunstein EM, Mih AD (1994) Occult dorsal carpal ganglion : comparison of US and MR imaging. Radiology 193:259–262
12. Cardinal E, Buckwalter KA, Braunstein EM, Raymond-Tremblay D, Benson MD (1996) Amyloidosis of the shoulder in patiens on chronic hemodialysis : sonographic findings. Am J Roentgenol 166:153–156
13. Cardinal E, Chem RK, Beauregard CG (1998) Ultrasound-guided interventional procedures in the musculoskeletal system. Radiol Clin North Am 36:597–604
14. Chinn DH, Filly RA, Callen PW (1982). Unusual ultrasonographic appearance of a solid schwannoma. J Clin Ultrasound 10:243–245
15. Choi H, Varma DGK, Fornage BD, Kim EE, Johnston DA (1991) Soft tissue sarcoma: MR imaging vs sonography for detection of local recurrence after surgery. Am J Roentgenol 157:353–358
16. Chiou HJ, Chou YH, Chiou SY, Liu JB, Chang CY (2003) Peripheral nerve lesions: role of high-resolution US. Radiographics. 2003 23(6):e15. Epub 2003 Aug 25
17. Christensen RA, Van Sonnenberg E, Casola G, Wittich GR (1988) Interventional ultrasound in the musculoskeletal system. Radiol Clin North Am 26:145–156
18. Daly BD, Cheung H, Gaines PA, Bradley MJ, Metreweli C (1992) Imaging of alveolar soft part sarcoma. Clin Radiol 46:253–256
19. De Clercq H, De Man R, Van Herck G, Tanghe W, Lateur L (1993) Case report 814: fibrolipoma of the median nerve. Skeletal Radiol 22:610–613
20. De Flaviis L, Nessi R, Del Bo P, Calori G, Balconi G (1987) High-resolution ultrasonography of wrist ganglia. J Clin Ultrasound 15:17–22
21. Derchi LE, Balconi G, De Flaviis L, Oliva A, Rosso F (1989) Sonographic appearances of hemangiomas of skeletal muscle. J Ultrasound Med 8:263–267
22. Fornage BD (1987) Tuberculoid leprosy. J Ultrasound Med 6:105–107
23. Fornage BD (1988) Peripheral nerves of the extremities: imaging with US. Radiology 167:179–182
24. Fornage BD (1988) Glomus tumors in the fingers: diagnosis with US. Radiology 167:183–185
25. Fornage BD, Lorigan J (1989) Sonographic detection and fine-needle aspiration biopsy of nonpalpable recurrent or metastatic melanoma in subcutaneous tissues. J Ultrasound Med 8:421–424

26. Fornage BD, Rifkin MD (1988) Ultrasound examination of the hand and foot. Radiol Clin North Am 26:114–129

27. Fornage BD, Tassin GB (1991) Sonographic appearances of superficial soft tissue lipomas. J Clin Ultrasound 19:215–220

28. Fornage BD, Schernberg FL, Rifkin MD, Touche DH (1984) Sonographic diagnosis of glomus tumor of the finger. J Ultrasound Med 3:523–524

29. Fornage BD, Schernberg FL, Rifkin MD (1985) Ultrasound examination of the hand. Radiology 155:785–788

30. Fornage BD, Richli WR, Chuapetcharasopon C (1991) Calcaneal bone cyst: sonographic findings and ultrasound-guided aspiration biopsy. J Clin Ultrasound 19:360–362

31. Fornage BD, McGavran MH, Duvic M, Waldron CA (1993) Imaging of the skin with 20-MHz US. Radiology 189:69–76

32. Friedman AP, Haller JO, Goodman JD, Nagar H (1983) Sonographic evaluation of non-inflammatory neck masses in children. Radiology 147:693–697

33. Graif M, Seton A, Nerubai J, Horoszowski H, Itzchak Y (1991) Sciatic nerve : sonographic evaluation and anatomic-pathologic considerations. Radiology 181:405–408

34. Greenspan A, Mc Gahan JP, Vogelsang P, Szabo RM (1992) Imaging strategies in the evaluation of soft-tissue hemangiomas of the extremities: correlation of the findings of plain radiography, angiography, CT, MRI and ultrasonography in 12 histologically proven cases. Skeletal Radiol 21:11–18

35. Griffith JF, Chan DP, Kumta SM, Chow LT, Ahuja AT (2004) Does Doppler analysis of musculoskeletal soft-tissue tumours help predict tumour malignancy? Clin Radiol 59(4):369–375

36. Gritzmann N, Schratter M, Traxler M, Helmer M (1988) Ultrasonography and computed tomography in deep cervical lipomas and lipomatosis of the neck. J Ultrasound Med 7:451–456

37. Harcke HT, Grissom LE, Finkelstein MS (1988) Evaluation of the musculoskeletal system with ultrasonography. Am J Roentgenol 150:1253–1261

38. Hashimoto BE, Kramer DJ, Wiitala L (1999) Applications of musculoskeletal sonography. J Clin Ultrasound 27:293–318

39. Heckmatt JZ, Dubowitz V (1985) Diagnostic advantage of needle muscle biopsy and ultrasound imaging in the detection of focal pathology in a girl with limb girdle dystrophy. Muscle Nerve 8:705–709

40. Hoddick WK, Callen PW, Filly RA, Mahony BS, Edwards MB (1984) Ultrasound evaluation of benign sciatic nerve sheath tumors. J Ultrasound Med 3:505–507

41. Hoglund M, Muren C, Engkvist O (1997) Ultrasound characteristics of five common soft-tissue tumours in the hand and forearm. Acta Radiologica 38:348–354

42. Hughes DG, Wilson DJ (1986) Ultrasound appearances of peripheral nerve tumors. British J Radiol 59:1041–1043

43. Jacobson JA (1999) Musculoskeletal sonography and MR imaging. A role for both imaging methods. Radiol Clin North Am 37:713–735

44. Inampudi P, Jacobson JA, Fessell DP, Carlos RC, Patel SV, Delaney-Sathy LO, Holsbeeck MT van (2003) Soft-tissue lipomas: accuracy of sonography in diagnosis with pathologic correlation. Radiology 233(3):763–767. Epub 2004 Oct 14

45. Jain R, Bandhu S, Sawhney S, Mittal R (2002) Sonographically guided percutaneous sclerosis using 1% polidocanol in the treatment of vascular malformations. J Clin Ultrasound 30(7):416–423

46. Kaufman RA, Towbin RB, Babcock DS, Crawford AH (1982) Arthrosonography in the diagnosis of pigmented villonodular synovitis. Am J Roentgenol 139:396–398

47. Kaushik S, Miller TT, Nazarian LN, Foster WC (2003) Spectral Doppler sonography of musculoskeletal soft tissue masses. J Ultrasound Med 22(12):1333–1336

48. Kay J, Benson CB, Lester S, Corson JM, Pinkus GS, Lazarus JM, Owen WF (1992) Utility of high-resolution ultrasound for the diagnosis of dialysis-related amyloidosis. Arthritis Rheum 35:926–931

49. Kraus R, Bokyung KH, Babcock DS, Oestreich AE (1986) Sonography of neck masses in children. Am J Roentgenol 146:609–613

50. Lang CJG, Neubauer U, Quaiyumi S, Fahlbusch R (1994) Intraneural ganglion of the sciatic nerve: detection by ultrasound (letter). J Neurol Neurosurg Psychiatry 57:870–871

51. Leijten FS, Arts WF, Puylaert JBC (1992) Ultrasound diagnosis of an intraneural ganglion cyst of the peroneal nerve. J Neurosurg 76:538–540

52. Levey DS, Park YH, Sartoris DJ (1995) Radiologic review: imaging of pedal soft tissue neoplasms. J Foot Ankle Surg 34 413–415

53. Lin EC, Middleton WD, Teefey SA (1999) Extended field of view sonography in musculoskeletal imaging. J Ultrasound Med 18:147–152

54. Liu JC, Chiou HJ, Chen WM, Chou YH, Chen TH, Chen W, Yen CC, Chiu SY, Chang CY (2004) Sonographically guided core needle biopsy of soft tissue neoplasms. J Clin Ultrasound 32(6):294–298

55. Marzano L, Failoni S, Gallazzi M, Garbagna P (2004) The role of diagnostic imaging in synovial sarcoma. Our experience. Radiol Med (Torino) 107(5–6):533–540

56. McMahon LP, Radford J, Dawborn JK (1991) Shoulder ultrasound in dialysis related amyloidosis. Clin Nephrol 35:227–232

57. Morris SJ, Adams H (1995) Case report: paedriatic intramuscular haemangiomata – don't overlook the phlebolith! Br J Radiol 68:208–211

58. Moss GD, Dishuk W (1984) Ultrasound diagnosis of osteochondromatosis of the popliteal fossa. J Clin Ultrasound 12:232–233

59. Obayashi T, Itoh K, Nakano A (1987) Ultrasonic diagnosis of schwannoma. Neurology 37:1817

60. Ogino T, Minami A, Fukuda K, Sakuma T, Kato H (1988) The dorsal occult ganglion of the wrist and ultrasonography. J Hand Surg 13B:181–183

61. Pai VR, Holsbeeck M van (1995) Synovial osteochondromatosis of the hip: role of ultrasonography. J Clin Ultrasound 23:199–203

62. Pathria MN, Zlatkin M, Sartoris DJ, Scheible W, Resnick D (1988) Ultrasonography of popliteal fossa and lower extremities. Radiol Clin North Am 26:77–85

63. Patten RM, Shuman WP, Teefey S (1989) Subcutaneous metastases from malignant melanoma : prevalence and findings on CT. Am J Roentgenol 152:1009–1012

64. Quinn TJ, Jacobson JA, Craig JG, Holsbeeck MT van (2000) Sonography of Morton's neuroma. Am J Roentgenol 174:1723–1728

65. Redd RA, Peters VJ, Emery SF, Branch HM, Rifkin MD (1989) Morton neuroma: sonographic evaluation. Radiology 171:415–417

66. Reuter KL, Raptopoulos V, De Girolami U, Akins CM (1982) Ultrasonography of plexiform neurofibroma in the politeal fossa. J Ultrasound Med 1:209–211

67. Richardson ML, Selby B, Montana MA, Mack LA (1988) Ultrasonography of the knee. Radiol Clin North Am 26:63–75

68. Richman JA, Gelberman RH, Engber WD, Salamon PB, Bean DJ (1987) Ganglions of the wrist and digits: results of treatment by aspiration and cyst wall puncture. J Hand Surg 12A:1041–1043

69. Rowley VA, Cooperberg PL (1987) Ultrasound guided biopsy in interventional ultrasound. Clin Diagn Ultrasound 21:59–76

70. Rubens DJ, Fultz PJ, Gottlieb RH, Rubin SJ (1997) Effective ultrasonographically guided intervention for diagnosis of musculoskeletal lesions. J Ultrasound Med 16:831–842

71. Sherman NH, Rosenberg HK, Heyman S, Templeton J (1985) Ultrasound evaluation of neck masses in children. J Ultrasound Med 4:127–134

72. Sheth S, Nussbaum AR, Hutchins GM, Sanders RC (1987) Cystic hygromas in children: sonographic-pathologic correlation. Radiology 1987:821–824

73. Silvestri E, Bertolotto RP, Neumaier CE, Derchi LE (1994) Case report: US detection of tendinous metastasis from malignant melanoma. Clin Radiol 49:288–289

74. Silvestri E, Martinoli C, Derchi LE, Bertolotto M, Chiaramondia M, Rosenberg I (1995) Echotexture of peripheral nerves: correlation between US and histologic findings and criteria to differentiate tendons. Radiology 197:291–296

75. Singson RD, Feldman F, Slipman CW, Gonzalea E, Rosenberg ZS, Kiernan H (1987) Postamputation neuromas and other symptomatic stump abnormalities: detection with CT. Radiology 162:743–745

76. Skirving AP, Kozak TKW, Davis SJ (1994) Infraspinatus paralysis due to spinoglenoid notch ganglion. J Bone Joint Surg 76B:588–591
77. Takagishi K, Maeda K, Ikeda Toshiaki, Itoman M and Yamamoto M (1991) Ganglion causing paralysis of the suprascapular nerve. Acta Orthop Scand 62:391–393
78. Takagishi K, Saitoh A, Tonegawa M, Ikeda T, Itoman M (1994) Isolated paralysis of the infraspinatus muscle. J Bone Joint Surg 76B:584–587
79. Vincent LM (1988) Ultrasound of soft tissue abnormalities of the extremities. Radiol Clin North Am 26:140–143
80. Weng L, Tirumalai AP, Lowery CM, Nock LF, Gustafson DE, Von Behren PL, Kim JH (1997) Extended-field-of-view imaging technology. Radiology 203:877–880
81. White EA, Filly RA (1980) Cholesterol crystals as the source of both diffuse and layered echoes in a cystic ovarian tumor. J Clin Ultrasound 8:241–243
82. Wilson DJ (1989) Ultrasonic imaging of soft tissues. Clin Radiol 40:341–342
83. Zornoza. Zornoza J, Bernardino ME, Ordonez NG, Thomas JL, Cohen MA (1982) Percutaneous needle biopsy of soft tissue tumors guided by ultrasound and computed tomography. Skeletal Radiol 9:33–36

Color Doppler Ultrasound

2

H.-J. van der Woude, K.L. Verstraete, J.L. Bloem

Contents

2.1 Introduction

Ultrasound (US), being a readily available, noninvasive and relatively inexpensive imaging modality, plays a significant part in the diagnostic workup of soft tissue masses. Owing to the nonspecific sonographic characteristics of most soft tissue masses, the particular roles of US are to confirm the presence of a suspected lesion, and to identify its size, volume and configuration, to determine its internal characteristics, to guide percutaneous biopsy and, in selected cases, to monitor response to chemotherapy. Furthermore, it may help in differentiating a localized mass from diffuse edema, and solid from cystic lesions.

After an initial US examination, the role of other imaging modalities can be determined. Magnetic resonance imaging (MRI) should be reserved for cases in which US fails to establish a specific diagnosis or fails to demonstrate the margins of a soft tissue mass accurately.

Advantages of US over MRI are the lack of partial volume averaging effects, the availability and low cost of the technique, and the short examination time. Moreover, motion artifacts, which may occur in noncooperative patients and children, are of less relevance when US is used. A limitation of US is encountered in the evaluation of the extension of a soft tissue tumor, in particular to adjacent bony structures. For specific tissue diagnosis, US-guided percutaneous needle biopsies are generally less time-consuming and less expensive than those using computed tomography (CT) or MRI, with easier patient access.

The use of color Doppler US (CDUS) as an additional means of describing the biological activity, structure, and extension of bone and soft tissue tumors and the blood supply to them has been described only incidentally. This chapter aims to summarize the potential value of this technique in the diagnosis and treatment of soft tissue tumors.

2.2 Color Doppler Ultrasound

2.2.1 Technique

CDUS is a noninvasive method of detecting blood flow and assessing flow direction simultaneously. The anatomical flow information is superimposed on all or part of the grayscale image. Backscattered signals in CDUS are displayed in color as a function of the motion of the erythrocytes toward or away from the transducer. Lower flow velocities are characterized by higher saturation of colors. The color-coded information is distinct from that yielded by spectral duplex Doppler imaging, which is useful when more detailed information about flow velocity or spectral analysis, of a kind that may aid in tissue characterization, is important [1]. As such, color flow US and spectral Doppler are complementary techniques. The ability of CDUS to provide a global view of flow in real time minimizes the chance of missing flow in an unexpected area and facilitates comparison of flow in different anatomical locations. To avoid diagnostic error, however, color flow mapping, which is solely a qualitative method, should be supported by spectral analysis [2–4].

The choice of the insonating frequency in pulsed Doppler measurements is a compromise between selection of higher frequencies, resulting in improved resolution and increased amplitude of the returned Doppler signal, versus attenuation. High frequencies are attenuated more strongly than low frequencies. For instance, superficial soft tissue masses can be well documented using a high insonating frequency of 7.5 MHz or more, whereas deeper lesions require frequencies of 5 MHz or less.

Another important phenomenon is aliasing: the lower the insonating frequency used, the higher the velocity that can be measured without aliasing. Aliased frequencies misrepresent high-velocity flow in a forward direction as a low-velocity reverse flow. Higher velocities can also be measured when the pulse repetition frequency (PRF, the sampling rate at which sequential tone bursts are transmitted by a pulse Doppler instrument) is higher, or when the angle between US beam and blood flow direction is increased. Commonly, angles between 30° and 60° are employed. Increase in PRF is limited by the distance to the target. In addition, inappropriate gain setting may cause either loss of flow information or degradation of spectral quality [5–11]. The highest signal amplification that does not introduce artifacts is best.

Power color Doppler flow images have the advantage of better signal-to-noise characteristics than conventional color Doppler techniques. Although this method cannot demonstrate flow direction, it is also less angle sensitive [12–14].

The application of newly developed US (microbubble) contrast agents may improve the strength of Doppler signals received from vascular structures, including tumor neovascularization [15–18]. These agents enhance the visualization of jets and may increase the echogenicity of the neovascular bed associated with malignant tumors [16].

2.2.2 Clinical Applications

CDUS has been proposed as a tool to document the biological behavior of malignant tumors, including soft tissue tumors, and to monitor regression of neovascularization induced by therapy [19–22]. One clinical application of CDUS is the identification of tumor vascularity [13, 23–27].

2.2.2.1 Presence of Tumor Vascularization

Increased vascularity, vascular changes, and abnormal Doppler signals have been noted in tumors arising from various organs and in superficially and deeper-located soft tissue masses [5, 13, 21, 24, 25, 28–37]. By depicting abnormal flow patterns, CDUS may add specificity in the US evaluation of soft tissue masses. It can be useful in the assessment of the degree of intratumoral blood flow in solid masses (Figs. 2.1, 2.2, 2.3, 2.4) and in the determination of the origin and pattern of vascular supply. Hence, CDUS can be helpful in selecting the preferential site for biopsy by differentiating areas that will

most likely represent (vascularized) viable tumor from (avascular) necrosis (Figs. 2.1, 2.2, 2.7, 2.8) [38]. As such, color Doppler-controlled needle biopsy assists in making the diagnosis of malignancy with an accuracy of 97% and of 94% for the diagnosis of soft tissue sarcoma. These results are comparable with those of incisional biopsy [39].

Absence of intratumoral blood flow may be real, or it may indicate that flow velocities present are below the minimal threshold of detection [17, 20, 22]. Furthermore, because the tumor vessels are microscopic, absence of flow may be due to sampling errors in large, heterogeneous tumors [22]. Initial screening of a mass with CDUS is therefore very useful in this setting, since the Doppler frequency shifts arising from the microvascular network give rise to various color patterns that can subsequently be examined with pulsed spectral Doppler [32]. Thus, color Doppler flow imaging and spectral analysis are complementary techniques and should be routinely used as a useful adjunct to conventional US in soft tissue masses [5].

As stated above, inappropriate machine settings (transducer frequency, gain, pulse-repetition frequency) are another cause of failure to detect intratumoral flow [22].

2.2.2.2 Pattern of Vascularization

Abnormal, newly formed vessels are most prevalent at the tumor periphery [22], but can also be encountered centrally within a mass, or seen in a mixed pattern (flow running into and around a mass) [32]. On the other hand, the center of a rapidly growing soft tissue mass may become necrotic as it outgrows its blood flow and thus contains no vessels (Fig. 2.1) [8, 16, 22]. The presence of three or more vascular hila and tortuous and irregular internal vessels making a soft tissue mass reinforces the suspicion of malignancy [25]. Other vessel characteristics that can be assessed and combined with conventional US features include stenoses, occlusions, vessel loops, and shunts [13]. On this subject, the reader is also referred to Chap 11, which deals with grading and characterization.

In malignant tumors, two different Doppler signals have been identified that may coexist in the same tumor [18, 23, 40]. One is a high-systolic Doppler shift with or without enhanced diastolic flow, and one is a low-impedance signal with little or no systolic/diastolic variation (Figs. 2.1, 2.2, 2.3, 2.5, 2.6, 2.7, 2.8). These Doppler signals seem to relate to the histological structure and hemodynamic properties of the tumor circulation [20, 41]. The former signal may arise from arteriovenous shunting, whereas the latter signal corresponds histologically to the presence of thin-walled sinusoidal spaces, lacking normal arteriolar smooth muscle [29, 41].

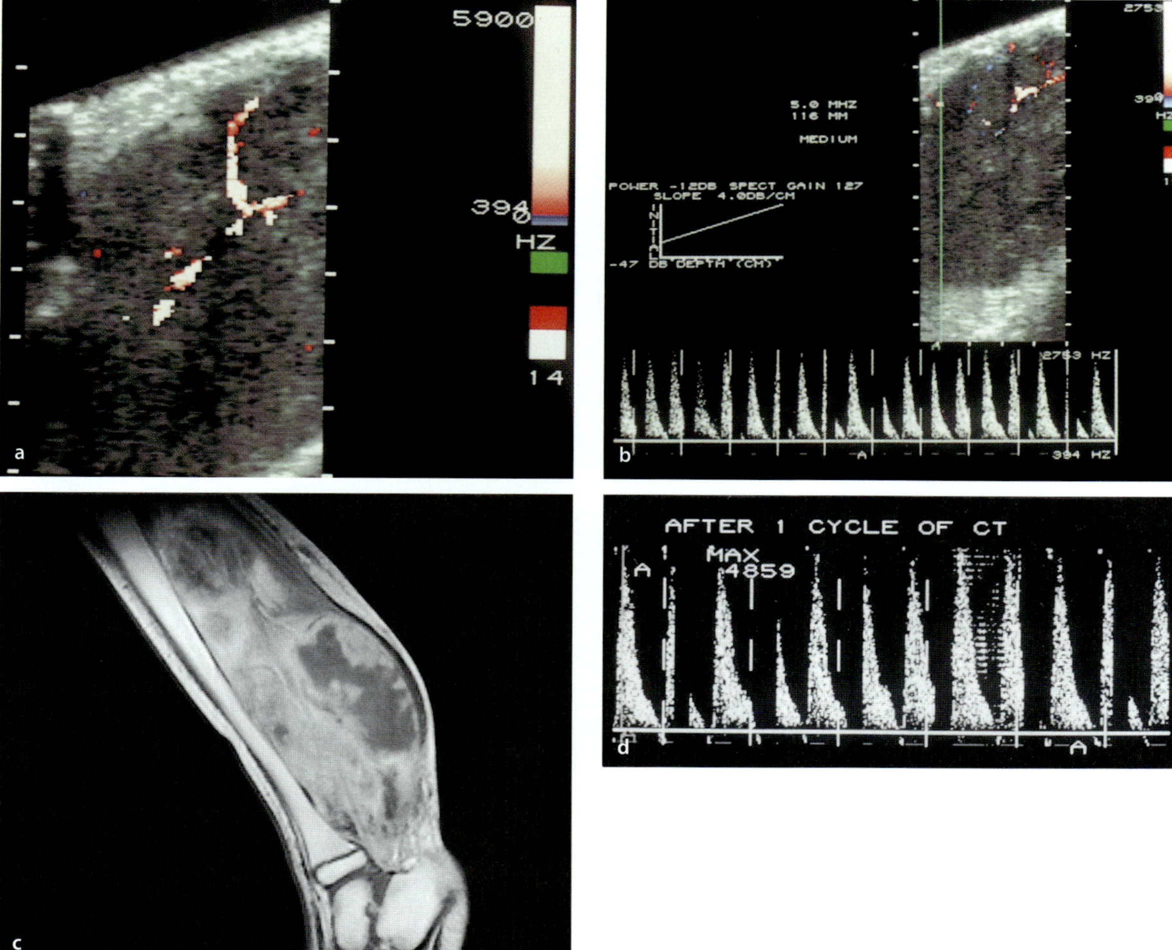

Fig. 2.1 a–d. Rhabdomyosarcoma invading the muscle compartments of the lower leg in a 10-year-old boy. **a** Longitudinal color Doppler (CD) image (5-MHz insonating frequency) before chemotherapy. **b** Color flow image with intramural spectrum. **c** Corresponding longitudinal, T1-weighted, contrast-enhanced MR image. **d** CD ultrasonography (US) spectral display after one cycle of chemotherapy (CT). A large, hypoechoic, partially well defined mass is appreciated in the calf. Tumor vessels are present at the tumor periphery (**a, b**). Spectral Doppler reveals arterial, high-frequency Doppler shifts arising from the tumor vessels (**b**). Peripheral enhancement is also seen on Gd-enhanced MR images (**c**). Persistent, intratumoral, abnormal high-frequency Doppler signals (maximum, 5 kHz) have been noted after chemotherapy (**d**), reflecting poor response. This was confirmed histologically after surgery.

2.2.2.3 Diagnostic Specificity

Solid lesions may show increased blood flow. High-frequency Doppler shifts have been described in high-grade malignant bone tumors with an associated soft tissue mass (Figs. 2.5, 2.6) [23] and in soft tissue Ewing's sarcoma, rhabdomyosarcoma (Fig. 2.1), synovial sarcoma, myxofibrosarcoma (formerly "malignant fibrous histiocytoma"), and other soft tissue tumors (Fig. 2.2) [17, 22, 29, 32, 33, 40], but there may be overlap with certain benign solid soft tissue tumors (Figs. 2.4, 2.7).

In one prospective study including 56 patients with a soft tissue mass, sensitivity and specificity were 60% and 55%, respectively, only for differentiation between benign and malignant tumors. When combined with color Doppler and spectral wave analysis, sensitivity and specificity increased to 90% and 91%, resulting in a correct diagnosis in 51 of 56 patients [5]. It has been suggested that Doppler features encountered in malignant soft tissue tumors may be different from those seen in tumors that are carcinomatous in nature [33].

Although various malignant neoplasms had partly very high and partly very low flow signals, a minimum intratumoral threshold velocity of 0.4 m/s has been shown to be best suited to the distinction of benign from malignant tumors [26]. Absence of flow was found to be nonspecific, but occurred only in benign lesions such as lipoma, neurofibroma, and cysts [32].

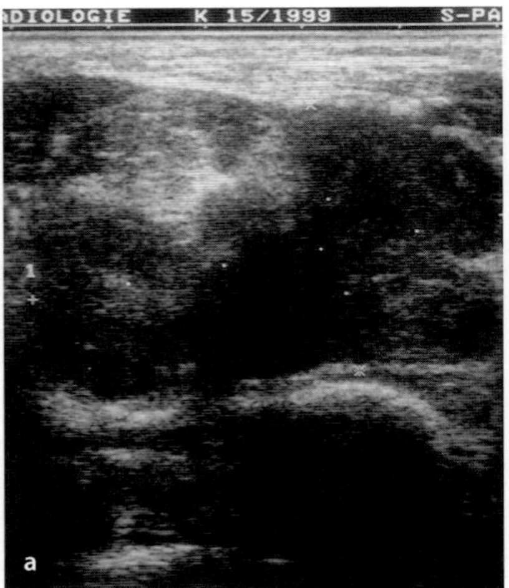
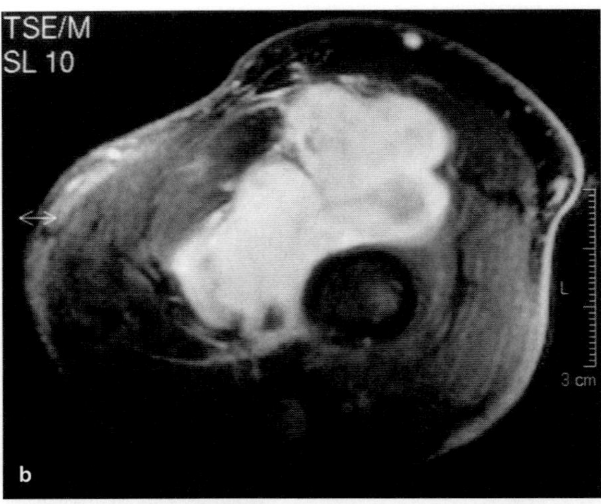
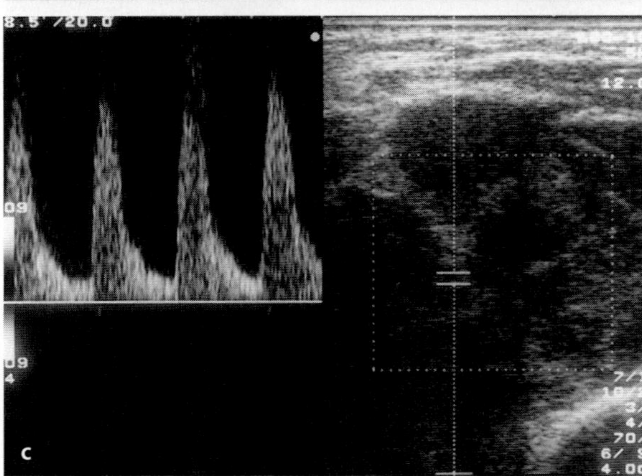

Fig. 2.2 a–c. Malignant peripheral nerve sheath tumor in a 60-year-old man after isolated limb perfusion with tumor necrosis factor (TNF). **a** Axial US image. **b** Axial T2-weighted turbo spin-echo MR image with fat-selective presaturation. **c** Spectral display obtained in central, solid tumor parts. A large, inhomogeneous mass is visible in the soft tissues of the upper arm, anterior to the humerus, with a lobulated border. There are areas with enhanced and decreased echogenicity (**a**). The tumor has a similar lobulated configuration and a predominantly high signal intensity on the axial MR image (**b**). High-velocity arterial Doppler signals are obtained from solid parts of the tumor, consistent with poor response to the TNF therapy (**c**). This was confirmed after surgical resection of the tumor

Power Doppler ultrasonography can be utilized to evaluate increased vascularity in lipomatous tumors and thus to differentiate between lipoma and well-differentiated liposarcoma [15]. Therefore, absence of detectable vessels on color Doppler studies performed on equipment sensitive to low-flow favors a benign lesion. Other authors stress the unreliability of CDUS in differentiating between malignant and benign soft tissue lesions on the basis of maximum systolic and end-diastolic velocity and intralesional resistive index [33]. Up to 2005, literature available on this subject is scarce and controversial. Nevertheless, negative findings permit no valid conclusions on this, but tumors with a benign appearance on US with high flow signals should prompt further assessment [28, 29, 41]. Color Doppler criteria, including vessel density, peak systolic Doppler shifts, resistive index and signs of arteriovenous shunting, have also been used to distinguish soft tissue hemangiomas (with high vessel density and high peak arterial Doppler shifts of more than 2 kHz) from other soft tissue masses and to distinguish hemangioma from vascular malformations [25, 30, 42].

The identification of a vascularized rim is also of value in making the diagnosis of an acute abscess, as differentiating a complicated cystic structure from a relatively hypoechoic solid structure with isolated grayscale US can be quite difficult. In a series of 50 soft tissue masses, a peripheral flow pattern surrounding suppurated areas was noted in almost all abscesses [32].

The highly vascularized periphery of masses can also be differentiated from the surrounding tissues by using CDUS. Although peritumoral, nonmalignant inflammatory or posttraumatic tissues may show marked vascularity [8, 23, 32, 33, 43], flow velocities are usually relatively low in these conditions [41]. In patients with hematoma and seroma, no flow has been demonstrated within or around the lesion.

Probably very early granulation tissue, with or without the presence of residual or recurrent tumor after surgery and/or radiation therapy, may yield signal characteristics that are similar to those seen in vascularized sarcomatous tissue.

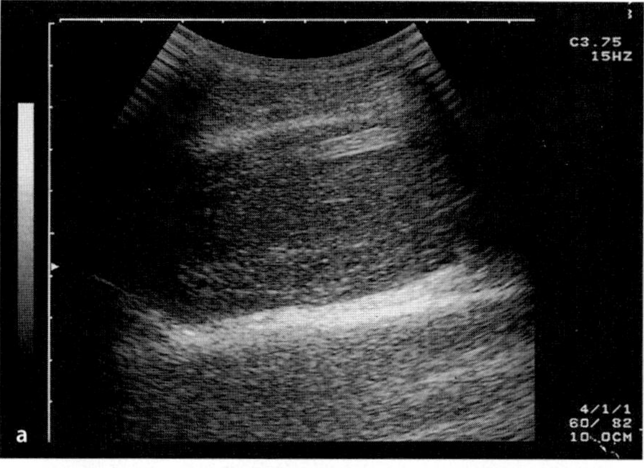

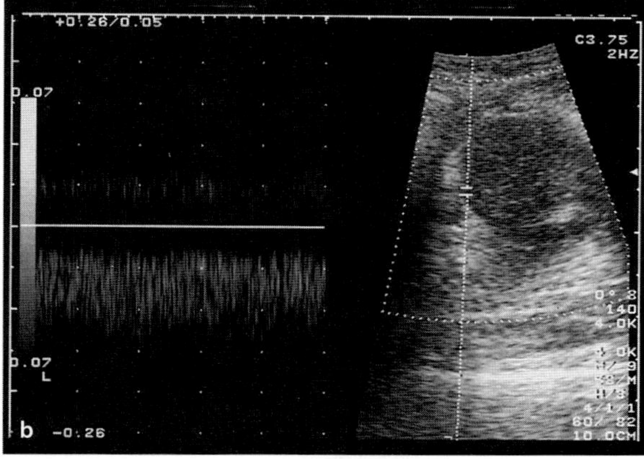

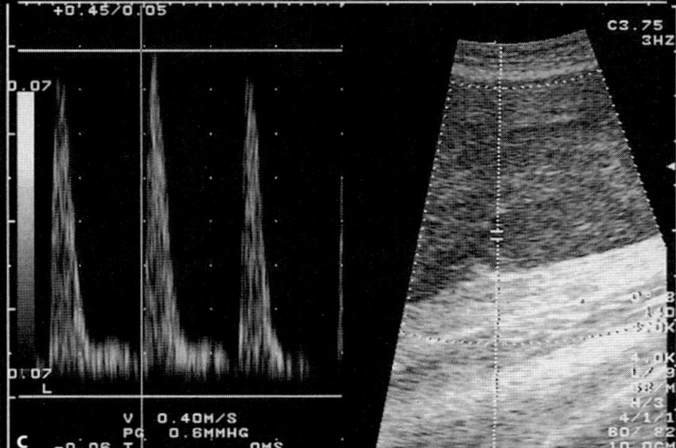

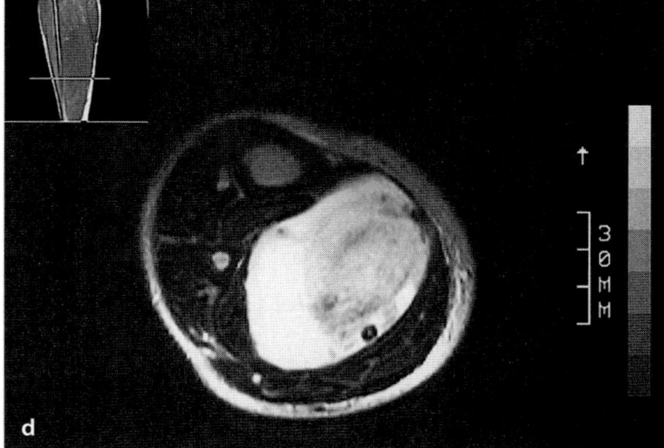

Fig. 2.3 a–d. Myxoid liposarcoma in the calf of a 43-yearold man. **a** Longitudinal sonographic image. **b** Spectral display obtained at tumor periphery. **c** Spectral display obtained in tumor center. **d** Longitudinal T2-weighted MR image. A large, relatively well defined hypoechoic mass is noted in the calf. The cortex of the tibia is seen posteriorly. Anteriorly, a longitudinal structure is depicted within the contours of the tumor, consistent with the tibial nerve (**a**). Arterial high-frequency shifts were measured mainly at the periphery of the mass (**b**). Elsewhere in the tumor, venous sig-nals were acquired (**c**). A biphasic pattern was seen at the popliteal artery feeding the tumor-bearing limb, in contrast to a normal triphasic pattern at the contralateral artery. This may reflect the presence of a mass with a low-resistance vascular network. The high signal intensity on the T2-weighted MR image (**d**) reflects the predominant myxoid matrix of the tumor. Notice the low signal intensity structure anteriorly, presumed to be the nerve. Probable flow voids are seen posteriorly

2.2.3 Evaluation of Therapy

CDUS has proved to be an appropriate modality for monitoring the effect of neoadjuvant chemotherapy in patients with high-grade bone sarcoma [23, 44, 45]. The presence of an associated soft tissue mass is a precondition of the use of CDUS as a tool for monitoring chemotherapy in such patients (Figs. 2.5, 2.6). In selected cases, CDUS can also be applied in patients with a malignant soft tissue tumor treated with systemic chemotherapy or with isolated limb perfusion with alpha tumor necrosis factor (Fig. 2.2). This may occur in patients with rhabdomyosarcoma, myxofibrosarcoma, synovial sarcoma, or undifferentiated spindle cell sarcomas.

CDUS has a critical advantage over other imaging modalities in monitoring the efficacy of therapy in patients with bone and soft tissue sarcomas, since it can provide both qualitative and quantitative flow informa-tion. In addition, it is a readily available and noninvasive method and its cost is low.

B-mode real-time imaging (5-MHz insonating frequency) can be used to locate the soft tissue mass and to identify the US features of the tumor, in particular the tumor margins, destruction of cortical bone, and the presence of areas of very high and very low echogenicity. Two-color Doppler imaging parameters are of interest in analysis of the results of therapy in sarcomas, being focused on changes in tumor perfusion: intratumoral blood flow and tumor blood supply.

2.2.3.1 Changes in Intratumoral Blood Flow

Prior to therapy, a qualitative impression of the amount of intratumoral blood flow can be obtained with color-coded (power) US. This "survey" color flow imaging allows scanning of a large area relatively quickly to detect

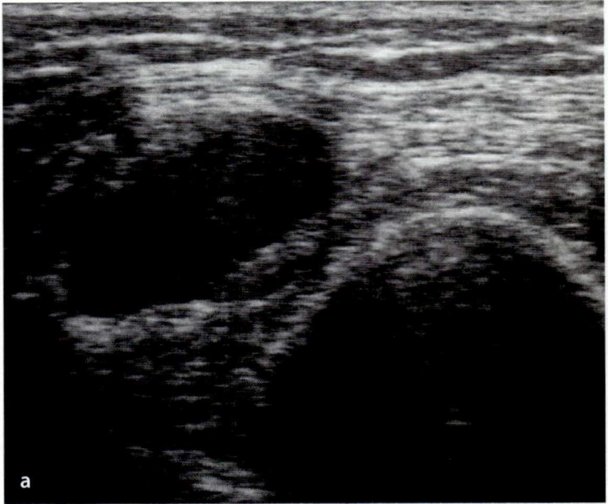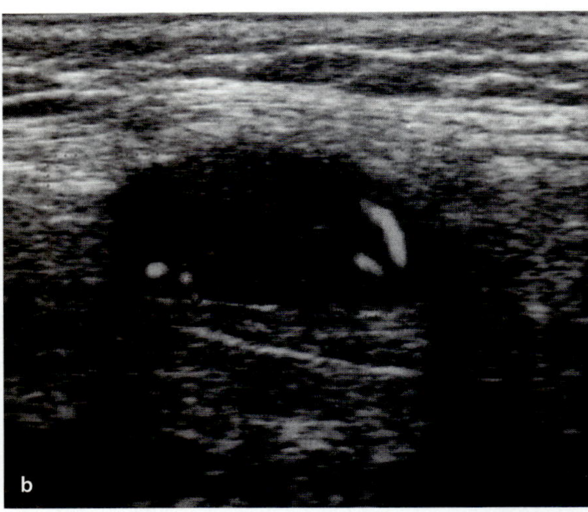

Fig. 2.4 a, b. Schwannoma in the lower leg of a 45-year-old woman. **a** Axial sonographic image. **b** Longitudinal sonographic image with peripheral flow signals. There is an oval, well-defined solid mass located lateral to the tibia (**a**). Despite the presence of (peripheral) flow signals, this is a benign schwannoma (**b**)

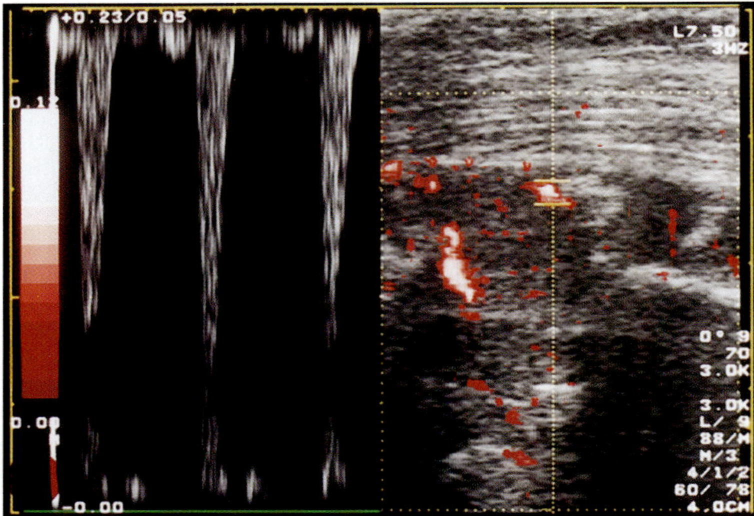

Fig. 2.5. Soft tissue extension of an osteosarcoma in the proximal tibia in a 14-year-old boy. CD flow image reveals predominantly peripheral flow within the soft tissue mass. Spectral display shows high-velocity signal with little or no diastolic flow

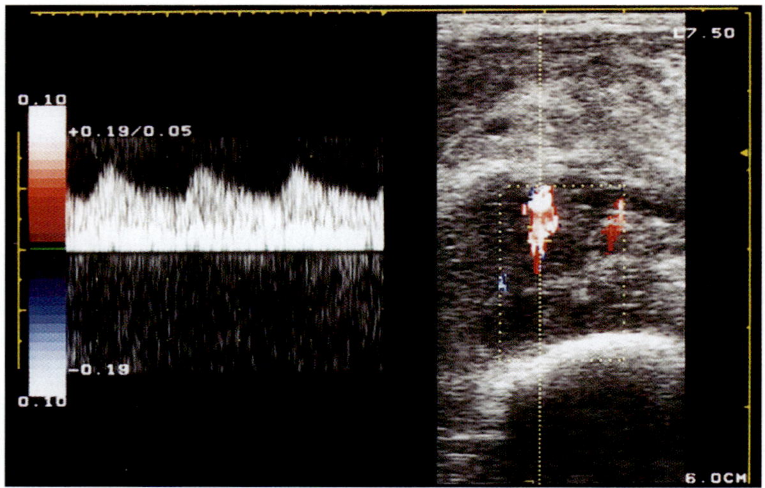

Fig. 2.6. Soft tissue extension of a Ewing's sarcoma in the proximal tibia in a 17-year-old male patient. Axial color-coded image shows soft tissue mass anterior to the tibia with peripheral slow signals. Spectral display shows low-resistance signal with little differentiation between systole and diastole

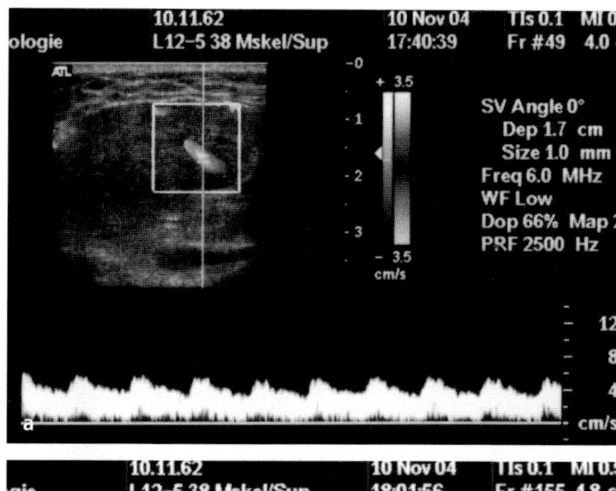

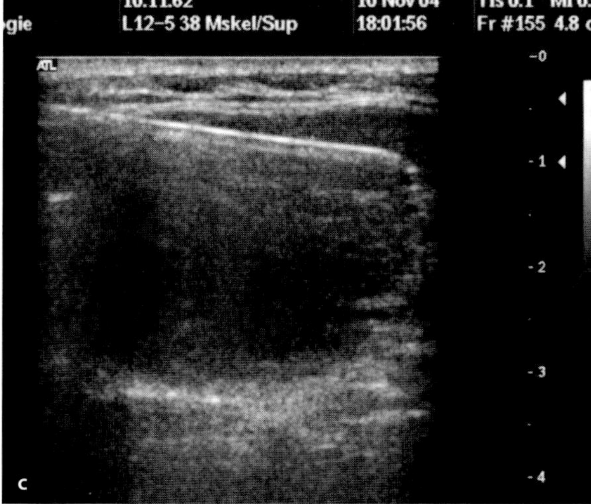

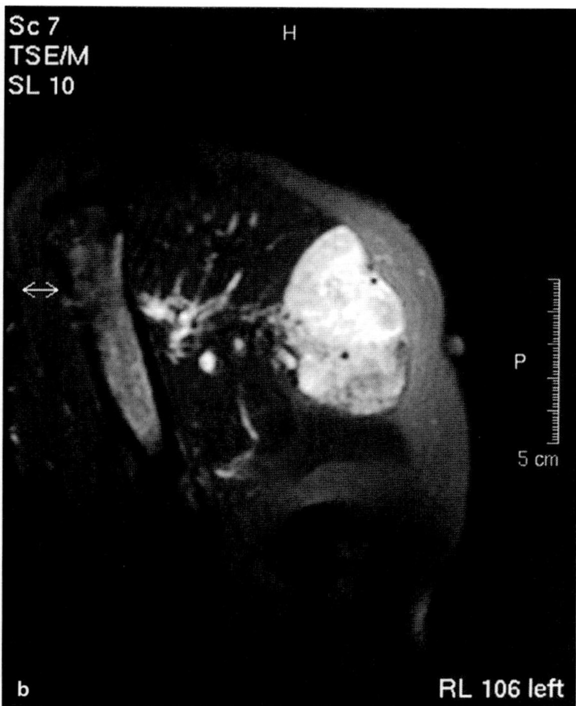

Fig. 2.7 a–c. Soft tissue mass in the upper arm of a 42-year-old woman. **a** Axial sonographic image with spectral display. **b** Corresponding sagittal, T2-weighted turbo spin-echo MR image with fat-selective presaturation. **c** Axial sonographic image with 14-gauge biopsy needle in situ. A low-resistance spectrum is displayed in one of numerous abnormal intratumoral vessels (**a**). High signal intensity mass with prominent flow voids (**b**). Ultrasound-guided biopsy reveals hemangiopericytoma (**c**)

areas of unsuspected flow or to quickly differentiate vascular from nonvascular structures. The amount of flow can be graded on a four-point scale: no flow, no pixels of color detected; little flow, scattered pixels of color present within the tumor mass; intermediate flow, presence of a vascularized rim, with scattered pixels or small areas of flow in the central portions of the soft tissue mass; high flow, flow present diffusely throughout the soft tissue mass [21, 23, 46]. Before, during, and after (chemo)therapy, pulsed duplex Doppler can be performed to examine the tumor (particularly the periphery of the mass) for abnormal signals. Initially, a low or intermediate pulse repetition frequency should be used. A higher PRF is necessary when aliasing occurs. Complete disappearance of intratumoral flow and abnormal Doppler signals after therapy is indicative of a favorable histological response [45]. Persistence of intratumoral Doppler shifts makes a poor or incomplete response more likely (Figs. 2.1, 2.2).

2.2.3.2 Changes in Blood Supply

The biological behavior of the mass in question can be monitored with Doppler scanning by analyzing the flow velocities. In the case of tumors arising from the soft tissues of an extremity, flow velocity measurements can easily be performed in the artery feeding the tumor-bearing limb (e.g., the common femoral artery or popliteal artery in the lower extremity) and compared with those in the corresponding contralateral artery (Fig. 2.8). Flow velocities can be assessed directly from the Doppler frequency shift by adjusting the angle between the axis of the flow vector and the direction of the US beam. The angle should always be less than 60°. A triphasic pattern with a distinct reverse flow component in diastole is to be expected in the normal artery during rest. Higher peak systolic velocities have been found on the side with the tumor, whereas no reversed flow is found in diastole in most extremities with tumors, re-

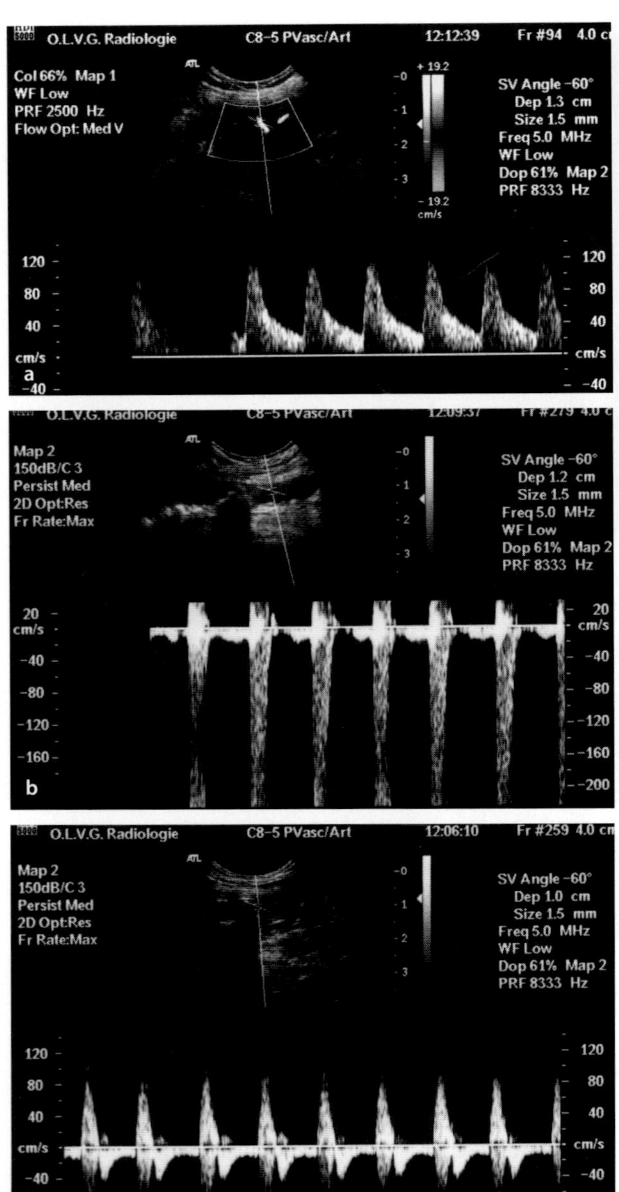

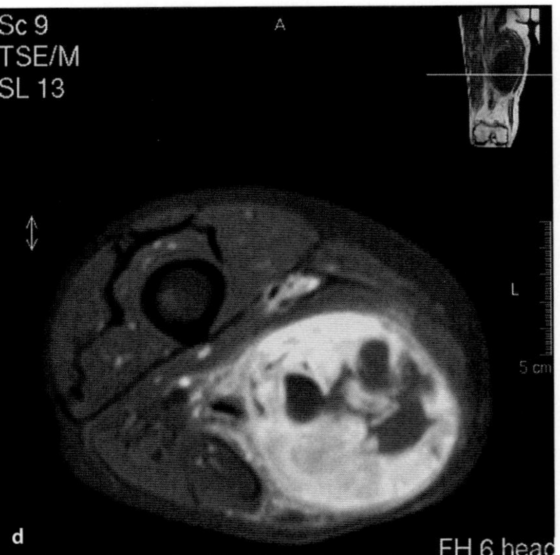

Fig. 2.8 a–d. Soft tissue mass in the upper leg of a 71-year-old male patient. **a** Axial sonographic image with spectral display of intratumoral flow. **b** Spectral display in femoral artery feeding the tumor-bearing leg. **c** Corresponding spectral display feeding the opposite (normal) leg. **d** Axial, T1-weighted turbo spin-echo MR image with fat-selective presaturation and after gadolinium contrast administration. High-velocity, low-resistance signals are encountered predominantly at the tumor periphery. Areas without flow and low echogenicity consistent with necrosis were found centrally (**a**). A high-velocity, low-resistance flow pattern with forward flow in diastole is appreciated. Aliasing occurs because of the high velocity (**b**). A normal triphasic pattern is found in the contralateral femoral artery (**c**). In accord with US, areas of necrosis are shown in a strongly enhancing mass (**d**). Biopsy reveals high-grade liposarcoma.

sulting in lower resistive indices [23, 45]. Presumably these findings are based on reduced peripheral resistance in the vascular bed of a metabolically active tumor relative to normal striated muscle with increased attraction of blood flow from the host's circulation [23]. A decreased or unaltered resistive index in the arteries that feed tumors, as a consequence of chemotherapy, suggests a poor histological response, particularly when it is associated with persistent intratumoral flow. An increase in the index to normal values in addition to a substantial decrease in intratumoral Doppler shifts is indicative of a good response [45]. In a study of bone sarcomas using CDUS, the histopathological response after surgery could be predicted after two cycles of chemotherapy, but not prior to or after the first cycle of chemotherapy.

The potential to noninvasively predict response to chemotherapy allows CDUS to contribute to decision making on the optimal treatment schedule for individual patients with high-grade sarcomas: whether or not chemotherapy should he continued, whether additional radiation therapy is required, etc. A major disadvantage of US in this connection is the operator expertise required; in addition, follow-up studies may be adversely affected by inter- and intraobserver variation.

Those soft tissue tumors that are intended to be surgically treated after systemic therapy should be accurately locoregionally staged prior to surgery with (contrast-enhanced) MRI. Besides thorough discernment of the real tumor extension with or without invasion of bone and optimal discrimination of tumor relative to critical neurovascular structures, MRI and dynamic contrast-enhanced MRI in particular allows the identification and localization of clusters of residual viable tumor [46].

Follow-up after surgery is important. Thorough history and physical examination still contribute to detection of the vast majority of recurrent soft tissue sarcomas. Routine surveillance imaging seems to be of benefit when the risk of asymptomatic recurrent disease is high or otherwise clinical assessment is difficult [47]. Local recurrences of soft tissue sarcomas occur frequently after surgery, and not all early recurrent (superficially located) soft tissue malignancies are detected by clinical examination [48]. US (including CDUS) is an accessible imaging tool that can be used to search for these (small) soft tissue recurrences. Seventy-seven percent of early local recurrences (minimum size 5 mm) of soft tissue sarcoma were correctly identified with US using high-frequency probes (5–7.5 MHz or higher)

[49]. In contrast, CT sensitivity was 69%, but CT detected only lesions that were greater than 5 cm [50]. CT (but preferably MRI) should therefore be proposed only as a presurgical procedure to assess the anatomical relationships between the recurrent tumor and the adjacent structures [50]. Moreover, US can be used in addition to MRI when susceptibility artifacts caused by orthopedic hardware prevent the evaluation of specific areas [50]. Sonographic imaging of a mass suggestive of recurrent sarcoma can immediately be followed by needle biopsy [49].

In conclusion, CDUS with spectral analysis is a powerful diagnostic modality and useful adjunct to conventional US that can yield information about the vascular heterogeneity and quantitative characterization of flow in soft tissue masses. As such, it may indicate representative sites for guiding diagnostic needle biopsy in large heterogeneous tumors and assist in monitoring the biological behavior of soft tissue sarcomas as a result of systemic or local therapy. Its role in differentiating between malignant benign and inflammatory lesions is still controversial.

Things to remember:
1. By depicting abnormal flow patterns, CDUS may add specificity in the US evaluation of soft tissue masses.
2. In malignant soft tissue sarcomas, both high-systolic Doppler shifts with or without enhanced diastolic flow and low-impedance signals with little systolic-diastolic variation can be encountered.
3. One should take care of inappropriate machine settings, including transducer frequency, gain, and pulse repeat frequency (PRF), which may cause false-negative findings regarding intratumoral flow.
4. Parameters based on changes in intratumoral blood flow and tumoral blood supply can be used for monitoring the effect of preoperative systemic chemotherapy or isolated-limb perfusion in soft tissue sarcomas.
5. CDUS is a low-threshold technique which can be easily used in the follow-up of patients with soft-tissue sarcoma, particularly when orthopedic hardware hampers optimal physical examination.
6. Color Doppler flow imaging and spectral analysis are complementary techniques and should be used routinely as an adjunct to conventional US in soft tissue tumors of unknown origin.

References

1. Scoutt LM, Zawin ML, Taylor KJ (1990) Doppler US. II. Clinical applications. Radiology 174(2):309–319
2. Orr NM, Taylor KJ (1990) Doppler detection of tumor vascularity. In: Tailor KJ, Strandness DE (eds) Duplex Doppler US. Churchill Livingstone, New York, pp 149–163
3. Zwiebel WJ (1990) Color duplex imaging and Doppler spectrum analysis: principles capabilities, and limitations. Semin Ultrasound CT MR ll:84–96
4. Belli P, Constantini M, Mirk P, Maresca G, Priolo F, Marano P (2000) Role of color Doppler sonography in the assessment of musculoskeletal masses. J Ultrasound Med 19:823–830
5. Burns PN (1987) The physical principles of Doppler and spectral analysis. J Clin Ultrasound 15:567–590
6. Kremkau FW (1992) Doppler principles. Semin Roentgenol 27:6–16
7. Mitchell DG (1990) Color Doppler imaging: principles, limitations, and artifacts. Radiology 177:1–10
8. Pozniak MA, Lagzebski JA, Scanlan KA (1992) Spectral and color Doppler artifacts. Radiographics 12:35–44
9. Rubin JM (1994) Spectral Doppler US. Radiographics 141:139–150
10. Taylor KJ, Holland S (1990) Doppler US. I. Basic principles, instrumentation, and pitfalls. Radiology 174:297–307
11. Zwiebel WJ (1990) Color duplex imaging and Doppler spectrum analysis: principles, capabilities, and limitations. Semin Ultrasound CT MR ll:84–96
12. Bodner G, Schocke MF, Rachbauer F et al (2002) Differentiation of malignant and benign musculoskeletal tumors: combined color and power Doppler US and spectral wave analysis. Radiology 223:410–416
13. De Marchi A, De Petro P, Faletti C et al (2003) Echo color power Doppler with contrast medium to evaluate vascularization of lesions of the soft tissues of the limbs. Chir Organi Mov 88:225–231
14. Futani H, Yamagiwa T, Yasojimat H, Natsuaki M, Stugaard M, Maruo S (2003) Distinction between well-differentiated liposarcoma and intramuscular lipoma using power Doppler ultrasonography. Anticancer Res 23:1713–1718
15. Brown JM, Quedens-Case C, Alderman JL, Greener Y, Taylor KJ (1998) Contrast-enhanced sonography of tumor neovascularity in a rabbit model. Ultrasound Med Biol 24:495–501
16. Taylor GA, Perlman EJ, Scherer LR, Gearhart JP, Leventhal BG, Wiley J (1991) Vascularity of tumors in children: evaluation with color Doppler imaging. AJR Am J Roentgenol 157:1267–1271
17. Taylor KJ, Wells PN (1989) Tissue characterisation. Ultrasound Med Biol 15:421–428
18. Wells PN (1990) Future developments in Doppler US. In: Taylor KJ, Strandness DE (eds) Duplex Doppler US. Churchill Livingstone, New York, pp 165–173
19. Ramos I, Fernandes LA, Morse SS, Fortune KL, Taylor KJ (1988) Detection of neovascular signals in a 3-day Walker 256 rat carcinoma by CW Doppler US. Ultrasound Med Biol 14:123–126
20. Shimamoto K, Sakuma S, Ishigaki T, Makino N (1987) Intratumoral blood flow: evaluation with color Doppler echography. Radiology 165:683–685.
21. Van Campenhout I, Patriquin H (1992) Malignant microvasculature in abdominal tumors in children: detection with Doppler US. Radiology 183:445–448
22. Van der Woude HJ, Bloem JL, Schipper J, et al (1994) Changes of tumor perfusion in bone sarcomas induced by chemotherapy: color Doppler flow, imaging compared with contrast-enhanced MRI and three-phase bone scintigraphy. Radiology 191:421–431
23. Adler RS, Bell DS, Bamber JC, Moscovic E, Thomas JM (1999) Evaluation of soft tissue masses using segmented color Doppler velocity images: preliminary observations. AJR Am J Roentgenol 172:781–788
24. Lagalla R, Iovane A, Caruso G, Lo Bello M, Derchi LE (1995) Color Doppler ultrasonography of soft tissue masses. Acta Radiol 39:421–426
25. Merrit CR (1987) Doppler color flow imaging. J Clin Ultrasound 15:591–597
26. Zwiebel WJ (1988) Color-encoded blood slow imaging. Semin Ultrasound CT MR 9:320–325
27. Griffith JF, Chan DP, Kumta SM, Chow LT, Ahuja AT (2004) Does Doppler analysis of musculoskeletal soft tissue tumours help prediction of malignancy? Clin Radiol 59:369–375
28. Dock W, Grabenwoger F, Metz V, Eibenberger K, Farres MT (1991) Tumor vascularization: assessment with Duplex sonography. Radiology 181:1–244
29. Dubois J, Patriquin HB, Garel L, et al (1998) Soft tissue hemangiomas in infants and children: diagnosis using Doppler sonography. AJR Am J Roentgenol 171:247–252
30. Giovagnorio F, Andreoli C, De Cicco ML. (1999) Color Doppler sonography of focal lesions of the skin and subcutaneous tissue. J Ultrasound Med 18:89–93
31. Latifi HR, Siegel MJ (1994) Color Doppler flow imaging of pediatric soft tissue masses. J Ultrasound Med 13:165–169
32. Özbek SS, Arkun R, Killi R, et al (1995) Image-directed color Doppler ultrasonography in the evaluation of superficial solid tumors. J Clin Ultrasound 23:233–238
33. Ramos IM, Taylor KJ, Kier R, Burns PN, Snower DP, Carter D (1985) Tumor vascular signals in renal masses: detection with Doppler US. Radiology 168:633–637
34. Schoenberger SG, Sutherland CM, Robinson AE, (1988) Breast neoplasms: duplex sonographic imaging as an adjunct in diagnosis. Radiology 168:665–668
35. Taylor KJ, Ramos I, Morse SS, Fortune KL, Hammers L, Taylor CR (1987) Focal liver masses: differential diagnosis with pulsed Doppler US. Radiology 164:643–647
36. De Marchi A, De Petro P, Faletti C et al (2003) Echo color power Doppler with contrast medium to evaluate vascularization of lesions of the soft tissues of the limbs. Chir Organi Mov 88:225–231.
37. Futani H, Yamagiwa T, Yasojimat H, Natsuaki M, Stugaard M, Maruo S (2003) Distinction between well-differentiated liposarcoma and intramuscular lipoma using power Doppler ultrasonography. Anticancer Res 23:1713–1718
38. Paltiel HJ, Birrows PE, Kozakewich HP, Zurakowski D, Mulliken JB (2000) Soft-tissue vascular anomalies: utility of US for diagnosis. Radiology 21:747–754
39. Schulte M, Heymer B, Sarkar MR, Negri G, Von Baer A, Hartwig E (1998) Color Doppler controlled needle biopsy in diagnosis of soft tissue and bone tumors. Chirurg 69:1059–1067
40. Taylor KJ, Ramos I, Carter D, Morse SS, Snower D, Fortune K (1988) Correlation of Doppler US tumor signals with neovascular morphologic features. Radiology 166:57–62
41. Kaushik S, Miller TT, Nazarian LN, Foster WC (2003) Spectral Doppler sonography of musculoskeletal soft tissue masses. J Ultrasound Med 22:1333–1336
42. Paltiel HJ, Burrows PE, Kozakewich HP, Zurakowski HP, Zurakowski D, Mulliken JB (2000) Soft-tissue vascular anomalies: utility of US for diagnosis. Radiology 214:747–754.
43. Hernanz-Schulman M (1993) Applications of Doppler sonography to diagnosis of extracranial pediatric disease. Radiology 189:1–14
44. Van der Woude HJ, Bloem JI, Oostayen JA van, et al (1995) Treatment of high-grade bone sarcomas with neoadjuvant chemotherapy: the utility of sequential color Doppler sonography in predicting final histopathologic response. AJR Am J Roentgenol 165:125–133

45. Van der Woude HJ, Vanderschueren G (1999) Ultrasound in musculoskeletal tumors with emphasis on its role in tumor follow-up. Radiol Clin North Am 37:753–766

46. Van der Woude HJ, Bloem JL, Verstraete KL, Taminiau AHM, Nooy MA, Hogendoorn PCW (1995) Osteosarcoma and Ewing's sarcoma after neoadjuvant chemotherapy: value of dynamic MRI in detecting viable tumor before surgery. AJR Am J Roentgenol 165:593–598

47. Kane JM 3rd (2004) Surveillance strategies for patients following surgical resection of soft tissue sarcomas. Curr Opin Oncol 16:328–332.

48. Alexander AA, Nazarian LN, Feld RI (1997) Superficial soft-tissue masses suggestive of recurrent malignancy: sonographic localization and biopsy. AJR Am J Roentgenol 169:1449–1451

49. Pino G, Conzi GF, Murolo C, et al (1993) Sonographic evaluation of local recurrences of soft tissue sarcomas. J Ultrasound Med 12:23–26

50. Hodler J, Yu JS, Steinert HC, Resnick D (1995) MRI versus alternative techniques. Magn Reson Imaging Clin N Am 3:591–608

Plain Radiography, Angiography, and Computed Tomography

3

A.M. Davies

Contents

3.1 Introduction

The imaging evaluation of a patient with a suspected soft tissue tumor requires a methodical approach that recognizes the benefits and limitations of the numerous imaging techniques that are available today. Consideration must be given to the financial costs and invasiveness of each technique balanced against the diagnostic reward. The temptation to routinely employ every technique in all patients should be resisted. Similarly, no examination should be reported in isolation without knowledge of relevant clinical details and results of prior investigations. Where possible, the prior investigations themselves should be available for review, as the appreciation of the significance of a new observation may well depend on a retrospective review of the previous studies [20].

In this chapter we discuss the role of plain radiography, angiography, and computed tomography (CT) in the management of a patient with a soft tissue mass, from detection and diagnosis through to the ultimate aim of medical management, a cure. It is beyond the scope of this book to discuss in detail the technology behind each technique. The reader is referred to subsequent chapters for an in-depth discussion of each type of soft tissue tumor.

3.2 Plain Radiography

Despite the undoubted technological advances in imaging over the past two decades, the evaluation of a suspected soft tissue mass should always commence with the plain radiograph [19]. It is cheap, universally available, and easy to obtain. The importance of this single piece of advice cannot be overemphasized. It is stated in virtually every textbook on the subject, but is all too frequently overlooked in day-to-day practice. Indeed it denigrates its value to call it "plain" radiography. In most cases two views at right angles are mandatory to delineate soft tissue planes and the integrity of adjacent cortical bone.

The lack of contrast resolution is a well-recognized limitation of plain radiography, but the value of the examination should not be underestimated. It may not identify the precise diagnosis in any but a minority of cases, but can still provide valuable information, e.g., the presence of calcification and bone involvement. Too often the humble radiograph is denigrated as noncontributory because it has failed to identify features that might be termed "positive." The absence of said features, however, can be just as significant. The absence, for example, of any bony abnormality immediately indicates that the primary pathology is of soft tissue origin, with a large differential diagnosis. Myositis ossificans, as a more specific example, can be effectively excluded from the differential diagnosis of a mass if there is no radiographic evidence of calcification, in all but the earliest of cases. The radiographic features that should be assessed in each case are discussed below [36].

3.2.1 Location

The identification of the location of a tumor is primarily clinical and will dictate which area is initially imaged. Whilst almost all true soft tissue tumors can occur anywhere in the musculoskeletal system, some have a predilection for certain areas, which will be highlighted in later chapters. Many non-neoplastic processes presenting with a soft tissue mass arise at characteristic locations; for example, gouty tophi in the hands and feet, and synovial cysts in the popliteal fossa [22]. Multiple soft tissue masses should suggest neurofibromatosis, lipoma, and occasionally metastatic deposits and Kaposi sarcoma [24, 25, 36]. The vast majority of soft tissue sarcomas, if given the opportunity to metastasize, will do so first to the lungs. It is for this reason that a chest radiograph is a mandatory early investigation in all cases of suspected soft tissue malignancy.

3.2.2 Size

Although the size of a soft tissue mass can have a bearing on subsequent management, the actual size is of limited diagnostic value [24]. Malignant lesions tend to be larger than benign ones [29], but this is rarely helpful in individual cases. Soft tissue masses, irrespective of their tissue of origin, arising in small anatomical areas such as the hands and feet typically are found relatively early. They therefore tend to be smaller than those arising in large anatomical areas such as the buttocks. It can be anticipated that tumors will be larger at presentation in those countries where access to medical facilities remains poorly developed.

3.2.3 Rate of Growth

Alterations in the size of a soft tissue tumor can be crudely estimated clinically and by comparing serial radiographs. Procrastination in advocating follow-up with serial radiographs should only be employed when the clinical and imaging features indicate a benign lesion with a considerable degree of certainty. Failure to promptly diagnose and treat a soft tissue sarcoma can only prejudice the outcome for the patient. Absent or slow growth is typical of a benign neoplasm, whereas malignant tumors frequently show a rapid rate of growth. It should be noted, however, that hemorrhage and infection will also produce rapidly enlarging soft tissue masses.

3.2.4 Shape and Margins

As with the size of a soft tissue tumor, the shape reveals little diagnostic information [36]. Malignant lesions are more commonly irregularly shaped, distorting and obscuring tissue planes. Benign lesions will tend to displace but not obliterate normal tissue planes [25]. Once again, infective lesions can mimic malignancy, as they are also frequently poorly defined due to fluid infiltration of the adjacent soft tissues. The definition of the margins of a lesion depends on a number of factors. These include the anatomical location relative to normal fat planes and bones, and the radiodensity of the constituents of the tumor relative to normal muscle.

3.2.5 Radiodensity

The muscle compartments of the extremities can be visualized radiographically as separated by low-density fat planes. The majority of soft tissues tumors are of a density similar to that of muscle and are, therefore, only revealed by virtue of mass effect. This includes displacement or disruption of the adjacent fat planes (Fig. 3.1), distortion of the skin contour, and involvement of bone.

In a minority of cases, part or all of the tumor may exhibit a radiodensity sufficiently different to that of water for the tumor to be visualized directly. Only fat and gas will give a radiodensity less than that of muscle. Lipomas, the commonest of all the soft tissue tumors, produce a low radiodensity between that of muscle and air. For this reason lipomas are well demarcated from the surrounding soft tissues and can be diagnosed with moderate confidence [17, 25] (Fig. 3.2). It should be noted that low-grade liposarcomas may contain variable amounts of lipomatous tissue, which also appears relatively radiolucent on radiography (Fig. 3.3). A low-kilovoltage technique can be used to accentuate the density differences between fat and muscle [25, 26, 33].

Air in the soft tissues is said to be specific to infection [24]. While infection is certainly the commonest cause, it may also be seen in necrotic fungating tumors, albeit with secondary infection (Fig. 3.4), as well as being a normal feature following open biopsy or other surgical procedures. Air in the soft tissues of the thoracic wall and neck always suggests the possibility of surgical emphysema.

Increased radiodensity may be seen in the tissues due to hemosiderin, calcification, or ossification. Hemosiderin deposition typically occurs in synovial tissues exposed to repeated hemorrhage, such as pigmented villonodular synovitis and hemophiliac arthropathy. Radiographs can distinguish between calcification and ossification and the differing patterns [49]. Mineralization in the soft tissues is a feature of a large spectrum of disorders including congenital, metabolic, endocrine,

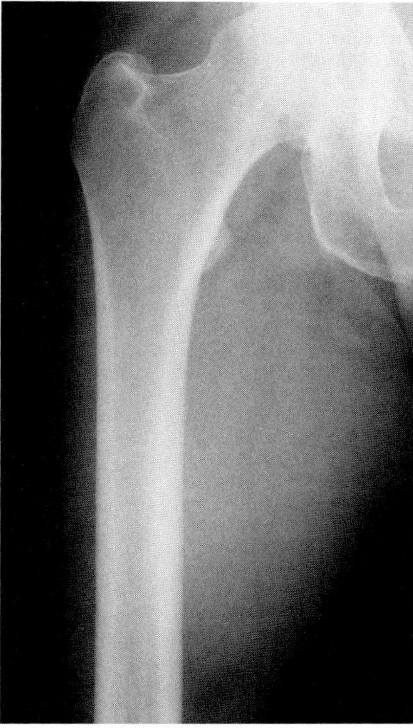

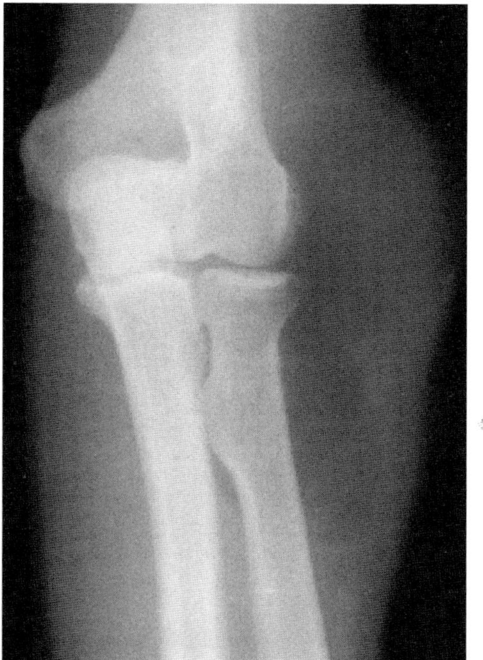

Fig. 3.1. Myxofibrosarcoma arising in the adductors of the upper thigh in a 75-year-old man. Plain radiograph. The tumor is only visible by virtue of its mass effect on tissue planes

Fig. 3.2. Lipoma arising on the radial aspect of the elbow. Plain radiograph. The tumor is sharply marginated with the uniform low density of fat

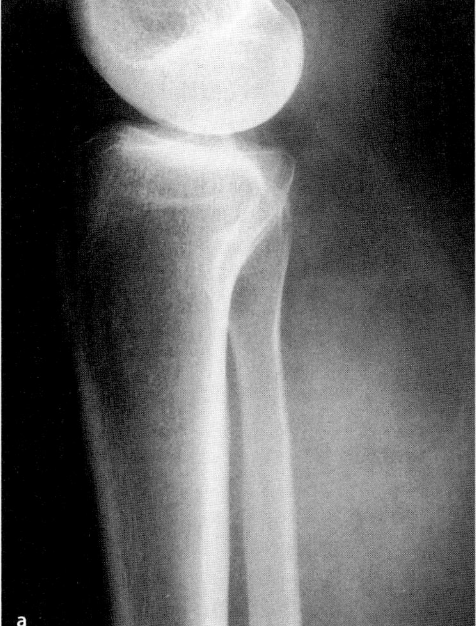

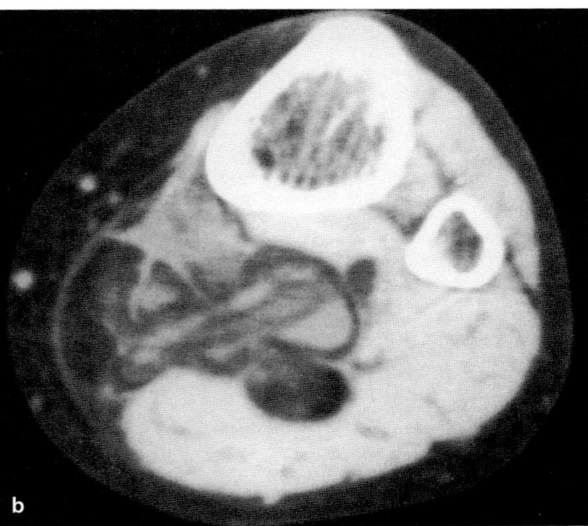

Fig. 3.3 a, b. Low-grade liposarcoma arising behind the knee joint in a 55-year-old woman. **a** Plain radiograph. **b** Computed tomography (CT). Fat density areas are visible on the radiograph (**a**) with mixed fat and soft tissue attenuation on CT (**b**)

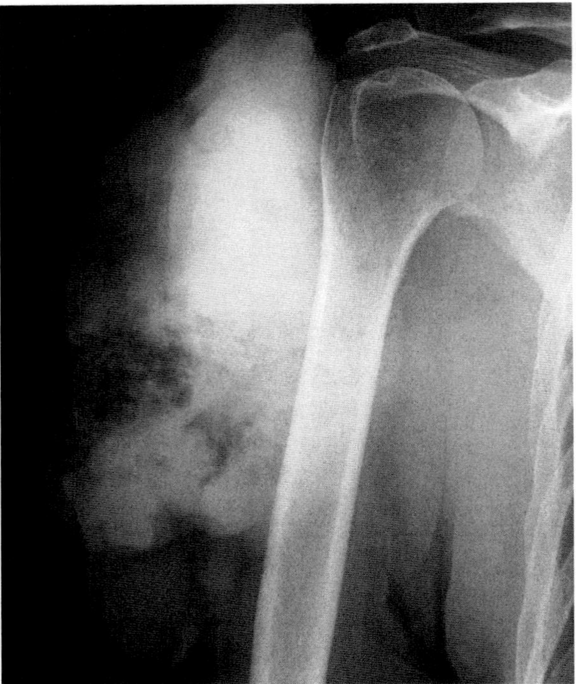

Fig. 3.4. Necrotic, fungating clear cell sarcoma in a 62-year-old woman. Plain radiograph. The loculi of gas within the tumor indicate secondary infection

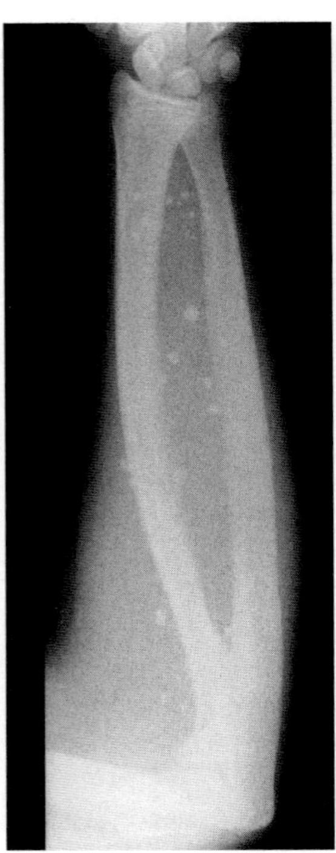

Fig. 3.5. Extensive hemangioma of the forearm in an adolescent male. Plain radiograph. Note the presence of multiple phleboliths

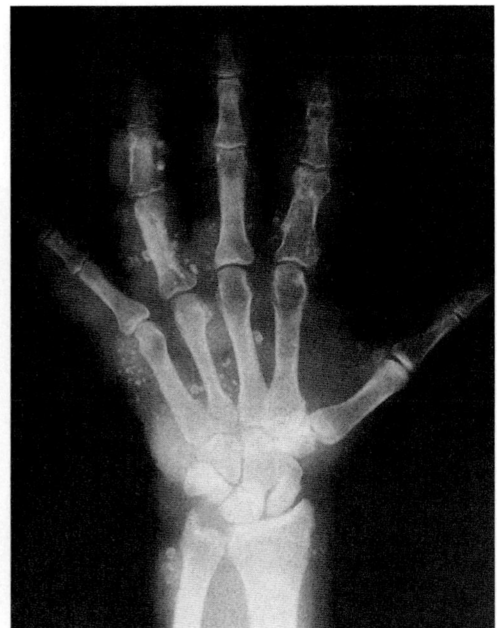

Fig. 3.6. Maffucci syndrome in a 32-year-old man. Plain radiograph. Multiple enchondromas and soft tissue hemangiomas indicated by the phleboliths

traumatic, and parasitic infections [35]. Primary soft tissue tumors are one of the less common causes of calcification that the general radiologist can expect to see in his or her routine practice. Close attention to the clinical details and location will exclude many of the non-neoplastic causes. For example, soft tissue calcifications in the hands and feet are rarely associated with neoplasia, and many of the multifocal lesions will be either due to a collagen vascular disorder or the residuum of a parasitic infection. Again, the clinical details and country of origin of the patient should be pointers to the correct diagnosis. Occasionally certain normal variants, including companion shadows and the fascia lata, may simulate soft tissue calcification or periosteal new bone formation and should not be mistaken for a neoplastic process [18].

Analysis of the pattern of calcification within a soft tissue tumor can indicate the tissue type. Circular foci with a lucent center representing a phlebolith, when identified outside the pelvis, is diagnostic of a hemangioma (Fig. 3.5). Phleboliths are not usually apparent until adolescence, so that conditions such as Maffucci syndrome (Fig. 3.6) in the child may not be radiographically distinguishable from multiple enchondromatosis (Ollier disease).

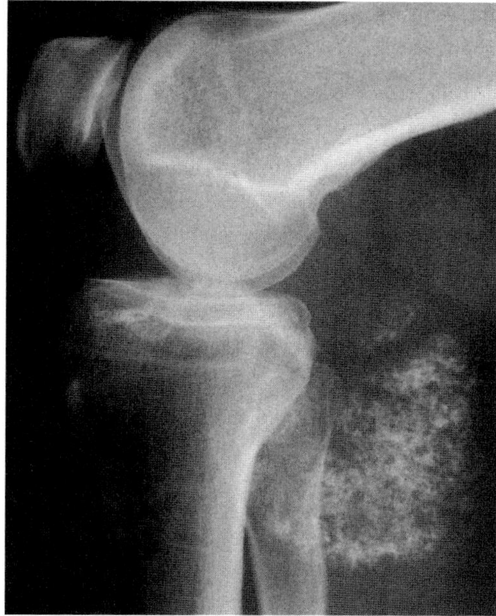

Fig. 3.7. Soft tissue mass in a 62-year-old man. Plain radiograph. Characteristic chondroid calcifications arising from the posterior aspect of the knee joint due to synovial chondromatosis

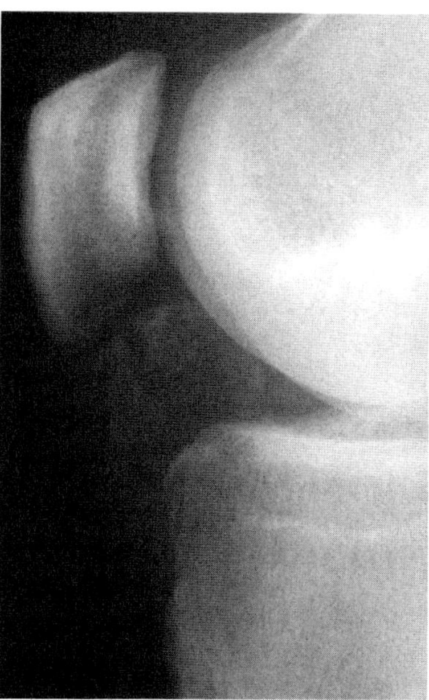

Fig. 3.8. Para-articular osteochondroma in a 44-year-old man. Plain radiograph. Minor ossification arising in the Hoffa fat pad

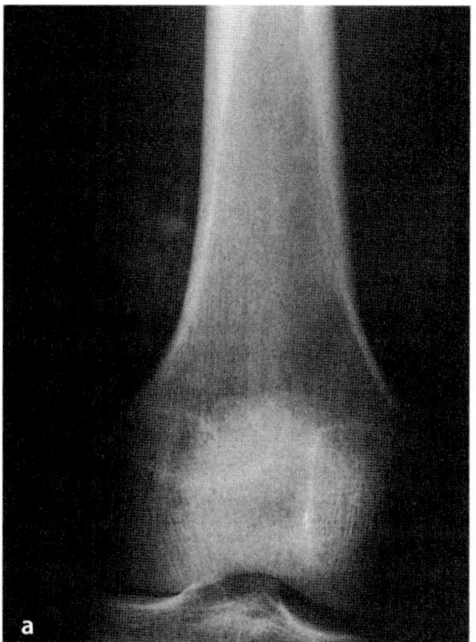

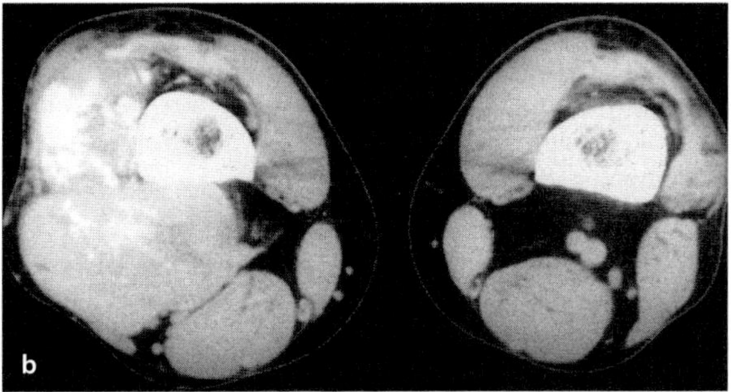

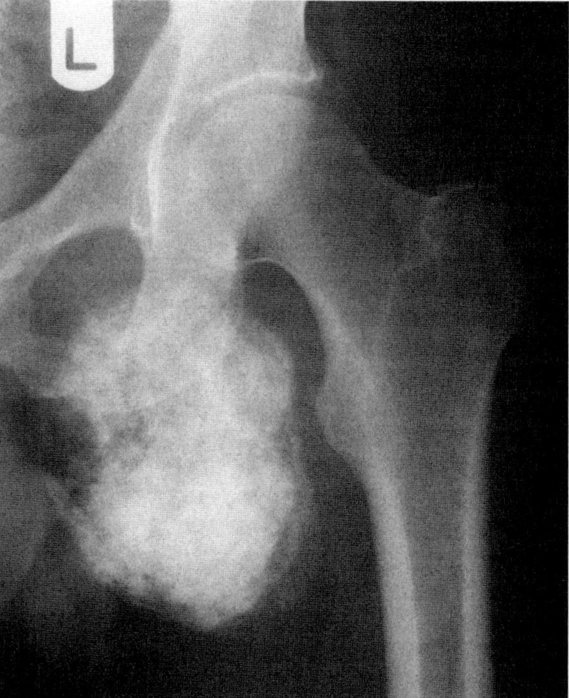

Fig. 3.10. Extraskeletal osteosarcoma in a 50-year-old man. Plain radiograph. Densely mineralized lesion arising in the adductors

Fig. 3.9 a, b. Synovial sarcoma arising in the vastus lateralis in a 66-year-old man. **a** Plain radiograph. **b** CT. Both imaging techniques demonstrate amorphous calcification

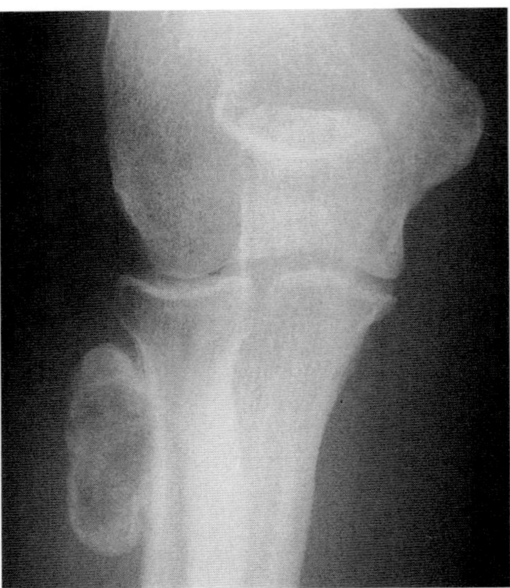

Fig. 3.11. Myositis ossificans of the forearm in a 38-year-old woman. Plain radiograph. Soft tissue mass lying on the surface of the proximal radius showing typical peripheral mineralization

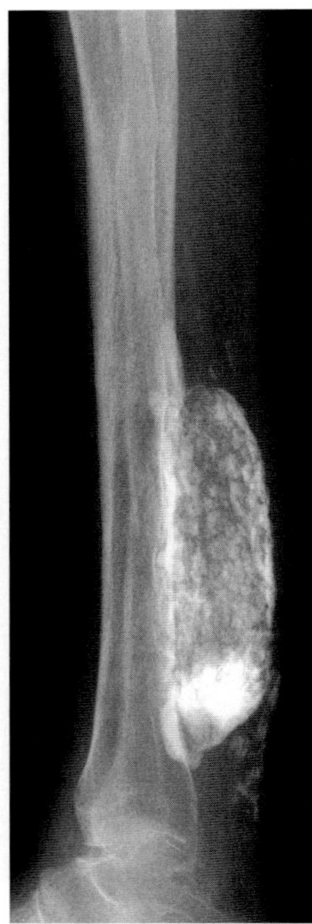

Fig. 3.12. Calcific myonecrosis in an 87-year-old woman. Plain radiograph. Soft tissue mass with peripheral mineralization causing pressure erosion on the adjacent tibia

Chondroid tissue reveals ring-and-arc calcification. While this does not distinguish between benign or malignant cartilage formation, the majority of soft tissue masses with this feature, in the vicinity of a joint, will arise from synovial chondromatosis [34] (Fig. 3.7), and in the hands and feet will be soft tissue chondromas. Calcification or ossification in the infrapatellar (Hoffa) fat pad is typical of a para-articular chondroma/osteochondroma (Fig. 3.8) [13].

Osteoid mineralization may occur as "cloud-like" densities or mature trabecular bone. The latter suggests a slow-growing lesion such as a lipoma, low-grade liposarcoma, or hemangioma [24]. Poorly defined, amorphous calcification is found in up to 30% of synovial sarcomas (Fig. 3.9) [4, 14, 27] and approximately 50% of extraskeletal osteosarcomas (Fig. 3.10). This is an extremely useful distinguishing feature from the tumor mimic myositis ossificans, which exhibits marginal calcification (Fig. 3.11) [9, 30]. Another traumatic condition that presents with a peripherally mineralized mass, almost exclusively in the calf, many years after a major injury, is calcific myonecrosis (Fig. 3.12) [7].

3.2.6 Bone Involvement

It may be difficult to differentiate a primary soft tissue tumor with osseous involvement from a bone tumor with soft tissue extension [24, 25]. As a rule, the site of the more extensive abnormality, be it bone or soft tissue, represents the primary focus [36]. Only a minority of soft tissue tumors involve bone. The degree of bone involvement may vary from cortical hyperostosis, as seen in a parosteal lipoma (Fig. 3.13), through the pressure erosion seen in slow-growing masses (Fig. 3.14), to direct invasion, as seen in aggressive lesions (Fig. 3.15). The presence of ill-defined cortical destruction is strongly indicative of malignancy, although it may also occur with paraosseous infections. The converse does not apply in that well-defined pressure erosion may occur with both benign and malignant soft tissue tumors (Fig. 3.11). Aggressive fibromatosis (extra-abdominal desmoid tumor) is a benign, but locally invasive condition which can cause irregular adjacent bone erosion in one-third of cases (Fig. 3.16).

Cortical destruction with an outer, saucer-like configuration, "saucerization," occurs in Ewing's sarcoma and bony metastatic disease and should not be mistaken for secondary bone invasion from a large soft tissue sarcoma [21].

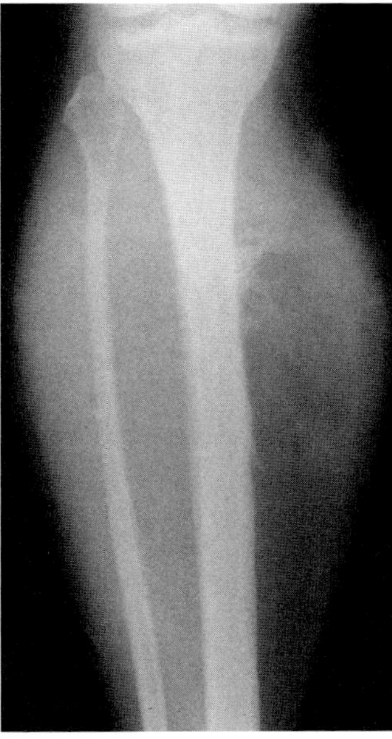

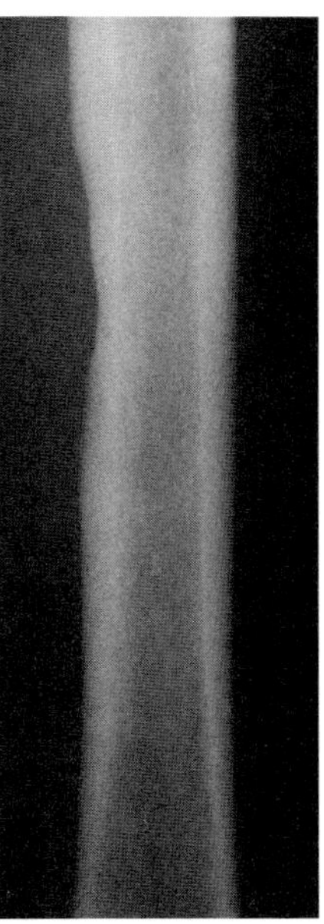

Fig. 3.13. Parosteal lipoma arising on the surface of the tibia in a 67-year-old woman. Plain radiograph. Lobulated fat density mass with typical periosteal new bone formation

Fig. 3.14. Myxofibrosarcoma of the upper leg in a 65-year-old man. Plain radiograph. Soft tissue mass causing pressure erosion on the medial cortex of the femoral diaphysis

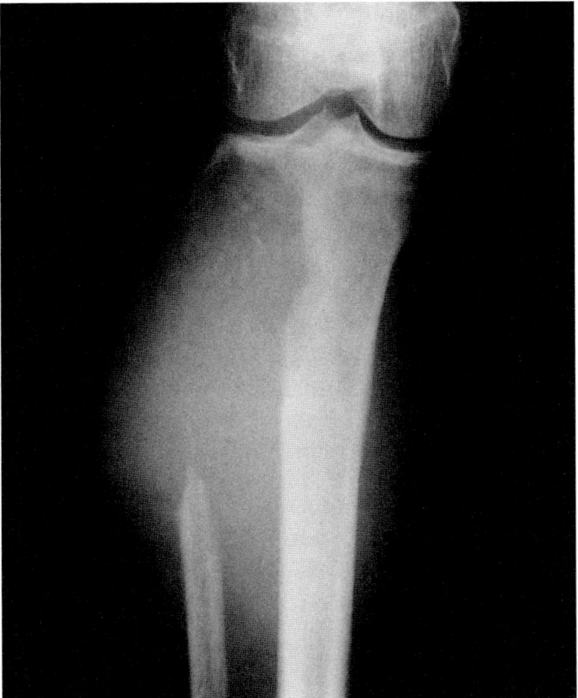

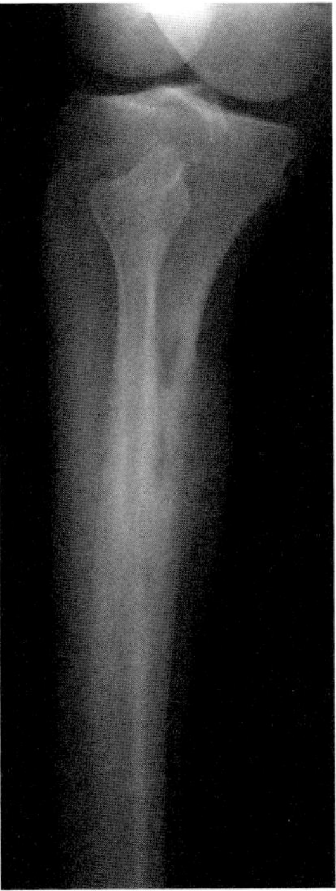

Fig. 3.15. Spindle cell sarcoma of the calf in a 78-year-old woman who refused medical treatment for 2 years. Plain radiograph. The tumor has destroyed the proximal fibula, with extensive invasion of the tibial metaphysis

Fig. 3.16. Aggressive fibromatosis in a 37-year-old woman. Plain radiograph. There is erosion of the proximal tibia

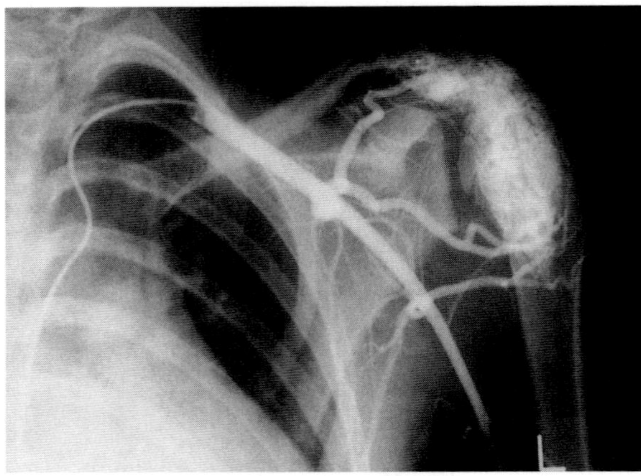

Fig. 3.17. Cavernous hemangioma of the soft tissues over the shoulder in an adolescent male. Angiography. An early film from a selective subclavian angiogram shows feeding via the thoracoacromial and circumflex humeral arteries

3.3 Angiography

Prior to the introduction of cross-sectional imaging, angiography was the most useful imaging technique for the demonstration of soft tissue sarcomas. For many years it was considered an important adjunct to conventional radiography in patient management [15, 23]. The angiographic features of soft tissue malignancies are similar to those at other sites [10]: tumor stain/blush, vessel encasement, and early venous filling. There is an association between increasing vascularity of a tumor and the degree of malignancy [2]. Despite this, it can be difficult to differentiate benign from malignant soft tissue tumors by angiography [15, 16, 44]. Inflammatory lesions such as myositis ossificans appear hypervascular, thereby being easily mistaken for malignancy [50]. Angiography currently has little role in the diagnosis and staging of most soft tissue tumors.

Decreased vascularity is considered a good indicator of tumor response to therapy [10]. It is difficult to justify angiography for this purpose because of its cost and invasiveness. Digital vascular imaging has improved image quality and reduced the radiation dose and contrast-medium load to the patient, but has not fundamentally altered the role of angiography in this patient group.

Angiography can delineate the full extent of feeding and draining vessels of vascular malformations, but has been largely superseded by CT angiography or magnetic resonance (MR) angiography. Preoperative angiography may continue to be employed in planning surgery in difficult cases or as a prelude to embolotherapy [47, 51].

Angiography can differentiate between the two histological types of hemangioma, capillary and cavernous (Fig. 3.17). MR angiography can be a useful adjunct to MRI in selected cases. This includes the differentiation of a soft tissue tumor from an aneurysm.

Controversy exists as to whether the use of adjuvant chemotherapy significantly improves the prognosis for most patients with a high-grade soft tissue sarcoma. In some of the treatment centers in which chemotherapy is given to patients, an intra-arterial route is advocated. In this situation prior angiography is required to ensure optimal siting of the catheter through which the chemotherapy will be administered.

3.4 Computed Tomography

The introduction of CT proved a revolution in the detection and preoperative management of soft tissue tumors [12, 15, 23, 41]. For the first time, a degree of precision was applied to preoperative staging that had previously not been possible. The improving spatial resolution of CT allows for tumors as small as 1–2 cm to be detected, depending on differential attenuation between the tumor and the surrounding soft tissues. The superior contrast sensitivity and cross-sectional ability of CT will reveal masses that are not visible on conventional radiography. Conversely, the demonstration of normal anatomy will exclude all but the smallest lesions.

3.4.1 Technical Considerations

Attention to technique is important. Contiguous slices should be obtained, no more than 5 mm thick. If an interslice gap is employed, there is the potential for understaging involvement of the neurovascular structures, as part of the tumor will not be imaged. Of equal importance are the cranial and caudal margins, which should be clearly demonstrated. In the lower limbs, both sides should be included in the scan field to allow comparison of the normal and abnormal anatomy. In this way subtle abnormalities may be more easily detected. This is not possible with the upper limbs because of the loss of resolution resulting from a scan field that is adequate to include the thorax and both upper limbs. Beam-hardening artifacts can be a particular problem in the upper limb and can be minimized by raising the unaffected arm above the head when positioning the patient on the examination couch.

The images should be assessed using both bone and soft tissue window settings. The window levels utilized will depend on personal preference and the type of scanner. Narrow window settings will be required if density differences are small. The full craniocaudal extent of the tumor can be displayed by performing sagittal or coronal reconstructions. The slice thickness used impacts on reconstruction resolution. The

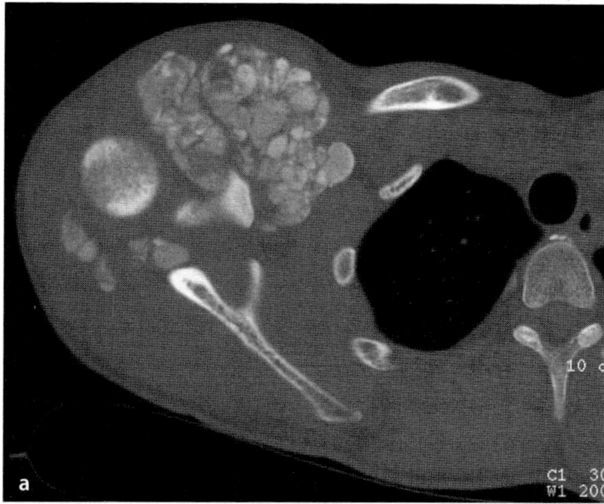

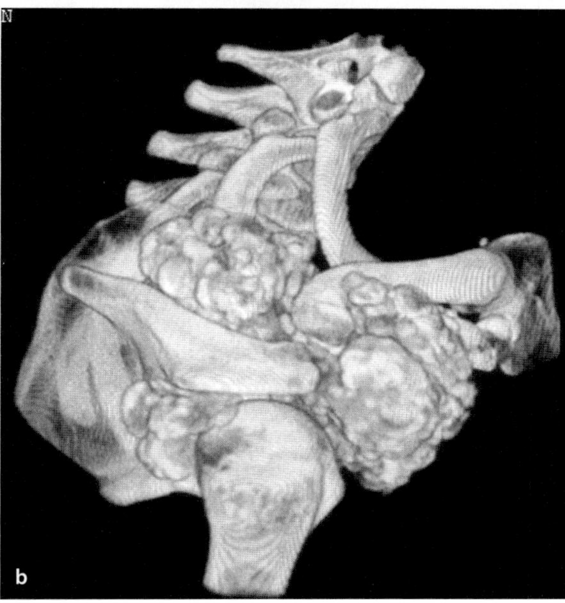

Fig. 3.18 a, b. Tumoral calcinosis associated with chronic renal failure. **a** Computed tomography. **b** Surface-rendered 3D reconstruction. Soft tissue masses with amorphous calcification. The distribution is readily appreciated on the reconstruction (**b**)

introduction in the last 10 years of multislice CT or multidetector-row CT has lead to a renaissance in this technique. Very fast image-acquisition times of large volumes with submillimeter section thickness have become the norm. Although there are some concerns regarding the potential for increasing the radiation dose, thin-section scanning allows for different types of postprocessing, such a multiplanar reconstructions, volume rendering, and surface-shaded display (Fig. 3.18) [38].

3.4.2 CT Features

The CT features that should be assessed in each case are similar to those described above for evaluating the conventional radiograph. This reflects the fact that both are radiographic techniques relying on the attenuation of an X-ray source. The principal advantages of CT over the radiograph are the improved soft tissue resolution and the axial, in contrast to longitudinal, imaging plane. The first feature to assess is the attenuation value of the mass. Fat will show the lowest attenuation of any tissue, and a benign lipoma can be diagnosed on CT by the uniformly low attenuation (–70 to –130 HU; Fig. 3.19) [11, 17]. It is not possible to reliably differentiate on CT a simple lipoma from an atypical lipoma (well-differentiated liposarcoma). In the peripheries this is rarely a management problem, as the treatment of the two conditions is the same. A few fibromuscular septa of soft tissue density traversing the lipoma are acceptable (Fig. 3.19). A tumor comprising a combination of fat and solid component is suggestive of a low-grade liposarcoma (Fig. 3.3b) [6]. Only air will show an attenuation less that that of fat (Fig. 3.20).

Fluid-filled structures, seromas, old hematomas, and synovial cysts have an attenuation value less than that of muscle and more than that of fat (Fig. 3.21) [39, 40, 43]. Such fluid collections are usually homogeneous and well-defined. Abscesses typically have an attenuation value slightly higher than that of simple fluid (Fig. 3.20) [32, 48].

The majority of soft tissue sarcomas have an attenuation value slightly less than that of normal muscle (Fig. 3.22). The highest attenuation found in the soft tissues on CT is that of calcification and ossification, approximating to that of cortical bone. CT exquisitely demonstrates calcification more clearly than conventional radiography (Figs. 3.9, 3.23) and can easily distinguish between calcification and ossification (Figs. 3.9, 3.24) [49]. A peripheral ring of calcification is a characteristic CT feature of myositis ossificans (Fig. 3.25) [1, 19]. The differential diagnosis should include the rare soft tissue aneurysmal bone cyst which also shows peripheral calcification [45].

Tumor margins can easily be defined on CT in most cases provided there is sufficient mass effect or attenuation difference. As might be expected, slow-growing lesions tend to be better defined than aggressive lesions. The margin is an indicator of the rate of growth rather than whether it is benign or malignant. As on conventional radiographs, infective lesions will tend to be poorly defined due to fluid infiltration in the surrounding soft tissues (Fig. 3.20) [32, 48]. The conspicuity of tumor margins and the relationship to adjacent vessels can be improved following enhancement with iodinated contrast medium (Fig. 3.22) [46]. Contrast medium is helpful in those cases where there is doubt as to whether

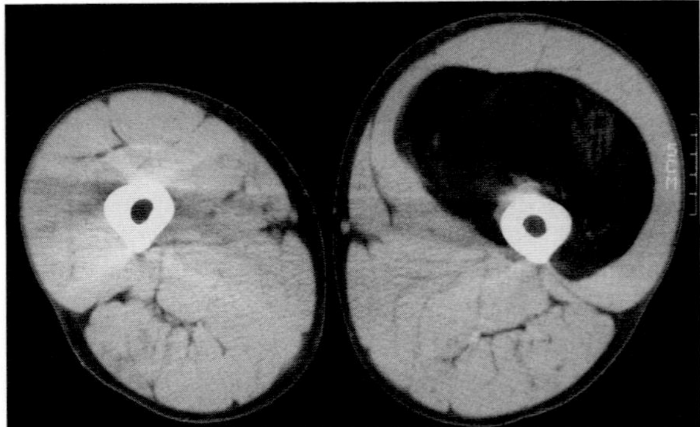

Fig. 3.19. Benign lipoma in the left anterior thigh of a 26-year-old man. Using computed tomography, a few fibromuscular septa can be identified traversing the lipoma

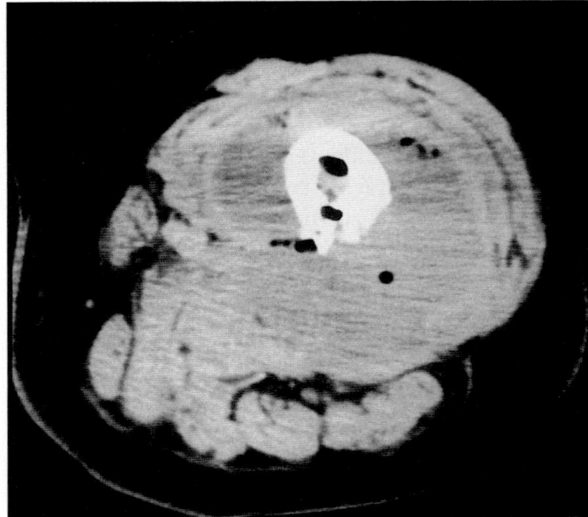

Fig. 3.20. Gas-forming clostridial osteomyelitis of the femur in a 59-year-old man. Computed tomography. Loculi of gas are present within the bone and surrounding abscess

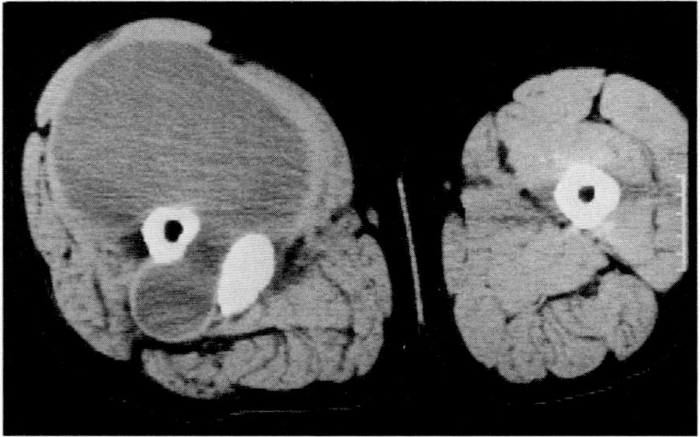

Fig. 3.21. Chronic hematoma in the thigh of a 28-year-old man at the site of nonunion of an old femoral fracture. Computed tomography. The overlapping fracture ends are seen as two separate bony structures. The attenuation of the hematoma measures 20 HU surrounded by a higher attenuation pseudocapsule

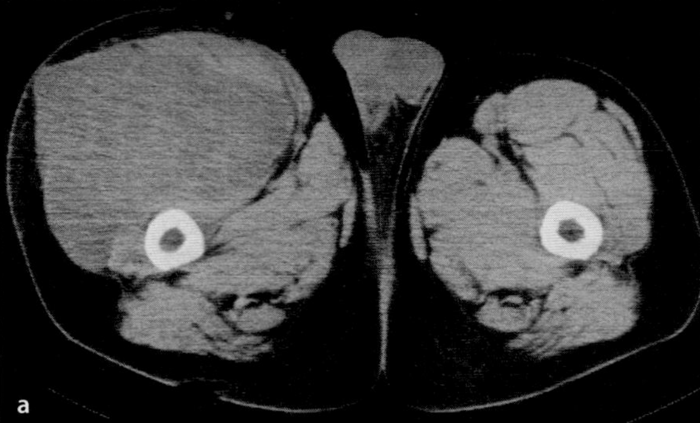

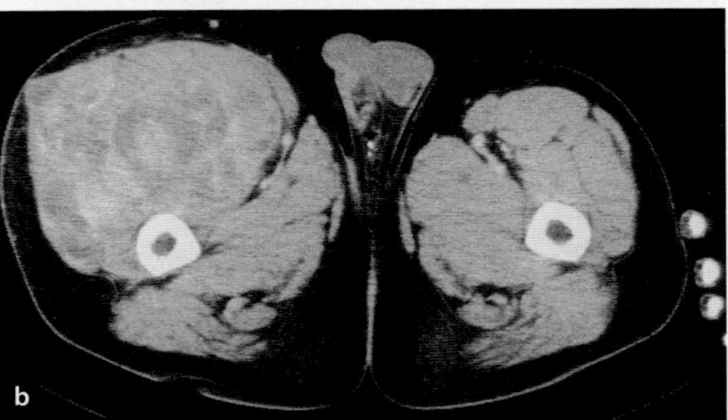

Fig. 3.22 a, b. Liposarcoma of the thigh in a 68-year-old man. **a** Computed tomography (CT) scan. **b** After intravenous contrast medium. Mass arising in the right vastus intermedius muscle slightly hypodense to muscle on unenhanced CT (**a**) and irregularly enhancing after contrast administration (**b**)

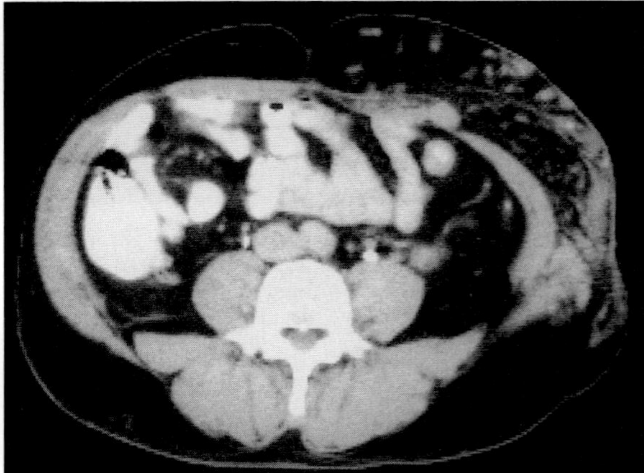

Fig. 3.23. Arteriovenous malformation of the abdominal wall in a 28-year-old woman. Computed tomography. Tiny phleboliths within the subcutaneous tissues of the anterior abdominal wall, not visible on plain radiography, help to confirm the diagnosis

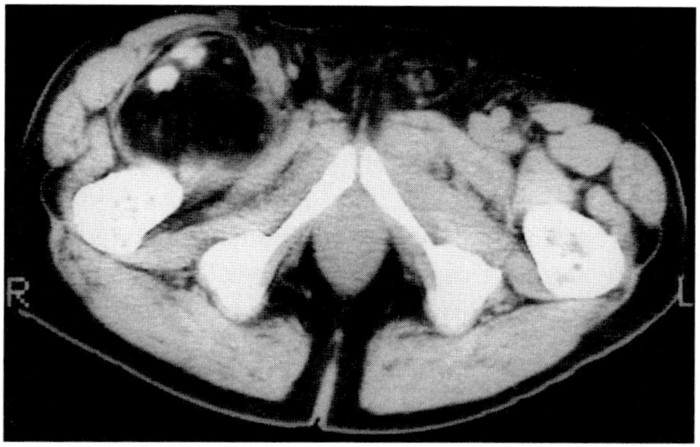

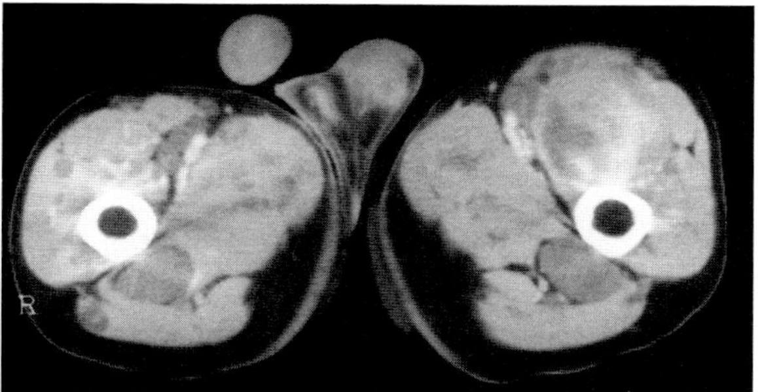

Fig. 3.24. Lipoma of the right thigh in a 51-year-old man. Computed tomography. Hypodense mass arising in the right adductor compartment containing fibromuscular septa and several foci of ossification

Fig. 3.26. Neurofibromatosis in the proximal thighs of a 23-year-old man. Computed tomography (CT) after iodinated contrast injection. Enhancement of the neurofibrosarcoma in the left anterior thigh. The numerous remaining neurofibromata, particularly involving the sciatic nerves, show no significant enhancement

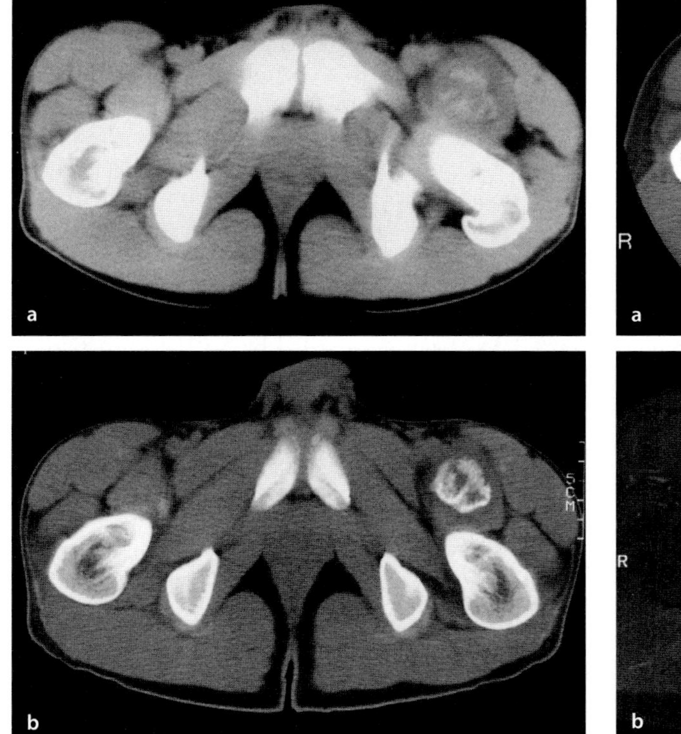

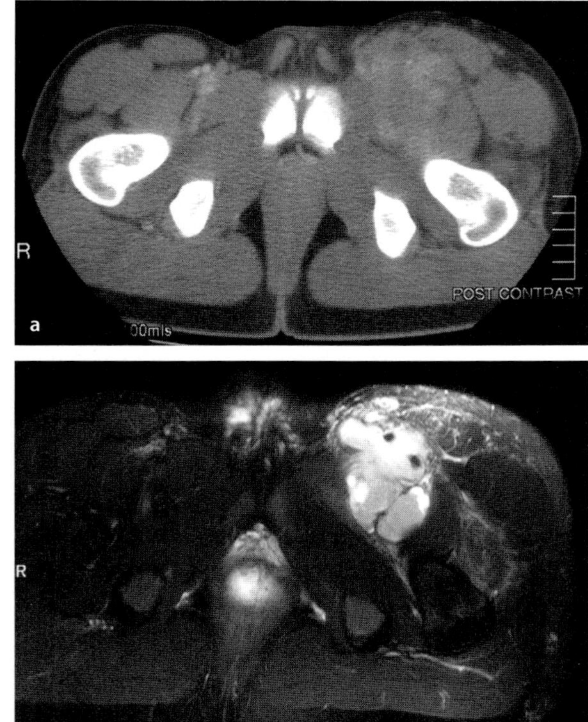

Fig. 3.25 a, b. Myositis ossificans of the proximal thigh in a 12-year-old girl. **a** Computed tomography (CT). **b** CT 6 weeks later. Mass with early peripheral calcification in the left iliopsoas muscle (**a**) and the signs of maturation 6 weeks later (**b**)

Fig. 3.27 a, b. Synovial sarcoma in a 19-year-old man. **a** Computed tomography (CT) with intravenous contrast medium. **b** Axial T2-weighted, fast spin-echo image with fat suppression. Both show the tumor arising in the left groin with involvement of the femoral vessels, but the features are more conspicuous on the MR image (**b**)

a mass is solid or cystic. Very occasionally a soft tissue tumor will be isodense with muscle on a precontrast CT scan and only be revealed on a postcontrast examination [23]. In this situation, the presence of mass effect will usually be sufficient to alert the wary observer. Contrast enhancement will also give an indication of the vascularity of a tumor, which can be of value in selected cases (Figs. 3.26, 3.27).

CT gives an excellent demonstration of the relationship of a soft tissue tumor to the adjacent bones. It is more accurate than conventional radiography, but less so than MRI, revealing medullary bone involvement. It can be useful in assessing the relationship of a tumor to bone in anatomically complex areas such as the spine and pelvis.

3.4.3 CT Compared with MRI

Studies have suggested that CT tends to overestimate the extent of a soft tissue sarcoma [8, 28], presumably due to local lymphatic obstruction. This is not a problem for management, as curative surgery will require excision of the whole compartment, edema and all. It would be a matter of more concern were CT to underestimate the true tumor extent, as this would prejudice attempts at curative surgery.

With limb-salvage surgery, the aim in most patients, there is always a risk of local recurrence, particularly in patients with a high-grade sarcoma. The risk is increased considerably if the excision is found to be marginal or even intralesional. MRI is the preferred technique to detect early recurrences, but both techniques are of comparable accuracy if the recurrence is greater than 15 cm^3 in volume [37]. CT is unable to reliably differentiate residual tumor from hematoma and granulation tissue following excisional biopsy [16].

Twenty years ago it was being claimed that MRI would supersede CT as the primary imaging technique in the evaluation of soft tissue tumors [3, 5]. In the developed world, this prediction has been fulfilled, but where access to MRI remains limited or contraindicated, CT will continue to provide an adequate alternative for the majority of patients with a soft tissue mass. Indeed, one study comparing CT and MRI in the local staging of primary malignant musculoskeletal neoplasms yields the conclusion that both techniques are equally accurate in the local staging of bone and soft tissue neoplasms (Fig. 3.27) [31]. In fairness, this study has been the subject of some controversy since its publication, as critics argue that many of the MR examinations were obtained on older machines, without the use of an intravenous gadolinium chelate [42].

CT remains preeminent in the investigation of chest metastases, revealing nodules several millimeters in diameter that are not visible on a chest radiograph. A CT examination of the chest should be performed as part of the initial preoperative staging of patients with a soft tissue sarcoma. Multislice CT, by eliminating respiratory motion and minimizing partial volume errors, results in a high rate of detection of smaller nodules than are detected with conventional CT. Routine follow-up of patients with serial chest CT examinations is of doubtful value, particularly in view of the considerable radiation dose involved. CT of the chest is indicated if a follow-up chest radiograph suggests early metastatic disease. Metastatic spread to regional lymph nodes is uncommon in soft tissue sarcomas and is usually present only in the later stages of the disease. CT identifies abnormally enlarged nodes but cannot reliably distinguish reactive change from metastatic involvement.

CT can be used to facilitate biopsy of soft tissue tumors, particularly utilizing CT fluoroscopy [52]. It is usually reserved for those cases in which tumors are either small (i.e., impalpable) or situated in a relatively inaccessible location.

Things to remember:
1. Evaluation of a suspected soft tissue mass should always commence with plain radiography. Valuable information may be derived from the presence of calcifications or ossifications, internal fatty components, and air and bone involvement.
2. Angiography has been largely replaced by MRI for soft tissue tumor characterization. It may still be used to preclude embolotherapy or in the case of isolated-limb perfusion with chemotherapy.
3. CT has been superseded by MRI for soft tissue tumor characterization, but it remains valuable for guiding biopsy and for the detection of distant tumor spread in the lungs.

References

1. Amendola MA, Glazer GM, Agha FP, Francis IR, Weatherhouse L, Martel W (1983) Myositis ossificans circumscripta: computed tomographic diagnosis. Radiology 149:775–779
2. Angervall L, Kindblom LG, Rydholm A, Stener B (1986) The diagnosis and prognosis of soft tissue tumors. Semin Diagn Pathol 3:40–258
3. Bland K, McCoy DM, Kinard RE, Copeland EM (1987) Application of magnetic resonance imaging and computed tomography as an adjunct to the surgical management of soft tissue tumors. Ann Surg 205:473–480
4. Cadman NL, Soule EH, Kelly PJ (1965) Synovial sarcoma: analysis of 134 tumors. Cancer 18:613–627
5. Chang AE, Matory YL, Dwyer AJ, Hill SC, Girton ME, Steinberg SM, Knop RH, Frank YA, Hyams D, Doppman YL (1987) Magnetic resonance imaging versus computed tomography in the evaluation of soft tissue tumors of the extremities. Ann Surg 205:340–348
6. deSantos LA, Ginaldi S, Wallace S (1981) Computed tomography in liposarcoma. Cancer 47:46–54
7. Dhillon M, Davies AM, Benham J, Evans N, Mangham DC, Grimer RJ (2004) Calcific myonecrosis: a report of ten new cases. Eur Radiol 14:1974–1979

8. Egund N, Ekeland L. Sako M, Persson B (1981) CT of soft tissue tumors. AJR Am J Roentgenol 137:725–729

9. Goldman AB (1976) Myositis ossificans circumscripta: a benign lesion with a malignant differential diagnosis. AJR Am J Roentgenol 126:32–40

10. Greenfield GB, Arrington JA (1995) Imaging of bone tumors. Lippincott, Philadelphia

11. Halldorsdottir A, Ekelund L, Rydholm A (1982) CT diagnosis of lipomatous tumors of the soft tissues. Arch Orthop Trauma Surg 100:211–216

12. Heiken JP, LeeJKT, Smathers RL, Totty WG, Murphy WA (1984) CT of benign soft tissue masses of the extremities. AJR Am J Roentgenol 142:575–580

13. Helpert C, Davies AM, Evans N, Grimer RJ Differential diagnosis of tumors and tumor-like lesions of the infrapatellar (Hoffa's) fat pad. Eur Radiol 14:2337–2346

14. Horowitz AL, ResnickD, Watson RC (1973) The roentgen features of synovial sarcoma. Clin Radiol 24:481–484

15. Hudson TM, Hass G, Enneking WF (1975) Angiography in the management of musculoskeletal tumors. Surg Gynecol Obstet 141:11–21

16. Hudson TM, Schakel M, Springfield DS (1985) Limitations of computed tomography following excisional biopsy of soft tissue sarcomas. Skeletal Radiol 13:49–54

17. Hunter JC, Johnston WH, Genant HK (1979) Computed tomography evaluation of fatty tumors of the somatic soft tissues: clinical utility and radiology-pathologic correlation. Skeletal Radiol 4:79–91

18. Keats TE (1992) Atlas of normal variants that may simulate disease, 5th edn. Mosby Year Book, St. Louis

19. Kransdorf MJ, Meis JM, Jelinek JS (1991) Myositis ossificans: MR appearance with radiologic-pathologic correlation. AJR Am J Roentgenol 157:1243–1248

20. Kransdorf MJ, Jelinek JS. Moser RP Jr (1993) Imaging soft tissue tumors. Radiol Clin North Am 31:359–372

21. Kricun ME (1983) Radiographic evaluation of solitary bone lesions. Orthop Clin North Am 14:39–64

22. Lec KR, Cox GC, Neff JR, Arnett GR, Murphy MD (1987) Cystic masses of the knee; arthrographic and CT evaluation. AJR Am J Roentgenol 148:329–334

23. Levine E, Lec KR, Neff JR, Maklad NF, Robinson RG, Preston DF (1979) Comparison of computed tomography and other imaging modalities in the evaluation of musculoskeletal tumors. Radiology 131:431–437

24. Madewell JE, Moser RPJr (1995) Radiologic evaluation of soft tissue tumors. In: Enzinger FM, Weiss SW (eds) Soft tissue tumors, 3rd edn. Mosby, St Louis, pp 39–88

25. MartelW, Abell MR (1973) Radiologic evaluation of soft tissue tumors: a retrospective study. Cancer 32:352–366

26. Melson GL, Staple TW, Evens RG (1973) Soft tissue radiographic techniques. Semin Roentgenol 8:9–24

27. Murray JA (1977) Synovial sarcoma. Orthop Clin North Am 8:963–972

28. Neifield JP, Walsh JW, Lawrence W (1983) Computed tomography in the management of soft tissue tumors (abstract). Radiology 147:911

29. Nessi R, Gattoni F, Mazzoni R, Coopmans Y de, Veronesi U (1981) Xeroradiography of soft tissue tumors. Fortschr Rontgenstr 134:669–673

30. Norman A, Dorfman HD (1970) Juxtacortical circumscribed myositis ossificans: evolution and radiographic features. Radiology 96:301–306

31. Panicek DM, Gatsonis CG, Rosenthal DI, et al (1997) CT and MRI in the local staging of primary malignant musculoskeletal neoplasms: report of the Radiology Diagnostic Oncology Group. Radiology 202:237–246

32. Patel RB, Barton P, Salimi Z, Molitor J (1983) Computed tomography of complicated psoas abscess with intraabscess contrast medium injection. J Comput Assist Tomogr 7:911–913

33. Pirkey EL, Hurt J (1959) Roentgen evaluation of the soft tissues in orthopedics. AJR Am J Roentgenol 82:271–276

34. Pope TL, Keats TE, Lange EE de, Fechner RE, Harvey YW (1987) Idiopathic synovial chondromatosis in two unusual sites: inferior radioulnar joint and ischial bursa. Skeletal Radiol 16:205–208

35. Reeder MM (1993) Gamuts in bones, joints and spine radiology. Springer, Berlin Heidelberg New York, pp 365–373

36. Resnick D (1995) Diagnosis of bone and joint disorders, 3rd edn. Saunders, Philadelphia, pp 4491–4500

37. Resther G, Mutscher W (1990) Detection of local recurrent disease in musculoskeletal tumors: magnetic resonance imaging versus computed tomography. Skeletal Radiol 19:85–90

38. Rydberg J, Liang Y, Teague SD (2004) Fundamentals of multichannel CT. Semin Musculoskel Radiol 8:137–146

39. Sartoris DJ, Danzig L, Gilula LA, Greenway G, Resnick D (1985) Synovial cysts of the hip joint and iliopsoas bursitis: a spectrum of imaging abnormalities. Skeletal Radiol 14:85–94

40. Schwimmer M, Edelstein G, Heiken JP, Gilula LA (1983) Synovial cysts of the knee: CT evaluation. Radiology 154:175–177

41. Soye I, Levine E, DeSmet AA, Neff YR (1982) Computed tomography in the preoperative evaluation of masses arising in or near the joints of the extremities. Radiology 143:727–732

42. Steinbach LS (1998) CT and MRI in the local staging of primary malignant musculoskeletal neoplasms: comments. Sarcoma 2:57–58

43. Steinbach LS, Schneider R, Goldman AB (1985) Bursae and abscess cavities communicating with the hip: diagnosis using arthrography and CT. Radiology 156:303–307

44. Viamonte MM, Roen S, LePage J (1973) Nonspecificity of abnormal vascularity in the radiographic diagnosis of malignant neoplasms. Radiology 106:59–69

45. Wang XL, Gielen JL, Salgado R, Delrue F, De Schepper AMA (2004) Soft tissue aneurysmal bone cyst: case report. Skeletal Radiol 33:477–480

46. Weekes RG, McLeod RA, Reiman HM, Pritchard DJ (1985) CT of soft tissue neoplasms. AJR Am J Roentgenol 144:355–360

47. Widlow DM, Murray RR, White RI, Osterman FA Jr, Schrieber ER, Satre RW, Mitchell SE, Kaufman SL, Williams GM, Weiland AJ (1988) Congenital arteriovenous malformations: tailored embolotherapy. Radiology 169:511–516

48. Wolverson MK, Jaggannadharao B, Sundaram M, Heiberg E, Grider R (1981) Computed tomography in the diagnosis of gluteal abscess and other peripelvic collections. J. Comput Assist Tomogr 5:34–38

49. Wybier M, Laredo JD (2004) Place et limites de la radiographie et du scanner dans le diagnostic des tumeurs et pseudotumeurs des parties molles. In: Laredo JD, Tomeno B, Malghem J, Drape JL, Wybier M, Railhac JJ (eds) Conduite á tenir devant une image osseuse ou des parties molles d'allure tumorale. Sauramps Medical, Montpelier, pp 285–295

50. Yaghmai I (1979) Angiography of bone and soft tissue lesions. Springer, Berling Heidelberg New York, pp 365–366

51. Yakes WF, Pevsner R, Reed M, Donohue HJ, Ghaed W (1986) Serial embolization of an extremity arteriovenous malformation with alcohol via direct percutaneous puncture. AJR Am J Roentgenol 146:1038–1040

52. Zornoza J, Bernardino ME, Ordonez NG, Cohen MA, Thomas YL (1982) Percutaneous needle biopsy of soft tissues guided by ultrasound and computed tomography. Skeletal Radiol 9:33–36

Nuclear Medicine Imaging

4

L. Carp, P.P. Blockx

Contents

4.1 Introduction

Until the 1990s, the role of nuclear medicine procedures in the workup of soft tissue tumors had been quite modest, for various reasons. Firstly, soft tissue tumors are not a common type of tumor; they only account for about 1% of all malignances [91].

Secondly, nuclear medicine procedures attempted in the past for this type of tumor yielded rather disappointing results, among other reasons due to technical limitations and a limited choice of appropriate radiopharmaceuticals [59].

Clinicians then gradually abandoned nuclear medicine examinations for this application and relied more and more upon the increasing armamentarium of nonradioactive imaging modalities: ultrasonography, computed tomography (CT), and magnetic resonance imaging (MRI).

However, a comeback of nuclear medicine procedures in the study of soft tissue tumors has been observed. This is mainly due to the introduction of positron emission tomography (PET) into clinical diagnosis, resulting in a sensitivity and a specificity that are unattained by other imaging modalities.

There are two main reasons to perform scintigraphic procedures in the management of soft tissue tumors:

1. If the tumor takes up the radiopharmaceutical, metastases and recurrences will generally also do so. This, combined with the possibility of performing total body imaging and as many additional spot views as may appear necessary without increasing the radiation burden leads naturally to the use of radiotracer techniques in staging procedures and in follow-up.

2. Some radiopharmaceuticals appear to be taken up only by viable tumor cells, which makes it possible to distinguish between scar tissue and residual tumor in post-therapeutic follow-up.

4.2 Radiopharmaceuticals

Some radiopharmaceuticals have been used extensively in the workup of soft tissue tumors ([67Ga]gallium citrate, 99mTc-labeled sestamibi, 99mTc-MIBI, skeletal imaging agents).

More specific radiopharmaceuticals are increasingly being used: [123I]iobenguane (MIBG), 111In-labeled octreotide, and in particular [18F]fluorodeoxyglucose ([18F]FDG).

4.2.1 Radiopharmaceuticals for General Use

4.2.1.1 Lesser-Used Radiopharmaceuticals

Lesser-used radiopharmaceuticals in the diagnosis of soft tissue tumors include 99mTc-labeled red blood cells (RBC; restricted to the diagnosis of hemangiomas) [3, 8, 20, 52, 73, 77], 99mTc-labeled diethyltriamine pentaacetic acid (DTPA) [29], 99mTc-labeled pentavalent dimercaptosuccinic acid [DMSA(V)] [11, 48, 49, 69], and 111In-labeled antimyosin monoclonal antibodies or fragments, which have been used especially in muscle tumors [17, 36, 37, 38, 45, 75]. None of these have become widely used, owing to the introduction of other imaging techniques with better sensitivity and/or specificity, in particular MRI and PET.

4.2.1.2 [^{67}Ga]Gallium Citrate

The mechanism of ^{67}Ga uptake by tumors is still not completely understood. Larson et al. have suggested that ^{67}Ga uptake in tumors is mediated by a cell-surface transferrin receptor [57].

However, soft tissue sarcomas have been reported to show a high avidity for ^{67}Ga: sensitivities as high as 96% have been reported [80, 86]. Specificity (i.e., detecting only tumoral processes) is generally very good, except in patients with inflammation.

For a few weeks after radiotherapy or chemotherapy, ^{67}Ga uptake in the tumor may be artificially decreased, perhaps through increased binding of iron to transferrin, displacing ^{67}Ga [68]. Iron therapy, as well as scandium and gadolinium contrast agents, have been reported to decrease ^{67}Ga uptake [33, 42, 97].

In a prospective study on 55 patients to evaluate the efficacy of gallium scintigraphy in detecting malignancy in any soft tissue mass, Schwartz et al. have reported a sensitivity of 96% and a specificity of 87%. Large and small sarcomas, irrespective of their fascial location, are identifiable by gallium imaging [80].

In a series of 56 patients with metastatic or recurrent soft tissue sarcoma, Southee et al. have reported ^{67}Ga avidity to be closely associated with tumor grade, with the exception of mesothelioma. No relationship has been found between ^{67}Ga avidity and cell type, lesion size, or disease site. The sensitivity for detection of metastases and recurrences is similar to that for the primary tumor (93% versus 91%). Tumor size is not a determining factor: high-grade lesions as small as 3×3 mm have been detected, while low-grade lesions of more than 1 cm remain undetected. Due to liver and bowel activity, however, sensitivity in these areas is substantially lower (e.g., 56% for intrahepatic lesions) [86].

Kaposi sarcoma, which biologically behaves differently from other sarcomas, generally does not show ^{67}Ga uptake. This feature may be used to distinguish Kaposi sarcoma from infection [76].

Imaeda et al. have conducted a study on 90 patients with soft tissue tumors of the extremities (19 malignant, 55 benign, 16 tumor-like lesions). Increased uptake of ^{67}Ga was found in 78% of patients with malignant tumors, 25% of patients with benign tumors, and 31% of patients with other disorders. High uptakes were observed in liposarcoma, leiomyosarcoma, malignant lymphoma, neurinoma, extraabdominal desmoid, and sarcoidosis [41].

In 1994, Cogswell et al. published a 10-year review of bone and gallium scintigraphy in children with rhabdomyosarcoma. With respect to detection of metastatic disease in all tissues, gallium scans had a sensitivity of 84% (specificity 95%) and bone scans a sensitivity of 70% (specificity also 95%). When only patients with gallium-avid primary tumors were considered, gallium scan sensitivity for detecting metastases was 94% [16].

Lin et al. studied the value of bone and gallium imaging in 34 patients with malignant fibrous histiocytoma. Gallium scintigraphy sensitivity was 93% with respect to primary tumors and 100% for metastases [60].

From these studies, we can conclude that ^{67}Ga imaging can have an adjunctive role in the staging of patients with soft tissue sarcomas and in identifying foci unsuspected clinically or radiographically, which are reported to be present in 9% [86] to 13% [80] of the patients. In particular, foci of active tumor within residual, posttreatment masses can be detected. Moreover a ^{67}Ga-positive site that reverts to negative is indicative of a favorable response to therapy [86].

4.2.1.3 ^{201}Tl Chloride

^{201}Tl is a monovalent cationic radionuclide with biological properties similar to those of potassium [26]. The mechanism of intracellular uptake is one of active transport, which makes thallium chloride a more accurate indicator of the viability of the tumor cells and of metabolic activity than radiotracers that are more flow dependent [66].

^{201}Tl in particular appears to reflect tumor activity more accurately than ^{67}Ga, because of the larger nonspecific uptake of the latter, due to uptake by inflammatory lesions [40]. ^{201}Tl can play a role in differentiating post-therapy changes from residual viable tumor tissue, local recurrence, or necrosis [95].

^{201}Tl chloride has been shown to have an affinity for a variety of soft tissue sarcomas [40, 51]. Terui et al. have reported a sensitivity of 81.2% for ^{201}Tl and 68.8% for ^{67}Ga in a group of 78 patients with soft tissue sarcomas and 22 patients with benign soft tissue tumors [90]. In a series of 29 patients previously treated for musculoskeletal sarcomas, Kostakoglu et al. found no correlation between different tumor types and ^{201}Tl uptake [51]. However, a relationship was found between the tumor grade, the number of viable cells, and the vascular supply. The presence of necrosis decreased ^{201}Tl uptake. The highest tumor-to-background ratio (TBR) was found in a patient with rhabdomyosarcoma and the lowest in one with low-grade osteosarcoma. The authors suggest that ^{201}Tl is particularly valuable in distinguishing benign from malignant tissue. In their series, ^{201}Tl scintigraphy performed better than other imaging modalities (CT, MRI, or angiography): sensitivity of

100% versus 95%, specificity of 87.5% versus 50%, and accuracy of 96.5% versus 82.7%.

In a series of 62 patients with bone and soft tissue tumors, Goto et al. evaluated sequential ^{201}Tl scans on both early images and delayed images. Sensitivity, specificity, and accuracy in detecting malignant tumors was 94%, 65%, and 82% for early imaging and 94%, 85%, and 90%, respectively, for delayed imaging. They concluded that ^{201}Tl scintigraphy, although showing some false-positive and false-negative findings, is a useful tool in differentiating malignant tumors from benign lesions [30].

4.2.1.4 ^{99m}Tc-Labeled Sestamibi

Because of its similarity to ^{201}Tl, and also because of its better imaging characteristics, ^{99m}Tc-MIBI has been proposed as a suitable radiotracer for use in imaging malignant tumors. In the specific area of soft tissue sarcomas, a few reports are available that explore these possibilities.

Taki et al. have compared the ability of ^{201}Tl and ^{99m}Tc-MIBI to detect and assess tumor response to chemotherapy in malignant and benign bone and soft tissue lesions. They studied 42 patients with various bone and soft tissue pathologies (29 malignant and 13 benign lesions). In quantitative analysis, the uptake ratios obtained with ^{201}Tl and ^{99m}Tc-MIBI were similar. In 11 patients with malignant tumors, ^{201}Tl and ^{99m}Tc-MIBI scintigraphy was repeated after chemotherapy, and the uptake of both tracers was significantly suppressed in patients with complete response confirmed by histological evaluation. The ability of ^{99m}Tc-MIBI to detect malignant and benign bone and soft tissue lesions and to assess tumor response to chemotherapy was comparable with that of ^{201}Tl. In addition blood flow was assessed by means of radionuclide angiography with ^{99m}Tc-MIBI [88].

Nagaraj et al. studied the usefulness of serial ^{99m}Tc-MIBI scans in evaluating the tumor response to preoperative chemotherapy in 28 patients with bone ($n=10$) and soft tissue sarcomas ($n=18$). They concluded that ^{99m}Tc-MIBI is an excellent indicator of tumor viability. Serial scans provide an accurate correlation between MIBI uptake and histological response to treatment, which allows optimization of chemotherapy prior to limb salvage [67].

Garcia et al. compared the diagnostic accuracy of FDG-PET and ^{99m}Tc-MIBI single-photon emission CT (SPECT) in 48 patients with clinically suspected recurrent or residual musculoskeletal sarcomas. The diagnostic sensitivities and specificities were 98% and 90% using [^{18}F]FDG, and 82% and 80% using ^{99m}Tc-MIBI, respectively. Four of nine patients with positive FDG but negative MIBI scans failed to respond to multidrug

therapy (see also Comparison with Other Radiotracers, Sect. 4.2.4.1) [25].

^{99m}Tc-MIBI has also been proposed as an indicator for multidrug resistance, both in vitro [6] and in vivo [13]. Multidrug resistance, which is a major limitation in chemotherapy, has been associated with amplification or increased expression of the *ABCB1* [*ATP-binding cassette, sub-family B (MDR/TAP), member 1*]*multidrug* gene and overproduction of its product, the transporter glycoprotein Pgp (P-glycoprotein), which causes washout of intracellular cytostatic drugs [46]. Several reports suggest that intracellular MIBI is also eliminated by Pgp, so that MIBI could be used for multidrug resistance scintigraphy in vivo.

Taki et al. studied ^{99m}Tc-MIBI as a functional imaging agent that reflected Pgp expression in malignant bone and soft-tissue tumors in 30 patients. The washout ratio of ^{99m}Tc-MIBI was higher in patients with a high Pgp expression than in patients without. They concluded that ^{99m}Tc-MIBI scintigraphy with washout analysis may be a useful method for evaluating Pgp overexpression and its function (washout of intracellular cytostatic drugs) [89].

De Moerloose et al. evaluated the usefulness of ^{99m}Tc-MIBI scintigraphy in the screening of neural crest tumors for the presence of Pgp. They studied ten children suffering from proto-oncogene *MYCN*-negative neuroblastoma, ganglioneuroblastoma or ganglioneuroma. In nine of ten patients they found that the intratumoral ^{99m}Tc-MIBI activity was comparable with the background activity, suggesting the presence of Pgp. In one patient ^{99m}Tc-MIBI enhancement was seen in the primary tumor and the bone marrow metastases, and this result was concordant with a negative Pgp status [19].

4.2.1.5 Skeletal Imaging Agents

^{99m}Tc-labeled phosphate compounds, which were originally intended for skeletal imaging, are also known to be taken up by a wide variety of soft tissue abnormalities, including various soft tissue tumors [14]. Several authors have suggested radiophosphate uptake to correlate with blood flow, hypervascularity, and microscopic calcification in the tumor [7, 71].

In a series of 113 patients with soft tissue masses, Chew et al. found that all but one of the patients with normal scans (28 of 29) had benign processes or no identifiable lesion at all. However, many other benign lesions did demonstrate radionuclide uptake (e.g., some angiolipomas, hematomas, lipomas, neurofibromas, myxomas; Figs. 4.1, 4.2) [12]. Moreover, soft tissue trauma, including surgical incisions, can produce focal uptake on the scan. Therefore confusion can arise if the patient has recently undergone biopsy.

Bone metastases from primary soft tissue sarcomas are unusual. Felix et al. [24] detected no metastases on

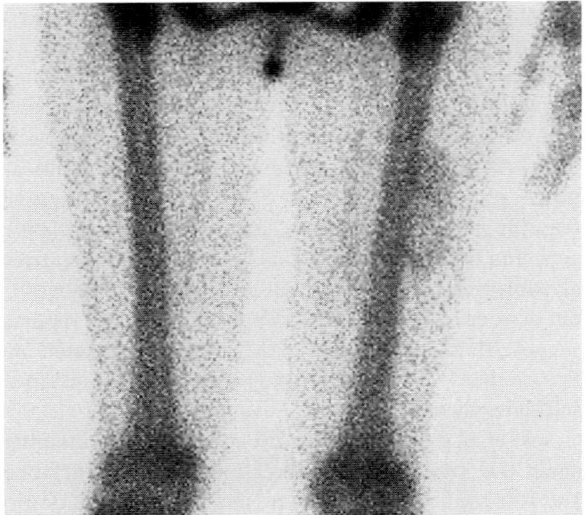

Fig. 4.1. Intramuscular myxoma of the left musculus vastus lateralis in a 38-year-old woman. Anterior view (planar scintigraphy). Scintigraphy with the skeletal imaging agent ^{99m}Tc-labeled methylene diphosphonate shows a large oval zone of slightly increased tracer uptake, lateral from the left femur, at about mid-shaft. The tumor shows a relatively less pronounced uptake in the center of the distal half, corresponding to a glazy substance found at biopsy

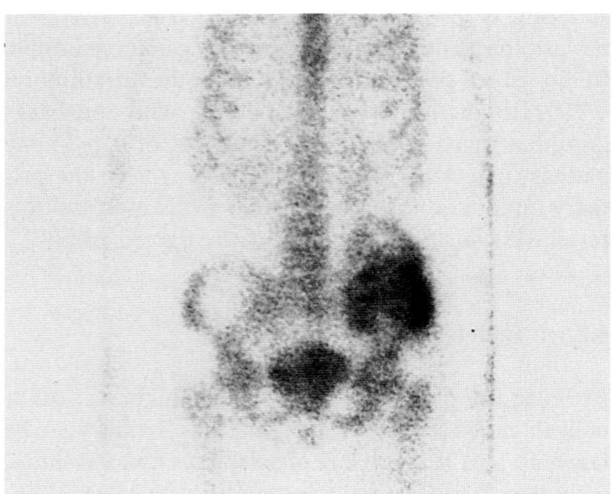

Fig. 4.2. Low-grade hemangiopericytoma within the greater pelvis of a 53-year-old woman. Anterior view (from total body scintigraphy). This very large soft tissue tumor invaded the bone structures of the left iliac wing. Scintigraphy with ^{99m}Tc-labeled methylene diphosphonate revealed a very intense, but inhomogeneous uptake in the tumor itself

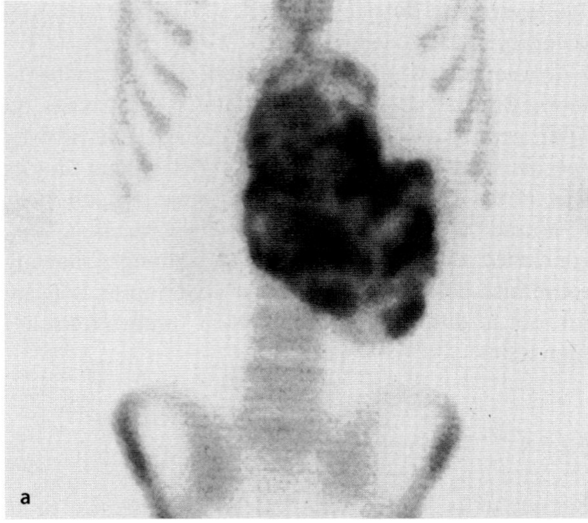

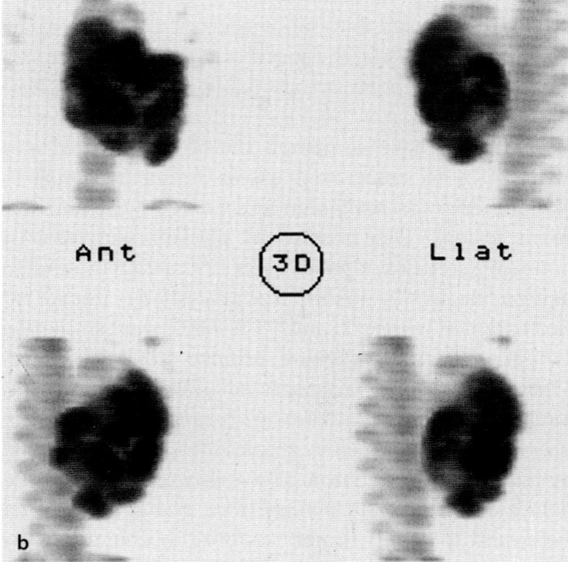

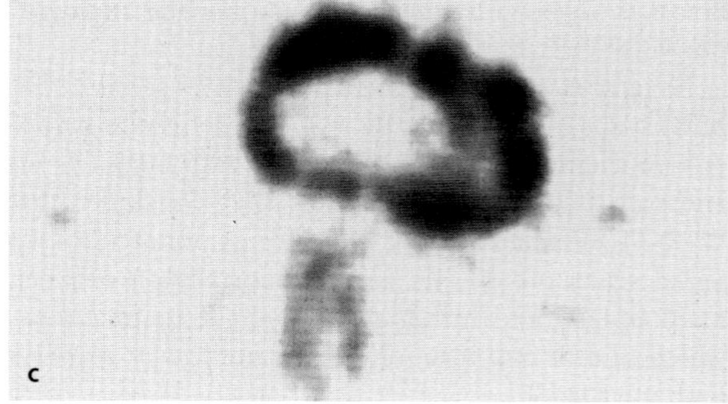

Fig. 4.3a–c. Soft tissue metastasis of an osteosarcoma in a 21-year-old man. **a** Anterior view (planar scintigraphy). **b** Three-dimensional reconstruction viewed from four different angles: anterior, left lateral, right posterior oblique, and right lateral (single-photon emission computed tomography, SPECT). **c** Transverse slice (SPECT) showing the large central uptake defect. An enormous abdominal soft tissue metastasis of a resected osteosarcoma of the left knee was found on follow-up bone scintigraphy images with ^{99m}Tc-labeled methylene diphosphonate (**a, b**). The uptake is very intense but also very inhomogeneous, with a large central uptake defect (necrosis) (**c**)

the radionuclide bone scans of 59 patients with sarcomas, and Chew et al. [12] found metastases on the bone scans of only 5 of 80 sarcoma patients (Fig. 4.3). The value of the radionuclide bone scan in the preoperative workup of soft tissue tumors lies therefore in the evaluation of the relationship of the primary tumor to adjacent bone rather than in the detection of metastases.

Enneking has shown that increased uptake in bone adjacent to a soft tissue sarcoma indicates bone involvement [22]. Such involvement may also be present when the bone tracer accumulation in the soft tissue lesion itself is contiguous with the bone and cannot be separated even on appropriate multiple scan views. Because adequate surgical resection of aggressive tumors requires complete removal of all involved structures, the bone scan may be useful when knowledge of the tumor's relationship to bone is critical for planning the appropriate operative treatment.

4.2.2 Specific Radiopharmaceuticals

4.2.2.1 Iobenguane

Iobenguane (MIBG), a norepinephrine analog, radiolabeled with either ^{123}I or ^{131}I, accumulates in neural crest-derived tumors [96]. Since MIBG uptake depends on the active transport of the radiopharmaceutical into viable tumor cells, it is a highly specific test to assess tumor activity. Normal uptake sites of MIBG are salivary glands, myocardium, liver, gut, and bladder. Normal adrenal glands are frequently seen when ^{123}I-MIBG is used, but seldom visualized with ^{131}I-MIBG.

The high sensitivity and specificity of this tracer have been well established for the detection of primary and metastatic neuroblastoma sites [34, 64, 70]. In a series of 745 scintigraphic studies on 150 patients with neuroblastoma (of whom 143 were children), Hoefnagel et al. found a sensitivity of 96%, detecting multiple tumor sites regardless of the location [35]. When analyzing the results of the major series of ^{131}I-MIBG scanning reported in the world literature involving 776 patients, they found a cumulative sensitivity of 91.5% (range 76.6–96.3%) with very high specificity (range 88–100%). In four studies, totaling 300 patients, the specificity was found to be 100%.

A report by Rufini showed that SPECT imaging may identify additional sites of disease and allow better anatomical localization in patients with neuroblastoma [78].

MIBG has also been used in the detection of paragangliomas. Maurea et al. compared MIBG, CT, and MRI in the preoperative and postoperative evaluation of paragangliomas in 36 patients [65]. Preoperatively, CT and MRI were more sensitive (100% for both) than MIBG (82%), but MIBG was more specific (100% versus 50% for both CT and MRI). Postoperatively, MIBG and MRI were more sensitive (83% for both) than CT (75%), but again MIBG was more specific (100% versus 67% for both CT and MRI).

MIBG scintigraphy provides an additional method of locating paragangliomas, which can be effective even when anatomy has been distorted by tumor growth or previous surgery [84]. MIBG is also useful for assessing extra-adrenal or unexpected disease [65].

As well as in tumor detection, MIBG also has an important role to play in therapy: when a tumor accumulates MIBG, it may be treated with therapeutic doses of ^{131}I-MIBG, with encouraging results [92].

4.2.2.2 Somatostatin-Receptor Scanning

Somatostatin membrane receptors have been identified on many cells and tumors of neuroendocrine origin, including neuroblastomas and paragangliomas [56]. The somatostatin analog octreotide has been shown to bind to somatostatin receptors on both tumorous and nontumorous tissues.

As a result, ^{111}In-labeled octreotide (Octreoscan) scintigraphy is a simple and specific technique with which to demonstrate somatostatin receptor-positive localizations.

Using ^{111}In-labeled octreotide scintigraphy, Kwekkeboom et al. reported a sensitivity of 94% in 25 patients with 53 known paraganglioma lesions [55]. Moreover, in 9 of these 25 patients (36%), unexpected additional paraganglioma sites undetected by conventional imaging techniques were found. This finding is of special interest, since multicentricity and distant metastases have each been reported to occur in only 10% of patients based on information from conventional imaging techniques [31]. The true frequency of multifocality may therefore have been underestimated previously. In this respect, one of the major advantages of octreotide scintigraphy is in identifying multiple tumor sites in one whole body examination. Krenning therefore advocates the use of octreotide scanning as a screening test, to be followed by CT, MRI, or ultrasonography at the sites at which abnormalities are found (Fig. 4.4) [53].

Apart from its merit in tumor localization, in vivo somatostatin receptor imaging, as a result of its ability to demonstrate somatostatin receptor-positive tumors, can be used to select those patients who are likely to respond favorably to octreotide treatment. In addition, octreotide scintigraphy may be used to monitor the efficacy of therapy.

In 2002, Lebtahi et al. compared the sensitivity of ^{111}In-labeled octreotide and ^{99m}Tc-P829, a new ^{99m}Tc-labeled somatostatin analog, in 43 patients with neuroendocrine tumors. They concluded that, for the detection of neuroendocrine tumors, ^{111}In-labeled octreotide clearly remained the most sensitive tracer [58].

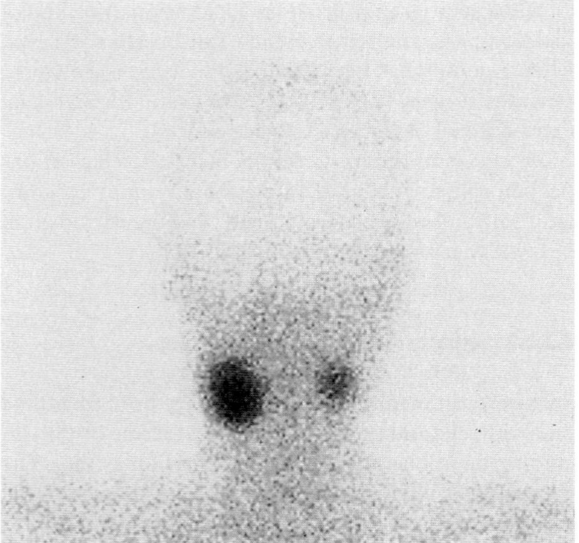

Fig. 4.4. Paraganglioma in the neck of a 27-year-old woman. Posterior view (planar scintigraphy, 6 h post injection). This patient was referred for staging of a known bilateral cervical paraganglioma. Somatostatin-receptor scintigraphy with [111]indium-labeled octreotide revealed only the two cervical tumors, with much more intense uptake in the left mass, which was also larger. Other sites of abnormal uptake were not found

4.2.3 Positron-Emitting Radiopharmaceuticals

The use of PET in oncology is increasing at a very rapid rate, primarily thanks to the increased use and widespread availability of [18F]FDG. FDG-PET does not replace other imaging modalities such as CT or MRI, but appears to be very helpful in specific situations in which CT or MRI have known limitations, such as differentiation of benign from malignant lesions, differentiation of posttreatment changes from residual or recurrent tumor, differentiation of benign from malignant lymph nodes, monitoring of therapy, and detection of unsuspected distant metastases [18]. The unique capability of PET to perform an easy whole body survey adds significant value to this technique. Besides [18F]FDG, other radiopharmaceuticals are being used, albeit mainly in research settings so far.

4.2.3.1 [18F]Fluorodeoxyglucose

■ **Detection of Soft Tissue Neoplasms and Differentiation of Benign from Malignant Lesions.** The substantial elevation of glucose uptake and retention by tumors compared with most nonneoplastic tissue is fundamental to FDG-PET imaging in oncology [94]. In 2003 Aoki et al. studied 114 soft tissue masses (80 benign and 34 malignant) with FDG-PET. They evaluated the standardized uptake value (SUV) of [18F]FDG for preopera-

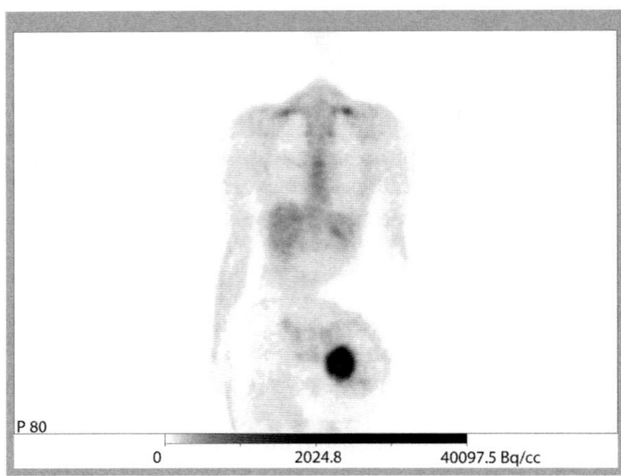

Fig. 4.5. Extrarenal rhabdoid sarcoma in the left gluteus maximus muscle of a 24-year-old woman. Coronal image of a [18F]fluorodeoxyglucose (FDG) PET scan. A focus of intense FDG uptake was seen in the left gluteal region. There were no other sites of abnormal FDG accumulation

tive differentiation between benign and malignant soft tissue masses. There was a statistically significant difference in SUV between benign and malignant soft tissue masses in total, although a considerable overlap in SUV was observed. Liposarcomas and synovial sarcomas did not show significantly higher SUV than any benign lesions, while some benign lesions such as sarcoidosis and giant cell tumors of the tendon sheath, showed an SUV as high as that of high-grade soft tissue sarcomas [2].

Feldman et al. studied the usefulness of FDG-PET in detection, analysis, and management of musculoskeletal lesions. From the 45 lesions studied, 19 cases were soft tissue tumors. Overall sensitivity, specificity, and accuracy for differentiating malignant from benign osseous and nonosseous lesions were 91.7%, 100%, and 91.7% (Fig. 4.5) [23].

Schwarzbach et al. investigated the use of FDG-PET in 42 patients with suspected liposarcomas. Pathology investigations revealed 11 primary liposarcomas, 14 locally recurrent liposarcomas, 5 other sarcomas, 1 lymphoma, and 11 benign lesions. [18F]FDG uptake was increased in higher-grade liposarcomas, while most low-grade liposarcomas presented a low [18F]FDG uptake. Pleomorphic, mixed, and myxoid liposarcomas showed an increased [18F]FDG uptake [83].

Cardona et al. investigated the use of FDG-PET to assess the nature of neurogenic soft tissue tumors in 25 patients (13 malignant peripheral nerve sheath tumors and 12 benign lesions). [18F]FDG uptake was significantly higher in malignant peripheral nerve sheath tumors than in benign lesions. They concluded that FDG-PET allows discrimination of benign from malignant neurogenic tumors (Fig. 4.6) [10].

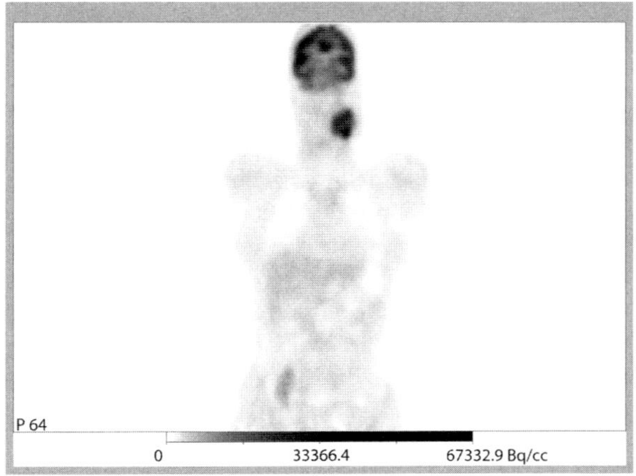
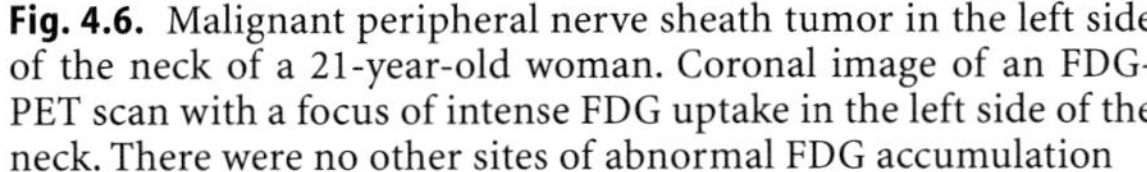

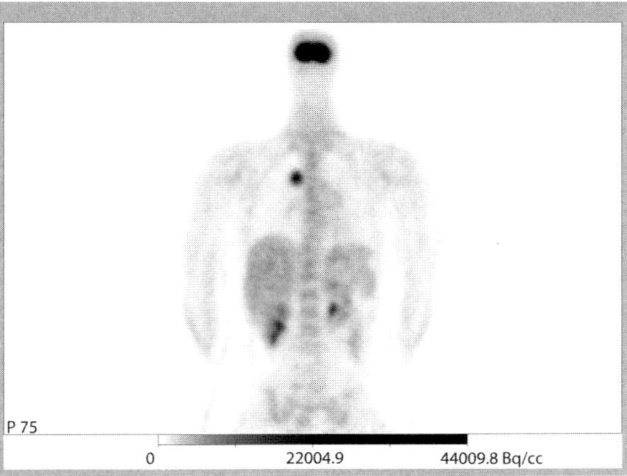

Fig. 4.6. Malignant peripheral nerve sheath tumor in the left side of the neck of a 21-year-old woman. Coronal image of an FDG-PET scan with a focus of intense FDG uptake in the left side of the neck. There were no other sites of abnormal FDG accumulation

Fig. 4.7. Nonmalignant schwannoma on the right side at thoracic level T3-4 in a 27-year-old woman. Coronal image of an FDG-PET scan. A focus of intense FDG uptake was seen in the right paravertebral region. There were no other sites of abnormal FDG accumulation

Beaulieu et al. studied the use of FDG-PET in nine patients with schwannomas. They concluded that schwannomas often have a high level of [^{18}F]FDG uptake and distinguishing schwannomas from malignant peripheral nerve sheath tumors before biopsy or surgery is not possible (Fig. 4.7) [4].

In a report by Schulte et al., an evaluation is given of the usefulness of FDG-PET in patients with suspected soft tissue neoplasms. In 102 patients the uptake of [^{18}F]FDG was evaluated semiquantitatively by determining the TBR. All patients underwent biopsy, resulting in the histological detection of 39 high-grade sarcomas, 16 intermediate-grade sarcomas, 11 low-grade sarcomas, 25 benign tumors, 10 tumor-like lesions such as spontaneous myositis ossificans (in 6 patients), and 1 non-Hodgkin lymphoma. All lesions except 2 lipomas showed an increased [^{18}F]FDG uptake. Using a TBR cut-off level of 3.0 for malignancy, the sensitivity of FDG-PET was 97.0%, the specificity 65.7%, and its accuracy 86.3%. Except for patients with pseudotumoral myositis ossificans, lesions with a TBR of more than 3 were sarcomas (91.7%) or aggressive benign tumors (8.3%). Tumors with a TBR of less than 1.5 were latent or active benign lesions exclusively. The group with intermediate TBR values (less than 3 and more than 1.5) had primarily latent or active benign lesions, but also 4 aggressive benign tumors and 2 low-grade sarcomas [79].

Lucas et al. studied the value of FDG-PET in patients presenting with soft tissue masses. Thirty-one masses were removed from 30 patients: 12 were benign and 19 were malignant soft tissue sarcomas. Using qualitative assessment of the FDG-PET images, all the high-grade soft tissue sarcomas (n=12) were correctly identified, but low-grade soft tissue sarcomas (n=7) could not be differentiated from benign lesions. Using a quantitative assessment, there was 95% sensitivity and 75% specificity in diagnosis of soft tissue sarcoma [63].

Adler et al. studied 25 patients with mass lesions involving the musculoskeletal system. There were 6 benign lesions and 19 malignant lesions of various grades. The high-grade malignancies had significantly greater uptake of [^{18}F]FDG than the benign lesions and low-grade malignancies combined [1]. Because soft-tissue sarcomas are often heterogeneous, with large areas of necrosis and hemorrhage, FDG-PET can guide the biopsy to a region with the highest-grade tumor [18, 32].

■ **Detection of Residual or Recurrent Soft Tissue Tumors and Differentiation of Posttreatment Changes.** Johnson et al. studied the role of FDG-PET in the detection of local recurrent and distant metastatic sarcoma in 28 patients. FDG-PET detected all 25 cases of local and distant recurrences with 100% sensitivity, while CT was able to detect 18 of the 22 cases of recurrent disease and MRI detected 5 of 7 cases of recurrence. FDG-PET was particularly useful in patients with extensive histories of surgery and radiation therapy, precisely the setting in which CT and MRI have the lowest specificity and sensitivity (Fig. 4.8) [43].

Schwarzbach et al. reported 50 patients with 59 masses that were potentially either suspicious primary or locally recurrent soft tissue sarcomas. FDG-PET was performed and SUV was calculated in tumor and normal muscle. Local recurrence was detected with a sensitivity of 88% and a specificity of 92%. All intermediate-grade and high-grade soft tissue sarcomas were clearly visual-

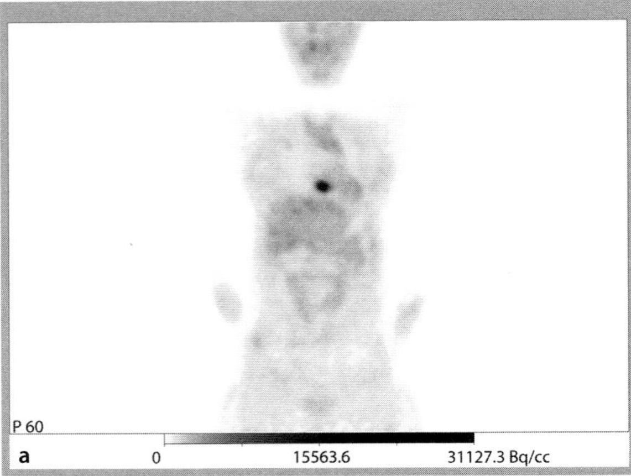

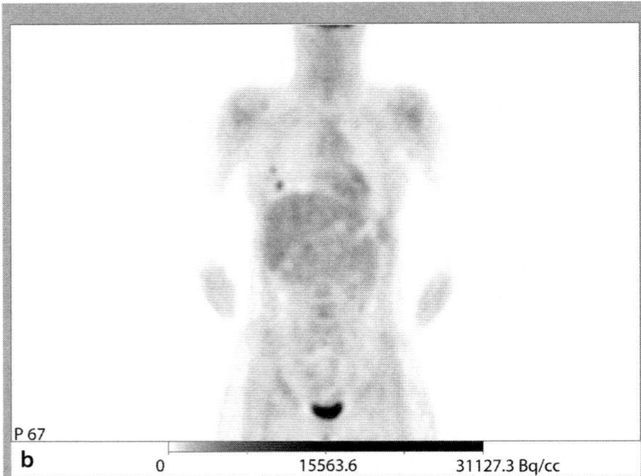

Fig. 4.8 a, b. Metastases of an extrarenal rhabdoid sarcoma in the heart and the right lung of a 24-year-old woman (same patient as in Fig. 4.5). **a** Coronal image of an FDG-PET scan with one focus of intense FDG uptake in the right side of the heart, confirmed as metastasis in the right ventricle on postmortem examination. **b** Coronal image of an FDG-PET scan with two hot spots in the right lung, confirmed as lung metastases on postmortem examination

ized, while 50% of low-grade sarcomas showed a [18F]FDG uptake equivalent to muscle. Benign soft tissue tumors did not accumulate [18F]FDG [82].

Bredella et al. studied the potential of FDG-PET to distinguish viable tumor from changes caused by therapy in areas with equivocal MRI findings in patients with musculoskeletal sarcomas. They evaluated 12 patients

with a history of bone or soft tissue sarcoma who had undergone various treatments and who presented with clinically suspected recurrent or residual tumor. In 9 patients MRI was equivocal and in 5 of these patients PET images showed increased [18F]FDG uptake, suggestive of recurrent tumor, which was confirmed by biopsy. In 4 patients FDG-PET showed no increased uptake and no tumor recurrence was found [9].

Lucas et al. compared the results of FDG-PET with those of MRI for the detection of local recurrence, and with CT of the chest for the detection of pulmonary metastases. They studied 62 patients who had 15 types of soft tissue sarcoma. For the detection of local disease, the sensitivities for FDG-PET and MRI were 74% and 88%, respectively, while the specificities for both techniques were 94% and 96%, respectively. For the identification of lung metastases, the sensitivities for FDG-PET and CT were 87% and 100%, respectively, while the specificities for both techniques were 100% and 96%, respectively [62].

Kim et al. reported on a prospective study in 43 patients with previously treated musculoskeletal sarcoma, in which they tried to distinguish between residual or recurrent tumors and posttreatment nonmalignant changes [47]. FDG-PET appeared to be useful in detecting metabolically active musculoskeletal sarcomas (sensitivity 98%, specificity 89%, positive predictive value 98%, negative predictive value 89%).

In a large group of 81 patients with proven musculoskeletal sarcomas, Korkmaz et al. compared the value of FDG-PET, [11C]methionine PET, and MRI and CT in differentiating recurrent or residual tumor from posttherapy changes [50]. FDG-PET showed a better overall performance than MRI and CT, which in turn both performed better than [11C]methionine (Table 4.1).

■ **Monitoring of Therapy.** Stroobants et al. evaluated whether FDG-PET can be used for the early evaluation of response to imatinib mesylate treatment in soft tissue sarcomas. They performed FDG-PET in 21 patients (17 gastrointestinal stromal tumors, 4 other soft tissue sarcomas) prior to and 8 days after the start of treatment. PET response was observed in 13 gastrointestinal stromal tumors (11 complete responders, 2 partial responders), followed by CT response in 10 of these patients af-

Table 4.1. Performance of [18F]fluorodeoxyglucose (FDG) PET, [11C]methionine (MET) PET, and magnetic resonance imaging (MRI) or computed tomography (CT) in musculoskeletal sarcomas [50]

	[18F]Fluorodeoxyglucose PET (%)	MRI/CT (%)	[11C]Methionine PET (%)
Sensitivity	93	93	77
Specificity	97	70	87
Accuracy	94	88	82
Positive predicted value	98	83	83
Negative predicted value	87	74	82

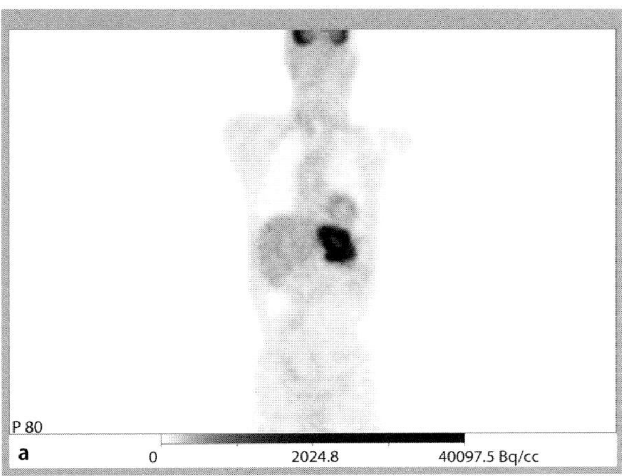

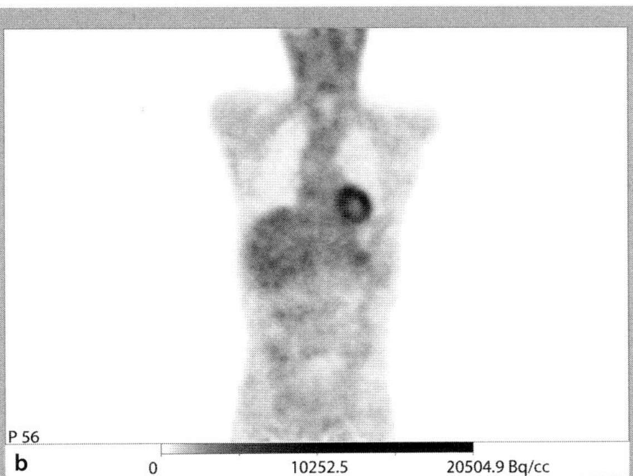

Fig. 4.9 a, b. Gastrointestinal stromal tumor (GIST) in the stomach of a 74-year-old man. **a** Coronal image of an FDG-PET scan with an intense uptake of FDG in the stomach. **b** Same patient 17 days later, after imatinib mesylate (Glivec) treatment. The intense focus of FDG uptake is no longer visible

ter a median follow-up of 8 weeks. Stable or progressive disease was observed on PET in 8 patients and none of them achieved a response on CT. PET response was also associated with a longer progression-free survival (Fig. 4.9) [87].

Vernon et al. reported on a patient with a pleomorphic high-grade sarcoma and discrepant results between the final histological diagnosis (tumor response after chemotherapy) and the percentage change in SUV by FDG-PET imaging, due to the heterogeneity of the tumor and heterogeneity in its response to treatment. They state that FDG-PET images present the metabolic activity of the entire tumor and are not subject to the sampling error which can occur in biopsy and histopathological sectioning [93].

Jones et al. showed changes in [18F]FDG uptake during and after neoadjuvant therapy in soft tissue and muscu-loskeletal sarcomas. The changes depended on the type of neoadjuvant therapy administered (chemotherapy or combined radiotherapy and hyperthermia): in the tumors treated with combined radiotherapy and hyperthermia, well-defined regions of absent [18F]FDG uptake developed within responsive tumors. Pathological examination showed that this was due to necrosis. In tumors treated with chemotherapy, [18F]FDG accumulation decreased more homogeneously throughout the tumor in responsive cases. Despite 100% tumor-cell kill in some patients, persistent tumor [18F]FDG uptake was observed which correlated with uptake within benign therapy-related fibrous tissue at pathological examination [44].

Similar findings have been reported by another group of investigators, who performed FDG-PET to evaluate the response to hyperthermic isolated limb perfusion for locally advanced soft tissue sarcomas. On the basis of the pretreatment glucose consumption in soft tissue sarcomas, they could predict the probability of a patient's achieving complete response confirmed at pathological examination after hyperthermic isolated limb perfusion. FDG-PET findings gave an indication of the tumor response to hyperthermic isolated limb perfusion, although the lack of specificity of [18F]FDG, in terms of differentiation between an inflammatory response and viable tumor tissue, hampered the discrimination between complete response and partial response at pathological examination [27].

■ **Assessment of Prognosis.** Eary et al. studied tumor maximum [18F]FDG uptake (SUVmax) for its ability to predict patient survival and disease-free interval. They imaged 209 patients with sarcoma prior to treatment with neoadjuvant chemotherapy or resection. The multivariate analyses showed that SUV_{max} information is a statistically significant independent predictor of patient survival and disease progression. In general, tumors that are more metabolically active (with high SUV_{max}) are more aggressive, as this increased metabolism reflects cell proliferation, vascularity increase, and cell activity [21].

■ **Methodological Factors Affecting the Ability of FDG-PET to Assess Tumor Malignancy.** Lodge et al. studied 29 patients with soft tissue masses, using a 6-h scanning protocol, and various indices of glucose metabolism were compared with histological grade. High-grade sarcomas were found to reach a peak activity concentration approximately 4 h after injection, whereas benign lesions reached a maximum within 30 min. This translated to improved differentiation between these two tumor types using a standardized uptake value derived from images acquired at later times. A standardized uptake value measured 4 h after injection was found to be as useful an index of tumor malignancy as the metabolic rate of [18F]FDG determined by means of either Patlak or nonlinear regression techniques. These indices each had a sensitivity and specificity of 100% and 76%, respectively, for the discrimination of high-grade sarcomas from benign tumors [61].

■ **Comparison with Other Radiotracers.** Kushner et al. studied the utility of FDG-PET in 51 patients with high-risk neuroblastoma. FDG-PET was equal or superior to MIBG for identifying neuroblastoma in soft tissue and extracranial skeletal structures, for revealing small lesions, for delineating the extent of disease and for localizing disease sites. FDG-PET and MIBG scans showed more skeletal lesions than bone scans, but the normally high physiological brain uptake of [18F]FDG blocked PET visualization of cranial vault lesions [54].

Shulkin et al. reported on a study on seven patients with neuroblastoma, using [11C]-hydroxyephedrine (HED) PET. They showed that HED uptake in neuroblastomas was rapid: tumors were evident on images within 5 min following i.v. injection. Such imaging is limited, however, by the short half-life of the 11C label (20.3 min). In addition, these tumors were also visualized using [123I]MIBG. The advantage of HED over MIBG is the possibility of very early imaging after administration (5 min versus 18–24 h) [85].

Garcia et al. compared the diagnostic accuracy of FDG-PET and 99mTc-MIBI SPECT in 48 patients with clinically suspected recurrent or residual musculoskeletal sarcomas. The diagnostic sensitivities and specificities were 98% and 90% with [18F]FDG, and 82% and 80% using MIBI, respectively. The tumors were demonstrated better in [18F]FDG studies, which produced higher visual grades (2.1 versus 1.6), and the tumors showed increasing standardized uptake values with time (from 6.3 to 7.3). Four of nine patients with tumors evident on FDG-PET images but not visible on 99mTc-MIBI SPECT images failed to respond to multidrug therapy [25].

Schwarzbach et al. evaluated three different PET radiotracers ([18F]FDG, [11C]aminoisobutyric acid, AIB, and 15O-labeled water) for imaging and detection of local recurrence of soft tissue sarcomas. They studied 21 patients, who had: 9 primary soft tissue sarcomas, 5 recurrent soft tissue sarcomas, and 10 lesions suspicious for local recurrence. All tracers accumulated in soft tissue sarcomas with no difference between primary and locally recurrent tumors. Of 10 patients with suspected recurrence, 6 presented neither PET criteria for recurrence nor confirmation of recurrence in the specimens or during follow-up, while 4 patients with positive PET scans were ultimately diagnosed with local failure [81].

4.2.3.2 18F-Labeled Dihydroxyphenylalanine

Becherer et al. studied the use of 18F-labeled dihydroxyphenylalanine ([18F]-DOPA) as PET tracer in 23 patients with histologically verified neuroendocrine tumors in advanced stages. FDOPA-PET was most accurate in detecting skeletal lesions (sensitivity 100%, specificity 91%) but was insufficient in the lung (sensitivity 20%, specificity 94%). Somatostatin-receptor scintigraphy was less accurate than [18F]-DOPA-PET in all organs. In about 40% of patients, initial CT failed to detect bone metastases shown by PET that were later verified by radiological follow-up [5].

Hoegerle et al. reported on a patient with metastasizing carcinoid in whom various imaging procedures were not successful in detecting the primary tumor. PET with [18F]-DOPA enabled localization of a potential primary tumor in the ileum. Moreover it detected an unknown mediastinal lymph node metastasis and a pulmonary metastasis [39].

4.2.3.3 [18F]Fluorodeoxythymidine

Cobben et al. studied the feasibility of [18F]-3'-fluoro-3'-deoxy-L-thymidine PET (FLT-PET) for the detection and grading of soft tissue sarcomas of the extremities in 19 patients. FLT uptake resulted in visualization of the tumors and facilitated differentiate between low-grade and high-grade soft tissue sarcomas. The uptake of FLT correlated with the proliferation of soft tissue sarcoma [15].

4.2.3.4 [11C]Choline

The use of short-lived PET tracers such as [11C]choline depends on the availability of a cyclotron near to a PET center (the half-life of 11C is 20 min). Zhang et al. compared the usefulness of [11C]choline PET with FDG-PET for the differentiation between benign and malignant bone and soft tissue tumors. They studied 43 patients with 45 lesions. The sensitivity, specificity, and accuracy of [11C]choline-PET were 100%, 64.5%, and 75.6%, respectively. The sensitivity, specificity, and accuracy of FDG-PET were 85.7%, 41.9%, and 55.6%, respectively. The [11C]choline uptake in the lesions correlated with [18F]FDG uptake [98].

4.2.3.5 L-[1-11C]Tyrosine

Protein synthesis rate (PSR) can be assessed in vivo using PET with L-[1-11C]tyrosine (TYR-PET) [72]. Pruim et al. reported on a study in 13 patients with soft tissue tumors (9 sarcomas, 4 benign lesions) using dynamic

PET with L-[1-^{11}C]tyrosine for visualization of the tumors and quantification of the PSR before and after therapy [74]. All malignant lesions were correctly identified. After therapy the PSR appeared to distinguish the patients with large tumor necrosis from patients with lesser tumor necrosis, suggesting a possible use as an indicator of therapeutic success.

Van Ginkel et al. investigated the use of TYR-PET in 17 patients undergoing hyperthermic isolated limb perfusion (HILP) with recombinant tumor necrosis factor alpha (rTNFα) and melphalan for locally advanced soft tissue sarcoma and skin cancer of the lower limb. TYR-PET studies were performed before HILP and 2 and 8 weeks afterwards, and the PSRs were calculated. All tumors were depicted as hot spots on PET studies before HILP. In the complete response group, the PSR was significantly lower at 2 and 8 weeks after perfusion than before HILP. With a threshold PSR of 0.91, the sensitivity and specificity of TYR-PET were 82% and 100%, respectively. The predictive value of a PSR of more than 0.91 for having viable tumor after HILP was 100%, whereas the predictive value of a PSR of 0.91 or less for having nonviable tumor tissue after HILP was 75% [28].

4.2.3.6 Practical Use of PET Tracers

FDG-PET is a useful tool for the detection of soft tissue neoplasms and the differentiation of benign from malignant lesions. High-grade malignancies have significantly greater uptake of [^{18}F]FDG than the combination of benign lesions and low-grade malignancies. Rarely, certain benign lesions can show a high level of [^{18}F]FDG uptake, for example as in schwannomas. FDG-PET presents the metabolic activity of the entire tumor and can be used to prevent sampling error by guiding a biopsy to a region with the highest grade tumor.

For the detection of residual or recurrent soft tissue tumors, the reported results of FDG-PET range from slightly inferior to superior compared with MRI and CT. FDG-PET is particularly useful in patients with extensive histories of surgery and radiation therapy, precisely the setting in which CT and MRI have the lowest specificity and sensitivity. Additional value is added to the technique of FDG-PET by its capabilities of therapy-monitoring and the performance of an easy whole-body survey with the possibility of detection of unsuspected distant metastases.

The clinical role of other PET tracers in the initial staging and follow-up of soft tissue neoplasms remains to be determined and will be partially dependent on the availability of a cyclotron nearby a PET-center, in order to be able to use short-lived PET-tracers such as [^{11}C]choline and [^{11}C]tyrosine.

4.3 Clinical Applications

To summarize the preceding data, nuclear medicine procedures may have an important role in the clinical workup of soft tissue tumors. This role, however, has been greatly underestimated, owing to the rather disappointing results of previous nuclear medicine techniques.

The introduction of FDG-PET in clinical use has been a major step forward in nuclear medicine, and there is enough evidence for FDG-PET to be the nuclear medicine imaging modality of choice for detection, staging, and follow-up of soft tissue neoplasms. In addition, bone scintigraphy, MIBG scintigraphy, and somatostatin-receptor scanning maintain a specific role in clinical practice. The use of other tracers such as gallium, thallium chloride, and sestamibi will be restricted mostly to hospitals without a PET scanner or in more specific clinical situations, as with sestamibi for the evaluation of multidrug resistance.

4.3.1 Diagnosis

If PET is available, FDG-PET is the first choice for diagnosis, although [^{18}F]FDG does not seem to be able to differentiate between low-grade malignancies and benign lesions. Furthermore, certain benign lesions can show a high level of [^{18}F]FDG uptake, for example in certain inflammatory conditions and in schwannomas. FDG-PET presents the metabolic activity of the entire tumor and can prevent sampling error by guiding a biopsy to a region with the highest-grade tumor. If PET is not available, gallium, thallium chloride, or sestamibi can be used, preferably in the absence of inflammatory lesions. Histological diagnosis can be attempted, e.g., in tumors accumulating MIBG or somatostatin-receptor labels (neuroendocrine tumors), antimyosin (muscular tumors), or RBC (hemangiomas).

4.3.2 Staging

A generally very high sensitivity, combined with the possibility of total body scanning, makes nuclear medicine very helpful in the staging of tumors (evaluation of locoregional extension or search for unsuspected additional tumor sites not seen with other imaging modalities). Most radiopharmaceuticals ([^{18}F]FDG, ^{67}Ga, ^{201}Tl, MIBI, MIBG, octreotide, antimyosin) are suited for this purpose, provided they accumulate at the primary tumor site.

An advantage of PET over traditional SPECT and planar whole body scintigraphy is the improved image quality with higher resolution, three-dimensional whole body imaging, facilitating the detection of smaller tumoral lesions. The role of bone scintigraphy in the preoperative workup is to evaluate involvement of bone structures adjacent to soft tissue tumors and, hence, to assess whether a broader resection is necessary.

4.3.3 Prognosis

Some nuclear medicine procedures provide prognostic information:

- The uptake of [18F]FDG is reported to be an independent predictor of patient survival and disease progression. In general, tumors that are more metabolically active (with high [18F]FDG uptake) are more aggressive.
- The uptake of ^{201}Tl and [^{18}F]FDG is reported to correlate well with tumor grade.
- Accumulation of ^{111}In-octreotide is proof of the presence of somatostatin receptors, and hence a favorable prognostic factor for somatostatin treatment; conversely, absence of ^{111}In-octreotide uptake is associated with a poor prognosis for somatostatin treatment.
- Accumulation of MIBG enables the use of ^{131}I-MIBG as a form of treatment.
- Fast tracer wash-out on sequential MIBI scans may be indicative of future multidrug resistance.

4.3.4 Therapy

As stated before, MIBG-accumulating tumors may be treated with ^{131}I-MIBG and somatostatin receptor-positive tumors may be treated with radiolabeled octreotide.

4.3.5 Follow-up

Because they concentrate in viable cells only, some radiopharmaceuticals may be used to monitor the effect of the treatment. Moreover, they can be used to distinguish residual tumor masses and recurrence from nonmalignant posttreatment changes, such as fibrotic masses. This is reported to be the case with [^{18}F]FDG, ^{67}Ga, ^{201}Tl, MIBI, MIBG and octreotide. The increasing access to clinical PET facilities is resulting in a rapidly rising use of FDG-PET for this specific purpose.

4.4 Conclusion

After a rather long period of underutilization in the field of soft tissue tumors, nuclear medicine procedures have made a remarkable comeback. This is due to technical improvements, the introduction of newer, more specific radiopharmaceuticals, and the introduction of FDG-PET. As a result, nuclear medicine methods are now not only used in the more classic context of staging and follow-up, but also in diagnosis, therapy, and even prognosis of soft tissue tumors. The future availability of other specific radiopharmaceuticals (e.g., labeled monoclonal antibodies and more specific PET tracers) is likely to confirm and enhance the current evolution.

Things to remember:
1. If a primary tumor takes up a radiopharmaceutical, metastases and recurrences will generally also do so. This, combined with the possibility of performing easy total body imaging, forms the strength of nuclear medicine techniques in primary staging and in follow-up of soft tissue tumors.
2. The fact that some radiopharmaceuticals appear to be taken up only by viable tumor cells makes it possible to distinguish between scar tissue and residual tumor or tumor recurrence in post-therapeutic follow-up.
3. The introduction of FDG-PET in clinical use has been a major step forward in nuclear medicine, and there is enough evidence for FDG-PET to be the first-choice nuclear medicine imaging modality for detection, staging, and follow-up of soft tissue neoplasms.
4. FDG-PET does not replace other imaging modalities such as CT or MRI, but appears to be very helpful in specific situations in which CT or MRI have known limitations.
5. FDG-PET reveals the metabolic activity of the entire tumor and can prevent sampling error by guiding a biopsy to a region with the highest-grade tumor.
6. The uptake of FDG is reported to be an independent predictor of patient survival and disease progression.
7. Due to technical improvements and the introduction of newer, more specific radiopharmaceuticals, the role of nuclear medicine in the management of soft tissue tumors is likely to become more important in the future.

References

1. Adler LP, Blair HF, Makley JT, Williams RP, Joyce MJ, Leisure G, al-Kaisi N, Miraldi F (1991) Noninvasive grading of musculoskeletal tumors using PET. J Nucl Med 32(8):1508–1512
2. Aoki J, Watanabe H, Shinozaki T et al (2003) FDG-PET for preoperative differential diagnosis between benign and malignant soft tissue masses. Skeletal Radiol 32:133–138
3. Barton DJ, Miller JH, Allwright SJ, Sloan GM (1992) Distinguishing soft tissue hemangiomas from vascular malformations using technetium-labeled red blood cell scintigraphy. Plast Reconstr Surg 89(1):46–52
4. Beaulieu S, Rubin B, Djang D, Conrad E, Turcotte E, Eary JF (2004) Positron emission tomography of schwannomas: emphasizing its potential in preoperative planning. Am J Roentgenol 182(4):971–974
5. Becherer A, Szabo M, Karanikas G, Wunderbaldinger P, Angelberger P, Raderer M, Kurtaran A, Dudczak R, Kletter K (2004) Imaging of advanced neuroendocrine tumors with (18)F-FDOPA PET. J Nucl Med 45(7):1161–1167
6. Bender H, Friedrich E, Zamora PO, Biersack HJ (1995) Detection of multidrug resistance with Tc-99m sestamibi. J Nucl Med 36(5):129P (Abstract)
7. Blatt CJ, Hayt DB, Desai M et al (1977) Soft-tissue sarcoma: imaged with technetium-99m pyrophosphate. NY State J Med 77:2118–2119
8. Brant WE, Floyd JL, Jackson DE et al (1987) The radiological evaluation of hepatic cavernous hemangioma. JAMA 257:1063–1070
9. Bredella MA, Caputo GR, Steinbach LS (2002) Value of FDG positron emission tomography in conjunction with MRI for evaluating therapy response in patients with musculoskeletal sarcomas. Am J Roentgenol 179(5):1145–1150
10. Cardona S, Schwarzbach M, Hinz U et al (2003) Evaluation of F-18-deoxyglucose positron emission tomography (FDG-PET) to assess the nature of neurogenic tumours. Eur J Surg Oncol 29(6):536–541
11. Chauhan UPS, Babbar A, Kashyap R, Prakash R (1992) Evaluation of a DMSA kit for instant preparation of ^{99m}Tc-(V)-DMSA for tumour and metastasis scintigraphy. Nucl Med Biol 19:825–830
12. Chew FS, Hudson TM, Enneking WF (1981) Radionuclide imaging of soft tissue neoplasms. Semin Nucl Med XI(4):266–276
13. Ciarmiello A, Del Vecchio S, Potena MI, Mainolfi C, Carriero MV, Tsuruo T, Marone A, Salvatore M (1995) Tc-99m-sestamibi efflux and P-glycoprotein expression in human breast carcinoma. J Nucl Med 36(5):129P (Abstract)
14. Citrin DL, McKillop JH (1978) Atlas of technetium bone scans. Saunders, Philadelphia, pp 43–65
15. Cobben DC, Elsinga PH, Suurmeijer AJ, Vaalburg W, Maas B, Jager PL, Hoekstra HJ (2004) Detection and grading of soft tissue sarcomas of the extremities with (18)F-3'-fluoro-3'-deoxy-L-thymidine. Clin Cancer Res 10(5):1685–1690
16. Cogswell A, Howman-Giles R, Bergin M (1994) Bone and gallium scintigraphy in children with rhabdomyosarcoma: a 10-year review. Med Pediatr Oncol 22(11):15–21
17. Cox PH, Verweij J, Pillay M, Stoter G, Schonfeld D (1988) Indium-111 antimyosin for the detection of leiomyosarcoma and rhabdomyosarcoma. Eur J Nucl Med 14:50–52
18. Delbeke D (1999) Oncological applications of FDG PET imaging. J Nucl Med 40:1706–1715
19. De Moerloose B, Van de Wiele C, Dhooge C, Philippé J, Speleman F, Benoit Y, Laureys G, Dierckx RA (1999) Technetium-99m sestamibi imaging in paediatric neuroblastoma and ganglioneuroma and its relation to P-glycoprotein. Eur J Nucl Med 26:396–403
20. Drane WE (1991) Nuclear medicine techniques for the liver and biliary system. Radiol Clin North Am 29:1129–1151
21. Eary JF, O'Sullivan F, Powitan Y, Chandhury KR, Vernon C, Bruckner JD, Conrad EU (2002) Sarcoma tumor FDG uptake measured by PET and patient outcome: a retrospective analysis. Eur J Nucl Med Mol Imaging 29(9):1149–1154
22. Enneking WF, Chew FS, Springfield DS et al (1981) The role of radionuclide bone-scanning in determining the resectability of soft-tissue sarcomas. J Bone Joint Surg 63:249–257
23. Feldman F, van Heertum R, Manos C (2003) 18-FDG PET scanning of benign and malignant musculoskeletal lesions. Skeletal Radiol 32:201–208
24. Felix EL, Sindelar WF, Bagley DH et al (1975) The use of bone and brain scans as screening procedures in patients with malignant lesions. Surg Gynecol Obstet 141:867–869
25. Garcia R, Kim EE, Wong FC, Korkmaz M, Wong WH, Yang DJ, Podoloff DA (1996) Comparison of fluorine-18-FDG PET and technetium-99m-MIBI SPECT in evaluation of musculoskeletal sarcomas. J Nucl Med 37(9):1476–1479
26. Gehring PJ, Hammand PB (1967) The interrelationship between thallium and potassium in animals. J Pharmacol Exp Ther 155:187–201
27. Ginkel RJ van, Hoekstra HJ, Pruim J, Nieweg OE, Molenaar WM, Paans AM, Willemsen AT, Vaalburg W, Koop HS (1996) FDG-PET to evaluate response to hyperthermic isolated limb perfusion for locally advanced soft-tissue sarcoma. J Nucl Med 37(6):984–990
28. Ginkel RJ van, Kole AC, Nieweg OE, Molenaar WM, Pruim J, Koops HS, Vaalburg W, Hoekstra HJ (1999) L-[1-^{11}C]-tyrosine PET to evaluate response to hyperthermic isolated limb perfusion for locally advanced soft-tissue sarcoma and skin cancer. J Nucl Med 40(2):262–267
29. Goshen E, Meller I, Lantsberg S, Sagi A, Moses M, Fuchsbrauner R, Quastel MR (1991) Radionuclide imaging of soft tissue masses with Tc-99m DTPA. Clin Nucl Med 16(9):636–642
30. Goto Y, Ihara K, Kawauchi S, Ohi R, Sasaki K, Kawai S (2002) Clinical significance of thallium-201 scintigraphy in bone and soft tissue tumors. J Orthop Sci 7(3):304–312
31. Grufferman S, Gillman MW, Pasternak LR et al (1980) Familial carotid body tumors: case report and epidemiologic review. Cancer 46:2116–2122
32. Hain SF, O'Doherty MJ, Bingham J, Chinyama C, Smith MA (2003) Can FDG PET be used to successfully direct preoperative biopsy of soft tissue tumours? Nucl Med Commun 24(11):1139–1143
33. Hattner RS, White DL (1990) Gallium-67/stable gadolinium antagonism: MRI contrast agent markedly alters the normal biodistribution of gallium-67. J Nucl Med 31:1844–1846
34. Hattner RS, Huberty JP, Engelstad BL, Gooding CA, Ablin AR (1984) Localization of *m*-iodo (I-131) benzylguanidine in neuroblastoma. Am J Roentgenol 143:373–374
35. Hoefnagel CA, de Kraker F (1994) Childhood neoplasia. In: Murray IPC, Ell PJ (eds) Nuclear medicine in clinical diagnosis and treatment, vol 2. Churchill Livingstone, Edinburgh, p 765–777
36. Hoefnagel CA, Voûte PA, Kraker J de, Behrendt H (1987) Scintigraphic detection of rhabdomyosarcoma. Lancet i:921
37. Hoefnagel CA, Kraker J de, Voûte PA, Behrendt H (1988) Tumor imaging of rhabdomyosarcoma using radiolabeled fragments of monoclonal anti-myosin antibody. J Nucl Med 29:791
38. Hoefnagel CA, Kapucu Ö, de Kraker J, Voûte PA (1993) Radioimmunoscintigraphy using ^{111}In-antimyosin Fab fragments for the diagnosis and follow-up of rhabdomyosarcoma. Eur J Cancer 29A:2096–2100
39. Hoegerle S, Schneider B, Kraft A, Moser E, Nitzsche EU (1999) Imaging of a metastatic gastrointestinal carcinoid by F-18-DOPA positron emission tomography. Nuklearmedizin 38(4):127–130
40. Howman-Giles R, Uren RF, Shaw PJ (1995) Thallium-201 scintigraphy in pediatric soft tissue tumors. J Nucl Med 36(8):1372–1376
41. Imaeda T, Seki M, Sone Y, Iinuma G, Kanematsu M, Mochizuki R, Takeuchi S, Nishimoto Y, Shimokawa K (1991) Gallium-67 citrate scintigraphy in the pre-operative evaluation of soft tissue tumors of the extremities. Ann Nucl Med 5(4):127–132
42. Jackson GE, Byrne MJ (1996) Metal ion speciation in blood plasma: gallium-67-citrate and MRI contrast agents. J Nucl Med 37(2):379–386

43. Johnson GR, Zhuang H, Khan J, Chiang SB, Alavi A (2003) Roles of positron emission tomography with fluorine-18-deoxyglucose in the detection of local recurrent and distant metastatic sarcoma. Clin Nucl Med 28(10):815–820

44. Jones DN, McCowage GB, Sostman HD, Brizel DM, Layfield L, Charles HC, Dewhirst MW, Prescott DM, Friedman HS, Harrelson JM, Scully SP, Coleman RE (1996) Monitoring of neoadjuvant therapy resonse of soft-tissue and musculoskeletal sarcoma using fluorine-18-FDG PET. J Nucl Med 37(9):1438–1444

45. Kairemo KJA, Wiklund TA, Liewendahl L et al (1990) Imaging of soft tissue sarcomas with In-111-labeled monoclonal antimyosin Fab fragments. J Nucl Med 31:23–31

46. Kaye SB (1988) The multidrug resistance phenotype. Br J Cancer 58:691–694

47. Kim E, Garcia JR, Wong FC, Kim CG, Broussard W, Podoloff DA (1995) Comparison of fluorodeoxyglucose (FDG) PET and Sestamibi (MIBI) SPECT in detection of residual or recurrent musculoskeletal sarcoma. J Nucl Med 36(5):234P (Abstract)

48. Kobayashi H, Sakahara H, Hosono M, Shirato M, Konishi J, Kotoura Y, Yamamuro T, Endo K (1993) Scintigraphic evaluation of tenosynovial giant-cell tumor using technetium-99m(V)-dimercaptosuccinic acid. J Nucl Med 34(10):1745–1747

49. Kobayashi H, Sakahara H, Hosono M, Shirato M, Endo K, Kotoura Y, Yamamuro T, Konishi J (1994) Soft-tissue tumors: diagnosis with Tc-99m (V) dimercaptosuccinic acid scintigraphy. Radiology 190(1):277–280

50. Korkmaz M, Kim EE, Wong F, Haynie T, Wong WH, Tilbury R, Benjamin R (1993) FDG and methionine PET in differentiation of recurrent or residual musculoskeletal sarcomas from posttherapy changes. J Nucl Med 34(5):33P (Abstract)

51. Kostakoglu L, Manicek DM, Divgi CR, Botet J, Healy J, Larson SM, Abdel-Dayem HM (1995) Correlation of the findings of thallium-201 chloride scans with those of other imaging modalities and histology following therapy in patients with bone and soft tissue sarcomas. J Nucl Med 22(11):1232–1237

52. Krause T, Hauenstein K, Studier-Fischer B, Schuemichen C, Moser E (1993) Improved evaluation of technetium-99m-red blood cell SPECT in hemangioma of the liver. J Nucl Med 34(3):375–380

53. Krenning EP, Kwekkeboom DJ, Reubi JC, Lamberts SWJ (1994) Somatostatin receptor scintigraphy with (^{111}In-DTPA-d-Phe^1) octreotide. In: Murray IPC, Ell PJ (eds) Nuclear medicine in clinical diagnosis and treatment, vol 2. Churchill Livingstone, Edinburgh, pp 757–764

54. Kushner BH, Yeung HW, Larson SM, Kramer K, Cheung NK (2001) Extending positron emission tomography scan utility to high-risk neuroblastoma: fluorine-18 fluorodeoxyglucose positron emission tomography as sole imaging modality in follow-up of patients. J Clin Oncol 19(14):3397–3405

55. Kwekkeboom DJ, Van Urk H, Pauw KH et al (1993) Octreotide scintigraphy for the detection of paragangliomas. J Nucl Med 43:873–878

56. Lamberts SWJ, Krenning EP, Reubi JC (1991) The role of somatostatin and its analogs in the diagnosis and treatment of tumors. Endocrinol Rev 12:450–482

57. Larson SM, Radey JS, Allen DR et al (1980) Common pathway for tumour cell uptake of gallium-67 and iron-59 via a transferring receptor. J Natl Cancer Inst 64:41–53

58. Lebtahi R, Le Cloirec J, Houzard C et al (2002) Detection of neuroendocrine tumors: 99m-Tc-P829 scintigraphy compared with 111-In-pentetreotide scintigraphy. J Nucl Med 43(7):889–895

59. Lepanto PB, Rosenstock J, Littman P, Alavi A, Donaldson M, Kuhl DE (1976) Gallium-67 scans in children with solid tumours. Am J Roentgenol 126:176–186

60. Lin WY, Kao CH, Hsu CY, Liao SQ, Wang SJ, Ueh SH (1994) The role of Tc-99m MDP and Ga-67 imaging in the clinical evaluation of malignant fibrous histiocytoma. Clin Nucl Med 19(11):996–1000

61. Lodge MA, Lucas JD, Marsden PK, Cronin BF, O'Doherty MJ, Smith MA (1999) A PET study of 18FDG uptake in soft tissue masses. Eur J Nucl Med 26(1):22–30

62. Lucas JD, O'Doherty MJ, Wong JC, Bingham JB, McKee PH, Fletcher CD, Smith MA (1998) Evaluation of fluorodeoxyglucose positron emission tomography in the management of soft-tissue sarcomas. J Bone Joint Surg Br 80(3):441–447

63. Lucas JD, O'Doherty MJ, Cronin BF, Marsden PK, Lodge MA, McKee PH, Smith MA (1999) Prospective evaluation of soft tissue masses and sarcomas using fluorodeoxyglucose positron emission tomography. Br J Surg 86(4):550–556

64. Lumbroso JD, Guermazi F, Hartmann O et al (1988) Metaiodobenzylguanidine (mIBG) scans in neuroblastoma: sensitivity and specificity, a review of 115 scans. Prog Clin Biol Res 271:689–705

65. Maurea S, Cuocolo A, Reynolds JC, Tumeh SS, Begley MG, Linehan WM, Norton JA, Walther MM, Keiser HR, Neumann RD (1993) Iodine-131-metaiodobenzylguanidine scintigraphy in preoperative and postoperative evaluation of paragangliomas: comparison with CT and MRI. J Nucl Med 34(2):173–179

66. Menendez LR, Fideler BM, Mirra J (1993) Thallium-201 scanning for the evaluation of osteosarcoma and soft-tissue sarcoma. A study of the evaluation and predictability of the histological response to chemotherapy. J Bone Joint Surg Am 75:526–531

67. Nagaraj N, Ashok G, Waxman A, Kovalevsky M, Youssim C, Forscher C, Rosen G (1995) Clinical usefulness of serial Tc-99m sestamibi scintigraphy in evaluating tumor response to preop chemotherapy in patients with bone and soft tissue sarcomas. J Nucl Med 36(5):129P (Abstract)

68. Noujaim AA, Turner CJ, Van Nieuwenhuyze BM, Terner U, Lentle BC (1981) An investigation of the mechanism of cis-diamine dichloroplatinum (cis-pt) interference with radiogallium uptake in tumors. Aust NZJ Med 11:437

69. Ohta H, Endo K, Konishi J et al (1990) Scintigraphic evaluation of aggressive fibromatosis. J Nucl Med 31:1632–1634

70. Parisi MT, Green MK, Dykes TM, Moraldo TV, Sandler ED, Hattner RS (1992) Efficacy of metaiodobenzylguanidine as a scintigraphic agent for the detection of neuroblastoma. Invest Radiol 10:768–772

71. Pearlman AW (1977) Preoperative evaluation of liposarcoma by nuclear imaging. Clin Nucl Med 2:47–51

72. Plaat B, Kole A, Mastik M, Hoekstra H, Molenaar W, Vaalburg W (1999) Protein synthesis rate measured with L-[1-^{11}C]tyrosine positron emission tomography correlates with mitotic activity and MIB-1 antibody-detected proliferation in human soft tissue sarcomas. Eur J Nucl Med 26(4):328–332

73. Prakash R, Jena A, Behari V et al (1987) Technetium-99m red blood cell scintigraphy in diagnosis of hepatic hemangioma. Clin Nucl Med 12:235–237

74. Pruim J, Ginkel RJ van, Willemsen ATM, Paans AMJ, Nieweg OE, Kole AC, Hoekstra HJ, Molenaar WM, Visser GM, Schraffordt Koops H, Vaalburg W (1995) Protein synthesis rate (PSR) measured with L-(1-C-11)-tyrosine in soft tissue tumours. J Nucl Med 36(5):217P (Abstract)

75. Reuland P, Koscielniak E, Ruck P, Treuner J, Feine U (1991) Application of an anti-myosin for scintigraphic differential diagnosis of infantile tumors. Int J Rad Appl Istrum (B) 18:89–93

76. Rosso J, Guillon JM, Parrot A, Denis M, Akoun G, Mayaud Ch, Scherrer M, Meignan M (1992) Technetium-99m-DTPA aerosol and gallium-67 scanning in pulmonary complications of human immunodeficiency virus infection. J Nucl Med 33(1):81–87

77. Rubin RA, Lichtenstein GR (1993) Scintigraphic evaluation in liver masses: cavernous hepatic hemangioma. J Nucl Med 34(5):849–852

78. Rufini V, Giordano A, Di Giuda D, Petrone A, Deb G, De Sio L, Donfrancesco A, Troncone L (1995) 123-I MIBG scintigraphy in neuroblastoma: a comparison between planar and SPECT imaging. Q J Nucl Med 39:25–28

79. Schulte M, Brecht-Krauss D, Heymer B, Guhlmann A, Hartwig E, Sarkar MR, Diederichs CG, Schultheiss M, Kotzerke J, Reske SN (1999) Fluorodeoxyglucose positron emission tomography of soft tissue tumours: is a noninvasive determination of biological activity possible? Eur J Nucl Med 26(6):599–605

80. Schwartz HS, Jones CK (1992) The efficacy of gallium scintigraphy. Ann Surg 215:78–82
81. Schwarzbach M, Willeke F, Dimitrakopoulou-Strauss A, Straus LG, Zhang YM (1999) Functional imaging and detection of local recurrence in soft tissue sarcomas by positron emission tomography. Anticancer Res 19(2B):1343–1349
82. Schwarzbach MH, Dimitrakopoulou-Strauss A, Willeke F et al (2000) Clinical value of 18-F-fluorodeoxyglucose positron emission tomography imaging in soft tissue sarcomas. Ann Surg 231(3):380–386
83. Schwarzbach MH, Dimitrakopoulou-Strauss A, Mechtersheimer G et al (2001) Assessment of soft tissue lesions suspicious for liposarcoma by F18-deoxyglucose (FDG) positron emission tomography (PET). Anticancer Res 21(5):3609–3614
84. Shapiro B, Copp JE, Sisson JC, Eyre PL, Wallis J, Beierwaltes WH (1985) Iodine-131 metaiodobenzylguanidine for the locating of suspected pheochromocytoma: experience in 400 cases. J Nucl Med 26:576–585
85. Shulkin BL, Wieland DM, Baro ME, Ungar DR, Mitchell DS, Dole MG, Rawwas JB, Castle VP, Sisson JC, Hutchinson RJ (1996) PET Hydroxyephedrine imaging of neuroblastoma. J Nucl Med 37(1):16–21
86. Southee AF, Kaplan WD, Jochelson MS, Gonin R, Dwyer JP, Antman KH, Elias AD (1992) Gallium imaging in metastatic and recurrent soft-tissue sarcoma. J Nucl Med 33(9):1594–1599
87. Stroobants S, Goeminne J, Seegers M et al (2003) 18FDG-Positron emission tomography for the early prediction of response in advanced soft tissue sarcoma treated with imatinib mesylate (Glivec). Eur J Cancer 39(14):2012–2020
88. Taki J, Sumiya H, Tsuchiya H, Tomita K, Nonomura A, Tonami N (1997) Evaluating benign and malignant bone and soft-tissue lesions with technetium-99m-MIBI scintigraphy. J Nucl Med 38:501–506
89. Taki J, Sumiya H, Asada N, Ueda Y, Tsuchiya H, Tonami N (1998) Assessment of P-glycoprotein in patients with malignant bone and soft-tissue tumors using technetium-99m-MIBI scintigraphy. J Nucl Med 39:1179–1184
90. Terui S, Terauchi T, Abe H, Fukuma H, Beppu Y, Chuman K, Yokoyama R (1994) On clinical usefulness of TI-201 scintigraphy for the management of malignant soft tissue tumors. Ann Nucl Med 8:55–64
91. Thompson DE, Frost HM, Hendrick JW et al (1971) Soft tissue sarcomas involving the extremities and the limb girdles: a review. South Med J 64:33–44
92. Troncone L, Galli G (eds) (1991) The role of 131-I-MIBG in the treatment of neural crest tumor. Proceedings of an international workshop, Rome, September 6–7. J Nucl Biol Med 35:177–363
93. Vernon CB, Eary JF, Rubin BP, Conrad EU, Schuetze S (2003) FDG PET imaging guided re-evaluation of histopathological response in a patient with high-grade sarcoma. Skeletal Radiol 32(3):139–142
94. Wahl RL, Hutchins GD, Buchsbaum DJ, Liebert M Grossman HB, Fischer S (1991) Fluorine-18-2-deoxy-2-fluoro-D-glucose (FDG) uptake into human tumor xenografts: feasibility studies for cancer imaging with PET. Cancer 67:1544–1549
95. Wallner KE, Galieich JH, Malkin MG, Arbit E, Korl G, Rosenblum MK (1989) Inability of computed tomography appearance of recurrent malignant astrocytoma to predict survival following reoperation. J Clin Oncol 7:1492–1496
96. Wieland DM, Wu J, Brown LE, Mangner TJ, Swanson DP, Beierwaltes WH (1980) Radiolabeled adrenergic neuron-blocking agents: adrenomedullary imaging with ^{131}I metaiodobenzylguanidine. J Nucl Med 21:349–353
97. Wiggins J, Goldstein H, Weinmann H (1991) Gallium-67/stable gadolinium antagonism. J Nucl Med 32:1830–1831
98. Zhang H, Tian M, Oriuchi N, Higuchi T, Watanabe H, Aoki J, Tanada S, Endo K (2003) ^{11}C-choline PET for the detection of bone and soft tissue tumours in comparison with FDG PET. Nucl Med Commun 24(3):273–279

Magnetic Resonance Imaging

5

P. Brys, H. Bosmans

Contents

5.1 Introduction

Due to its unequaled soft tissue contrast and multiplanar imaging capability, magnetic resonance imaging (MRI) is the modality of choice to image soft tissue tumors. An impressive arsenal of sequence types has become available, especially with regard to fast MRI, fat-suppression techniques and contrast-enhanced studies. In this section, we make a distinction between what is essential in daily practice, what should be avoided, and what are useful additional techniques, taking into account the equipment available and the demands of the clinician. We address the following topics: appropriate choice of imaging planes and routine sequences, why and how to perform contrast-enhanced studies, and the choice of sequences, depending on the possible demands of tissue characterization and the assessment of tumor extent in the adjacent soft tissue or bone. Topics such as posttreatment imaging and dynamic contrast-enhanced imaging, which are highlighted in other chapters in this book, are briefly mentioned.

The strategy in designing the optimal MR examination will always depend on the location, the desired coverage of the anatomical region to be examined, the suspected abnormality, the available hardware (field strength, local coil), time constraints, and local preferences.

5.2 Imaging Planes and Routine MR Sequences

Careful assessment of the region of clinical concern should precede any imaging to ensure its complete coverage with the most appropriate coil and to avoid waste of time due to repositioning of the patient after the first imaging sequence. The placement of a lipid marker at the area of interest may be helpful in this regard. Unless no lesion is detected on the initial sequences, it is usually not necessary to examine the contralateral side for comparison when an extremity is being evaluated.

Multiplanar imaging is an important factor in tumor staging, as it is extremely helpful in determining the anatomical extent of the lesion and its relationship to adjacent structures. In planning the appropriate surgical procedure, it is of the utmost importance to determine whether a lesion is within a well-delineated anatomical compartment (e.g., intrafascial or intra-articular) or is diffusely infiltrating adventitial planes and spaces. Accurate staging information may also determine the necessity for preoperative treatment [36].

Imaging usually starts with a sequence in the most appropriate longitudinal plane. Anteriorly or posteriorly located lesions are best imaged in a sagittal plane. For medial or lateral localizations, coronal imaging is preferred. Care should be taken to respect the anatomical orthogonal planes since, with excessive rotation of a limb, inappropriate positioning of longitudinal scan planes results in images which are difficult to interpret and probably useless for surgical planning. Since this sequence should depict the lesion, together with eventually surrounding edema, with the highest conspicuity and over its entire cephalocaudal extent, fat-suppressed, fast spin-echo (FSE) T2-weighted or short-tau inversion recovery (STIR) imaging with a large field of view (FOV) is recommended. Inclusion of the nearest joint serving as a reference in at least one of the longitudinal imaging planes is well appreciated by all surgeons, since especially deeply situated masses can be hard to localize based on clinical examination alone.

This first sequence in the longitudinal plane is usually followed by imaging in the axial plane. Most anatomical and functional compartments of the extremities are

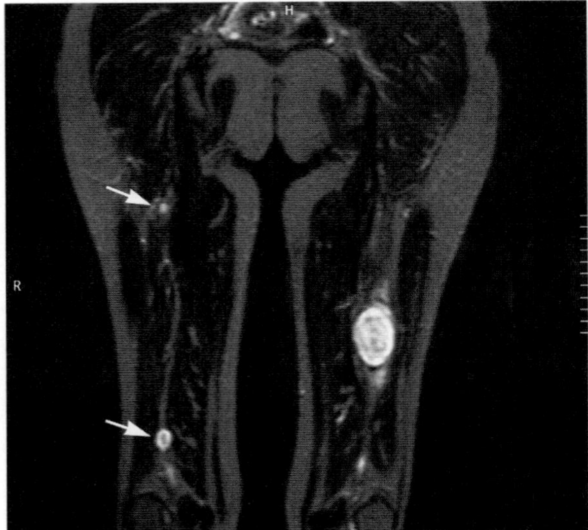

Fig. 5.1. Coronal spin-echo (SE) T2-weighted image (TE 110 ms). In this patient, known to have neurofibromatosis, a painful mass was palpated halfway down the posterior part of the left thigh. Here lower-resolution body-coil imaging was used to search for additional neurofibromata besides the one suspected along the course of the left sciatic nerve, which were demonstrated proximally and distally along the right sciatic nerve (*arrows*)

oriented longitudinally. This requires imaging in the axial plane for adequate evaluation of the tumor extent and its relation to vessels and nerves [2, 26]. Not only the entire tumor but also the peritumoral edema at its proximal and distal poles should be covered by these axial sequences. As a rule, the most proximal and distal slices should show no pathology in the tissues. Usually T1- and T2-weighted acquisitions are obtained in the axial plane at exactly the same location, thus allowing an image-by-image comparison. Contrast-enhanced images have to be acquired at least in the axial and the most useful longitudinal plane and at the same positions as the precontrast images. The choice of an additional imaging plane depends on the location of the lesion and the clinical questions to be answered (Fig. 5.1). Oblique planes may also be useful. Typical examples are oblique sagittal images for optimal depiction of a lesion's relation to the scapula or the iliac wing.

The use of spin-echo MR sequences is recommended. It is the most reproducible technique, the one with which we are most familiar for tumor evaluation, and the most often referenced in tumor-imaging literature [29].

The main disadvantage of classic, double-echo T2-weighted sequences remains the relatively long acquisition times [29]. For its increased lesion conspicuity and shorter acquisition times, fat-suppressed, FSE T2-weighted MRI is frequently preferred. Fat-suppressed, FSE T2-weighted images also show a higher signal-to-noise ratio compared with STIR imaging [12]. However, since fat appears bright on all FSE sequences [3, 16],

with subsequent decrease in conspicuity of tumors or edema in bone marrow or juxtaposed to fat [29], FSE T2-weighted sequences without fat suppression should not be used in tumor imaging. After i.v. administration of gadolinium (Gd), STIR type sequences should not be used, since not only fat but also enhancing tissue will be shown with a reduced signal intensity.

5.3 Contrast-Enhanced MRI

Contrast-enhanced MR studies lead to a prolonged examination time and high costs. In routine musculoskeletal MRI, routine i.v. Gd administration is not a requirement and should be reserved for cases in which the results would influence patient care [18].

Characterization and delineation of, e.g., lipomas and vascular malformations are easily performed on unenhanced sequences. However, contrast administration is certainly helpful in MR characterization and the clinical management of most of the soft tissue tumors.

The superior diagnostic performance of contrast enhancement, compared with unenhanced MRI, improving the diagnosis of benign lesions but also the detection of malignant ones, has been well established [43]. Contrast-enhanced imaging helps to narrow down differential diagnosis, facilitating clinical management. Lesions in which the observer is highly confident of a benign diagnosis at MRI may not require histological biopsy [43]. Although contrast-enhanced MRI is not able to reliably differentiate between benign and malignant soft tissue tumors, it helps to increase the suspicion of malignant lesions, in which inappropriate excisional biopsies should be avoided because of the risk of tumor-positive, surgical section margins.

5.3.1 Static Enhanced MRI

Compared with unenhanced T1-weighted imaging (WI), enhanced T1-WI improves the delineation of a lesion in terms of tumor-to-muscle contrast but without improvement of this contrast compared with T2-WI [10, 46]. On the other hand, enhanced T1-WI decreases or even obscures the tumor-to-fat contrast (Figs. 5.2b, c, 5.3, 5.4), which can be counteracted by the use of fat-suppressed T1-WI (Fig. 5.5c). Since fat-suppressed T1-weighted images after i.v. administration of gadolinium show areas of contrast enhancement with a greater conspicuity than T1-WI without fat suppression, subsequently resulting in images that are easier to interpret, the use of this sequence has become very popular.

However, one should be aware of the risk of misinterpretation of fat-suppressed, enhanced T1-weighted images, since a high signal intensity of a lesion can be the consequence of two variables: real Gd enhancement or

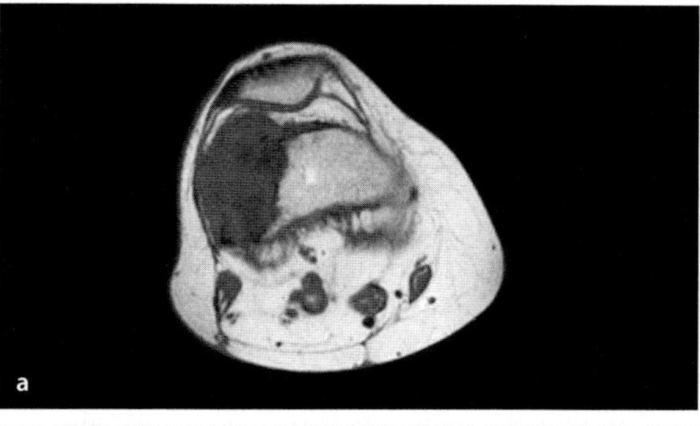

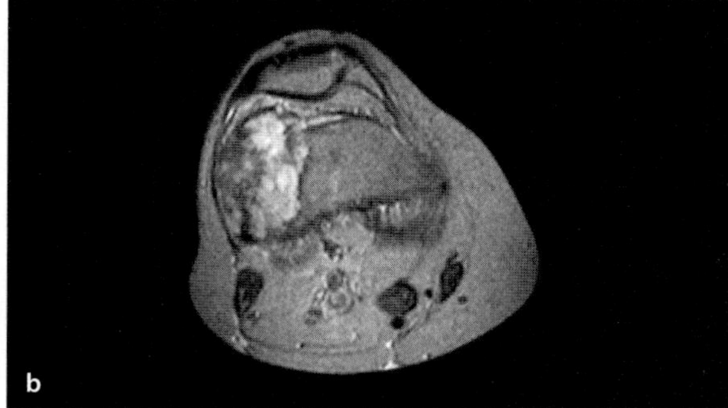

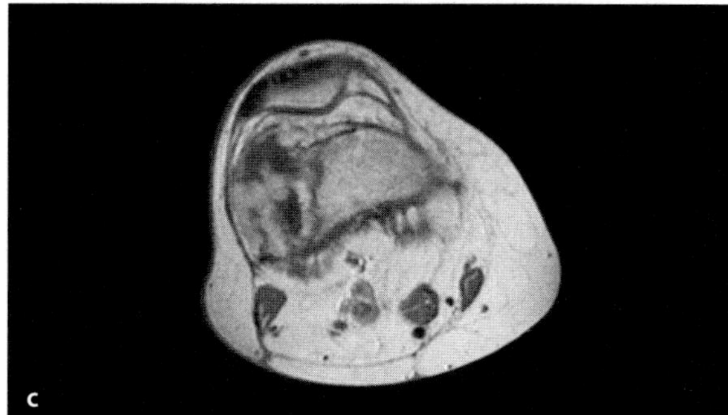

Fig. 5.2. a Axial, unenhanced SE T1-weighted image. **b** Axial, SE T2-weighted image. **c** Axial, Gd-enhanced SE T1-weighted image. Patient with a leiomyosarcoma. For local tumor staging, the unenhanced T1-weighted image provides the most useful information, showing high tumor-to-fat contrast at the extraosseous side, as well as a sharp delineation between tumor-invaded and normal bone marrow. The conventional T2-weighted SE image (with TE 80 ms) shows a poor tumor-to-fat contrast at the extraosseous side and a moderate contrast between tumor and normal bone marrow. As for tumor staging, the worst result is obtained with the Gd-enhanced, SE T1-weighted image. Both this and the T2-weighted acquisition would benefit from fat suppression

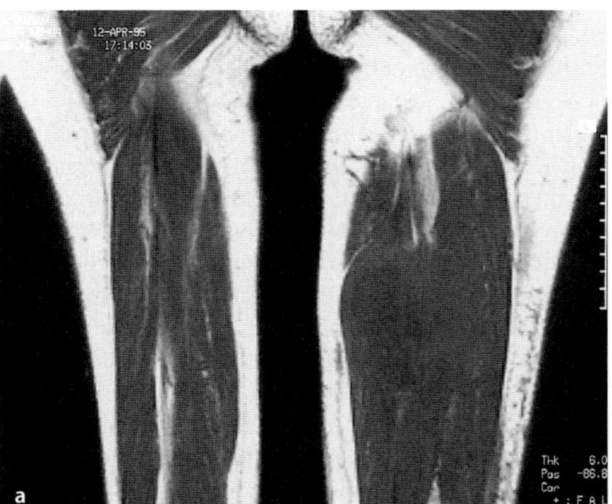

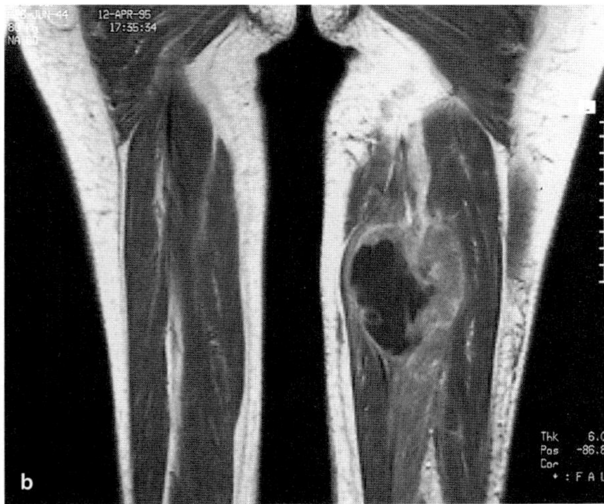

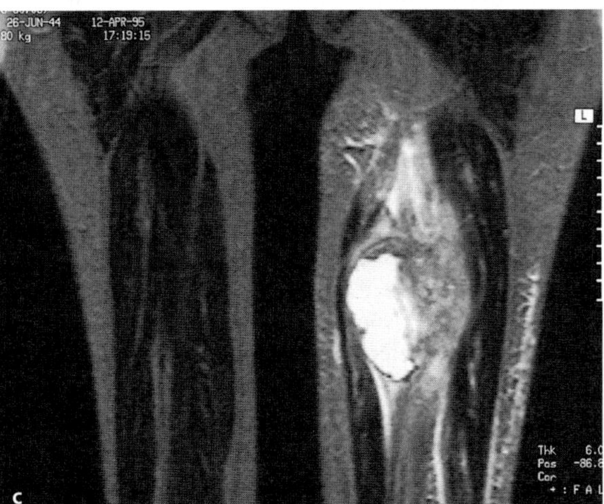

Fig. 5.3 a–c. Dedifferentiated liposarcoma in the posterior compartment of the thigh. **a** Coronal, unenhanced T1-weighted image. A mass lesion is shown in the hamstrings muscles. However, tumor-to-muscle contrast is very low, resulting in impossibility of analysis of the soft tissue extent. **b** Coronal, Gd-enhanced T1-weighted image. In this patient, additional coronal imaging demonstrates marked extent of tumor or peritumoral edema distally in the semitendinosus muscle, which is information of major value when the field of preoperative radiotherapy has to be delineated or the width of surgical resection has to be determined. Since the medial half of the lesion shows extensive necrosis, a biopsy should be obtained from the viable later part. **c** Coronal, T2-weighted image (heavily T2-weighted with TE of 120 ms), showing peritumoral brightening (edema and/or tumor spread) in the adjacent semitendinosus muscle

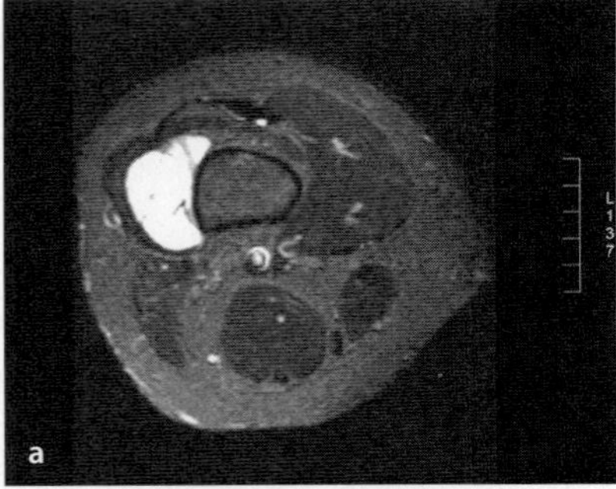

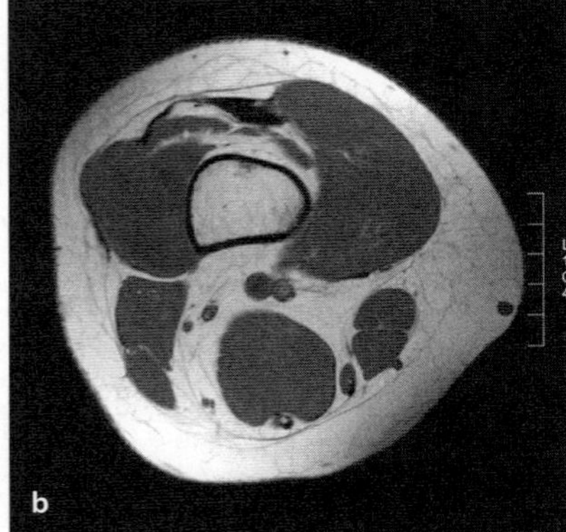

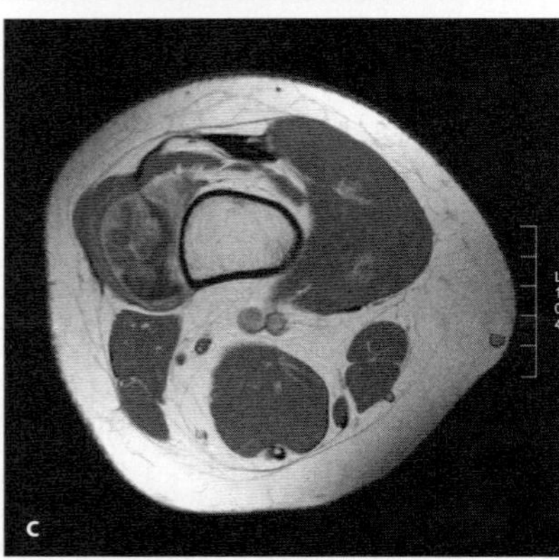

Fig. 5.4a–c. Patient with a myxoid liposarcoma. **a** Axial STIR sequence shows a sharply margined mass lesion with homogeneous high-signal intensity interposed between the vastus lateralis muscle and the distal femur. **b** Axial, unenhanced T1-weighted image. A very low tumor-to-muscle contrast is shown, with the lesion's signal intensity slightly lower than muscle. In combination with the high signal intensity on STIR sequence, this lesion could be mistaken for a cyst based on unenhanced sequences alone. Also note the very high tumor-to-fat contrast, typical for unenhanced T1-weighted images. **c** Axial, Gd-enhanced T1-weighted image shows a definite and very heterogeneous enhancement, inconsistent with a cystic origin of the lesion. Although there is a decreased tumor-to-fat contrast, delineation of the tumor from the adjacent fat still is perfectly possible. In addition, due to a clear increase in tumor-to-muscle contrast, this sequence is very suitable for surgical planning. Besides the adequate delineation of the tumor, this enhanced T1-weighted sequence improves the evaluation of the internal structure of the tumor. It helps to differentiate viable tumor from a cyst, with a totally different surgical approach, and helps to select an appropriate biopsy site. Because it mainly consists of less well-vascularized and myxoid or necrotic tissue, a biopsy in the posterior part of the lesion should be avoided

apparent Gd uptake due to the scaling effect caused by the fat-suppression technique. Suppression of the high signal intensity of fat induces a rescaling, a redistribution of gray levels, so that minor differences in signal intensity between tissues on non-fat-suppressed T1-WI are magnified (Figs. 5.7a, b, 5.8). The same rescaling effect of fat suppression is responsible for an apparently obvious Gd enhancement of tissue that only shows minimal enhancement on non-fat-suppressed T1-weighted images [14, 15]. As a consequence, reliable interpretation of fat-suppressed T1-weighted images after i.v. administration of gadolinium is only possible if also unenhanced fat-suppressed T1-WI and enhanced non-fat-suppressed T1-WI sequences are obtained. This results in a longer examination time. However, the use of fat-suppressed, enhanced T1-WI certainly is not a routine requirement [15].

One example in which enhancement conspicuity does not increase with addition of a chemical shift-based fat-suppression technique is when, on unenhanced T1-weighted images, the lesion is hyperintense due to the presence of methemoglobin. Since there is little or no contrast between Gd-enhancing areas and hemorrhage, differentiation between a subacute hematoma and a hemorrhagic tumor can be quite difficult. Here enhancement conspicuity is only obtained from subtraction images on which hyperintensity is only consistent with enhancement (Fig. 5.6). Unenhanced images are, by means of a postprocessing tool, subtracted from the enhanced ones. To obtain useful subtraction images, the patient should not change position during the examination and i.v. access should be acquired before the start of the examination.

Enhanced T1-WI not only improves the delineation but also the evaluation of the internal structure of a tumor (Figs. 5.3a, b, 5.4b, c, 5.6, 5.7). It helps to differentiate well-perfused, viable tumor from tumor necrosis, cysts or cystic parts of a tumor from myxoid ones, and intratumoral hemorrhage from hematoma. This is essential for deciding whether to perform a biopsy, and planning of the biopsy site, the field of preoperative radiotherapy, or the area of surgical resection.

Since every additional procedure increases the risk of inadvertent tumor cell contamination, the selection of the biopsy site should be well considered. A biopsy containing vascularized viable tumor will be of greater value than a nondiagnostic specimen with hemorrhage, edema, or necrotic tissue. Well-vascularized viable tumor will be of greater value for determination of the tumor type and grade. If only static enhanced MR images are used, the area showing the most intense enhancement should be selected as biopsy site [44] (Figs. 5.3b, 5.4c).

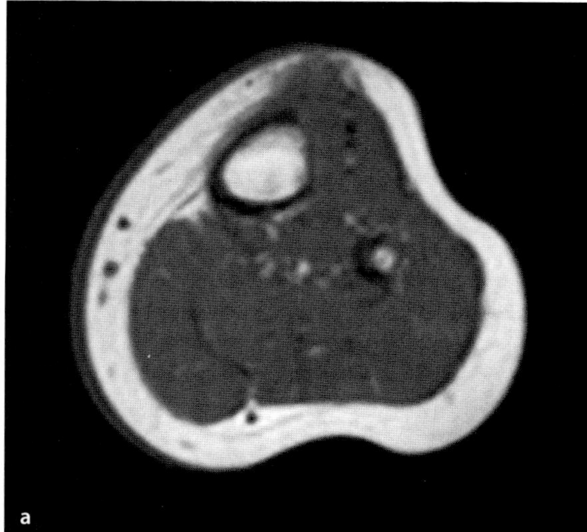

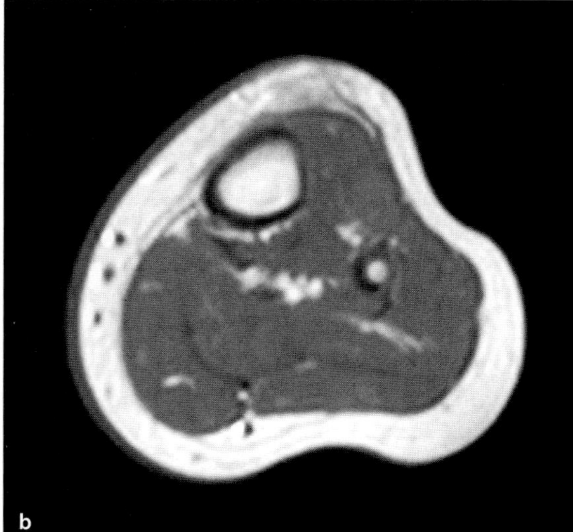

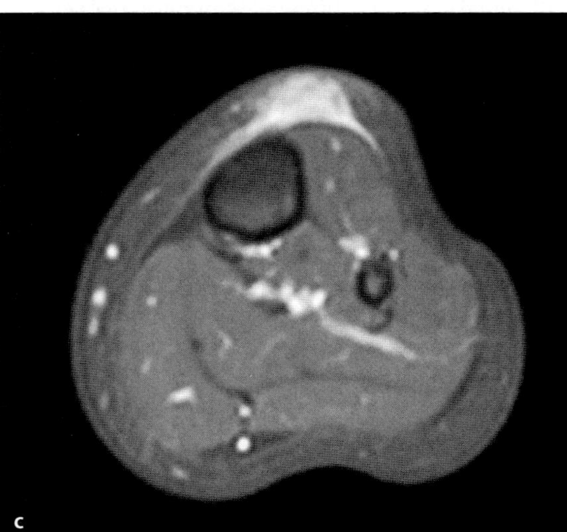

Fig. 5.5a–c. Patient with a pretibial, subcutaneous soft-tissue mass in the left lower leg, most probably of inflammatory origin. **a** Axial, unenhanced T1-weighted images shows high lesion-to-fat contrast but a poor lesion-to-muscle contrast. **b** Axial, Gd-enhanced T1-weighted image. Increasing signal intensity due to T1-shortening results in a poor lesion-to-fat contrast, but, on the other hand, a much better lesion-to-muscle contrast than on the unenhanced image. **c** Axial, fat-suppressed, Gd-enhanced T1-weighted image. Because of fat suppression, maximal lesion-to-fat and lesion-to-muscle contrast is obtained in one sequence. Moreover, additional information of the lesion's extension along the fascial plane is clearly provided

Since static enhanced MRI is performed in the equilibrium state when the Gd concentration in the interstitium equals that of plasma, it is not able to distinguish among the various simultaneously enhancing tissues [33]. Examples are differentiation between tumor extension through a pseudocapsule and peritumoral edema [31] (Fig. 5.3b, c), between highly vascularized and less well vascularized viable tumor tissue [33], between viable tumor and inflammation or granulation tissue after chemotherapy [11], and between tumor recurrence and an inflammatory pseudotumor. Static MR is also unable to provide accurate quantitative measurement of tumor response to chemotherapy [17, 21, 30, 37]. Since the spatial resolution and hence the anatomical detail of dynamic enhanced MR images is suboptimal, even an "advanced" dynamic enhanced MR study should be completed by the more "classic" static enhanced MR sequences.

5.3.2 Dynamic Enhanced MRI

Dynamic contrast-enhanced MRI provides physiological information such as tissue perfusion and vascularization, capillary permeability, and the volume of the interstitial space, which is not available on static contrast-enhanced MRI [45, 47].

The analysis of the tumor structure by dynamic contrast-enhanced studies improves differentiation between highly vascularized, less well vascularized, and necrotic tumor areas, which is important in the selection of the most highly vascularized, highest-grade part of the tumor for the biopsy site, in differentiation of tumor from peritumoral edema, in the assessment of good and poor responders to preoperative chemo- and radiation therapy, and in the assessment of possible tumor recurrence [33, 44]. It further narrows down the differential diagnosis and helps to increase the suspicion of malignant lesions in addition to unenhanced and static enhanced MRI [43]. Dynamic MRI should be done when conventional MRI results in indeterminate findings [33]. The role of dynamic MR studies is discussed more extensively in Chap. 6.

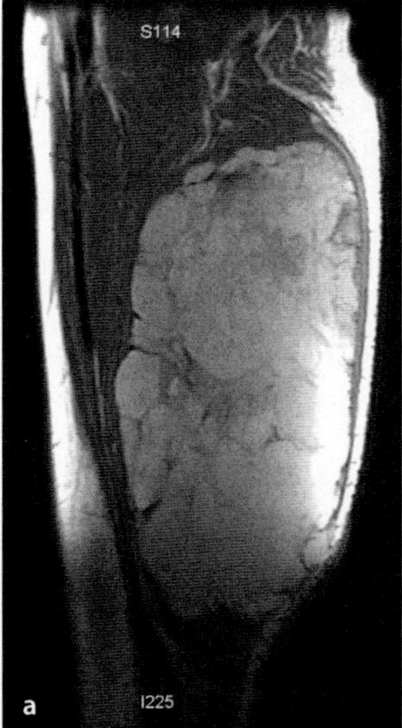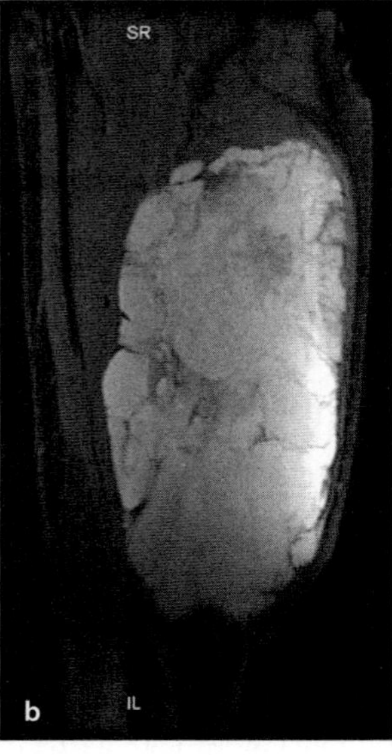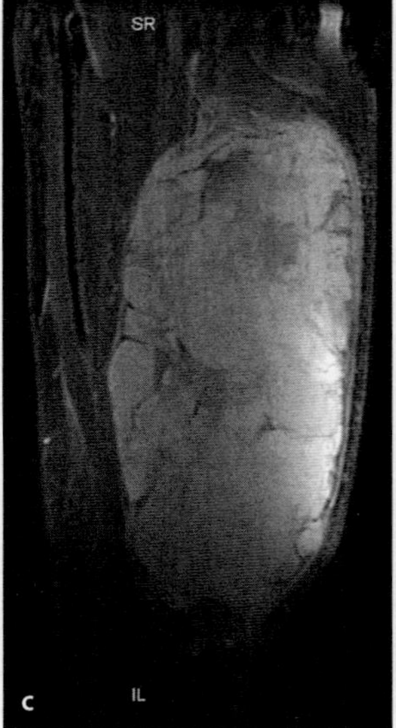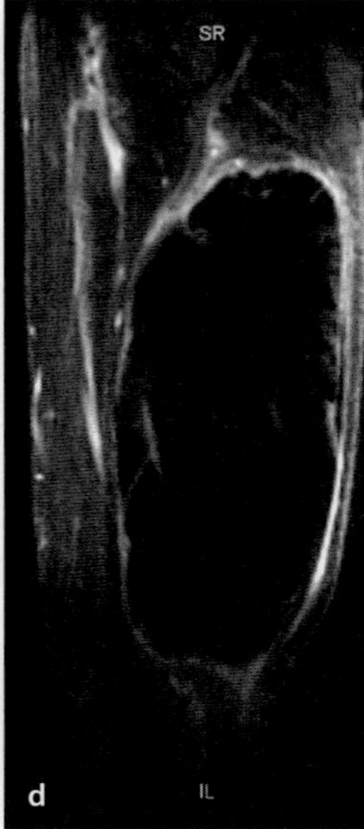

Fig. 5.6 a–d. Patient with a necrotic, hemorrhagic high-grade pleiomorphic sarcoma of the posterior thigh compartment. **a** Sagittal, unenhanced T1-weighted image. The large mass lesion is showing an inhomogeneous high signal intensity, possibly of lipomatous origin. **b** Sagittal, fat-suppressed, unenhanced T1-weighted image. Persistence of the high signal intensity despite fat suppression is inconsistent with the hypothesis of a fatty tumor, and suggests the presence of methemoglobin in a large hematoma or hemorrhagic tumor. **c** Sagittal, fat-suppressed, Gd-enhanced T1-weighted image. Differentiation between hematoma and hemorrhagic tumor needs Gd administration. Unfortunately, because of the presence of intralesional methemoglobin, the conspicuity of Gd enhancement does not benefit from the fat-suppression technique. Based on this sequence, it is virtually impossible to differentiate enhancement from methemoglobin. **d** Sagittal subtraction image (**b** subtracted from **c**). Subtraction of pre- from post-Gd, fat-suppressed, T1-weighted images permits isolation of the areas of Gd enhancement, showing a thin rim-enhancement and only some small foci of mural enhancement in the upper-posterior part of the lesion

5.4 Characterization

Tissue characterization is based on several imaging parameters [4]. Some of them are signal-intensity related: signal homogeneity, changing pattern of homogeneity, and the presence of hemorrhage and peritumoral edema. This information is obtained by comparison of the signal characteristics on T1- and T2-weighted sequences.

Extra information can be derived from the addition of a fat-suppression technique to a T1- as well as a T2-weighted sequence. Chemical shift-based fat-suppression should be used in these cases.

Fat-suppressed T2-WI is used to increase not only the conspicuity of a lesion and its surrounding edema/reactive zone but also of nonlipomatous components in lipomatous tumors, the latter helping in distinguishing lipoma from well-differentiated liposarcoma [13]. Fat-suppressed T1-WI is well known for its capacity to differentiate between fatty tissue and melanin or methemoglobin, which all show a high signal intensity on conventional T1-weighted images. A chemical shift-based, fat-suppressed T1-weighted sequence decreases the signal intensity of fatty tissue, while melanin and methemoglobin remain hyperintense on this sequence [25, 35] (Figs. 5.6b, 5.7b, 5.8b)

The additional value of this spin-echo T1-weighted sequence with fat-suppression in characterization has been established. The sequence facilitates characterization and differentiation of fat and melanin/methemoglobin and fibrous or hemosiderotic parts versus highly cellular parts in tumors. It also enhances confidence in the characterization of neurogenic tumors and hemangiomas. In addition, because of the magnification of small signal-intensity differences, nonhomogeneity, an important parameter in characterization and staging, is also better evaluated [14].

Static Gd-enhanced MRI has only a limited value in the characterization of soft tissue tumors and the differentiation of benign from malignant lesions. The application of dynamic Gd-enhanced MR studies yields information about the malignant potential of a tumor, but with a certain degree of overlap between benign and malignant tumors [10, 45]. In dynamic enhanced MRI, the enhancement pattern only reflects tissue vascularity and perfusion. Especially in fast-enhancing lesions, this overlap is too high to be of practical value in most cases [44]. On the other hand, slowly enhancing malignant tumors are rare but do exist [43].

Gradient echo (GRE) techniques are not routinely used for tissue characterization. However, in some selected applications they can be very useful. In the absence of calcifications or gas on radiographs and computed tomography (CT), a marked signal loss on GRE sequences is almost pathognomonic for hemosiderin. (Fig. 5.9)

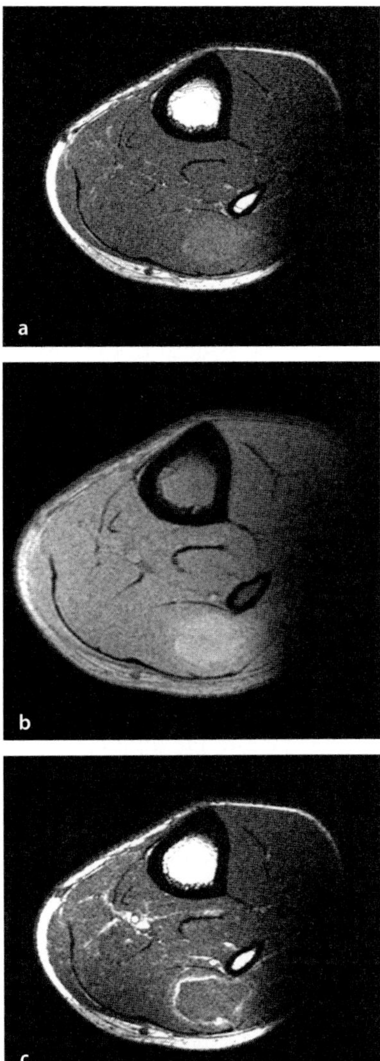

Fig. 5.7 a–c. Soccer player with a subacute hematoma after direct contact trauma of his left calf. **a** Axial, unenhanced T1-weighted image. In the lateral part of the soleus muscle, a lesion with a slightly higher signal intensity than muscle is shown. **b** Axial, fat-suppressed, unenhanced T1-weighted image. Due to suppression of the high signal intensity of fat, a rescaling effect is induced, with subsequent magnification of the difference in signal intensity between muscle and lesion. **c** Axial, Gd-enhanced, T1-weighted image. After Gadolinium contrast administration, only a thin enhancing rim is shown, consistent with the presence of an intramuscular hematoma

Some centers have investigated the possible role of diffusion-weighted MRI in tumor characterization. Apparent diffusion coefficient (ADC) values of benign soft tissue tumors and sarcomas overlap and cannot be used to differentiate between the bulk of benign and malignant tumors [6,42]. True diffusion coefficients (perfusion-corrected diffusion-WI) are reported to be significantly lower in malignant than in benign soft tissue masses; however, there is still a substantial overlap between both [42].

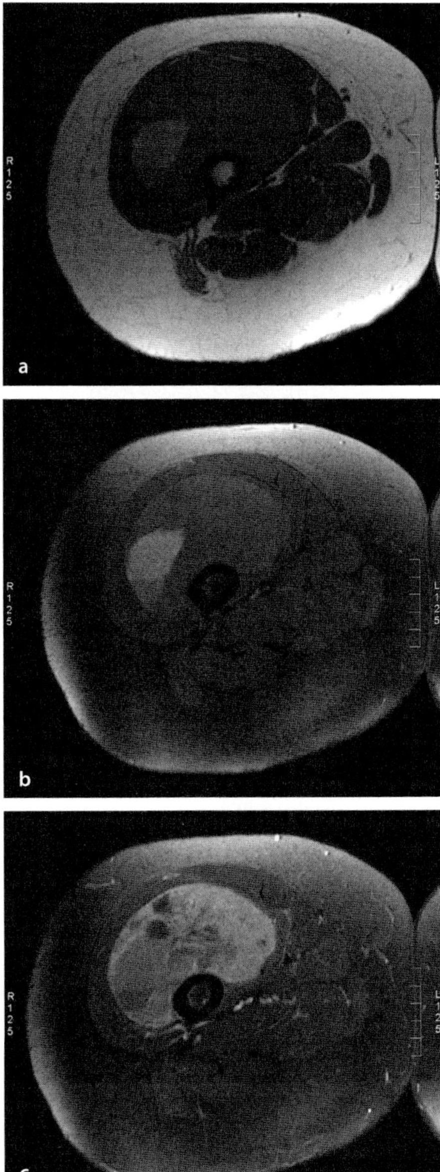

Fig. 5.8 a–c. Patient with a high-grade sarcoma of the anterior thigh compartment. **a** Axial, unenhanced, T1-weighted image. This unenhanced T1-weighted sequence typically shows a poor tumor-to-muscle contrast, the lesion showing a signal intensity only slightly higher than muscle. Note a hemorrhagic area with fluid-fluid level in the lateral part of the lesion, with a high signal-intensity upper level and a dependent part with a signal intensity slightly hyperintense to the tumor. **b** Axial, fat-suppressed, unenhanced T1-weighted image. This sequence does not contribute to characterization or delineation of the lesion but illustrates the rescaling effect caused by the fat-suppression technique: The upper level, which was the second most hyperintense area after the fatty tissue on the non-fat-suppressed image, now becomes strongly hyperintense. The slight differences in signal intensity between tumor and muscle and between dependent part and tumor now get clearly magnified. **c** Axial, fat-suppressed, Gd-enhanced T1-weighted image. The addition of Gd enhancement induces a new rescaling effect: As the tumor strongly enhances with its signal intensity higher than the upper level, the signal intensity from the latter gets rescaled to a lower gray level. The rescaling of the dependent part and the slight normal enhancement of muscle tissue results in both areas being isointense to each other

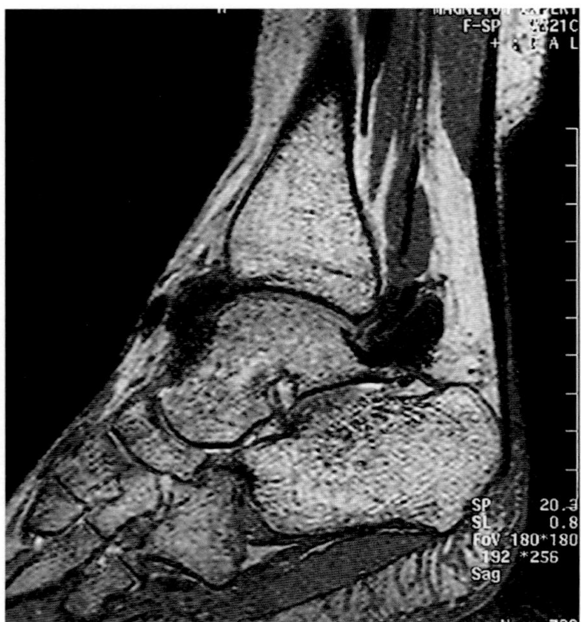

Fig. 5.9. Patient with pigmented villonodular synovitis (PVNS) of the ankle joint. Plain films showed joint distension without intra-articular calcifications. With this DESS gradient-echo technique, the presence of hemosiderin results in susceptibility artifacts and profound signal loss of the hypertrophic synovium, being almost pathognomonic for PVNS. This sagittal image shows extension in the anterior and posterior recess of the joint and along the tendon sheath of the flexor hallucis longus muscle

5.5 Soft Tissue Extent

The most important variable for predicting local recurrence is the quality of surgery [22]. Accurate depiction of the local extent of disease is important, since this is an indispensable factor in determining the extent of surgical resection and the need for preoperative chemotherapy or radiation therapy.

In delineation of a soft tissue tumor, distinction must be made between tumor-to-muscle and tumor-to-fat contrast.

On T1-weighted images, with exception of fat-containing tumors, soft tissue tumors are generally isointense to muscle, resulting in low tumor-to-muscle contrast, but have a high contrast with the hyperintense fat (Figs. 5.2a, 5.3a, 5.4b, 5.5a, 5.8a). As a consequence, T1-weighted images are essential in the delineation of a tumor from intermuscular fat planes, fat surrounding neurovascular structures, subcutaneous fat, and fatty bone marrow. A fat plane between a tumor and an adjacent anatomical structure is sufficient to exclude invasion or encasement [28].

T2-weighted or STIR imaging allows differentiation of hyperintense tumors and their surrounding edema from the hypointense surrounding muscles (Figs. 5.3c, 5.4a). The reactive edema around a tumor, as visualized on T2-weighted sequences, often contains satellite tumor micronodules, is considered as an integral part of the lesion, and therefore is removed en bloc with the tumor [23, 36] (Fig. 5.3c). If the reactive zone extends beyond the compartment, a tumor is considered extracompartmental even if the tumor itself is confined to the compartment [8, 9]. Fat-suppressed T2-weighted sequences and STIR sequences increase the conspicuity of this peritumoral edema and hence enable the detection of a greater volume of tissue at risk for malignancy, although this may result in overestimation [24]. This may have important implications for local staging and planning of surgery and radiation therapy [34]. MRI should always precede biopsy, as blood and edema that follow a biopsy can be difficult to separate from tumor or the peritumoral reactive zone, with or without Gd administration. An appropriate decision about whether to perform limb-salvaging surgery based on a postbiopsy MR examination may be impossible.

Reliable differentiation between tumor and peritumoral edema cannot be made by means of T2-weighted nor by static enhanced T1-WI. Dynamic enhanced MR studies can contribute to the differentiation of tumor from edema, because edema always shows a much more gradual increase in signal intensity than the tumor tissue. Improved differentiation of tumor from edema can change the preoperative strategy (e.g., help the surgeon in deciding whether to perform amputation or a limb-salvage procedure) [19]. However, he precise role of dynamic enhanced MRI in this topic has not yet been established.

On T1-weighted sequence images, tumor-to-muscle contrast increases markedly after i.v. administration of gadolinium diethyltriamine pentaacetic acid (Gd-DTPA; Figs. 5.3a, b, 5.4b, c, 5.5a, b, 5.8a–c). Although there is no improvement of this tumor-to-muscle contrast when compared with T2-WI [10, 46], the static enhanced T1-weighted sequence without fat-suppression is a very useful one. As an "almost-all-in-one-sequence," it has the anatomical detail, fat planes inclusive, typical for T1-weighted images, a tumor-to-muscle contrast equal to that of T2-weighted images, and it provides useful information on tumor content due to the Gd-administration (Fig. 5.4c). Most surgeons use these images for planning their interventions.

A disadvantage of enhanced T1-WI is a decreased tumor-to-fat contrast (Figs. 5.2c, 5.5b). The use of a chemical-shift type of fat-suppression technique decreases the signal intensity of fat, with consequently an excellent tumor-to-fat contrast (Fig. 5.5c). However, this fat suppression results in obscured fat planes, which is a disadvantage in planning surgery. Although very popular among radiologists because of the very high conspicuity of enhancement, this FSE enhanced T1-weighted sequence should never be acquired without its non-fat-suppressed equivalent and is only recommended when tumor abuts or infiltrates adjacent fat. When time constraints are a consideration, enhancement conspicuity can also be obtained by the use of image subtraction (Fig. 5.6).

5.6 Neurovascular Involvement

In a series of 133 soft tissue sarcomas, the frequency of encasement was reported as 4.5% for major vessels and 6.8% for major nerves [27]. A neurovascular bundle is encased when surrounded with tumor for at least half of its circumference, with associated obliteration of its fat plane [28].

On MR images, the appearance of blood vessels can be highly variable (low signal intensity flow void, high signal intensity entry slice phenomenon, target-like patterns of signal intensity). Their appearance depends on several parameters, such as the pulse sequence used, the position of the slice, and the flow velocity. Knowledge of the appearance of flow effects on MR images is needed for the accurate evaluation of blood vessels.

Neurovascular involvement is assessed best by axial images. Tumor-to-vessel contrast is demonstrated better on regular T1- and T2-weighted spin-echo images than on STIR-based acquisitions, whereas both ultrafast contrast-enhanced and plain "time-of-flight" techniques can be used to image blood vessels [1].

5.7 Bone Invasion

Osseous invasion by soft tissue sarcomas is uncommon, with a frequency of 9% reported in a series of 133 sarcomas [27]. Bone invasion is defined as extension of a tumor into the bone cortex. Periosteal contact alone is not considered sufficient to diagnose bone involvement [28].

T1-weighted and fat-suppressed T2-weighted sequences are equally highly accurate in the assessment of cortical invasion, showing cortical signal intensity changes and/or cortical destruction [7]. In sites of predominantly fatty bone marrow, T1-WI and fat-suppressed T2-WI are equally highly sensitive in the assessment of medullary invasion, with T1-WI being more specific [7]. Since, on unenhanced T1-weighted images, the contrast between tumor/edema and hematopoietic marrow is poor, one should rely on FSE T2-weighted sequences to assess tumor invasion in this type of bone marrow.

5.8 Imaging After Preoperative Chemotherapy or Radiation Therapy

The aim of monitoring of preoperative chemotherapy is to predict the percentage of tumor necrosis in order to differentiate responders from nonresponders [44].

It should be performed in chemotherapy-sensitive tumors because of impact on modification of neoadjuvant treatment protocols, selection of postoperative chemotherapy regimens, patient selection for performance and timing of limb-salvage surgery, and planning of radiation therapy [32, 39].

Unenhanced MR images cannot be used to evaluate tumor necrosis after chemotherapy, mainly because signal intensities of viable tumor, tumor necrosis, edema, and hemorrhage overlap on T2-WI. Static enhanced MRI also has been unable to provide an accurate quantitative measure of tumor response after chemotherapy [17, 21, 30, 37]. After preoperative radiotherapy, static enhanced MR could not reliably differentiate between viable tumor, tumor necrosis, inflammation, and granulation tissue [5]. Reliable differentiation between viable tumor and necrosis is possible with dynamic enhanced MRI, which is now the method of choice to monitor preoperative therapy [32, 38, 40, 41, 47].

Diffusion-weighted MRI has been used successfully to assess tumor necrosis in rats with osteosarcoma [20]. In soft tissue sarcomas, an increase in ADC values after radiotherapy has been demonstrated [6]. Although further studies are needed to establish the role of diffusion-weighted imaging (DWI) in the evaluation of response to chemotherapy, this technique is promising, as DWI is performed with fast sequences and does not require contrast media injection, so it can be repeated frequently during therapy [6]. This technique may be applicable in the future to monitor tumor viability during treatment. The MRI strategy developed for the assessment of postoperative tumor recurrence is discussed in Chap. 28.

Things to remember:

1. MRI should always precede biopsy, since tumor staging based on a postbiopsy MR examination may be impossible.
2. Adequate evaluation of tumor extent requires multiplanar imaging, invariably including the axial plane, and should depict all peritumoral edema.
3. Don't use FSE T2-weighted sequences without fat suppression in tumor imaging.
4. Routine i.v. Gd-contrast administration is not a requirement but is helpful in MR characterization and the clinical management, including the choice of biopsy site, of most of the soft tissue tumors.
5. The use of fat-suppressed, enhanced T1-WI is not a routine requirement and is only recommended when tumor abuts or infiltrates adjacent fat. Gd-enhancement conspicuity can also be obtained from subtraction images.
6. Do not use fat-suppressed T1-WI without their non-fat-suppressed equivalent, since they obscure surgically important fat planes, and the risk of misinterpretation of Gd enhancement.
7. Static enhanced MRI is unable to provide accurate quantitative measurement of tumor response to chemotherapy. This requires dynamic MR studies.

References

1. Arlart PI, Bongartz G, Marchal G (1995) Magnetic resonance angiography. Springer, Berlin Heidelberg New York
2. Bongartz G, Vestring T, Peters PE (1992) Magnetresonanztomographie der Weichteiltumoren. Radiologe 32:584–590
3. Constable RT, Anderson AW, Zhong J, Gore JC (1992) Factors influencing contrast in fast spin-echo MRI. Magn Reson Imaging 10:497–511
4. De Schepper AM (2001) Grading and characterization of soft tissue tumors. In: De Schepper AM, Parizel PM, De Beukeleer L, Vanhoenacker F (eds) Imaging of soft tissue tumors, 2nd edn. Springer, Berlin Heidelberg New York, pp 123–141
5. Einarsdottir H, Wejde J, Bauer H (2001) Pre-operative radiotherapy in soft tissue tumors. Assessment of response by static post-contrast MRI compared with histopathology. Acta Radiologica 42(1):1–4
6. Einarsdottir H, Karlsson M, Wejde J, Bauer H (2004) Diffusion-weighted MRI of soft tissue tumours. Eur Radiol 14:959–963
7. Elias DA, White LM, Simpson DJ, Kandel RA, Tomlinson GT, Bell RS, Wunder JS (2003) Osseous invasion by soft tissue sarcoma: assessment with MRI. Radiology 229:145–152
8. Enneking E (1985) Staging of musculoskeletal neoplasms. Skeletal Radiol 13:183–194
9. Enneking W (1989) Principles of musculoskeletal oncology surgery. In: Evrats C (ed) Surgery of the musculoskeletal system, Chap 175. Churchill Livingstone, New York
10. Erlemann R, Reiser MF, Peters PE, Vasallo P, Nommensen B, Kusnierz-Glaz CR, Ritter J, Roessner A (1989) Musculoskeletal neoplasms: static and dynamic Gd-DTPA-enhanced MRI. Radiology 171:767–773
11. Erlemann R, Sciuk J, Bosse A, et al (1990) Response of osteosarcoma and Ewing sarcoma to preoperative chemotherapy. Assessment with dynamic and static MRI and skeletal scintigraphy. Radiology 175:791–796
12. Fleckenstein JL, Archer BT, Barker BA, Vaughan JT, Parkey RW, Peshock RM (1991) Fast short-tau inversion-recovery MRI. Radiology 179: 499–504
13. Galant J, Marti-Bonmati L, Saez F, Soler R, Alcala-Santaella R, Navarro M (2003) The value of fat-suppressed T2 or STIR sequences in distinguishing lipoma from well-differentiated liposarcoma. Eur Radiol 13:337–343
14. Gielen J., De Schepper A., Parizel P., Wang X., Vanhoenacker F (2003) Additional value of magnetic resonance with spin echo T1-weighted imaging with suppression in characterization of soft tissue tumors. J Comput Assist Tomogr 27(3):434–441
15. Helms CA (1999) The use of fat suppression in gadolinium-enhanced MRI of the musculoskeletal system: a potential source of error. AJR Am J Roentgenol 173:234–236
16. Henkelman RM, Hardy PA, Bishop JE, Poon CS, Piewes DB (1992) Why is fat bright in RARE and fast spin-echo imaging. J Magn Reson Imaging 2:533–540
17. Kauffman WM, Fletcher BD, Hanna SL, Meyer WH (1994) MRI findings in recurrent primary osseous Ewing sarcoma. Magn Reson Imaging 12(8):1147–53
18. Kransdorf MJ, Murphey MD (2000) Radiologic evaluation of soft tissue masses: a current perspective. AJR Am J Roentgenol 175:575–587
19. Lang P, Honda G, Roberts T, Vahlensieck M, Johnston JO, Rosenau W, Mathur A, Peterfy C, Gooding Ca, Genant HK (1995) Musculoskeletal neoplasm-perineoplastic edema versus tumor on dynamic post-contrast MR images with spatial-mapping of instantaneous enhancement rates. Radiology 197(3):831–9
20. Lang P, Wendland MF, Saeed M, Gindele A, Rosenau W, Mathur A, Gooding CA, Genant HK (1998) Osteogenic sarcoma: non-invasive in vivo assessment of tumor necrosis with diffusion-weighted MRI. Radiology 206(1):227–35
21. Lawrence JA, Babyn P, Chan HSL, Thorner PS, Pron GE, Krajbich IJ (1993) Extremity osteosarcoma in childhood: prognostic value of radiologic imaging. Radiology 189:43–47
22. Mandard AM, Petiot JF, Marnay J, et al (1989) Prognostic factors in soft tissue sarcomas: a multivariate analysis of 109 cases. Cancer 63:1437–1451
23. McDonald DJ (1994) Limb-salvage surgery for treatment of sarcomas of the extremities. AJR Am J Roentgenol 163:509–513
24. Mirowitz SA (1993) Fast scanning and fat-suppression MRI of muscloskeletal disorders. Review. AJR Am J Roentgenol 161(6):1147–1157
25. Mirowitz SA, Apicella P, Reinus WR, Hammerman AM (1994) MRI of bone marrow lesions: relative conspicuousness on T1-weighted, fat-suppressed T2-weighted, and STIR-images. AJR Am J Roentgenol 162:215–221
26. Olson PN, Everson LI, Griffiths HJ (1994) Staging of musculoskeletal tumors. Radiol Clin North Am 32:151–162
27. Panicek DM, Gatsonis C, Rosenthal DI, et al (1997) CT and MRI in the local staging of primary malignant musculoskeletal neoplasms: report of the Radiology Diagnostic Oncology Group. Radiology 202:237–246
28. Panicek DM, Go SD, Healey JH, Leung DH, Brennan MF, Lewis JJ (1997) Soft tissue sarcoma involving bone or neurovascular structures: MRI prognostic factors. Radiology 205:871–875

29. Rubin DA, Kneeland JB (1994) MRI of the musculoskeletal system: technical considerations for enhancing image quality and diagnostic yield. AJR Am J Roentgenol 163:1155–1163
30. Sanchez RB, Quinn SF, Walling A, Estrada J, Greenberg H (1990) Musculoskeletal neoplasms after intraarterial chemotherapy: correlation of MR images with pathologic specimens. Radiology 174(1)237–40
31. Seeger LL, Widoff BE, Bassett LW, Rosen G, Eckardt JJ (1991) Preoperative evaluation of osteosarcoma: value of gadopentetate dimeglumine-enhanced MRI. AJR Am J Roentgenol 157(2):347–351
32. Shapeero LG, Vandel D, Verstraete KL, Bloem JL (1999) Dynamic contrast-enhanced MRI for soft tissue sarcomas. Semin Musculoskeletal Radiol 3(2):101–113
33. Shapeero LG, Vanel D, Verstraete KL, Bloem JL (2002) Fast magnetic resonance imaging with contrast for sof tissue sarcoma viability. Clin Orthop 397:212–227
34. Shuman WP, Patten RM, Baron RI, Liddell RM, Conrad EU, Richardson ML (1991) Comparison of STIR and spin-echo MRI at 1.5 T in 45 suspected extremity tumors: lesion conspicuity and extent. Radiology 179:247–252
35. Soulie D, Boyer B, Lescop J, Pujol A, Le Friant G, Cordoliani YS (1995) Liposarcome myxoide. Aspects en IRM. J Radiol 1:29–36
36. Stark D, Bradley W (1992) Magnetic resonance imaging, 2nd edn. Mosby Year Book, St.Louis
37. Van der Woude HJ, Bloem JL, Holscher HC, Nooy MA, Taminiau AHM, Hermans J, Falke THM, Hogendoorn PCW (1994) Monitoring the effect of chemotherapy in Ewing's sarcoma of bone with MRI. Skeletal Radiol 23(7):493–500
38. Van der Woude HJ, Bloem JL, Verstreate KL, Taminiau A, Nooy M, Hogendoorn P (1995) Osteosarcoma and Ewing's sarcoma after neoadjuvant chemotherapy: value of dynamic MRI in detecting viabl tumor before surgery. AJR Am J Roentgenol 165:593–98
39. Van der Woude HJ, Bloem JL, Pope TL Jr (1998) Magnetic resonance imaging of the musculoskeletal system. 9. Primary tumors. Clin Orthop 347:272–286
40. Van der Woude HJ, Verstraete KL, Hogendoorn PCW, Taminiau AHM, Hermans J, Bloem JL (1998) Musculoskeletal tumors: Does fast dynamic contrast-enhanced subtraction MRI contribute to characterization? Radiology 208:821–8
41. Van der Woude HJ, Bloem JL, Hogendoorn PCW (1998) Preoperative evaluation and monitoring chemotherapy in patients with high grade osteogenic and Ewing's sarcoma: review of current imaging modalities. Skeletal Radiol 27:57–71
42. van Rijswijk CS, Kunz P, Hogendoorn PC, Taminiau AH, Doornbos J, Bloem JL (2002) Diffusion-weighted MRI in the characterization of soft tissue tumors. J Magn Reson Imaging. 15(3):302–307
43. van Rijswijk CS, Geirnaerdt MJ, Hogendoorn PC, Taminiau AH, van Coevorden F, Zwinderman AH, Pope TL, Bloem JL (2004) Soft tissue tumors: value of static and dynamic Gadopentetate dimeglumine-enhanced MRI in prediction of malignancy. Radiology 233:493–502
44. Verstraete KL, Lang P (2000) Bone and soft tissue tumors: the role of contrast agents for MRI. Eur J Radiol 34:229–246
45. Verstraete KL, De Deene Y, Roels H, Dierick A, Uyttendaele D, Kunnen M (1994) Benign and malignant musculoskeletal lesions: dynamic contrast-enhanced MRI – parametric "first-pass" images depict tissue vascularization and perfusion. Radiology 192:835–43
46. Verstraete KL, Vanzieleghem B, De Deene Y, Palmans H, De Greef D, Kristoffersen DT, Uyttendaele D, Roels H, Hamers J, Kunnen M (1995) Static, dynamic and first-pass MRI of musculoskeletal lesions using gadodiamide injection. Acta Radiol 36(1):27–36
47. Verstraete KL, Van der Woude HJ, Hogendoorn PC, De Deene Y, Kunnen M, Bloem JL (1996) Dynamic contrast-enhanced MRI of musculoskeletal tumors: basic principles and clinical applications. J Magn Reson Imaging 6(2):311–321

Dynamic Contrast-Enhanced Magnetic Resonance Imaging

6

K.L. Verstraete, J.L. Bloem

Contents

6.1 Introduction

The purpose of this chapter is to review the basic principles and clinical applications of dynamic contrast-enhanced magnetic resonance imaging (MRI) of soft tissue tumors. Dynamic contrast-enhanced MRI is a method of physiological imaging, based on fast or ultrafast imaging, with the possibility of following the early enhancement kinetics of a water-soluble contrast agent after intravenous bolus injection. This technique provides clinically useful information, by depicting tissue vascularization and perfusion, capillary permeability, and composition of the interstitial space [1–3]. The most important advantages of this technique are its abilities to monitor response to preoperative chemotherapy, to identify areas of viable tumor before biopsy, and to provide physiological information for improved tissue characterization and detection of residual or recurrent tumor tissue after therapy.

6.2 Basic Principles

In patients with tumors and tumor-like lesions of the musculoskeletal system, MRI is performed with (fast-) spin-echo sequences, before and after administration of a water-soluble chelate of gadolinium, at a dose of 0.1 mmol/kg and a concentration of 0.5 M. As these sequences last for minutes, tissues are imaged in a quasi-equilibrium state of the water-soluble contrast agent between the blood and interstitial space [1, 3–5]. Therefore, this type of imaging is referred to as "static MRI," in which spatial resolution is emphasized over temporal resolution, in order to define anatomy.

This is in contrast to "dynamic MRI," where imaging is performed during and immediately after bolus injection, to study a dynamic physiological phenomenon, i.e., the initial distribution of the contrast agent in the capillaries and into the interstitial space of the tissues. This type of physiological imaging requires attention to a sufficiently high temporal resolution and serial imaging. According to the Nyquist theorem limit, in physiological imaging the process of interest must be sampled at twice the frequency of the dynamic event being measured [3]. After bolus injection (0.2 ml/kg) at an injection rate of 5 ml/s, the first pass of a contrast agent through a tissue generally lasts for about 7–15 s [2]. An imaging frequency of at least one image per 3.5–7 s is thus mandatory.

The extracellular distribution of fluid MR contrast agents is among blood plasma and the interstitial spaces. When such a contrast agent is administered intravenously by a rapid bolus injection, it is first diluted in the blood of the peripheral vein and the right heart, before it passes through the lungs and the left heart into the peripheral circulation (Fig. 6.1a). During the first pass of the contrast agent through the capillaries, a net unidirectional, fast diffusion occurs into the tissue, due to the high concentration gradient between the intravascular and the interstitial space: in normal tissues, approximately 50 % of the circulating contrast agent diffuses from the blood into the extravascular compartment during the first pass [1, 4–7]. This first-pass diffu-

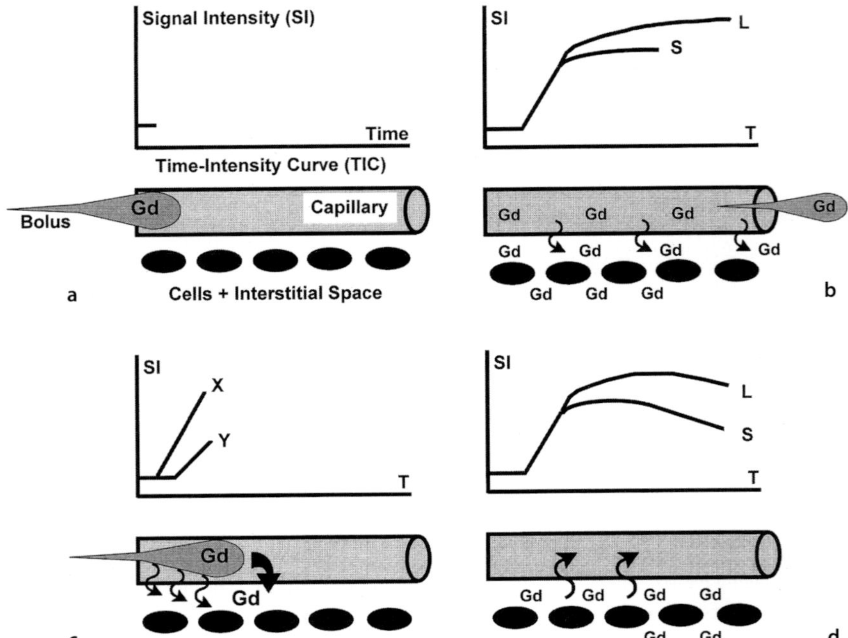

Fig. 6.1 a–d. Factors determining early tissue enhancement. The *lower parts* of **a–d** show what occurs at the level of the capillary and the interstitial space after intravenous bolus injection; the *upper parts* graphically display the changes in signal intensity (*SI*) in a time-intensity curve. **a** The time interval between the intravenous bolus injection and arrival of the bolus in the capillary is determined by the injection rate, the heart rate, the localization of the lesion, and the local capillary resistance (tissue perfusion). **b** The enhancement rate during the first pass of the contrast agent is determined by number of vessels (tissue vascularization), local capillary resistance (tissue perfusion), and capillary permeability. Tissues with high vascularization, perfusion, and capillary perme-ability (*X*) will enhance earlier and faster than tissues with a lower number of vessels, higher capillary resistance, and lower capillary permeability (*Y*). **c** After the first pass of the bolus, the SI increases further until the concentration of the gadolinium (*Gd*) contrast medium in the blood and the interstitial space of the tissue are equal. In tissues with a small (*S*) interstitial space, this equilibrium is reached earlier than in tissues with a larger (*L*) interstitial space. **d** As the arterial concentration of the contrast medium decreases, the SI drops while the Gd is progressively washed out from the interstitial space. This process occurs faster in tissues with a small (*S*) interstitial space than in tissues with a large (*L*) interstitial space

sion is essentially different from that during the second pass and later: at this initial moment, there is no contrast agent in the interstitial space, and the agent has its highest possible plasma concentration, because it is diluted in only a very small part of the total plasma volume, namely that volume that enters into the right side of the heart at the same time as the bolus, i.e., approximately 300 ml for a person weighing 75 kg at an injection rate of 5 ml/s (Fig. 6.1b). After the first pass, the diffusion rate immediately drops, because the concentration of the recirculating contrast medium has decreased owing to further dilution in the blood and partial accumulation in the interstitial space throughout the body (Fig. 6.1c). The length of the time interval between the end of the first pass and the equilibrium state, with equal concentrations of contrast medium in plasma and interstitial space, depends on the size of the interstitial space (Fig. 6.1c). This time interval may vary from less than 20 s in lesions with a small interstitial space to more than 3–5 min in tissues with a larger interstitial space [4, 5, 8]. After this equilibrium phase, the contrast medium is progressively washed out from the interstitial space as the arterial concentration decreases (Fig. 6.1d). Only in highly vascular lesions with a small interstitial space does early washout occur within the first minutes after bolus injection [8]. The aim of dynamic contrast-enhanced MRI is to detect and depict differences in early intravascular and interstitial distribution, as this process is influenced by pathological changes in tissues [2, 4, 5, 9–14].

6.3 Imaging Techniques

To study the early enhancement characteristics of a lesion with dynamic MRI, several factors have to be taken into account: type of sequence, selection and orientation of the imaging plane, number of slices, temporal resolution of the dynamic sequence, and spatial resolution of the images.

6.3.1 Sequence Parameters

As a rule, dynamic contrast-enhanced imaging has to be performed within the first 3 min after contrast injection: in this period of early intravascular and interstitial distribution, and large concentration gradients between these two compartments, important physiological information on tissue vascularization, perfusion, capillary permeability, and interstitial composition can be obtained. Due to the short distribution half-life of all water-soluble contrast agents and extravascular leakage of about 50% of the contrast agent during the first pass, most of this information is not available after a few recirculations, when capillary and interstitial space concentrations reach equilibrium[1, 4–7].

In ideal circumstances, a multislice sequence, covering the whole lesion, with a high spatial and temporal resolution should be used. With the current techniques, however, this is not possible, so that compromises are necessary: imaging with a high temporal resolution (e.g., one image per 3 s or less) is preferable in order to obtain at least three or four images during the first pass, but this is at the cost of spatial resolution and number of slices.

In the past, single- or double-slice, T1-weighted gradient-echo sequences, such as fast low-angle shot (FLASH; Siemens; Erlangen, Germany) and gradient-recalled acquisition in the steady state (GRASS; General Electric, Milwaukee, USA), with a temporal resolution between 7 and 23 s, and single or mostly multislice (3–11 slices), T1-weighted rapid spin-echo (RASE) sequences, with a temporal resolution between 18 and 90 s, have been used [9–13, 15–30]. However, as mentioned previously, an imaging frequency of at least one image per 3–5 s is preferable to study the physiological phenomena which occur during the first pass and which provide important information on tissue vascularization and perfusion [2, 8, 31–34].

Fast or ultrafast MRI sequences using gradient echos such as turbo FLASH (Siemens; Erlangen, Germany), turbo field echo (TFE; Philips, Best, The Netherlands), inversion recovery (IR) prepared fast GRASS and fast (multiplanar) spoiled GRASS [F(M)SPGR; General Electric, Milwaukee, USA] permit study of the earliest contrast-enhancement kinetics with a sufficiently high temporal and satisfactory spatial resolution by rapid acquisition in the order of 1–3 s per image [35–37]. These so-called snapshot-imaging techniques are based on a gradient-echo sequence with a very short repetition and echo time (less than 10 ms). The present generation of MR units permit single- and even double-slice snapshot dynamic studies with a temporal resolution of less than 3 s per image and a matrix of at least 128×128 (Table 6.1) [2, 31–34, 38, 39].

In dynamic MRI, the use of more than one average per acquisition should be avoided, as this decreases temporal resolution. Imaging with two (or more) averages per acquisition instead of one would lead to a loss of important temporal physiological information, which is now available on two (or more) images, obtained in the same time interval. Although fat saturation might be useful, e.g., by use of a selective-preparation radiofrequency pulse, in practice this is not done, as fat is adequately suppressed by most postprocessing techniques, e.g., in subtraction and first-pass images.

6.3.2 Selection of the Imaging Plane

The main disadvantage of the snapshot dynamic technique is that after bolus injection only one dynamic examination can be performed in the same patient (the examination cannot be repeated before all contrast is excreted from the body, i.e., at least 12 h), and that images for analysis are usually obtained at only one level

Table 6.1. Selection of pulse sequence parameters

Field strength (tesla)	Sequence	TR (ms)	TE (ms)	TI (ms)	Flip angle (degrees)	Matrix	Number of slices	Acquisition time (s)	Reference
1.5	Turbo FLASH	9	4	200	8	128×128	1	1.41	3
1	Turbo-FLASH	8.5	4	200	8	128×128	1	1.33	40
1.5	TFE	5.4	1.4	–	30	128×95	1	3	41
0.5	TFE	15	6.8	741	30	128×256	1–2	1.5–3	38
1.5	Fast MPGR	39	5	–	60	–	1	3.5	69

The dynamic study should last for at least 3 min after bolus injection, with only one average per acquisition, a section thickness of 5–10 mm, and a field of view between 200 and 500 mm

FLASH fast, low-angle shot, *TFE* turbo field echo, *MPGR* multiplanar GRASS

[2, 42]. It is presumed that this section represents the contrast enhancement behavior of the entire lesion. Nevertheless, significant variations in enhancement have been described in different regions within musculoskeletal lesions [25]. Due to this nonuniform contrast enhancement, the single-slice technique is subject to sampling error. To minimize this inevitable sampling error, the different components of the lesion should be thoroughly evaluated on the precontrast T1- and T2-weighted images, to find an imaging plane which includes most components of the lesion. This preselection may provide a representative imaging plane in small and uniformly enhancing lesions. Nevertheless, the nonuniform contrast enhancement must be considered an important motivation for development of new, faster techniques that permit sampling the entire lesion [25, 42]. Inclusion of an artery in the imaging plane is useful to evaluate differences in time of onset of enhancement in various parts of the lesion, compared with the time of arrival of the bolus.

6.3.3 Imaging Procedure

In practice, one test snapshot image should be obtained after preselection of a representative imaging plane (Table 6.1). If the lesion and the regional artery are displayed well on this image, the dynamic snapshot sequence can be started simultaneously with the bolus injection. During all acquisitions of the dynamic study, the transmitter and receiver gains should be held constant. Overall, the dynamic study should last for at least 3 min after bolus injection. The whole procedure lengthens the MR examination for about 5–10 min [2, 41]. To obtain high concentrations of contrast medium during the first pass, the bolus injection should be performed at an injection rate of 3–5 ml/s in the *right* antecubital vein, which is easily accessible and nearer to the heart than the left one: this causes less dilution of the bolus. To empty the contrast medium completely from the infusion line, the bolus should be followed immediately by a saline flush of about 20 ml at the same injection rate. At this rapid injection rates, no serious side effects have been observed [2, 33, 34, 39, 43]. As reproducibility is dependent on the injection rate and on the patient's cardiovascular status, use of a power-injector is preferable whenever repeat examinations are considered; e.g., for monitoring the effect of chemotherapy, a dynamic study should be performed before biopsy, during chemotherapy and just before surgery [2, 33, 39, 44–46].

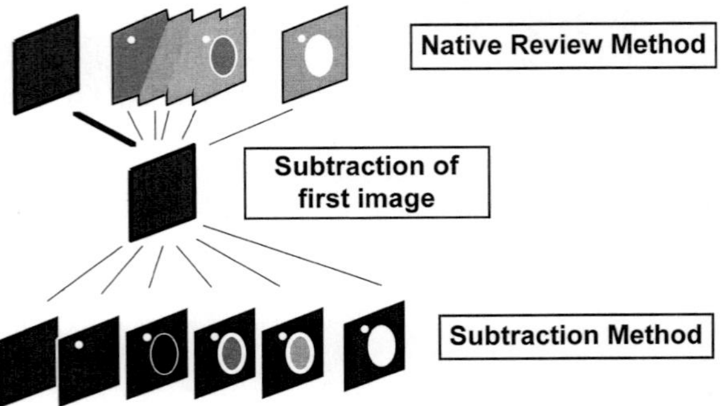

Fig. 6.2. Evaluation and postprocessing of a dynamic study with the "native review" and the "subtraction" method. In the native review method (*top*), the observer examines contrast enhancement sequentially on all images of the dynamic sequence. In the subtraction method (*bottom*), contrast enhancement is easily detected, as the first image (i.e., before bolus injection) is subtracted from all subsequent images of the dynamic study. In this way, only enhancing areas will be displayed on subtraction

6.4 Evaluation and Postprocessing Techniques

After performing a dynamic study, a large number of images (up to 180) have to be evaluated qualitatively and/or quantitatively. Evaluation of a series of images obtained with dynamic contrast-enhanced MRI can be performed in different ways. Each technique has its own advantages and disadvantages.

6.4.1 Native Review Method

A simple, fast, but subjective, qualitative method is the "native review method," in which an observer examines contrast enhancement sequentially on all images of the dynamic sequence. This can be done by viewing all images in "cine-mode" on a console, or simply by printing all images on a film and reviewing them one by one on a viewing box (Fig. 6.2). With this method, detection of small areas of enhancement or of areas with discrete enhancement may be difficult. Moreover, delineation of enhancing areas from fat and hemorrhage may be very difficult (Fig. 6.3). Therefore, it is preferable that the physiological information behind the dynamic MR images is extracted by postprocessing.

6.4.2 Subtraction Method

A readily available qualitative method is the "subtraction method," in which the first image (i.e., before contrast injection) is subtracted from all subsequent images of the dynamic study [9, 30, 38] (Fig. 6.2). In this way, all (especially discrete, early, and small) enhancing

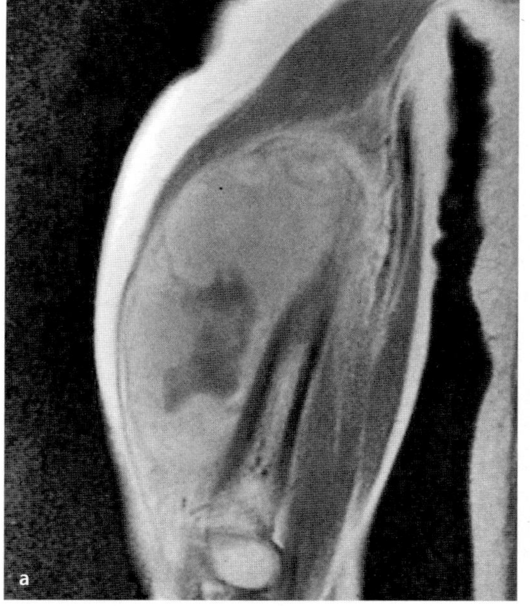

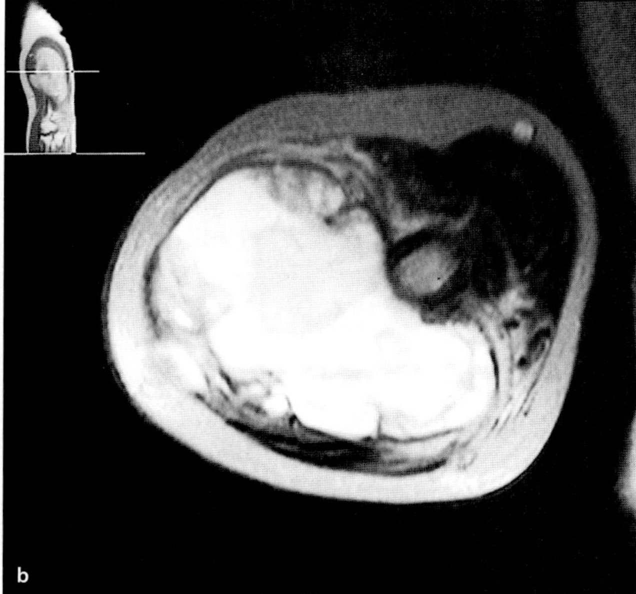

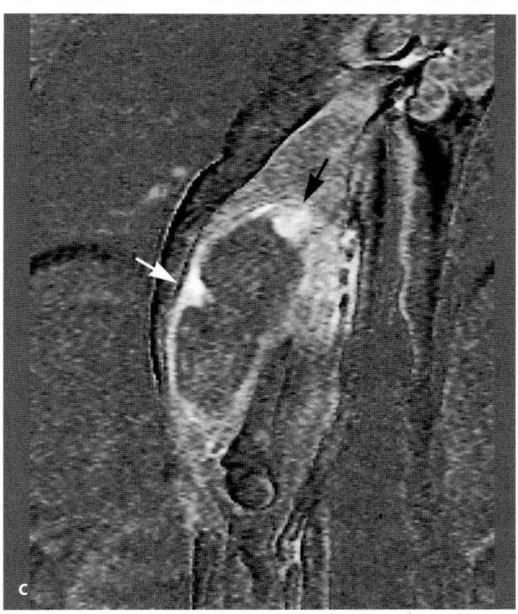

Fig. 6.3a–c. Indication of biopsy site on subtraction images. A 50-year-old woman with large soft tissue mass of the upper arm. Histological diagnosis of myxofibrosarcoma. **a** The coronal contrast-enhanced, spin-echo T1-weighted image (TR 600 ms, TE 20 ms) shows a soft tissue mass, predominantly of high signal intensity. There is an area of low signal intensity in the central part. **b** On the axial turbo spin-echo T2-weighted image (TR 3,873 ms, TE 150 ms), the mass has an inhomogeneous appearance and consists of areas of high and very high signal intensity. **c** Fast gradient-echo, dynamic contrast-enhanced subtraction image (turbo field echo; 0.5 T; TR 15 ms, TE 6.8 ms, TI 741 ms, flip angle 30°) reveals that only the periphery of the tumor shows (early) enhancement, whereas the central part lacks enhancement due to recent hemorrhage and necrosis. The solid areas at the periphery (*arrows*) should be attacked selectively to obtain a representative biopsy

areas are easily detected, and high signals from fat and hemorrhage are nullified (Figs. 6.3, 6.4). Subtraction images are evaluated in cine-mode on a console, or printed on film and reviewed one by one on a viewing box. Using this method, it is easy to evaluate the time interval between the onset of arterial and tumoral enhancement, and to detect the most "active" parts in tumors, e.g., in order to indicate the best site for biopsy or to determine the degree of response to preoperative chemotherapy qualitatively [9, 30, 38] (Fig. 6.3). However, late-enhancing tissues such as fat and connective tissue may be hardly recognizable on early subtraction images (Fig. 6.3).

6.4.3 Region-of-Interest Method

Another, operator-dependent and more time-consuming but quantitative method is the region-of-interest (ROI) method [13, 19–21, 34]. In this method, signal intensities (SI) in one or more circular or freely determined ROIs are measured and plotted against time in a time-intensity curve (TIC; Figs. 6.4–6.7). Most often, ROIs encircling the whole lesion and the quickest-enhancing area are evaluated [13, 19–21, 34] (Fig. 6.8). The area enhancing fastest can often be delineated easily after review of the native or subtraction images, or from other postprocessing methods. Several types of TICs

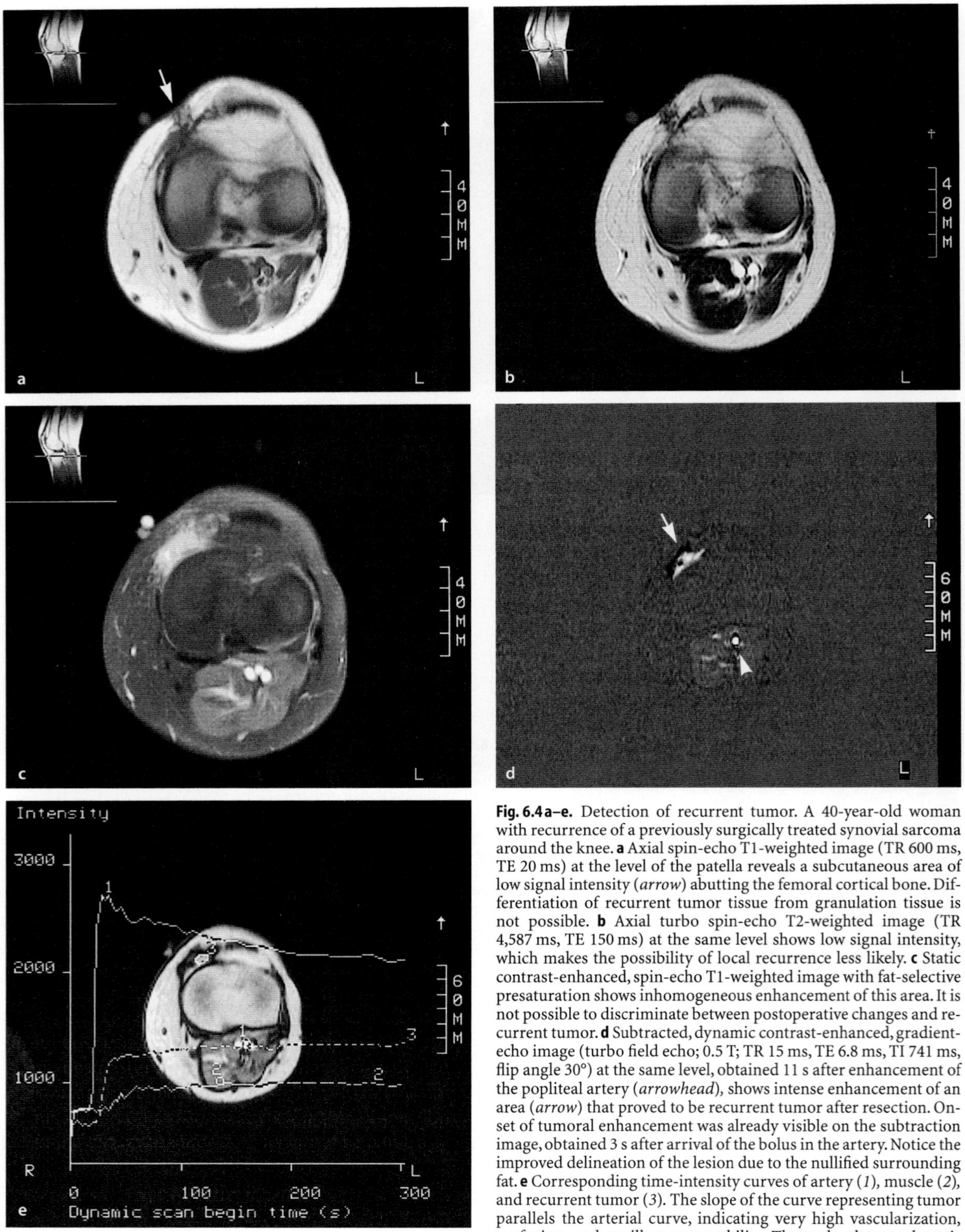

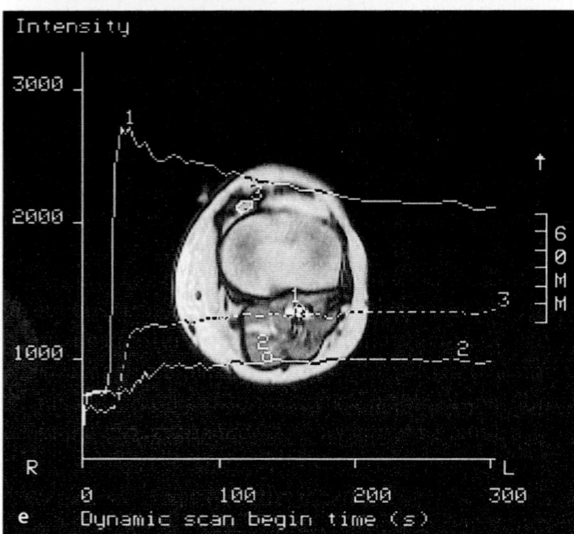

Fig. 6.4a–e. Detection of recurrent tumor. A 40-year-old woman with recurrence of a previously surgically treated synovial sarcoma around the knee. a Axial spin-echo T1-weighted image (TR 600 ms, TE 20 ms) at the level of the patella reveals a subcutaneous area of low signal intensity (*arrow*) abutting the femoral cortical bone. Differentiation of recurrent tumor tissue from granulation tissue is not possible. b Axial turbo spin-echo T2-weighted image (TR 4,587 ms, TE 150 ms) at the same level shows low signal intensity, which makes the possibility of local recurrence less likely. c Static contrast-enhanced, spin-echo T1-weighted image with fat-selective presaturation shows inhomogeneous enhancement of this area. It is not possible to discriminate between postoperative changes and recurrent tumor. d Subtracted, dynamic contrast-enhanced, gradient-echo image (turbo field echo; 0.5 T; TR 15 ms, TE 6.8 ms, TI 741 ms, flip angle 30°) at the same level, obtained 11 s after enhancement of the popliteal artery (*arrowhead*), shows intense enhancement of an area (*arrow*) that proved to be recurrent tumor after resection. Onset of tumoral enhancement was already visible on the subtraction image, obtained 3 s after arrival of the bolus in the artery. Notice the improved delineation of the lesion due to the nullified surrounding fat. e Corresponding time-intensity curves of artery (*1*), muscle (*2*), and recurrent tumor (*3*). The slope of the curve representing tumor parallels the arterial curve, indicating very high vascularization, perfusion, and capillary permeability. The early plateau phase is indicative of a small interstitial space in the tumor

Fig. 6.5. Time-intensity curve (TIC). In a TIC, the temporal change of the signal intensity in a region of interest (ROI; or pixel) is plotted against time. At T_{start}, when the bolus enters the ROI, the signal intensity rises above the baseline signal intensity (SI_{base}). The steepest slope represents the highest enhancement rate during the first pass (wash-in rate) and is mainly determined by tissue vascularization, perfusion, and capillary permeability. At T_{max}, the time of maximum enhancement, capillary and interstitial concentrations reach equilibrium. The time period between the end of the first pass and the maximum enhancement is mainly determined by the volume of the interstitial space. The washout rate can be calculated from the negative slope of the curve. (*a.u.* arbitrary units, T time interval between SI_{end} and SI_{prior})

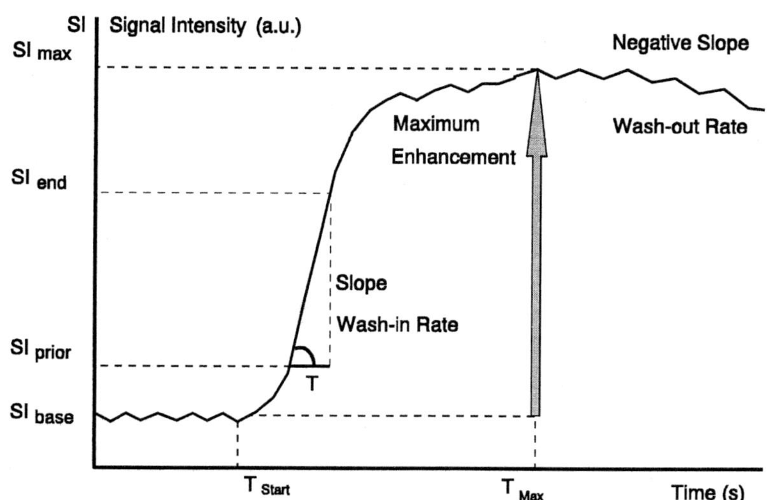

have been described [8, 31]. These TICs provide a graphic display of the early pharmacokinetics of the contrast agent during and immediately after the first pass (Figs. 6.1, 6.5, 6.8). From these curves, quantitative information can be obtained: time of onset of enhancement (T_{start}), slope (enhancement rate during the first pass, FP), maximum enhancement (E_{max}), and eventually negative slope (i.e., washout rate; Figs. 6.5, 6.8). The time of onset of enhancement in a lesion (T_{start}) can be measured relative to arterial enhancement. The difference in time between local arterial enhancement and tissue enhancement is mainly determined by tissue perfusion, and thus indirectly by the local capillary resistance [34, 47]. The slope represents the maximum enhancement rate during the first pass and is mainly determined by tissue vascularization (i.e., number of vessels) and perfusion [2, 8]. However, capillary permeability may also play an important role [48]. During the first pass, approximately 50% of the contrast agent (or even more in pathological tissues) enters the interstitial space [1, 4–7]. After the first pass, the concentration gradient and diffusion rate of the contrast agent drop immediately. The change in signal intensity is now mainly determined by the capillary permeability and the composition of the interstitial space (Fig. 6.1c). In tissues with a small interstitial space, a rapid equilibrium and even a washout of contrast will occur; whereas, in tissues with a larger interstitial space, a further wash-in will still be going on (Fig. 6.1d) [8].

The main advantage of the ROI method is that quantitative data are available and that the early pharmacokinetics of the contrast agent in the lesion are visually displayed in a TIC (Figs. 6.1. 6.5–6.8). The ROI method has, however, some disadvantages: it is operator dependent, and only the selected regions are studied. Moreover, it is a time-consuming procedure, especially when several areas have to be investigated (Fig. 6.8). To overcome the main disadvantages of the ROI method, several groups of investigators have tried to develop fast, operator-independent postprocessing techniques that evaluate the physiological information on a pixel-by-pixel basis [2, 16, 31, 33, 49].

6.4.4 First-pass Images

Another, rapid, largely operator-independent postprocessing technique that creates "first-pass images" focuses on the maximum enhancement rate during the first pass of the contrast agent, by calculating the first-pass slope value on a pixel by pixel basis, according to the equation (Fig 6.9) [2, 32–34]:

$$\text{steepest slope} = \frac{(SI_{\text{end}} - SI_{\text{prior}})}{(SI_{\text{baseline}} \times t)} \times 100 \ (\%/s) \quad (\text{Eq.1})$$

In this equation, SI_{baseline} represents the mean signal intensity in a pixel before arrival of the bolus; t is the time interval between the acquisition of two consecutive images with the largest change in signal intensity in a pixel (i.e., from SI_{prior} to SI_{end}) and corresponds to the temporal resolution of the dynamic sequence. By displaying the steepest slope value of all pixels with a grayscale value identical to the fastest enhancement rate, this method simultaneously provides quantitative and qualitative information in a new parametric image, the first-pass image (Figs. 6.6, 6.10). In this way, the operator-dependent selection of different ROIs with the subsequent time-consuming calculation of the slope value from the TIC can be avoided. It was shown by radiological-pathological and angiographic correlation that these images depict tissue (micro)vascularization

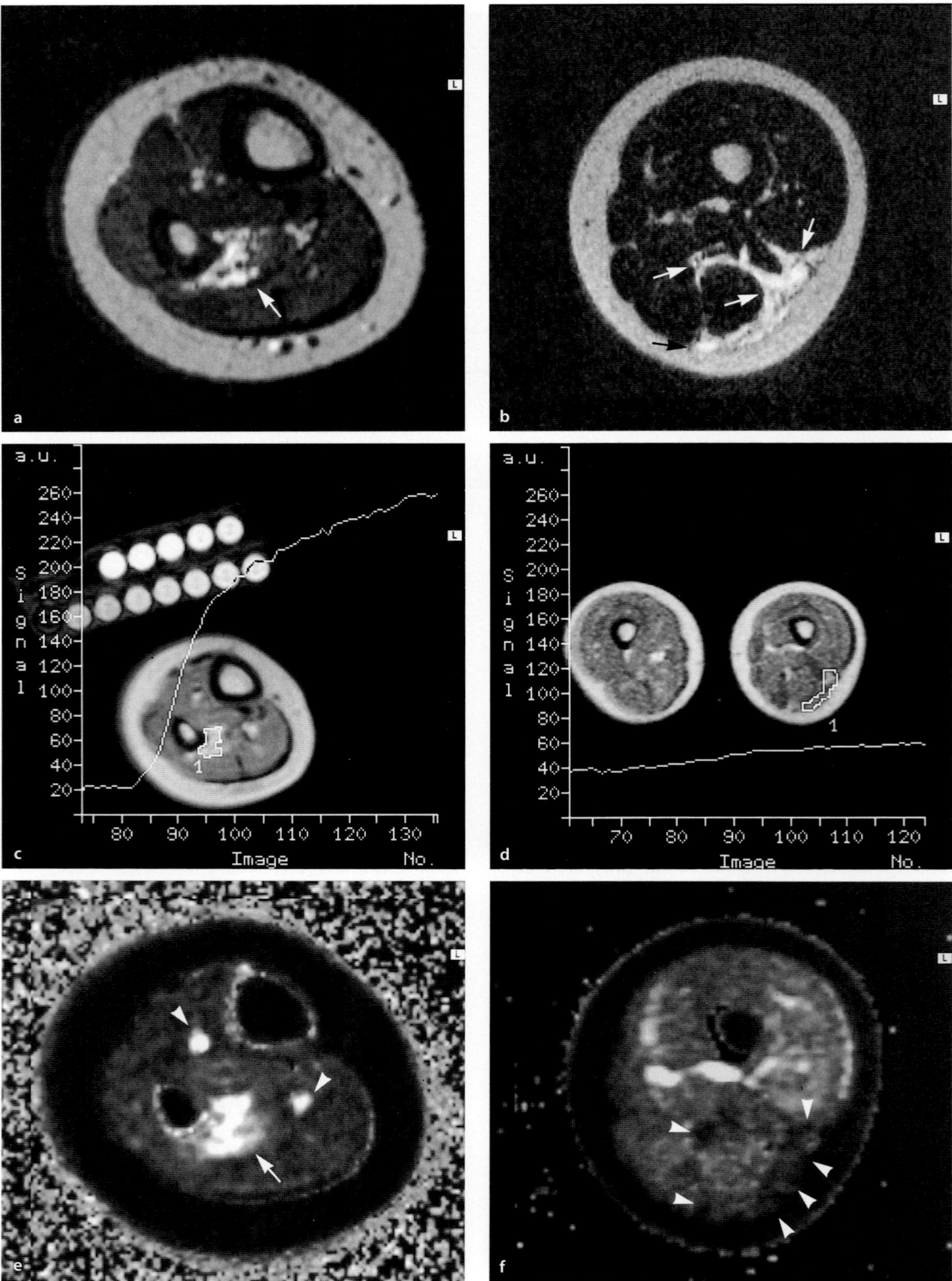

Fig. 6.6 a–h.

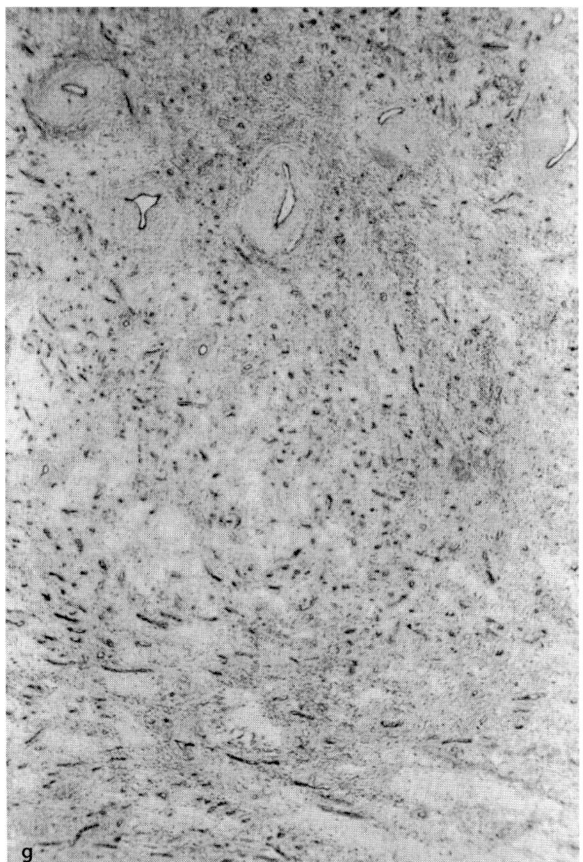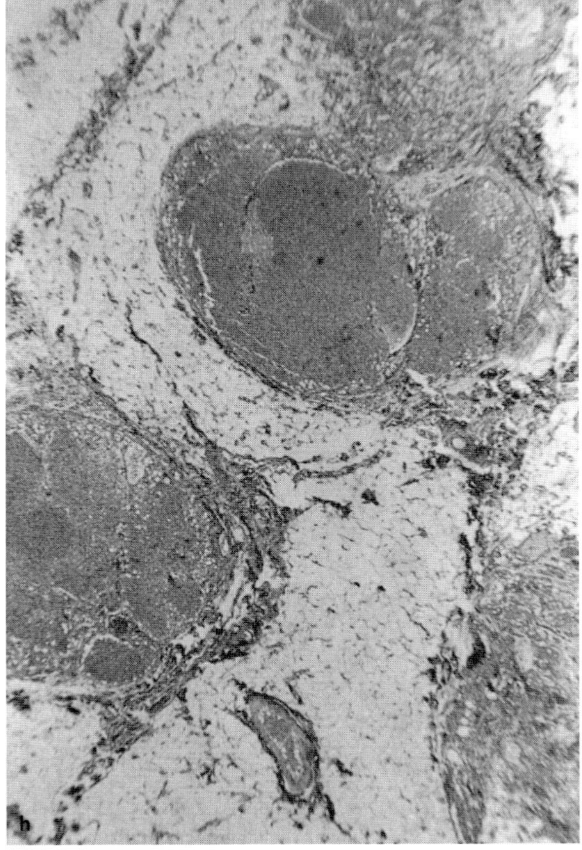

Fig. 6.6 g, h. Differentiation of capillary (high-flow) from cavernous (slow-flow) hemangioma with dynamic MRI. **a** On the T2-weighted spin-echo image of the right lower leg in a 10-year-old girl, the hemangioma is visible as a high signal-intensity mass against the fibula (*arrow*). **b** The T2-weighted image of the left thigh in a 14-year-old boy shows a soft tissue lesion with a high signal intensity, corresponding to a large hemangioma (*arrows*). The spin-echo images do not allow differentiation of highly and slowly perfused hemangiomas. **c, d** On the TIC, the capillary hemangioma (**c**) has a high first-pass enhancement, indicating high perfusion, whereas the cavernous hemangioma (**d**) has a slow per-

fusion. **e** On the first-pass image (turbo FLASH; 1.5 T; TR 9 ms, TE 4 ms, TI 200 ms, flip angle 8°), the capillary hemangioma (*arrow*) appears as bright as the major arteries (*arrowheads*) due to high perfusion. **f** The cavernous hemangioma appears dark on the first-pass image due to slow perfusion (*arrowheads*). **g** A photomicrograph of the capillary hemangioma shows numerous capillaries in the highly perfused hemangioma (factor VIII stain, specific for endothelial cells). **h** A photomicrograph of the cavernous hemangioma shows numerous red blood cells in the large lumina of the cavernous vessels, indicative of slow perfusion. (H&E)

and perfusion very well [2]. However, a visual display of the early pharmacokinetics of the contrast agent, as observed on a TIC, obtained with the ROI method, is not available with this method (Fig. 6.6).

A variant of this postprocessing method, "spatial mapping of instantaneous enhancement rates," applies an exponential-fitting algorithm on a pixel-by-pixel basis to allow derivation of the initial slope of the TIC, in order to create parametric "slope images" [50].

6.4.5 Discrete Signal Processing

Discrete signal processing of dynamic contrast-enhanced MR images is another, analogous postprocessing method which displays the initial and delayed rate of contrast-agent accumulation, and the maximum enhancement on a pixel-by-pixel basis in three parametric images, with a gray scale proportional to those three parameters [49]. The combination of these three parameters provides information on the pharmacokinetics of the contrast agent, otherwise available in a TIC.

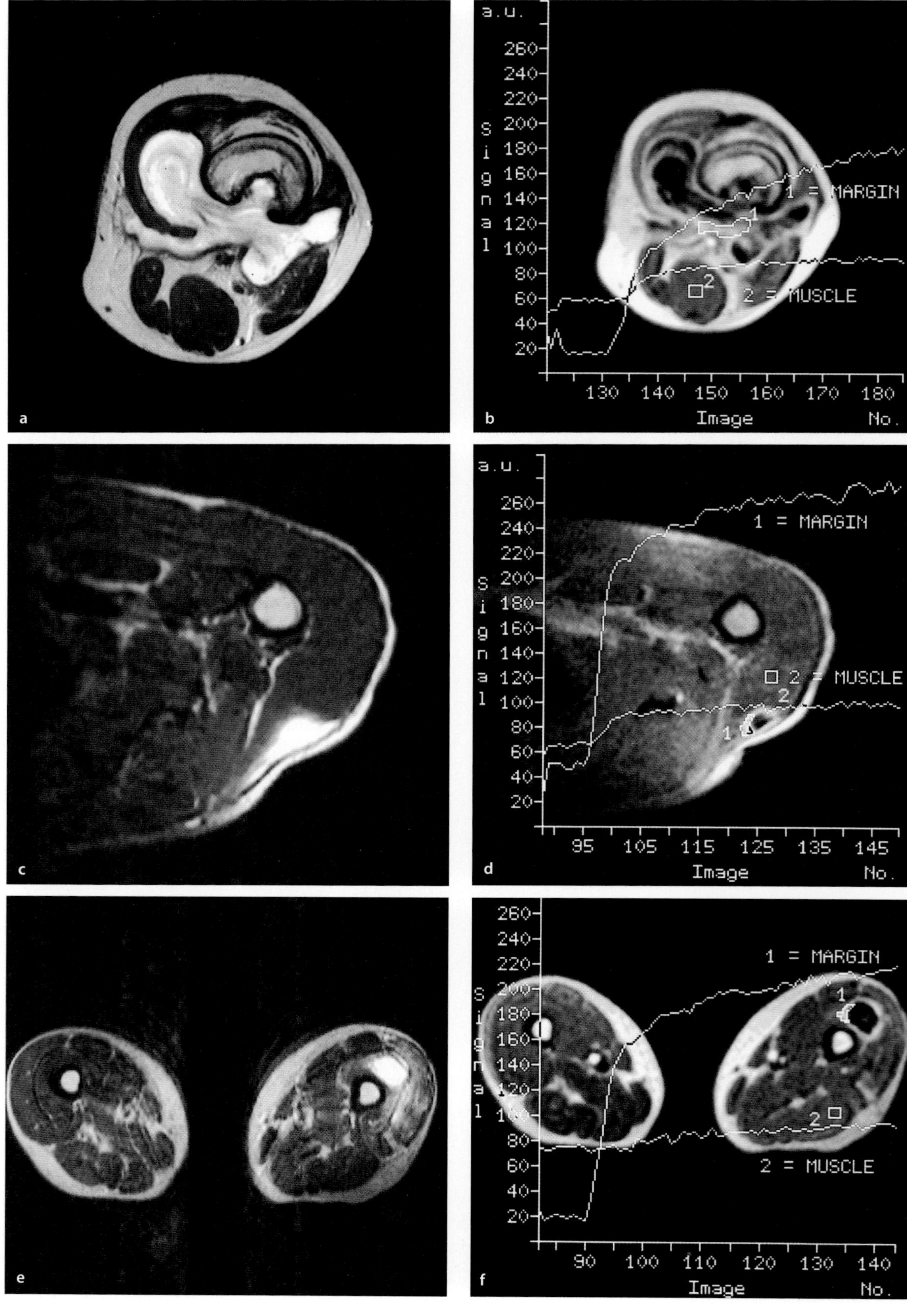

Fig. 6.7 a–f. Tissue characterization with dynamic MRI. T2-weighted image (**a, c, e**) and TIC (**b, d, f**) in a 23-year-old woman with chronic osteomyelitis and a soft tissue abscess in the left thigh (**a, b**), in a 23-year-old woman with posttraumatic myonecrosis of the left deltoid muscle (**c, d**), and in a 77-year-old man with a myxofibrosarcoma of the left quadriceps muscle (**e, f**). Dynamic MRI does not allow differentiation of benign and malignant lesions, as some highly vascularized and perfused benign lesions [such as granulation tissue at the periphery of an abscess (**b**) or of posttraumatic myonecrosis (**d**)] have slope values in the same range as malignant tumors, such as malignant fibrous histiocytoma (**f**). All three lesions show an early and fast enhancement at the periphery, where the most "active" part of the lesion is located

6.4.6 Practical Guidelines

In practice, review of the native images, or preferentially of subtracted images, in cine mode or on a viewing box, quickly provides information on the vascularization and perfusion of the lesion (e.g., to help characterize a lesion, to indicate the best site for biopsy, or to detect residual nests of viable tumor; Figs. 6.3, 6.4, 6.11–13). TICs can be obtained by delineating the whole lesion, the fastest-enhancing area, a feeding artery, and a reference tissue (e.g., muscle; Figs. 6.4, 6.6, 6.7, 6.13). These curves provide graphic information on perfusion, the wash-in rate, and eventually the washout rate. They can be used to calculate the steepest slope and to monitor chemotherapy. First-pass images and other pixel-by-pixel postprocessing techniques such as subtraction can be performed to evaluate all physiological information in one or only a few images, and therefore seem to have the greatest potential (Figs. 6.4, 6.6, 6.10–13).

6.5 Clinical Applications

Dynamic contrast-enhanced MRI has been used as an additional imaging technique in various clinical applications, such as: differentiation of benign from malignant lesions, tissue characterization by narrowing down the differential diagnosis, identification of areas of viable tumor before biopsy, differentiation of tumor from perineoplastic edema, early detection of avascular necrosis and inflammatory sacroiliitis, and evaluation of rheumatoid arthritis and carpal tunnel syndrome [2, 11, 12, 15, 18, 19, 24, 25, 27, 28, 33, 34, 41, 50]. In all these applications, this technique provides global information on tissue vascularization, perfusion, capillary permeability, and composition of the interstitial space. The most important applications in the musculoskeletal system, however, are monitoring of chemotherapy and detection of residual or recurrent tumor tissue after therapy [9, 10, 16, 17, 20–22, 29, 30, 49, 51].

6.5.1 Monitoring Chemotherapy

The most important application of dynamic MRI in the musculoskeletal system is evaluation of response to preoperative chemotherapy in bone tumors and soft tissue tumors, because plain radiography, CT, and static MRI are not reliable means of solving this problem [52]. The aim of monitoring is to predict the percentage of tumor necrosis in order to differentiate responders from nonresponders. Moreover, response to initial chemotherapy is one of the most reliable predictors of outcome [53–57]. Assessment of the effect of preoperative chemotherapy is important, because a poor response may affect the feasibility of future conservative surgery and change the postoperative (adjuvant) chemotherapy [55, 57, 58]. In contrast, a good responsive tumor that was considered inoperable at the time of first presentation can conceivably become operable [59].

Many studies have assessed the value of dynamic MRI in monitoring the response to preoperative chemotherapy in osteosarcoma, Ewing sarcoma, rhabdomyosarcoma, and synovial sarcoma [2, 9, 10, 16, 17, 20, 21, 33, 39, 42, 51, 60, 61]. The promising results, with accuracy levels to distinguish responders from nonresponders of 85.7–100 %, can largely be explained by the possibility of dynamic MRI to depict tissue vascularization. Other successful methods, such as angiography, color Doppler flow imaging, and blood-pool scintigraphy with technetium-99m diphosphonate (^{99m}Tc-labeled MDP), are also based on the demonstration of a significant decrease in tumor vascularization and perfusion in responders [47, 62–65].

In dynamic MRI, the ROI method allows creation of TICs from regions encircling the whole tumor [2, 20, 21, 33]. An increase in slope value during follow-up indicates poor response, whereas a decrease in type of curve and slope not always indicates good response, because small nests of residual tumor tissue may be missed. To detect these areas, smaller areas of interest should be investigated, e.g., by MR mapping [10, 42]. This is very time-consuming, and therefore computerized, pixel-by-pixel postprocessing techniques are preferable.

The most easy, qualitative postprocessing method to evaluate dynamic contrast-enhanced images is subtraction MR [9, 39] (Figs. 6.6, 6.8, 6.11). Subtraction images display areas with remaining viable tumor cells as high signal-intensity nodules and allow a good differentiation between viable tumor and inflammation (Figs. 6.8, 6.11).

In first-pass images, all structures are displayed with a gray scale equal to the highest enhancement rate (i.e., during the first pass; Figs. 6.9, 6.10) [2, 32]. In this way, quantitative evaluation of the effect of chemotherapy is possible by measuring the first-pass enhancement rate of the whole tumor (i.e., the mean value of all pixels in the tumor) in consecutive examinations during preop-

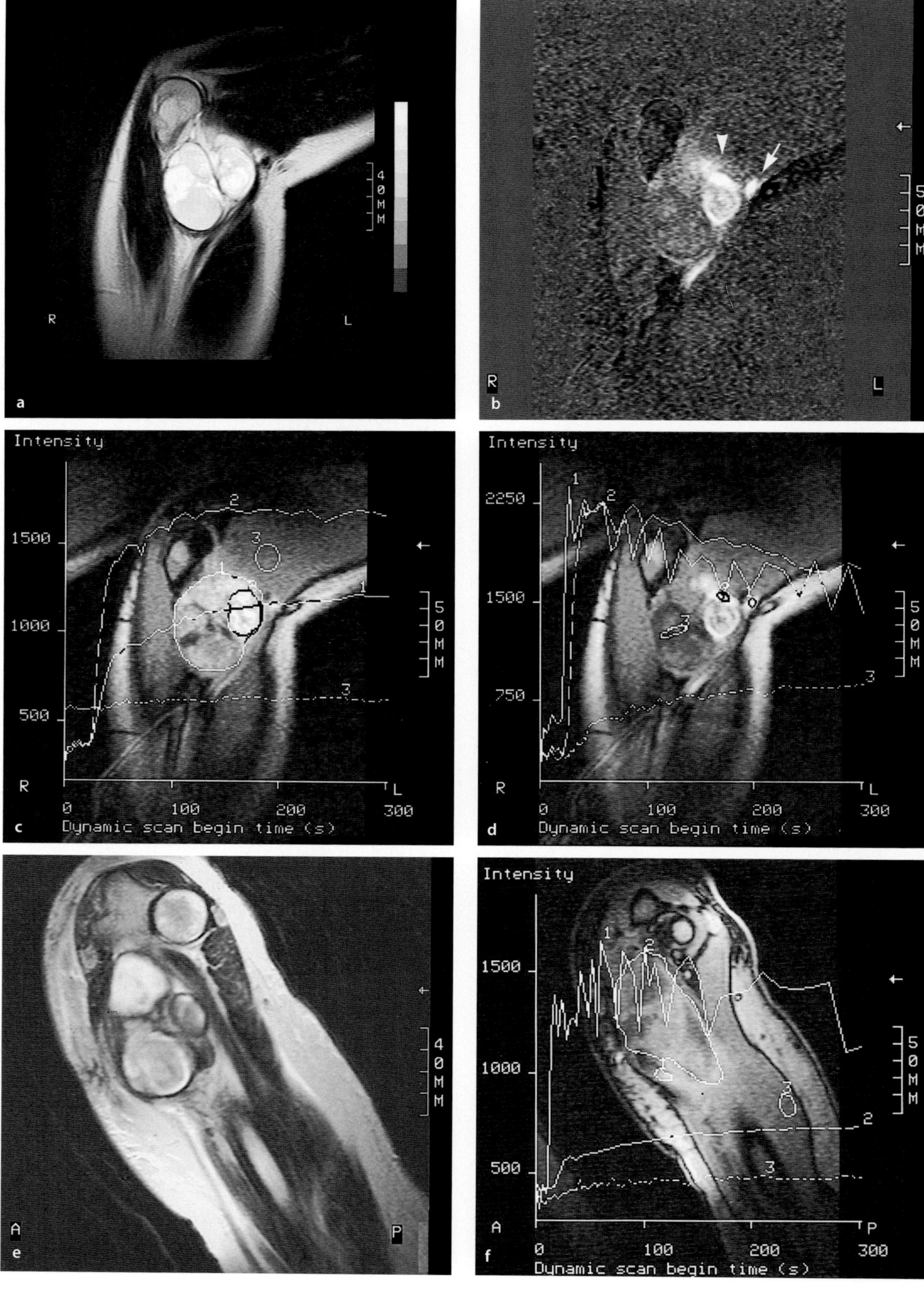
Intensity
1500
1000
500
R
L
0   100   200   300
Dynamic scan begin time (s)
c
Intensity
2250
1500
750
R
L
0   100   200   300
Dynamic scan begin time (s)
d
Intensity
1500
1000
500
A
P
0   100   200   300
Dynamic scan begin time (s)
f
a
b
e
R
L
R
L
A
P

Fig. 6.8a–f. Monitoring chemotherapy with dynamic MRI. A 51-year-old man with inflammatory myxofibrosarcoma of the soft tissues in the cubital fossa before (**a–d**) and after (**e, f**) isolated perfusion with tumor necrosis factor-alpha. Histological response was good. **a** Sagittal turbo spin-echo T2-weighted image (TR 3,873 ms, TE 150 ms) before treatment shows a lobulated mass with a predominantly high signal intensity. **b** Fast, dynamic gradient-echo, gadolinium-diethyltriamine pentaacetic acid (DTPA)-enhanced subtraction image (turbo field echo; 0.5 T; TR 15 ms, TE 6.8 ms, TI 741 ms, flip angle 30°) acquired 3 s after arrival of the bolus of contrast medium in the artery (*arrow*). Early peripheral enhancement of the tumor is clearly shown (*arrowhead*). **c** TIC of the whole tumor (*1*), a fast-enhancing nodule within the tumor (*2*), and the brachial muscle (*3*). **d** TIC of the brachial artery (*1*), a peripheral, very fast, and early enhancing tumor nodule, with early washout (*2*), and a central, more slowly enhancing area within the tumor (*3*). Note that the curve of the peripheral tumor nodule (*2*) parallels the arterial curve (*1*), indicating a very high vascularization, perfusion, and capillary permeability. **e** After therapy, there is an inhomogeneous residual mass with high signal-intensity areas on the turbo spin-echo T2-weighted images. The degree of response to chemotherapy cannot be assessed on spin-echo images. **f** The dynamic contrast-enhanced gradient-echo images show delayed onset of enhancement of the tumor relative to the artery and to the first examination. No focal areas of early enhancement consistent with viable tumor can be seen. The corresponding TICs now show gradual enhancement of the whole tumor (*2*) relative to the artery (*1*), with absence of an early plateau phase or early washout, indicating decreased vascularization, perfusion, and capillary permeability. Histological response to chemotherapy was good

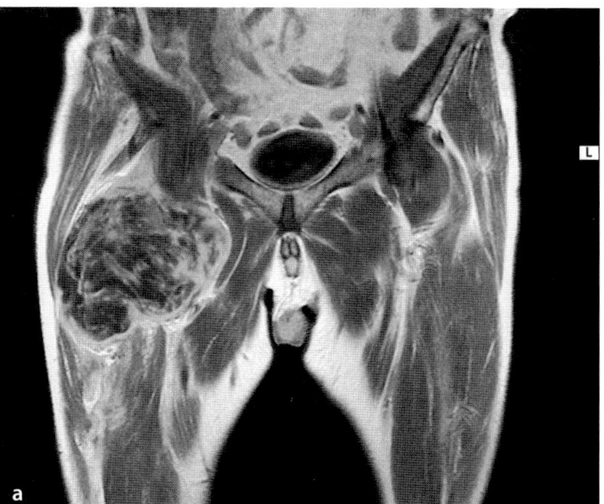

a

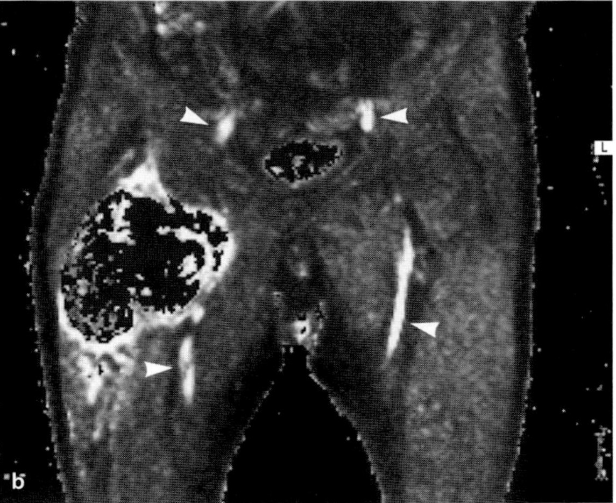

b

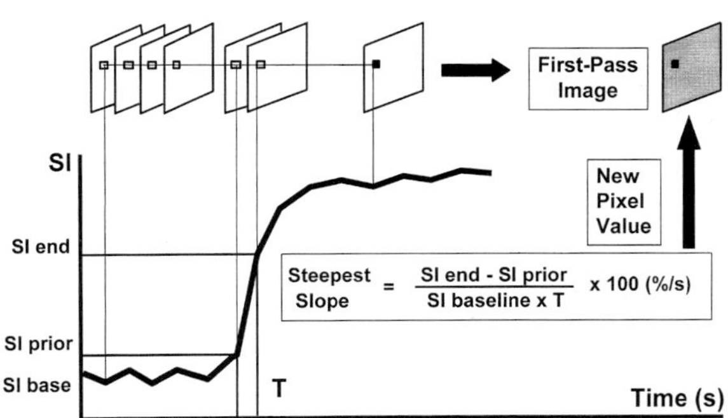

Fig. 6.9. First-pass images: postprocessing procedure. For each pixel of the dynamic image, the steepest slope of the TIC is calculated. This value represents the highest enhancement rate during the first pass. Subsequently, a single new image with the same matrix can be composed. The value of each pixel in this image is equal to the spatially corresponding first-pass slope value. This parametric image is therefore called the first-pass image [65, 66, 68]

Fig. 6.10a, b. Monitoring chemotherapy with first-pass images. **a** The coronal contrast-enhanced T1-weighted image shows inhomogeneous enhancement in a large myxofibrosarcoma after two cycles of chemotherapy. The degree of response cannot be assessed on the spin-echo images. **b** The first-pass image (turbo FLASH; 1.5 T; TR 9 ms, TE 4 ms, T1 200 ms, flip angle 8°) shows high first-pass enhancement rates in the arteries (*arrowheads*) and at the periphery of the tumor. Histologically, these fast-enhancing areas corresponded to residual viable tumor

erative chemotherapy. Direct visual inspection (qualitative evaluation) of these images allows easy detection of highly vascular and/or highly perfused viable tumor tissue. This is useful for the qualitative assessment of tumor response (Fig. 6.10). Whenever areas with a bright appearance are detected, poor response, with more than 10% of tumor tissue remaining vital should be suspected. In such cases, the first-pass image was useful to guide a new biopsy or to focus the attention of the pathologist on those areas in the resected specimen, in which tumor cells might have survived chemotherapy [2] (Figs. 6.10, 6.11). However, with this and other postprocessing techniques, young granulation tissue replacing tumor necrosis may mimic vital tumor areas, especially in the early phase of chemotherapy.

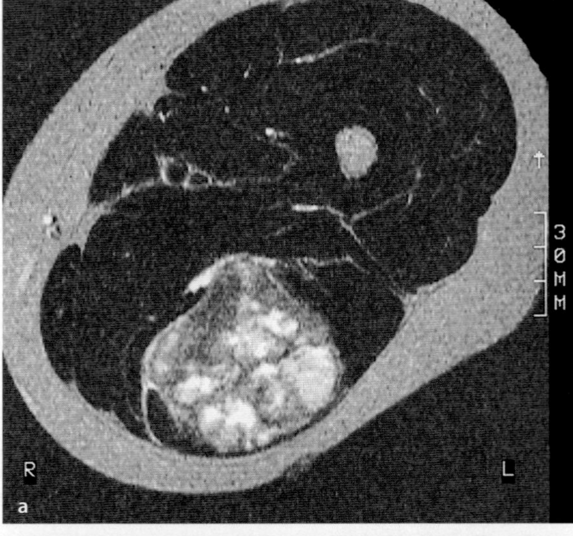

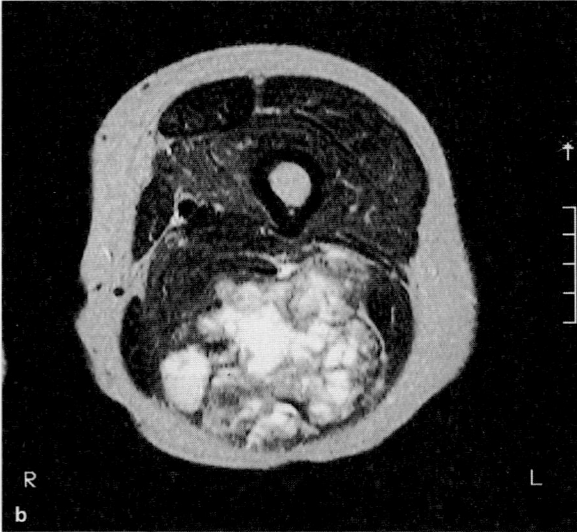

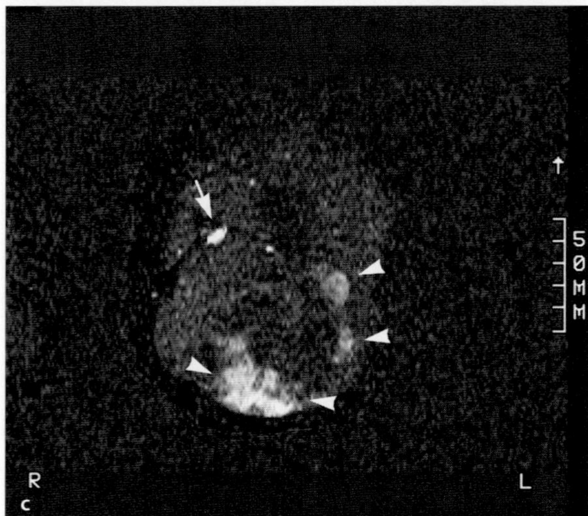

Fig. 6.11a–c. Monitoring chemotherapy with dynamic MRI. A 23-year-old woman with soft tissue metastasis of an osteosarcoma in the thigh before (**a**) and after (**b, c**) treatment with isolated limb perfusion with tumor necrosis factor-alpha. Histological response to chemotherapy was poor. **a** Axial turbo spin-echo T2-weighted image (TR 4,598 ms, TE 150 ms) shows inhomogeneous mass with areas of intermediate and high signal intensity. **b** Axial turbo spin-echo T2-weighted image (TR 4,590 ms, TE 150 ms) after therapy displays a large heterogeneous mass, mainly composed of high signal-intensity areas with fluid levels compatible with hemorrhage and/or necrosis. However, the degree of response cannot be assessed on the spin-echo images. **c** Early dynamic gadolinium-enhanced, gradient-echo subtraction image (turbo field echo; 0.5 T; TR 15 ms, TE 6.8 ms, TI 741 ms, flip angle 30°) shows rapidly progressive enhancing areas (*arrowheads*) at the periphery of the mass, starting within 3 s after arterial enhancement (*arrow*). These early-enhancing foci corresponded to areas of highly cellular, residual viable tumor. The central part of the tumor lacked enhancement, corresponding to necrosis

6.5.2 Tissue Characterization – Differentiation of Benign from Malignant Lesions

Attempts have been made to use the slope of a TIC as a differential diagnostic criterion to differentiate benign (low-slope) from malignant (high-slope) lesions (Table 6.2; Figs 6.5, 6.7) [2, 19–21, 33, 34, 51]. In these studies, evaluation of the malignant potential of musculoskeletal lesions with the slope of TICs was possible with levels of sensitivity and specificity ranging from 72% to 83%, and 77% to 89%, respectively. Although there was a highly statistically significant difference in slope values of benign and malignant lesions, there was some overlap: some highly vascularized or perfused benign lesions, such as: aneurysmal bone cyst, eosinophilic granuloma, giant cell tumor, osteoid osteoma, acute osteomyelitis, myositis ossificans, and occasionally aggressive fibromatosis, fibrous dysplasia,

neurinoma, and neurofibroma, had slope values in the same range as malignant tumors (Figs. 6.6, 6.7; Table 6.2). The highest slope values were found in synovial sarcoma and fibrosarcoma. On the other hand, low slope values seemed to have a high predictive value in favor of a benign lesion. (Fig. 6.12, Table 6.2). Due to this overlap between benign and malignant lesions, TICs and slope values should only be used in conjunction with conventional spin-echo images and other radiological, anatomical, and clinical data to narrow down the differential diagnostic possibilities, by providing physiological information on the vascularization and perfusion of the lesion, rather than to predict the benignity or malignancy of a lesion. A recent study evaluating the value of static and dynamic gadopentetate dimeglumine-enhanced MRI in prediction of malignancy showed that contrast-enhanced MRI parameters that favored malignancy were liquefaction, early dynamic

Table 6.2. Slope values of soft tissue tumors

Slope value	3–40%/s	40–96%/s	>100%/s
Benign lesions	Lipoma Lipoblastoma Elastofibroma Organizing old hematoma Ganglion Dermoid Fat necrosis Cavernous hemangioma (slow flow) Angiolipoma Synovial chondromatosis Pigmented villonodular synovitis Neurofibroma Rheumatoid nodule Calcifying tendinitis Schwannoma	Myositis Capillary (high-flow) hemangioma Abscess Granulation tissue Myositis ossificans	
Malignant lesions		Epithelioid sarcoma Lymphoma Liposarcoma Fibrosarcoma	Malignant fibrous histiocytoma Synoviosarcoma

The slope values were obtained using a single-slice turbo-FLASH sequence on a 1.5-T magnet, with the following parameters: TR 9 ms; TE 4 ms; TI 200 ms; flip angle 8°; matrix 128×128; one average per acquisition; slice thickness 6–10 mm; acquisition time 1.41 s/image; linear view order

enhancement (within 6 s after arterial enhancement), peripheral or inhomogeneous dynamic enhancement, and rapid initial dynamic enhancement followed by a plateau or washout phase [41]. The slope of the TIC, the time of onset of enhancement (relative to the onset of enhancement in a local artery) and the type of curve are not helpful to differentiate benign from malignant lesions, although curves with a high slope, early equilibrium phase, and early washout seem to occur more frequently in malignant fibrous histiocytoma and synoviosarcoma [8, 38] (Fig. 6.13).

Dynamic contrast-enhanced MRI has been used successfully to differentiate capillary and arteriovenous (high-flow) hemangiomas from cavernous (slow-flow) hemangiomas [2, 31, 34] (Fig. 6.6). Identification of viable areas in a tumor is important for biopsy, as, on histopathological examination, well-vascularized viable tumor will be of greater value for determining the tumor type and grade than a biopsy specimen containing a mixture of poorly vascularized tumor tissue, edema, or necrotic material. Dynamic contrast-enhanced MRI may provide useful information for guiding the biopsy needle toward representative areas, as areas with well-vascularized viable tumor tissue will be depicted considerably better than on contrast-enhanced spin-echo images [34] (Fig. 6.3). During the first pass of the contrast agent in the tumor, the most highly vascular areas will appear brighter than other tumor components and peritumoral edema, due to a faster enhancement (Figs. 6.3, 6.4, 6.8, 6.13) [50].

6.5.3 Detection of Residual or Recurrent Tumor

After resection of a musculoskeletal tumor, regular follow-up studies are mandatory. Whenever a mass is detected with high signal intensity on T2-weighted images, dynamic contrast-enhanced MRI is indicated, as differentiation between inflammatory changes, hygromas, and residual or recurrent tumor tissue is not possible with static MRI [30, 66–70]. According to Vanel et al., no or slow increase observed with dynamic contrast-enhanced MRI indicates pseudomass, whereas early and fast increase indicates recurrence [29, 30] (Figs. 6.4, 6.13).

6.6 Conclusions

Dynamic MRI is a promising method of physiological imaging which provides clinically useful information, by depicting tissue vascularization and perfusion, capillary permeability, and composition of the interstitial space. The most important applications in the musculoskeletal system are an indication of the biopsy site, tissue characterization, monitoring of preoperative chemotherapy, and detection of residual or recurrent tumor tissue.

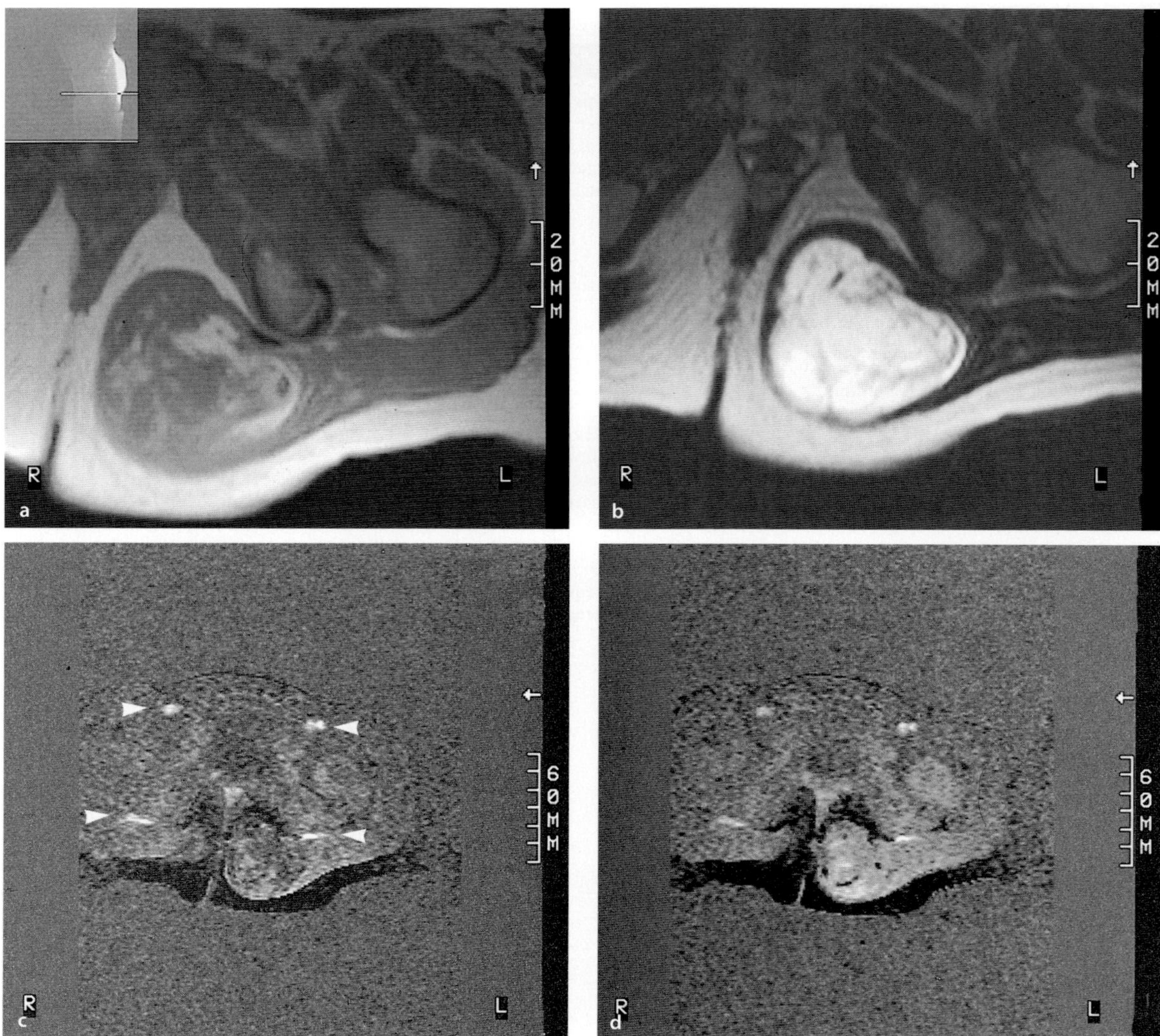

Fig. 6.12 a–d. Tissue characterization with dynamic MRI. A 5-year-old boy with painful swelling of the buttocks. **a** The axial spin-echo T1-weighted image shows a poorly defined mass in the left gluteus maximus muscle. The tumor is heterogeneous, with both ill-defined areas of intermediate signal intensity and areas of high signal intensity corresponding to fat. **b** On the turbo spin-echo T2-weighted image, the mass is well defined and predominantly of very high signal intensity, with some serpentine areas of intermediate signal intensity corresponding to fatty tissue. **c** Early dynamic, gadolinium-enhanced gradient-echo subtraction image (turbo field echo; 0.5 T; TR 15 ms, TE 6.8 ms, TI 741 ms, flip angle 30°), acquired 3 s after enhancement of the arteries (*arrowheads*), shows no enhancement in the tumor. **d** Late dynamic, gadolinium-enhanced gradient-echo subtraction image, acquired 112 s after arterial enhancement, shows only discrete enhancement in the tumor. The late and low enhancement makes the diagnosis of a high-grade soft tissue sarcoma (e.g., liposarcoma or rhabdomyosarcoma) less likely. Biopsy and subsequent tumor resection in this patient revealed a (benign) lipoblastoma

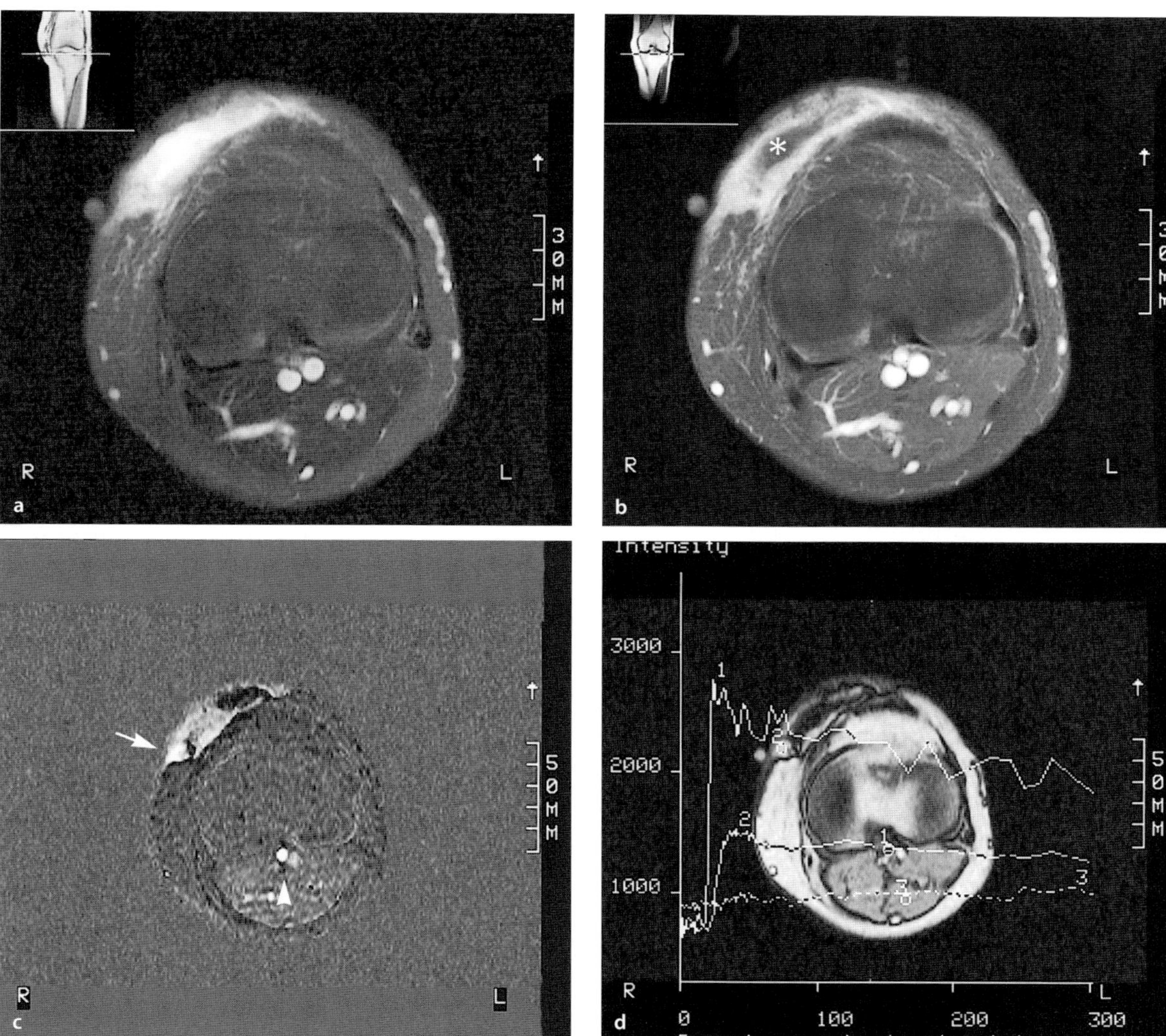

Fig. 6.13 a–d. Detection of residual tumor with dynamic MRI. A 58-year-old woman referred for an MRI examination after marginal resection of what was originally thought to be a lipoma but proved to be a myxofibrosarcoma. **a** Axial fat-saturated, turbo spin-echo T2-weighted image (1,901 ms/100 ms) at the level of the scar, which is marked with a vitamin A pearl. There is a nonspecific area of high signal intensity within the subcutaneous tissue; differentiation of residual tumor tissue and granulation tissue is not possible. **b** Static T1-weighted, contrast-enhanced image with fat-selective presaturation displays nonspecific enhancement of the scar region: differentiation of residual tumor tissue and granulation tissue is not possible. The nonenhancing area (*asterisk*) represents a postoperative fluid collection (seroma). **c** Subtracted dynamic contrast-enhanced gradient-echo image (turbo field echo; 0.5 T; TR 15 ms, TE 6.8 ms, TI 741 ms, flip angle 30°) at the same level, obtained 30 s after bolus injection. There is a small, nodular area of very high signal intensity (*arrow*) abutting the seroma cavity. Enhancement started 6 s after arrival of the bolus in the artery (*arrowhead*). The early and intense enhancement are more suggestive of residual tumor tissue than postoperative granulation tissue. **d** The TIC of this small nodular area (*2*) parallels the arterial curve (*1*) and an early plateau phase is seen, followed by a gradual washout. Histology of the biopsy revealed residual myxofibrosarcoma

Things to remember:

1. Dynamic contrast-enhanced imaging is a method of physiological imaging.
2. The first pass of contrast medium provides information on tissue vascularization, perfusion, and capillary permeability
3. The enhancement after the first pass provides information on the interstitial space
4. Dynamic contrast-enhanced imaging does not reflect benignity or malignancy of a lesion
5. Dynamic contrast-enhanced imaging is useful to monitor chemotherapy
6. Dynamic contrast-enhanced imaging is useful to indicate the best site for biopsy
7. Dynamic contrast-enhanced imaging is useful to detect tumor recurrence and differentiate recurrence from reactive tissue
8. In selected cases dynamic contrast-enhanced imaging can be helpful to narrow the differential diagnosis
9. The procedure of dynamic contrast-enhanced imaging can be performed in less than 5 min
10. Interpretation of a dynamic contrast-enhanced imaging study can be performed by reviewing the native images in cine mode, by subtraction or pixel-by-pixel postprocessing techniques, and by drawing TICs from selected regions of interest (e.g., whole tumor, fastest-enhancing area, muscle and artery)

References

1. Brasch RC (1992) New directions in the development of MR imaging contrast-media. Radiology 183:1–11
2. Verstraete KL, Dedeene Y, Roels H, Dierick A, Uyttendaele D, Kunnen M (1994) Benign and malignant musculoskeletal lesions – dynamic contrast-enhanced MR-imaging – parametric first-pass images depict tissue vascularization and perfusion. Radiology 192:835–843
3. Wolf GL (1991) Contrast agents in spine and body MRI: introduction. In:Hasso AN, Stark DD (ed) American Roentgen Ray Society – categorical course syllabus: spine and body magnetic resonance imaging. Reston, VA, pp 111–115
4. Dean PB, Kormano M (1977) Intravenous bolus of ^{125}I-labeled meglumine diatrizoate. Early extravascular distribution. Acta Radiol Diagn (Stockh) 18:293–304
5. Kormano M, Dean PB (1976) Extravascular contrast material: the major component of contrast enhancement. Radiology 121:379–382
6. Tong CY, Prato FS, Wisenberg G, et al (1993) Measurement of the extraction efficiency and distribution volume for Gd-DTPA in normal and diseased canine myocardium. Magn Reson Med 30:337–346
7. Tong CY, Prato FS, Wisenberg G, et al (1993) Techniques for the measurement of the local myocardial extraction efficiency for inert diffusible contrast agents such as gadopentate dimeglumine. Magn Reson Med 30:332–336
8. Verstraete KL et al (1992) Dynamic contrast enhanced MRI of musculoskeletal neoplasms: different types and slopes of TICs (abstract). Proceedings of Society of Magnetic Resonance in Medicine. Berkely, p 2609
9. Debaere T, Vanel D, Shapeero LG, Charpentier A, Terrier P, Dipaola M (1992) Osteosarcoma after chemotherapy – evaluation with contrast material enhanced subtraction MR imaging. Radiology 185:587–592
10. Hanna SL, Parham DM, Fairclough DL, Meyer WH, Le AH, Fletcher BD (1992) Assessment of osteosarcoma response to preoperative chemotherapy using dynamic flash gadolinium-DTPA-enhanced magnetic-resonance mapping. Invest Radiol 27:367–373
11. Konig H, Sieper J, Wolf KJ (1990) Rheumatoid arthritis – evaluation of hypervascular and fibrous pannus with dynamic MR imaging enhanced with Gd-DTPA. Radiology 176:473–477
12. Konig H, Sieper J, Wolf KJ (1990) Dynamic MRI for the differentiation of inflammatory joint lesions. Rofo Fortschr Geb Rontgenstr Neuen Bildgeb Verfahr 153:1–5
13. Ross JS, Delamarter R, Hueftle MG et al (1989) Gadolinium-DTPA-enhanced MRI of the postoperative lumbar spine: time course and mechanism of enhancement. AJR Am J Roentgenol 1989;152:825–834
14. Verstraete KL, Dierick A, De Deene Y et al (1994) First-pass images of musculoskeletal lesions: a new and useful diagnostic application of dynamic contrast-enhanced MRI. Magn Reson Imaging 12:687–702
15. Bollow M, Braun J, Hamm B et al (1995) Early sacroiliitis in patients with spondyloarthropathy – evaluation with dynamic gadolinium-enhanced MR-imaging. Radiology 194:529–536
16. Bonnerot V, Charpentier A, Frouin F, Kalifa C, Vanel D, Dipaola R (1992) Factor-analysis of dynamic magnetic-resonance-imaging in predicting the response of osteosarcoma to chemotherapy. Invest Radiol 27:847–855
17. Charpentier E et al (1990) Factor analysis processing of dynamic MRI: new method to assess osteosarcoma preoperative chemotherapy response (abstract). Radiology 177 [Suppl] p 221
18. Cova M, Kang YS, Tsukamoto H et al (1991) Bone-marrow perfusion evaluated with gadolinium-enhanced dynamic fast MR imaging in a dog-model. Radiology 179:535–539
19. Erlemann R, Reiser MF, Peters PE et al (1989) Musculoskeletal neoplasms – static and dynamic Gd-DTPA enhanced MR imaging. Radiology 171:767–773
20. Erlemann R, Sciuk J, Bosse A et al (1990) Response of osteosarcoma and Ewing sarcoma to preoperative chemotherapy – assessment with dynamic and static MR imaging and skeletal scintigraphy. Radiology 175:791–796
21. Fletcher BD, Hanna SL, Fairclough DL, Gronemeyer SA (1992) Pediatric musculoskeletal tumors – use of dynamic contrast-enhanced MR imaging to monitor response to chemotherapy. Radiology 184:243–248
22. Hanna SL, Fletcher BD, Fairclough DL, Le A (1990) Use of dynamic Gd-DTPA enhanced MRI in musculoskeletal malignancies (abstract). Proceedings of Society of Magnetic Resonance Imaging, p 9
23. Lang P, Stevens M, Vahlensieck M (1991) Rheumatoid arthritis of the hand and wrist: evaluation of soft-tissue inflammation and quantification of inflammatory activity using unenhanced and dynamic Gd-DTPA enhanced MRI (abstract). Proceedings of Society of Magnetic Resonance in Medicine p 66
24. Mirowitz SA Totty WG, Lee JKT (1990) Evaluation of musculoskeletal masses with dynamic Gd-DTPA enhanced rapid-acquisition spin-echo imaging (abstract). Radiology 177[Suppl] p 221
25. Mirowitz SA, Totty WG, Lee JKT (1992) Characterization of musculoskeletal masses using dynamic Gd-DTPA enhanced spin-echo MRI. J Comput Assist Tomogr 16:120–125
26. Reiser MF, Bongartz GP, Erlemann R et al (1989) Gadolinium-DTPA in rheumatoid-arthritis and related diseases – first results with dynamic magnetic-resonance imaging. Skeletal Radiol 18:591–597
27. Sugimoto H, Miyaji N, Ohsawa T (1994) Carpal-tunnel syndrome – evaluation of median nerve circulation with dynamic contrast-enhanced MR-imaging. Radiology 190:459–466
28. Tsukamoto H, Kang YS, Jones LC et al (1992) Evaluation of marrow perfusion in the femoral-head by dynamic magnetic-resonance-imaging – effect of venous occlusion in a dog-model. Invest Radiol 27:275–281

29. Vanel D et al (1993) Dynamic contrast-enhanced subtraction MRI in follow-up of aggressive soft-tissue tumors: a prospective study of 74 patients (abstract). Radiology 189 [Suppl] p 205

30. Vanel D, Shapeero LG, Debaere T et al (1994) MR-imaging in the follow-up of malignant and aggressive soft-tissue tumors – results of 511 examinations. Radiology 190:263–268

31. Verstraete K (1994) Dynamic contrast-enhanced MRI of tumor and tumor-like lesions of the musculoskeletal system, pp 63–185. Thesis, University of Gent, Gent, Belgium

32. Verstraete KL, Dierick A, De Deene Y et al (1993) First-pass images of musculoskeletal lesions: a new and useful diagnostic application of dynamic contrast-enhanced MRI. Proceedings of Society of Magnetic Resonance Imaging, p 869

33. Verstraete KL, Dierick A, Dedeene Y et al (1994) First-pass images of musculoskeletal lesions – a new and useful diagnostic application of dynamic contrast-enhanced mri. Magn Reson Imaging 12:687–702

34. Verstraete KL, Vanzieleghem B, De Deene Y et al (1995) Static, dynamic and first-pass MRI of musculoskeletal lesions using gadodiamide injection. Acta Radiol 36:27–36

35. Chien D, Edelman RR (1991) Ultrafast imaging using gradient echos. Magn Reson Q 7:31–56

36. Haase A, Matthaei D, Bartkowski R, Duhmke E, Leibfritz D (1989) Inversion Recovery Snapshot Flash Mr Imaging. J Comput Assist Tomogr 13:1036–1040

37. Haase A (1990) Snapshot FLASH MRI – applications to T1, T2, and chemical-shift imaging. Magn Reson Med 13:77–89

38. Van der Woude H et al (1995) Double slice dynamic contrast-enhanced subtraction MR images in 60 patients with musculoskeletal tumors or tumor-like lesions (abstract). Eur Radiol [Suppl 5] 181

39. Vanderwoude HJ, Bloem JL, Verstraete KL, Taminiau AHM, Nooy MA, Hogendoorn PCW (1995) Osteosarcoma and Ewings-sarcoma after neoadjuvant chemotherapy – value of dynamic MR-imaging in detecting viable tumor before surgery. Am J Roentgenol 165:593–598

40. Verstraete KL, Lang P (2000) Bone and soft tissue tumors: the role of contrast agents for MRI. Eur J Radiol 34:229–246

41. Rijswijk CS van, Geirnaerdt MJ, Hogendoorn PC et al (2004) Soft-tissue tumors: value of static and dynamic gadopentetate dimeglumine-enhanced MRI in prediction of malignancy. Radiology 233:493–502

42. Shapeero LG, Henry-Amar M, Vanel D (1992) Response of osteosarcoma and Ewing sarcoma to preoperative chemotherapy: assessment with dynamic and static MRI and skeletal scintigraphy. Invest Radiol 27:989–991

43. Kashanian FK, Goldstein HA, Blumetti RF, Holyoak WL, Hugo FP, Dolker M (1990) Rapid bolus injection of gadopentetate dimeglumine: absence of side effects in normal volunteers. AJNR Am J Neuroradiol 11:853–856

44. Chambers TP, Baron RL, Lush RM, Dodd GD, Miller WJ, Confer SR (1993) Hepatic CT enhancement – a method to demonstrate reproducibility. Radiology 188:627–631

45. Chambers TP, Baron RL, Lush RM (1994) Hepatic CT enhancement. 1. Alterations in the volume of contrast material within the same patients. Radiology 193:513–517

46. Chambers TP, Baron RL, Lush RM (1994) Hepatic CT enhancement. 2. Alterations in contrast material volume and rate of injection within the same patients. Radiology 193:518–522

47. Vanderwoude HJ, Bloem JL, Schipper J et al (1994) Changes in tumor perfusion induced by chemotherapy in bone sarcomas – color Doppler flow imaging compared with contrast-enhanced MR-imaging and 3-phase bone-scintigraphy. Radiology 191:421–431

48. Vaupel P, Kallinowski F, Okunieff P (1989) Blood-flow, oxygen and nutrient supply, and metabolic microenvironment of human-tumors – a review. Cancer Research 49:6449–6465

49. Reddick WE, Langston JW, Meyer WH et al (1994) Discrete signal-processing of dynamic contrast-enhanced MR-imaging – statistical validation and preliminary clinical-application. J Magn Reson Imaging 4:397–404

50. Lang P, Honda G, Roberts T et al (1995) Musculoskeletal neoplasm: perineoplastic edema versus tumor on dynamic post-contrast MR images with spatial mapping of instantaneous enhancement rates. Radiology 197:831–839

51. Erlemann R (1993) Dynamic gadolinium-enhanced MR imaging to monitor tumor response to chemotherapy. Radiology 186:904

52. Lawrence JA, Babyn PS, Chan HSL, Thorner PS, Pron GE, Krajbich IJ (1993) Extremity osteosarcoma in childhood – prognostic value of radiologic imaging. Radiology 189:43–47

53. Glasser DB, Lane JM, Huvos AG, Marcove RC, Rosen G (1992) Survival, prognosis, and therapeutic response in osteogenic-sarcoma – the Memorial Hospital Experience. Cancer 69:698–708

54. Hudson M, Jaffe MR, Jaffe N et al (1990) Pediatric osteosarcoma – therapeutic strategies, results, and prognostic factors derived from a 10-year experience. J Clin Oncol 8:1988–1997

55. Meyers PA, Heller G, Healey J et al (1992) Chemotherapy for nonmetastatic osteogenic-sarcoma – the Memorial Sloan-Kettering experience. J Clin Oncol 10:5–15

56. Oberlin O, Patte C, Demeocq F et al (1985) The response to initial chemotherapy as a prognostic factor in localized Ewing sarcoma. Eur J Cancer Clin Oncol 21:463–467

57. Rosen G, Caparros B, Huvos AG et al (1982) Preoperative chemotherapy for osteogenic-sarcoma – selection of postoperative adjuvant chemotherapy based on the response of the primary tumor to preoperative chemotherapy. Cancer 49: 1221–1230

58. Winkler K, Beron G, Delling G et al (1988) Neoadjuvant chemotherapy of osteo-sarcoma – results of a randomized cooperative trial (Coss-82) with salvage chemotherapy based on histological tumor response. J Clin Oncol 6:329–337

59. Raymond AK, Chawla SP, Carrasco CH et al (1987) Osteosarcoma chemotherapy effect – a prognostic factor. Semin Diagn Pathol 4:212–236

60. Erlemann R, Sciuk J, Wuisman P et al (1992) Dynamic MR tomography in diagnosis of inflammatory and tumorous space-occupying growths of the musculoskeletal system. Rofo Fortschr Geb Rontgenstr Neuen Bildgeb Verfahr 156:353–359

61. Fletcher B, Hanna S (1989) Musculoskeletal neoplasms: dynamic Gd-DTPA-enhanced MRI (letter). Radiology 177:287–288

62. Carrasco CH, Charnsangavej C, Raymond AK et al (1989) Osteo-sarcoma – angiographic assessment of response to preoperative chemotherapy. Radiology 170:839–842

63. Chuang VP, Benjamin R, Jaffe N et al (1982) Radiographic and angiographic changes in osteosarcoma after intraarterial chemotherapy. AJR Am J Roentgenol 139:1065–1069

64. Knop J, Delling G, Heise U, Winkler K (1990) Scintigraphic evaluation of tumor-regression during preoperative chemotherapy of osteosarcoma – correlation of Tc-99m-methylene diphosphonate parametric imaging with surgical histopathology. Skeletal Radiol 19:165–172

65. Kumpan W, Lechner G, Wittich GR et al (1986) The angiographic response of osteosarcoma following pre-operative chemotherapy. Skeletal Radiol 15:96–102

66. Biondetti PR, Ehman RL (1992) Soft-tissue sarcomas: use of textural patterns in skeletal muscle as a diagnostic feature in postoperative MRI. Radiology 183:845–848

67. Bloem JL, Reiser MF, Vanel D (1990) Magnetic resonance contrast agents in the evaluation of the musculoskeletal system. Magn Reson Q 6:136–163

68. Maas R (1992) Radiological-diagnosis of recurrent soft-tissue sarcoma. Radiologe 32:597–605

69. Reuther G, Mutschler W (1990) Detection of local recurrent disease in musculoskeletal tumors – magnetic-resonance-imaging versus computed-tomography. Skeletal Radiol 19:85–90

70. Vanel D, Lacombe MJ, Couanet D, Kalifa C, Spielmann M, Genin J (1987) Musculoskeletal tumors – follow-up with MR imaging after treatment with surgery and radiation-therapy. Radiology 164:243–245

Cytogenetics and Molecular Genetics of Soft Tissue Tumors and Bone Tumors

7

A.A. Sandberg

Contents

7.1 Introduction

This chapter presents the genetic changes (cytogenetic and molecular) in bone tumors and soft tissue tumors applicable to fuller understanding and evaluation of their in the clinical setting. Thus, in keeping with the aims and nature of this volume, the genetic changes are addressed primarily to radiologists, but also to orthopedists, oncologists, and surgeons.

The genetic changes in tumors can be established by a number of methodologies: cytogenetics, fluorescence in situ hybridization (FISH), and molecular approaches [1, 2]. Chromosomal (karyotypic, cytogenetic) changes in human tumors are confined to the involved tissues and cells and are not reflected in other somatic cells, e.g., blood cells. The establishment of chromosomal changes in a tumor requires fresh (not fixed) tissue; following short-term culture, dividing cells can be examined in late prophase or metaphase, when the chromosomes are morphologically well defined and readily recognized. These chromosomal changes may be either numerical (gain or loss or chromosomes) or structural (morphological; Fig. 7.4).

Since space limitations for this chapter preclude detailed presentations of cytogenetic terminology (Figs. 7.1–7.4) and of the genetics of soft tissue and bone tumors, proportionally more space has been given to pictorial presentations (Figs. 1–10). The salient cytogenetic changes in these tumors are listed in Tables 1 and 2, accompanied by short discussions of particular tumors.

Human tumors are primarily caused by anomalies affecting two types of genes: (1) Dominantly acting oncogenes, whose protein products serve to accelerate cell growth and whose functions are altered by increased gene dosage (amplification) or by activating mutations or participation in fusion genes, resulting from chromosomal translocations, inversions, or insertions; and (2) tumor-suppressor genes (TSG), whose products normally serve as brakes on cell growth and runaway cell proliferation and whose inactivation leads to uncontrolled cell proliferation and downregulation of apoptosis (programmed cell death). Such inactivation is typically altered by physical elimination of TSG or by inactivating mutations (Fig. 7.7).

The recurrent and specific translocations in many soft tissue and bone tumors are unique in that they are diagnostic of the tumor and usually affect the oncogenes that have been identified in almost all of these conditions (Table 7.1). The translocations lead to the genesis of abnormal fusion genes of varying parts of the oncogenes involved and result in the mutation and/or overexpression of components of the fused genes.

The occurrence of specific chromosome changes in benign tumors (e.g., lipoma, leiomyoma; Table 7.2), i.e., translocations, as well as nonspecific changes in a number of others, bears witness to the role of genetic events in cellular proliferation but without malignant aspects. In

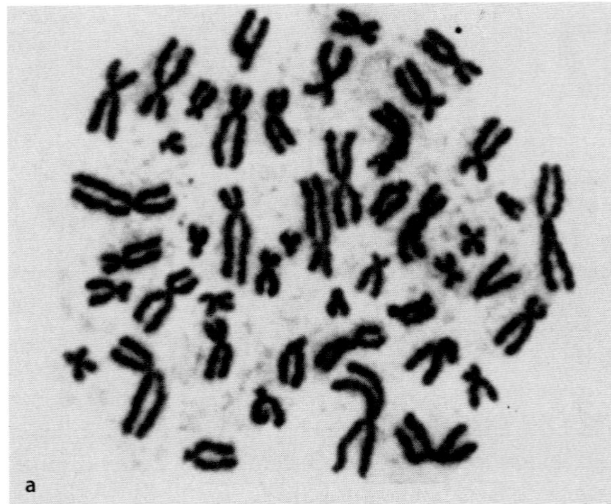

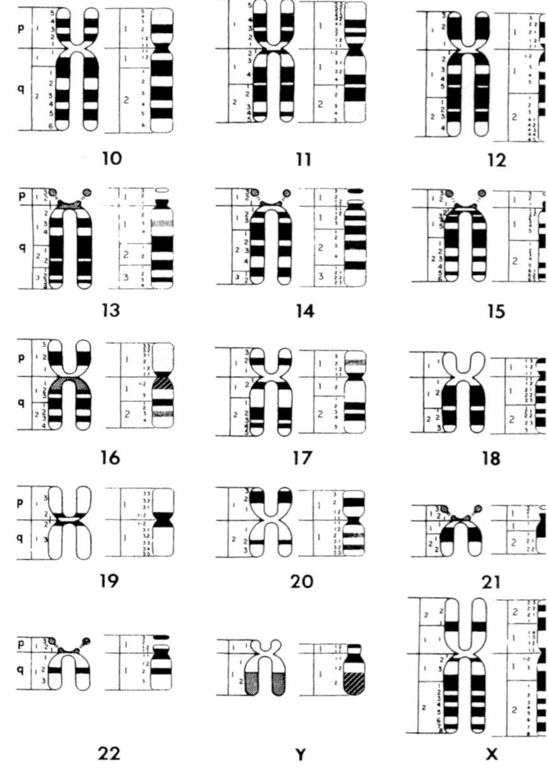

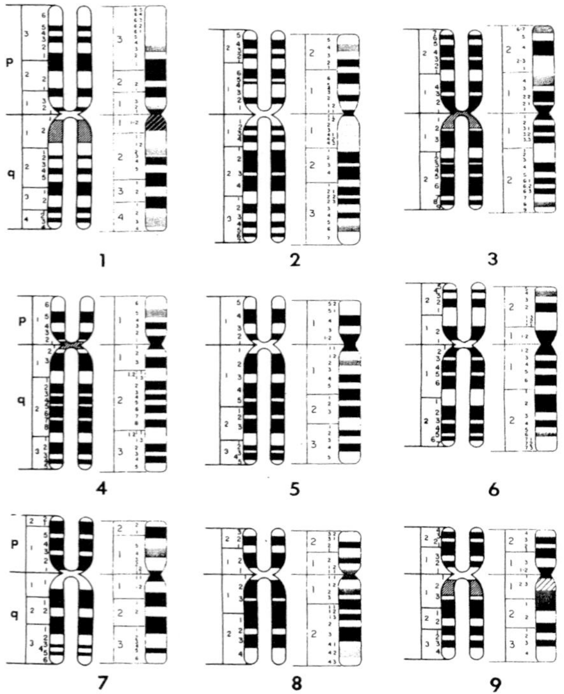

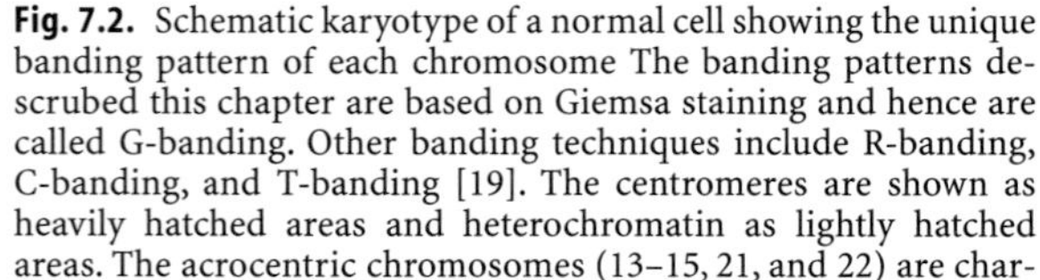

Fig. 7.1 a, b. Metaphase spread (**a**) consisting of 46 unbanded chromosomes (22 pairs of somatic chromosomes or autosomes and 1 pair of sex chromosomes, XY in males and XX in females). The variations in chromosome length, location of the centromere (structures holding the two chromatids together prior to cell division into daughter cells), and particularly the banding pattern of the chromosomes (see Fig. 7.2) are used to arrange and identify individual chromosomes (**b**). The normal set of the 46 chromo- somes is called diploid. Cells with less than 46 chromosomes are hypodiploid and those with a higher number than 46 are hyper- diploid. Cells with 69 or 92 chromosomes are triploid and tetraploid, respectively. Cells with the above numbers of chromo- somes but with numerical or structural anomalies are labeled pseudodiploid, etc. **b** Shown is a karyotype of a normal male cell, containing 22 pairs of autosomes and one set of sex chromosomes (XY)

Fig. 7.2. Schematic karyotype of a normal cell showing the unique banding pattern of each chromosome The banding patterns de- scrubed this chapter are based on Giemsa staining and hence are called G-banding. Other banding techniques include R-banding, C-banding, and T-banding [19]. The centromeres are shown as heavily hatched areas and heterochromatin as lightly hatched areas. The acrocentric chromosomes (13–15, 21, and 22) are char- acterized by satellites. Chromosomes with the centromeres located centrally are called metacentric, those with the centromere away from the center are called submetacentric, and those with the cen- tromeres at the end are called telocentric or acrocentric. For fur- ther information and details regarding cytogenetic terms, nota- tions, definitions, etc., the reader should consult ISCN 1995 [19]

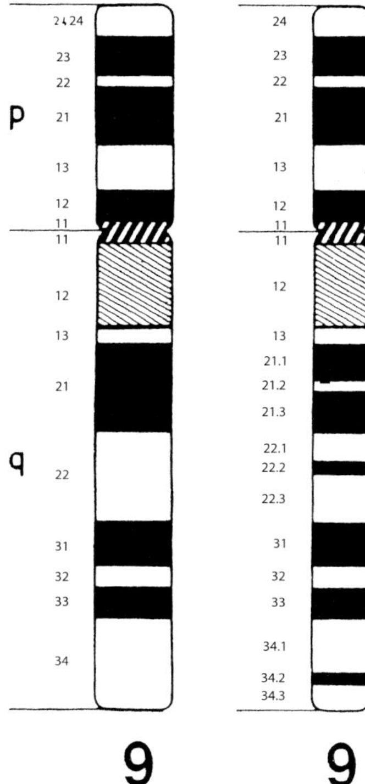

Fig. 7.3. For a full appreciation of the chromosome changes in tumors, one must understand the nomenclature used to describe normal and abnormal chromosomes. The nomenclature for banded chromosomes is based on a system in which each chromosome (chromosome 9 is used as an example here) is divided in relation to the centromere (*heavily hatched area*) into its *upper* (usually short) *arm* labeled *p* and *lower* (usually long) *arm* labeled *q*. Each arm is divided into regions: in chromosome 9 into two regions in the p arm and into three regions in the q arm. The bands are then assigned to each region, the numbering system consisting of the region and then band number . Thus, for example, 9q23 refers to band number 3 on chromosome 9 in region 2. In the higher-resolution system, the sub-band number is shown following a period. A band overlapping two regions is assigned to the more distal region. The centromere per se is designated as 10. The total set of chromosomes contains about 400 bands (chromosome 9 on the *left*) demonstrated with usual banding techniques; more refined banding increases the number to 550, so that sub-bands can be visualized, as shown with the chromosome 9 on the *right* [19]

fact, the specific chromosome alterations in benign tumors not only serve diagnostic purposes, but also serve as a means of differentiating them from their malignant counterparts (e.g., liposarcomas, leiomyosarcoma).

Some of the genes (particularly TSG) affected in malignant tumors may be involved in the genesis of benign tumors. In fact, the same genes can be altered in a number of different tumors, but apparently at varying

chronologies in tumor development and associated with different genetic changes and milieus (Fig. 7.10).

The preponderant number of human cancers, including tumors of the bones and soft tissues, are not characterized by specific translocations affecting oncogenes, but develop through a stepwise and orchestrated sequence of genetic events, primarily loss of heterozygosity (LOH) of TSG (Fig. 7.10). Some of these losses are evident as deletions of chromosomal material established microscopically, ranging from partial loss of a band to loss of the whole arm of a chromosome or a whole chromosome. Other LOH changes are submicroscopic.

Advantage has been taken of the composition and structure of fusion genes by tailoring therapies affecting the function of these genes, e.g., blocking of expression of the mutated tyrosine kinase present in the fusion gene of chronic myelocytic leukemia and in the mutated *KIT* gene in gastrointestinal stromal tumors (GIST). The uniqueness of such therapy is reflected by the successful treatment of GIST with imatinib, which inhibits the tyrosine kinase of *KIT*, but only if the mutation occurs at exon 11 and not, for example, at exon 17.

In many tumors specific translocations may be the only alterations; however, in a significant number of cases, additional karyotypic changes appear and are possibly responsible (or at least associated with) progression of the disease. This is also reflected by alterations in the expression of a number of genes (not evident microscopically and hence cytogenetically) aside from those involved in the translocation. The exact cause(s) for these alterations is not known, i.e., whether the translocation per se is responsible or the process leading to the translocation or other factors. In some of these conditions, e.g., Ewing-type tumors (Table 7.1), variant translocations may occur, but they always involve the *EWS* gene located on chromosome 22.

The genetic and molecular consequences of inversions and insertions, quite rare events in soft tissue tumors and bone tumors, are probably similar to those associated with translocations in that they lead to the genesis of fusion genes.

The specific translocations shown in Table 7.1 are diagnostic of the tumors in which they are found; they have not been observed in other tumor types and can be of crucial value in establishing the correct diagnosis in confusing cases. As mentioned above, fresh tumor tissue is required for cytogenetic analysis and, hence, both the surgeon and pathologist must be alert to the possibility of a tumor requiring cytogenetic analysis and obtain appropriate tissue for such an analysis. Such an alert could originate with the radiologist (see Things to remember).

Having failed to obtain fresh tissue for cytogenetic analysis, the presence of specific translocations can be established by several interphase FISH techniques, par-

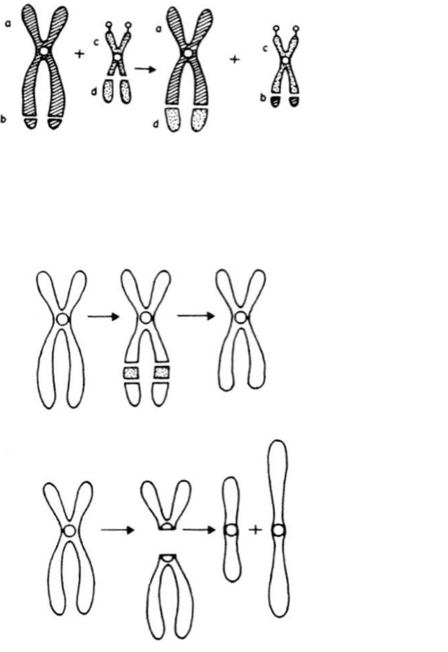

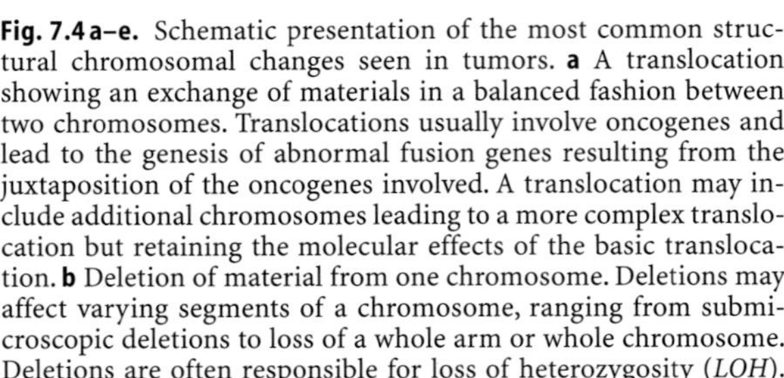

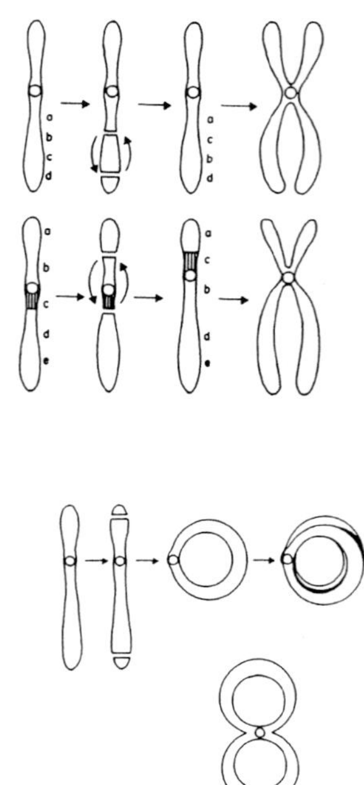

Fig. 7.4 a–e. Schematic presentation of the most common structural chromosomal changes seen in tumors. **a** A translocation showing an exchange of materials in a balanced fashion between two chromosomes. Translocations usually involve oncogenes and lead to the genesis of abnormal fusion genes resulting from the juxtaposition of the oncogenes involved. A translocation may include additional chromosomes leading to a more complex translocation but retaining the molecular effects of the basic translocation. **b** Deletion of material from one chromosome. Deletions may affect varying segments of a chromosome, ranging from submicroscopic deletions to loss of a whole arm or whole chromosome. Deletions are often responsible for loss of heterozygosity (*LOH*).

c Formation of isochromosomes consisting of two identical arms. Thus, i(17q) would describe an isochromosome of the long arm of chromosome 17. **d** Paracentric inversions (*top*) do not involve the centromere, e.g., inv(3)(q21q26); pericentric inversion (*bottom*) include the centromere, e.g., inv(3)(p13q21). Note that, in contrast to the notation of translocations, no semicolons are placed between the two breakpoints in inversions. As in translocations, inversions may result in fusion genes resulting from the juxtaposition of parts of genes. **e** Ring chromosomes. Though shown as originating from one chromosome, rings may contain material from a number of chromosomes. A r(12) would describe a ring chromosome originating from chromosome 12

ticularly with cosmid probes, which can be applied to frozen or archival tissues. In fact, results have been obtained in fixed specimens a number of years old.

The presence of translocations may also be ascertained by molecular analysis (usually reverse transcriptase polymerase chain reaction, RT-PCR), based on messenger ribonucleic acid (mRNA) or deoxyribonucleic acid (DNA) extracted from fresh or archival tissues and in which the products of fusion genes can be identified. This approach may also detect varying transcripts of such fusion genes.

Examples of genetic changes not reflected in recognizable cytogenetic anomalies but determinable with molecular techniques or FISH are the *KIT* mutation in GIST, amplification of *HER2/neu* in breast cancer, and *NMYC* in neuroblastoma.

The genetic findings in Ewing tumors based on a number of techniques (Figs. 7.5 and 7.6) are examples of the approaches available in the diagnosis of the tumors associated with specific translocations shown in Table 7.1. The translocation t(11;12)(q24;q12) in Ewing sarcoma and related tumors leads to the genesis of an abnormal fusion gene containing elements of the *EWS*

and *FUL* genes involved by the breaks in the t(11;12). However, the products of this translocation show variability in the breaks in these genes occurring at different exons (but still in the chromosomal bands indicated), leading to variable transcripts. The clinical consequences of such variability is the demonstration that patients with tumors with type 1 transcript do much better than those with type 2. Though as many as 18 different transcripts have been identified as a result of the *EWS-FUL* fusion gene, insufficient numbers of cases with the other fusion products have been examined and hence clinical significance of these varying transcripts is unknown.

The appearance of chromosomal changes, numerical and/or structural, in addition to the translocations seen in bone tumors and soft tissue tumors is usually associated with biological progression, manifested by invasion and metastases. These additional changes are usually variable from tumor to tumor, even those with the same diagnosis. With or without additional chromosome changes, tumors with specific translocations may show a variety of anomalies at the molecular level which may involve a number of genes.

Fig. 7.5 a–c. The cytogenetic changes in Ewing sarcomas will be presented as examples for the range of genetic tests available in diagnosing certain tumors. **a** A translocation, t(11;22)(q24;q12), seen in most Ewing tumors and involving the oncogenes *EWSR1* on 22q12 and *FLI1* on 11q24. The notation for translocations consists of two sets of parentheses: the first shows the chromosomes involved, and the second, the breakpoints. As shown here for Ewing tumors and based on the ISCN guidelines, e.g., in the notation t(11;12)(q24;q12), t indicates a translocation with involvement of chromosomes 11 and 12 shown in the first set of parentheses and the breakpoints on chromosome 11 at q24 and on chromosome 12 at q12 in the second set of parantheses. All the translocations shown in Table 7.1 follow this notation. The resulting fusion chromosome shown in **b**, i.e., *EWSR1/FLI1*, and its protein products are probably responsible for the genesis of Ewing tumors. An "alternative splice" area is shown in the *EWSR1* gene associated with variability in the breakpoints and leading to the genesis of fusion products of varying nature and of clinical significance regarding tumor aggressiveness. **c** A karyotype (containing 50 chromosomes) of a Ewing tumor with the t(11;22) (*horizontal arrows*). Four extra chromosomes are indicated by *vertical arrows*. The presence of chromosomes (normal and/or abnormal) in addition to the translocation is usually associated with more aggressive tumors [20, 21]

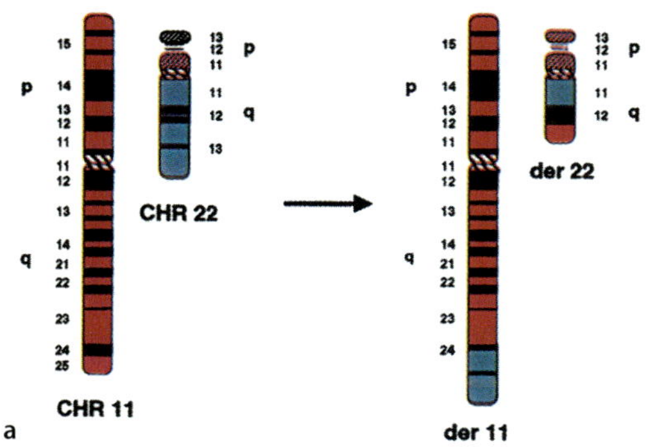

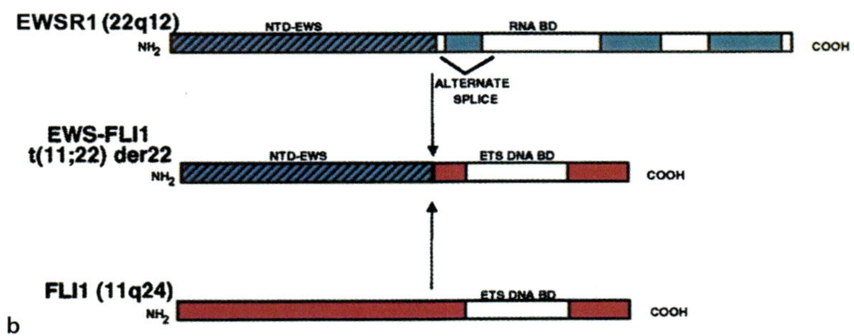

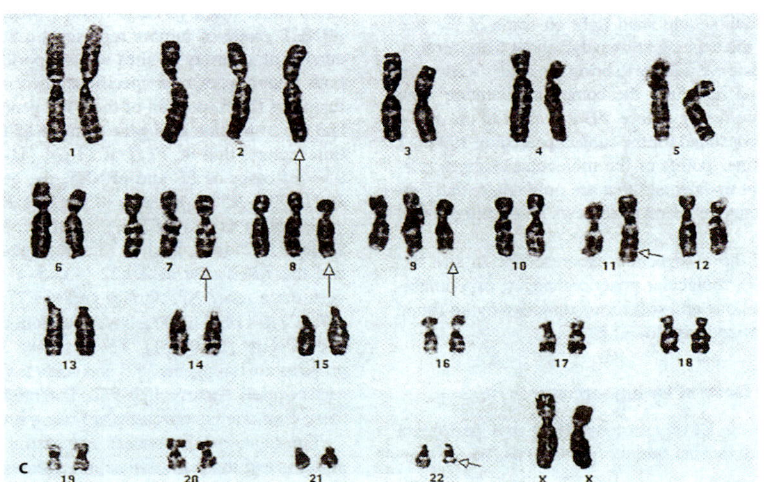

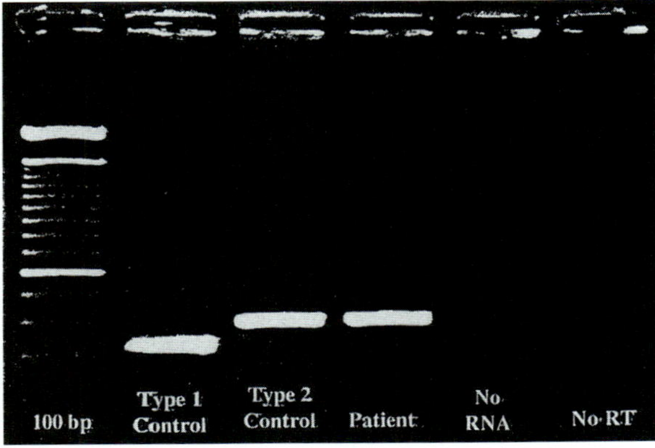

Fig. 7.6. Results obtained with reverse transcriptase polymerase chain reaction (RT-PCR) on the DNA of Ewing tumors. The difference in the mobility of type 1 and type 2 tumors is due to the differences (mentioned in Fig 7.5) in the breakpoint in the *EWSR1* gene. Patients with type 1 have a more favorable prognosis than those with other types of translocation breaks. Note that the patient tested here had the unfavorable type 2 results [21]

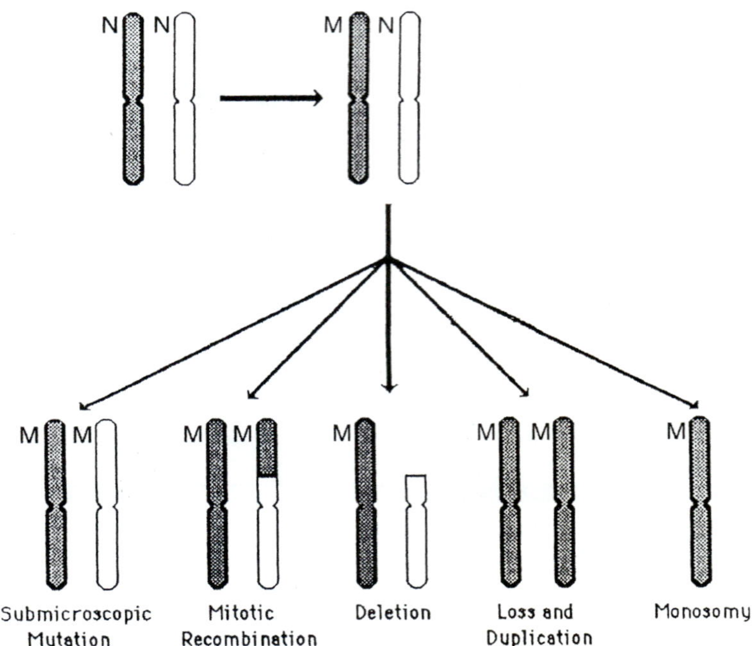

Fig. 7.7. Schematic presentation of loss of heterozygosity (*LOH*) often affecting tumor suppressor genes and responsible for the genesis of most human tumors. *M*, a mutated normal gene; *N*, a normal gene. The various mechanisms responsible for LOH are shown: submicroscopic mutation and chromosomal deletion are the two most common mechanisms

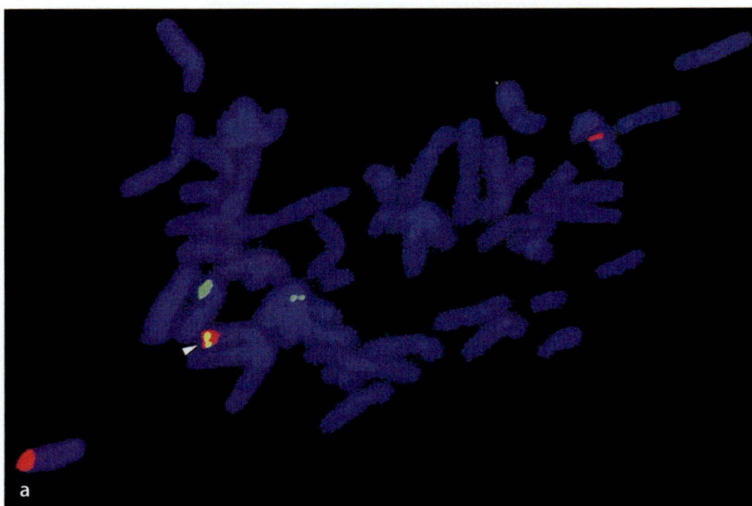

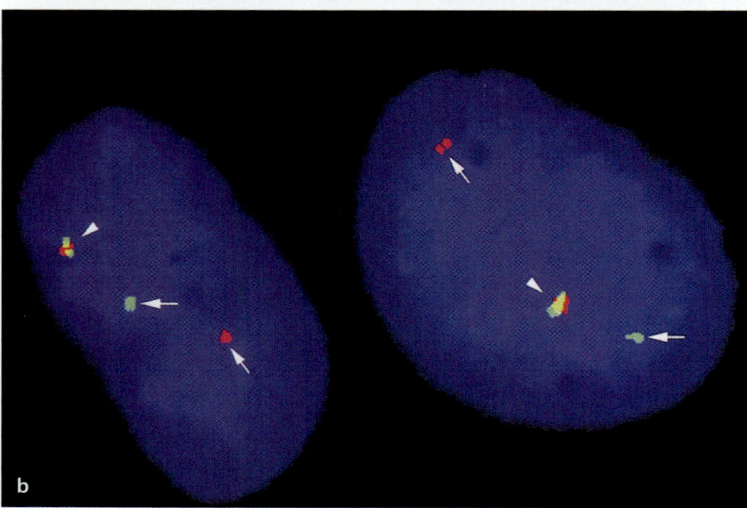

Fig. 7.8 a, b. An example of the use of FISH with cosmid probes in a metaphase (**a**) and two interphase nuclei (**b**) for ascertaining a translocation. The green probe includes one gene and the red probe another gene. *Arrowheads* point to the fusion gene. The findings in **B** show the feasibility of ascertaining translocations in interphase nuclei, such as in archival tissues [22]

7.2 Soft Tissue Tumors and Bone Tumors with Specific and Diagnostic Translocations

Emphasis is put on those tumors for which the cytogenetic and/or molecular changes are diagnostic (Table 7.1); though the changes shown in Table 7.2 may not be specific in most of these tumors, these can be of diagnostic help in confusing and complicated cases [2].

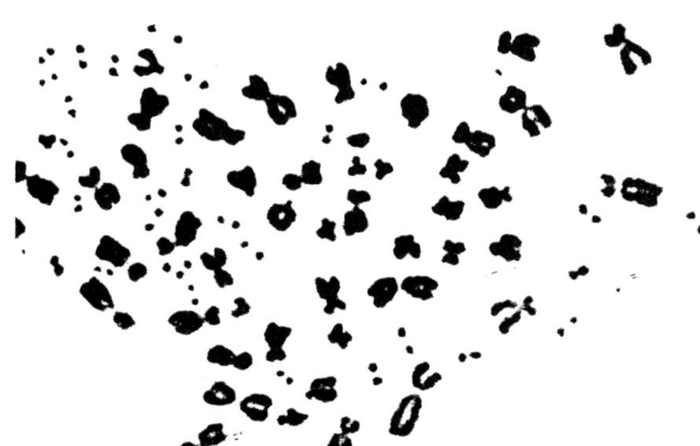

Fig. 7.9. Metaphase of a tumor cell containing double minutes (dms), a finding usually associated with gene amplification and a poor prognosis, e.g., in neuroblastoma

7.2.1 Synovial Sarcoma

Histologically, synovial sarcoma (SS) can be either monophasic (containing preponderantly spindle cells) or biphasic (containing both spindle cell and epithelial elements), and the molecular findings seen in SS bear a distinct relationship to the tumor histology [3]. A specific and diagnostic translocation in SS consists of t(X;18)(p11.2;q11.2) (Table 7.1), seen in almost all of these tumors. An oncogene at 18q11.2 (*SS18*) is either fused to the *SSX1* or to its neighboring *SSX2* gene. Cytogenetically, it is not possible to distinguish *SS18-SSX1* from *SS18-SSX2*; however, these fusions can be demonstrated with either FISH or RT-PCR.

SS with the *SS18-SSX1* are invariably biphasic, whereas SS with *SS18-SSX2* can be either biphasic or monophasic and have a longer metastasis-free survival than patients with the *SS18-SSX1* fusion gene.

The t(X;18)(p11.2;q11.2) translocation is unique to SS and serves to differentiate it from confusing tumors such as hemangiopericytoma, mesothelioma, leiomyosarcoma, or malignant peripheral nerve sheath tumors.

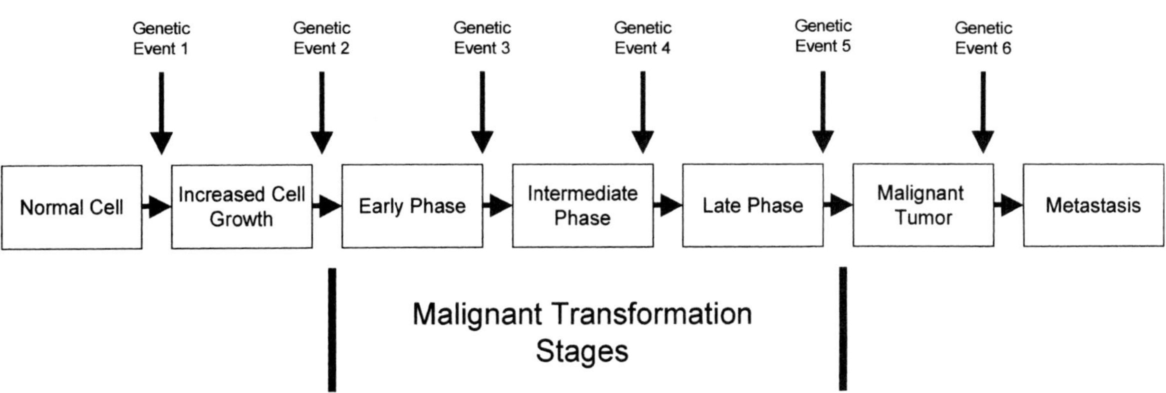

Fig. 7.10. Stepwise process of genetic changes leading to full tumor development. Thus, an initial genetic change affects cell proliferation, followed by further stepwise changes which lead to neoplastic transformation and ultimately to an aggressive tumor. This process probably accounts for the bulk of tumors, particularly cancers of epithelial origin. Most of the genetic changes consist of LOH (Fig. 7.7), often through chromosomal deletions seen microscopically, but may also consist of translocations and mutations of varying origin as well as of altered expression of some genes. The same genes may be involved in different types of tumors. For examples, the step at which the *p53* gene is involved may be genetic event 2 in one type of tumor and genetic event 5 in another type. Furthermore, in one tumor the *p53* may be overexpressed, whereas in another it may be underexpressed or totally silent. This process of involvement of multiple genes in an orchestrated and progressive succession is quite different from the process of fusion genes resulting from a translocation and apparently sufficient by itself to cause tumor development

Table 7.1. Specific chromosomal translocations established cytogenetically and the corresponding gene changes in bone and soft tissue tumors

Tumors	Translocation	Gene changes
Aggressive angiomyxoma	t(8;12)(p12;q15)	*HMGA2*
Alveolar rhabdomyosarcoma	t(2;13)(q35;q14) t(1;13)(p36;q14)	*PAX3-FOXO1A* *PAX7-FOXO1A*
Alveolar soft part sarcoma	t(X;17)(p11.2;q25)	*ASPSCR1-TFE3*
Aneurysmal bone cyst	t(16;17)(q22;p13)	*CDH11-DUSP6*
Angiomatoid fibrous histiocytoma[a]	t(12;16)(q13;p11)	*FUS-ATF1*
Clear cell sarcoma (malignant melanoma of soft parts)	t(12;22)(q13;q12)	*ATF1-EWSR1*
Congenital fibrosarcoma and mesoblastic nephroma	t(12;15)(p13;q25)	*ETV6-NTRK3*
Dermatofibrosarcoma protuberans (giant cell fibroblastoma)	t(17;22)(q22;q13)	*COL1A1-PDGFB*
Desmoplastic round cell tumor	t(11;22)(p13;q12)	*WT1-EWSR1*
Endometrial stromal sarcoma	t(7;17)(p15;q21) t(10;17)(q22;p13)	*JAZF1-SUZ12*
Ewing tumor and peripheral primitive neuroectodermal tumors	t(11;22)(q24;q12) t(21;22)(q22;q12) t(7;22)(p22;q12) t(17;22)(q12;q12) t(2;22)(q33;q12)	*EWSR1-FLI1* *EWSR1-ERG* *EWSR1-ETV1* *EWSR1-ETV4* *FEV-EWSR1*
Hemangioendothelioma, epithelioid[a]	t(1;3)(p36.3;q25)	
Hemangiopericytoma[a]	t(12;19)(q13;q13)	
Inflammatory myofibroblastic tumor	t(2;19)(p23;p13.1) t(1;2)(q22–23;p23)	*ALK-TPM4* *TPM3-ALK*
Low-grade fibromyxoid sarcoma	t(7;16)(q34;p11)	*CREB3L2-FUS*
Myxoid chondrosarcoma, extraskeletal	t(9;22)(q22;q12) t(9;17)(q22;q11) t(9;15)(q22;q21)	*EWSR1-NR4A3* *TAF15-NR4A3* *TEC-TCF12*
Myxoid liposarcoma	t(12;16)(q13;p11) t(12;22)(q13;q12)	*FUS-DDIT3* *EWSR1-DDIT3*
Synovial sarcoma	t(X;18)(p11;q11)	*SS18-SSX1* *SS18-SSX2*

[a] Small number of cases analyzed

7.2.2 Liposarcoma

Liposarcoma (LPS) is characterized by cytogenetic anomalies unique to each histological type [4]. Myxoid or round cell LPS is associated with a recurrent and diagnostic chromosomal change consisting of t(12;16) (q13;p11.2) and much less frequently t(12;22)(q13;q12). The t(12;16) translocation results in the fusion of the *DDIT3* gene at 12q13 to the *FUS* gene at 16p11.2. In t(12;22) the *DDIT3* gene is fused with the *EWSR1* gene. These translocations are retained in myxoid LPS acquiring round-cell features. The translocations just described have not been found in any other types of LPS or in other types of myxoid tumors.

Well-differentiated LPS are characterized by large to giant marker and/or ring chromosomes [4], which are usually comprised of chromosome 12 material, as well as that from several other chromosomes. The abnormal chromosomes in well-differentiated LPS contain various amplified genes which are retained when these LPS progress to the much more aggressive dedifferentiated LPS.

Lipomas, tumor types which may on occasion present diagnostic dilemmas in differentiating from LPS, are associated with several distinct cytogenetic profiles. A significant proportion of lipomas show involvement of 12q14-q15, often as translocations with one of the other chromosomes [5]. These translocations involve the *HMGA2* gene, resulting in fusion genes. Another group of lipomas is associated with rearrangements of the short arm of chromosome 6 or deletion of the long arm of chromosome 13. Lipomas with deletions of the long arm of chromosome 16, often accompanied by deletions of the long arm of chromosome 13, often have a spindle-cell or pleomorphic histology.

Lipoblastomas contain translocations involving the long arm of chromosome 8 at bands 8q11–12, leading to rearrangement of the *PLAG1* oncogene. Hibernomas, consisting of brown fat, usually have rearrangements of the long arm of chromosome 11. Angiolipomas usually have normal karyotypes.

Table 7.2. Recurrent but not specific chromosome changes in soft tissue tumors and bone tumors

Tumors	Chromosome changes	Molecular findings
Atypical fibroxanthomas		*TP53* mutations (due to UV radiation?)
Cardiac myxoma	12p12 rearrangements; telomeric association	
Chondromatous, synovial	Chromosome 6 and 1p abnormalities	
Chondromyxoid fibroma	del(6q)	
Collagenous fibroma (desmoplastic fibroblastoma)		11q12 involvement
Elastofibroma	1p rearrangements	
Fibroma of tendon sheath	11q12 involvement	
Gastrointestinal stromal tumor	del(1p), –14, –22	*KIT* mutations
Giant cell tumor of bone	Telomere association	
Giant cell tumor of tendon sheath		Cathepsins B and K expressed
Hamartoma		
Pulmonary	12q14-q15 rearrangements	
	6p21	*HMGA1* rearrangement
	t(6;14)(p21;q23-q24)	*RAD51L1* involvement
Hepatic	19q13.4 rearrangements	
Hibernoma	11q13 rearrangements	
Inflammatory myofibroblastic tumors	2p23 rearrangements	*ALK* fusion genes
Leiomyoma, extrauterine	del(1p)	
Uterine	t(12;14)(q15;q24) or del(7q)	*HMGA2* rearrangement
Leiomyosarcoma	del(1p)	
Lipoblastoma	8p12 rearrangement, polysomy 8	*PLAG1* oncogene changes
Lipoma	12q14-q15 rearrangements (often translocations with various chromosomes)	*HMGA2* rearrangement
Spindle cell or pleomorphic	del(13q) or del(16q)	
Chondroid	t(11;16)(q13;p12–13)	
Parosteal	12q14 rearrangements	
Malignant fibrous histiocytoma myxofibrosarcoma		r(12)
Malignant mesenchymoma	Ring markers containing amplified 1q21-q23 and 12q14-q15 sequences	
Mesothelioma	del(1p), del(9p)	*BCL10* inactivation, CDKN2A inactivation
Neurinoma	–22	
Neuroblastoma	Hyperdiploid, no del(1p)	*MYCN* amplification
Poor prognosis	del(1p), dms	
Neurofibroma	–22 and other changes	
Osteochondroma	del(8q)	*EXT1* inactivation
Osteosarcoma		
Low-grade	Ring chromosomes	
High-grade		*RB1* and *TP53* inactivation
Paraganglioma (nonfamilial)	–11	*SDHD* mutations
Pigmented villonodular synovitis	+5, +7	
Rhabdoid tumor	del(22q)	*SMARCB1* inactivation
Rhabdomyosarcoma, embryonal	+2q, +8, +20, LOH at 11p15	
Schwannoma, benign	del(22q)	*NF2* inactivation
Sclerosing epithelioid fibrosarcoma	Amplification of 12q13 and 12a15	
Sclerosing hemangioma of lung and other hemangiomas	Possible TSG at 5q	TTF1 expression

The notation del(1q) or any other chromosome arm means that the deletion may involve varying sections of the arms. Extra chromosomes are designated by the + sign, e.g., +5, and loss by a – sign, e.g., –22. The terms "rearrangements," "abnormalities," and "involvement" refer to a variety of chromosomal changes, which may include translocations, deletions, inversions, additional material on a chromosome, and other structural changes. Telomeric association results from the fusion of the telomere ends of two or more chromosomes

7.2.3 Ewing Tumors

Ewing sarcomas contain chromosome translocations involving the Ewing sarcoma gene (*EWSR1*), located at 22q12 with a number of partner genes (Table 7.1). The most common rearrangement is t(11;22)(q24;q12), which leads to the fusion of the *EWSR1* with the *FLI1* gene located at 11q24, i.e., the *EWSR1-FLI1* abnormal fusion gene, diagnostic of and probably responsible for Ewing sarcoma [6]. In the other types of translocations, other genes fuse with *EWSR1*; these belong to the *ETS* family of transcription factor genes (Table 7.1). The *EWSR1* gene is apparently essential to the development of Ewing tumors, with the varying partner genes playing roles which have not been clearly defined. When tumor material is not available for cytogenetic analysis, FISH studies using cosmid probes for *EWSR1* and partner genes, most often *FLI1*, or RT-PCR analysis readily establish the diagnosis of Ewing sarcoma. Clinical correlates with the various translocations seen in Ewing tumors have not been established. On the other hand, variability in the breakpoint location in the exons, particularly of the *EWSR1* gene, as determined by RT-PCR, may have a prognostic significance.

Askin tumor of the thoracopulmonary region has the same cytogenetic changes as those seen in Ewing sarcoma; esthesioneuroblastoma only rarely shows such changes.

7.2.4 Rhabdomyosarcoma

Cytogenetic findings have revealed specific and diagnostic translocations in alveolar rhabdomyosarcoma (RMS), t(2;13)(q35;q14) being the most common and t(1;13)(p36;q14) much less common [2]. The former translocation results in a fusion gene of the *FOXO1A* gene located at 13q14 and of the *PAX3* gene located at 2q35. The translocation t(1;13) results in a fusion gene involving the *PAX7* gene at 1p36 with the *FOXO1A* gene. The *PAX7-FOXO1A* fusion gene is often highly amplified, particularly in the form of double minutes (dms) (Fig. 7.9.).

Embryonal RMS lack specific translocations, but do have a recurrent cytogenetic profile, including extra copies of chromosomes 2, 8, and 20. The role of 11p deletions in embryonal RMS has not been clearly defined. Clinical or pathological correlates with these two types of diagnostic translocations in RMS have not been published.

7.2.5 Clear Cell Sarcoma (Malignant Melanoma of Soft Parts)

The bulk of clear cell sarcomas are associated with a diagnostic translocation, t(12;22)(q13;q12) [7]. Though clear cell sarcoma may resemble malignant melanoma phenotypically and histologically, the t(12;22) translocation has not been seen in malignant melanomas and serves as a means of differentiating these two entities. The t(12;22) translocation leads to the creation of a fusion gene consisting of *ATF1* located at 12q13 and the *EWSR1* located at 22q12, i.e., *ATF1-EWSR1*.

7.2.6 Desmoplastic Round-Cell Tumor

These tumors are usually found in intra-abdominal soft tissues and are quite aggressive in nature. Almost all cases are associated with a diagnostic translocation, t(11;22)(p13;q22) [8]. This results in the fusion gene *WT1-EWSR1*, which upregulates the expression of platelet-derived growth factor-α (PDGFA), the latter being an activator of mitogenic signaling pathways in fibroblasts.

7.2.7 Dermatofibrosarcoma Protuberans

Dermatofibrosarcoma protuberans (DFSP) and Bednar tumors may be characterized by a diagnostic translocation, t(17;22)(q23;q13), or by ring chromosome containing sequences of chromosomes 17 and 22 related to multiple copies of the fusion gene *COL1A1-PDGFB*, the former located at 17q22 and the latter at 22q13 [9]. The *COL1A1-PDGFB* fusion results in the overexpression of PDGFB (platelet-derived growth factor-β), which is a growth factor that activates platelet-derived growth factor-β receptor and platelet-derived growth factor receptor-α. The drug imatinib is an inhibitor of the PDGFB receptor and has been used successfully in the treatment of DFSP.

7.2.8 Congenital (Infantile) Fibrosarcoma and Mesoblastic Nephroma

These two tumors are characterized by the diagnostic translocation t(12;15)(p13;q25), which may be difficult to ascertain cytogenetically [10]. However, the fusion gene *ETV6-NTRK3* is readily determined by RT-PCR or FISH. Those tumors that do not contain the t(12;15) translocation may have trisomies of chromosomes 8, 11, 17, and 20.

7.2.9 Inflammatory Myofibroblastic Tumor

Some of these tumors are characterized by either a t(2;19)(p23;p13.1) or t(1;2)(q22–23;p23) translocation. The former results in the fusion gene *ALK-TPM4* and the latter in the fusion gene *TPM3-ALK*, where *ALK* is located at 2p23, *TPM4* at 19p13.1, and *TPM3* at 1q21–22. Cytogenetic or FISH analysis for *ALK* rearrangements is helpful in differentiating inflammatory myofibroblastic tumors from other similar spindle-cell proliferations [2].

7.2.10 Chondrosarcoma

Only extraskeletal myxoid chondrosarcoma (CS) is characterized by a diagnostic translocation, t(9;22) (q22;q12), including less common variants thereof, i.e., t(9;17)(q22;q11) and t(9;15)(q22;q21) [11]. Since extraskeletal myxoid CS, often occurring in the deep tissues of the extremities, particularly the musculature of the thigh and popliteal fossa, is not associated with a distinctive radiographic picture to separate it from other types of soft tissue tumors, the chromosome changes mentioned above may be of diagnostic help. The t(9;22) translocation results in the fusion of the *EWSR1* gene located at 22q12 and the *NR4A3* gene located at 9q22. The t(9;22) translocation and the variants mentioned above can be ascertained in extraskeletal myxoid CS by cytogenetics or FISH and spectrokaryotyping (SKY) and the products of the fusion gene by RT-PCR. In other types of CS there is considerable heterogeneity in the cytogenetic findings, ranging from simple numerical changes to very complex karyotypes with many numerical and structural changes.

7.2.11 Alveolar Soft-Part Sarcoma

This is a rare, malignant neoplasm found predominantly in adolescents and young adults with a rather poor prognosis. Cytogenetically it has been established that alveolar soft-part sarcoma (ASPS) is characterized by a specific change, i.e., der(17)t(X;17)(p11.2;q25) [12]. The translocation fuses the *TFE3* gene at Xp11 to a gene at 17p25 designated as *ASPSCR1*; the fusion gene leads to transcriptional deregulation in the pathogenesis of ASPS. It should be remembered that a small group of renal cell carcinomas (primarily in infants and children) display a t(X;17)(p11.2;q25) translocation and molecular findings identical to those seen in ASPS.

Several kinds of tumor in Table 7.1 (aggressive angiomyxoma, angiomatoid fibrous histiocytoma, epithelioid hemangioendothelioma) are probably associated with specific chromosome changes (translocations), but these remain to be more firmly established, as are the molecular aspects of these changes. Low-grade fibroid sarcoma and its closely related hyalinizing spindle-cell tumor, both thought to be distinct variants of fibrosarcoma, have been described to be associated with t(7;16)(q34;p11.2) [13].

7.3 Soft Tissue Tumors and Bone Tumors Without Specific Cytogenetic Changes

The genetic events shown in Table 7.2 are related to tumors of the bone and soft tissues which are not characterized by specific translocations (or other karyotypic changes) but may contain some anomalies which are more frequent than others [2, 14, 15]. In some tumors the changes shown in Table 7.2 are part of complex karyotypes seen in these tumors, e.g., skeletal chondrosarcoma, osteosarcoma, leiomyosarcoma, malignant fibrous histiocytoma (MFH), and malignant peripheral nerve sheath tumors, in which the malignant process probably developed through a stepwise mechanism (Fig. 7.10).

7.3.1 Malignant Peripheral Nerve Sheath Tumor

Malignant peripheral nerve sheath tumors (MPNST) often have a deletion of the *NF1* gene, which can be demonstrated with FISH, and are usually accompanied by complex karyotypes. Characterization of the neurofibromatoses genes (*NF1* located on 17q/1.2 and *NF2* on 22q/2.2) has shed light on MPNST pathogenesis. Both these genes encode tumor-suppressor proteins. Neurofibromas and MPNST are common in individuals with neurofibromatosis type 1, whereas schwannomas are associated with type 2 [2].

7.3.2 Gastrointestinal Stromal Tumors

These tumors deserve special attention because of molecular facets that have played a key role in their therapy. GIST contain activating mutation of the *KIT* or *BGFRA* oncogenes [16]. If the mutation is in exon 13 (present in approx. 70% of cases) therapy with imatinib is quite effective; whereas if the mutation is in exon 17 (present in approx. 30% of cases) the drug is ineffective. These point mutations can only be ascertained by RT-PCR, since they are not detectable cytogenetically. GIST is probably caused by a *KIT* mutation; cytogenetic changes, when present, may play a role in tumor progression. Loss of 14q, often accompanied by loss of 1p, 9p, 11p, or 22q, is common in GIST of various stages, though 9p deletion, 8q amplification, and 17 amplification are seen only in malignant tumors.

7.3.3 Desmoid Tumors

Desmoid tumors (deep fibromatoses) may be associated with a number of cytogenetic changes [2], e.g., trisomies 8 and 20, and del(5q). Mutations of *APC* and the β-catenin genes may precede the chromosome changes. The latter would then be responsible for, or at least be associated with, progression.

7.3.4 Rhabdoid Tumors

Rhabdoid tumors of various locations (kidney, CNS, or soft tissue) usually have a deletion of 22q, involving a TSG, *SMARCB1*, which encodes a protein involved in chromatin remodeling. The 22q deletion is often the only anomaly in rhabdoid tumors, suggesting that *SMARCB1* inactivation is an early event in rhabdoid tumorigenesis.

7.3.5 Leiomyosarcomas

Leiomyosarcomas (LMS) usually have a complex karyotype, with deletion of 1p occurring with some consistency [17]. Since a similar deletion may occur in other tumors (MFH, MPNST, and GIST), the finding of del(1p) lacks specificity for LMS. Karyotypic complexity is present even in low-grade LMS.

Leiomyomas, benign counterparts of LMS, often have translocations and deletions with rather simple karyotypes, though 50% of leiomyomas lack evident karyotypic abnormalities [18]. A distinctive cytogenetic abnormality in uterine leiomyoma is a translocation, t(12;14)(q15;q23), seen in about 20% of these tumors. This translocation leads to overexpression of the *HMGA2* gene, located at 12q15, through its fusion with the *RAD51* gene, located at 14q23.

7.3.6 Neuroblastoma

Cytogenetics and molecular studies can be of considerable clinical value in evaluating the prognosis in neuroblastoma [2]. The tumors prompting a favorable prognosis are usually near-triploid, without 1p deletions or *N-MYCN* amplification. Neuroblastomas carrying an unfavorable prognosis have near-diploid or near-tetraploid karyotypes, 1p deletion and *MYCN* amplification, often manifest as dms (Fig. 7.9). In cases where cytogenetic results are not obtained, the *MYCN* amplification and the del(1p) can be determined in interphase cells by FISH with appropriate probes.

7.3.7 Chondroma

The chromosome changes seen in chondroma cannot differentiate those tumors which arise in bone from those in the periosteum or soft tissues [11]. Rearrangements of chromosome 6 and 12p(q13-q15) appear to be recurrent. Maffucci syndrome and Ollier disease, mentioned elsewhere in this book, are conditions associated with multiple enchondromatosis.

Plantar fibromatosis (Ledderhose disease) has been shown to be associated with +8 and +14 as has been shown for other fibromatosis subtypes, e.g., Dupuytren contracture. Though clonal chromosome abnormalities have been reported for nodular fasciitis, proliferative myositis, Dupuytren contracture, Kaposi sarcoma, and Peyronie disease, no convincing recurrent changes have been described in these conditions.

Things to remember:
1. The radiologist is in a unique position for determining which soft tissue tumor or bone tumor may require cytogenetic and/or molecular diagnostic studies.
2. When the radiological findings are confusing and raise uncertainty regarding the exact diagnosis, the radiologist is in a position to alert the responsible surgeons and physicians before surgical or therapeutic procedures are initiated to the possibility that genetic studies may be indicated. This is particularly true if cytogenetic analysis is contemplated, since fresh (not fixed) tissue is required for such an analysis and may be obtained at the time of surgery or biopsy. Though a similar uncertainty regarding the exact diagnosis may be encountered by the pathologist, usually fresh tissue is not available at that time, though interphase FISH and/or molecular studies can be performed on fixed specimens.
3. Emphasis must be placed again on the combined use of cytogenetic (including various FISH methodologies) and molecular techniques in obtaining an optimal and full picture of diagnostic value of the genetic changes in tumors, due to the fact that tumors may have molecular changes exceeding in number that of the cytogenetic anomalies and at the same time present cytogenetic changes not reflected in the molecular abnormalities. Particularly useful in that regard are FISH and RT-PCR.
4. FISH can be based on a number of methodologies, depending on the probes employed, i.e., centromeric probes unique for the centromeric area of each chromosome are hence very useful in establishing numerical changes of individual chromosomes. This approach is applicable not only to

metaphase but also to interphase chromosomes; cosmid dual-color probes for unique genetic or chromosomal sequences (of genes or various chromosome bands or areas) are particularly useful in establishing the presence of translocations both in metaphase and interphase nuclei; and SKY and M-FISH by which each chromosome is uniquely labeled and hence are useful in the establishment of esoteric or complex translocations or changes not deciphered by cytogenetics.

5. For diagnostic purposes, the use of FISH in interphase nuclei, i.e., in fixed or archival tissues, must be stressed, since this approach affords an opportunity to establish genetic changes when cytogenetic studies are not available.

6. A number of methodologies are available for the determination of genetic molecular changes in tumors, e.g., PCR amplification of tumor DNA, RT-PCR in which tumor mRNA is converted to cDNA, which is then amplified, and nested PCR, which can effectively amplify low copy-number templates.

7. Molecular studies are useful when cytogenetics and FISH have yielded inconclusive results. Furthermore, the molecular techniques require small amounts of tissue, can be performed on archival specimens, and require a relatively short time for analysis.

References

1. Sandberg AA (1990) The chromosomes in human cancer and leukemia, 2nd edn. Elsevier Science, New York
2. Sandberg AA, Bridge JA (1994) The cytogenetics of bone and soft tissue tumors. Landes, Austin
3. Sandberg AA, Bridge JA (2002) Updates on the cytogenetics and molecular genetics of bone and soft tissue tumors. Synovial sarcoma. Cancer Genet Cytogenet 133:1–23
4. Sandberg AA (2004). Updates on the cytogenetics and molecular genetics of bone and soft tissue tumors. Liposarcoma. Cancer Genet Cytogenet 155:1–24
5. Sandberg AA (2004) Updates on the cytogenetics and molecular genetics of bone and soft tissue tumors. Lipoma. Cancer Genet Cytogenet 150:93–115
6. Sandberg AA, Bridge JA (2000) Updates on the cytogenetics and molecular genetics of bone and soft tissue tumors. Ewing sarcoma and peripheral primitive neuroectodermal tumors. Cancer Genet Cytogenet 123:1–26
7. Sandberg AA, Bridge JA (2001) Updates on the cytogenetics and molecular genetics of bone and soft tissue tumors. Clear cell sarcoma (malignant melanoma of soft parts). Cancer Genet Cytogenet 130:1–7
8. Sandberg AA, Bridge JA (2002) Updates on the cytogenetics and molecular genetics of bone and soft tissue tumors: desmoplastic small round-cell tumors. Cancer Genet Cytogenet 138:1–10
9. Sandberg AA, Bridge JA (2003) Updates on the cytogenetics and molecular genetics of bone and soft tissue tumors: dermatofibrosarcoma protuberans and giant cell fibroblastoma. Cancer Genet Cytogenet 140:1–12
10. Sandberg AA, Bridge JA (2002) Updates on the cytogenetics and molecular genetics of bone and soft tissue tumors: congenital (infantile) fibrosarcoma and mesoblastic nephroma. Cancer Genet Cytogenet 132:1–13
11. Sandberg AA, Bridge JA (2003) Updates on the cytogenetics and molecular genetics of bone and soft tissue tumors. chondrosarcoma and other cartilaginous neoplasms. Cancer Genet Cytogenet 143:1–31
12. Sandberg AA, Bridge JA (2002) Updates on the cytogenetics and molecular genetics of bone and soft tissue tumors: alveolar soft part sarcoma. Cancer Genet Cytogenet 136:1–9
13. Reid R, Chandu de Silva MV, Paterson L, Ryan E, Fisher C (2003) Low-grade fibromyxoid sarcoma and hyalinizing spindle cell tumor with giant rosettes share a common t(7;16)(q34;p11) translocation. Am J Surg Pathol 27:1229–1236
14. Sandberg AA, Bridge JA (2003) Updates on the cytogenetics and molecular genetics of bone and soft tissue tumors. osteosarcoma and related tumors. Cancer Genet Cytogenet 145:1–30
15. Sandberg AA, Bridge JA (2001) Updates on the cytogenetics and molecular genetics of bone and soft tissue tumors. Mesothelioma. Cancer Genet Cytogenet 127:93–110
16. Sandberg AA, Bridge JA (2002) Updates on the cytogenetics and molecular genetics of bone and soft tissue tumors: gastrointestinal stromal tumors. Cancer Genet Cytogenet 135:1–22
17. Sandberg AA (2005) Updates on the cytogenetics and molecular genetics of bone and soft tissue tumors. Leiomyosarcoma. Cancer Genet Cytogenet 161:1–19
18. Sandberg AA (2005) Updates on the cytogenetics and molecular genetics of bone and soft tissue tumors. leiomyoma. Cancer Genet Cytogenet 158:1–26
19. Mitelman F (ed) (1995) ISCN: an international system for human cytogenetic nomenclature. Karger, Basel
20. Alava E de, Gerald WL (2000) Molecular biology of the Ewing's sarcoma/primitive neuroectodermal tumor family. J Clin Oncol 18:204–213
21. Alava E de, Kawai A, Healey JH, Fligman I, Meyers PA, Huvos AG, Gerald WL, Jhanwar SC, Argani P, Antonescu CR, Pardo-Mindán FJ, Ginsberg J, Womer R, Lawlor ER, Wunder J, Andrulis I, Sorensen PHB, Barr FG, Ladanyi M (1998) *EWS-FLI1* fusion transcript structure is an independent determinant of prognosis in Ewing's sarcoma. J Clin Oncol 16:1248–1255
22. Knezevich SR, McFadden DE, Tao W, Lim JF, Sorenson PHB (1998) A novel *ETV6-NTRK3* gene fusion in congenital fibrosarcoma. Nature Genet 18:184–187

Soft Tissue Tumours: the Surgical Pathologist's Perspective

8

Roberto Salgado, Eric Van Marck

Contents

Recently, using transcriptional gene profiling complemented with, e.g. tissue microarrays, new potential therapeutic markers of histiotype-specific soft tissue tumours have emerged, e.g. CD117 (c-kit) and DOG1 for gastrointestinal stromal tumours, PDGFRβ in dermatofibrosarcoma protuberans and EGFR1 for synovial sarcomas, which in some cases might even be able to predict therapy response and prognosis [1–3]. These advances have led to an increased appreciation of the importance that histological typing might have in predicting natural history and treatment sensitivity of soft tissue tumours.

Tumour tissue procurement and exact tissue handling are critical issues to provide the pathologist with adequate and well preserved tissue, in order to perform the necessary ancillary studies for making an exact diagnosis. Cross-talk between pathologists, radiologists and clinicians is crucial in obtaining this goal.

8.1 Introduction

The diagnosis of soft tissue tumours has always been difficult and controversial. This was mainly due to the rarity of these lesions, comprising <1 % of all malignant tumours. Nevertheless, according to the Surveillance, Epidemiology, and End Results (SEER) database, about 15,000 cases of both bone and soft tissue tumours are diagnosed annually in the US. This puts soft tissue and bone tumours in the same order of magnitude as myeloma, gliomas and cervical carcinoma.

Previously, the clinical importance of the exact histological typing of soft tissue tumours by the pathologist was limited, knowing that grade and stage, and not histological type determined treatment options. The pathologist merely served to grade the lesion and to exclude malignant non-sarcomatous, benign or pseudotumoral lesions. The small number of lesions – in particular of single histological types – and the poorly defined pathological criteria are the major sources of discordances in diagnostic soft tissue pathology. Even in specialist centres about 5–10 % of soft tissue lesions remain unclassified.

8.2 When Pathology Meets Radiology

The importance for the pathologist of both clinical and radiological information cannot be overemphasised. Some tumours merely occur in children, e.g. rhabdomyosarcomas, while others are rare in children and are mostly found in adults, e.g. pleiomorphic liposarcoma [4].

Magnetic Resonance Imaging (MRI) and Computed Tomography (CT) give the pathologist information about the size, consistency, homogeneity, location, presence or absence of necrosis, infiltration pattern, interface with adjacent structures, etc.

Anatomic pathologists rendering a diagnosis on mostly limited material without having the advantages of clinical and radiological information might be in a disadvantageous position in many cases. It is imperative that pathologists with a special interest in soft tissue tumours do at least have a rudimentary knowledge of the radiological and clinical features of the tumours, in analogy with pathologists interested in bone tumours. On the other hand, it is equally important to have a radiologist and clinicians with a keen interest in soft tissue tumour pathology.

Some soft tissue tumours such as liposarcomas are quite heterogeneous. Therefore, the pathologist might aid in choosing which area of the tumour is best suited for sampling, considering that sampling in areas of overt necrosis is best avoided. Sampling near necrotic areas, however, can be meaningful since the presence or absence of necrosis is considered an integral part of grading schemes [5]. Meanwhile, in analogy with bone tumours, e.g. osteosarcoma and chondrosarcoma, imaging features might provide the pathologist with spatial features of soft tissue lesions that are highly suggestive of being the high grade areas of the tumour. For example, chondrosarcomatous tumours having myxoid areas juxtaposed to cartilaginous areas are highly suggestive of being of high grade malignancy [6]. Sampling in these areas might be necessary for arriving at an exact diagnosis, meanwhile trying to avoid underestimation of the malignant potential of the tumour when sampling of non-high grade areas occurs. Sampling is also imperative for performing additional studies such as cytogenetic analysis, as will be explained later.

Estimating the percentage of necrosis preoperatively by the radiologist might also be important, since some tumours, e.g. Ewing's sarcoma and extra-renal rhabdoid tumours, are treated preoperatively, and the pathologist is asked to estimate the percentage of viable tumour tissue left after treatment, as a measure of tumour response. This is quite elaborate and subjective since it is quite impossible, histologically, to distinguish between spontaneous or therapy-induced necrosis.

Close collaboration between radiologists and pathologists is important, not only to decide where to sample but also in determining how to sample.

8.3 When Pathology Meets the Clinics

Once the lesion is localised, obtaining a biopsy in the appropriate tumour area is the next logical step. Ideally, the biopsy should occur in the centre where the patient will be treated. It is not surprising that a pathologist often requests larger tumour samples or asks for a second opinion when being confronted with a soft tissue tumour. This is mainly due to the rarity of the lesions, the lack of adequately defined diagnostic criteria and the "unearthing" of new entities. There are some 50 different subtypes of soft tissue tumours. Considering the rarity of the lesions and the difficulties associated in obtaining an adequate biopsy from representative tumour areas, which can only occur once the tumour has been investigated thoroughly by adequate imaging means (MRI and CT), biopsy procedures in the primary care settings should be discouraged. Biopsy procedures without having adequate radiological information given by CT or preferable by MRI, should be avoided, unless the lesion is small and superficially located. Exci-

sion biopsies should only be performed on superficial or subcutaneous tumours which are usually smaller than 2–3 cm in size. Excision biopsies of larger and/or deep seated masses are best avoided.

Open, incisional biopsies are performed in most centres. Open biopsies enable the pathologist to have enough tissue, not only with a preserved architecture of the tumour which is crucial for histological subtyping, but also for performing ancillary studies, e.g. immunohistochemistry, cytogenetic and gene expression profiling-studies, when deemed necessary.

Recently, more emphasis is being placed on the ability of pathologists to make a reliable diagnosis on relatively smaller amounts of tissues. This is mainly due to economic reasoning and patient comfort. Core Needle Biopsies (CNB) and Fine Needle Aspiration Biopsies (FNAB) are temporarily quite popular [7, 8]. The main advantages of both these methods include the feasibility in performing these kinds of biopsies in outpatient clinical settings, the minimal risk of complications, the cost-effectiveness and the acceptability of the patient. Moreover, the reduced risk of spilling tumour cells during the biopsy procedure and the lack of compromising the subsequent surgical management are considered additional features in favour of FNAC or CNB vs open biopsy. Spilling of tumour cells and compromising herewith the surgical bed and subsequent therapeutic measures are often the case when open, incisional biopsies are performed by inexperienced surgeons. This urges that for soft tissue lesions suspicious of being malignant, biopsy procedures should be decided on after intense cross-talk between pathologists, radiologists and clinicians, and should preferable be performed in reference centres.

Nevertheless, despite the above-mentioned obvious advantages of sampling limited material, this does not imply that pathologists are willing or able to make a specific diagnosis on small amounts of material. Limited sampling might make grading and exact subtyping quite difficult. Moreover, preoperative chemo- and/or radiotherapy for some tumours, e.g. Ewing sarcoma, might make adequate and reliable histological typing and grading evaluation of resected specimens extremely difficult, if not impossible.

Preoperatively, with limited material, especially after FNAC, the pathologist is in some cases only able to provide diagnoses such as "malignant soft tissue tumour, not otherwise specified" or "spindle" or "round cell" tumour. This would imply in some cases that it would even not be possible to know exactly which tumour was treated, since preoperative therapy might distort morphology considerably.

Deep seated lesions, however, are amenable for CNB, avoiding the discomfort of open, incisional biopsy in these specific circumstances. FNAC is indicated mostly for assessing local recurrence or metastasis or in cases where incisional biopsy is difficult to perform. Nevertheless, in some specialised centres, with extensive expertise in soft tissue tumour pathology, reliable subtyping might be possible in most of the (untreated) cases using FNAC or CNB. Similarly, distinguishing between benign and malignant lesions can be done in these specialist centres, which, as mentioned before, is currently considered sufficient to initiate treatment. Failure of exact subtyping does not in all instances withhold initiating therapy, since quite limited information is needed by the clinician. This information might be rendered by limited samples, with FNAB yielding less material than CNB. Obviously, when both FNAB and CNB are inadequate, an open and incisional biopsy is mandatory. Nevertheless, an open, incisional biopsy is recommended in centres without explicit experience in FNAC or CNB.

As already mentioned, in this era of targeted therapy, histological subtyping is crucial. Since imaging modalities cannot reliably distinguish between benign and definitely malignant lesions, morphology has the last word. This can only be accomplished in a reliable manner with substantial material.

8.4 When Morphology is not Enough

Considering the increased importance of histological typing and the presence/absence of molecular markers for diagnostic, predictive or prognostic purposes, adequate handling of biopsy material is mandatory.

It is imperative that radiologists and clinicians need to be aware of not only the total amount of material they (need to) sample, but also on the handling of soft tissue tumour tissue by the pathologist. The tissue needs to be transported fresh in an unfixed state to the pathology department. This allows an accurate and exact orientation of the specimen by, ideally, both the surgeon and the pathologist who is going to diagnose the lesion. This cross-talk is also important for assessing the often complex resection margins of soft tissue tumour specimens. Resection margins, be it other than fascia or periosteum, less than 1 cm are associated with a substantial risk of recurrence, prompting additional treatment such as. e.g. radiotherapy or wider surgical excision.

When the tissue arrives at the pathology department, critical decisions are made with respect to how the tissue is handled. With limited amounts of material, as obtained by FNAC and CNB, the pathologist is deemed to include all tissue for, e.g. formalin fixation and subsequent paraffin embedding. Yet, as mentioned before, histological typing of the tumour should be the main objective of the pathologist. With small amounts of tissue, it is sometimes quite difficult, even impossible to asses the histology of the tumour. Moreover, differentiating between benign and low grade malignant lesions is not always possible. Snap-frozen tissue, tissue samples stored in culture media for subsequent cytogenetic analysis and fixing tissue in glutaraldehyde for electron microscopic investigation are necessary when morphologic features on haematoxylin and eosin slides are deemed insufficient. Tumour tissue stored in this manner is never wasted and can be consulted later on for diagnostic and research purposes, when appropriate.

Yet, in most cases the pathologist does not have the luxury of having enough material to be stored in a way as mentioned before.

Immunohistochemistry might be beneficial in these circumstances. Immunohistochemistry is the use of antibodies specific to epitopes located on the cells of interest. A range of immunohistochemical markers are available nowadays. These antibodies should be applied according to the morphology of the tumour (Table 8.1), which should enable the pathologist to arrive at an accurate diagnosis. The rationale of the use of these antibodies lies with the assumption that antigens expressed by the tumour cells are the same as those expressed by their normal counterparts. For example, myogenin and MyoD-1 seem to be specific for muscle cells, since foetal muscle cells do express these proteins. Similarly, blood vessels are CD31 and CD34 immunoreactive (Figs. 8.1 and 8.2), and consequently their tumoral counterparts, the angiosarcomas, are immunoreactive for both these proteins. In a number of cases, however, this simplification does not hold. Some soft tissue tumours, e.g. angiosarcomas might have an anomalous expression of proteins pointing to another lineage, e.g. cytokeratin. For example, only two soft tissue tumours do have "true" cytokeratin expression, namely epitheloid sarcoma and synovial sarcoma. These two tumours have so far an undetermined origin. The example of the synovial sarcoma is interesting in another respect. Although the name might imply a synovial origin, most synovial tumours do not arise in or near joints. Using transcriptional gene profiling experiments it has been shown that these tumours might have a neuroectodermal (stem cell?) origin [9]. Another example illustrative of the incongruent relation between a normal cell and its tumoral counterpart are the rhabdomyosarcomas. Some rhabdomyosarcomas are located in bladder and gall bladder, yet in these organs no striated muscle cells are found. Expression of a single marker should therefore not be considered in all cases as indicative of the origin of a specific tumour. The example mentioned before of the synovial sarcoma might also be applied to the gastrointestinal soft tissue tumours (GIST), of which a plethora of publications have arisen during the past years. One of the criteria to diagnose GIST-tumours is the presence of the membrane protein c-kit (Figs. 8.3 and 8.4). Since this protein is detected on the interstitial cells of Cajal in the intestine, it has been speculated that these cells might be the origin of these tumours. However, some tumours are c-kit negative and

Table 8.1. Immunohistochemical panel according to the morphology of the tumour

Immunohistochemical panels	
Spindle cell tumours	Cytokeratin, epithelial membrane antigen (EMA), desmin, smooth muscle actin (SMA), h-caldesmon, S-100
Round-cell tumours	CD99, myogenin, desmin, cytokeratin, EMA, synaptophysin, FLI-1
Epitheloid tumours	Cytokeratin, EMA, CD34, CD31, S-100, FLI-1

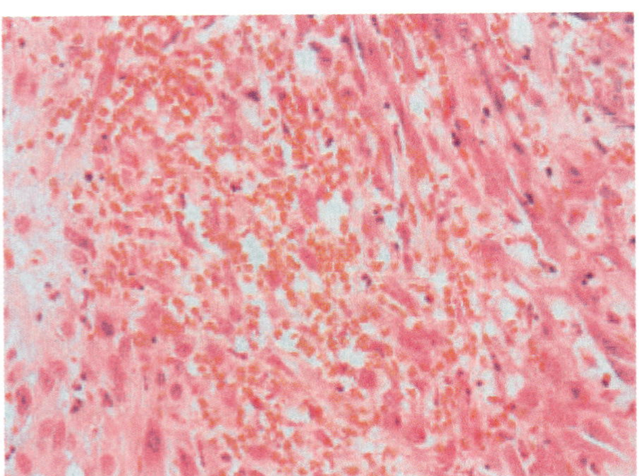

Fig. 8.1. Angiosarcoma (magnification: ×200)

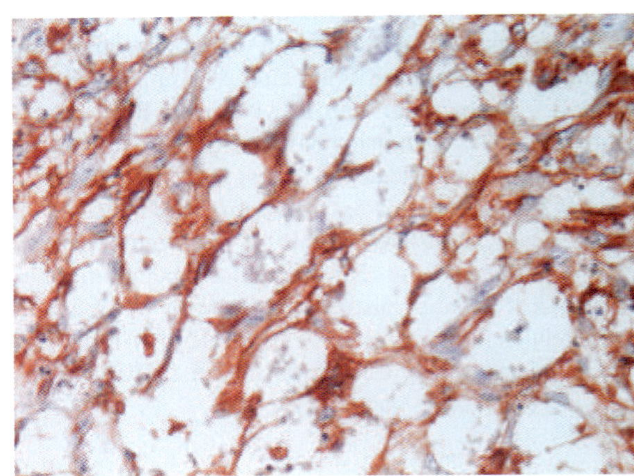

Fig. 8.2. Angiosarcoma tumour cells staining for CD31 (magnification: ×200)

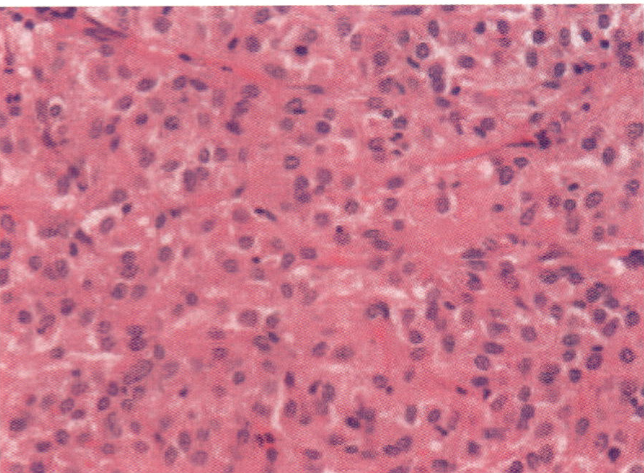

Fig. 8.3. Gastrointestinal stromal tumour (GIST) (magnification: ×200)

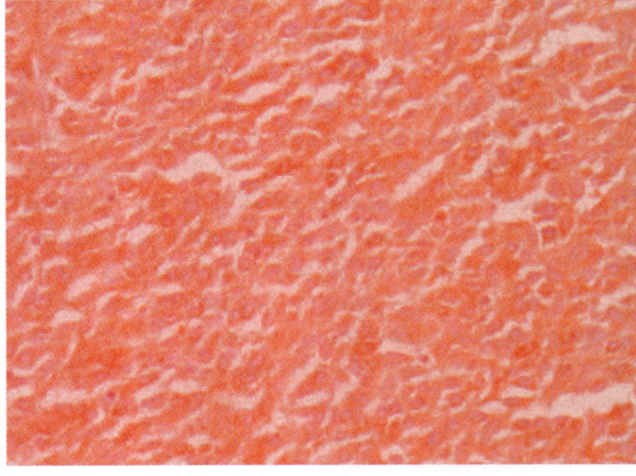

Fig. 8.4. GIST-tumour cells staining for CD117 (c-kit) (magnification: ×200)

some do not at all arise in the gastrointestinal tract, e.g. the extra-gastrointestinal GIST. C-kit expression in most of these cases is related to an acquired gain of function mutation of the c-kit gene. C-kit expression in GIST-tumours is also related to the therapeutic effectiveness of imatinib mesylate (Glivec). Intriguingly, GIST-tumour cells expressing the protein without having the corresponding mutation have less response to imatinib mesylate (Glivec) therapy.

Considering that GIST-tumours were previously categorised as being of smooth muscle cell or neural origin, the comments above illustrate that identification of genetic alterations in histiotype-specific tumours is able to change the morphological classification of soft tissue tumours.

If sufficient tissue is available, additional investigations can be performed such as cytogenetic analysis and electron microscopic studies.

Cytogenetic analysis is the identification of specific molecular alterations thought to be specific for certain tumours. This concept will be discussed elsewhere by A. Sandberg.

Performing electron microscopic investigations for soft tissue tumours is not routine in most pathology departments. This might be due to the pathologists themselves who are unwilling to embrace and further develop or invest in "old" techniques such as electron microscopy. In any branch of medicine any technique which might offer additional clinical information is difficult to be discarded, in contrast to electron microscopy for soft tissue tumour diagnostics.

It is argued that electron microscopy does not add much to the diagnosis of soft tissue tumours.

Specific examples highlight the importance electron microscopy might have in soft tissue tumours:

1. Distinguishing between malignant peripheral nerve sheath tumours and monophasic synovial tumours. Monophasic synovial sarcomas are much more chemosensitive than malignant peripheral nerve sheath tumours.
2. Distinguishing between mimics of soft tissue tumours such as sarcomatous carcinoma and metastatic melanoma.
3. Diagnosing alveolar soft tissue sarcoma in an aspecific clinical or metastatic setting.

All the above-mentioned features highlight a few issues:

1. The pathologist needs to have sufficient material to perform the ancillary studies which he seems necessary to arrive at a diagnosis as accurate as possible.
2. Without sufficient material it is difficult to distinguish between benign, low grade and sometimes even high grade malignant lesions.
3. Ancillary immunohistochemical techniques might help the pathologist in arriving at a diagnosis.
4. The expression of molecules on soft tissue tumour cells does not always imply a corresponding normal counterpart.
5. The expression of molecules on tumour cells, is sometimes not merely diagnostic, but might in some cases also have prognostic and predictive information.
6. It might be argued that the classification of soft tissue tumours by the corresponding normal counterpart of the tumours should be abandoned, considering the anomalous expression of proteins by some tumour cells. Some (all?) soft tissue tumours seem to arise from somatic stem cells, and not from its normal counterpart.

8.5 World Health Classification of Soft Tissue Tumours 2002 [10]

Once a specific diagnosis is reached the lesion should be categorized accordingly. Recent advances in cytogenetic and molecular genetic information, the recognition of new entities and the enhanced understanding of the biological behaviour have prompted a new morphological classification of soft tissue tumours.

It is recommended to categorise the lesions in a benign, intermediate (locally aggressive), intermediate (rarely metastasizing) or a malignant category:

1. Benign lesions: e.g. lipoma. These tumours mostly do not recur and if recurrence occurs it is most of the time in a non-destructive fashion. In exceptional circumstances metastasis might occur, as in e.g. benign fibrous histiocytoma.
2. Intermediate (locally aggressive): e.g. kaposiform haemangioendothelioma and desmoid fibromatosis. These tumours are infiltrative and might recur locally, sometimes in a destructive fashion when incompletely excised.
3. Intermediate (rarely metastasizing): e.g. retiform haemangioendothelioma. These tumours are locally aggressive, recur if incompletely excised and may give rise to metastasis. Histological features are not, in most cases, predictive for metastasis.
4. Malignant: e.g. round cell liposarcoma. These tumours are infiltrative, recur locally if incompletely excised and have a significant risk of metastasis.

Significant changes have occurred in the new WHO-classification compared with the previous classification published in 1994. Major adaptations include:

1. Adipocytic tumours: new entities include myolipoma and chondroid lipoma. Four types of liposarcoma occur:

   a) Atypical lipomatous tumour/ well differentiated liposarcoma: these terms are synonyms, although the term well differentiated liposarcoma is preferable in retroperitoneal and paratesticular areas, due to its higher morbidity and mortality in these specific areas.

   b) Dedifferentiated liposarcoma: previously were these tumours categorised as being definitively high grade. In the current classification a low-grade variant is included. These tumours, although being of the dedifferentiated type, do have a more protracted clinical course compared with other dedifferentiated soft tissue tumours.

   c) Myxoid liposarcoma: both round-cell liposarcoma and myxoid liposarcoma are considered to be one entity, with the round-cell liposarcoma type being at the less dedifferentiated spectrum of this tumour.

d) Pleiomorphic liposarcoma: these are the rarest lipomatous tumours and are considered to have a worse prognosis.

2. Fibroblastic/myofibroblastic tumours: keloid is not longer regarded as a soft tissue tumour. New benign entities include, e.g. giant cell fibroblastoma, Gardner fibroma and angiomyofibroblastoma. New malignant entities include, e.g. sclerosing epitheloid fibrosarcoma and low-grade fibromyxoid sarcoma. Importantly, the term "hemangiopericytoma" is included in the chapter of the solitary fibrous tumours considering the lack of morphological dissimilarities between these two tumour types.

3. Fibriohistiocytic tumours: pleiomorphic malignant fibriohistiocytic tumour (MFH) is considered to be a high grade undifferentiated tumour.

4. Smooth muscle tumours: inclusion of GIST-tumours in different organs, e.g. in the gastrointestinal tract is considered in the respective WHO-volumes.

5. Pericytic/perivascular tumours: only glomus and myopericytoma are included in this category.

6. Skeletal muscle tumours: the embryonal, alveolar and pleiomorphic subtypes are included.

7. Vascular tumours: in this category is only the epitheloid haemangioendothelioma included as a malignant subtype of the haemangioendotheliomas.

8. Chondro-osseous: myositis ossificans and fibro-osseous pseudotumours are considered to be variants of nodular fasciitis. Since extra-skeletal myxoid chondrosarcoma does not seem to have chondroid differentiation, this lesion is placed in the category "tumours of uncertain differentiation".

8.6 To Grade or not to Grade?

The purpose of grading is to segregate tumours in those with a favourable prognosis, amenable to surgical excision only, and in those with an unfavourable prognosis, amenable to surgical treatment and additional chemotherapeutic and/or radiotherapeutic treatment. Moreover, adequate grading is considered to be more reproducible than histological typing, might even circumvent diagnostic disagreement between pathologists and might triage unclassified sarcoma in a low or high risk category. As a matter of fact, most contemporary oncologists triage their patients for subsequent treatment by merely relying on the tumour grade provided by the pathologist. Relying in a way that grading is in all circumstances able to distinguish between benign, low grade and high grade lesions, irrespective of histiotype.

Currently, two grading classifications exist: the National Cancer Institute (NCI)-grading system (Table 8.2) and the Fédération Nationale des Centres de Lutte Contre le Cancer (FNCLCC)-grading system, the so called "Trojani system" (Table 8.3). The FNCLCC-

Table 8.2. National Institute of Cancer grading system

Common histological types		
Grade 1	Grade 2	Grade 3
Well-differentiated liposarcoma	Pleiomorphic liposarcoma	Alveolar rhabdomyosarcoma
Myxoid liposarcoma	Fibrosarcoma	Soft tissue osteosarcoma
Deep-seated dermatofibrosarcoma protuberans	Malignant fibrous histiocytoma	Primitive neuroectodermal tumour
Some leioymyosarcomas		Alveolar soft part sarcoma
Epitheloid haemangioendothelioma	Synovial sarcoma	Mesenchymal chondrosarcoma
Spindle cell haemangioendothelioma	Leiomyosarcoma	
Infantile fibrosarcoma	Neurofibrosarcoma	
Subcutaneous myxofibrosarcoma	or 0–15% necrosis	or >15% necrosis

Table 8.3. Fédération Nationale des Centres de Lutte Contre le Cancer grading system

Differentiation score		Mitosis score (per 10 HPF)	Necrosis
Score 1	Sarcomas resembling adult mesenchymal tissue	0–9	No necrosis
Score 2	Sarcomas of certain histiotype	>9; <20	<50% necrosis
Score 3	Embryonal/undifferentiated sarcomas and sarcomas of uncertain histiotype	20 or more	>50% necrosis

HPF: high power field.
The total scores for each grade are as follows: grade 1, 2–3; grade 2, 4–5; grade 3; 6–8

grading system is considered to be more reproducible and more apt to classify patients in either grade 1 or grade 3, avoiding more frequently the inclusion of patients in the "indeterminate" grade 2 category, compared with the NCI-system. Both systems are included in the latest WHO Soft Tissue Tumour Classification. Both are three-tiered systems, assigning different weights to histiotype, necrosis, mitotic figures, cellularity, pleiomorphism and differentiation.

Grading should be performed on untreated tumours on representative and well preserved tissue. This should be the case for all tumours, be it sarcomatous or non-sarcomatous. Previous therapy, whether be it chemotherapy or radiotherapy, precludes grading in all circumstances since both mitotic figures and the extent of necrosis can be affected. It is also well known that soft tissue tumours acquire a higher grade in local recurrence or metastatic lesions. Grading of visceral sarcomas should also be avoided.

It is a genuine fact that some soft tissue tumours are not amenable at all to exact histological grading. Histological typing does not in all cases provide the necessary prognostic and/ or predictive information. Some soft tissue tumours should not at all be graded, especially considering the inherent malignant potential of these tumours. According to the WHO 2002 Classification of Soft Tissue Tumours grading should not be performed on malignant peripheral nerve sheath tumours, angiosarcomas, extraskeletal myxoid chondrosarcoma, alveolar soft part sarcoma, clear cell sarcoma and epithelioid sarcoma.

Considering both grading systems it is quite clear that some histological typing is crucial for grading soft tissue tumours. As previously mentioned, exact histological typing should be the main aim of the pathologist, yet, it is not always possible, as is the case when having only small amounts of tissue. On the other hand, if a pathologist wants to use one of the grading systems, an attempt at histological typing is necessary, despite the inherent difficulties of soft tissue diagnostics. It is even elaborated that both tumour type and tumour size are able to adequately predict survival, withholding grading in these cases [11].

Mitotic counts are inherently associated with the FNLCC-grading system. However, as mentioned before, histological typing is mandatory because some tumours behave in a benign fashion despite having many mitoses, e.g. cellular schwannoma and atypical fibroxanthoma. Some tumours are considered low grade despite the presence of mitotic figures, e.g. infantile fibrosarcoma. Conversely, some tumours are inherently malignant despite the lack of mitotic figures and/ or necrosis, e.g. the round-cell liposarcoma.

Grading systems can thus not be meaningfully applied to all soft tissue tumours. Some tumours are definitively malignant, e.g. Ewing sarcoma/MPNET and angiosarcomas. Some tumours are definitively of low malignant potential, e.g. infantile fibrosarcoma and well differentiated liposarcoma. Some tumours are not yet amenable for grading, e.g. malignant giant cell tumour and hemangiopericytoma. Conversely, some tumours are amenable for grading, e.g. leiomyosarcoma, myxoid liposarcoma and fibrosarcoma.

When looking at both grading systems it is obvious that some subjectivity in applying these parameters is unavoidable. Although, e.g. mitotic figure counting should be performed rigidly in soft tissue tumours, the inter-observer reproducibility, equally as e.g. in breast carcinoma, is in the range of 60–70%, even among soft tissue specialists. Cellularity, mitotic figure counting and, e.g. extent of necrosis are all influenced by sampling, fixation, section thickness, the number of blocks taken and microscopic field size. Also, as previously mentioned, having small amounts of material precludes grading in most cases. Considering the intra-tumoral heterogeneity of soft tissue tumours, sampling error is likely to occur, especially when trying to avoid highly necrotic areas. It is also difficult to asses macroscopically the extent of necrosis since myxoid and hyalinized areas might mimic necrosis. There is also no consensus as whether the mere presence or the extent of necrosis determines prognosis. Similarly, how to measure necrosis, micro- or macroscopically, is not at all defined.

Counting mitoses is, as previously mentioned, inherently subjective. Distinguishing mitotic figures from pyknosis is sometimes difficult. There is also no universal consensus on which cut-off and microscopic field size to use.

Some have argued that intra-tumoral (lympho)vascular invasion should also be searched for. In analogy with epithelial tumours, there is considerable difficulty in distinguishing artefactual retraction from "true" lymphatic or blood vessels. Immunohistochemistry might be helpful in this respect.

In the FNCLCC-system differentiation is one the parameters to asses. As previously mentioned, no normal counterpart exists for some tumours, e.g. epithelioid sarcoma.

Also, some tumours, e.g. GIST-tumours do have their own grading system including tumour size, mitotic figure counting and location [12]. Here also, estimating mitotic figure counting is subjected to the same inherent subjectivity as mentioned before. Size should be assessed by the pathologist on a fresh resected specimen.

It is argued that the FNCLCC- and the NCI-grading system should be restricted to adult tumours, considering the unique features of childhood soft tissue tumours. For example, childhood rhabdomyosarcomatous tumours are graded according to the system provided by the Intergroup Rhabdomyosarcoma Study Group where risk assignment, rather than grading is performed by a combination of both exact histology and the location of the tumour. A modified TNM staging system has even developed for these tumours, with sites being defined as unfavourable (e.g. bladder, prostate) and favourable (e.g. orbit, head and neck) [13].

Importantly, currently no method, e.g. DNA flow cytometry, other than histological subtyping and grading provides more prognostic information in soft tissue tumours. It is clear that there is no single universal parameter applicable to all tumours. In ideal circumstances should grading systems be developed and applied for each histological subtype.

8.7 Reporting Soft Tissue Tumours (Table 8.4)

A template for reporting soft tissue tumours should include the following:
1. Histological type.
2. Grade (1–3) or risk assessment, when applicable.
3. Size, assessed by the pathologists on fresh, unfixed tissue.
4. Location, cross-talk with radiologist and surgeon is crucial, especially when trying to identify infiltration in critical structures, e.g. blood vessels and nerves.
5. Margins, especially mentioning those margins <1 cm and whether there is a surrounding fascia or periosteum.
6. Necrosis, if assessed macroscopically it should ideally be on fresh, unfixed and untreated tissue.
7. Additional investigations, e.g. karyotyping.

Table 8.4. Template for soft tissue tumour reporting

Template
a) Histological type
b) Grade (1–3), or risk assessment
c) Size
d) Location
e) Margin status
f) Necrosis
h) Additional investigations

8.8 Gene Expression Profiling and Tissue Microarrays in Soft Tissue Tumours

Soft tissue tumours are heterogeneous, both with respect to the morphology and the clinical behaviour. Although grade and histiotype currently determine treatment options and prognosis, prediction of clinical behaviour remains elusive in most circumstances, especially in individual cases. Tumour growth, even within the same subtype, ranges from slow growing with low risk of metastasis, to fast growing lesions with considerable morbidity and mortality. This precludes adequate morphological classification.

Furthermore, progress in the adequate identification of molecules that might be useful for therapeutic targeting is hampered by the examination of only a small set of genes by the more conventional methods such as, e.g. Northern and Southern blotting.

Gene expression profiling might be useful in this respect. The basis of microarray studies is the labelling of cDNA of the tumour with a fluorescent dye. This labelled cDNA is hybridised together with a reference fluorescent labelled cDNA onto a microarray chip. The slide is scanned after hybridisation on a gene specific probe and the ratio values of the intensity of the sample cDNA vs the reference cDNA is measured and calculated. Thousands of mRNA transcripts can be analysed in this manner.

A number of different array technologies are available, each with its advantages and disadvantages. A main review of all aspects of gene expression profiling is beyond the scope of this review. These are covered more extensively in excellent reviews ([14] and references therein).

Sample preparation is crucial for these kinds of experiments. This method measures the abundance of gene transcripts (mRNA). One caveat is the fragility of mRNA by its rapid degradation by RNAses present in cells and tissues. Thus, it is crucial that the tissue is stored as rapid as possible at −80 °C when sampling the tissue. Although formalin fixed and paraffin embedded tissue might also be useful for RNA extraction, this is more laborious and the risk of not having substantial RNA is considerable. This is mainly due to the slow inactivation of RNAses by the fixative.

Gene expression profiling has revealed novel subtypes in other tumours, e.g. in breast cancer and malignant lymphoma. An illustrative example of the application of gene expression profiling in soft tissue tumours include a study performed by Nielsen and colleagues. Unsupervised analysis of a set of 5500 genes demonstrated that synovial sarcomas, GIST-tumours, malignant peripheral nerve sheath tumours and some leiomyosarcomas clustered in separate groups, in support of the morphological classification of these tumours. When applying a supervised analysis, several transcripts were found to be specifically upregulated in the respective subgroups. For GIST-tumours this included c-kit, for synovial sarcomas EGFR-1 and SSX-transcripts were upregulated [15].

Importantly, the identification of these transcripts in specific tumour histiotypes prompted the development of agents directed specifically at these molecules (Glivec directed at c-kit positive GIST-tumours and Iressa at EGFR-1 positive synovial sarcoma). Clinical trials are in progress.

Moreover, using gene expression profiling it has also been shown that synovial sarcomas clustered on the one hand separately from other tumours, but on the other hand clustered closely to malignant peripheral nerve sheath tumours and expressed genes that are involved in the migration of neural crest cells, such as, e.g. ephrin-3 and endothelin-3, raising suspicion that synovial sarcomas might be of neuroectodermal origin.

Considering the plethora of data provided by gene expression profiling, many new markers have emerged which need to be tested and validated on large tumour sets.

Tissue microarrays might be useful in this respect. Tissue microarrays utilises 0.6-mm core needle biopsies of representative areas of the tumour on a paraffin block. This core is subsequently re-embedded in a novel paraffin block. With this method a large number of tumour samples, ranging to 1000 samples on a single slide, can be analysed at the RNA, DNA or protein level. The GIST-marker DOG-1 was evaluated and validated in such a manner, following identification by gene expression profiling [1].

8.9 Conclusions and Future Perspectives

Soft tissue tumours are rare tumours. Pathological diagnosis is difficult. This is mainly due to the poorly defined pathological criteria and the more than 50 different histological subtypes. Second opinion or, even preferable, a centralised pathological review should be mandatory for difficult cases. The Belgian Soft Tissue Neoplasm Registry (BSTNR) is worth mentioning in this respect. The BSTNR is composed partly of experienced soft tissue tumour pathology- and radiology experts confirming or even providing an alternative diagnosis in submitted cases. Biopsy and diagnosis should be performed in the centre were the patient will be treated. It is imperative that cross-talk between radiologists, clinicians and pathologists occurs at all phases of patient management. Preoperatively, when choosing the biopsy technique and the area to sample and postoperatively, at the bench side. Clinicians and radiologist need to be aware of the amount of tissue the pathologist needs for an accurate diagnosis. Adequate sampling is mandatory, not only for diagnostic purposes, but also

for ancillary studies, such as karyotyping and electron microscopy. Pathologists should aim at trying to histiotype and grade soft tissue tumours, whenever considered adequate. Clinicians need to be aware that grade does not replace histology. It is mandatory that soft tissue tumoral specimens should always be stored in liquid nitrogen for future diagnostic and research purposes. Gene expression profiling and tissue microarrays refine the morphological classification and are currently the best ways to identify new diagnostic, prognostic and predictive molecules in soft tissue tumours. Clinical trials with target specific compounds are ongoing. Centralised pathological review is considered critical in these circumstances.

Things to remember:
1. Pathological diagnosis of soft tissue tumours is difficult. Second opinion or even preferable a centralised pathological review should be mandatory for difficult cases.
2. Biopsy and diagnosis should be performed in the centre were the patient will be treated.
3. Cross-talk between radiologists, clinicians and pathologists should occur at all phases of patient management.
4. Clinicians and radiologist need to be aware of the amount of tissue the pathologist needs for an accurate diagnosis.
5. Grading does not replace histology.
6. Pathologists should aim at trying to histiotype and grade soft tissue tumours.
7. It is mandatory that soft tissue tumoral tissue should always be stored in liquid nitrogen for future diagnostic and research purposes.

References

1. West RB, Corless CL, Chen X, Rubin BP, Subramanian S, Montogomery K, Zhu S, Ball CA, Nielsen TO, Patel R, Goldblum JR, Brown PO, Heinrich MC, van de Rijn M (2004) The novel marker, DOG1, is expressed ubiquitously in gastrointestinal stromal tumors irrespective of KIT or PDGFRA mutation status. Am J Pathol 165(1):107–113
2. Blay JY, Ray-Coquard I, Alberti L, Ranchere D (2004) Targeting other abnormal signalling pathways in sarcoma; EGFR in synovial sarcoma, PPAR-gamma in liposarcoma. Cancer Treat Res 120:151–167
3. McArthur G (2004) Molecularly targeted treatment for dermatofibrosarcoma protuberans. Semin Oncol 31(2 Suppl 6): 30–36
4. Enzinger and Weiss's soft tissue tumors. Fourth Edition (2001)
5. Guillou L, Coindre JM, Bonichon F, Binh Bui N, Terrier P, Collin F, Vilain M, Mandard A, Le Doussal V, Leroux A, Jacquemier J, Duplay H, Sasttre-Garau X, Costa J (1997) Comparative study of the National Cancer Institute and French Federation of Cancer Centers Sarcoma Group Grading Systems in a population of 410 adult patients with soft tissue sarcoma. J Clin Oncol 15:350–362
6. Dahlin's Bone Tumors. Sixth Edition (1996)

7. Sing H, Kilpatrick S, Silverman J (2004) Fine needle aspiration biopsy of soft tissue tumours. Adv Anat Pathol 11(1):24–36
8. Gielen J (2004) Magnetic resonance imaging of soft tissue tumours. A prospective study of malignancy and tumor phenotype on MRI. Epidemiological studies and evaluation of characterization parameters. Thesis, University of Antwerp
9. Allander SV, Illei PB, Chen Y, Antonescu CR, Bittner M, Ladanyi M, Meltzer PS (2002) Expression profiling of synovial sarcoma by cDNA microarrays: association of ERBB2, IGFBP2, and ELF3 with epithelial differentiation. Am J Pathol 161(5):1587–1595
10. Fletcher CDM, Krishnan U, Mertens F (2002) Pathology and genetics. Tumours of soft tissue and bone. World Health Organization Classification of Tumours
11. Evans HL (1995) Classification and grading of soft-tissue sarcomas: a comment. Hematol Oncol Clin North Am 9:653–656
12. Miettinen M, El-Rifai W, Sobin HL, Lasota J (2002) Evaluation of malignancy and prognosis of gastrointestinal stromal tumors: a review. Hum Pathol 33(5):478–483
13. Meyer W, Spunt S (2004) Soft tissue sarcoma of childhood. Cancer Treatment Rev 30:269–280
14. Yang YH, Speed T (2002) Design issues for cDNA microarray experiments. Nat Rev Genet 3(8):579–588
15. Nielsen TO, West RB, Linn SC, Knowling MA, O'Connel JX, Zhu S, Fero M, Sherlock G, Pollack JR, Botstein D, van de Rijn M (2002) Molecular characterisation of soft tissue tumours: a gene expression study. Lancet 359(9314):1301–1307

Biopsy of Soft Tissue Tumors

9

J. Gielen, A. De Schepper

Contents

9.1 Introduction

Staging of soft tissue tumors frequently includes a biopsy that is mostly performed percutaneously using imaging guidance (ultrasound, computed tomography CT, or magnetic resonance imaging, MRI). A biopsy is necessary when the orthopedic surgeon and the radiologist believe they are dealing with a progressive process, requiring intervention [1]. Otherwise, unexpected manipulation of a soft tissue sarcoma (STS) can influence its biological behavior and prognosis [2]. Moreover, biopsy of soft tissue tumors with large needles involves a risk of seeding malignant cells along the needle track. Because biopsy is considered part of the surgical therapy, en bloc resection of tumor and needle track is usually needed [3].

9.2 Intracompartmental Compared with Extracompartmental Spread

Determination of whether the location and/or extension of a tumor is intracompartmental or extracompartmental is an important element in staging. Extracompartmental spread and inadvertent tumor spread can be due to a poorly planned biopsy [4]. If uninvolved anatomical compartments are crossed to obtain the biopsy specimen, the result may be a more radical resection or even amputation. Therefore, knowledge of compartmental anatomy is mandatory for planning and performance of a percutaneous needle biopsy [5, 6]. For treatment of the different compartments of the upper and lower extremities, the reader is referred to the excellent article of Anderson et al. [6], whose cross-sectional diagrams of the different compartments are reprinted here (Figs. 9.1–9.5).

Generally, skin and subcutaneous fat, bone, paraosseous spaces, and joint spaces are regarded as intracompartmental. For the upper extremity, the periclavicular region, axilla, antecubital fossa, wrist, and dorsum of the hand, and for the lower extremity the groin, popliteal fossa, ankle and dorsum of the foot are considered extracompartmental.

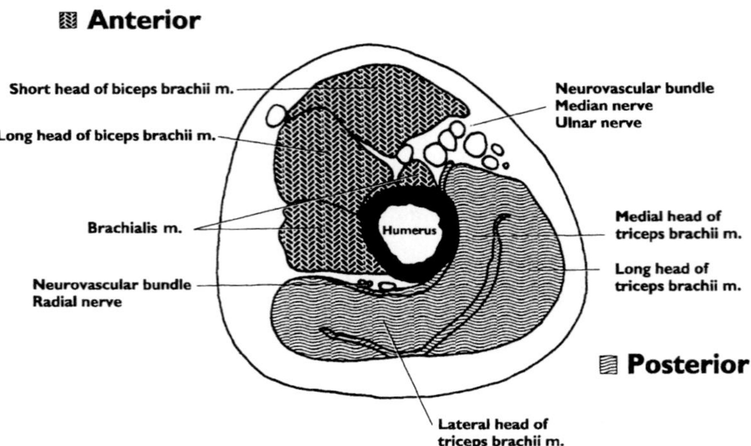

Fig. 9.1. Cross section of mid-upper arm shows contents of anterior and posterior compartments. (Reprinted from [6] with permission)

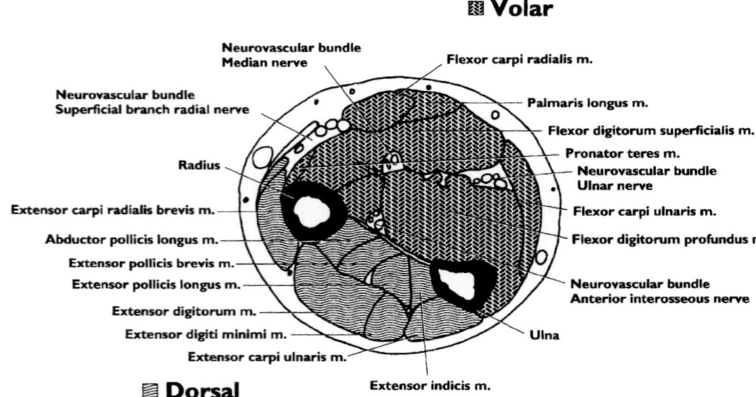

Fig. 9.2. Cross section of mid-forearm shows contents of volar and dorsal compartments. (Reprinted from [6] with permission)

Fig. 9.3 a–c. Cross section of thigh shows contents and relative positions of anterior, medial, and posterior compartments at these levels. **a** Proximal thigh; **b** mid-thigh; **c** distal thigh. (Reprinted from [6] with permission)

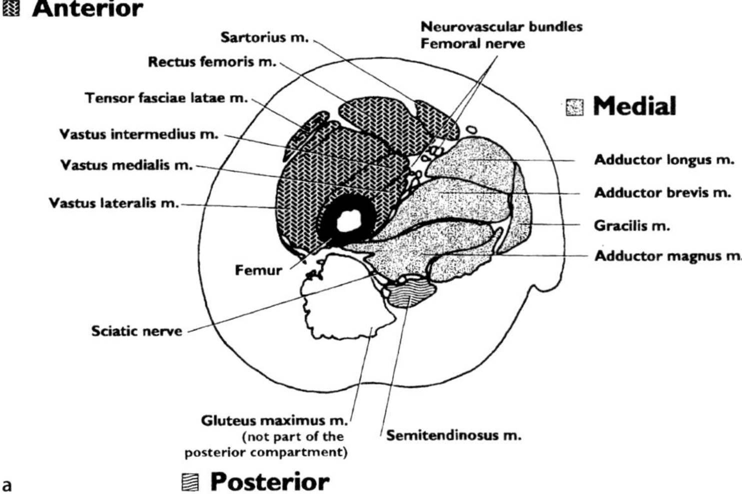

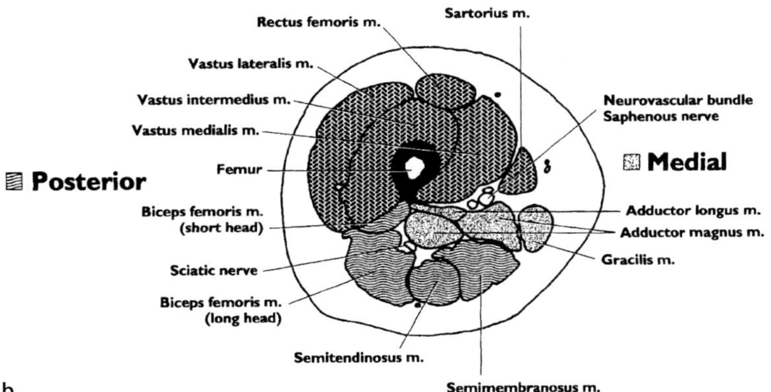

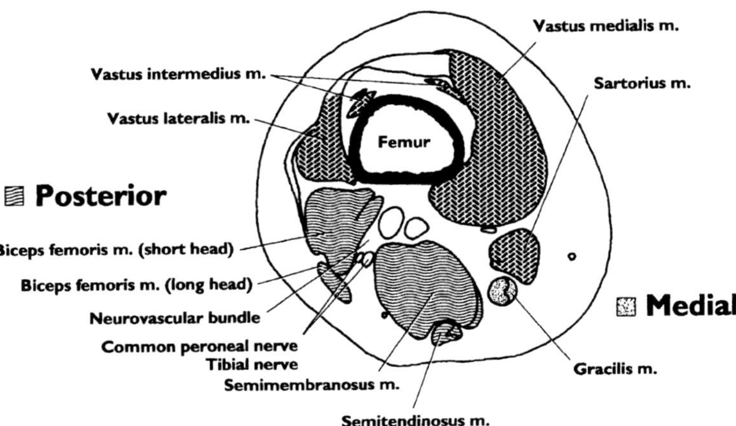

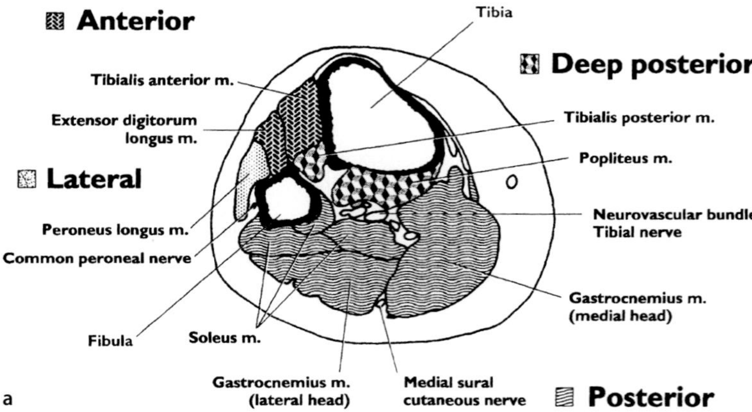

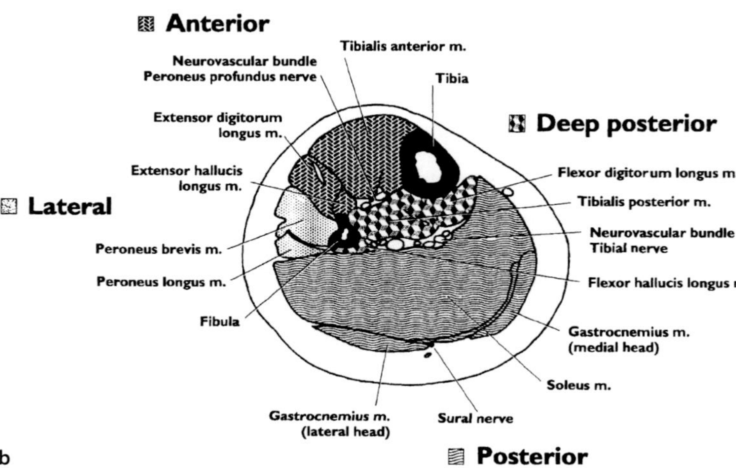

Fig. 9.4 a, b. Lower leg. Cross section of **a** proximal calf and **b** mid-calf show contents of anterior, deep posterior, posterior, and lateral compartments. (Reprinted from [6] with permission)

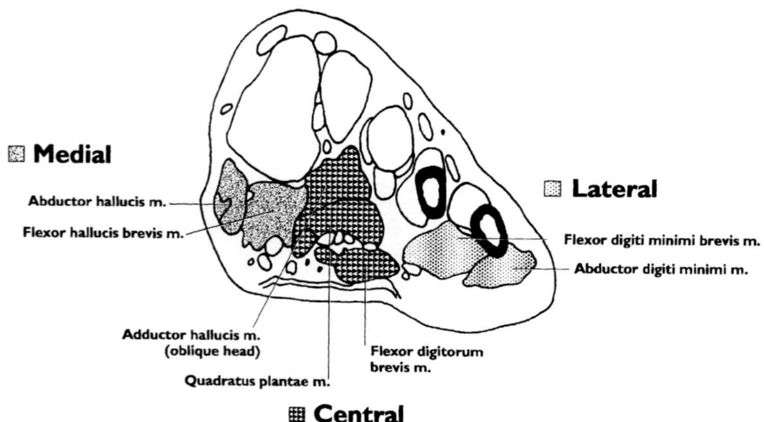

Fig. 9.5. Cross section of foot shows contents of medial, central, and lateral compartments. (Reprinted from [6] with permission)

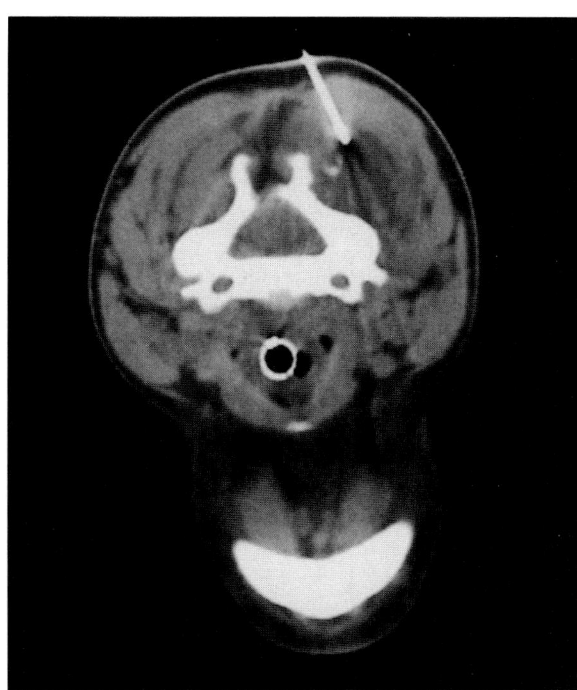

Fig. 9.6. Percutaneous core-needle biopsy, with CT guidance, of a deeply seated mass lesion with intralesional calcification. Histological examination revealed a myositis ossificans. Control examination after conservative therapy showed more typical, zonal calcification of the lesion

9.3 General Rules for Biopsy Safety

A CT scan is performed to localize the lesion precisely. Ultrasound may be used in superficial lesions. The entry point and the pathway are determined, avoiding nerve, vascular, and visceral structures (Figs. 9.6–9.7).

General principles for safe percutaneous biopsy:
1. The shortest path between skin and the lesion should be chosen.
2. The needle should not traverse an uninvolved compartment.
3. The joint or neurovascular bundle and the anticipated needle path should be discussed with the surgeon who will be performing the definitive surgery (Fig. 9.6).

9.4 Diagnostic Accuracy

Percutaneous musculoskeletal biopsy (PMSB) can be performed by fine-needle aspiration (FNAB), core-needle biopsy (CNB), or open (incisional) biopsy. Excisional biopsy should be used only for small lesions (less than 3 cm) or when the radiologist is convinced that the lesion is benign [7, 8].

Open surgical biopsy is advocated by Huvos [9], who claims that only an adequate amount of removed tissue will allow for a maximal diagnostic benefit.

Kilpatrick et al. [10] have used FNAB and obtained a histogenetically specific diagnosis in 93% of cases of pediatric bone and soft tissue tumors, all of which were correctly recognized as either benign or malignant. In adults fine-needle aspiration biopsy is recommended for diagnosis of tumors in the head and neck region [11] and whenever direct incisional biopsy is contraindicated [7, 12]. Gonzalez [12, 13] have reported a specificity of FNAB of more than 90%, the method being most effective when performed by an experienced pathologist. Agreement between FNAB histopathological and cytological grading in musculoskeletal sarcomas treated by FNAB has been studied by Jones et al. [14] Although a statistically significant correlation between cytologically assigned grade and final histo-pathological grade is found, statistical analysis reveals only a moderate correlation between the two, with an overall r value of approximately 0.57. Cytological analysis tends to undergrade in comparison with final histopathological grading. FNAB is moderately successful at predicting histopathological grading. Only analysis of nuclear atypia shows good correlation with final surgical grade [14].

Skrzynski et al. [15] have performed a prospective study on the value of closed CNB in 62 patients with soft tissue tumors or bone tumors with soft tissue extension. The diagnostic accuracy is 84% or 96%, respectively, for groups of patients who have undergone open biopsy performed by the same surgeon. Disadvantages include a nondiagnostic biopsy, indeterminate biopsy, and potential errors in histological grade. The hospital charges for a closed core biopsy are much less than those for an open biopsy! Comparable results are reported by Hodge [16], with a diagnostic accuracy of 76.9%.

Bennert [17] has evaluated the diagnostic yield of FNAB relative to that of CNB in 117 patients with soft tissue lesions. FNAB was unsatisfactory in 44 patients, 22 of whom were correctly diagnosed with CNB. The author's conclusion is that FNAB gives a yield identical to that of CNB and that unsatisfactory FNAB should prompt further evaluation by CNB.

Hau et al. [18] have studied the accuracy of CT-guided FNAB relative to CNB in a large number of patients (n=359) with musculoskeletal lesions. They found an overall accuracy of 71%, i.e., 63% for FNAB (n=101) and 74% for CNB (n=258). Biopsies of 81 pelvic lesions had a higher rate of diagnostic accuracy (81%) than nonpelvic sites (68%). The lowest accuracies (61% and 50%, respectively) have been noted in lesions of the spine and infectious diseases [18].

The best results have been reported by Dupuy et al. [19], who performed 176 CNB and 45 FNAB of musculoskeletal neoplasms under CT guidance. They obtained

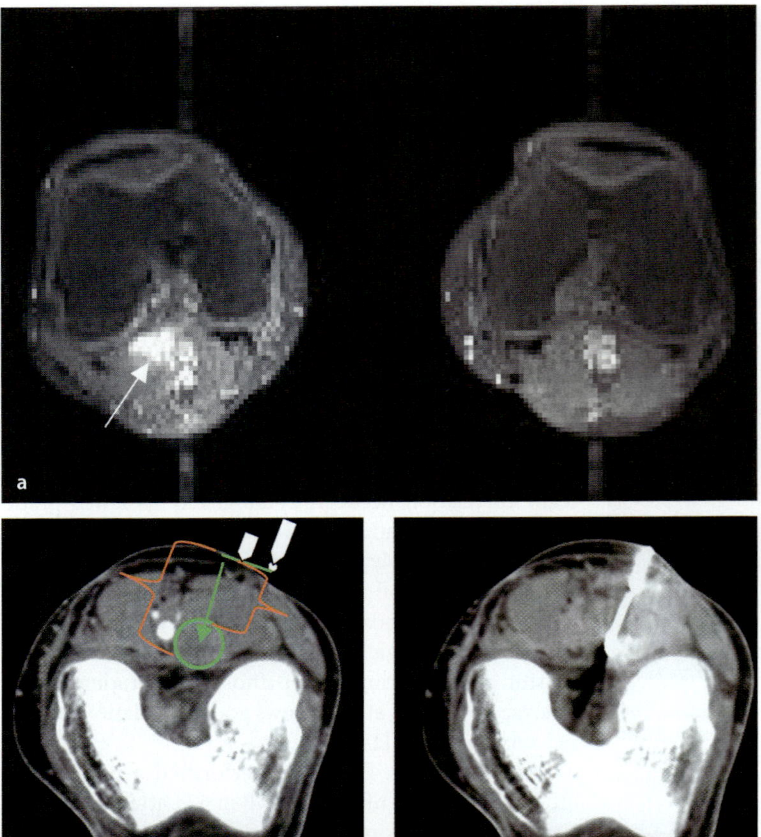

Fig. 9.7 a–c. Small, pigmented villonodular synovitis (PVNS) in a young female patient at the right popliteal space. **a** MRI of both knees in supine position, axial spin-echo T1-weighted image with fat suppression (FS) and after intravenous gadolinium-DTPA administration. A small, markedly enhancing mass lesion at the left popliteal space adjacent to the popliteal neurovascular structures is seen (*white arrow*). **b** Computed tomography of the left knee, axial plane in prone position with soft tissue window and level settings and after intravenous administration of iodinated contrast material. The nonenhancing, hypointense mass lesion is seen at the lateral aspect of the enhancing popliteal neurovascular bundle (*circle*). Entry point in relation to an external radioopaque marker is measured (*arrowheads*), biopsy pathway (*arrow*), and skin-to-lesion interval and skin to deepest margin of the lesion (*braces*) are determined. **c** Computed tomography of the left knee after insertion of biopsy needle, comparable axial plane, verification of needle position before cut

an accuracy of 93% for CNB and 80% for FNAB. Complication rate was less than 1%.

Ray-Coquard et al. have evaluated CNB in 110 STS patients. They found lower sensitivity in low-grade sarcomas (85%) than in high-grade sarcomas (100%). Histological grading on CNB seems hardly feasible, except for grade III tumors [21].

In cases of impalpable soft tissue tumors, a needle containing a hookwire with an overbent hook that springs open when protruded beyond the needle top and anchors the wire in the lesion is positioned under ultrasound guidance and will facilitate excisional biopsy [20]. As a consequence, diagnostic accuracy of PMSB is not only dependent on the specific sampling technique but also on the location and the ultimate histological diagnosis of the lesion [21].

9.5 Immunohistochemistry

Considerable progress has been made in the clinical and biological understanding of soft tissue sarcomas. This led to the launch of a new WHO classification of soft tissue tumors in 2002, which integrates morphological data with tumor-specific (cyto-)genetics. Worldwide consensus has grown on how to predict clinical behavior based on a specific grading system and which specific types of tumors seem not to obey these rules. Immunohistochemical characterization plays a key role in the diagnostic workup of STS. The determination line is crucial in order not only to ensure proper classification, but also to provide predictive information. The recent identification of tumor-specific drug targets by immunohistochemistry has had impact on specimen requirements and handling as well as laboratory standards [22]. Thus these new insights influence sampling technique. Tissue-sample fixation is adapted to permit immunohistochemical characterization. Acetic acid solutions are avoided because mitotic components are hardly visible after treatment with 70% acetic acid. Thus the formerly used technique with alcohol-formalin-acetic acid (AFA) fixation has been abandoned [23]. A buffered 4% dilution of formalin (NF4) is recommended for tissue samples (CNB), and an alcoholic solution (Saccomano) is used for cell samples (FNAB) [24, 25].

9.6 Technique and Choice of Needle

In STS not only cytology but also matrix, architectural structure, and immunohistochemistry may add to the pathological diagnostic clues. FNAB essentially obtains cells without revealing its tissue architecture or matrix. It is able to study cytonuclear disturbances but not tumor differentiation and matrix components. The pathologist is often only able to differentiate malignant from benign lesions [26, 27]. It gives good results in tumors at the soft tissues in patients with known adenocarcinoma or myeloma and lymphoma or if the MRI characteristics are suggestive for lymphoma. In bone lesions it gives also good results in cases of Langerhans cell histiocytosis, chondroblastoma, chordoma, and giant cell tumor [28].

CNB is able to provide tissue in which matrix is disclosed and the architectural structure may be preserved. It is evident that 14-gauge needles produce better results than 20-gauge needles. Open incisional or excisional biopsy also provides information of the reactive processes around the lesion. These latter techniques (CNB and open biopsy) show best diagnostic accuracy in cases of primary soft tissue tumors.

Moreover nonhomogeneity of tumors also may influence CNB technique. Highest-graded zones in a tumor predict outcome, lowest-graded zones are best differentiated, may produce matrix, and help to characterize lesions. As a consequence location of the biopsy trajectory in the lesion itself depends on its imaging characteristics. In homogeneous lesions, the trajectory is only determined according to its compartmental anatomy. Best results in nonhomogeneous lesions are gained if also the lesion's inner architecture is taken into account. If possible a single long trajectory which encompasses evolving segments with imaging characteristics of high grade, i.e., cellular or lytic parts avoiding necrotic parts and parts that produce more differentiated matrix (calcified). Two or more slightly angled trajectories that involve the same anatomical compartments may be necessary.

For these reasons, consensus is growing to centralize tissue sampling to dedicated centers and to prefer CNB over FNAB.

9.7 Conclusion

Although the choice of biopsy type largely depends on the particular clinical setting and the experience of the clinician, radiologist, orthopedic surgeon, and pathologist, CNB is recommended as the procedure of first choice for obtaining representative specimens of soft tissue tumors for histological and immunohistochemical examination because of its high diagnostic accuracy and low complication rate. It allows planning for single surgery or neoadjuvant chemotherapy when combined with appropriate imaging. Except for FNAB, it is less time-consuming, less painful, and cheaper than other procedures. It can be performed under CT or ultrasound guidance, CT being preferred for deep-seated lesions or those that are difficult to reach. There are only few reports of MR guidance. The entry point and the pathway are determined in cross talk with the managing surgeon, avoiding nerve, vascular, and visceral structures. Two or more slightly angled trajectories that involve the same anatomical compartments may be necessary in radiologically nonhomogeneous lesions. Tissue-sample fixation is adapted to permit immunohistochemical characterization. Open biopsy is mandatory if CNB is inadequate.

> **Things to remember:**
> 1. The shortest path between skin and the lesion should be chosen and the anticipated needle path should be discussed with the surgeon who will be performing the definitive surgery.
> 2. The needle should not traverse an uninvolved compartment.
> 3. Compared with FNAB, CNB is able to provide a tissue sample in which matrix is disclosed with preservation of the tumor's architectural structure.
> 4. Soft tissue tumors often are spatially heterogeneous with respect to tumor grade and characterization features, and tumor necrosis may be widespread. Thus two or more slightly angled biopsy trajectories may be necessary.
> 5. Tissue-sample fixation is adapted to permit immunohistochemical characterization. A buffered 4% dilution of formalin (NF4) is recommended for tissue samples (CNB), and an alcoholic solution (Saccomano) is used for cell samples (FNAB).

References

1. Peabody TD, Simon MA (1996) Making the diagnosis: keys to a successful biopsy in children with bone and soft-tissue tumors. Orthop Clin North Am 27(3):453–459
2. Van Geel AN, Van Unnik JA, Keus RB (1995) Consensus soft tissue tumors. Dutch Workgroup Soft-Tissue Tumors. Ned Tijdschr Geneeskd 139(6):833–837
3. Laredo JD (1999) Percutaneous biopsy of primary soft tissue tumors. Semin Musculoskeletal Radiol 3:139–144
4. Aboulafia AJ (1999) Biopsy. Instr Course Lect 48:587–590
5. Bickels J, Jelinek JS, Shmookler BM, Neff RS, Malawer MM (1999) Biopsy of musculoskeletal tumors. Current concepts. Clin Orthop 368:212–219
6. Anderson MW, Temple HT, Dussault RG, Kaplan PA (1999) Compartmental anatomy: relevance to staging and biopsy of musculoskeletal tumors. AJR Am J Roentgenol 173:1663–1671
7. Frassica FJ, McCarthy EF, Bluemke DA (2000) Soft-tissue masses: when and how to biopsy. Instr Course Lect 49:437–442
8. Iwamoto Y (1999) Diagnosis and treatment of soft tissue tumors. J Orthop Sci 4(1):54–65

9. Huvos AG (1995) The importance of the open surgical biopsy in the diagnosis and treatment of bone and soft-tissue tumors. Hematol Oncol Clin North Am 9(3):541–544

10. Kilpatrick SE, Ward WG, Chauvenet AR, Pettenati MJ (1998) The role of fine-needle aspiration biopsy in the initial diagnosis of pediatric bone and soft tissue tumors: an institutional experience. Mod Pathol 11(10):923–928

11. Skoog L, Pereira ST, Tani E (1999) Fine-needle aspiration cytology and immunocytochemistry of soft-tissue tumors and osteo/chondrosarcomas of the head and neck. Diagn Cytopathol 20(3):131–136

12. Gonzalez Campora R (2000) Fine needle aspiration cytology of soft tissue tumors. Acta Cytol 44(3):337–343

13. Gonzalez Campora R, Munoz Arias G, Otal Salaverri C et al (1992) Fine needle aspiration cytology of primary soft tissue tumors. Morphologic analysis of the most frequent types. Acta Cytol 36(6):905–917

14. Jones C, Liu K, Hirschowigz S, Klipfel N, LayfieldLJ (2002) Concordance of histopahtologic and cytologic grading in musculoskeletal sarcomas: can grades obtained from analysis by the fine-needle aspirates serve as the basis for therapeutic decisions? Cancer 96(2):83–91

15. Skrzynski MC, Biermann JS, Montag A, Simon MA (1996) Diagnostic accuracy and charge-savings of outpatient core needle biopsy compared with open biopsy of musculoskeletal tumors. J Bone Joint Surg Am 78(5):644–649

16. Hodge JC (1999) Percutaneous biopsy of the musculoskeletal system : a review of 77 cases. Can Assoc Radiol J 50(2):121–125

17. Bennert KW, Abdul Karim FW (1994) Fine needle aspiration cytology vs. needle core biopsy of soft tissue tumors. A comparison. Acta Cytol 38(3):381–384

18. Hau MA, Kim JI, Kattapuram S, Hornicek FJ, Rosenberg AE, Gebhardt MC, Mankin HJ (2002) Accuracy of CT-guided biopsies in 359 patients with musculoskeletal lesions. Skeletal Radiol 31:349–353

19. Dupuy DE, Rosenberg AE, Punyaratabandhu T, Tan MH, Mankin HJ (1998) Accuracy of CT-guided needle biopsy of musculoskeletal neoplasms. Am J Roentgenol 171(3):759–762

20. Rutten MJ, Schreurs BW, van Kampen A, Schreuder HW (1997) Excisional biopsy of impalpable soft tissue tumors. US-guided preoperative localization in 12 cases. Acta Orthop Scand 68(4):384–386

21. Ray-Coquard I, Ranchere-Vince D, Thiesse P, Ghesquieres H, Biron P, Sunyach MP, Rivoire M, Lancry L, Meeus P, Sebban C, Blay JY (2003) Evaluation of core needle biopsy as a substitute to open biopsy in the diagnosis of soft-tissue masses. Eur J Cancer 39(14):2021–2025

22. Hogendoorn PCW, Collin F, Daugaard S, Dei Tos PA, Fisher C, Schneider U, Sciot R/Pathology and Biology Subcommittee of the EORTC Soft Tissue and Bone Sarcoma Group (2004) Changing concepts in the pathological basis of soft tissue and bone sarcoma treatment. Eur J Cancer 40(11):1644–1654

23. Bettio D, Rizzi N, Colombo P, Bianchi P, Gaetani P (2004) Unusual cytogenetic findings in a synovial sarcoma arising in the paranasal sinuses. Cancer Genet Cytogenet 155(1):79–81

24. Werner M, Chott A, Fabiano A, Battifora H (2000) Effect of formalin tissue fixation and processing on immunohistochemistry. Am J Surg Pathol 24(7):1016–1019

25. Kurtycz DF, Logrono R, Leopando M, Slattery A, Inhorn SL (1997) Immunocytochemistry controls using cell culture. Diagn Cytopathol 17(1):74–79

26. Amin MS, Luqman M, Jamal S, Mamoon N, Anwar M (2003) Fine needle aspiration biopsy of soft tissue tumors. J Coll Physicians Surg Pak 13(11):625–628

27. Nagira K, Yamamoto T, Akisue T, Marui T, Hitora T, Nakatani T, Kurosaka M; Ohbayashi C (2002) Reliability of fine-needle aspiration biopsy in the initial diagnosis of soft-tissue lesions. Diagn Cytopathol 27(6):354–361

28. Gangi A, Guth S, Dietemann J-L, Roy C (2001). Interv Musculoskeletal Procedures Radiographics 21:E1-e1 (online only)

Part 2
Staging, Grading, and Tissue Specific Diagnosis

Staging

S.M. Levine, R.M. Terek, T.J. Hough, G.A. Tung

10

Contents

10.1 Staging Rationale

Staging of a neoplasm refers to the clinical, radiological, and pathological evaluation of local extent and distant spread. Medical imaging has assu0med an increasingly important role in the staging of the known or suspected neoplasm because of the relative insensitivity of the physical examination. Staging serves several important roles in the optimal management of the patient with a soft tissue tumor. The stage of the tumor gives a prognosis for the patient and guides treatment. The staging variables that can be assessed by imaging modalities are size and location of the primary tumor and presence or absence of metastatic disease. Staging of local extent is used by the oncology surgeon or interventional radiologist to plan the optimal approach to biopsy, the tissues that need to be removed for the definitive resection, and in some cases the field for radiation therapy. For soft tissue malignancies, distant metastases confers a particularly poor prognosis for long-term survival and usually indicates the need for systemic chemotherapy and metastasectomy. Finally, staging systems permit medical personnel to communicate meaningfully with one another about a disease and its prognosis. This facilitates the understanding of the natural history of a disease as well as the design of clinical trials. For these reasons, it is essential to appreciate the implications of inaccurate staging.

The accuracy of a staging procedure is determined by both its sensitivity and specificity. A sensitive test is one which has a low false-negative value. Therefore, an insensitive test is one which underestimates the extent of disease. If a staging examination for local or regional disease is insensitive, surgery or local radiation may leave residual tumor and this may compromise the chance for long-term, disease-free survival. In addition, residual tumor may be misinterpreted at a later date as recurrent disease and thereby create a false impression of local treatment failure. A test with high specificity has a relatively low false-positive value and thus a nonspecific staging test would tend to overestimate the extent of disease. This could result in unnecessary morbidity for the patient due to overly aggressive therapy. Thus there are consequential penalties of an inaccurate staging examination, and it is important for the diagnostic radiologist to understand the operational characteristics of the test that is chosen for staging.

Staging studies may be repeated several times in the course of managing a patient with a soft tissue tumor. Initial imaging of a deep soft tissue mass and larger superficial masses should be performed before the biopsy. One of the common errors in the management of suspected soft tissue neoplasm is to perform a biopsy before the assessment of local disease. Hematoma, reactive changes, and edema distort the appearance of a soft tissue mass after biopsy and can reduce the specificity of an imaging test performed subsequently for local staging [34, 58] (Fig. 10.1). It is imperative that an evaluation of local extent be completed before biopsy for this reason. In addition, imaging may be used to plan the type and approach of the biopsy. Restaging of local disease or surveillance for local recurrence is performed after neoadjuvant chemotherapy, surgery, and periodically thereafter. Monitoring for development of metastatic disease is performed with chest radiographs and chest CT scanning.

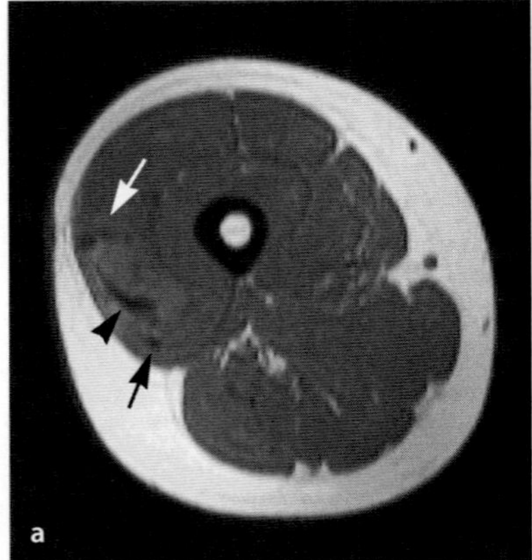
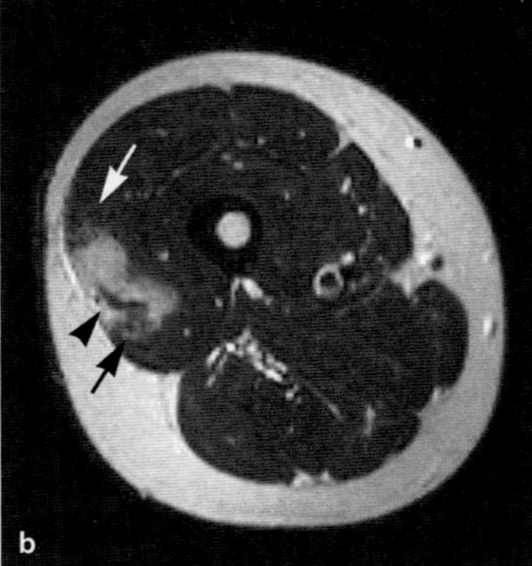
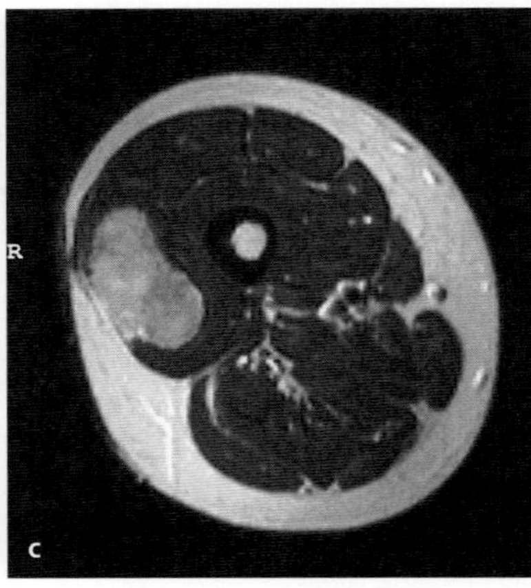

Fig. 10.1a-c Distorted tissue planes 3 months after a false-negative open biopsy. **a** Axial spin-echo (SE) T1-weighted MR image. **b, c** Axial turbo SE T2-WI (WI). Presence of a soft tissue mass in the vastus lateralis muscle. Nodular (*arrow*) and linear (*arrowhead*) hypointense areas that are consistent with chronic blood products at the site of an open biopsy (**a, b**). In contrast to a part of the tumor which had not been biopsied (**c**), these biopsy-related changes distort the margins of the tumor. Pathological diagnosis: alveolar soft part sarcoma

10.2 Staging Systems for Soft Tissue Sarcoma

The most well accepted staging system for soft tissue sarcoma is the American Joint Commission on Cancer (AJCC) system (Table 10.1). Others are summarized in Tables 10.2–10.4. All of these staging schemes are based on evaluation of tumor grade, local extent, and distant metastases [1, 28].

The single variable which best predicts the likelihood of local recurrence after surgery, development of distant metastases, and long-term survival is tumor grade [25]. In the AJCC system, histopathological grade is stratified into good (G1), moderate (G2), poor (G3), and undifferentiated (G4). Operationally G1 and G2 are combined, as are G3 and G4, so that grade is distilled down to low and high grade. In the other staging systems, a neoplasm is graded as low grade (G1) or high grade (G2). This pathological assessment is based on features such as cellular atypia and pleomorphism, cellularity, infiltration, frequency of mitoses, presence of necrosis, matrix immaturity, and vascularity [16]. The specific histopathological type of tumor does not seem to influence prognosis except as it relates to tumor grade.

In addition to pathological grade, the "T" stage of a tumor is defined by its local extent and size. The size of the neoplasm is represented in the T stage of the AJCC, Memorial Sloan-Kettering Cancer Center (MSKCC), and Hajdu systems [28]. Tumor size is a continuum. Patients with large tumors have the worst prognoses. Tumors are arbitrarily grouped into greater or less than a diameter of 5 cm [25]. In the Musculoskeletal Tumor Society (MSTS) staging system, the size of the tumor is only an indirect variable. Tumors are grouped into "intracompartmental" and "extracompartmental." Larger tumors tend to be extracompartmental; however, small tumors arising in sites such as the popliteal fossa are also extracompartmental. The MSTS system has been found to be less useful than the other systems [67]. Another variable which has come out of multivariate analysis of tumor variables is location relative to the in-

Table 10.1. American Joint Commission on Cancer (AJCC) staging system for soft tissue malignancy [1]

Stage	Grade	Tumor	Node	Metastases
IA	1–2	1a-b	0	0
IB	1–2	2a	0	0
IIA	1–2	2b	0	0
IIB	3–4	1a-b	0	0
IIC	3–4	2a	0	0
III	3–4	2b	0	0
IV	Any	Any	0	1
IV	Any	Any	1	0

Grade (G):
- G1   Well differentiated
- G2   Moderately differentiated
- G3   Poorly differentiated
- G4   Undifferentiated

Tumor (T):
- T1   Diameter ≤5 cm
  - T1a   Superficial tumor
  - T1b   Deep tumor
- T2   Diameter >5 cm
  - T2a   Superficial tumor
  - T2b   Deep tumor

Node (N):
- N0   No regional lymph node involvement
- N1   Histopathological lymph node involvement

Metastases (M):
- M0   No evidence of metastases
- M1   Distant metastases

Table 10.2. Musculoskeletal Tumor Society/Enneking staging system for malignant musculoskeletal lesions [28]

Stage	Grade	Site	Metastases
IA	1	1	0
IB	1	2	0
IIA	2	1	0
IIB	2	2	0
III	1 or 2	1 or 2	1

Grade (G):
   G0   Benign
   G1   Low-grade malignant
   G2   High-grade malignant

Site (T):
   T1   Intracompartmental
   T2   Extracompartmental

Metastases:
   M0   No evidence of regional or distant metastases
   M1   Regional or distant metastases

Table 10.3 Memorial Sloan-Kettering Cancer Center staging scheme [28]

Stage	Grade	Site	Size (cm)
0	1	Sp	<5
1	1	Dp	<5
1	1	Sp	>5
1	2	Sp	<5
2	1	Dp	>5
2	2	Dp	<5
2	2	Dp	<5
III	2	Dp	>5

Criteria:

Grade:
   1   Low histopathological grade
   2   High histopathological grade
Site:
   Sp   Superficial
   Dp   Deep to fascia

Size: the maximum diameter of the lesion in centimeters

Table 10.4. Hajdu staging system [30]

	Grade	Size	Depth
Favorable	Low	<5 cm	Superficial[a]
Unfavorable	High	>5 cm	Deep

Stage:

0	All three favorable signs are present
I	Two favorable signs; one unfavorable sign
II	One favorable sign and two unfavorable signs
III	All three unfavorable signs are present
IV	Regional lymph node or distant metastases

[a] Location relative to muscle fascia

vesting fascia. Deep tumors, those that arise deep to the muscle fascia, are assigned a higher stage in the AJCC, MSKCC, and Hajdu systems [29]. The accurate determination of tumor extent is important not only for staging, but also for presurgical planning. The primary determinants of the surgical margins and the type of local treatment are the anatomical location of the tumor, and the proximity of the tumor to bone, joint, and neurovascular structures.

Metastases can either be to lymph nodes (N) or other sites (M). The presence of any type of metastases results in a stage IV tumor. Hematogenous spread to the lung parenchyma may be seen in approximately 10% of musculoskeletal neoplasms at the time of diagnosis [50] and occurs in approximately 50% of the highest-risk tumors: large, deep, and high grade. Eighty percent of delayed metastases occur within 2 years of diagnosis.

10.2.1 Staging System for Rhabdomyosarcoma

The most common pediatric soft-tissue sarcoma is rhabdomyosarcoma. In addition to the variables discussed above, resectability, anatomical location, and histological subtype are important prognostic factors. In general, extremity tumors and the alveolar histological type have a more grave prognosis than genitourinary and head and neck tumors or nonalveolar histological types of rhabdomyosarcoma [31, 32]. Regional lymph node metastases and distant metastases advance the stage of rhabdomyosarcoma in all systems [45].

10.3 Imaging of the Primary Tumor

The variables in staging the local extent of a tumor include:
1. Tumor size
2. Confinement to or extension beyond the anatomical compartment of origin
3. Location relative to the deep fascia

The four most commonly used staging systems place slightly different emphasis on each of these T staging criteria. The AJCC, MSKCC, and Hajdu systems utilize size and depth, whereas the MSTS staging system is more surgically oriented, placing particular emphasis on whether the tumor extends beyond the anatomical compartment of origin or both. A brief discussion of the pathological and anatomical basis of compartments and tumor growth is warranted (see also Chap 9).

Soft tissue neoplasms of the extremities tend to grow along anatomical paths of least resistance. They preferentially extend longitudinally within soft tissues rather than transversely through the fascial septa [14] (Fig. 10.2). A tumor is considered "intracompartmen-

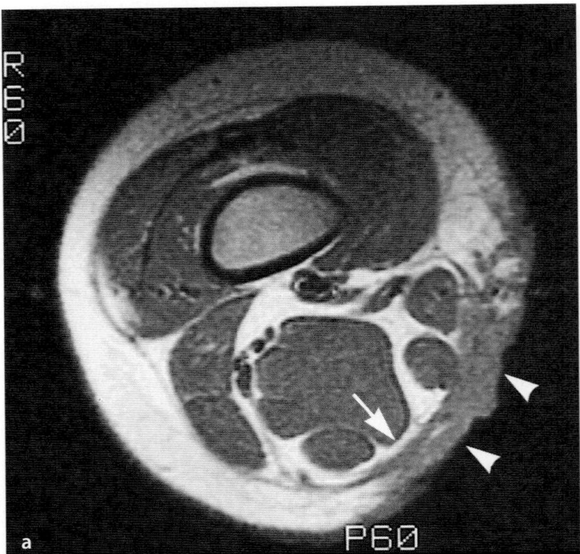
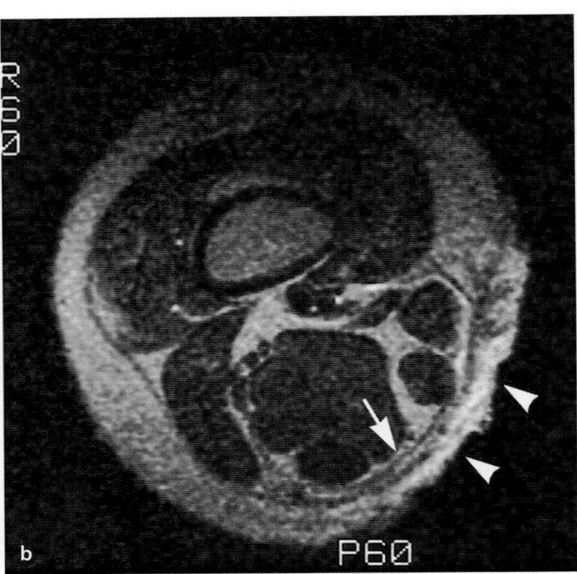

Fig. 10.2 a, b. Superficial, infiltrative growth pattern of tumor arising from the subcutaneous compartment. **a** Axial SE T1-weighted MR image. **b** Axial SE T2-weighted MR image. Both images show a cutaneous ulcer (*arrowheads*) associated with an infiltrative lesion (**a, b**). Although there is thickening of the fascia (*arrow*), the tumor grows circumferentially and longitudinally without invading the muscular compartment of the lower thigh. Pathological diagnosis: fibrous histiocytoma

tal" if the outermost margin is bounded by natural anatomical barriers. Such barriers include cortical bone, articular cartilage, joint capsule, fascial septa, tendon, and ligament. The boundaries of the compartment may be *distorted* by a tumor that is still considered intracompartmental. An extracompartmental tumor can arise de novo or result from direct extension from an intracompartmental lesion. Tumors are still considered intracompartmental even if they invade more than one muscle within a muscular compartment, the best example being the anterior compartment of the thigh. The relationship of the soft tissue tumor and the superficial fascia may help characterize the mass. Malignant subcutaneous tumors tend to either cross or form obtuse angles with the superficial fascia compared with benign neoplasms [24]. Finally, the skin and subcutaneous tissues are considered to be a single compartment which is bounded transversely by the deep fascia [13] (Fig. 10.2). There is no longitudinal boundary to the superficial compartment.

As the tumor grows, a peripheral zone of reactive tissue containing chronic inflammatory cells, proliferating mesenchymal cells, and capillaries forms. As this reactive zone is compressed and fibrous tissue matures, a pseudocapsule develops around the tumor. Low-grade tumors tend to form thin, mature fibrous pseudocapsules, whereas high-grade tumors incite more vascular and edematous reactive zones, making differentiation >from adjacent normal tissue difficult. If the *reactive zone* extends beyond the compartment, a tumor is considered "extracompartmental" even if the tumor itself is

confined to the compartment [13, 14]. On the other hand, some high-grade sarcomas can appear to have a distinct capsule and not have surrounding edema, so that a well-marginated mass on MR images does not confer benignity.

Thus, by the MSTS staging system, A T1 lesion is contained within a compartment. A T2 tumor is extracompartmental. The crucial factors in planning definitive surgery, and specifically the type of surgical margin, are the anatomical compartments involved, encasement of the adjacent major neurovascular bundle, and invasion of cortical bone.

There are four possible oncological surgical margins: intralesional, marginal, wide, and radical. An intralesional margin leaves behind gross tumor at the surgical margin. With a "marginal" surgical margin, the plane of dissection is extracapsular but within the reactive zone and therefore leaves microscopic disease in the surgical bed. A "wide" margin includes a rim of normal tissue around the specimen, which contains the tumor in toto. Finally, a "radical" margin includes the entire compartment containing the tumor.

These four types of surgical margins can be used to describe both limb-salvage surgery and amputation. Thus, there are eight possible surgical procedures, as Enneking has described [13]. Radical margins are no longer ordinarily performed for soft tissue sarcoma. Accurate preoperative staging is essential to planning the most appropriate surgical procedure.

The main radiological objectives in the preoperative T staging of soft tissue neoplasms are:

1. To distinguish abnormal from normal tissue for biopsy planning
2. To define precisely the anatomical extent for the planning of definitive surgery and radiation.

It is important to reiterate that it is imperative to complete the imaging evaluation of local extent *prior* to biopsy of a suspected neoplasm. A poorly executed biopsy may preclude a limb-salvage procedure, since the biopsy tract is usually removed with the surgical specimen. The radiological arsenal is extensive; however, MRI has clearly emerged as the single most valuable imaging modality in determining the locoregional extent of disease. Other imaging modalities supplement MRI and are occasionally useful in the evaluation of local disease. These examinations include CT, plain film radiography, ultrasound, angiography, and nuclear medicine studies.

10.3.1 Magnetic Resonance Imaging

MRI is now the preferred modality for the evaluation of soft tissue tumors. The salient advantages of MRI over other imaging modalities for local staging of soft tissue tumors are direct multiplanar imaging capability and unequaled soft tissue contrast. High soft tissue contrast enables tumor detection. The MRI examination is tailored to the individual patient and requires the proper selection of multiple imaging parameters. These include the choice of the appropriate coil, scan plane, pulse sequence, and use of contrast. In general, a surface coil is used for all soft tissue tumors of the extremities. Images are obtained in the transverse (axial) plane and at least one longitudinal plane for optimal definition of extent. It is essential that the entire cephalocaudal extent of the tumor be imaged and that the nearest joint be included in a long-axis scan (Fig. 10.3).

For optimal detection, the lesion must have a significantly different signal intensity from surrounding normal tissue and from noise. The goal in selecting the appropriate pulse sequence is to maximize tumor conspicuity, by increasing signal-intensity contrast between the tumor and normal tissue. For the detection and staging of a soft tissue mass, several pulse sequences are utilized: spin-echo T1-weighted, spin-echo T2-weighted, or fast spin-echo T2-weighted with fat saturation, short-tau inversion recovery (STIR) and contrast-enhanced spin-echo T1-weighted or gradient echo. Pre-gadolinium (Gd) contrast spin-echo T1-weighted images with fat suppression have been shown to improve tumor conspicuity as well as improve characterization of fibrous and hemosiderotic parts from cellular components of lesions [26]. Therefore, this sequence should be part of the standard imaging protocol. Shuman et al. have compared STIR and spin-echo sequences for the

detection of 26 malignant and 19 benign musculoskeletal neoplasms [57]. Although the sensitivity of T2-weighted spin-echo is not significantly less than that of STIR, 78% of the lesions were more conspicuous on STIR images. For lesion conspicuity, the advantages of STIR are due to the additive effect of long T1 and T2 relaxation on tissue signal intensity and the inherent nulling of fat signal [63]. However, both tumor and associated reactive changes such as edema and inflammation can prolong T1 and T2 relaxation times. Consequently, the volume of abnormal signal is twice as large on STIR images for one-third of lesions and similar for the remainder. Histological *sampling* of tissue where the discrepant signal abnormality is more extensive on STIR images has identified tumor in 25% and edema without tumor in 75% of cases [57]. Mirowitz et al. have compared the conspicuousness of bone marrow lesions using T1-weighted, fast spin-echo T2-weighted, and STIR images [42]. It has been concluded that all sequences provide a high sensitivity for depiction of bone marrow lesions. While MR is the optimal modality for soft tissue tumor detection and staging, its ability to accurately characterize masses and suggest a tissue-specific diagnosis remains controversial [4, 8, 35].

The role of Gd contrast in the evaluation of soft tissue tumors also is controversial. Conventional and dynamic contrast-enhanced imaging has been utilized. Typically, contrast agents enhance the signal intensity on T1-weighted spin-echo MR images of many tumors. The use of Gd-enhanced MRI has been investigated for lesion detection and for identification of nonnecrotic tissue. Erlemann et al. have found that static Gd-enhanced T1-weighted images show improved tumor-muscle contrast when compared with native T1-weighted images [19]. However, lesion conspicuity is superior on native T2-weighted images [53]. Benedikt et al. have concluded that contrast-enhanced MRI has not been shown to increase lesion conspicuity, nor does it replace conventional T2-weighted imaging [3, 36]. Necrosis within a lesion has a high (97%) positive predictive value in predicting malignancy; however, necrosis can occasionally be seen in benign lesions [12] (Fig. 10.3). Also, non-necrotic cystic areas within a tumor can mimic tumor necrosis. Static, enhanced images have also been shown to aid in distinguishing tumor necrosis from viable tumor with areas of necrosis showing virtually no enhancement [12]. However, myxoid lesions and hyaline cartilage lesions may show little enhancement and may mimic cysts or lesions with cystic components. It has been suggested that ultrasound is more reliable than MRI in differentiating solid and cystic lesions [36]. Another potentially valuable use of Gd-enhanced imaging includes evaluation of hematomas. Gd may reveal small nodules of tumor within thrombus or necrosis on conventional imaging. Cystic or necrotic areas within solid tumor do not enhance. Conventional T2-weighted

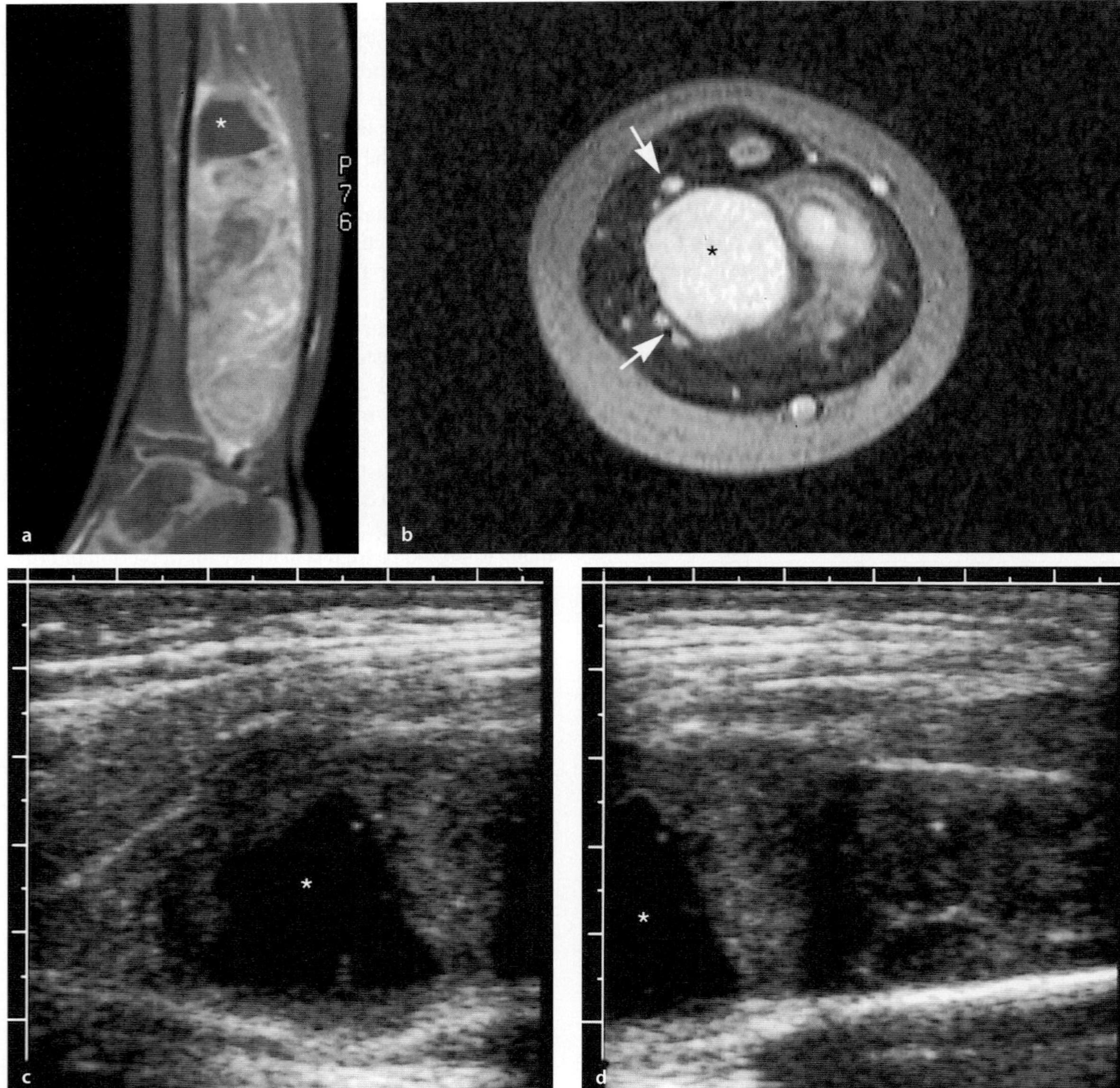

Fig. 10.3 a-d Local tumor extent on MR and ultrasound images. **a** Sagittal, fat-suppressed T1-weighted MR image. **b** Axial TSE T2-weighted MR image. **c, d** Contiguous sagittal ultrasound scans. Delineation of the cephalocaudal extent of the tumor as well as its proximity to the tibial cortex and the tibiotalar joint is shown on the sagittal image (**a**). Areas of abnormal enhancement in the tibial marrow are consistent with nests of tumor. A large necrotic area of the tumor (*asterisk*) does not enhance. Displacement of the anterior and posterior tibial neurovascular bundles (*arrows*) is seen on the axial T2-WI (**b**). Contiguous sagittal images from an ultrasound examination (**c, d**) show the mass and the necrotic area (*asterisk*) but, when compared with MRI, tissue contrast is poorer and the relationship of the tumor to the tibia cannot be determined. Using a hand-held transducer, the field of view of ultrasound is also a limitation for local staging. Pathological diagnosis: rhabdomyosarcoma

images may not make this distinction when both tumor and fluid show increased signal intensity, well-circumscribed margins, and homogeneous signal intensity [36].

Dynamic contrast-enhanced MRI has been investigated for distinguishing benign from malignant soft tissue masses [17, 21]. These studies have shown that both malignant and benign aggressive tumors enhance more rapidly than less aggressive lesions and peritumoral edema. However, the accurate distinction between tumor and edema is possibly of little clinical value, since edema is considered part of the reactive zone surrounding the neoplasm and is therefore removed en bloc with the tumor [36, 41]. Since enhancement is a reflection of both tissue vascularity and perfusion, generally speaking, malignant tumors have a greater rate of enhancement than benign lesions. However, the overlap between

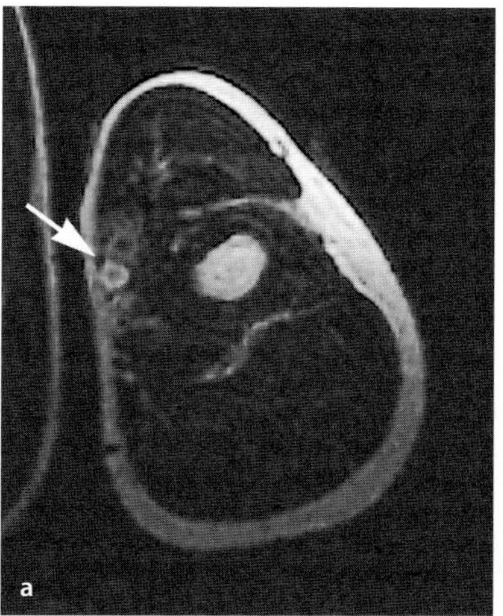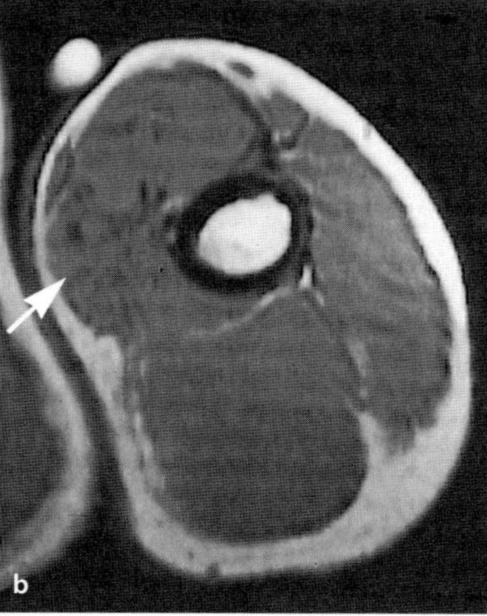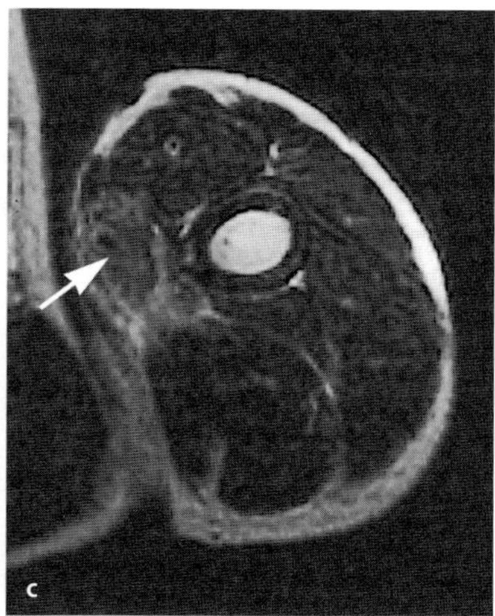

Fig. 10.4 a-c Neurovascular encasement. **a** Axial TSE T2-weighted MR image. **b** Axial SE T1-weighted MR image at a more cephalad level. **c** Axial TSE T2-weighted MR image at a more cephalad level. The normal brachial artery and vein (*arrow*) can be identified on a T2-WI at the level of the mid-humerus (**a**). At a more cephalad level, the neurovascular bundle is encased by a soft tissue mass that is isointense compared with normal muscle on a T1-WI (**b**) and slightly hyperintense relative to muscle (*arrow*) on a T2-WI (**c**). Pathological diagnosis: granular cell tumor

benign and malignant is great enough that the difference is of little practical value [36, 43]. Dynamic contrast-enhanced MRI has also been studied to evaluate tumor response to chemotherapy [18, 22]. These studies show a high correlation between the histological response and enhancement slopes (percentage of increase in signal intensity per minute) postchemotherapy and no correlation with tumor size.

In conclusion, Gd-enhanced MRI may be valuable in distinguishing vascularized and, by extension, viable areas of tumor >from those that are necrotic. This is important when selecting an optimal site to biopsy. Gd enhancement may also play a role in evaluating hematomas and assessing response to chemotherapy. Its role in the evaluation of tumor recurrence will be discussed in Chap 28 (MRI in the Follow-up of Malignant and Aggressive Soft Tissue Tumors). In terms of defining lesion margin, however, contrast-enhanced MRI does not increase lesion conspicuity compared with STIR, spin-echo T2-weighted, or fast spin-echo T2-weighted with fat-saturation sequences. Likewise, it has not been shown to increase the diagnostic specificity of MRI and hence does not differentiate benign from malignant lesions.

The location of a tumor relative to major neurovascular structures can be assessed accurately with MRI. A soft tissue tumor may either abut, displace, or encase a major neurovascular bundle. Demas et al. have found MRI to be highly accurate in defining the extent of bone and soft tissue tumor relative to the neurovascular bundle [11]. However, *adherence* of tumor to the neurovascular bundle cannot be predicted preoperatively unless there is encasement. Encasement of the neurovascular sheath necessitates its removal if definitive surgery is attempted with a wide surgical margin (Fig. 10.4). If the neurovascular bundle is abutting or being displaced by the mass, the oncology surgeon may attempt to spare the neurovascular bundle with a marginal surgical margin (Fig. 10.3).

More recently, the role of magnetic resonance angiography (MRA) in preoperative staging has been assessed. Swan et al. have compared conventional angiography with two-dimensional (2D) time-of-flight and phase-contrast MRA in the preoperative evaluation of 23 musculoskeletal neoplasms [61]. MRA is adequate for delineating the major vascular structures in the tumor bed but is inaccurate for assessing feeder vessels and tumor neovascularity compared with conventional angiography. In this study the failure of MRA to identify a secondary vessel as branch feeder was linked to its inability to detect a neovascular blush. A more recent study by Lang et al. has concluded that standard projection MRI and 3D reconstructions of raw angiographic MRI data provide adequate visualization of tumor neovascularity and peripheral vascular branches in the presurgical evaluation of primary bone tumors [39] (Fig. 10.5).

The destruction of cortical bone and the invasion of bone marrow by a soft tissue malignancy can be evaluated by MRI. The sensitivity of MRI for detecting cortical erosion by an adjacent soft tissue mass is debated. Some hold that CT is superior to MRI for depicting cortical destruction, whereas others believe MRI is comparable [9]. MRI is superior to CT for staging the intramedullary extent of tumor [66]. Where conversion to fatty marrow is complete, normal yellow bone marrow

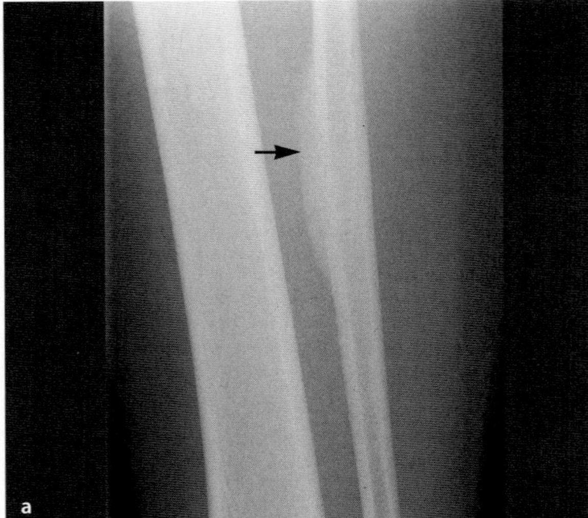

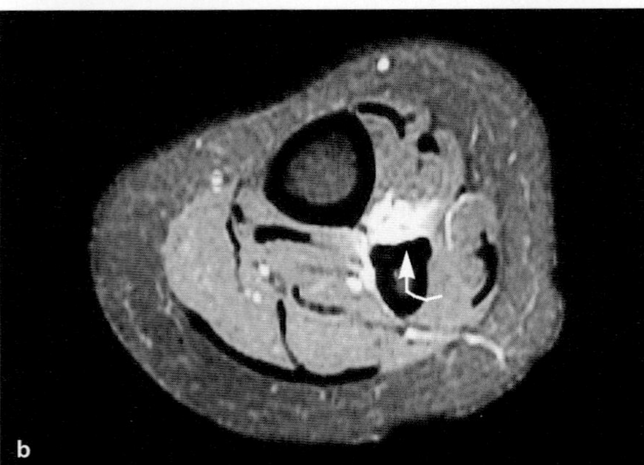

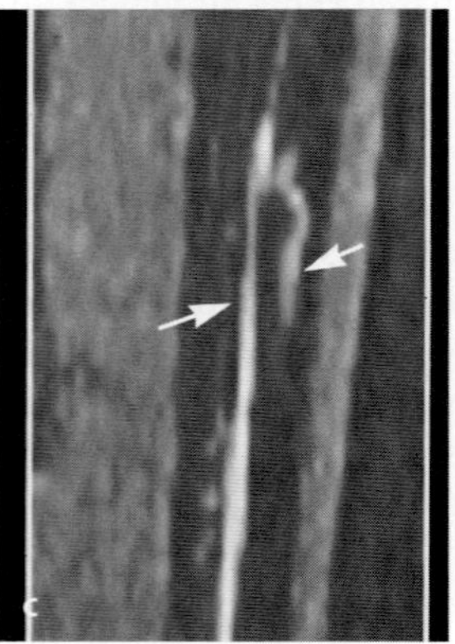

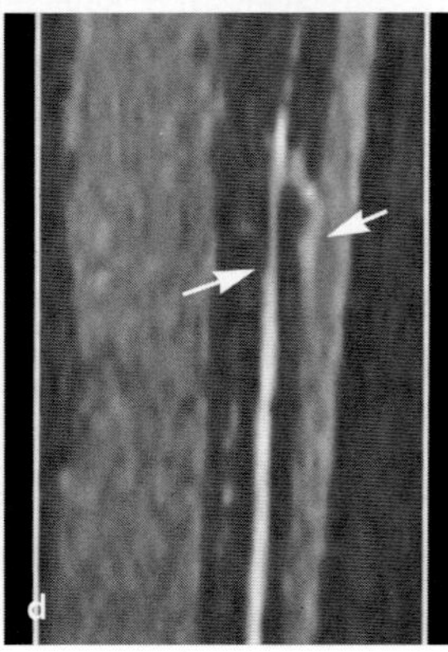

Fig. 10.5 a-d Feeding arterial vessel demonstrated on MR angiography. **a** Plain radiograph. **b** Axial SE T1-weighted MR image. **c, d** MR angiograms. In a patient with leg pain, the plain film demonstrates focal, thick periostitis (*arrow*) of the mid-fibula (**a**). T1-WI after contrast administration and with fat saturation demonstrates homogeneous, intense enhancement of a mass with lobulated margins. The mass abuts the fibula at the site of the periosteal reaction (*curved arrow*) (**b**). Projection MR angiograms show a small vessel (*arrow*) from the anterior tibial artery (*arrow*) which feeds the juxtacortical mass (**d**). Pathological diagnosis: - juxtacortical hemangioma

appears homogeneously hypointense on a STIR pulse sequence. Medullary infiltration appears as focal or confluent areas of increased signal intensity. In a study of MRI with pathological correlation, Golfieri et al. have found that the combined use of T1-weighted spin-echo and STIR sequences is accurate in assessing intramedullary tumor extent [27].

10.3.2 Plain Film Radiography, Computed Tomography, Conventional Angiography, Nuclear Medicine, Ultrasound

The role of other imaging modalities in staging soft tissue tumors is highlighted in the chapters on ultrasound, Doppler echography, radiography and CT, nuclear medicine examinations, and molecular biology and genetics. See Figs. 10.3–10.7 for cases illustrating the role of different imaging techniques in staging soft tissue tumors. See the following references regarding the value of imaging modalities other than MRI in staging of soft tissue tumors:

Angiography	23
CT	6, 11, 33, 40, 46–48, 59, 62, 66
Nuclear medicine	2, 15, 20, 37, 38, 48
Ultrasound	7, 36

10.4 Metastatic Disease

The lung is the most frequent site of distant hematogenous spread by malignant soft tissue tumors and bone is the second most common site. CT is the most sensitive imaging modality available to detect pulmonary metastases. Routine chest CT can reveal peripheral nodules as small as 2–3 mm [10] (Fig. 10.6). However, benign nodules can be mistaken for metastatic disease. Peuchot et al. report radiological-surgical correlation in 84 patients with extrathoracic malignancies and 173 resected pulmonary parenchymal nodules. Approximately 75% of the nodules were detected on CT scan and 82% proved to be metastatic lesions [49]. Any patient with a primary malignant soft tissue neoplasm should undergo chest CT as part of the initial staging evaluation.

Metastatic disease rather than local recurrence is the major cause of death in patients with soft tissue malignancy of the extremities, and hence the detection of metastatic disease has important prognostic and therapeutic implications. The distinction between regional lymph node or distant viscera as the site of metastasis is not as critical, since the prognosis is uniformly poor for both.

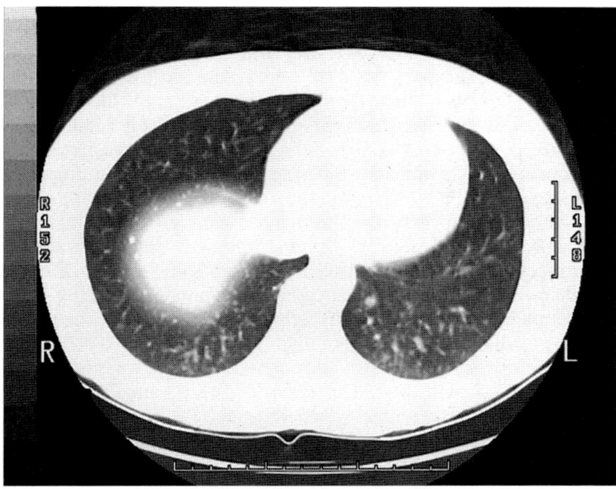

Fig. 10.6. Miliary metastases. CT scan. Multiple tiny, noncalcified nodules are seen at both lung bases on chest CT. The chest radiograph was normal. Wedge biopsy of the lung showed alveolar soft part sarcoma

Metastatic spread of sarcoma to regional nodes is infrequent. A review of 12 series by Mazeron et al. has found that 3.9% of patients develop regional lymph node metastases during the course of disease [44]. For certain histologic types of soft tissue sarcoma, regional lymph node involvement is relatively more prevalent. These subtypes are rhabdomyosarcoma, vascular sarcoma, epithelioid sarcoma, clear cell sarcoma, and synovial sarcoma. For detecting lymph node spread, contrast-enhanced abdominal and pelvic CT can be beneficial. Today there is little use for gallium in this setting. Fluorodeoxyglucose (FDG)-positron-emission tomography (PET) may play a role in the future [2].

10.5 Surveillance and Repeat Staging

After primary treatment of a soft tissue malignancy, periodic evaluation of the operative site is performed to evaluate tumor recurrence. Several studies have reported an association between the development of a local recurrence and a higher subsequent rate of death. The development of a recurrence was found to be as important a prognostic predictor as baseline predictors such as tumor grade and size in some studies [52, 60], whereas others have found it to be significant only if poor prognostic baseline variables such as high grade, deep location, and size (more than 5 cm) are not present [25]. This debate has clearly important implications for decisions about the use of adjuvant treatment that may reduce the risk of local recurrence.

Since the majority of recurrences occur within the first 2 years, it seems prudent to concentrate surveillance in this period [50, 52, 55] (Table 10.5). We obtain a baseline, contrast-enhanced MRI examination of the

Table 10.5. Surveillance imaging

Protocol
Pre- and postgadolinium-enhanced SE T1-weighted images with fat suppression in the axial and longitudinal planes Fast SE T2-weighted images with fat suppression in the axial and longitudinal planes
Frequency: 3-month baseline examination with subsequent examinations dictated by clinical presentation

surgical site 3 months after primary resection. It is then available as a baseline if a recurrence is suspected. Thereafter, clinical presentation dictates the frequency of surveillance with MRI. The MRI protocol includes a transaxial T1-weighted spin-echo sequence before and after the administration of contrast. The precontrast spin-echo T1-weighted images should include fat suppression. The postcontrast T1-weighted image is performed with frequency-selective fat saturation. In addition, a fast or turbo spin-echo T2-weighted sequence is performed in both a longitudinal and the transaxial plane. It is important to mark the cephalic and caudal margins or the entire length of the scar, since the operative site is the most likely area for tumor to recur. Recurrent tumor typically appears as a discrete mass or nodule with decreased signal intensity on T1-weighted images and increased signal intensity on T2-weighted images.

The differential diagnosis of an area of abnormal signal intensity in the operative bed can be divided into mass lesions and areas of abnormal muscle swelling (edema) without a discrete mass. When a mass is detected on surveillance imaging, tumor recurrence must be excluded. However, a variety of nonneoplastic masses may be identified on the follow-up MRI examination. The differential diagnosis of a nonneoplastic mass includes focal fluid collection due to seroma or lymphatic cyst, hematoma, and an infectious mass such as an abscess or phlegmon. A *seroma* is a discrete fluid collection in the operative bed, which may be proteinaceous and thus similar in signal intensity to normal muscle on precontrast, T1-weighted images. Contrast enhancement is variable but when present is peripheral, thin, and regular [65]. Unlike recurrent tumor with central necrosis, these fluid-filled pseudocysts remain stable in appearance or resolve on follow-up imaging tests. An *abscess* is a very unusual complication of excisional surgery and quite often clinical clues are present. Unlike a simple seroma, an abscess may contain areas of hemorrhage, have a thicker wall, and the enhancement pattern is more extensive and irregular than the seroma. We have encountered cases of hematoma in which the appearance on MRI mimics abscess and tumor recurrence.

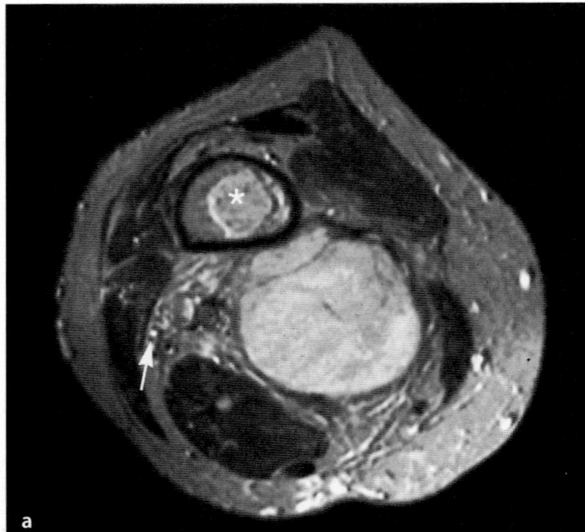

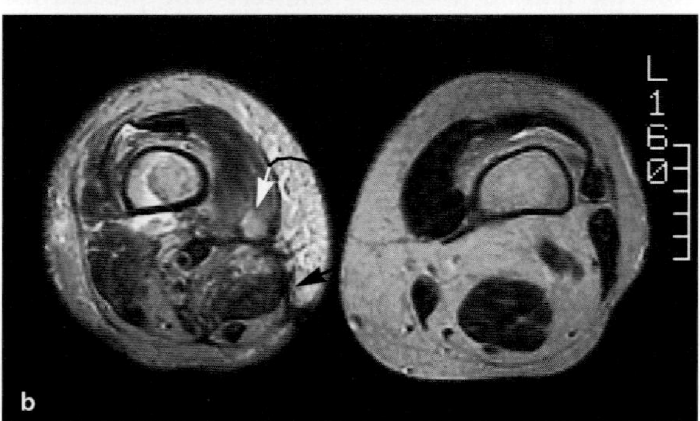

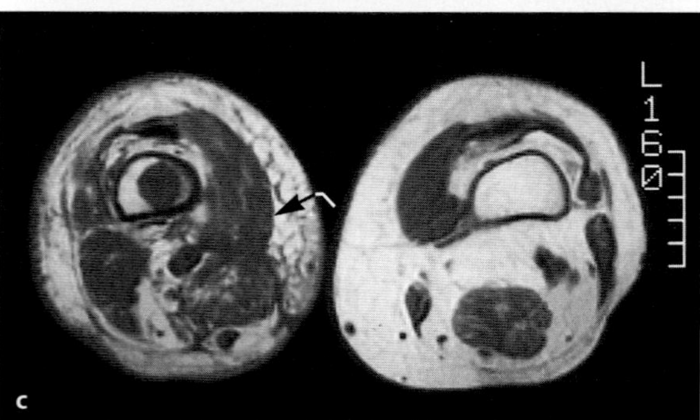

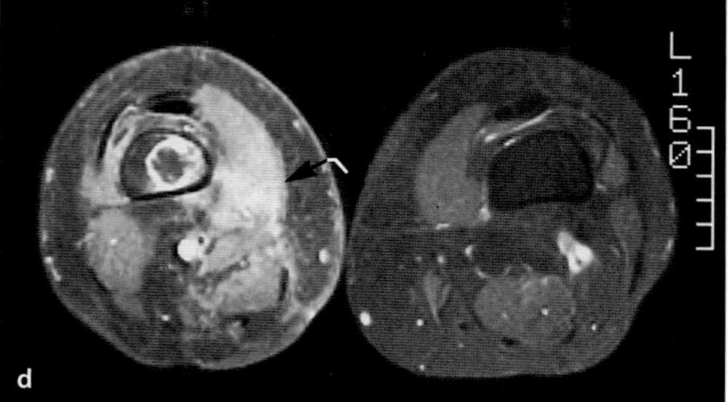

Fig. 10.7 a-d Small recurrent tumor following marginal resection and radiation therapy. **a** Axial SE T2-weighted MR image. **b** Axial SE T2-weighted MR image 6 months later. **c** Axial SE T1-weighted MR image. **d** Axial fat-suppressed T1-weighted MR image after Gd-contrast injection. Presurgical T2-WI shows a large, heterogeneous mass arising in the popliteal space. There is displacement of the popliteal vessels (*arrow*) and the mass abuts but does not erode the posteromedial cortex of the distal femur. Incidental enchondroma is present (*asterisk*) (**a**). Pathological diagnosis: mixed pleomorphic and myxoid liposarcoma At the 6-month follow-up, there is atrophy and postradiation change, including subcutaneous edema and areas of high signal intensity in the semimembranosus and vastus medialis muscles on the T2-WI. A hypointense scar (*arrow*) is also seen. A 1-cm nodule (*curved arrow*) is seen in the posteromedial aspect of the vastus medialis muscle (**b**). When compared with the noncontrast T1-WI (**c**), there is enhancement of the vastus medialis muscle and partial enhancement of the nodule (*curved arrow*) on the postcontrast T1-WI with fat saturation (**d**). Pathological diagnosis: recurrent liposarcoma

Areas of abnormal signal in muscle or intercompartmental soft tissues in the absence of a mass may be due to acute postoperative edema, scarring or granulation tissue, and radiation change. *Scar* appears as an ill-defined area of low signal intensity on T1-weighted images [5] and decreased signal intensity on proton density- and T2-weighted images. Fiber bundles and fascicles create a recognizable parenchymal pattern in skeletal muscle on T1-weighted images. This normal, "marbled" textural pattern of muscle on T1-weighted images is often disrupted at sites of postsurgical scarring, and enhancement may also be observed [51]. *Postradiation change* may have a similar appearance to scar, but in many cases the textural pattern of muscle is changed less dramatically. Furthermore, reticular subcutaneous edema is often more marked in radiation-associated inflammation and soft tissue changes are restricted to the portals of treatment (Fig. 10.7). The enhancement kinetics of radiation-induced changes in the soft tissues has been reported to be distinctive from that of recurrent tumor. Using dynamic, contrast-enhanced MRI, Vanel et al. have shown that there is more gradual enhancement of radiation-induced inflammation compared with recurrent tumor [65]. Furthermore, when conventional MRI cannot distinguish between local recurrence and postsurgical change such as hygroma, dynamic contrast-enhanced imaging may be helpful. Recurrent tumor demonstrates early enhancement, whereas peripheral rim enhancement or no enhancement at all will be seen in hygromas [49].

Although long-term survival is more dependent on the control of distant metastases, the early detection of local recurrence is important, because it may create morbidity and its treatment may impact on the development of metastases. The majority of recurrences, whether local or distant, occur during the first 2 years after treatment of the primary tumor [50, 55]. Local recurrences present as a discrete soft tissue nodule or mass, frequently in the operative bed. Both the sensitivity and specificity of MRI for the detection of recurrent sarcoma have been reported to range from 85 to 95% [9, 51, 64, 65], and recurrences as small as 1 cm can be detected. On noncontrast MRI, recurrences have longer T1 and T2 relaxation times than that of muscle and, in the absence of high signal intensity on T2-weighted images, a recurrent sarcoma is unlikely [65]. In addition, homogeneous contrast enhancement of a nonnecrotic mass is more typical for recurrent sarcoma and this homogeneous pattern of enhancement should be compared with that of the ring enhancement pattern of a seroma or hematoma (Fig. 10.7). Soft tissue inflammatory masses may rarely exhibit signal intensity or an enhancement pattern similar to that of recurrent sarcoma and, in these cases, needle aspiration or biopsy may be necessary. In general, the absence of either a region of high signal intensity on T2-weighted images or enhancing tissue on T1-weighted images suggests that tumor has not recurred.

Things to remember:
1. Staging means clinical, radiological, and pathological evaluation of local extent and distant spread.
2. Biopsy has to be performed after evaluation of local disease.
3. Staging systems are based on evaluation of tumor grade, local extent, and distant metastases.
4. Pediatric rhabdomyosarcomas have a separate staging system.
5. Tumor size, compartmental anatomy, relationship to deep fascia, and reactive zone are major staging parameters, defining oncosurgical margins.
6. MRI is the best staging modality. Grading capability will be discussed in Chap 11 (Grading and Tissue-Specific Diagnosis).
7. Chest CT is the most sensitive imaging modality to detect pulmonary metastases.
8. MRI has a high sensitivity and specificity for the detection of recurrent tumor for guidelines concerning post-therapy surveillance (see Chap 28).

References

1. American Joint Commission on Cancer (2002) Soft tissues. In: Greene FL, Balch CM, Fleming ID et al (eds) AJCC Cancer Staging Manual, 6th edn. Springer, New York, pp 193–197
2. Bastiaannet E, Groen H, Jager PL et al (2003) The value of FDG-PET in the detection, grading and response to therapy of soft tissue and bone sarcomas; a systematic review and meta-analysis. Cancer Treat Rev 30:83–101
3. Benedikt RA, Jelinek JS, Kransdorf MJ et al (1994) MRI of soft-tissue masses: role of gadopentetate dimeglumine. J Magn Reson Imag 4:485–490
4. Berquist TH, Ehman RL, King BF et al (1990) Value of MRI in differentiating benign from malignant soft tissue masses: Study of 95 lesions. AJR Am J Roentgenol 155:1251–1255
5. Biondetti PR, Ehman RL (1992) Soft tissue sarcomas: use of textural patterns in skeletal muscle as a diagnostic feature in postoperative MRI. Radiology 183:845
6. Bland KI, McCoy DM, Kinard RE et al (1987) Application of MRI and CT as an adjunct to the surgical management of soft tissue sarcomas. Ann Surg 205:473–481
7. Choi H, Varma DGK, Fornage BC et al (1991) Soft tissue sarcoma: MRI versus sonography for detection of local recurrence after surgery. AJR Am J Roentgenol 157:343
8. Crim JR, Seeger LL, Yao L et al (1992) Diagnosis of soft tissue masses with MRI: can benign masses be differentiated from malignant ones? Radiology 185:581–586
9. Dalinka M, Zlatkin M, Chao P, Kricun M, Kressel H (1990) The use of magnetic resonance imaging in the evaluation of bone and soft-tissue tumors. Radiol Clin North Am 28(2):461
10. Davis S (1991) CT evaluation for pulmonary metastases in patients with extrathoracic malignancy. Radiology 180:1
11. Demas B, Heelan R, Lane J, Marcove R, Hadju S, Brennan M (1988) Soft-tissue sarcomas of the extremities: comparison of MR and CT in determining the extent of disease. Radiology 150:615
12. De Schepper A, Ramon F, Degryse H (1992) Statistical analysis of MRI parameters predicting malignancy in 141 soft tissue masses. Rofo Fortschr Rontg 155(6):587
13. Enneking E (1985) Staging of musculoskeletal neoplasms. Skeletal Radiol 13:183
14. Enneking W (1990) Principles of muskuloskeletal oncologic surgery. In: Evarts C (ed) Surgery of the musculoskeletal system. Churchill Livingston, New York
15. Enneking W, Chew F, Springfield D, Hudson T, Spanier S (1981) The role of radionuclide bone-scanning in determining the resectability of soft-tissue sarcomas. J Bone Joint Surg 63A:249
16. Enzinger RM, Weiss SW. General considerations. In Enzinger FM, Weiss SW (eds) (1988) Soft tissue tumors, 2nd edn. Mosby, Saint Louis, pp 1–18
17. Erlemann R, Reiser M, Perers P et al (1989) Musculoskeletal neoplasms: static and dynamic Gd-DTPA-enhanced MRI. Radiology 171:767
18. Erlemann R, Sciuk J, Bosse A et al (1990) Response of osteosarcoma and Ewing sarcoma to preoperative chemotherapy: assessment with dynamic and static MRI and skeletal scintigraphy. Radiology 175:791–796
19. Erlemann R, Vassallo P, Bongartz G et al (1990) Musculoskeletal neoplasms: fast low-angle shot MRI with and without Gd-DTPA. Radiology 176:489
20. Finn H, Simon M, Martin W, Darakjian H (1987) Scintigraphy with gallium-67 citrate in staging of soft-tissue sarcomas of the extremity. J Bone Joint Surg 69A:886
21. Fletcher B, Hanna S (1990) Letter: musculoskeletal neoplasms: dynamic Gd-DTPA-enhanced MRI. Radiology 177:287
22. Fletcher BD, Hanna SL, Fairclough DL, Gronemeyer SA (1992) Pediatric musculoskeletal tumors: use of dynamic, contrast-enhanced MRI to monitor response to chemotherapy. Radiology 184:243–248
23. Fujii J, Ozaki T, Kawai A, Kunisada T, Sugihara S, Inoue H (1999) Angiography for assessment of preoperative chemotherapy in musculoskeletal sarcomas. Clin Orthop 360:197–206
24. Galant J, Marti-Bonmati L, Soler R, Saez F, Lafuente J, Bonmati C, Gonzalez I (1998) Grading of subcutaneous soft tissue tumors by means of their relationship with the superficial fascia on MRI. Skeletal Radiol 27(12):657–663
25. Gaynor JJ, Tan CC, Casper ES et al (1992) Refinement of clinicopathological staging for localized soft tissue sarcoma of the extremity: a study of 423 adults. J Clin Oncol 10:1317–1329
26. Gielen JL, De Schepper AM, Parizel PM, Wang XL, Vanhoenacker F (2003) Additional value of magnetic resonance with spin-echo T1-weighted imaging with fat suppression in characterization of soft tissue tumors. J Comput Assist Tomogr 27(3):434–441

27. Golfieri R, Baddeley H, Pringle J, Souhami R (1990) The role of the STIR sequence in magnetic resonance imaging examination of bone tumours. Br J Radiol 63:251

28. Greer RJ, Woodruff J, Casper ES et al (1992) Management of small soft tissue sarcoma of the extremity in adults. Arch Surg 127:1285–1289

29. Hahn PF, Saini S, Stark DD et al (1987) Intra-abdominal hematoma: the concentric ring sign in MRI. Am J Roentgenol 148:115

30. Hajdu S (1979) Pathology of soft tissue tumors. Lea and Febiger, Philadelphia

31. Hays DM, Newton W, Soule EH et al (1983) Mortality among children with rhabdomyosarcomas of the alveolar histological subtype. J Pediatr Surg 18:412

32. Hays DM, Soule EH, Lawrence W et al (1982) Extremity lesions in the inter-group rhabdomyosarcoma study (IRS-1): a preliminary report. Cancer 48:1

33. Hogeboom WR, Hoekstra HJ, Mooyaart EL et al (1991) MRI and CT in the preoperative evaluation of soft tissue tumors. Arch Orthop Trauma Surg 110:162–164

34. Hudson T, Schakel MI, Springfield D (1985) Limitations of computed tomography following excisional biopsy of soft tissue masses. Skeletal Radiol 13:49–54

35. Kransdorf MJ, Jelinek JS, Moser RP et al (1989) Soft tissue masses: Diagnosis using MRI. AJR Am J Roentgenol 153:541–547

36. Kransdorf MJ, Murphey MD (1997) The use of gadolinium in the MR evaluation of soft tissue tumors. Sem Ultrasound CT MR 18:251–268

37. Kirchner P and Simon M (1984) The clinical value of bone and gallium scintigraphy for soft-tissue sarcomas of the extremities. J Bone Joint Surg 66A:319

38. Kole AC, Nieweg OE, Van Ginkel RJ et al (1997) Detection of local recurrence of soft-tissue sarcoma with positron emission tomography using [18F]fluorodeoxyglucose. Ann Surg Oncol 4:57–63

39. Lang P, Grampp S, Vahlensieck M et al (1995) Primary bone tumors: value of MR angiography for preoperative planning and monitoring response to chemotherapy. Am J Roentgenol 165:135

40. Majeron J, Suit H (1987) Lymph nodes as sites of metastases from sarcomas of soft tissue. Cancer 60:1800

41. McDonald DJ (1994) Limb-salvage surgery for treatment of sarcomas of the extremities. AJR Am J Roentgenol 163:509–513

42. Mirowitz SA, Apicella P, Reinus WR, Hammerman AM (1994) MRI of bone marrow lesions: relative conspicuousness on T1-weighted, fat-suppressed T2-weighted, and STIR images. AJR Am J Roentgenol 162:215–221

43. Mirowitz SA, Totty WG, Lee JKT (1992) Characterization of musculoskeletal masses using dynamic Gd-DTPA enhanced spin-echo MRI. J Comput Assist Tomogr 16:120–125

44. Musculoskeletal Tumor Society (1985) Staging of musculoskeletal neoplasms. Skeletal Radiol 13:183–194

45. Neville HL, Andrassy RJ, Lobe TE et al (2000) Preoperative staging, prognostic factors, and outcome for extremity rhabdomyosarcoma: a preliminary report from the Intergroup Rhabdomyosarcoma Study IV (1991–1997). J Pediatr Surg 35(2):317–321

46. Panicek DM, Gatsonis C, Rosenthal DI et al (1997) CT and MRI in the local staging of primary malignant musculoskeletal neoplasms: report of the radiology diagnostic oncology group. Radiology 202:237–246

47. Petasnick J, Turner D, Charters J, Gitelis S, Zacharias C (1986) Soft-tissue masses of the locomotor system: comparison of MRI with CT. Radiology 160:125

48. Pettersson H, Thurman III G, Hamlin D et al (1987) Primary musculoskeletal tumors: examination with MRI compared with conventional modalities. Radiology 164:237

49. Peuchot M, Libshitz H (1987) Pulmonary metastatic disease: radiological-surgical correlation. Radiology 164:7–19

50. Potter DA, Glenn J, Kinsella T et al (1985) Patterns of recurrence in patients with high grade soft tissue sarcomas. J Clin Oncol 3:353

51. Reuther G, Mutschler W (1990) Detection of local recurrent disease in musculoskeletal tumors: magnetic resonance imaging versus computed tomography. Skeletal Radiol 19:85

52. Rooser B, Attevell R, Berg NO et al (1987) Survival in soft tissue sarcoma – prognostic variables identified by multivariate analysis. Acta Orthop Scand 58:516–522

53. Rosenthal R, Wozney P (1991) Diagnostic value of gadopentetate dimeglumine for 1.5 T MRI of musculoskeletal masses: comparison with unenhanced T1- and T2-weighted imaging. J Magn Reson Imaging 1:547

55. Sauter ER, Hoffman JP, Eisenberg BL (1993) Part I: Diagnosis and surgical management of locally recurrent soft tissue sarcomas of the extremity. Semin Oncol 20:451

56. Schwartz H, Jones C (1992) The efficacy of gallium scintigraphy in detecting malignant soft tissue neoplasms. Ann Surg 215:78

57. Shuman W, Patten R, Baron R, Liddell R, Conrad E, Richardson M (1991) Comparison of STIR and spin-echo MRI at 1.5 T in 45 suspected extremity tumors: lesion conspicuity and extent. Radiology 179:247

58. Simon M (1982) Biopsy of musculoskeletal tumors. J Bone Joint Surg Am 64:1253–1257

59. Sundaram M, McGuire MH, Herbold DR (1988) Magnetic resonance imaging of soft tissue masses: an evaluation of 53 histologically proven tumors. J Magn Reson Imag 6:237–248

60. Stotter AT, A'Hern RP, Fisher C et al (1990) The influence of local recurrence of extremity soft tissue sarcoma on metastases and survival. Cancer 65:1119–1129

61. Swan JS, Grist T, Sproat I, Heiner J, Wiersma S, Heisey D (1995) Musculoskeletal neoplasms: preoperative evaluation with MR angiography. Radiology 194:519

62. Totty W, Murphy W, Lee J (1986) Soft tissue tumors: MRI. Radiology 160:135

63. Tung G, Davis L (1993) The role of magnetic resonance imaging in the evaluation of the soft tissue mass.Crit Rev Diagn Imaging 34(5):239

64. Vanel D, Lacombe MR, Couanet D et al (1987) Musculoskeletal tumors: followup with MRI after treatment with surgery and radiation therapy. Radiology 164:243

65. Vanel D, Shapeero LG, Baere TD et al (1994) MRI in the follow-up of malignant and aggressive soft tissue tumors: results of 511 examinations. Radiology 190:263–268

66. Wetzel L, Levin E, Murphey M (1987) A comparison of MRI and CT in the evaluation of musculoskeletal masses. Radiographics 7(5):851

67. Wunder JS, Healey JH, Davis AM, Brennan MF (2000) A comparison of staging systems for localized extremity soft tissue sarcoma. Cancer 88(12):2721–2730

Grading and Tissue-Specific Diagnosis

11

A.M. De Schepper

Contents

11.1 Introduction

Characterization consists of both grading and tissue-specific diagnosis.

While tissue specific diagnosis implies pathological typing, grading implies a differentiation between benign and malignant tumors and definition of malignancy grade. Although pathology will always remain the gold standard in the diagnosis of soft tissue tumors, prediction of a specific histologic diagnosis remains one of the ultimate goals of each new imaging technique [34]. Moreover, decisions regarding biopsy and treatment could be simplified if a specific diagnosis or a limited differential diagnosis could be provided on the basis of imaging [1, 36].

Sundaram stressed the importance of "naming" soft tissue masses based on MR imaging criteria, working on the premise that one's inability to "name", or provide a succinct differential diagnosis requires the lesion to be considered "indeterminate" and biopsied. The approach to such indeterminate lesions is that they are sarcomas until microscopically proven otherwise [38].

Benign soft tissue tumors outnumber their malignant counterparts by about 100 to 1. Otherwise most cutaneous and subcutaneous masses are very small and are often excised without imaging studies. As a consequence 60% of the soft tissue tumors in adults who are referred for evaluation by medical imaging are benign, this proportion increasing to 75% in the pediatric age group. The major role of grading consists merely in recognizing benign soft tissue tumors which will be excluded from further invasive diagnostic and therapeutic procedures.

The statement that disease stage and grade are more important than tumor type with respect to five-year survival (American Joint Committee of Soft Tissue Sarcomas) [23] was discussed at the 20th anniversary meeting of the Soft Tissue and Bone Sarcoma Group of the European Organization for Research and Treatment of Cancer (EORTC) in Amsterdam (April 11–13, 1996). There was a broad consensus that staging and grading systems should always be based on tumors of one specific histological type, because conventional staging and grading parameters are of different importance in different tumor types. Also the significance and the predictive value of the various histologic parameters vary in different types of sarcoma. And because of morphologic variations in different portions of the tumor, the grade is determined on the basis of the least differentiated area and its extent [19, 24, 53]. The pathologist's perspective on grading is well described in Chap. 8.

11.2 Grading

Grading refers to differentiation between benign and malignant tumors and definition of malignancy grade. Moreover tumor grading is also an important staging parameter as already discussed. Well known histological grading parameters are cellularity, cellular pleomorphism, mitotic rate, matrix and presence of necrosis. In this regard presence of necrosis, tumor size and most importantly mitotic count are significantly correlated with the duration of survival or the time to distant metastases [48]. Since most of these parameters influence signal intensity on MRI, the grading capacity of this imaging method seemed promising. Nevertheless, there is still much controversy regarding the value of imaging, in particular of MRI in the differentiation of benign and malignant soft tissue tumors [10]. However, although the signal characteristics of both benign and malignant tumors overlap frequently, certain benign lesions, because of a certain contained tissue type or material, a characteristic shape, or a favored location can

Table 11.1. Soft tissue tumor (STT) grading parameters

Origin (subcutaneous, fascial, intramuscular, mixed)
Location

Distribution
    Intracompartmental
    Extracompartmental

Size
Shape
Margins
Relationship with superficial fasciae
Neurovascular bundle displacement/encasement
Bone involvement
Signal intensity on different pulse sequences
Signal homogeneity
Changing pattern of homogeneity
Low signal intensity septations
Peritumoral edema
Hemorrhage

Contrast enhancement
    Static studies (type, intensity)
    Dynamic studies (ratio, slope)

Diffusion-weighted MRI

be accurately diagnosed on MR imaging. Initially though to be limited to a handful, the list of soft-tissue conditions that can be diagnosed on MR imaging continues to grow. Soft tissue masses that do not demonstrate distinguishing features on MR imaging should be considered indeterminate and will require biopsy [39]. These items will be discussed in depth in the part devoted to characterization in this same chapter.

A variety of imaging-grading parameters have been described in the literature, and are listed in Table 11.1.

11.2.1 Individual Parameters

Examples of commonly used individual parameters for predicting malignancy are *intensity* and *homogeneity of the MR signal* with different pulse sequences. High signal intensity (SI) on T2-WI [40] and inhomogeneity on T1-WI are sensitive parameters but present with an unacceptable low specificity. Because 90% of the malignant lesions are inhomogeneous ("disorganized" or "hectic") absence of heterogeneity is a reliable negative predictive indicator for the presence of malignancy [51]. Otherwise smaller lesions tend to be more homogeneous, whether they are benign or malignant. Concerning signal intensity, high grade malignant soft tissue tumors may present with low to intermediate signal intensity on T2-WI as a consequence of hypercellularity, increased nucleocytoplasmatic index and an altered ratio between cellular and interstitial components both

resulting in a decreased amount of intra- and extracellular water [5, 7, 13]. In this regard lymphomas and non differentiated (high grade) sarcomas may present with low SI on T2-weighted images and have to be differentiated from tumors showing recurrent intralesional bleeding and hemosiderin loading causing shortening of the T2-relaxation time and consequently lower SI on T2-WI.

Clear cell sarcomas (deep seated melanomas) may present with increased SI on T1-weighted images, depending on their content on melanin which shortens the T1-relaxation time [12].

Changing homogeneity (from homogeneous on T1-WI to heterogeneous on T2-WI) and the presence of a lobular morphology with intervening low signal intratumoral septations were reported by Hermann respectively with a sensitivity of 72 and 80%, respectively, and a specificity of 87 and 91%, respectively, in predicting malignancy [26].

Galant et al. described a grading system of subcutaneous soft tissue tumors by means of their *relationship with the superficial fascia* on MRI. Obtuse angles between superficial fascia and a subcutaneous mass crossing the fascia indicate a probability of malignancy six to seven times that for lesions that do not cross the fascia or have contact with acute angles. Exceptions are vascular and neurogenic tumors, which can cross the fascia through preexisting anatomical channels and fibromatosis [21].

Location has a limited value in differentiating soft tissue tumors. In contradistinction to malignant tumors, benign ones frequently have a preferential location. In this regard elastofibroma has a predilection for the subscapular region, PVNS for the knee, nodular fasciitis for the forearm, desmoids for the deltoid and gluteal region, glomus tumors for the subungual soft tissues while soft tissue tumors of the hand and wrist are benign in more than 90% of the cases, and intra-articular tumoral lesions being almost always benign. Concerning malignant lesions, soft tissue sarcomas have a predilection for the thigh and in particular synovial cell sarcomas for the foot. In this same regard location can be a valuable parameter in differentiating between low-grade liposarcomas and benign lipomas. Subcutaneous fatty tumors are mostly benign lipomas and if they are of low grade malignancy they never metastasize [51]. The parameter location will be discussed further in the section "characterization" of this chapter.

Although the *size* and *shape* of the lesion at detection seem unlikely to contribute to tumor grading, Tung combined the data from three investigations and postulated that a diameter of less than 3 cm is a reasonable indicator that a lesion is benign, as this threshold is associated with a positive predictive value of 88%. Conversely, a diameter of 5 cm predicts the malignant nature of a soft tissue mass with a sensitivity of 74%, specificity of 59%, and an accuracy of 66% [44].

Although benign tumors tend to be well-delineated and, conversely, malignant tumors have rather ill-defined margins, several studies have concluded that the *margin* (well-defined versus infiltrating) of a soft tissue mass on MRI is of no statistical relevance in predicting of malignancy. Moreover, Bongartz reported that aggressive sarcomas may have a pseudocapsule while benign lesions such as desmoid tumors may invade neighboring tissues [7, 49].

Peritumoral edema, shown on T2-weighted images as an ill-defined area of high signal intensity, can indicate infiltrative tumor, reparative inflammation, or both, and as a consequence is not helpful as a grading parameter [24].

Involvement of adjacent bone, extracompartmental distribution, and *encasement of the neurovascular bundle* are relatively uncommon findings that are specific but insensitive signs of malignancy. They are also seen in aggressive benign soft tissue lesions including desmoids, hemangiomas, and pigmented villonodular synovitis. Osseous invasion was studied by Elias et al. [16]. They found that cortical and medullary signal intensity changes and cortical destruction observed on MRI are highly sensitive and highly specific signs of osseous invasion by soft tissue sarcoma. Increasing maximal diameter and increasing circumference of osseous abutment by the tumor did not result in a statistically significant increase in the likelihood of osseous invasion. Moreover their study proved that observation of a completely preserved soft tissue interface on T1-weighted images, even in the presence of peritumoral edema and/or reactive changes extending to the bone surface, has a NPV of 100% for osseous invasion.

For compartmental anatomy we refer to the article of Anderson MW [2] which will be discussed in more detail in Chap. 9.

The parameter *"growth rate"* is related to the aggressiveness of a soft tissue tumor and not to its malignancy grade.

Intratumoral hemorrhage is a rare finding, which can be observed in both benign and malignant lesions, and is difficult to differentiate from nontumoral soft tissue hematoma. In a study by Moulton et al., intratumoral hemorrhage was observed in 23 benign and in 5 malignant tumors among a total number of 225 masses. Hemorrhage was diagnosed on the basis of high signal on T1-weighted images, coupled with low or high signal on T2-weighted images, provided the tissue was not isointense to fat on all sequences. A low signal hemosiderin rim was interpreted as evidence of prior hemorrhage [36].

Although malignant tumors show increased vascularity and have large extracellular spaces, depending on tumoral activity or aggressiveness, we found no correlation between *degree and pattern of enhancement* and malignancy grade.

Erlemann et al. showed that dynamic contrast-enhanced studies are valuable in distinguishing benign from malignant lesions. On time-intensity plots, the increase in signal intensity was always lower than 100% for benign tumors and between 80% and 280% for malignant tumors.

Slopes with a greater than 30% increase in signal intensity per minute were seen in 84% of malignant tumors, and slopes with a lower than 30% increase in signal intensity per minute were seen in 72% of benign tumors. However, some overlap was observed. Largely necrotic malignant tumors showed slopes similar to those of benign tumors, while rapidly growing benign lesions such as myositis ossificans showed slopes similar to those of malignant ones [17, 18].

Although a statistically significant difference was found between the "first pass" slope values of benign and malignant lesions, pathological and angiographic findings indicated that first pass images reflect tissue vascularization and perfusion rather than benignity or malignancy. In 25% of the cases, the dynamic MR images provide new information for diagnosis, choice of biopsy site, and follow up during chemotherapy [50].

Ma et al. demonstrated that intratumoral enhancement patterns of malignant and benign masses differ because of differences in neovascularity and interstitial pressure. Malignant lesions showing increased neovascularity at their periphery and increased interstitial pressure at their center. Their results suggest that the rim-to-center differential enhancement ratio has potential as an additional parameter for the MRI differentiation of indeterminate musculoskeletal masses [31].

More recently Van der Woude et al. [46] prospectively analyzed the value of fast, dynamic, subtraction MRI in grading soft tissue tumors. They assessed the interval between arterial and early tumor enhancement (sensitivity of 91% and specificity of 72%), peripheral or diffuse enhancement (sensitivity of 73% and specificity of 97%) and the progression of enhancement (time-signal intensity curves) (sensitivity of 86% and specificity of 81%) in differentiation of benign from malignant soft tissue tumors. Most malignant soft tissue tumors exhibited an early and peripheral enhancement with a steep slope, an early maximum followed by a transition to a stable level or a slight decrease of signal intensity.

Tacikowska found that determination of the enhancement rate coefficient in percent per second (erc %/s) on dynamic MRI had a high sensitivity (93%) and high specificity (73%) in differentiating benign and malignant STT while the pattern of enhancement better correlated with vascularization and perfusion and the size of the interstitial space rather than with tumor's histology [41, 42]. In a second study the same author assessed the value of total tumor enhancement expressed as percent and found it less accurate than the erc %/s [41, 42].

The best results are obtained by Van Rijswijk et al. [47] using a multivariate logistic regression to identify the best combination of MR imaging parameters that might be predictive of malignancy. This multivariate analysis of 140 soft tissue tumors revealed that combined nonenhanced static and dynamic contrast-enhanced MR imaging parameters were significantly superior to nonenhanced MR imaging parameters alone and to nonenhanced MR imaging parameters combined with static contrast-enhanced MR imaging parameters in prediction of malignancy. The most discriminating parameters were presence of liquefaction, start of dynamic enhancement (time interval between start of arterial and tumor enhancement), and lesion size (diameter) (Fig. 11.6).

One of the reasons for the controversy about the value of dynamic contrast enhanced MRI refers to the small molecular weight of commonly used gadolinium chelates. In a recent study about dynamic contrast-enhanced MR imaging of mammary soft tissue tumors Daldrup et al. demonstrated that quantitative tumor microvascular permeability assays generated with macromolecular MRI contrast medium correlate closely with histologic tumor grade while no significant correlation was found using small-molecular gadopentetate. Gadopentetate-enhanced MRI is highly sensitive for tumor detection but has been shown to lack specificity for cancer grading [11].

The potential value of diffusion-weighted MRI in characterizing STT was studied by Van Rijswijk et al. They found that true diffusion coefficients of malignant STT were significantly lower than those of benign masses whereas ADC values between both groups were not significantly different [47].

11.2.2 Combined Parameters

Although most investigators failed to establish reliable criteria for distinguishing benign from malignant lesions, a combination of individual parameters (MR signal characteristics, morphology, internal architecture, growth pattern and other anatomic features) yields higher sensitivity and specificity [51]. Berquist et al. reported important criteria (size, margins, and homo-

geneity of signal intensity) predicting malignancy with a specificity of 82–96%, a negative predictive value of 92–96%, and a positive predictive value of 88–90% [5].

In a prospective analysis of 36 consecutive cases of soft tissue tumors by Ma et al., MRI was 100% sensitive but only 17% specific, with an accuracy of 58% in predicting malignancy. These authors found a wide variability in the appearance of benign and malignant lesions on MR images, with a poor correlation between "benign characteristics" and the benignity of the lesion [32].

Moulton et al. analyzed the imaging features of 225 soft tissue tumors (179 benign, 46 malignant) to evaluate the efficacy of MRI in distinguishing benign from malignant lesions. Univariate analysis of individual features and stepwise logistic regression analysis of combinations of imaging features were performed. Quantitative analysis showed that no single imaging feature or combination of features could reliably be used to distinguish benign from malignant lesions. With subjective analysis, a correct and specific diagnosis of benignity could be made in 44% of the 225 tumors. For the entire cohort the sensitivity for diagnosis of malignancy by subjective analysis was 78%, while the specificity was 89%. When benign tumors were excluded, the specificity decreased to 76%, whereas the sensitivity remained the same. The authors concluded that the accuracy of MRI declines when typically benign tumors are excluded from analysis. A significant percentage of malignant lesions may appear deceptively benign with the currently used criteria [36].

We performed multivariate statistical analysis to determine the accuracy of ten parameters, individually and in combination, for predicting malignancy. When the following signs were observed together, malignancy was forecast with a sensitivity of 81% and a specificity of 81%: absence of low signal intensity on T2-weighted images, signal inhomogeneity on T1-weighted images, and mean diameter of the lesion greater than 33 mm (Fig. 11.1). Malignancy was predicted with the highest sensitivity when a lesion had high signal intensity on T2-weighted images, was larger than 33 mm in diameter, and had an inhomogeneous signal intensity on T1-weighted images. Signs that had the greatest specificity for malignancy included the presence of tumor necrosis, bone or neurovascular involvement, and a mean di-

Table 11.2. Diagram of the "grading" results in absolute numbers with statistical workup (95% "confidence intervals" within brackets)

	Histology malignant	Histology benign		
MRI malignant	115 (0.1778–0.2460)	76 (0.1121–0.1703)	82% (0.7324–0.8839	Specificity
MRI benign	8 (0.0069–0.0291)	349 (0.5958–0.6761)	98% (0.9256–0.9989)	NPV
	93% (0.8602–0.9680) Sensitivity	60% (0.5019–0.6907) PPV	548	Total p<0.0001

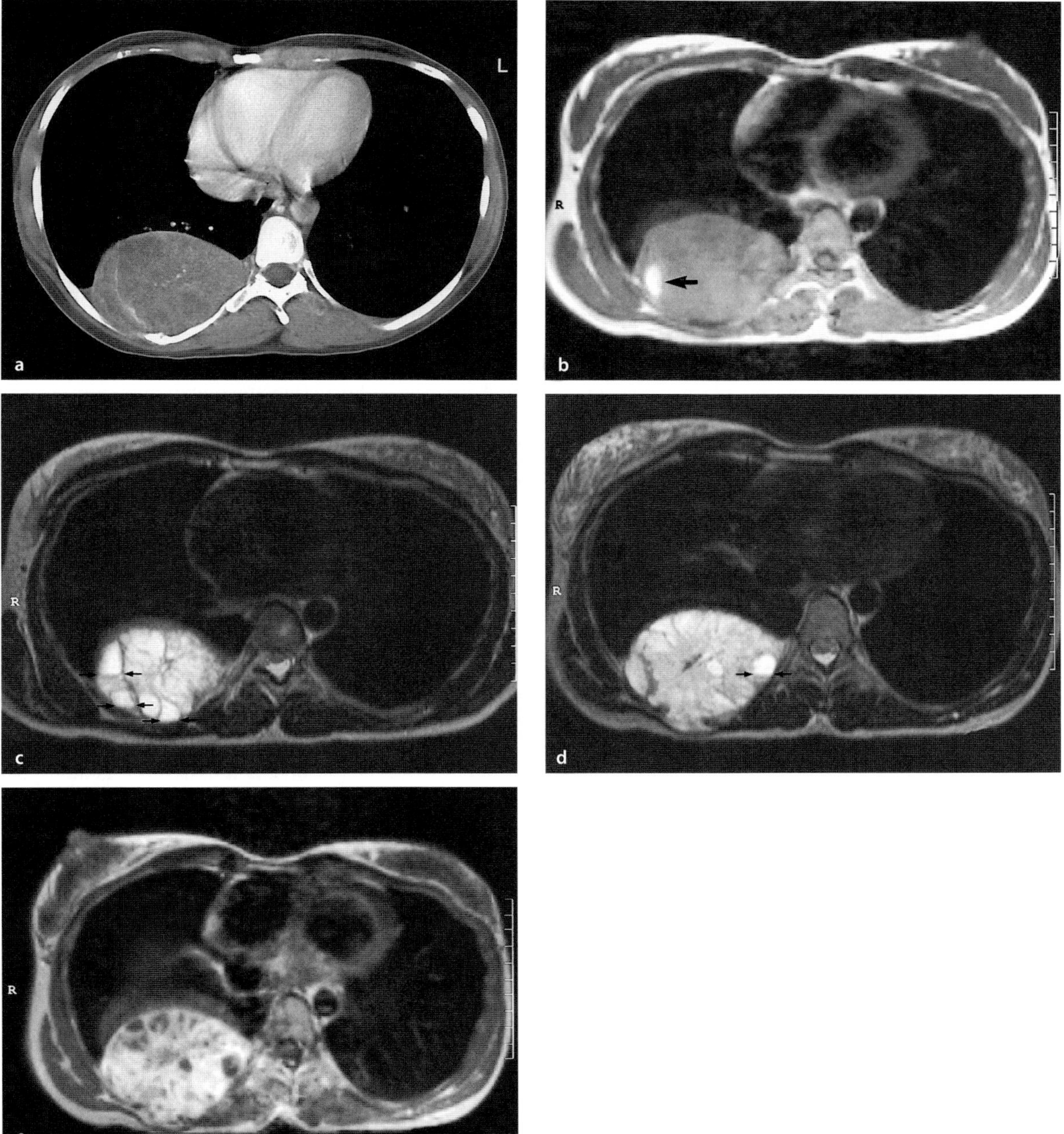

Fig. 11.1 a–e. Malignant peripheral nerve sheath tumor of the chest wall in a 29-year-old woman: **a** CT scan of the chest after I-contrast injection; **b** axial SE T1-weighted MR image; **c,d** axial SE T2-weighted MR image; **e** axial SE T2-weighted MR image after Gd-contrast injection. On CT scan of the chest there is a large, rounded and sharply demarcated mass located in the costovertebral gutter, with presence of intralesional calcifications and spoke-wheel-like enhancement after contrast injection (**a**). On T1-WI the lesion is inhomogeneous and of intermediate SI. There is a small area of high SI laterally within the mass (*arrow*) (**b**). On T2-WI there is again a spoke-wheel appearance of the lesion, there are multiple fluid-fluid levels, and rounded high SI areas (*small arrows*) on a background of intermediate to high SI (**c,d**). On T1-WI after contrast injection there is marked enhancement without enhancement of the rounded high SI areas on T2-WI (compare **d** with **e**). Large size (50×80×80 mm), extracompartmental extension and bone involvement, inhomogeneous distribution of SI and presence of amorphous calcifications within the lesion are parameters, predicting malignancy. Sharp margins and presence of intralesional hemorrhage are non-discriminatory parameters. Localization is in favor of a neurogenic tumor. Histologic diagnosis after resection confirmed the diagnosis of a malignant nerve sheath tumor (right 8th intercostal nerve)

ameter of more than 66 mm. Of the malignant lesions, 80% had irregular or partially irregular margins, while a similar percentage of benign masses had well-defined or partially irregular margins. The majority of both benign and malignant lesions showed moderate or strong enhancement, no predominant enhancement pattern emerged for either type of mass. In contrast to the study of Berquist et al., margin, signal homogeneity on T2-weighted images, signal intensity on T1-weighted images, shape, and enhancement pattern were statistically nondiscriminatory [14].

More recently we prospectively assessed the value of MRI in grading soft tissue tumors in a series of 548 untreated patients originating from a multi-institutional database, 123 with malignant and 425 with benign tumors. The thresholds to differentiate between malignant and benign STT are interpreted in a non quantitative way using grading parameters described in literature and mentioned before and, based on a fifteen year experience time of our research group. In this regard we obtained a sensitivity of 93%, a specificity of 82%, a negative predictive value of 98% and a positive predictive value of 60% in diagnosing malignancy (Table 11.2) [22].

11.3 Tissue Specific Diagnosis

Even though the primary concern of the referring physician is not histologic determination of tumor type but recognition of malignant features and distinction from benign counterparts, it was expected that MR imaging had great potential for the histological classification of soft tissue tumors because of its high intrinsic contrast resolution [8, 35, 36]. Unfortunately, the initial enthusiasm has not entirely been confirmed.

There are two reasons for this failure. First, MR images provide only indirect information about tumor histology by showing signal intensities related to some physicochemical properties of tumor components (e.g. fat, blood, water, collagen) and consequently reflect the gross morphology of the lesion rather than the underlying histology. Soft tissue tumors belonging to the same histological group may have a different composition or different proportions of tumor components resulting in different MR signals. This feature is well exemplified by the group of liposarcomas which can be well differentiated (lipomatous), myxoid, round cell or pleomorphic, or contain different proportions of these components.

Only well differentiated liposarcomas are predominantly fatty, while the other histologic subtypes have less than 25% fat or no fat at all. As a consequence, there are no specific MRI characteristics for liposarcomas as a total group.

The second reason for the poor performance of MR in characterizing tumors histologically is the fact of time-dependent changes during natural evolution or as a consequence of therapy. Young desmoid tumors have a high water content and are highly vascularized, which results in high signal intensity on T2-weighted images. With aging they become more collagenous, which results in decreasing signal intensity. The same transformation is described for many tumors of fibrous tissue and also for the formerly named malignant fibrous histiocytomas. Furthermore, the signal intensity of large malignant tumors undergoes changes as a consequence of intratumoral necrosis and/or bleeding.

These limitations have prompted Kransdorf to state that "a correct histologic diagnosis reached on the basis of imaging studies is possible in only approximately one quarter of cases" [30].

In an early retrospective study on characterization Balzarini [3] reported that most lesions have a non-specific MRI appearance, except for lipomatous and fibrous lesions. On the other hand, in a retrospective study of 134 masses and pseudo-masses of the hand and wrist Capelastegui et al. reported an accurate diagnosis with differentiation of tumor-like lesions from genuine tumor [8].

In their prospective study on grading and characterization of 95 lesions (50 benign and 45 malignant) Berquist et al. predicted the exact histology of the lesion in 22% and in 58% of the benign group. Predicting histology of malignant lesions was not successful at all [5].

In the largest, partially prospective study Moulton et al. were able to predict the diagnosis confidently and correctly in 44% of 225 cases of soft tissue tumors. The majority of these cases were benign lesions such as lipomas, hemangiomas and arteriovenous malformations, benign neural tumors, periarticular cysts, hematomas, pigmented villonodular synovitis (PVNS), giant cell tumors of tendon sheath, and abscesses [36].

More recently Gielen et al. [22] reported on a series of 548 histologically proven soft tissue tumors in which a correct tissue specific diagnosis on MRI was made in 294 out of 425 benign tumors and in 47 out of 123 malignant tumors.

Table 11.3. Statistical work-up of tissue specific diagnosis [22]

	Sensitivity	Specificity	PPV	NPV
Benign+malignant	67%	98%	70%	98%
Benign	75%	98%	76%	98%
Malignant	37%	96%	40%	96%

Statistical workup for the whole cohort of benign and malignant tumors are summarized in Table 11.3. A correct tissue specific diagnosis was included in the differential diagnosis made on MRI (maximum of three possibilities) in 367 (67%) of the cases.

To determine whether potential MR imaging features suggest a specific diagnosis, we reviewed the current literature and found a large number of specific features, most of which were unfortunately of poor sensitivity. As for grading, the evaluation of a combination of different parameters seems more useful than the evaluation of individual parameters.

The usefulness of the relative prevalence, age at presentation, sex distribution and zonal distribution of 18,677 benign and 12,370 malignant soft tissue tumors was studied by Kransdorf in a large referral population [27, 28]. Approximately 70% of benign lesions were classified into eight diagnostic categories : lipoma and lipoma variants (16%), fibrous histiocytoma (13%), nodular fasciitis (11%), hemangioma (8%), fibromatosis (7%), neurofibroma (5%), schwannoma (5%), and giant cell tumor of tendon sheath (4%). In total, 52 diagnostic categories were used for analysis. It was possible to group approximately 80% of all benign tumors in the seven most common diagnostic categories for each age and location.

More than 80% of the malignant lesions were classified into eight diagnostic categories: malignant fibrous histiocytoma (24%), liposarcoma (14%), leiomyosarcoma (8%), malignant schwannoma (6%), dermatofibrosarcoma protuberans (6%), synovial sarcoma (5%), fibrosarcoma (5%) and sarcoma, not classified further (12%). In total, 31 malignant diagnostic categories were used for analysis. It was possible to group approximately 79% of all malignant tumors under the five most common diagnoses for each age and location (Tables 11.4 and 11.5) [27, 28].

In this study there were inherent biases, which the author himself recognized. To begin with, there is a relatively high percentage of malignant tumors in this series. The consultative nature of the cases probably introduced a preference for difficult case material. Second, the reported data reflect lesions found at biopsy. Many small superficial lesions are excised or sampled without imaging. Lesions in this group include dermatofibrosarcoma protuberans, giant cell fibroblastoma and atypical fibroxanthoma. In our own series of more than 2500 soft tissue tumors, these lesions were indeed rarely seen. Nevertheless, the tables from Kransdorf's paper are highly useful and should be accessible to all radiologists interested in soft tissue tumor pathology.

Signal intensity on different pulse sequences may be helpful in making a more specific diagnosis. And although most tumors display intermediate signal, similar to that of muscle on T1-weighted images, intermediate to high with respect to fat on T2-weighted images [24], we found that a large number of soft tissue tumors can be classified into five diagnostic categories, according to their signal intensity on T1- and T2-weighted images [Table 11.9]. Combination of signal intensities have been described in neurofibromas where a central low signal on T2-weighted images is combined with a high signal of the surrounding periphery. This so called "target" pattern is characteristic for neurofibromas, rarely seen in schwannomas and almost never described in malignant nerve sheath tumors [9, 51].

We observed an inverted target sign (high signal intensity center combined with a low signal periphery) in nodular fasciitis and metastasis.

The use of intravenously injected paramagnetic contrast agents is valuable in the detection and staging of soft tissue tumors, but neither the intensity nor the pattern of enhancement contributes to further tissue specific diagnosis of these lesions [25]. Dynamic contrast studies are useful in assessing the response of soft tissue tumors to chemotherapy and in differentiating postoperative edema from recurrent tumor. First pass imaging introduced by Verstraete may aid in differentiating hemangioma from arteriovenous malformation [50].

Multi-institutional approach allows to gain the best experience of a rare pathology such as soft tissue tumors. In this regard Marti-Bonmati and coworkers introduced a STT decision support system based on web services architecture. The system uses a pattern recognition technology (artificial neural networks, support vector machine, k-nearest neighbor) and epidemiological information to discriminate between benign and malignant tumors. After the systems had learned by using training samples (with 302 cases), the clinical decision support system was tested in the diagnosis of 128 new STT cases with a 88–92% efficacy [33].

A comparable system was introduced by A. De Schepper and coworkers by organizing the "Belgian Soft Tissue Neoplasm Registry" (BSTNR), a multi-institutional database of soft tissue tumors with the cooperation of most MR centers in Belgium.

As a guideline for the reader we have summarized the value of different parameters such as preferential location (Table 11.6), shape (Table 11.7), presence of signal voids (Table 11.8), signal intensities on different pulse sequences (Table 11.9), concomitant diseases (Table 11.11), fluid-fluid levels (Table 11.12), and multiplicity (Table 11.10) in concise tables.

The above-mentioned and other morphological features characteristic for some specific tumors are highlighted and illustrated in Fig. 11.1 until 11.14 and described in the respective chapters.

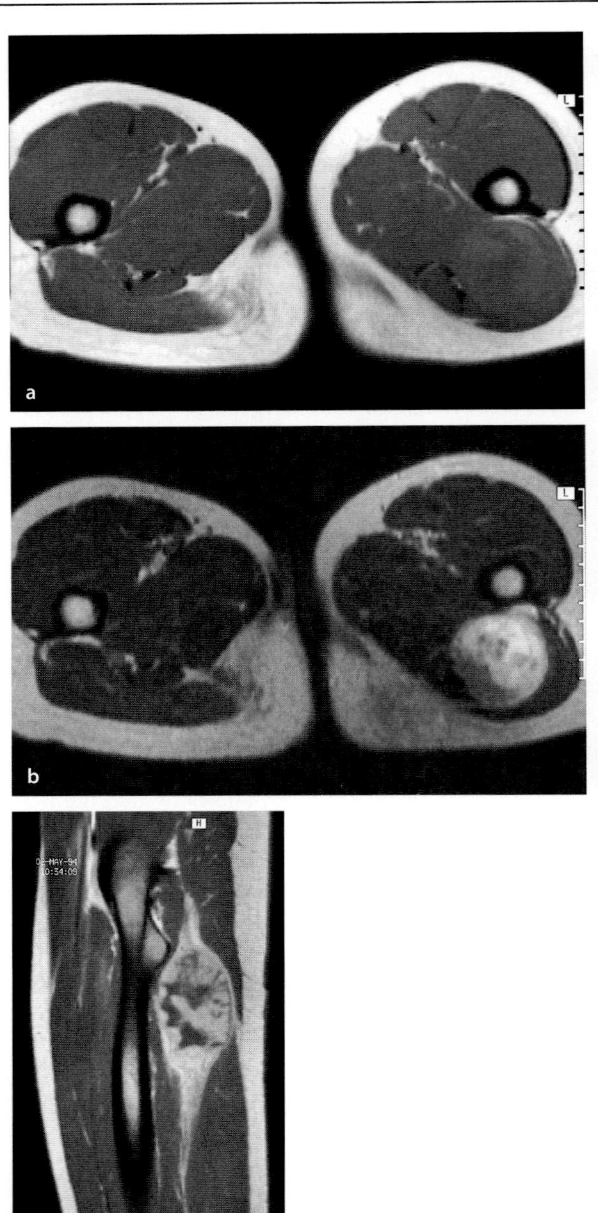

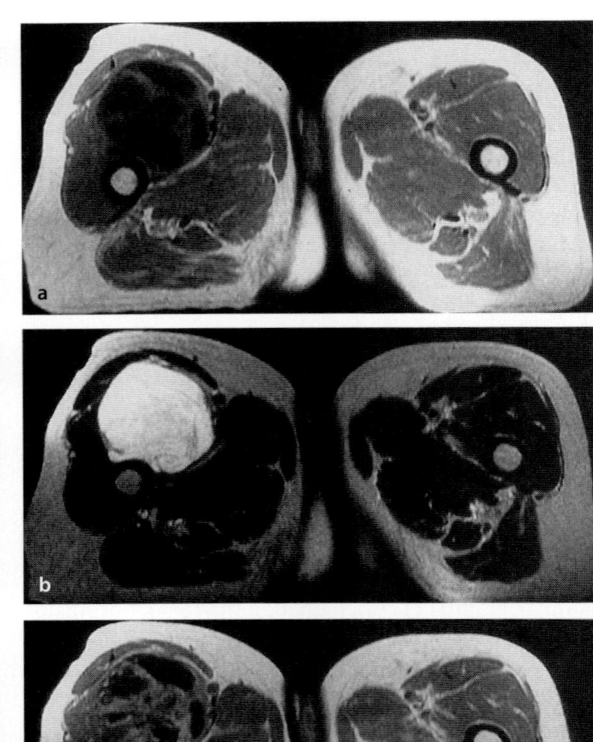

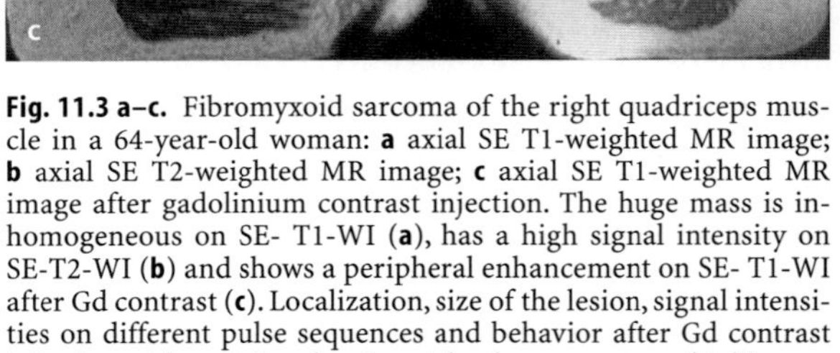

Fig. 11.3 a–c. Fibromyxoid sarcoma of the right quadriceps muscle in a 64-year-old woman: **a** axial SE T1-weighted MR image; **b** axial SE T2-weighted MR image; **c** axial SE T1-weighted MR image after gadolinium contrast injection. The huge mass is inhomogeneous on SE- T1-WI (**a**), has a high signal intensity on SE-T2-WI (**b**) and shows a peripheral enhancement on SE- T1-WI after Gd contrast (**c**). Localization, size of the lesion, signal intensities on different pulse sequences and behavior after Gd contrast injection with peripheral and septal enhancement, are highly suggestive of a malignant tumor

Fig. 11.2 a–c. Malignant peripheral nerve sheath tumor (MPNST) of the thigh in a 22-year-old woman: **a** axial SE T1-weighted MR image; **b** axial SE T2-weighted MR image; **c** sagittal SE T1-weighted MR image after Gd-contrast injection. There is a mass lesion in between the left adductor and gluteal muscles. The lesion is slightly inhomogeneous on T1-WI and definitely inhomogeneous on T2-WI. Sagittal image after contrast injection shows the fusiform shape of the lesion, the location on the course of the sciatic nerve and the presence of intratumoral necrosis. Imaging features are suggestive for a malignant (diameter of more than 80 mm, inhomogeneity, changing homogeneity, intratumoral necrosis) neurogenic (fusiform, along the course of a major nerve) tumor. Histologic examination after resection confirmed the diagnosis of MPNST

Table 11.4 Distribution of common benign soft tissue tumors by anatomic location and age

Age (years)	Hand and wrist	%	Upper extremity	%	Axilla and shoulder	%	Foot and ankle	%	Lower extremity	%
0–5	Hemangioma	15	Fibrous hamartoma of infancy	16	Fibrous hamartoma of infancy	29	Granuloma annulare	30	Granuloma annulare	23
6–15	Fibrous histiocytoma	14	Fibrous histiocytoma	23	Fibrous histiocytoma	34	Fibromatosis	23	Hemangioma	22
16–25	GCTTS	20	Nodular fasciitis	35	Fibrous histiocytoma	36	Fibromatosis	22	Fibrous histiocytoma	24
26–45	Fibrous histiocytoma	18	Nodular fasciitis	38	Lipoma	28	Fibromatosis	21	Fibrous histiocytoma	25
46–65	GCTTS	23	Nodular fasciitis	20	Lipoma	58	Fibromatosis	25	Lipoma	23
66 and over	GCTTS	21	Lipoma	22	Lipoma	58	Fibromatosis	14	Lipoma	26

Age (years)	Hip, groin & buttocks	%	Head and neck	%	Trunk	%	Retroperitoneum	%
0–5	Fibrous hamartoma of infancy	20	Nodular fasciitis	20	Hemangioma	18	Lipoblastoma	37
6–15	Nodular fasciitis	27	Nodular fasciitis	33	Nodular fasciitis	28	Lymphangioma	37
16–25	Neurofibroma	16	Nodular fasciitis	21	Nodular fasciitis	24	Fibromatosis	20
26–45	Lipoma	17	Lipoma	29	Lipoma	19	Schwannoma	23
46–65	Lipoma	35	Lipoma	46	Lipoma	44	Schwannoma	19
66 and over	Lipoma	21	Lipoma	50	Lipoma	42	Schwannoma	26

GCTTS, giant cell tumor of tendon sheath.
From Kransdorf [28].

Table 11.5 Distribution of common malignant soft tissue tumors by anatomic location and age

Age (years)	Hand and wrist	%	Upper extremity	%	Axilla and shoulder	%	Foot and ankle	%	Lower extremity	%
0–5	Fibrosarcoma	45	Fibrosarcoma	29	Fibrosarcoma	56	Fibrosarcoma	45	Fibrosarcoma	45
6–15	Epithelioid sarcoma	21	Angiomatoid MFH	33	Angiomatoid MFH	21	Synovial sarcoma	21	Synovial sarcoma	22
16–25	Epithelioid sarcoma	29	Synovial sarcoma	23	Synovial sarcoma	18	Synovial sarcoma	30	Synovial sarcoma	22
26–45	MFH	18	MFH	28	DFSP	33	Synovial sarcoma	26	Liposarcoma	28
46–65	MFH	19	MFH	46	MFH	35	MFH	25	MFH	43
66 and over	MFH	35	MFH	60	MFH	50	Kaposi's sarcoma	37	MFH	55

Age (years)	Hip, groin & buttocks	%	Head and neck	%	Trunk	%	Retroperitoneum	%
0–5	Fibrosarcoma	32	Fibrosarcoma	37	Fibrosarcoma	26	Fibrosarcoma	20
6–15	Angiomatoid MFH	21	Rhabdomyosarcoma	26	Angiomatoid MFH	15	Rhabdomyosarcoma	31
16–25	Synovial sarcoma	18	MFH	19	DFSP	23	Malignant schwannoma	20
26–45	Liposarcoma	18	DFSP	30	DFSP	30	Leiomyosarcoma	32
46–65	Liposarcoma	24	MFH	28	MFH	31	Liposarcoma	33
66 and over	MFH	46	MFH	34	MFH	44	Liposarcoma	39

DFSP, dermatofibrosarcoma protuberans; MFH, malignant fibrous histiocytoma (myxofibrosarcoma).
From Kransdorf [27].

Table 11.6. Preferential location of soft tissue tumors

Location		Tumor
Neck		Cystic hygroma – lymphangioma (infants)
		Capillary hemangioma (infants)
		Myofibroma (children)
		Infantile desmoid fibromatosis (children)
	Dorsal neck	Nuchal fibroma
	Sternocleidomastoid muscle	Fibromatosis colli (children)
	Carotid bifurcation	Glomus tumor
Trunk	Axilla	Cystic hygroma – lymphangioma
	Subscapular	Elastofibroma
	Spinoglenoid notch	Ganglion cyst
	Paraspinal gutter	Neurogenic tumor
Abdomen	Rectus abdominis muscle	Abdominal desmoid
	Costal gutter – paraspinal gutter	Neurogenic tumor
	Psoas muscle, parapsoatic	Plexiform neurofibroma
Pelvis	Presacral	Plexiform neurofibroma
	Buttock, lateral aspect	Desmoid
		Injection granuloma
	Coccyx	Extraspinal ependymoma
Upper limb	Deltoid, subcutaneous	Desmoid
		Injection granuloma
	Forearm, volar aspect	Nodular fasciitis
	Medial epitrochlear lymph node	Cat scratch disease
	Wrist	Ganglion cyst
	Wrist, volar aspect	Fibrolipohamartoma of median nerve
	Hand	Gouty tophi
	Hand, volar aspect	Palmar fibromatosis
		Fibrolipohamartoma of median nerve
	Hypothenar	Hypothenar hammer syndrome
	Finger	Macrodystrophia lipomatosa
	Finger, volar aspect	Giant cell tumor of tendon sheath
	Finger, dorsal aspect	Digital fibroma (children)
	Finger, tip	Epidermoid cyst
		Glomus tumor
Lower limb	Flexor aspect, along major nerves	Schwannoma
	Thigh	Fibrohamartoma of infancy (infants)
		Alveolar soft part sarcoma (adults)
		Sarcoma (liposarcoma) (older men)
	Knee	Synovial hemangioma
		Pigmented villonodular synovitis (young, middle aged men)
		Lipoma arborescens (older men)
	Knee, popliteal fossa	Pigmented villonodular synovitis
		Baker's cyst
		Synovial cyst
		Ganglion cyst
		Meniscal cyst
		Nerve sheath tumor
		Aneurysm of popliteal artery
	Knee, tibio-fibular joint	Ganglion cyst
	Ankle	Ganglion cyst
	Foot, extensor aspect	Ganglion cyst
	Sole	Synoviosarcoma (young adults)
		Plantar fibromatosis
	Heel	Clear cell sarcoma
	Metatarsals	Morton's neuroma (women)
	Toes	Giant cell tumor of tendon sheath
Upper and lower limb		Fibrous histiocytoma
		Myxofibrosarcoma
		Myositis ossificans
	Extensor aspect	Leiomyoma (young adults)
Joints, periarticular		Synovial hemangioma
		Amyloidosis
		Lipoma arborescens
		Pigmented villonodular synovitis
		Synoviosarcoma
Tendons	(Achilles tendon, bilateral)	Xanthoma
		Giant cell tumor of tendon sheath
Course of major nerves		Nerve sheath tumors
Cutis, subcutis		Desmoid
		Neurofibroma
		Nodular fasciitis
		Dermatofibrosarcoma protuberans
		Granular cell tumor

Table 11.7. Shape

Fusiform (ovoid)	Neurofibroma Lipoma
Dumbbell	Neurofibroma Desmoid
Moniliform	Neurofibroma Synovial – ganglion cyst
Round	Cyst Schwannoma
Serpiginous	Hemangioma
Soap bubbles – cauliflower	Lipoma arborescens
Nodular	Fibromatosis (plantaris, palmaris)
Branching (bilateral) Finger-like	Plexiform neurofibroma

Table 11.8. Intratumoral signal void

Flow	Hemangioma (capillary) Arteriovenous malformation

Calcification	Hemangioma (phlebolith)
	Lipoma (well-differentiated and
	   dedifferentiated)
	Desmoid
	Cartilaginous tumors
	Osteosarcoma of soft tissue
	Synoviosarcoma (poorly defined,
	   amorphous)
	Chordoma
	Alveolar soft part sarcoma
	Myositis ossificans (marginal-zonal)

High content of collagen	Desmoid

Table 11.9. Groups of STT according to their signal intensities on T1- and T2-weighted images

Group I High signal intensity on T1-weighted images, intermediate signal intensity on T2-weighted images	Lipoma Liposarcoma Lipoblastoma Hibernoma Elastofibroma Fibrolipohamartoma Metastasis of melanoma (melanin) Clear cell sarcoma (melanin)
Group II High signal intensity on T1-weighted images, high signal intensity on T2-weighted images	Hemangioma Lymphangioma Subacute hematoma Small arteriovenous malformation
Group III Low signal intensity on T1-weighted images, high signal intensity on T2-weighted images	Cyst Myxoma Myxoid liposarcoma Sarcoma
Group IV Intermediate signal intensity on T1-weighted images, high signal intensity on T2-weighted images	Neurogenic tumor Desmoid Tumors of muscular origin
Group V Low to intermediate signal intensity on T1-weighted images, low to intermediate signal intensity on T2-weighted images	Desmoid and other fibromatoses Pigmented villonodular synovitis Morton's neuroma Fibrolipohamartoma Giant cell tumor of tendon sheath Acute hematoma (few days) Old hematoma Xanthoma High flow arteriovenous malformation Mineralized mass Scar tissue Amyloidosis Granuloma annulare Lymphoma High grade malignancies

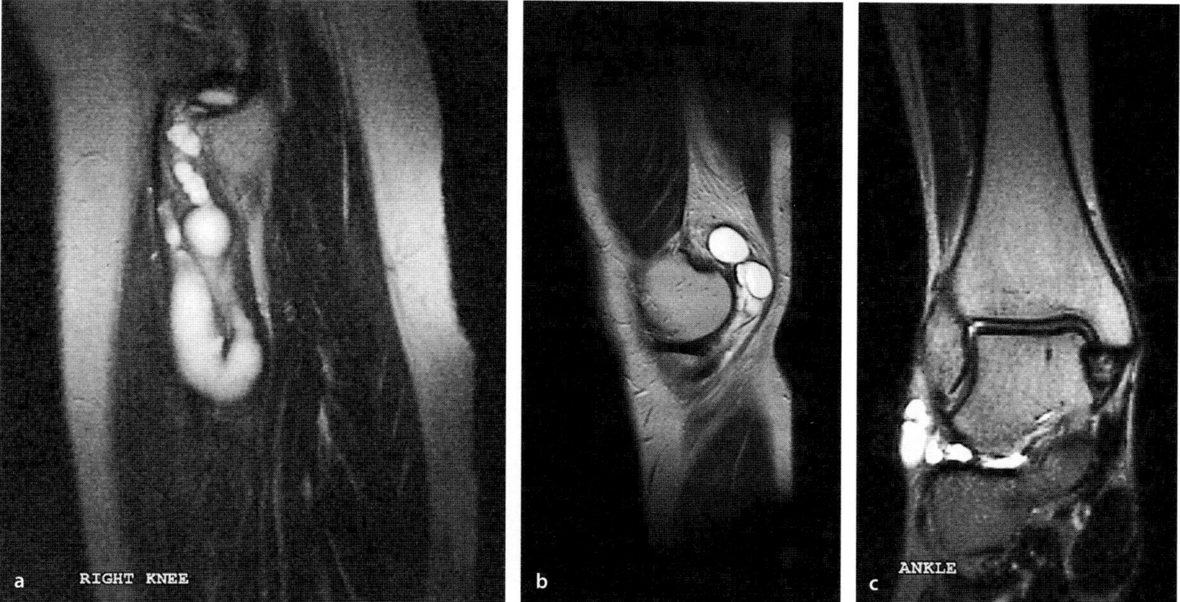

Fig. 11.4 a–c. Synovial cysts in three different patients: **a** sagittal SE T2-weighted MR image of the lower leg (34-year-old woman); **b** sagittal SE T2-weighted MR image of the knee (31-year-old woman); **c** coronal SE T2-weighted MR image of the ankle (46-year-old woman). All three lesions have a beaded appearance, very high SI on T2-WI and show connection with the neighboring joint. These imaging features make the diagnosis of a synovial cyst almost certain

Fig. 11.5 a–d. Four examples of soft tissue tumors having a characteristic localization and signal intensities on MRI: **a** giant cell tumor of the tendon sheath at the volar aspect of a finger with low signal intensity on SE- T1 and SE- T2-WI (not shown); **b** synovial hemangioma of the knee with intra-articular localization, characteristic serpiginous morphology and high signal intensity on fat suppressed T2-WI; **c** elastofibroma dorsi of the subscapular region with a characteristic lenticular shape, and mixed signal intensities (fat and fibrous tissue) on SE- T1-WI; **d** malignant nerve sheath tumor of the sciatic nerve with fusiform shape, "fat split" sign, localization on the course of a major nerve (neurogenic tumor) and peripheral enhancement and/or central necrosis (malignant lesion)

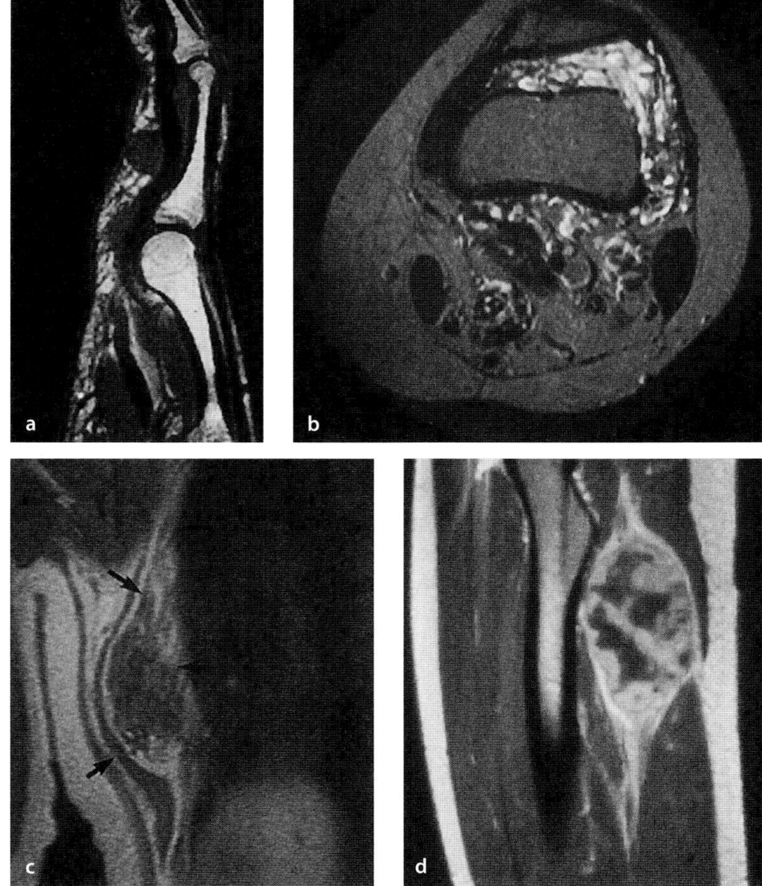

Table 11.10. Multiplicity

| Venous malformation |
| Lipoma 5–8% |
| Lipoma of tendon sheath (50%) |
| Desmoid |
| Neurofibroma |
| Myxoma |
| Metastasis |
| Dermatofibrosarcoma protuberans |
| Kaposi's sarcoma |

Table 11.12. Fluid-fluid levels

| Hemangioma |
| Cystic lymphangioma |
| Synoviosarcoma |
| Myxoma |
| Hematoma |
| Myositis |
| Metastasis |

Table 11.11. Concomitant diseases

Concomitant osseous involvement	Pigmented villonodular synovitis Lymphoma Desmoid Angiomatosis Parosteal lipoma Myofibromatosis (children) Juvenile hyalin fibromatosis (children)
Maffucci's disease	Cavernous hemangioma(s)
Fibrous dysplasia (Mazabraud)	Myxoma(s)
Neurofibromatosis	Schwannoma(s) Neurofibroma(s)
Gardner's syndrome	Fibromatosis
Dupuytren's disease (flexion contractures)	Palmar fibromatosis
Macrodystrophia lipomatosa of the digits	Fibrolipohamartoma of the median nerve
Familial hypercholesterolemia	Xanthoma
Normolipidemia+lymphoma or granuloma	Cutaneous xanthoma
Multiple myeloma	Amyloidosis
Turner's syndrome	Lymphangioma
Diabetes+degenerative joint disease+trauma	Lipoma arborescens

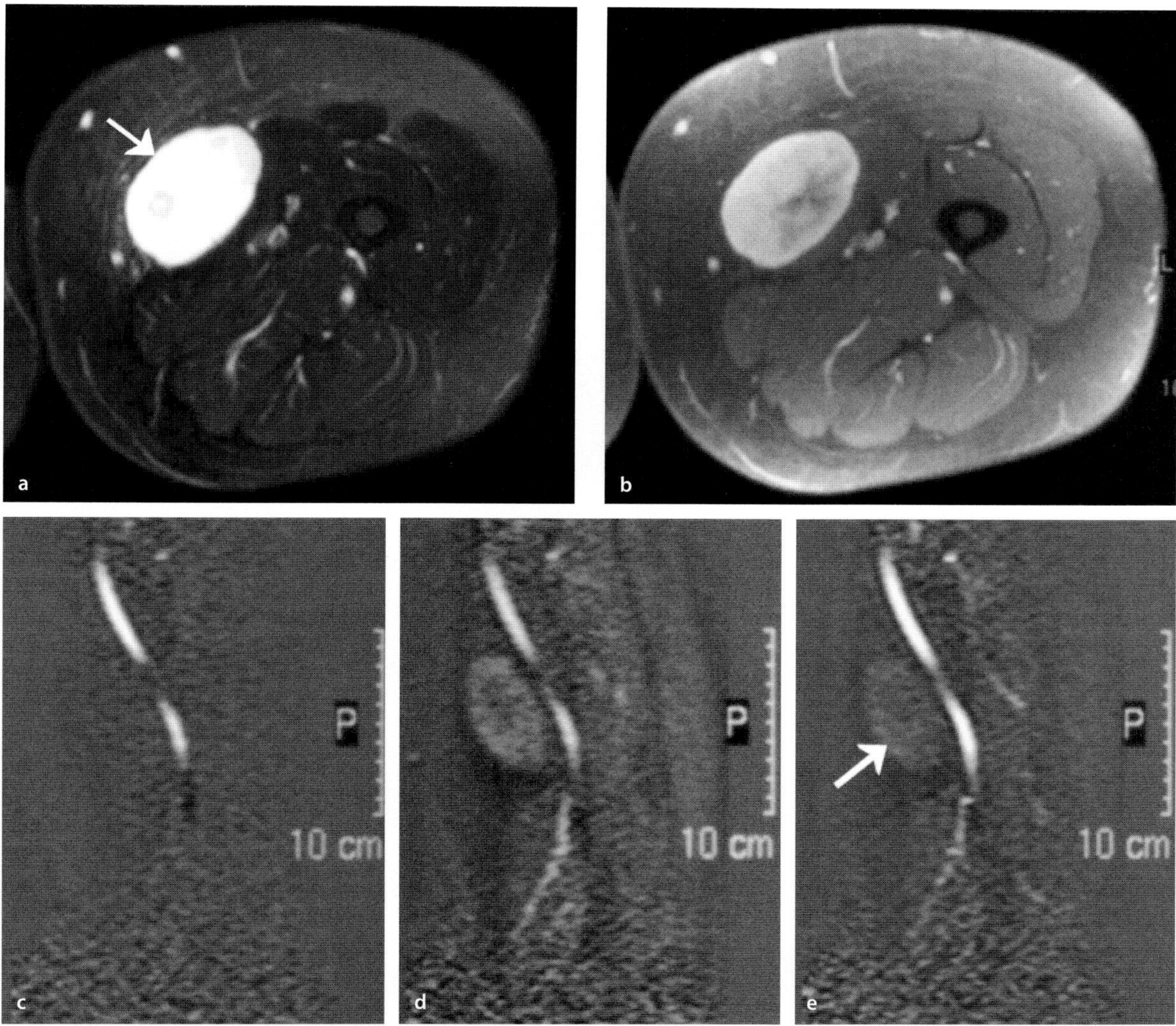

Fig. 11.6 a–e. Myxoid round cell liposarcoma: **a** axial SE T2-weighted MR image with fat suppression; **b** axial SE- T1-weighted MR image after Gd contrast administration with fat suppression; **c–e** dynamic MR sequence, subtraction images at the same level. **c.** Arrival of the bolus in the femoral artery. **d.** Image obtained 6 s later than **c. e.** Image obtained 30 s later than **d.** Early and intense enhancement in favor of a malignant soft tissue tumor [Courtesy of C.S.P van Rijswijk et al. Radiology (2004) 233:493–502]

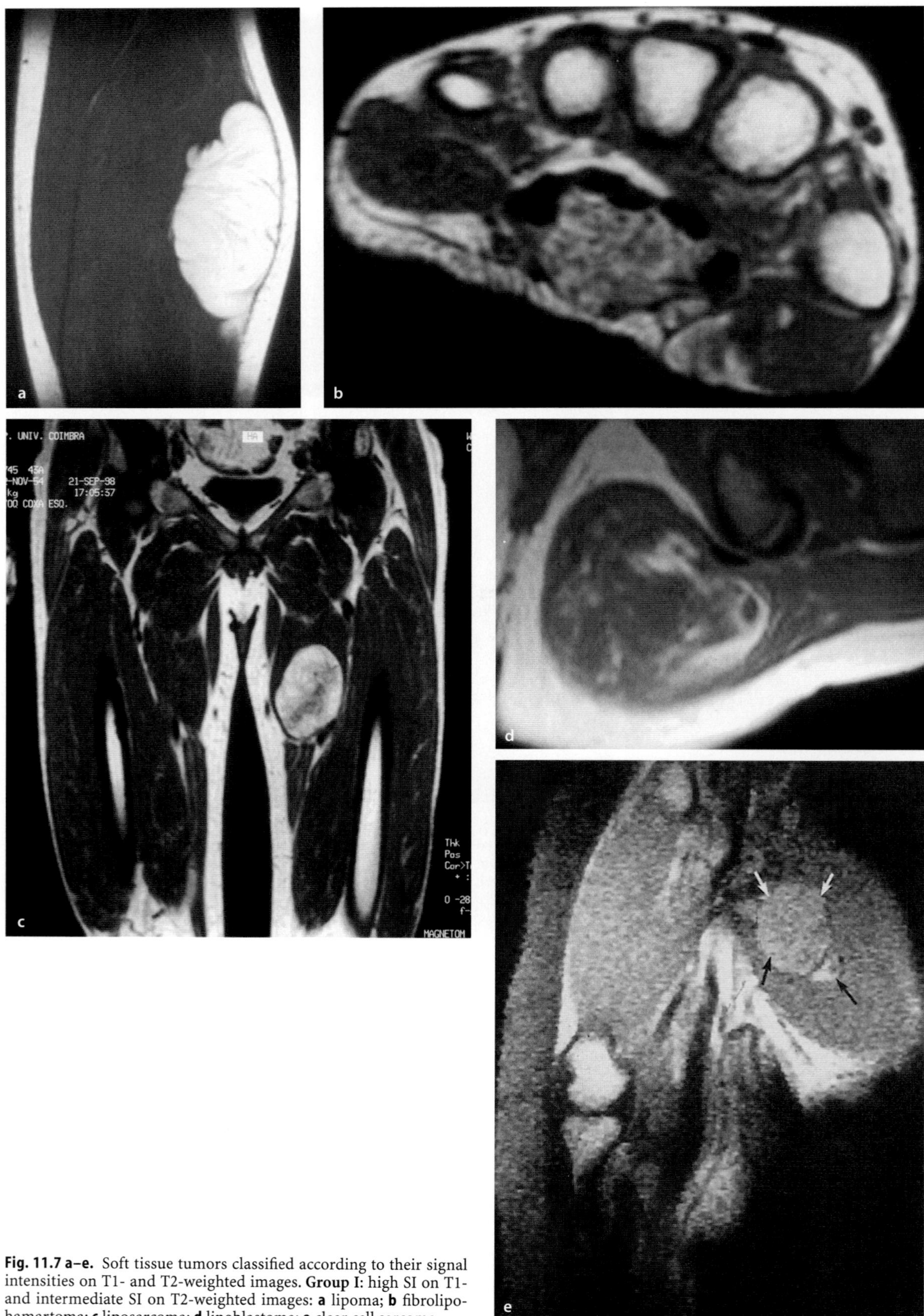

Fig. 11.7 a–e. Soft tissue tumors classified according to their signal intensities on T1- and T2-weighted images. **Group I**: high SI on T1- and intermediate SI on T2-weighted images: **a** lipoma; **b** fibrolipo-hamartoma; **c** liposarcoma; **d** lipoblastoma; **e** clear cell sarcoma

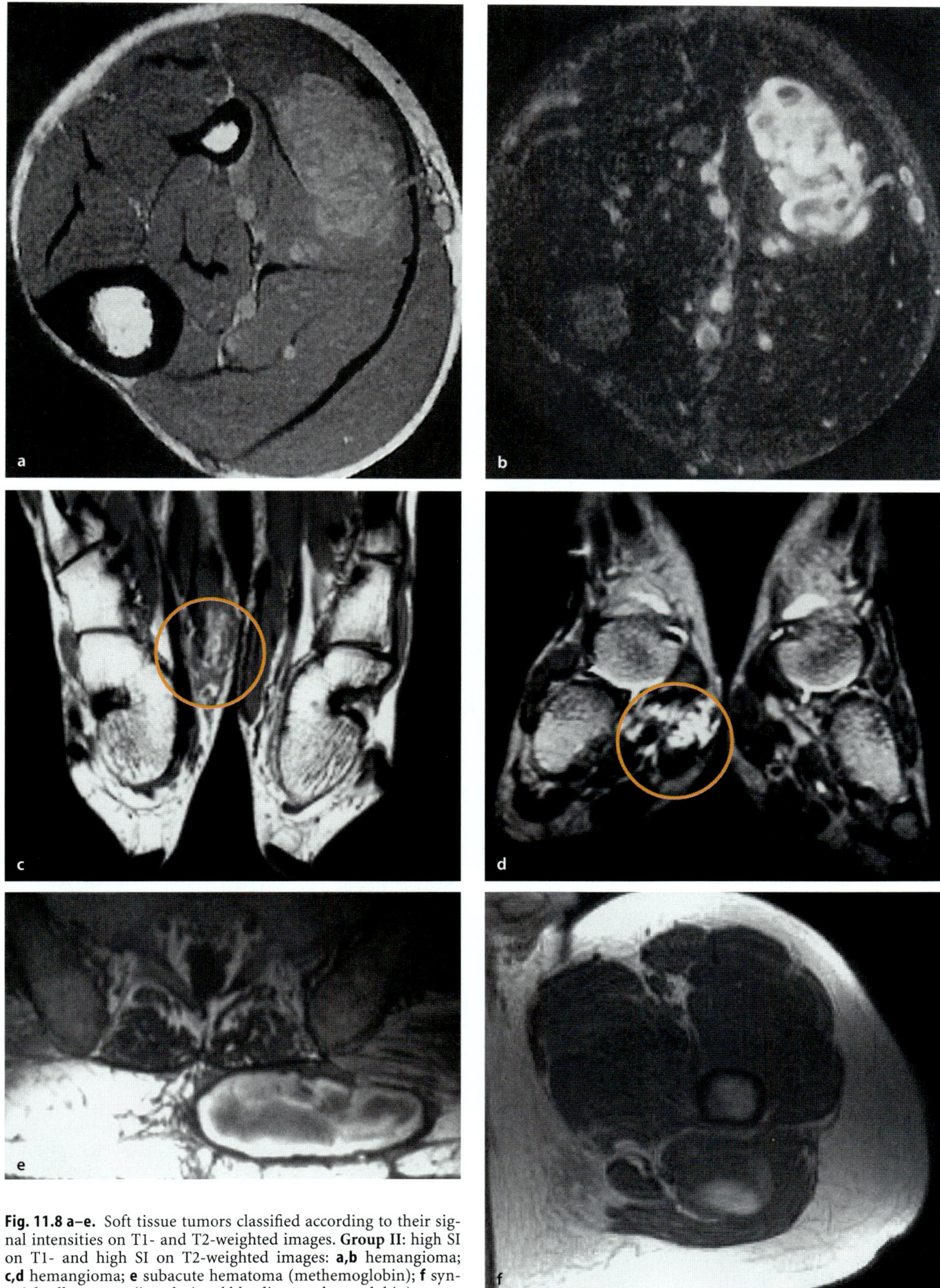

Fig. 11.8 a–e. Soft tissue tumors classified according to their signal intensities on T1- and T2-weighted images. **Group II**: high SI on T1- and high SI on T2-weighted images: **a,b** hemangioma; **c,d** hemangioma; **e** subacute hematoma (methemoglobin); **f** synovial cell sarcoma (intralesional bleeding-methemoglobin)

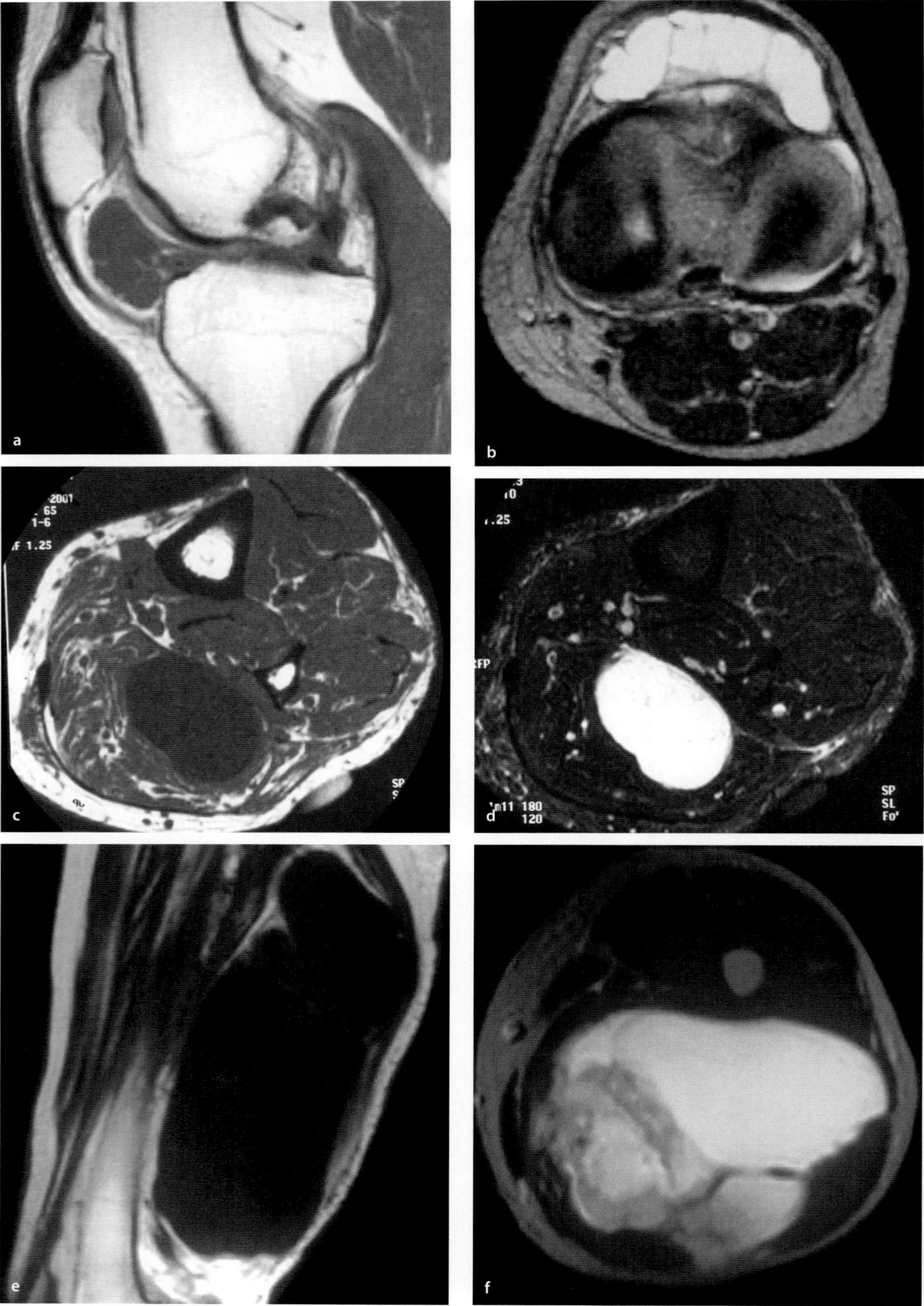

Fig. 11.9 e,f. Soft tissue tumors classified according to their signal intensities on T1- and T2-weighted images. **Group III:** low SI on T1- and high SI on T2-weighted images: **a,b** meniscal cyst; **c,d** myxoma; **e,f** myxoid liposarcoma

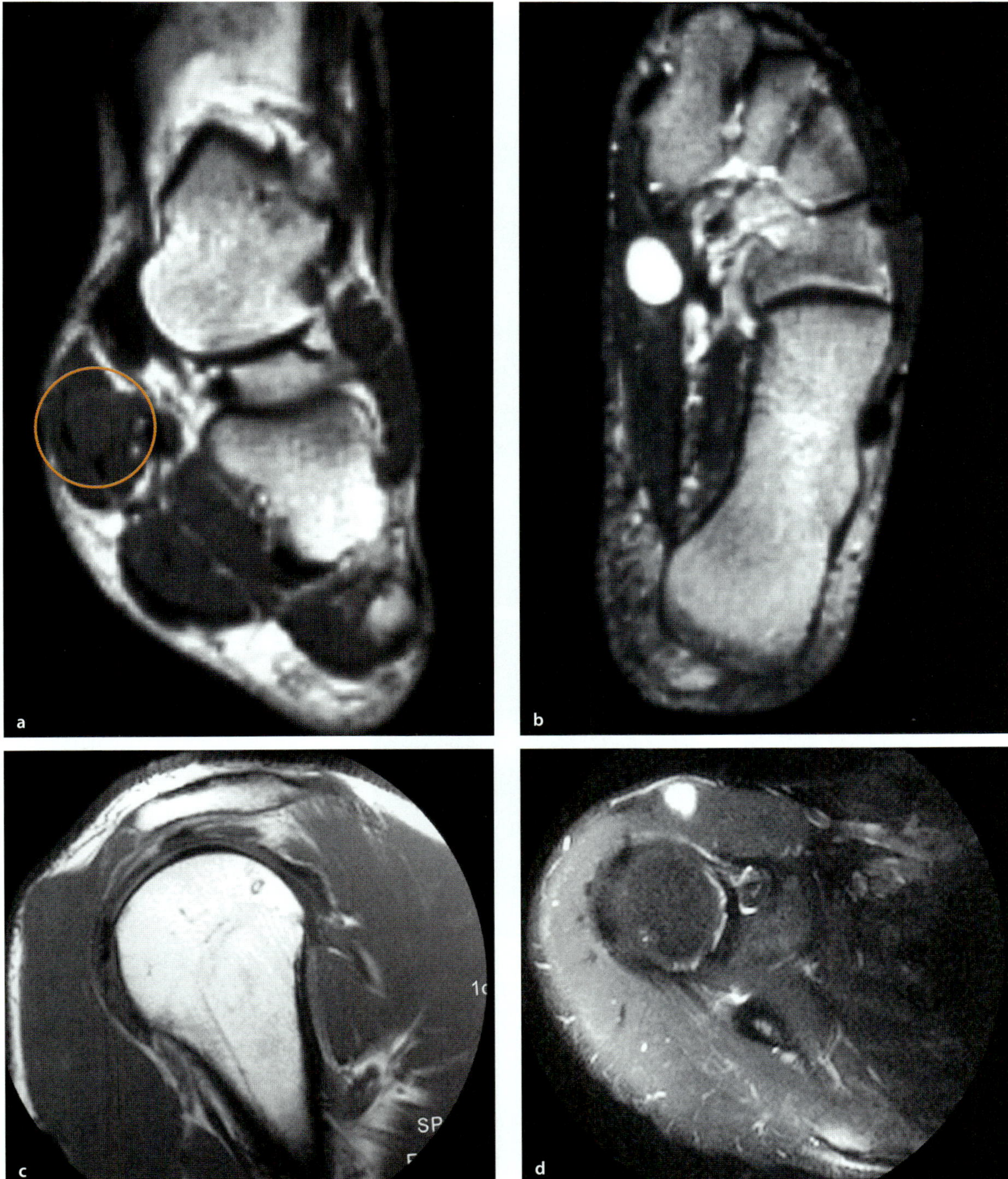

Fig. 11.10 a–d. Soft tissue tumors classified according to their signal intensities on T1- and T2-weighted images. **Group IV:** intermediate SI on T1- and high SI on T2-weighted images: **a,b** schwannoma (T1-WI / T2-WI); **c,d** nodular fasciitis (T1-WI/T2 WI)

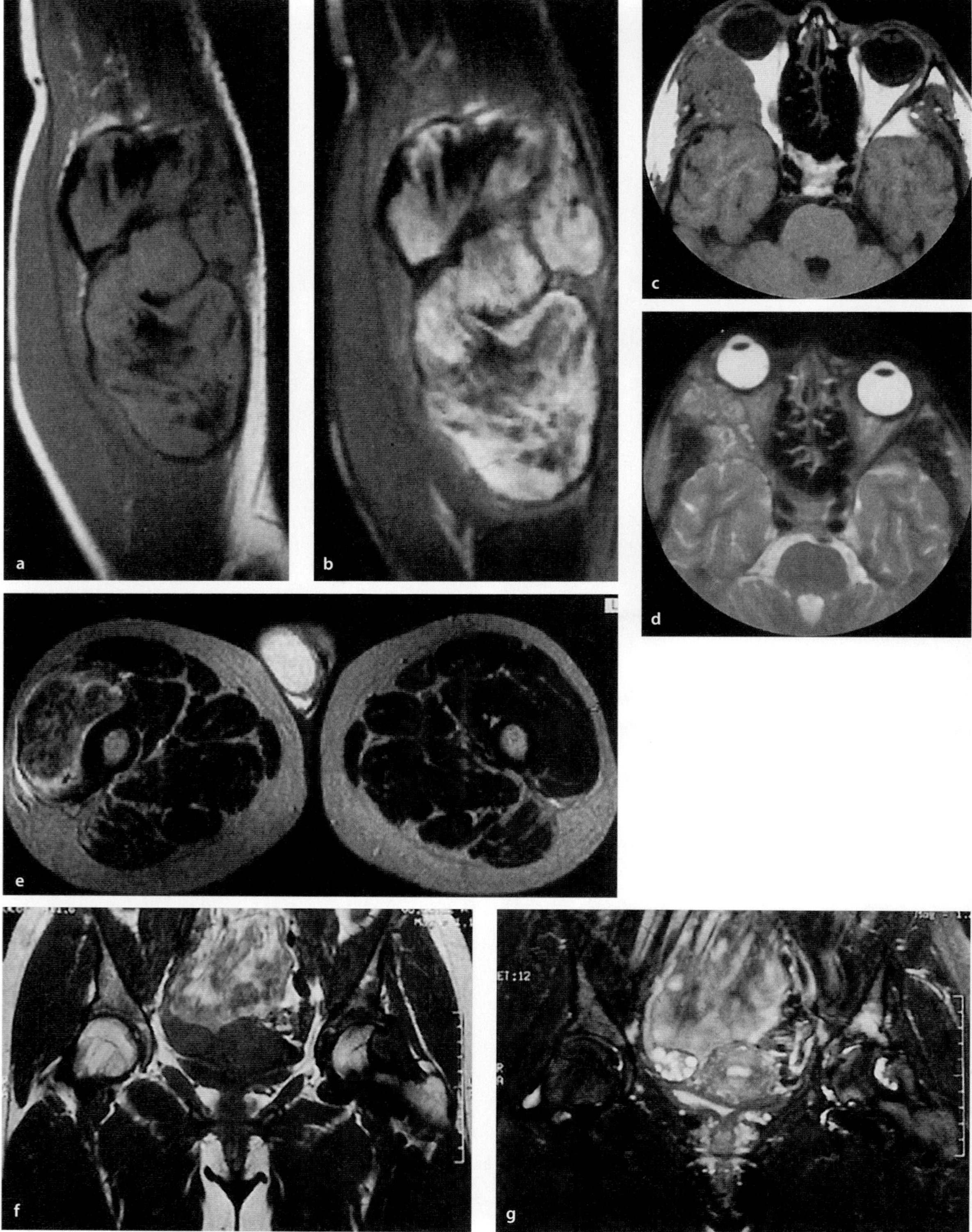

Fig. 11.11 a–i.

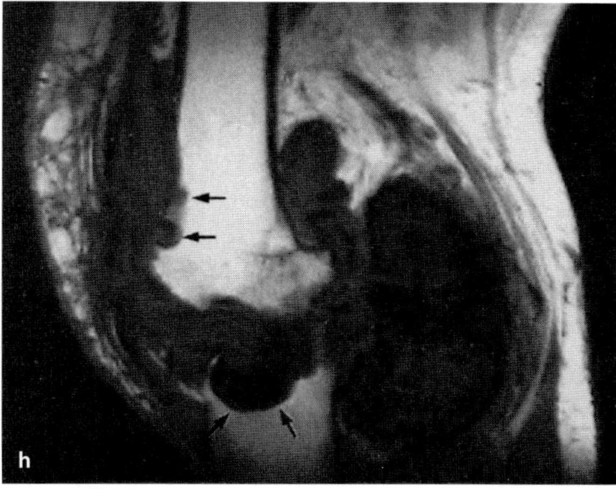

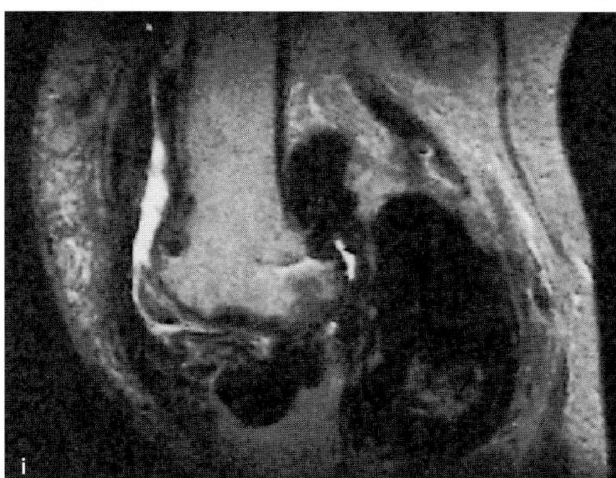

Fig. 11.11 h,i. Soft tissue tumors classified according to their signal intensities on T1- and T2-weighted images. **Group V**: low SI on T1- and low SI on T2-weighted images: **a,b** desmoid tumor (collagen); **c,d** rhabdomyosarcoma (high cellularity, decreased amount of intra- and extracellular water); **e** old hematoma (hemosiderin); **f,g** pigmented villonodular synovitis (hemosiderin); **h,i** pigmented villonodular synovitis (hemosiderin)

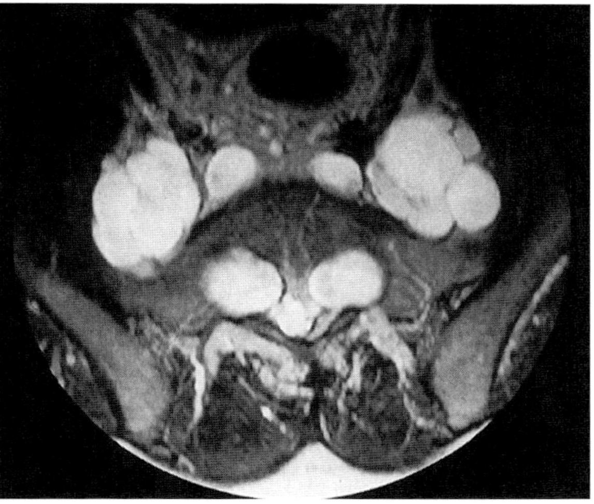

Fig. 11.12. Multiple neurofibromata of the presacral region and sacral spinal canal in a case of neurofibromatosis I presenting with a moniliform masses of high signal intensity on T2-WI.

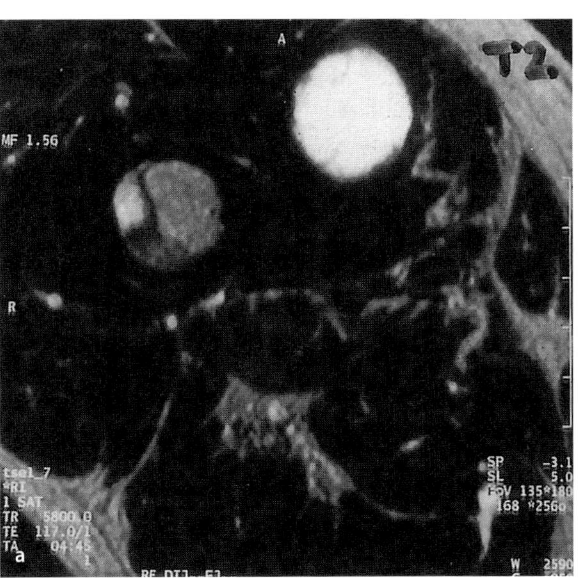

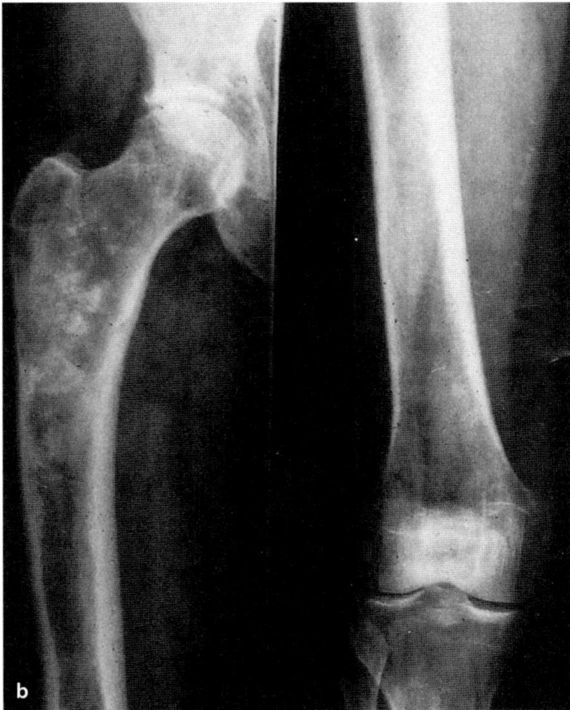

Fig. 11.13 a,b. Myxoma of the thigh (**a**) in a patient with fibrous dysplasia of the right femur (**b**) (Mazabraud's syndrome). Adjacent to the pathological right femur there is a rounded soft tissue mass with high signal intensity on SE-T2-WI

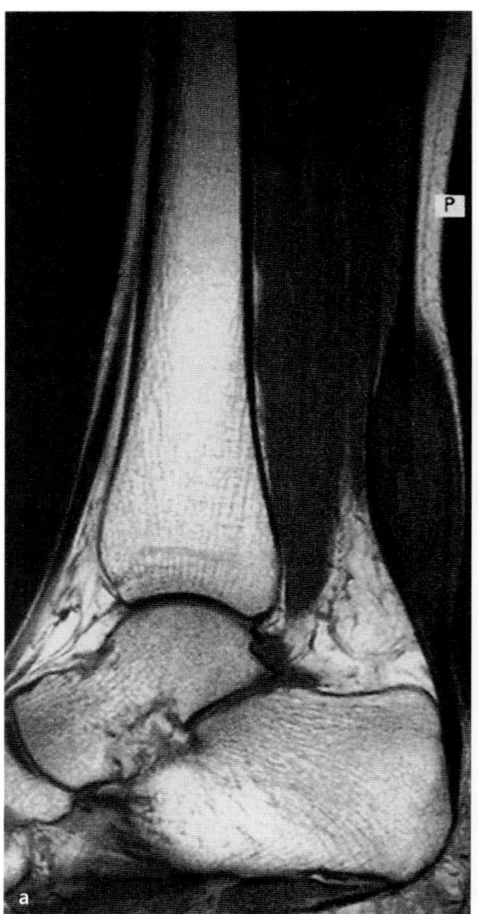

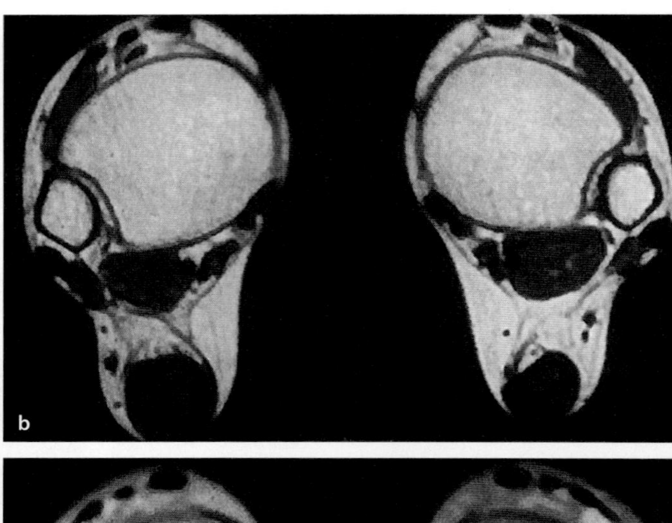

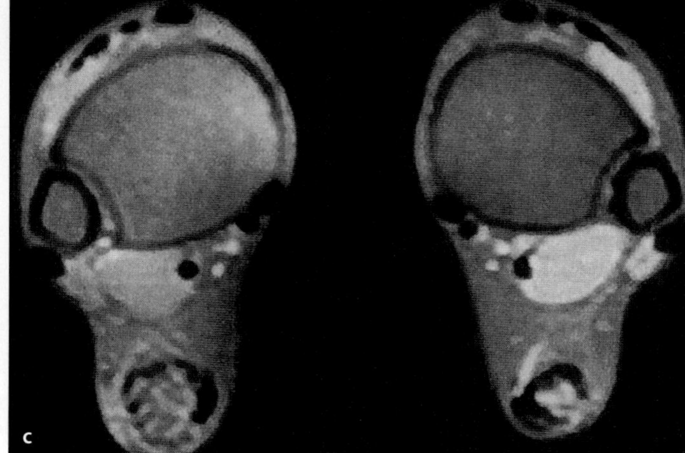

Fig. 11.14 a–c. Xanthoma of both Achilles tendons in a patient with familial hypercholesterolemia. Both lesions are fusiform on sagittal images (**a**), have a speckled appearance on axial SE- T1- WI (**b**) and the signal of intratendinous xanthomatous areas is not reduced on fat suppressed T1- WI (**c**)

Things to remember

1. Most soft tissue tumors are benign (60-75%). The major role of grading consists in recognizing benign soft tissue tumors, which will be excluded from further invasive diagnostic and therapeutic procedures.
2. Accuracy of individual (MR imaging-) parameters is low except for dynamic contrast-enhanced MR parameters which allow the best differentiation between benign and malignant soft tissue tumors.
3. Best results are obtained by combining individual grading parameters (sensitivity 93%/specificity 82%).
4. Besides age and location, shape, signal intensities on different pulse sequences, presence of signal voids, presence of fluid-fluid levels, multiplicity and knowledge of associated diseases, are major tissue specific parameters. Here also, combination of different parameters increases imaging performance.
5. Five groups of soft tissue tumors are defined, according to their signal intensities on T1- and T2-weighted MR images. High SI on T1- and low SI on T2-weighted images have the best predictive value concerning tissue specific diagnosis.
6. Multi-institutional approach of soft tissue tumors guarantees best diagnostic and therapeutic results.

References

1. Alexander A, Nazarian L, Feld R (1997) Superficial soft tissue masses suggestive of recurrent malignancy: sonographic localization and biopsy. AJR Am J Roentgenol 169:1449–1451
2. Anderson MW, Temple HT, Dussault RG, Kaplan PA (1999) Compartmental anatomy: relevance to staging and biopsy of musculoskeletal tumors. Am J Roentgenol 173:1663–1671
3. Balzarini L, Ceglia E, Petrillo R, Tesoro Tess JD, Reitano A, Musumeci R (1989) Magnetic resonance in neoplasms of the adipose, fibrous and muscular tissues. Radiol Med 77:87–93
4. Bass J, Korobkin M, Francis I, Ellis J, Cohan R (1994) Retroperitoneal plexiform neurofibromatosis: CT findings. AJR Am J Roentgenol 163:617–620

5. Berquist T, Ehman R, King B, Hodgman C, Ilstrup D (1990) Value of MR imaging in differentiating benign from malignant soft-tissue masses: study of 95 lesions. AJR Am J Roentgenol 155:1251–1255
6. Binkovitz L, Berquist T, McLeod (1990) Masses of the hand and wrist: detection and characterization with MR imaging. AJR Am J Roentgenol 154:323–326
7. Bongartz G, Vestring T, Peters P (1992) Magnetresonanztomographie der Weichteiltumoren. Radiology 32:584–590
8. Capelastegui A, Astigarraga E, Fernandez-Canton G, Saralegui I, Larena JA, Merino A (1999) Masses and pseudomasses of the hand and wrist: MR findings in 134 cases. Skeletal Radiol 28:498–507
9. Cerofolini E, Landi A, Desantis G, Maiorana A, Canossi G, Romagnoli R (1991) MR of benign peripheral nerve sheath tumors. J Comput Assist Tomogr 15:593–597
10. Crim J, Seeger L, Yao L, Chandnani V, Eckardt J (1992) Diagnosis of soft tissue masses with MR imaging: can benign masses be differentiated from malignant ones? Radiology 185:581–586
11. Daldrup H, Shames D, Wendland M, et al (1998) Correlation of dynamic contrast-enhanced MR imaging with histologic tumor grade. AJR Am J Roentgenol 171:941–949
12. De Beuckeleer LH, De Schepper AM, Vandevenne JE, Bloem (2000) MR imaging of clear cell sarcoma (malignant melanoma of the soft parts): a multicenter correlative MRI-pathology study of 21 cases and literature review. Skeletal Radiol 29(4):187–195
13. De Schepper A, Ramon F, Degryse H (1992) Magnetic resonance imaging of soft tissue tumors. J Belge Radiol 75:286–296
14. De Schepper A, Ramon F, Degryse H (1992) Statistical analysis of MRI parameters predicting malignancy in 141 soft tissue masses. Rofo Fortschr Geb Rontgenstr Neuen Bildgeb Verfahr 156:587–591
15. De Schepper A, De Beuckeleer L, Vandevenne J, Somville J (2000) Magnetic resonance imaging of soft tissue tumors. Eur Radiol 10:213–222
16. Elias DA, White LM, Simpson DJ, Kandel RA, Tomlinson G, Bell RS, Wunder JS (2003) Osseous invasion by soft-tissue sarcoma: assessment with MR imaging. Radiology 229(1):145–152
17. Erlemann R, Reiser M, Peters P, Vasallo P, Nommenson B, Kusnierz-Glaz C, Ritter J, Roessner A (1989) Musculoskeletal neoplasms: static and dynamic Gd-DTPA-enhanced MR imaging. Radiology 171:767–773
18. Erlemann R, Sciuk J, Wuisman P, Bene D, Edel G, Ritter J, Peters P (1992) Dynamische MR-Tomographie in der Diagnostik entzündlicher und tumoröser Raumforderungen des musculoskeletalen Systems. Rofo Fortschr Geb Rontgenstr Neuen Bildgeb Verfahr 156:353–359
19. Fleming I (1992) Staging of pediatric cancers. Semin Surg Oncol 8:94–97
20. Fletcher B, Hanna S, Fairclough D, Gronemeyer S (1992) Pediatric musculoskeletal tumors: use of dynamic contrast-enhanced MR imaging to monitor response to chemotherapy. Radiology 184:243–248
21. Galant J, Marti-Bonmati L, Soler R, et al (1998) Grading of subcutaneous soft tissue tumors by means of their relationship with the superficial fascia on MR imaging. Skeletal Radiol 27:657–663
22. Gielen JL, De Schepper AM, Vanhoenacker F, Parizel PM, Wang XL, Sciot R, Weyler J (2004) Accuracy of MRI in characterization of soft tissue tumors and tumor-like lesions. A prospective study in 548 patients. Eur Radiol 14(12):2320–2330
23. Greenfield G, Arrington J, Kudryk B (1993) MRI of soft tissue tumors. Skeletal Radiol 22:77–84
24. Hanna SL, Fletcher B (1995) MR Imaging of malignant soft tissue tumors. Magn Reson Imaging Clin N Am 3:629–650
25. Harkens K, Moore T, Yuh W, Kathol M, Hawes D, El-Khoury G, Berbaum K (1993) Gadolinium-enhanced MRI of soft tissue masses. Australas Radiol 37:30–34
26. Hermann G, Abdelwahab I, Miller T, Klein M, Lewis M (1992) Tumour and tumour-like conditions of the soft tissue: magnetic resonance imaging features differentiating benign form malignant masses. Br J Radiol 65:14–20
27. Kransdorf M (1995) Malignant soft tissue tumors in a large referral population: distribution of specific diagnoses by age, sex and location. AJR Am J Roentgenol 164:129–134
28. Kransdorf M (1995) Benign soft tissue tumors in a large referral population: distribution of specific diagnoses by age, sex and location. AJR Am J Roentgenol 164:395–402
29. Kransdorf M, Murphey M (1997) Imaging of soft tissue tumors. WB Saunders, Philadelphia
30. Kransdorf M, Jelinek J, Moser R (1993) Imaging of soft tissue tumors. Radiol Clin North Am 31:359–372
31. Ma L, Frassica F, Scott E, Fishman E, Zerhouni E (1995) Differentiation of benign and malignant musculoskeletal tumors: potential pitfalls with MR imaging. Radiographics 15:349–366
32. Ma L, Frassica F, McCarthy E, et al (1997) Benign and malignant musculoskeletal masses: MR imaging differentiation with rim-to-center differential enhancement ratios. Radiology 202:739–744
33. Marti-Bonmati L (2004) Benign/malignant classifier of soft tissue tumors using MR imaging. Mag Reson Mater Phys Biol Med 16(4):194–201
34. Meiss-Kindblom J, Enzinger F (1996) Color atlas of soft tissue tumors. Mosby-Wolfe, St Louis
35. Miller T, Potter H, McCormack R (1994) Benign soft tissue masses of the wrist and hand: MRI appearances. Skeletal Radiol 23:327–332
36. Moulton J, Blebea J, Dunco D, Braley S, Bisset G, Emery K (1995) MR imaging of soft tissue masses: diagnostic efficacy and value of distinguishing between benign and malignant lesions. AJR Am J Roentgenol 164:1191–1199
37. Petasnick J, Turner D, Charters J, Gitelis S, Zacharias C (1986) Soft tissue masses of the locomotor system: comparison of MRI with CT. Radiology 160:125–133
38. Sundaram M, McLeod R (1990) MR imaging of tumor and tumorlike lesions of bone and soft tissue. AJR Am J Roentgenol 155:817–824
39. Sundaram M, Sharafuddin M (1995) MR Imaging of benign soft tissue masses. Magn Reson Imaging Clin N Am 3:609–627
40. Sundaram M, McGuire M, Herbold D, Beshany S, Fletcher J (1987) High signal intensity soft tissue masses on T2-weighted pulse sequence. Skeletal Radiol 16:30–34
41. Tacikowska M (2002) Dynamic MR imaging of soft tissue tumors with assessment of the rate and character of lesion enhancement. Med Sci Monit 8(2):MT31–35
42. Tacikowska M (2002) Dynamic magnetic resonance imaging in soft tissue tumors- assessment of the diagnostic value of tumor enhancement rate indices. Med Sci Monit 8(4):MT53–57
43. Totty W, Murphy W, Lee J (1986) Soft tissue tumors: MR imaging. Radiology 160:135–141
44. Tung G, Davis L (1993) The role of magnetic resonance imaging in the evaluation of the soft tissue mass. Crit Rev Diagn Imaging 34:239–308
45. Vanel D, Shapeero L, Tardivon A, et al (1998) Dynamic contrast-enhanced MRI with subtraction of aggressive soft tissue tumors after resection. Skeletal Radiol 27:505–510
46. Van der Woude H, Verstraete K, Hogendoorn P, et al (1998) Musculoskeletal tumors : does fast dynamic contrast-enhanced subtraction MR imaging contribute to the characterization. Radiology 208:821–828
47. van Rijswijk Catharina SP, Geirnaerdt Maarje JA, Hogendoorn Pancras CW, Taminiau Antonie HM, van Coevorden Frits, Zwinderman Aeilko H, Pope Thomas L, Bloem Johan L (2004) Soft-tissue tumors: value of static and dynamic gadopentetae dimeglumine-enhanced MR imaging in prediction of malignancy. Radiology 233:493–502
48. van Unnik JA, Coindre JM, Contesso C, Albus-Lutter CE, Schiodt T, Sylvester R, Thomas D, Bramwell V, Mouridsen HT (1993) Grading of soft tissue sarcomas: experience of the EORTC Sc. Tissue and Bone Sarcoma Group. Eur J Cancer 29A(15):2089–2093
49. Vandevenne J, De Schepper AM, De Beuckeleer L, et al (1997) New Concepts in understanding evolution of desmoid tumors: MR imaging of 30 lesions. Eur Radiol 7:1013–1019
50. Verstraete K (1994) Dynamic contrast-enhanced magnetic resonance imaging of tumor and tumor-like lesions of the musculoskeletal system. Thesis, University of Ghent

51. Verstraete K, De Deene Y, Roels H, Dierick A, Uyttendaele D, Kunnen M (1994) Benign and malignant musculoskeletal lesions: dynamic contrast-enhanced MR imaging – parametric "first-pass" images depict tissue vascularization and perfusion. Radiology 192:835–843

52. Weatherall PT (1995) Benign and malignant masses. MR Imaging differentiation. Magn Reson Imaging Clin N Am 3: 669–694

53. Wetzel L, Levine E (1990) Soft tissue tumors of the foot: value of MR imaging for specific diagnosis. AJR Am J Roentgenol 155:1025–1030

54. Wolf R, Enneking W (1996) The staging and surgery of musculoskeletal neoplasms. Orthop Clin North Am 27:473–481

General Imaging Strategy of Soft Tissue Tumors

12

P. Van Dyck, J. Gielen, F.M. Vanhoenacker,
A. De Schepper

Contents

12.1 Introduction

The imaging evaluation of a patient with a suspected soft tissue tumor (STT) requires a methodological approach that recognizes the benefits and limitations of the numerous imaging techniques that are available. Consideration must be given to the individual experience of the investigator, and the financial costs, availability, and invasiveness of each technique balanced against the diagnosis. Therefore, an "optimal imaging pathway" that meets all these criteria probably does not exist, and the imaging pathway should be tailored to individual cases.

Whenever a patient presents with a soft tissue mass, a detailed history should be taken and a thorough clinical examination performed. Cardinal information is derived from the age of the patient and the location of the lesion. Patients may complain of (usually painless) local swelling, numbness, paresthesia, or irradiating pain due to neural entrapment, or they may have no complaints at all. Nevertheless, further imaging is often required early in the evaluation procedure to, in most instances, reassure both patient and clinician of the benign character of the lesion. The major role of imaging is detection, grading (characterization and tissue-specific diagnosis), staging, and follow-up.

12.2 Detection

The choice of the initial imaging technique used for *detection* of a STT is determined by whether the mass lesion is palpable or not. For a superficially located lesion, (high-frequency) ultrasound is used. In these instances, ultrasound will frequently establish the benign (e.g., lipoma) or "pseudotumoral" (e.g., ganglion cyst, tenosynovitis, hematoma, sebaceous cyst) nature of the mass lesion, obviating unnecessary and invasive imaging workup. A follow-up ultrasound examination can be scheduled in the near future, depending on the ultrasound characteristics and the clinical evolution of the lesion. If the lesion has not changed (e.g., lipoma), further investigation is not necessary. However, if ultrasound shows volume increase or changed echotexture, the patient is referred to the magnetic resonance imaging (MRI) unit.

Although Doppler/ultrasound is suitable for differentiation of cystic or solid components of a soft tissue mass and evaluation of vascularity, it often reveals nonspecific imaging findings, and therefore its role in lesion characterization is rather limited. For deeper-located and/or nonpalpable lesions, plain radiography (with two views at right angles) may be performed initially to detect associated bone involvement and intralesional calcification and/or ossification. Due to its high sensitivity, MRI must be performed in patients with clinical suspicion of a STT when other imaging techniques remain negative or inconclusive.

12.3 Grading and Local Staging

Because of its superior soft-tissue contrast resolution, MRI is regarded as the imaging modality of choice for *grading and local staging* of a STT. The use of a standardized MR-examination protocol (including a combination of T1- and T2-weighted images in different imaging planes, with and without fat suppression, and before and after gadolinium contrast administration) provides maximal information on the size, the local extent, and the "tissue" content of a STT. Furthermore, fast gradient sequences during administration of intravenous gadolinium can be used to determine the vascularization of a STT (dynamic MRI). For a detailed discussion of the MRI signs of benign or malignant STTs, the reader is referred to Chaps. 13–27.

Most benign lesions have signal characteristics highly suggestive of their diagnosis. In these cases, a follow-

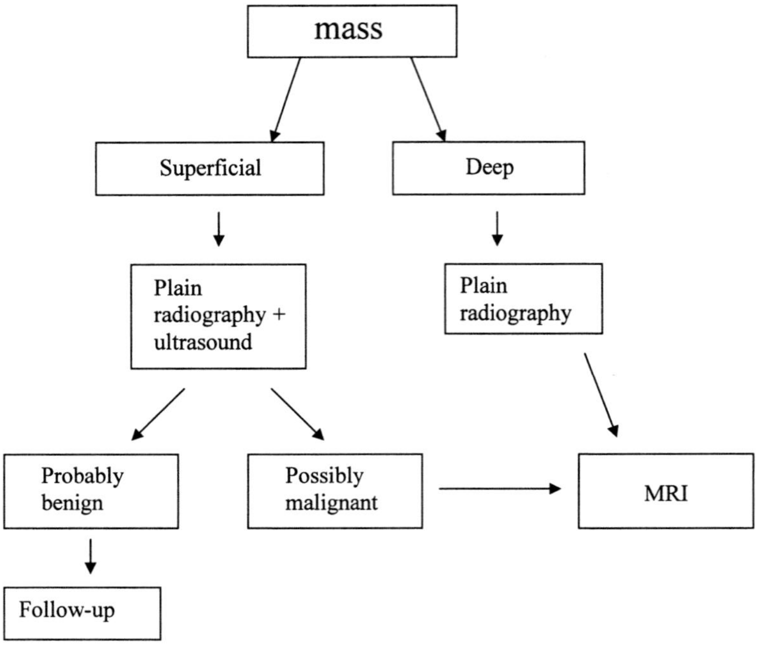

Fig. 12.1. Diagnostic imaging pathway for STT

up MR examination can be planned. Whenever MRI findings are not characteristic of a benign lesion or whenever equivocal MRI findings are displayed, biopsy is mandatory.

For grading and local staging of a STT, the other imaging modalities are of limited use but can be helpful to answer specific questions: the presence or absence of calcification, which plays a role in the characterization of a STT, or of adjacent bone involvement, which is important in the staging process, can be detected by plain radiography and even better by CT. However, the major role of a CT scan is twofold. Firstly, to investigate distant spread of (malignant) STT in the lungs or abdomen in a preoperative setting, and secondly, to guide biopsy.

The role of conventional angiography in characterization of a STT is limited but may provide (preoperative) vascular mapping, employed as a prelude to embolotherapy or isolated limb perfusion. Scintigraphy has a limited role to play and has to be reserved for detecting bone metastases.

12.4 Post-therapeutic Follow-up

Finally, MRI is of cardinal importance in the *post-therapeutic follow-up* of a STT. Due to the use of a specific MRI protocol (with fat-saturated T2-weighted images and dynamic contrast-enhanced sequences), post-therapeutic fibrosis can be differentiated from residual tumor or tumor recurrence.

12.5 Conclusion

Baseline imaging evaluation of a STT always starts with plain radiography. Ultrasound can be performed secondarily for superficially located lesions. However, MRI plays a central role in the medical imaging of a STT.

Our imaging algorithm is summarized in Fig. 12.1. If there is any suspicion for malignancy, biopsy should be performed.

Although pathology is still regarded as the gold standard, this does not obviate the need for a second opinion, after thorough discussion between orthopedic surgeons, pathologists, and radiologists, reaching a diagnosis in consensus in such rare pathologies. To meet this purpose, we have installed at our institution a peer review committee of pathologists and radiologists, all having extensive experience in pathology of STTs.

Things to remember:
1. Clinical information is of utmost importance in the diagnosis of STT.
2. Initial imaging evaluation of a patient presenting with a STT starts with plain radiography and/or ultrasound.
3. If the lesion has no definite benign characteristics on these imaging modalities, MRI has to be performed for further evaluation of the lesion.
4. If the mass suggests malignancy on MR images, biopsy is mandatory.
5. MRI is the best method for detecting recurrent tumor after therapy.
6. Close cooperation between radiologists and pathologists increases diagnostic accuracy.

Part 3
Imaging of Soft Tissue Tumors

Tumors of Connective Tissue

A. M. De Schepper, J. E. Vandevenne

13

Contents

13.1 Introduction

Fibrous tissue consists of fibroblasts and an extracellular matrix containing both fibrillary structures (collagen, elastin) and nonfibrillary, gel-like ground substance. Both fibroblasts (spindle-shaped cells) and myofibroblasts, which are modified fibroblasts showing features common to fibroblasts and smooth muscle cells, produce procollagen and collagen. Collagen is the main, noncontractile component of the extracellular matrix, elastin is the main, contractile component of elastic fibers. The amorphous ground substance of fibrous tissue contains glycosaminoglycans (mucopolysaccharides), the most common types being hyaluronic acid, chondroitin 4- and 6-sulfates, and proteoglycans. [56] Fibrous tissue can be loose or dense depending on the relative amount of the three components. Dense fibrous tissue is seen in tendons, ligaments, and aponeuroses.

Fibroblastic/myofibroblastic tumors represent a very large subset of mesenchymal tumors. Many lesions in this category contain cells with both fibroblastic and myofibroblastic features, which may in fact represent functional variants of a single cell type. The relative proportions of these cell types vary not only between individual cases but also within a single lesion over time (often in proportion to cellularity). A significant subset of spindle cell and pleomorphic sarcomas are probably myofibroblastic in type, but, to date, only low-grade forms have been reproducibly characterized. Among lesions formerly known as malignant fibrous histiocytoma (MFH), at least some represent pleomorphic myofibrosarcomas.

Principal changes and advances since the 1994 WHO classification have been the characterization of numerous previously undefined lesions, including ischemic fasciitis, desmoplastic fibroblastoma, mammary-type myofibroblastoma, angiomyofibroblastoma, cellular angiofibroma, Gardner fibroma, low-grade fibromyxoid sarcoma, acral myxoinflammatory fibroblastic sarcoma, sclerosing epithelioid fibrosarcoma, and low-grade myofibroblastic sarcoma.

Conceptual changes have included the clearer recognition of solitary fibrous tumor in soft tissue and the realization that most cases of so-called hemangiopericytoma belong in this category, as well as the reclassification of lesions formerly labeled "myxoid MFH" as "myxofibrosarcoma" and the definitive allocation of the tumors to the fibroblastic category.

The new (2002) WHO classification of fibroblastic/myofibroblastic tumors [20] contains a large number of new and modified lesions. They are categorized into four groups according to their degree of malignancy, i.e., (1) benign, (2) intermediate (locally aggressive), (3) intermediate (rarely metastasizing), and (4) malignant:

1. **Benign:**
   Nodular fasciitis
   Proliferative fasciitis
   Proliferative myositis
   Myositis ossificans
   Fibro-osseous pseudotumor of digits
   Ischemic fasciitis
   Elastofibroma
   Fibrous hamartoma of infancy
   Myofibroma/Myofibromatosis
   Fibromatosis colli
   Juvenile hyaline fibromatosis
   Inclusion-body fibromatosis
   Fibroma of tendon sheath
   Desmoplastic fibroblastoma
   Mammary-type myofibroblastoma
   Calcifying aponeurotic fibroma
   Angiomyofibroblastoma
   Cellular angiofibroma
   Nuchal-type fibroma
   Gardner fibroma
   Calcifying fibrous tumor
   Giant cell angiofibroma
2. **Intermediate (locally aggressive):**
   Superficial fibromatoses (palmar/plantar)
   Desmoid-type fibromatoses
   Lipofibromatosis
3. **Intermediate (rarely metastasizing):**
   Solitary fibrous tumor and hemangiopericytoma (including lipomatous hemangiopericytoma)
   Inflammatory myofibroblastic tumor
   Low-grade myofibroblastic sarcoma
   Myxoinflammatory fibroblastic sarcoma
   Infantile fibrosarcoma
4. **Malignant:**
   Adult fibrosarcoma
   Myxofibrosarcoma
   Low-grade fibromyxoid sarcoma hyalinizing spindle-cell tumor
   Sclerosing epithelioid fibrosarcoma

In the case of several fibroblastic proliferations (elastofibroma, fibroma of tendon sheath, extra-abdominal desmoids, fibromatosis colli), it is unclear whether these constitute reactive fibrosing processes or true neoplasms. Fibromatoses are aggressive, infiltrating lesions, despite their histologically benign character, and aggressive fibromatoses or musculoaponeurotic desmoid tumors are by far the largest group of tumors of fibrous tissue. The terminology of childhood fibromatosis is confusing, and there are many classification systems based on different clinicopathological parameters such

as age, localization, histology, and aggressiveness of the lesion [86]. Fibrous tumors of infancy and childhood and soft tissue fibrosarcomas are rare and have only sparsely been reported in the radiological literature. It is a constant finding that the majority of these tumors have a high recurrence rate after surgical resection, and recurrent lesions mostly have a more aggressive behavior than their primary counterparts. Another constant finding is the natural evolution of tumors of fibrous tissue, which are hypercellular in their initial stage and become more collagenous in later stages. Localization of the lesion and age of the patient are major diagnostic factors. Fibroma of tendon sheath, elastofibroma, all types of fibromatosis, and fibromatosis colli are characterized by typical localizations [30, 85].

13.2 Benign Fibroblastic Proliferations

Benign fibroblastic proliferations constitute a heterogeneous group of well-defined entities. Some of these, such as nodular fasciitis, grow rapidly and are richly cellular. Others, such as fibroma of the tendon sheath and elastofibroma, grow slowly, are much less cellular, and contain considerable amounts of collagen [17, 71].

13.2.1 Nodular Fasciitis

Nodular fasciitis, also called pseudosarcomatous fasciitis, infiltrative fasciitis, or proliferative fasciitis, is a benign soft tissue lesion composed of proliferating fibroblastic-myofibroblastic cells. It is characterized by rapid growth, which may arouse suspicion of sarcoma [47]. Although the cause is unknown, it is likely that it is triggered by local injury or a local inflammatory process. Most patients are asymptomatic or note only mild discomfort. Lesions are round to oval and mostly located in the upper extremity (48%), mostly the volar aspect of the forearm [83], trunk (20%), head and neck (17%), and lower extremity (5%) [42, 59]. Shimizu has reported on a series of 250 patients with a mean age of 39 years and a peak in the fourth decade, in whom 44% of the lesions are located in the upper extremity, which is followed in frequency by the lower extremity and the trunk [75]. Although no sex predilection for nodular fasciitis is mentioned in literature, we reported on a series of ten patients, nine of them being female [83]!

There are three subtypes of nodular fasciitis, defined according to their topography: the most common subcutaneous type, the intramuscular type, and the fascial type, which spreads along superficial fascial planes. Microscopically, younger lesions consist of fibroblasts embedded in a dense reticulin meshwork and birefringent collagen. There is a rich intervening myxoid matrix. Older lesions tend to be more fibrous. In this re-

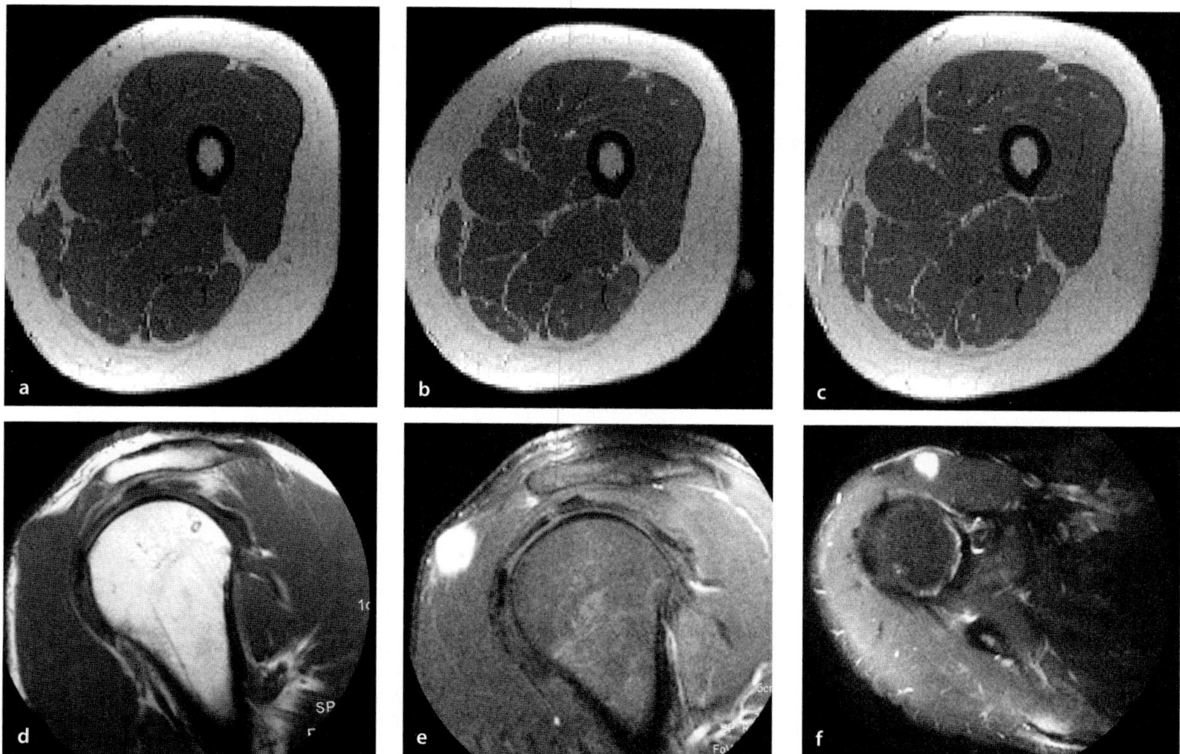

Fig. 13.1 a–f. Two cases of nodular fasciitis, fascial type: a first case (**a–c**) at the fascia of the sartorius muscle, a second case (**d–f**) at the fascia of pectoralis muscle. **a** Axial spin-echo T1-weighted MR image. **b** Axial spin-echo T1-weighted MR image after gadolinium contrast injection. **c** Axial spin-echo T2-weighted MR image. **d** Sagittal spin-echo T1-weighted MR image. **e** Sagittal spin-echo T1-weighted MR image after gadolinium contrast injection, with fat suppression. **f** Axial spin-echo T2-weighted MR image. Both lesions are in close contact with superficial fasciae. On T1-weighted images, both lesions are of slightly higher signal intensity (SI) when compared with SI of normal muscle (**a, d**). They both enhance markedly after contrast injection (**b, e**) and are of high SI on T2-weighted MR images (**c, f**)

gard, nodular fasciitis can be subdivided into three types based on the predominant histological features: myxoid (type 1), cellular (type 2), and fibrous (type 3). However, since many different features may coexist in one lesion, definition of a single fixed type is not always possible. There is no correlation between histological subtypes and the subtypes classified according to their anatomical location. Histological transformation from type 1 to type 2 and then to type 3 is indicative of the natural evolution of these lesions. Recurrence after excision is very rare and occurs in less than 2% of the cases.

On ultrasound images, lesions of this kind are mostly solid, and cystic change has been reported (Fig. 13.2a). On CT scans, nodular fasciitis has low attenuation values, reflecting the myxoid character of the lesions [59]. The appearance on MR images reflects the gross morphology of the tumor. Myxoid and cellular lesions are iso- to hyperintense compared with skeletal muscle on T1-weighted images and iso- to hyperintense compared with fat on T2-weighted images. Lesions with a more fibrous histology are markedly hypointense on all spin-

echo sequences [59]. Myxoid lesions show a marked and homogeneous enhancement, cellular lesions a nonhomogeneous enhancement, and fibrous lesions a moderate, nonhomogeneous enhancement [83]. Three cases in our own series had the same appearance on MR images: a central area of low signal intensity (SI) and a peripheral area of higher SI on T1-weighted images, and an inverted SI pattern (high SI of the center, and low SI of the periphery) on T2-weighted images. After gadolinium (Gd) contrast injection there is a marked enhancement of the peripheral zone, with poor enhancement of the center. This pattern was described in 1991 by Frei et al. [25]. On comparing these findings with the MR features of some neurogenic tumors (target sign), we named the pattern "the inverted target sign" (Figs. 13.1, 13.2).

The cellular type of nodular fasciitis is apt to be mistaken for a sarcoma (myxofibrosarcoma and fibrosarcoma), while the fibrous type must be differentiated from fibromatosis. Recurrent tumors have a more aggressive behavior than primary ones (Fig. 13.3).

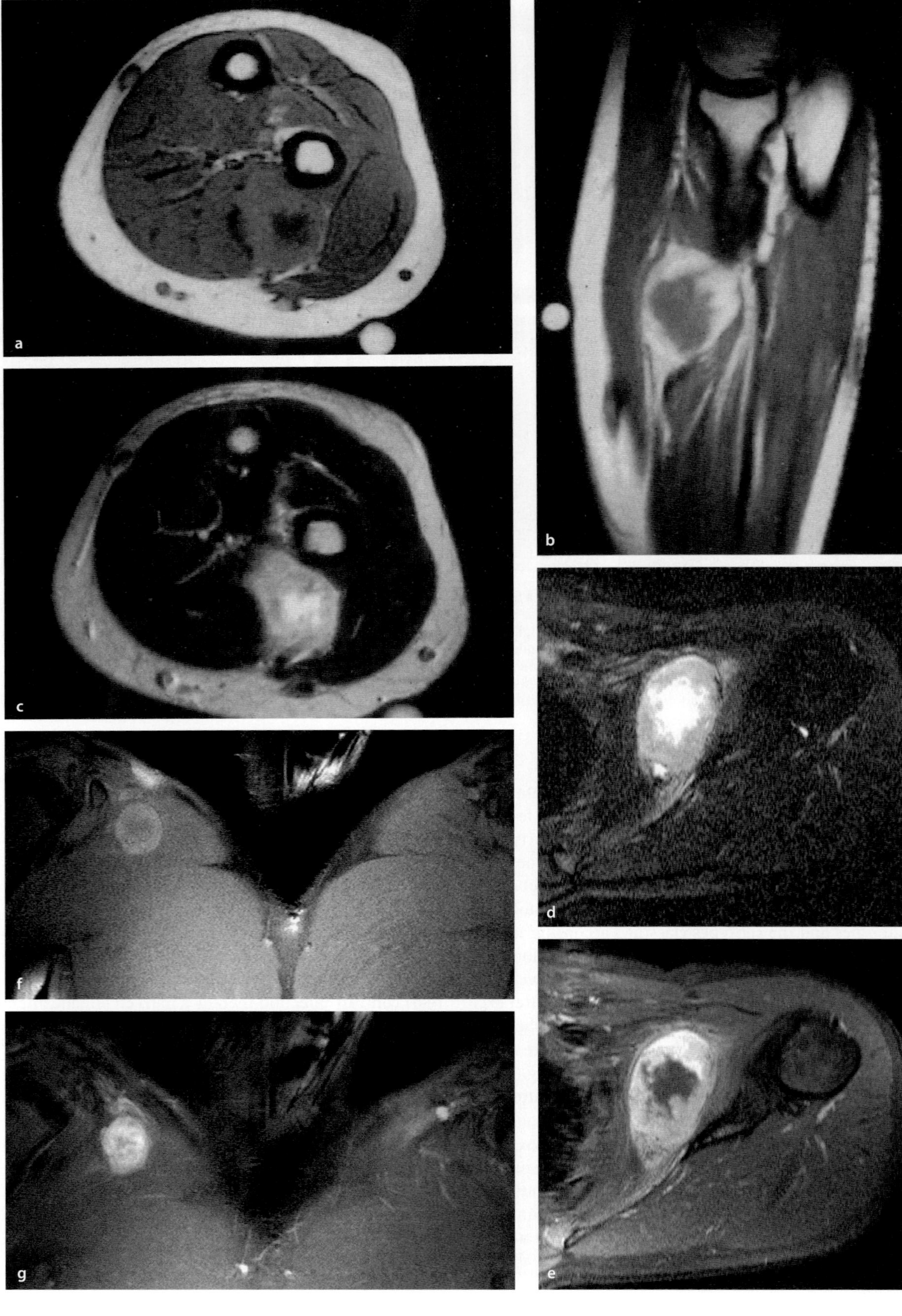

Fig. 13.2 a–g. Three cases of nodular fasciitis, intramuscular type: the first case (**a–c**) at the forearm, the second case (**d, e**) at the subscapularis muscle, and the third case (**f, g**) at the pectoralis muscle. **a** Axial spin-echo T1-weighted MR image. **b** Coronal spin-echo T1-weighted MR image after gadolinium contrast injection. **c** Axial spin-echo T2-weighted MR image. **d** Axial spin-echo T2-weighted MR image. **e** Axial spin-echo T1-weighted MR image after gadolinium contrast injection, with fat suppression. **f** Coronal spin-echo T1-weighted MR image, with fat suppression. **g** Coronal spin-echo T1-weighted MR image after gadolinium contrast injection, with fat suppression. All three cases present with the so called "inverted target" sign consisting of a peripheral zone of increased SI on T1-weighted MR images (**a, f**), decreased SI on T2-weighted MR images (**c, d**) and merely peripheral contrast enhancement (**b, e, g**)

13.2.2 Fibroma of Tendon Sheath

Fibroma of the tendon sheath consists of a benign, slow-growing, dense fibrous nodule (or multinodular mass) firmly attached to the tendon sheath and is found most frequently in the hands and feet (Fig. 13.4). The thumb, index finger, and middle finger together with lesions of

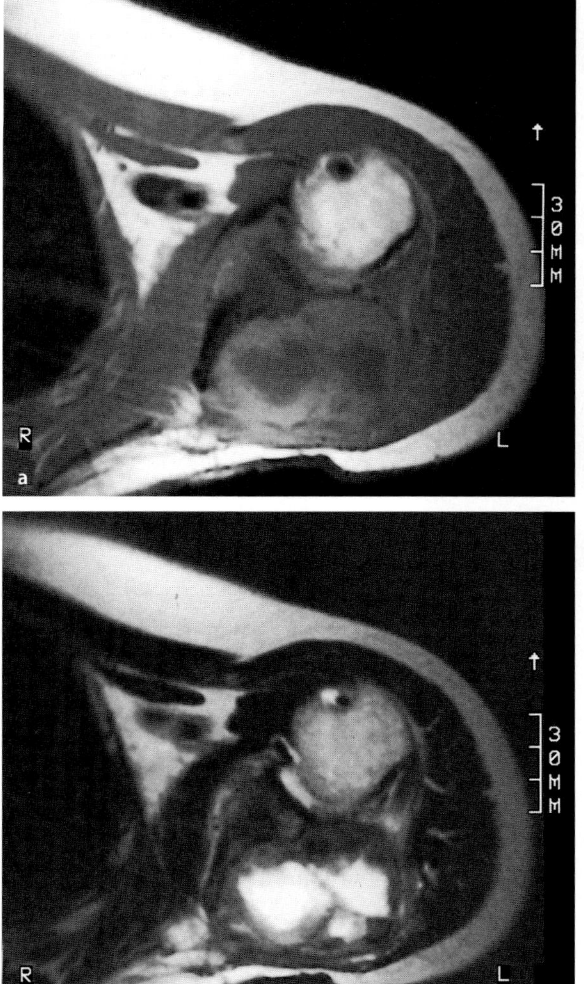

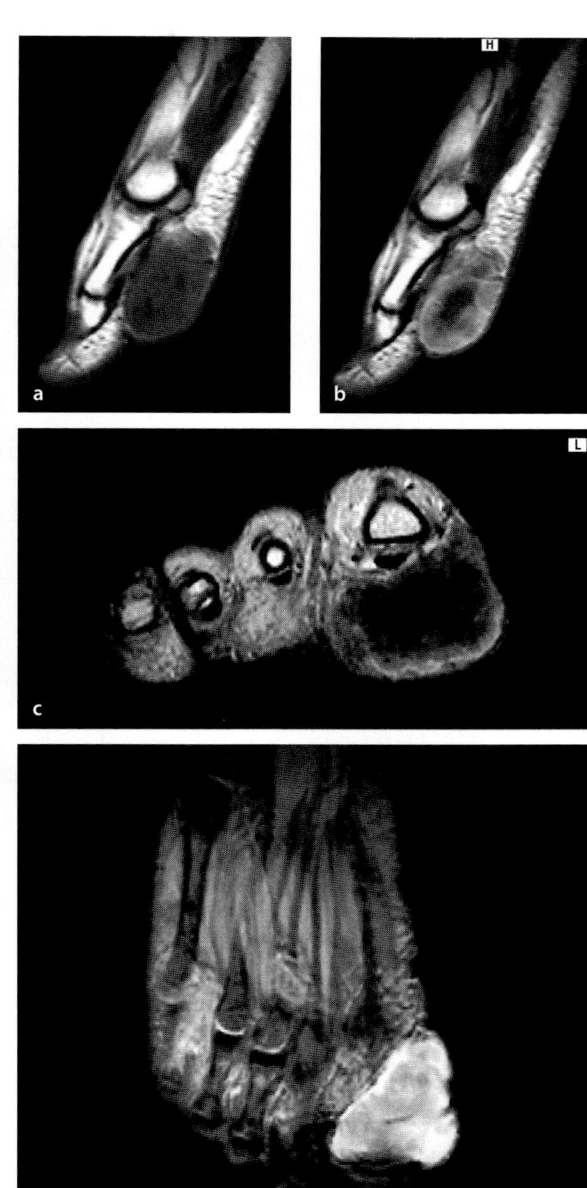

Fig. 13.3 a, b. Recurrent nodular fasciitis of the fascial type in a 37-year-old woman. **a** Axial spin-echo T1-weighted MR image. **b** Axial spin-echo T2-weighted MR image. Well-delineated, oval mass within the region of the infraspinatus muscle, adjacent to the scapula. The lesion is hyperintense to muscle on the T1-weighted image, with a central, bilobate area of lower signal intensity (**a**). Central parts of the lesion show high signal intensity on the T2-weighted image (**b**), while the peripheral component remains of lower signal intensity. This case also illustrates the "inverted target sign"

Fig. 13.4 a–d. Fibroma of tendon sheath in a 35-year-old woman. **a** Sagittal spin-echo T1-weighted MR image. **b** Sagittal spin-echo T1-weighted MR image after gadolinium contrast injection. **c** Axial spin-echo T2-weighted MR image. **d** Coronal gradient T2*-weighted image. Large, oval mass at the plantar aspect of the left great toe. The lesion is inhomogeneous and ill-defined at the proximal pole (**a**). After contrast injection there is marked enhancement at the periphery of the lesion (**b**). On the T2-weighted image, the whole lesion is of low signal intensity (**c**). On gradient-echo sequence, the periphery of the lesion is of extremely high signal intensity (**d**)

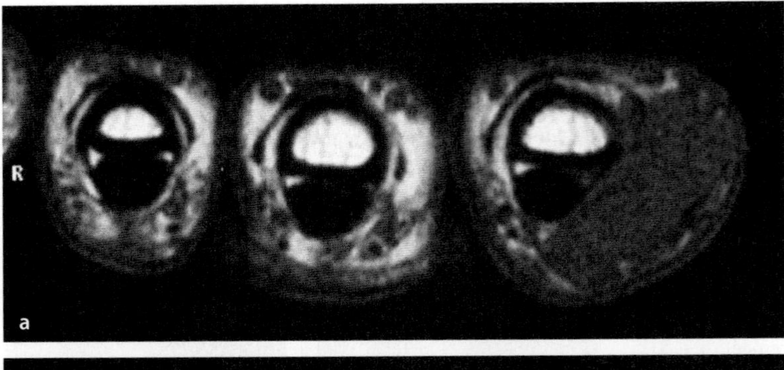

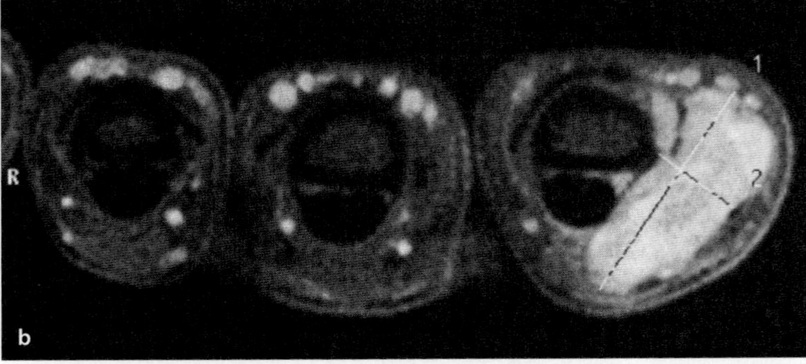

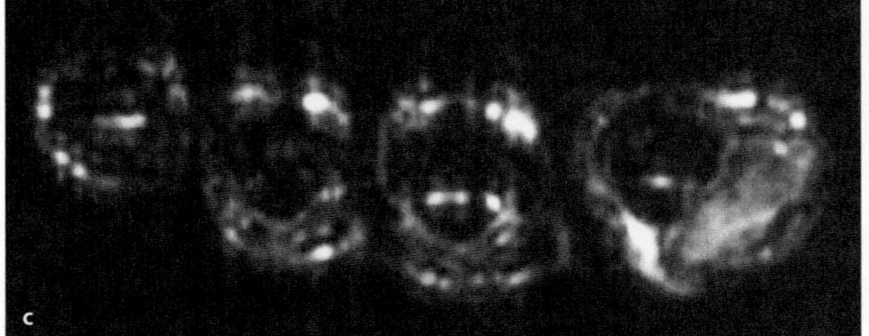

Fig. 13.5 a–c. Fibroma of tendon sheath at the volar aspect of the third finger adjacent to the flexor tendon. **a** Axial spin-echo T1-weighted MR image. **b** Axial spin-echo T1-weighted MR image after gadolinium contrast injection with fat suppression. **c** Axial spin-echo T2-weighted MR image with fat suppression. The lesion is of low SI on T2-weighted MR images (**c**) and enhances moderately after gadolinium contrast injection (**b**)

the volar aspect of the wrist account for 80% of cases. It is considered to be either a reactive fibrosing process or a benign neoplasm. It is found most commonly in adults and is more than twice as common in men as in women. The main symptom is a small mass that rarely measures more than 2 cm and is painless but may limit motion of the involved digit [52]. Macroscopically, it resembles the lobular configuration of the much more common giant cell tumor of the tendon sheath, but it is less cellular and there are no xanthoma cells or giant cells [17]. Microscopically this lobulated nodular lesion is composed of tightly packed spindle cells (fibroblasts), vessels, and large amounts of dense collagenous material, which is markedly hyalinized. Occasionally there is a gradual transition from the poorly cellular hyalinized collagenous areas to more cellular areas which are thought to be characteristic of the early stages of the tumor development. More cellular forms must be differentiated from nodular fasciitis, fibrous histiocytoma, and even fibrosarcoma.

Although fibromas of the tendon sheath may resemble nodular fasciitis histologically, they involve hands and feet almost exclusively and are slow-growing lesions, while lesions of nodular fasciitis appear suddenly, grow rapidly, and usually attain full size in 3–6 weeks. Moreover, they have a predilection for the volar aspect of the forearm [67].

Plain radiographic findings in a fibroma of tendon sheath eroding the third metatarsal have been reported by Lourie et al. [52].

Fox et al. [23] have reported on a series of six patients with fibroma of the tendon sheath. Findings from MRI were not at all specific, i.e., low to intermediate SI on both T1- and T2-weighted images and a variable enhancement (from none to markedly enhanced) after contrast administration. MR findings depend on and reflect the relative amount of different tumor components that are cellular, myxoid, vascular, or collagenous. As a consequence there can be overlap in MR findings with features of giant cell tumor of the tendon sheath (Fig. 13.5).

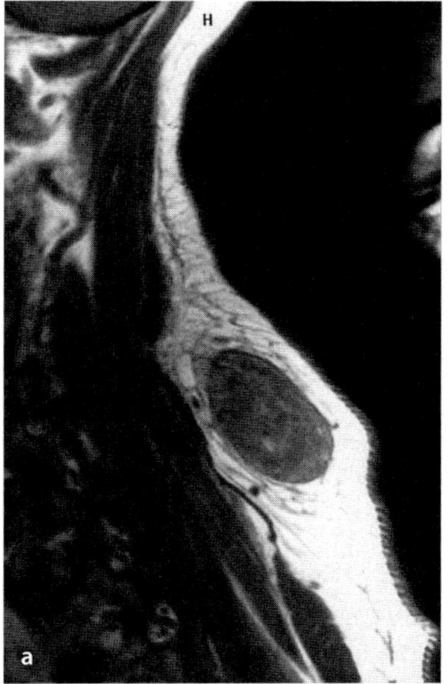
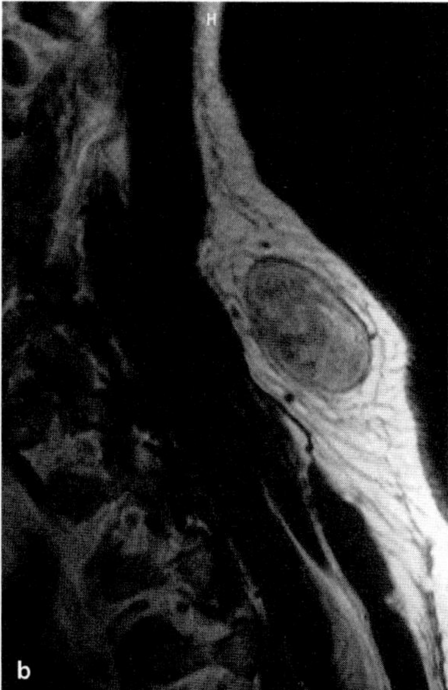
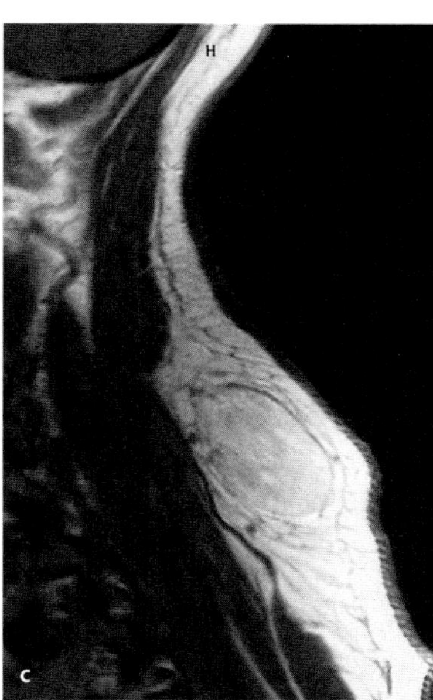

Fig. 13.6a–c. Nuchal fibroma in a 50-year-old man. **a** Sagittal spin-echo T1-weighted MR image. **b** Sagittal spin-echo T2-weighted MR image. **c** Sagittal spin-echo T1-weighted MR image after gadolinium contrast injection. Oval, well-delineated mass within the subcutaneous fatty tissue of the neck. There is an intermediate signal intensity on both spin-echo images owing to the mixed histological composition of entrapped fat within a collagenous mass (**a, b**). There is marked enhancement after contrast injection (**c**). Localization and MR presentation are characteristic of a nuchal fibroma

13.2.3 Nuchal Fibroma

Nuchal fibroma, or collagenosis nuchae, is a benign soft tissue tumor that arises from the posterior cervical subcutaneous tissue, with a predilection for the interscapular and paraspinal regions. Nuchal fibroma is significantly more common in men, with a peak incidence during the third to the fifth decades.

Microscopically, nuchal fibromas have a superficial (subcutaneous or dermal) component and consist of paucicellular, thick bundles of lobulated collagen fibers with inconspicuous fibroblasts. Entrapped adipose tissue and traumatic neuroma-like nerve proliferations are typically present. Skeletal muscle infiltration is also seen in a minority of cases. The process has a strong association with diabetes and also appears to be linked to Gardner's syndrome, fibromatosis, and dermatofibrosarcoma protuberans. Local recurrence probably reflects the persistence of local or systemic factors related to its pathogenesis [60, 72].

The MR appearance reflects the histological composition: collagen has a low SI both on T1- and T2-weighted images. Small foci of high SI on T1-weighted images are due to entrapped adipose tissue (Figs. 13.6, 13.7). In this regard there is a strong similarity to elastofibromas.

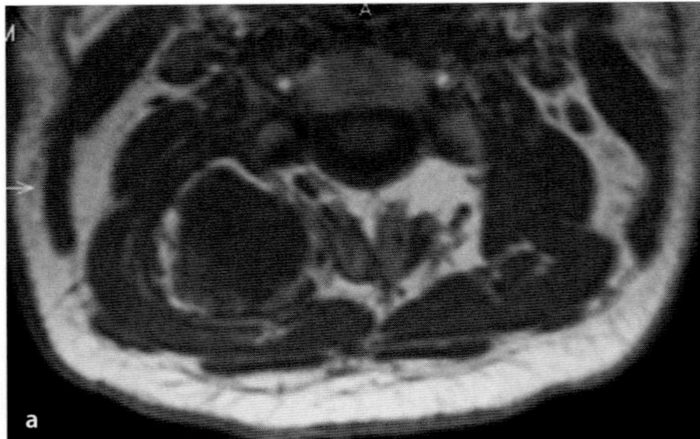

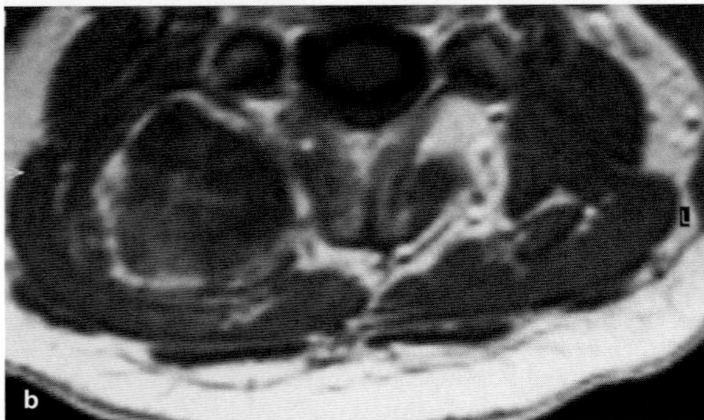

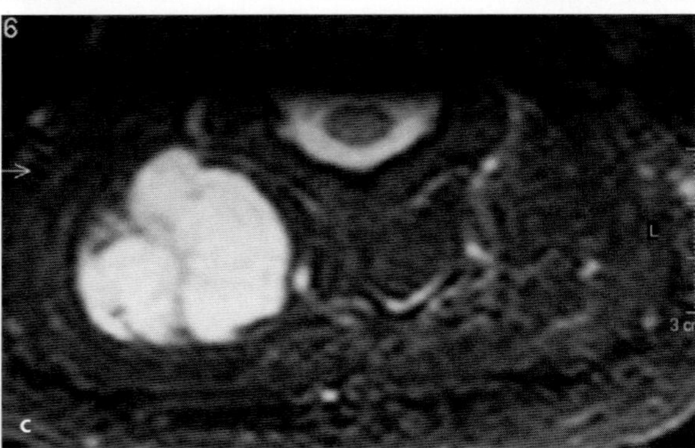

Fig. 13.7 a–c. Nuchal fibroma. **a** Axial spin-echo T1-weighted MR image. **b** Axial spin-echo T1-weighted MR image after gadolinium contrast injection. **c** Axial short-tau inversion recovery (STIR) MR image. Atypical presentation of a nuchal fibroma with high SI on STIR sequence (**c**) and minimal, cloudy enhancement after contrast injection (**b**)

13.2.4 Elastofibroma

Elastofibroma is generally considered to be a fibroelastic pseudotumor. It occurs almost exclusively in the subscapular region beneath the rhomboideus major and latissimus dorsi muscles adjacent to the inferior angle of the scapula. It is thought to be caused by repeated mechanical friction between the chest wall and the tip of the scapula, which was the site of the lesion in 99% of the reported cases. Other locations, albeit uncommon, include the infraolecranon, thoracic wall, axilla, and greater trochanter regions. Bilateral lesions are common and seen in 10–60% of patients. Most patients are older adults, and there is a definite predominance in women. Single cases have been reported in children [12]. Half of the patients are asymptomatic, and 50% have pain on arm motion. Chromosomal abnormalities and familial occurrences support a genetic predisposition to elastofibroma dorsi.

On gross examination, these lesions are firm and rubbery [12, 47, 50, 55]. Histologically, lesions are composed mainly of elastin-like fibers and entrapped islands of mature adipose tissue. Microscopic examination shows hypertrophy and degeneration of elastin with a background of mature collagen and fat. CT scans show attenuation similar to that of adjacent muscle. Sometimes there are strands of low density similar to that of subcutaneous fat [48] (Fig. 13.8a). MRI nicely reflects the histological composition of entrapped fat within a predominantly fibrous mass. On both T1- and T2-weighted images, the lesion presents as a lenticular, well-defined mass with an intermediate SI approximately equal to that of skeletal muscle. Interlaced areas have a SI similar to that of fat [45]. Areas of low SI on both T1- and T2-weighted images correspond histologically to fibroelastic tissue [48] (Fig. 13.8b–d).

Surgery should not be performed for diagnostic purposes in elderly individuals. Indeed, familiarity of the radiologist with this entity may make it possible to avoid some surgery [54]. Differential diagnosis is limited, but includes older desmoids, which are hypocellular, contain large amounts of collagen, and occur in younger patients.

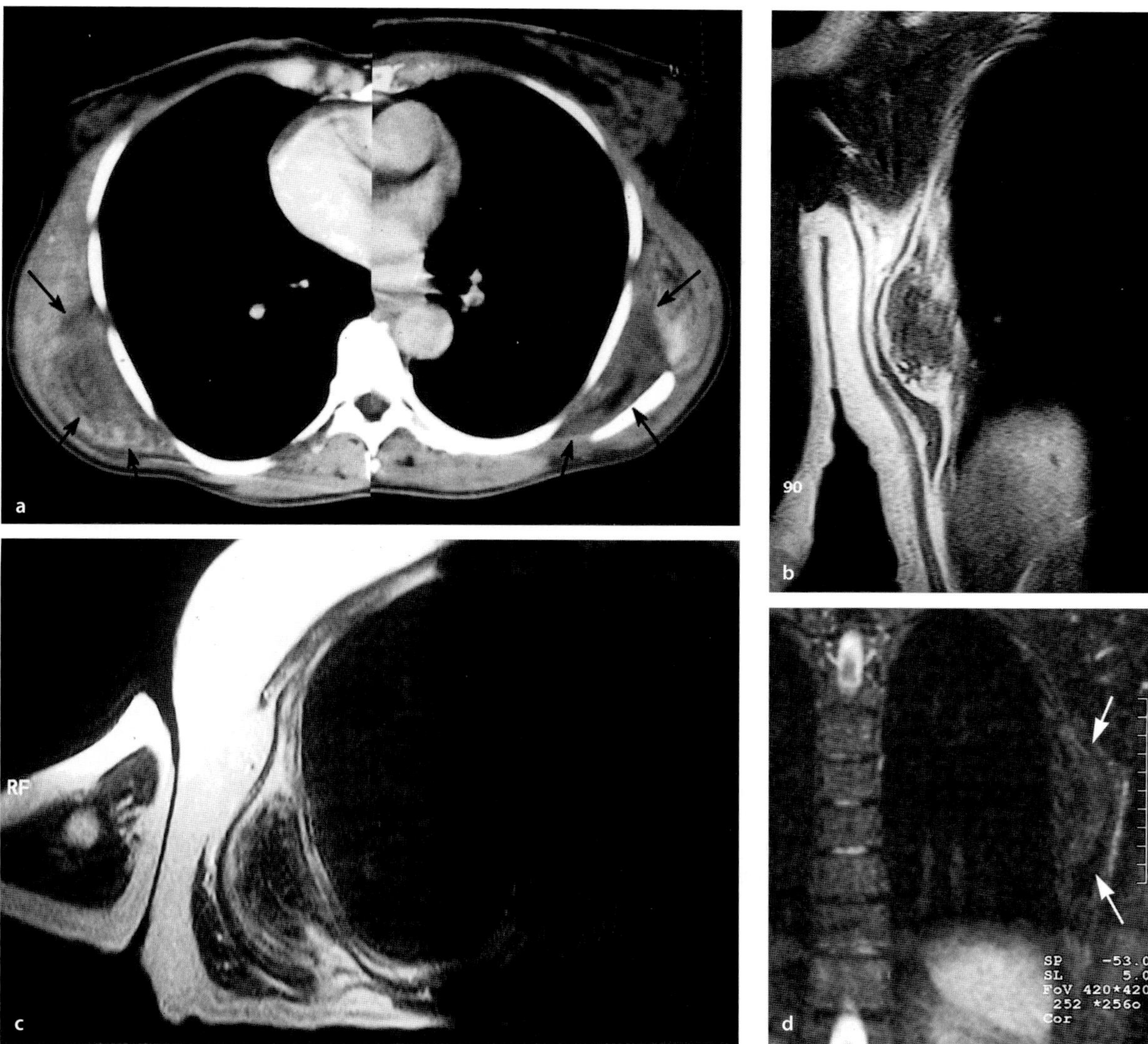

Fig. 13.8 a–d. Elastofibroma dorsi in a 60-year-old woman (**a**), in a 67-year-old woman (**b**, **c**), and in a 56-year-old woman (**d**). **a** CT scan after iodinated contrast injection. **b** Coronal spin-echo T1-weighted MR image. **c** Axial turbo spin-echo T2-weighted MR image. **d** Coronal STIR MR image. On the CT scan there is an oval mass between the rhomboid major and latissimus dorsi muscles on both sides (*arrows*). The lesions show mixed attenuation and enhancement after iodinated contrast injection (**a**). Oval mass within the subscapular region, showing signal intensity equal to that of fat and muscle on a T1-weighted image (**b**), and an overall low signal intensity on T2-weighted an on STIR images (**c**, **d**). Three cases of elastofibroma showing characteristic location, attenuation on CT scan, and signal intensity on MR images, reflecting the histological composition of entrapped fat within a fibrous mass

13.3 Fibromatoses

Fibromatoses cover a wide range of benign fibroblastic proliferations. They are classified according to Enzinger and Weiss into superficial and deep types, and are further subdivided according to anatomical location:

1. Superficial (fascial) fibromatosis
   a) Palmar fibromatosis (Dupuytren contracture)
   b) Plantar fibromatosis (Ledderhose disease)
   c) Penile fibromatosis (Peyronie disease)
   d) Knuckle pads
2. Deep (musculoaponeurotic) fibromatosis
   a) Extra-abdominal fibromatosis
   b) Abdominal fibromatosis
   c) Intra-abdominal fibromatosis:
      - Pelvic fibromatosis
      - Mesenteric fibromatosis
      - Gardner syndrome

Although both superficial and deep lesions have a similar microscopic appearance, superficial lesions are slow growing, while deep ones have a more aggressive biological behavior, between that of fibrosarcomas and fibromas [7]. Division into abdominal and extra-abdominal desmoids is arbitrary, since the lesions are histologically alike [5].

Fibromatoses are uncommon lesions, constituting 0.03% of all neoplasms. They are found in young adults, with a peak incidence at 30 years. There is no sex predominance, and most lesions are solitary, although synchronous multicentric lesions have been reported. A familial tendency has been observed. Local recurrence after surgery is seen in as many as 50% of patients [45].

Key criteria that establish the diagnosis are growth pattern, relationship with surrounding tissues, and cytological features. Lesions consist of uniform fibroblasts proliferating in a parallel way and intermingled with variable amounts of collagen. No atypical or hyperchromatic nuclei are found, while mitoses are infrequent. Generally, the most cellular areas are present in the center of the lesion, whereas the periphery has less numerous fibroblasts and greater amounts of dense collagen [24]. Although fibromatoses are histologically benign, their relationship to adjacent tissue is marked by interdigitating and infiltrative growth. Penile fibromatosis and intra-abdominal fibromatosis will not be discussed, since these do not belong to the locomotor system [68].

On ultrasound scans, fibromatoses appear as masses with low, medium, or high echogenicity and smooth, sharply defined borders. On CT images, the masses are either ill-defined or well circumscribed. Before contrast administration, desmoids show variable attenuation. After contrast administration, lesions usually have a higher attenuation than that of adjacent muscle [5].

In an attempt to explain the variable CT appearance of these lesions, Francis et al. have carried out a retrospective analysis of CT findings and histopathological features in nine patients with fibromatosis. In three of four patients who had precontrast CT scans, the tumors were hyperdense relative to muscle, while in one patient the lesion was hypodense. The postenhancement appearance was variable. The pathological specimens have been analyzed and graded for collagen content, cellular content, tumor necrosis, and tumor vascularity. No consistent relationship can be established between the CT appearance of these lesions and their histological appearance [24].

On MR images, most lesions demonstrate slightly increased SI relative to skeletal muscle on T1-weighted images and intermediate SI on T2-weighted images. The slight increase in SI on T1-weighted images is much less than that seen in lipomas and subacute hemorrhages. Enhancement pattern after contrast administration is variable.

Increased SI on T2-weighted images is seen in hypercellular lesions. Lesions that are hypointense or contain hypointense foci (linear or curvilinear) on both spin-echo sequences are found to be relatively hypocellular with abundant collagen. As a consequence, most lesions are rather inhomogeneous. Although usually well demarcated on MR images, microscopically fibromatosis is seen to invade adjacent structures [68].

The conditions that deserve consideration in the differential diagnosis of intra- and extra-abdominal desmoids are malignant lesions such as fibrosarcoma, rhabdomyosarcoma, synoviosarcoma, liposarcoma, myxofibrosarcoma, lymphoma, and metastases, and benign lesions such as neurofibroma, neuroma and leiomyoma, and acute hematoma of the rectus sheath and chest wall [5].

13.3.1 Palmar Fibromatosis

Palmar fibromatosis or Dupuytren contracture primarily involves palmar aponeurosis of the hand and its extensions. Usually the disease is diagnosed clinically on the basis of characteristic history and physical examination. The earliest clinical manifestation is the appearance of a subcutaneous nodule in the palm of the hand. As the disorder progresses, the overlying skin thickens and retracts, and a cord forms, producing progressive flexion contracture of the affected ray (Figs. 13.9, 13.10).

Palmar fibromatosis tends to affect adults, with a rapid increase in incidence with advancing age. It is bilateral in 40–60% of cases. The condition is by far more frequent in men and is most common in Northern Europe. Pathogenesis in both palmar and plantar

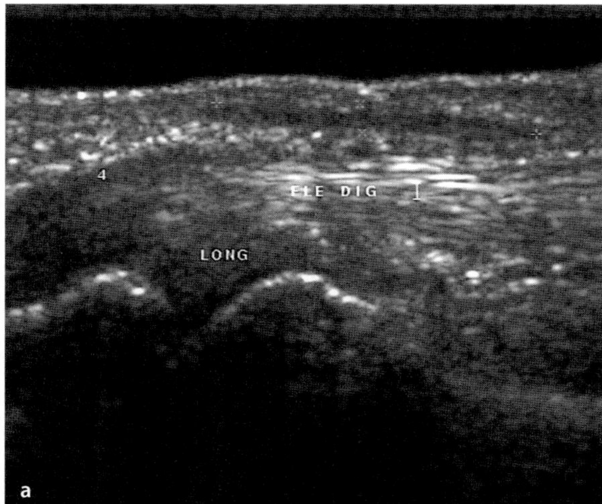

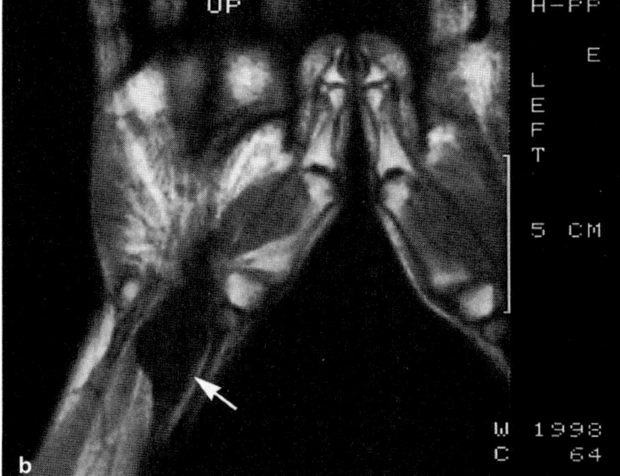

Fig. 13.9 a, b. Palmar fibromatosis in a 40-year-old man (ultrasound) (**a**) and in a 39-year-old woman (coronal spin-echo T1-weighted MR images) (**b**). In the first patient, the ultrasound image shows a cord- or plate-like hypoechoic lesion subcutaneously at the palmar aspect of the fourth metacarpophalangeal joint (**a**). In the second patient, there is a plate-like mass of low signal intensity within the carpal tunnel on the T1-weighted image (*arrow*; the lesion also had a low signal intensity on T2-weighted images, not shown) (**b**). Hypocellular type of cord- or plate-like palmar fibromatosis with characteristic location and imaging features on ultrasound and MR images

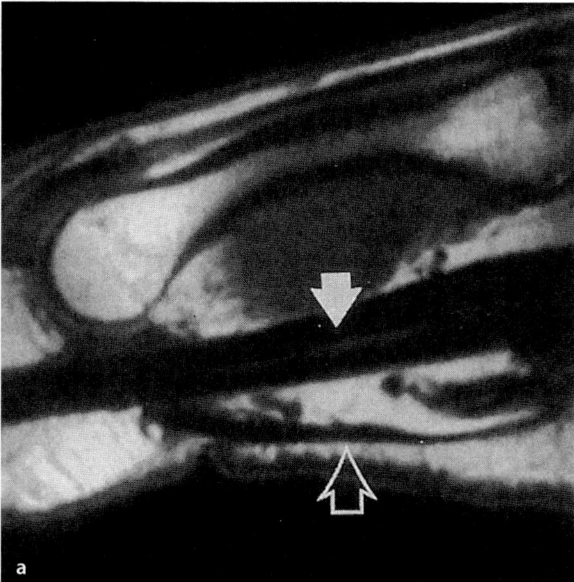

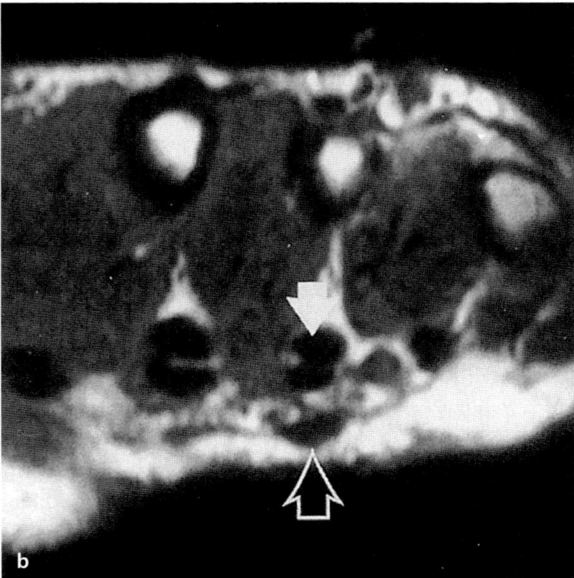

Fig. 13.10 a, b. Dupuytren contracture in a patient with palmar fibromatosis. **a** Sagittal spin-echo T1-weighted MR image. **b** Axial spin-echo T2-weighted MR image. There is a low signal intensity cord (*open arrows*) in the superficial palmar soft tissue at the level of the fourth metacarpal on the T1-weighted image (**a**) and a low signal intensity area superficial to the flexor tendon of the fourth ray (*white arrows*) on the T2-weighted image (**b**). This case illustrates the characteristic appearance of cord in Dupuytren contracture with signal intensity reflecting the hypocellular collagenous composition. (Reproduced from [87], with permission)

fibromatosis includes a genetic component, with family history and chromosome aberrations in 50% of cases.

Histologically, the nodules are quite cellular, composed of whorls of proliferative myofibroblasts. Cords contain a large amount of collagen and are hypocellular. The condition is treated surgically, but the recurrence rate is high (30–40%). The recurrence rate of lesions with mitotically active, cellular nodules is far higher (70%) than that of hypocellular lesions.

The appearance of the nodules and cords on MR images and the correlation between the SI and the lesion's degree of cellularity has been described by Yacoe et al. [87]. On MR images, the cords have a uniformly low SI (similar to the SI of tendon) on both T1- and T2-weighted images. In 18% of patients, nodules have a low to intermediate SI on T1-weighted images (slightly higher than that of tendon) and a low SI on T2-weighted images. Most nodules have an intermediate SI (similar to that of muscle) on both T1- and T2-weighted images. Only three nodules have a low SI on both T1- and T2-weighted images and were hypocellular on histological examination.

Signal characteristics of the lesions correlate with the degree of cellularity. The preoperative assessment of cellularity may be of prognostic significance, because highly cellular lesions tend to have a higher rate of recurrence after surgery than hypocellular lesions. As a consequence surgery may be delayed until the lesion matures and becomes more hypocellular and collagenous [23].

13.3.2 Plantar Fibromatosis

Plantar fibromatosis, also called Ledderhose disease, is a benign, fibroblastic, proliferative, and locally invasive disorder characterized by the replacement of elements of the plantar aponeurosis by abnormal fibrous tissue, which slowly invades the skin and the deep structures (Fig. 13.11)

The plantar aponeurosis is a strong band which originates at the inner tubercle of the calcaneus and contains two layers: a superficial layer which extends to the four smaller toes and a deeper layer which runs from lateral to medial and appears as a separate band to the great toe [49]. On ultrasound scans, the plantar aponeurosis is noted as a bright linear interface, approximately 5–8 mm from the surface of the sole [69]. On MR images the aponeurosis is seen as a thin linear strip of low SI that originates at the inferior border of the calcaneus and inserts into the distal flexor tendons near the metatarsophalangeal joints.

The etiology of plantar fibromatosis is unknown but, as in palmar fibromatosis, trauma, neuropathy, faulty development, alcoholism, and infection have been proposed as etiologic factors. Pathogenesis in both palmar and plantar fibromatosis includes a genetic component, with family history and chromosome aberrations in 50% of the cases. Most lesions are located at the medial aspect and just superficial to the aponeurosis. Involvement is bilateral in 19% of patients and multiple in 32%. There is a higher prevalence in white and middle-aged (fourth decade) male patients and in patients who have epilepsy. There is also an association with knuckle pads in 5%, with palmar fibromatosis in 10–50%, and

with penile fibromatosis (Peyronie disease) in 5–10% of patients. There are no reports of malignant transformation. Clinically, plantar fibromatosis presents as a non-mobile, irregular, single or multinodular lesion located in the longitudinal medial arch of the plantar surface of the foot. The lesion frequently consists of small nodules merged with each other and with the fascial bundles [4]. Although some authors report pain as a main symptom in one-third of patients, most lesions are asymptomatic and are discovered incidentally by palpation. Unlike palmar fibromatosis, this condition rarely causes contracture of the toes.

Microscopically, the lesion consists of a proliferation of well-differentiated hyperplastic, fibroblast-like cells or myofibroblasts with an infiltrative pattern of growth and usually an abundance of proliferating cells between the heavy strands of relatively hypocellular, mature collagen. Collagen is present in the actively growing foci in every specimen: quantitatively it usually is in an inverse ratio to the degree of cellularity [4]. Mitotic figures, necrosis, and vascular infiltration are uncommon. A cellular vascular cuffing and the presence of perivascular inflammatory cells have been described by Allen [4]. The natural history comprises a proliferative phase with increased fibroblastic activity and cellular proliferation, an involutional phase, and a residual phase in which fibroblastic activity is reduced and maturation of the collagen is noted.

If this condition is treated by simple excision, there is an recurrence rate of 50–65%, frequently resulting in a more aggressive form. Infiltration of neighboring structures is more frequently seen in recurrent lesions [4]. Wide, radical excision, encompassing 0.5 cm of surrounding, normal-appearing fascia is, therefore, the treatment of choice.

On ultrasound images, plantar fibromatosis is seen as a well-defined, hypoechoic nodule or mass superficial to the medial slip of the plantar aponeurosis. Plantar fibromatosis exhibits a consistent and characteristic appearance on MR images [61]. Most lesions are heterogeneous, with an overall SI equal to or slightly higher than that of muscle on both spin-echo T1- and (spin-echo and fast spin-echo) T2-weighted images (Fig. 13.11a, b). SI on T2-weighted images reflects the stage of the disease. The proliferative phase is characterized by higher cellularity, resulting in higher SI. The low SI on T2-weighted images of the involutional and residual phases is attributed to the hypocellularity and presence of abundant collagen. Lesions are slightly hyperintense to muscle on short-tau inversion recovery (STIR) sequences (Fig. 13.11c). After intravenous injection of Gd contrast, enhancement is inversely related to the stage of fibromatosis. "Burned out" lesions with abundant collagen fibers enhance to a lesser degree than lesions in the proliferative phase (Fig. 13.11e, f).

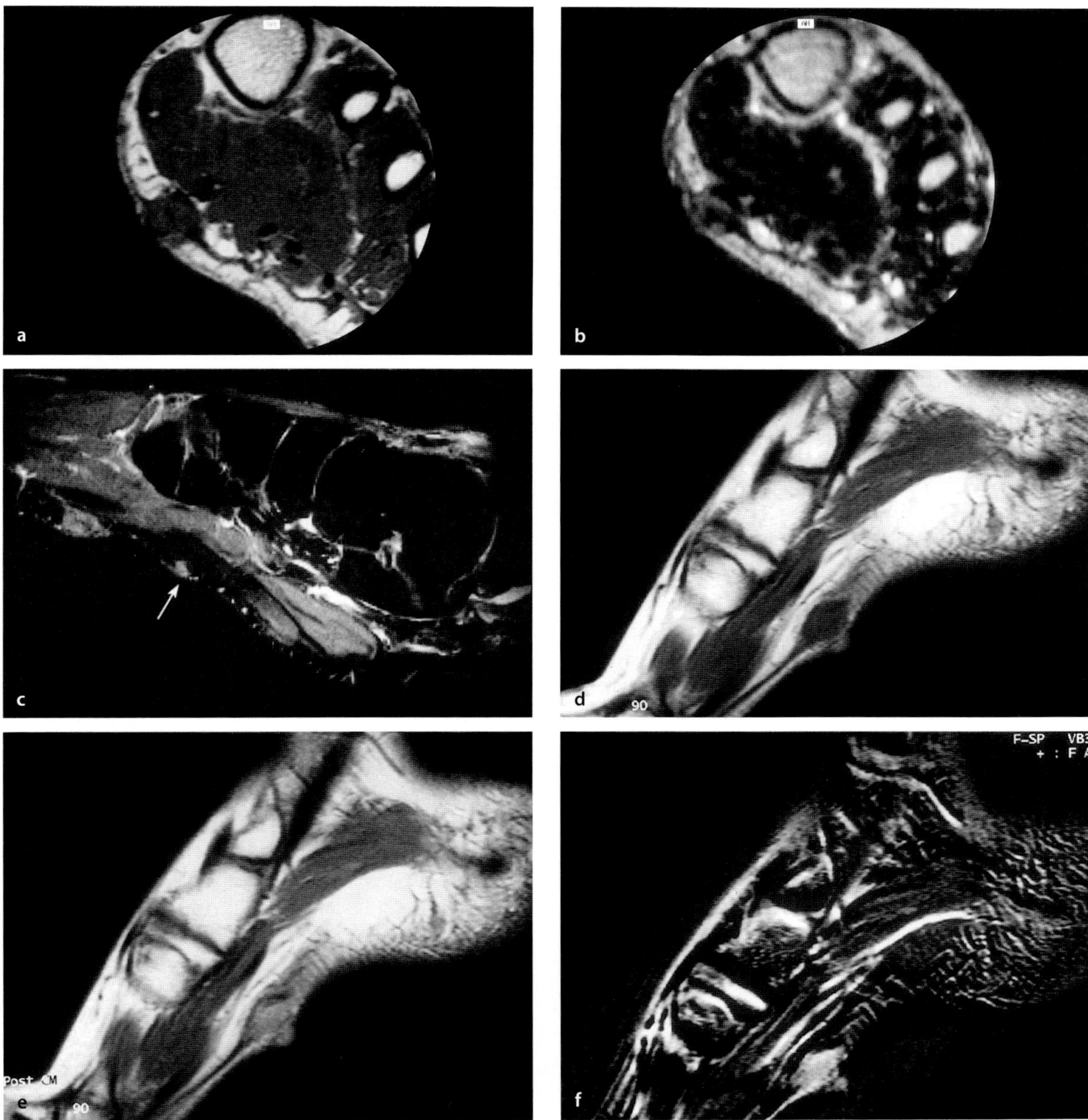

Fig. 13.11 a–f. Two cases of plantar fibromatosis in a 37-year-old-man (**a–c**) and in a 13-year-old girl (**d–f**). **a** Axial spin-echo T1-weighted MR image. **b** Axial turbo spin-echo T2-weighted MR image. **c** Sagittal STIR MR images. **d** Sagittal spin-echo T1-weighted MR image. **e** Sagittal spin-echo T1-weighted MR image after gadolinium contrast injection. **f** Sagittal subtraction MR image. Subcutaneous nodular lesion of intermediate signal intensity at the sole of the foot in apposition with the plantar aponeurosis. The lesion is isointense to muscle on the T1-weighted image (**a**), and of higher, variable signal intensity on the T2-weighted (**b**) and STIR (**c**) images. On the SRIR image, there is a smaller second lesion having similar signal characteristics (**c**; *arrow*). The second case reveals a lesion centered on the plantar fascia, isointense to muscle on the T1-weighted image (**d**), with marked enhancement after gadolinium contrast injection (**e**). This is also nicely demonstrated on the subtraction image (**f**)

Differential diagnosis has to be made between plantar fibromatosis in the residual phase, callus, and scarring. Since plantar fibromatosis in the proliferative phase may be an extremely cellular and infiltrative lesion, it has to be differentiated from aggressive fibromatosis and fibrosarcoma. If the lesion is associated with palmar fibromatosis or Peyronie disease, or if both feet are involved, the diagnosis is almost certain.

13.3.3 Knuckle Pads

Knuckle pads consist of a flat or dome-shaped fibrous thickening on the dorsal aspect of the proximal interphalangeal or metacarpophalangeal joints. They are frequently associated with palmar and plantar fibromatosis. Microscopically this condition resembles palmar fibromatosis, but there are no reports about knuckle pads in recent radiological literature.

13.3.4 Extra-abdominal Desmoid Tumors

Extra-abdominal desmoids are rare soft tissue tumors arising from connective tissue of muscle, overlying fascia, or aponeurosis. They have also been described as desmoid tumor, aggressive fibromatosis, or musculoaponeurotic fibromatosis. The term "desmoid" means band-like or tendon-like lesion [12].

The reported incidence of extra-abdominal desmoids is between three and four cases per million annually. The peak incidence is between ages 25 and 40 years. Although some authors report a predominance in women of childbearing age [16, 33], men and women are almost equally affected. Its cause is unknown, but surgical or accidental trauma, pregnancy, and estrogenic hormones are known associations. We have seen a recurrent desmoid tumor demonstrating an important increase in size (400%) during pregnancy, while most desmoids regress after the menopause [74].

The localization of a large number of extra-abdominal desmoids at the lateral aspect of the shoulder and the buttocks supports the idea of a posttraumatic etiology. The notion of an inherited defect in connective tissue formation is supported by some authors, and a genetic basis for at least some desmoid tumors is suggested by the familial Gardner syndrome, in which desmoid tumors, bony osteomas, dermoids and epidermoids, and/or nuchal fibromas coexist with abdominal wall desmoids, mesenteric desmoids, and intestinal polyposis [1, 78]. Some authors have hypothesized that an underlying mesenchymal defect may result in an imbalance in growth factors, resulting in multiple proliferative diseases, and may be responsible for the coexistence of desmoids, gastrointestinal polyps, and breast cancer [66].

Extra-abdominal desmoids arise most commonly in the lower limb or limb girdle and in the shoulder region. In cases of lower limb localization, a preference for the region of the sciatic nerve is reported [78]. Our own series consists of 30 extra-abdominal desmoid tumors in 26 patients. The localizations were as follows: head and neck region (n=1), upper limb (n=4), trunk (n=6), pelvis (n=8), and lower limb (n=11). Extra-abdominal desmoids never metastasize but multicentric, synchronous and metachronous presentation has been reported [77, 82]. In this condition, second tumor localizations generally develop proximally to the primary lesion. In our series, 5 of 26 patients had multiple localizations.

Bone involvement is not uncommon and has been reported in up to 37% of patients. In addition, primary intramedullary, juxtacortical, and periarticular desmoids are found, which are histologically indistinguishable from soft tissue desmoids. In the same way, bone desmoids can extend into the soft tissues just as soft tissue desmoids can involve bone [13].

Microscopically, extra-abdominal desmoids consist of elongated spindle-shaped cells (fibroblasts) of uniform appearance, surrounded and separated from each other by varying amounts of collagen. Dense collagen is found at the periphery, fibroblasts at the center [45]. Conversely, the center of the lesions may contain dense collagen, whereas the periphery may be composed of fibroblasts [78]. In addition, myxoid change, focal hemorrhage, increased vascularity, and focal inflammation may be seen [45]. Immunohistochemistry staining was positive for actin, consistent with myofibroblastic differentiation in extra-abdominal desmoid tumors [82] Despite their benign microscopic appearance, extra-abdominal desmoids have an aggressive behavior, which is expressed as large tumoral growth, infiltration of neighboring tissues, and a high incidence of postsurgical recurrence (between 25% and 68%). Most recurrent tumors have a different behavior and morphology. In our series they show an increased frequency of extracompartmental spread, grow considerably faster than primary tumors, and have a tendency to invade bone more frequently.

In a retrospective study of 138 patients with extra-abdominal desmoids, 11 died as a consequence of locally uncontrolled tumor growth [65]. Kim [40] has retrospectively analyzed the clinical records and MRI findings in 40 patients (8 juveniles, 32 adults) with proven desmoid tumor. In his series, recurrences in the juvenile patients were more often multiple (50% versus 12%) and appeared significantly earlier than in the adult patients.

On ultrasound scans, extra-abdominal desmoids may be well defined or poorly defined and may show variable echogenicity because of variable degrees of cellularity, matrix water content, and collagen. In many cases, marked shadowing from the surface of the lesion, a result of the large amount of dense collagen tissue in the tumor, totally obscures the mass [22].

Because of the variability in tumor composition, the lesions have variable attenuation and enhancement on CT scans [2]. Duda has reported that extra-abdominal desmoids are iso- or hypodense relative to muscle and enhance to 100–110 HU after injection of iodinated contrast material [14].

On MR images, the appearance of extra-abdominal desmoids varies [12, 64]. There are remarkable differences in shape in various patients as well as in different locations in a given patient with multicentric extra-ab-

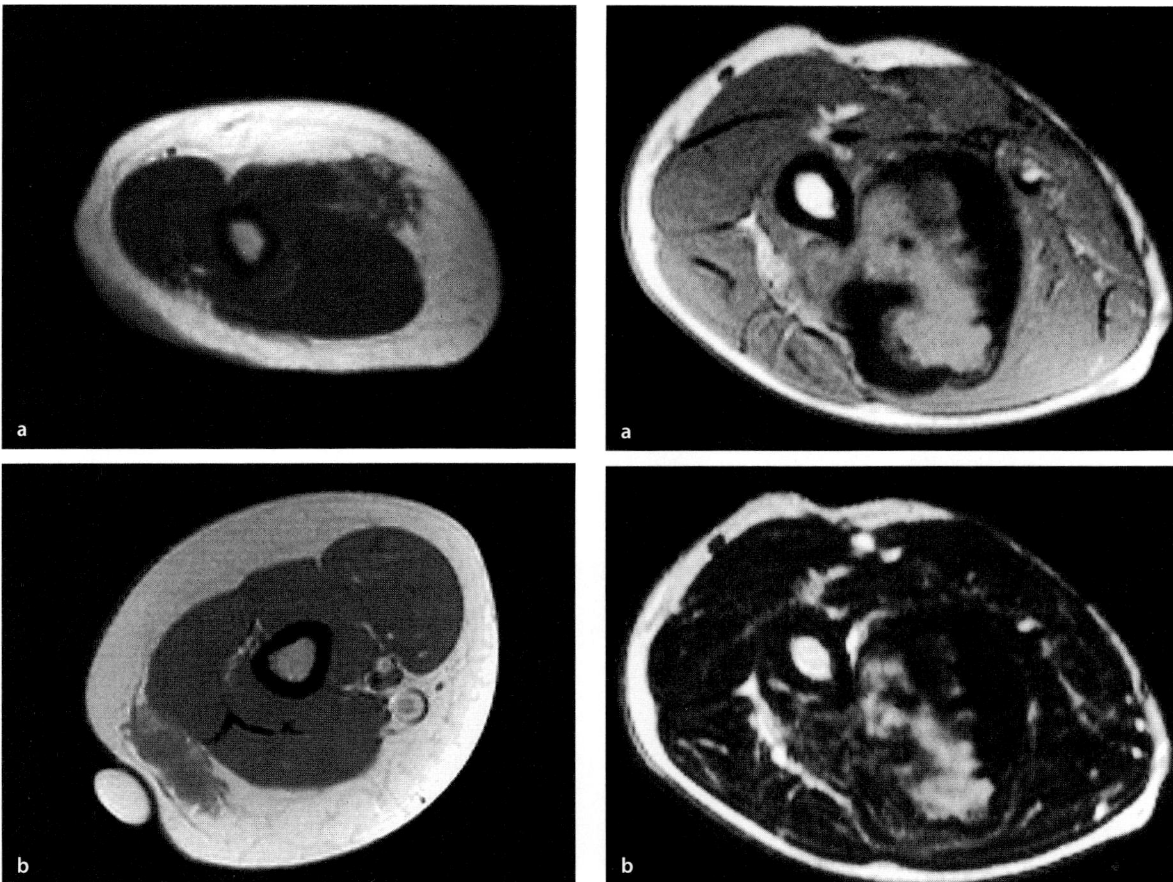

Fig. 13.12 a, b. Desmoid of the upper arm (**a**) in a 23-year-old woman and (**b**) in a 44-year-old woman. **a** Axial spin-echo T1-weighted MR image. **b** Axial spin-echo T1-weighted MR image after gadolinium contrast injection. In the first patient there is a stellar, infiltrating lesion within the subcutaneous fat of the deltoid region in close contact with the adjacent muscle fascia (**a**). In the second patient there is a stellar, nodular infiltrating lesion within the subcutaneous fat of the deltoid region. The fat plane between the lesion and the adjacent muscle fascia is blurred (**b**). These two cases of superficial, stellar desmoid in the deltoid region with infiltration of neighboring fat and muscle fascia illustrate the characteristic shape and location of superficial aggressive fibromatosis

Fig. 13.13 a, b. Desmoid of the forearm in a 71-year-old man. **a** Axial spin-echo T1-weighted MR image. **b** Axial spin-echo T2-weighted MR image. On the T1-weighted image, there is a large mass at the volar aspect of the forearm adjacent to the interosseous membrane, with a rim of low signal intensity at the periphery of the lesion (**a**). On the T2-weighted image, the peripheral rim remains hypointense while the central part is of higher signal intensity (**b**). This case illustrates a pattern of natural evolution where dense collagen is responsible for low signal intensity at the periphery of the lesion on all pulse sequences

dominal desmoids. Likewise, for a given lesion, shape may vary on follow-up examinations. The infiltrative pattern is significantly more common in juvenile patients (63%), whereas the nodular pattern is more frequent in the adult patients (81%) [40]. In our series, the shape of the lesions was fusiform-ovoid or dumbbell, and irregular or stellate when located in the subcutis (Fig. 13.12). The mean maximum diameter was 72 mm.

In the reported cases, extra-abdominal desmoids appear hypo- or isointense to muscle on spin-echo T1-weighted images. SI on T2-weighted images is mostly intermediate, although very low and extremely high signal intensities have been noted occasionally. Low-SI, patchy, linear or curvilinear areas on T2-weighted images correspond to hypocellular tissue and dense colla-

gen. On both spin-echo sequences, but predominantly on T2-weighted images, extra-abdominal desmoids are inhomogeneous, mostly with higher SI in the central part (cellular) than at the periphery (collagenous) [33, 45] (Figs. 13.13–13.16).

After a retrospective study of 36 patients with histologically proven extra-abdominal desmoids, Hartman et al. have concluded that on MR images, the desmoids showed inhomogeneous SI (97%), poor margination (89%), neurovascular involvement (58%), and bone involvement (37%). Fibrosis was present in 88% of primary desmoids and 90% of recurrent lesions, and intermediate SI (greater than that of muscle and lower than that of fat) was present in 75% and 50% of these, respectively [32].

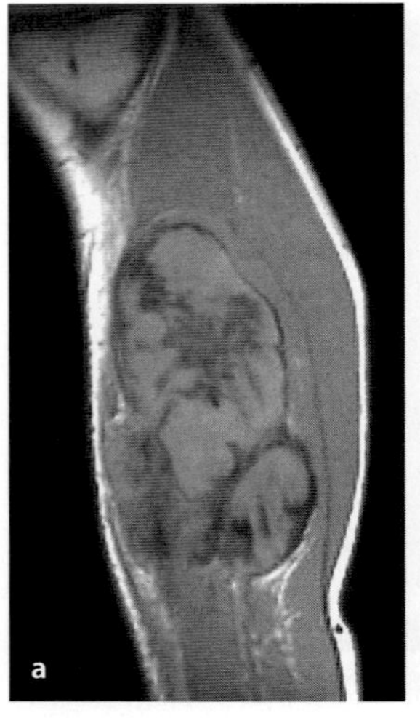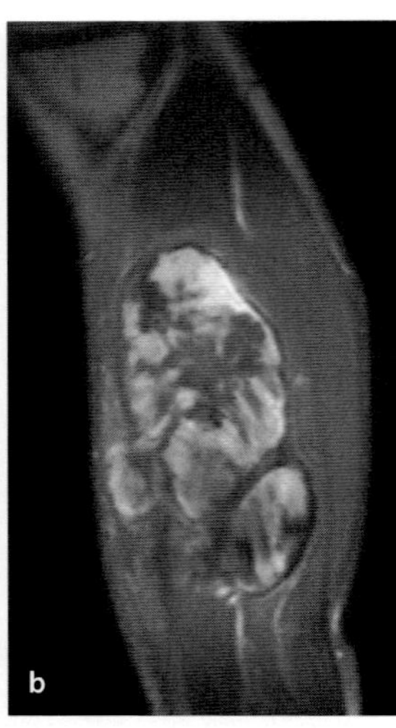

Fig. 13.14a, b. Desmoid of the calf in a 23-year-old man. **a** Sagittal spin-echo T2-weighted MR image. **b** Sagittal spin-echo T1-weighted MR image after gadolinium contrast injection. On the T2-weighted image, there is a polylobular mass with central areas of low signal intensity within each nodule and presence of a low signal-intensity capsule around the lesion (**a**). After contrast injection there is marked enhancement of the peripheral zones without enhancement of the central scar-like areas (**b**). This case of deeply seated juxtacortical desmoid (adjacent to the dorsal aspect of the tibial cortex) illustrates another pattern of natural evolution where collagen is found in the center and less collagenous parts at the periphery of the lesion. Furthermore, it illustrates a frequent finding that areas of higher signal intensity on T2-weighted images enhance after gadolinium administration, whereas areas of low signal intensity on T2-weighted images do not enhance and remain hypointense on all pulse sequences

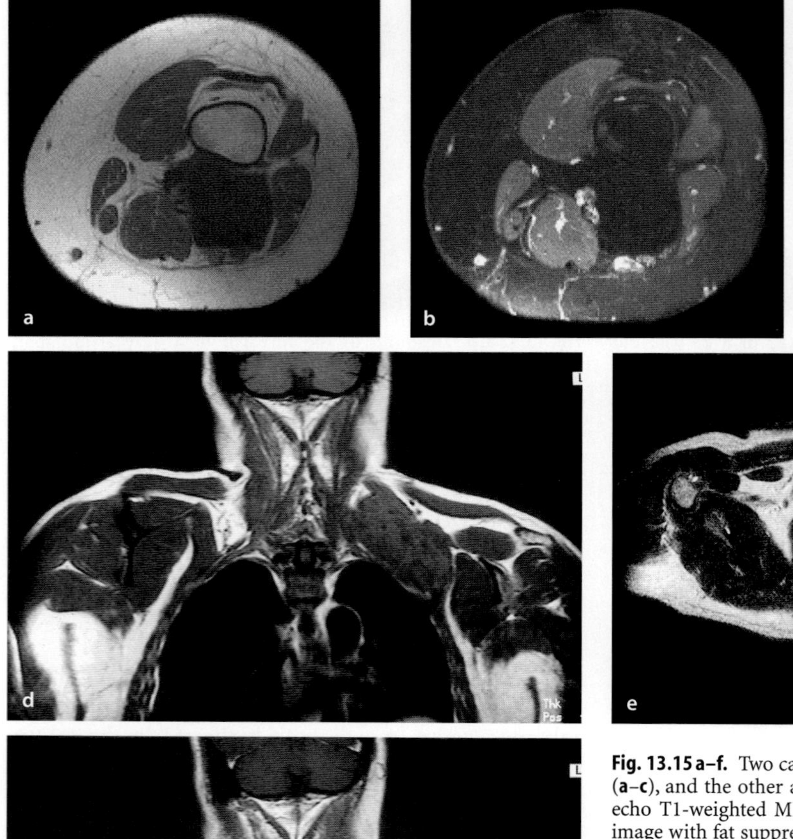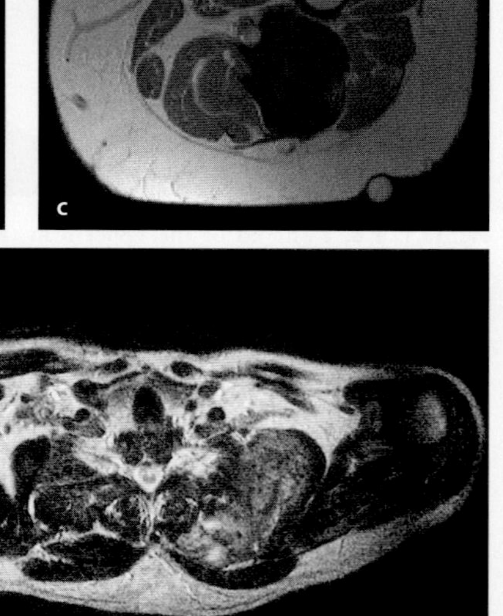

Fig. 13.15a–f. Two cases of desmoid, one located at the hamstrings (**a–c**), and the other at the left serratus muscle (**d–f**). **a** Axial spin-echo T1-weighted MR image. **b** Axial spin-echo T2-weighted MR image with fat suppression. **c** Axial spin-echo T1-weighted MR image, after gadolinium contrast injection. **d** Coronal spin-echo T1-weighted MR image. **e** Axial turbo spin-echo T2-weighted MR image with fat suppression. **f** Coronal spin-echo T1-weighted MR image after gadolinium contrast injection. The first case is an old, mature desmoid which has low SI on all pulse sequences (**a, b**) and does not enhance after contrast injection (**c**). The second case shows an ill-defined lesion, isointense to muscle on the T1-weighted image (**d**) and with a variable, mostly high SI on the T2-weighted image (**e**). In contrast with the first case, there is now a marked enhancement after gadolinium injection (**f**). These two cases demonstrate tumors of different age with different degrees of vascularity and collagen deposition having different features on MR images

Fig. 13.16 a–d. Four different cases of desmoid tumor showing their most characteristic feature, i.e., nonhomogeneity and low SI on T2-weighted MR images

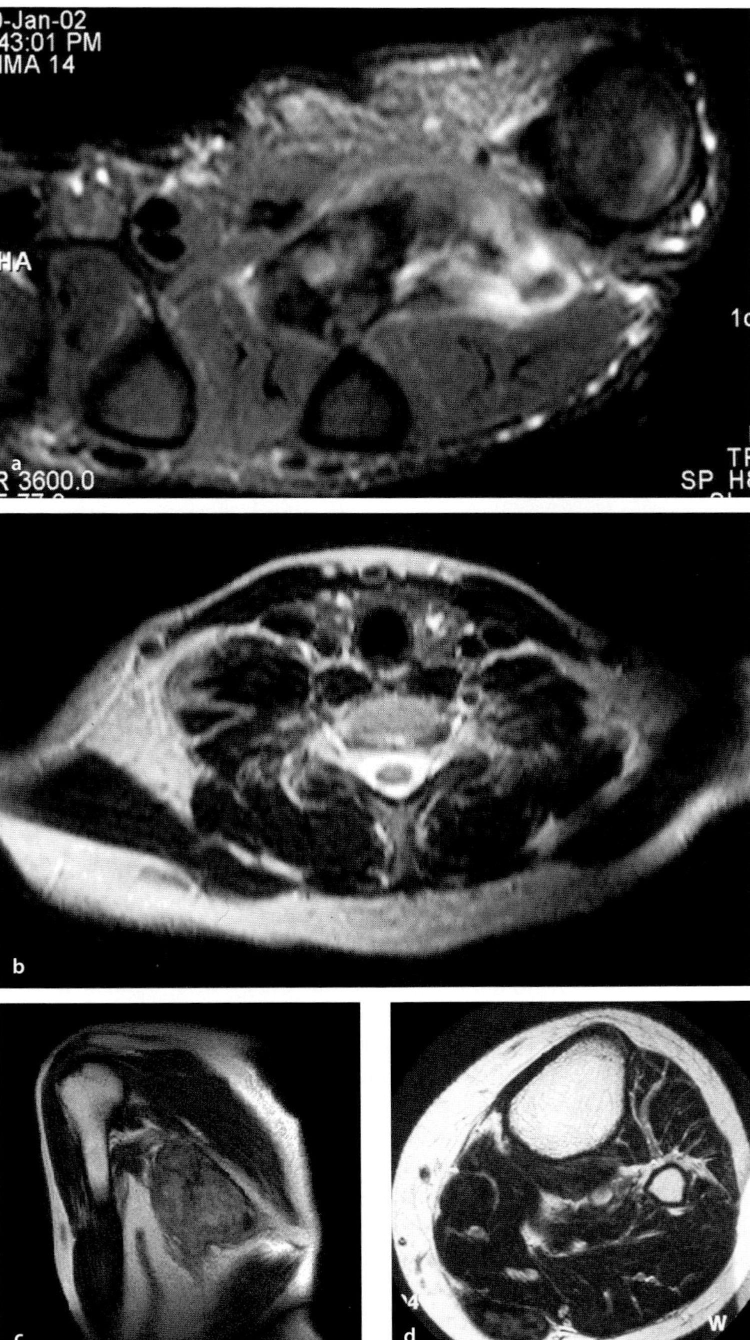

In our personal study of 30 desmoid tumors, MR signal characteristics were variable. On T1-weighted images, lesions were usually almost homogeneous or homogeneous ($n=25$). The overall SI was rated as equal to SI of muscle in 21 cases. The SIs on T2-weighted images mostly were heterogeneously distributed ($n=24$), with an overall SI slightly lower than ($n=15$) or equal to ($n=8$) fat. Hypointense areas were mostly curvilinear to irregular and may have a central ($n=4$) or peripheral ($n=3$) distribution within the lesion. Two cases with central low-intensity areas also show a low-SI peripheral band. The low-SI areas mostly comprise 0–20% of the lesion ($n=14$).

There are few reports regarding the use of contrast agents in extra-abdominal desmoids. In our series, all desmoid tumors showed a moderate to strong enhancement on spin-echo Gd T1-weighted images, except for the areas of low SI on T2-weighted images, which re-

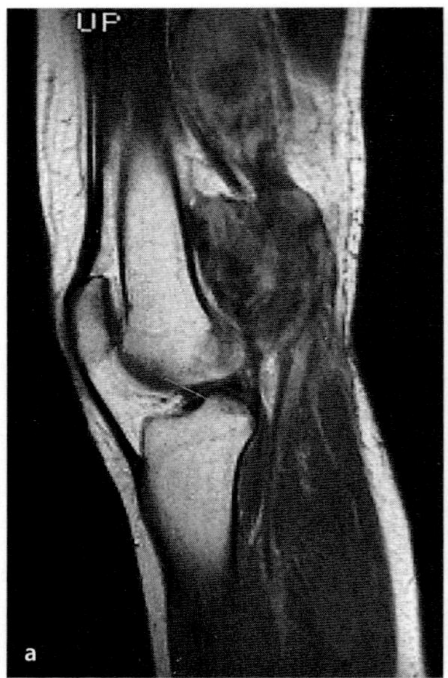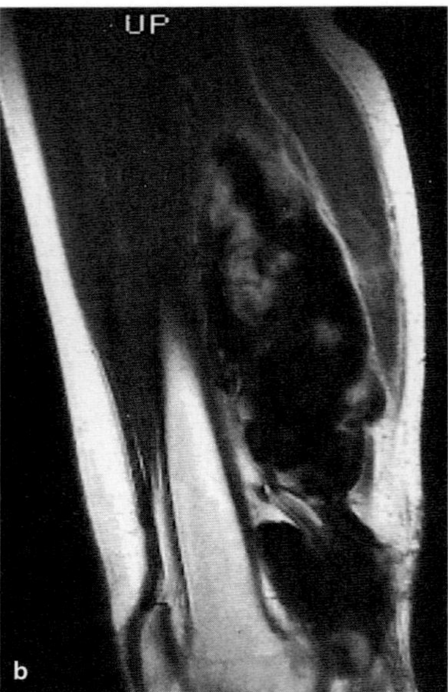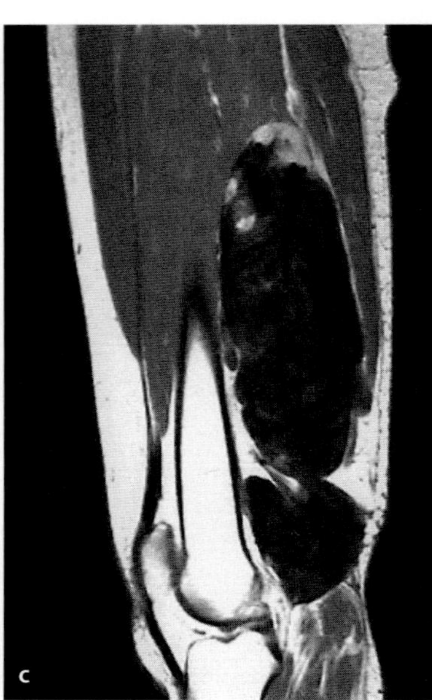

Fig. 13.17 a–c. Desmoid of the popliteal fossa in a 28-year-old woman. **a** Sagittal spin-echo T1-weighted MR image after gadolinium contrast injection (January 1989). **b** Sagittal spin-echo T1-weighted MR image after gadolinium contrast injection (November 1991). **c** Sagittal spin-echo T1-weighted MR image after gadolinium contrast injection (April 1994). The MRI examination from 1989 shows a large, dumbbell-shaped mass in the popliteal fossa with marked, nonuniform enhancement of 80% of the lesion (**a**). In 1991, the proximal part of the mass had increased in size, while the size of the distal part had decreased. Limited areas (20% of the lesion) of enhancement in the proximal part and no enhancement in the distal part (**b**). On the image from MRI performed in 1994, there is no further change in tumor size. Except for two small enhancing nodules within the top of the proximal lesion (5% of the lesion), the whole mass remains hypointense after contrast injection (**c**). This case illustrates the natural evolution of a primary desmoid tumor over a period of 6 years, showing the proximal migration of the lesion and the gradual decrease in enhancing cellular areas, together with an increase in nonenhancing collagenous components

mained unenhanced. Enhancement was more pronounced in the areas of high SI on spin-echo T2-weighted images. As a result, inhomogeneity was even better demonstrated on spin-echo Gd T1-weighted images (Figs. 13.12, 13.14, 13.15). On follow-up examinations, the inhomogeneous pattern of contrast enhancement became more evident and paralleled the changes in SI noted on spin-echo T2-weighted images.

In cases of multicentric presentation, the distal lesion tended to be more heterogeneous and hypointense on T2-weighted images than the proximal one. Since the low SI of extra-abdominal desmoids on spin-echo T2-weighted images is thought to be a consequence of an increased amount of collagen, we presume that in these cases the distal localization is more collagenous than the proximal one.

On follow-up MR examination, the distal lesions showed a tendency to shrink, as may be concluded from their size and progressive serration of their borders. In contrast, the proximal lesions increased with time and became more convex. Moreover, during follow-up examination, the extent of the hypointense areas in the distal lesions increased, and this was associated with a further decrease in SI on spin-echo T2-weighted images.

The same phenomenon has been described by Feld in a patient with multicentric involvement in which a gluteal lesion manifested low SI on T2-weighted images, whereas a lesion in the psoas muscle showed heterogeneous, increased SI on T2-weighted images. Histological examination of the gluteal lesion revealed dense collagenous bundles, with cellular areas comprising less than 20% of the tumor, while the lesion in the psoas muscle showed less collagenization and a more pronounced cellularity [19].

The amount of collagen in a given lesion may be reflected by SI on spin-echo T2-weighted images. This correlation between amount of collagen and SI on spin-echo T2-weighted images suggests that older localizations of extraabdominal desmoids (mature fibromatosis) show an increase in collagen that suggests progressive fibrosis, while, in cases of multicentric presentation, the proximal lesion seems to be less collagenous compared with the distal one (Fig. 13.17).

The relationship between cellularity and SI on T2-weighted images, as described by several authors [14, 19], could not be confirmed in our own series. Subtle changes in cellularity cannot explain substantial variance in SI on T2-weighted images, and, although there is a difference in cellularity between young and older desmoids and between primary and recurrent ones, the overall cellularity of desmoids is low. Differences in SI between different tumor components, between asynchronous multicentric desmoids, and between primary and recurrent desmoids will therefore be a consequence of a combination of variability in cellularity, amount of collagen, water content of the extracellular space, myxoid substance, and vascularity.

Periarticular desmoid tumors have to be differentiated from other lesions with low SI on T2-weighted images, such as pigmented villonodular synovitis, giant cell tumor of the tendon sheath, hemorrhagic synovitis, and hemophilic arthropathy [88]. Differential diagnosis of subcutaneous desmoids includes other superficial fibromatoses, such as nodular fasciitis, injection granulomas, granuloma annulare, pentazocine-induced myopathy with subcutaneous fibrosis, and postsurgical fibrosis [10, 80].

13.3.5 Abdominal Fibromatosis (Abdominal Desmoids)

Abdominal desmoids are rare fibroblastic lesions commonly found within the musculoaponeurotic fascia of the anterior abdominal wall, especially of the rectus and oblique external muscles. Occasionally they grow eccentrically and present as an intra-abdominal tumor. Seventy percent of cases occur in patients between the second and fourth decades, and they are common in women. There is a definite relationship with pregnancy (during or after), abdominal surgery, and trauma. It has been postulated that these tumors are estrogen sensitive. Abdominal desmoids may occur as isolated lesions or may be seen as a manifestation of Gardner syndrome.

Abdominal desmoid tumors are well-defined lesions, 5–15 cm in diameter, and in rare cases contain calcifications, necrotic or cystic changes, or hemorrhagic components. If they originate in the rectus muscle they do not cross the midline of the abdomen. On CT scans, most abdominal desmoids are well defined and homogeneous and appear isodense or slightly hypodense with respect to muscle. If lesions are hyperdense, this is due to the high density of abundant collagen and the rich capillary network [16]. The majority of lesions are either isodense or hyperdense when compared with muscle on contrast-enhanced scans.

On MR images, tumors show nonspecific high SI on T2-weighted images, while low-SI areas on T2-weighted images probably represent abundant fibrous tissue [36] (Fig. 13.18). Despite adequate resection with clear histological margins, the recurrence rate may be as high as 40%. Sifumba has reported a tumor recurrence during pregnancy in an old scar 9 years after resection of a first abdominal desmoid [76].

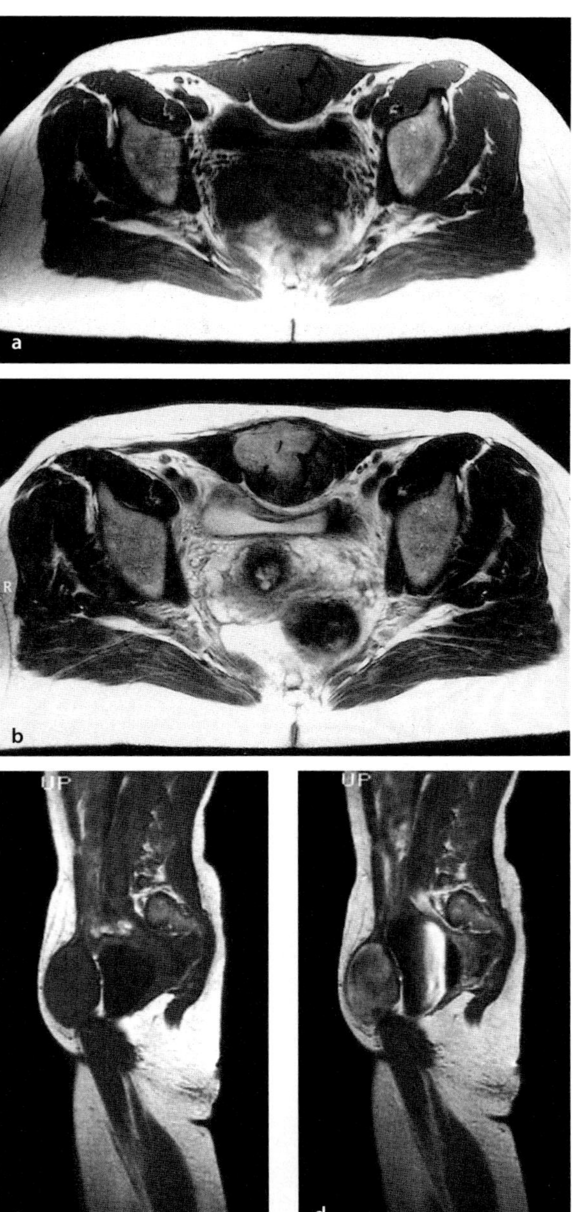

Fig. 13.18 a–d. Abdominal desmoid in a 50-year-old woman (**a, b**) and in a 22-year-old woman (**c, d**). **a** Axial spin-echo T1-weighted MR image. **b** Axial turbo spin-echo T2-weighted MR image. **c** Sagittal spin-echo T1-weighted MR image. **d** Sagittal spin-echo T1-weighted MR image after gadolinium contrast injection. A polylobular mass can be seen, isointense to muscle and with low signal intensity septations on the T1-weighted image (**a**). On the T2-weighted image, the lesion has a mixed, overall low signal intensity (**b**). The second case involves the rectus muscle in a woman in the postpuerperal period. On the T1-weighted image, there is a well-delineated fusiform, inhomogeneous mass within the rectus muscle, with signal intensity comparable with signal intensity of muscle (**c**). The lesion demonstrates marked, nonuniform enhancement (**d**). These cases are illustrative of abdominal desmoids with characteristic location, patient age, and time of onset (postpuerperal)

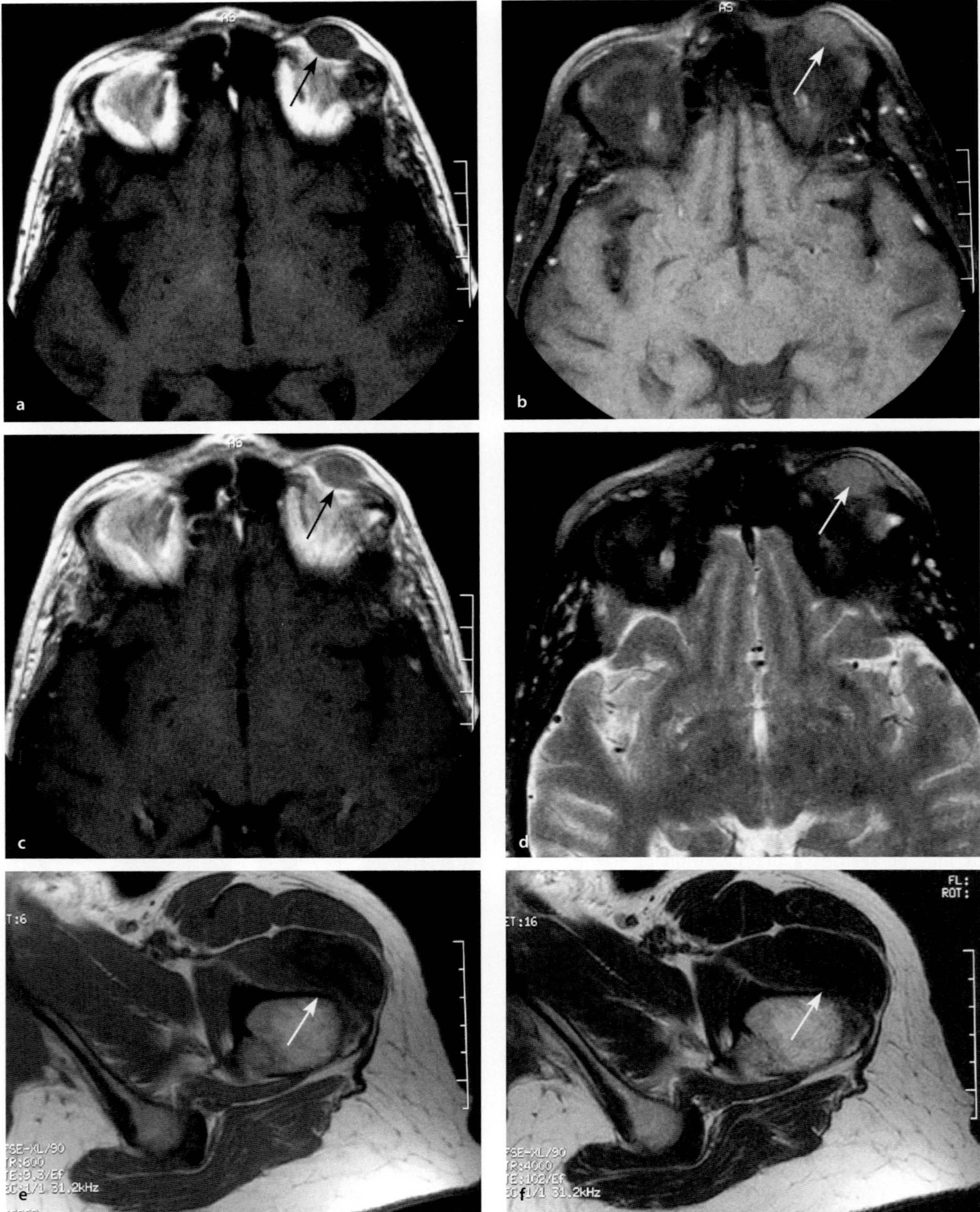

Fig. 13.19 a–g.

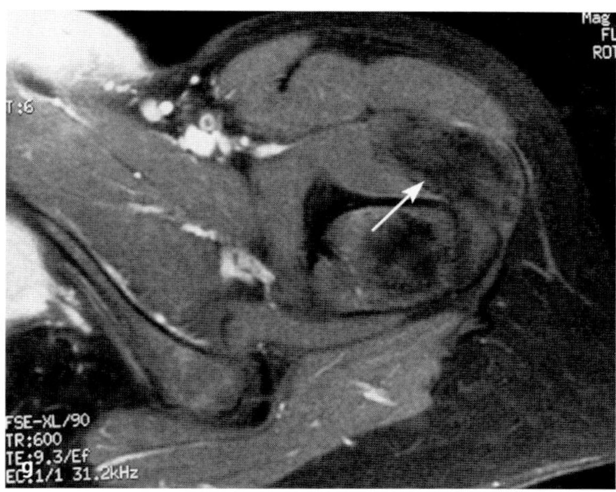

Fig. 13.19 g. Two cases of collagenous fibroma, one in the subcutis (**a–d**) and a second in the vastus muscle (**e–g**). **a** Axial spin-echo T1-weighted MR image. **b** Axial spin-echo T1-weighted MR image with fat suppression. **c** Axial spin-echo T1-weighted MR image, after gadolinium contrast injection. **d** Axial spin-echo T2-weighted MR image. **e** Axial spin-echo T1-weighted MR image. **f** Axial spin-echo T2-weighted MR image. **g** Axial spin-echo T1-weighted MR image, after gadolinium contrast injection. Morphology and MR presentation doesn't allow differentiation between collagenous fibroma and extra-abdominal desmoid

13.3.6 Collagenous Fibroma (Desmoplastic Fibroblastoma)

Collagenous fibroma commonly occurs in patients in the fifth and sixth decades of life, more frequent in men (75%). The tumor often manifests as a sharply demarcated, mobile, firm, solitary mass involving subcutaneous tissue, or skeletal muscle. The common locations of the tumor are the arm, shoulder, and posterior neck or upper back. The size of reported collagenous fibromas range from 1 to 20 cm in the largest dimension. Histologically, the tumors appear well marginated on low-power examination. The tumor cells are relatively bland stellate- and spindle-shaped fibroblastic cells separated by densely fibrous to fibromyxoid matrix. The cellularity is low or very low, mitotic figures are very rare or absent, and tumor necrosis is not seen. On MR images collagenous fibroma shows areas of decreased SI on T1- and T2-weighted images. Because both have a high collagen content, similar findings have been described in desmoid tumors (Fig. 13.19).

Nevertheless, collagenous fibromas are less cellular, less vascular, and less infiltrative at their periphery and as a consequence more mobile, better circumscribed, and easier to remove than desmoids. Moreover they occur in older (more than 40 years old) patients. Differential diagnosis is essential to prevent overtreatment in collagenous fibroma [63].

13.4 Fibrous Tumors of Infancy and Childhood

The following types of fibrous tumors of infancy and childhood are recognized:
1. Fibrous hamartoma of infancy
2. Infantile digital fibromatosis
3. Infantile myofibromatosis
4. Juvenile hyaline fibromatosis
5. Gingival fibromatosis
6. Fibromatosis colli
7. Infantile (desmoid-type) fibromatosis (aggressive infantile fibromatosis)

The term "fibromatosis" is used for fibroblastic-myofibroblastic proliferations with the following characteristics: (a) a tendency to invade surrounding tissues, (b) a tendency to recur after incomplete resection, (c) absence of metastases, (d) in some fibromatoses, spontaneous regression, and (e) presentation with multifocal tumors [15].

13.4.1 Fibrous Hamartoma of Infancy

Fibrous hamartoma of infancy is a solitary, benign, painless, subcutaneous tumor occurring before the age of 2 years and characterized by an organoid mixture of three components: trabeculae of dense fibrocollagenous tissue, areas of immature-appearing, small, rounded, primitive mesenchymal cells, and mature fat. The lesion occurs predominantly in males. The most common locations are the shoulder, axilla, and upper arm [17, 53]. There is a strong correlation between the imaging findings and the histological pattern showing fat and fibrous tissue (Fig. 13.20).

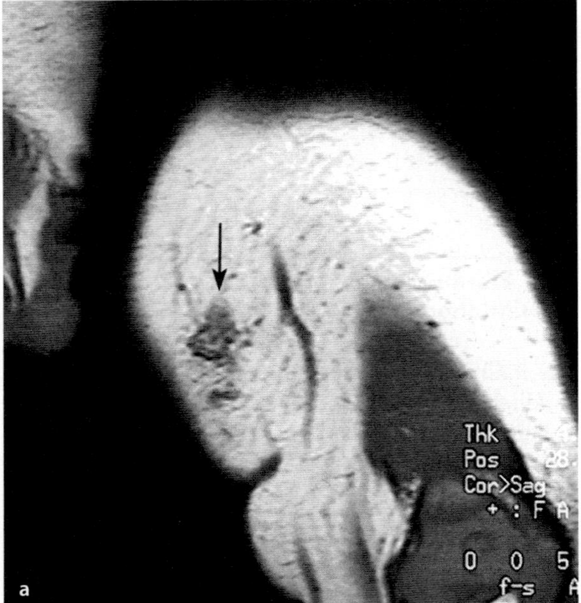

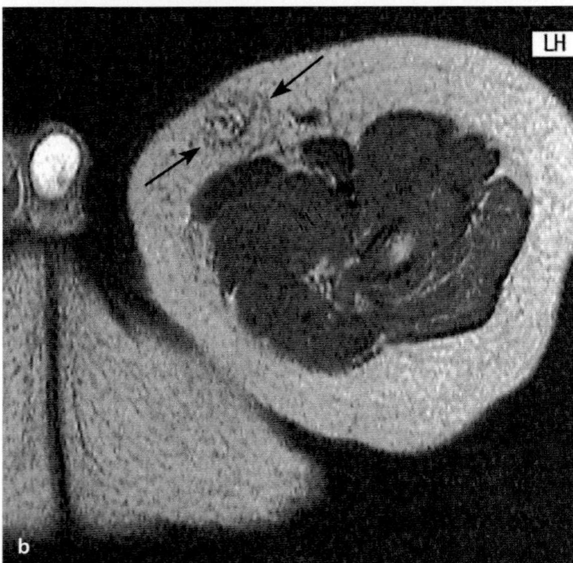

Fig. 13.20a,b. Fibrous hamartoma in a 6-month-old boy. **a** Coronal spin-echo T1-weighted MR image. **b** Axial spin-echo T2-weighted MR image. On the T1-weighted image, the lesion presents as an ill-defined, inhomogeneous mass of intermediate signal intensity within the subcutaneous tissue of the ventral aspect of the left thigh (**a**). On the T2-weighted image, the lesion is spider-like, with low to intermediate signal intensity (**b**). MRI demonstrates the histological composition with fatty and fibrous parts

13.4.2 Infantile Digital Fibromatosis – Inclusion-Body Fibromatosis

In infantile digital fibromatosis, single or multiple fibromatous lesions arise from the fingers and toes, affecting predominantly the dorsolateral aspect of the distal parts of adjacent digits. This rare entity mostly develops in patients under the age of 3 years, and histological examination typically reveals intracytoplasmatic inclusion bodies [37].

13.4.3 Infantile Myofibromatosis

Infantile myofibromatosis, also called congenital multiple or diffuse fibromatosis, is a rare mesenchymal disorder in newborns and infants, which is characterized by solitary or multiple nodular foci of myoblastic and fibroblastic tissue in the skin, musculoskeletal system, and visceral organs. The condition is also known as multiple mesenchymal hamartomas or multiple vascular leiomyomas of the newborn, and infantile hemangiopericytoma. Its etiology is unknown, although familial occurrence of the disease has been noted.

According to the anatomical distribution of the myofibroblastic lesions, two types of infantile myofibromatosis can be distinguished, each with a different clinical course. The first (solitary) type is limited to soft tissue and bone and has an excellent prognosis, since spontaneous regression with complete resolution of the lytic bone lesions may occur. It is mostly found in boys. Most solitary myofibromas occur in cutaneous/subcutaneous tissues of the head and neck region. The second (multicentric) type shows widespread visceral involvement, mainly of the lungs, myocardium, and gastrointestinal tract. This type of myofibromatosis is almost always lethal in early life. It is mostly found in girls [84].

Subcutaneous nodules are usually firm and encapsulated, and frequently contain calcifications. They are the most common manifestations of infantile myofibromatosis and are easily detectable at birth. Tumors measure from less than 1 cm to a few centimeters in diameter. They contain foci of hemorrhage, cystic degeneration, necrosis, calcification, ossification, and fat [15]. Histologically nodular lesions consist of fusiform spindle cells and cells of intermediate differentiation between fibroblasts and smooth muscular cells, called myofibroblasts. Immunocytochemical staining is positive for vimentin and smooth muscle actin, and negative for desmin.

Plain films and CT scans show a low-density soft tissue tumor developing within muscle or subcutaneous tissue and containing calcifications (Fig. 13.21). After contrast injection, there is a homogeneous enhancement [6]. Eich [15] describes the MR appearance of infantile myofibromatosis: they are isointense to muscle

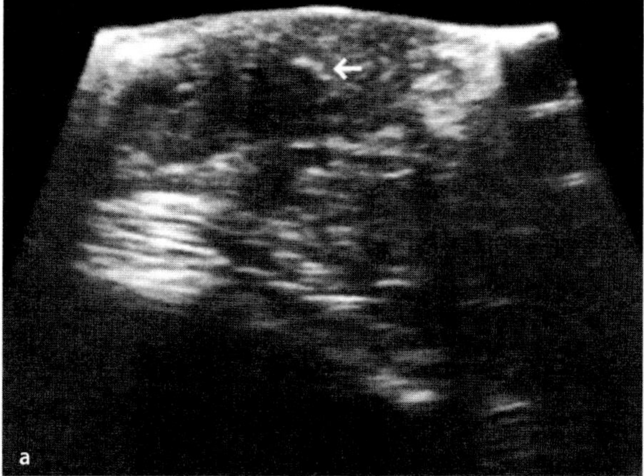
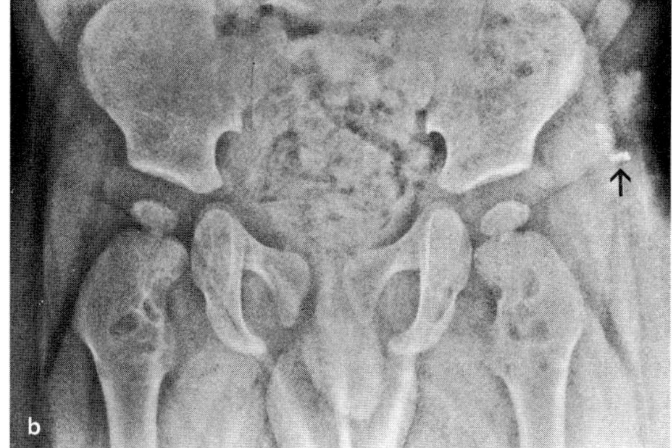
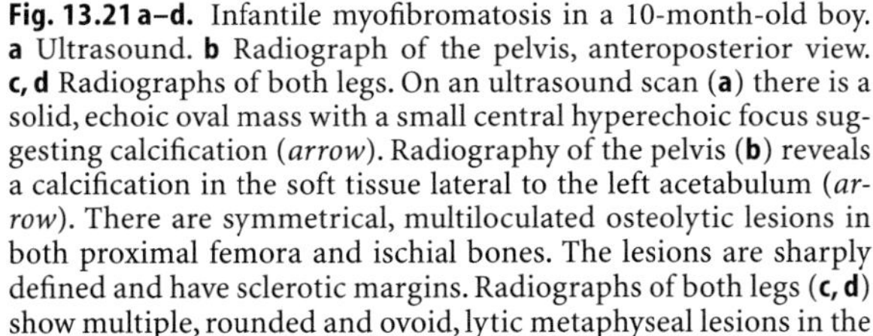
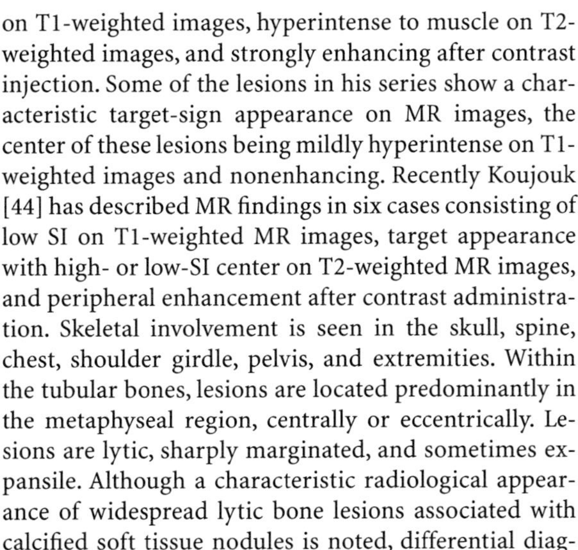
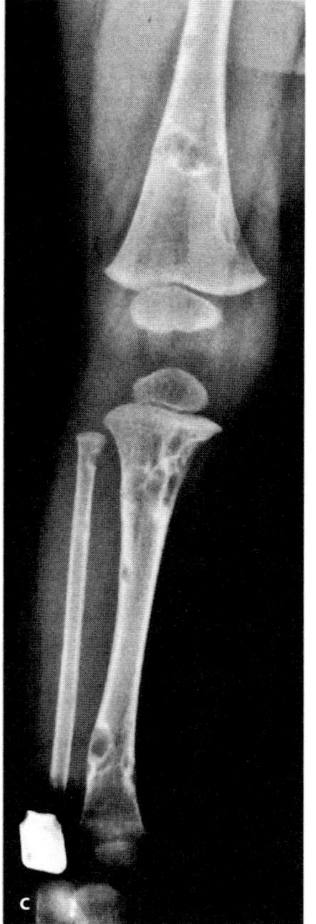
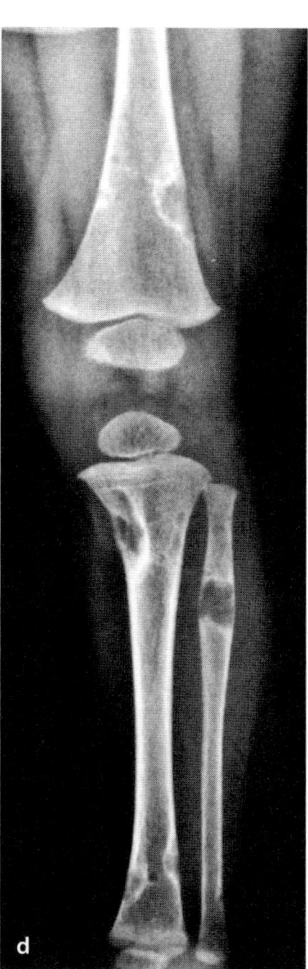

Fig. 13.21 a–d. Infantile myofibromatosis in a 10-month-old boy. **a** Ultrasound. **b** Radiograph of the pelvis, anteroposterior view. **c, d** Radiographs of both legs. On an ultrasound scan (**a**) there is a solid, echoic oval mass with a small central hyperechoic focus suggesting calcification (*arrow*). Radiography of the pelvis (**b**) reveals a calcification in the soft tissue lateral to the left acetabulum (*arrow*). There are symmetrical, multiloculated osteolytic lesions in both proximal femora and ischial bones. The lesions are sharply defined and have sclerotic margins. Radiographs of both legs (**c, d**) show multiple, rounded and ovoid, lytic metaphyseal lesions in the femur, tibia, and fibula bilaterally. They all have an intracortical localization and sclerotic margins. The lesion in the proximal left fibula is slightly expansile. In this case, the age of the patient and the coexistence of bone and soft tissue lesions are indicative of infantile myofibromatosis. Follow-up demonstrated spontaneous regression and even disappearance of the lesions. (By courtesy of W.G. Wassenaar, Afdeling Radiodiagnostiek, Academisch Ziekenhuis Nijmegen St. Radboud, Geert Grooteplein 18, Postbus 9101, 6500 HN Nijmegen, The Netherlands [84])

on T1-weighted images, hyperintense to muscle on T2-weighted images, and strongly enhancing after contrast injection. Some of the lesions in his series show a characteristic target-sign appearance on MR images, the center of these lesions being mildly hyperintense on T1-weighted images and nonenhancing. Recently Koujouk [44] has described MR findings in six cases consisting of low SI on T1-weighted MR images, target appearance with high- or low-SI center on T2-weighted MR images, and peripheral enhancement after contrast administration. Skeletal involvement is seen in the skull, spine, chest, shoulder girdle, pelvis, and extremities. Within the tubular bones, lesions are located predominantly in the metaphyseal region, centrally or eccentrically. Lesions are lytic, sharply marginated, and sometimes expansile. Although a characteristic radiological appearance of widespread lytic bone lesions associated with calcified soft tissue nodules is noted, differential diag-nosis of multiple myofibromas should include fibrous dysplasia, neurofibromatosis, and lymphangiomatosis; while solitary myofibroma should include traumatic myositis ossificans, juvenile aponeurotic fibroma, and soft tissue chondroma [79].

13.4.4 Juvenile Hyaline Fibromatosis

Juvenile hyaline fibromatosis is a rare condition that is thought to be a mesenchymal dysplasia, showing multiple subcutaneous tumors, hypertrophic gingiva, and flexion contractures of the extremities. Calcifications in soft tissue tumors, scoliosis, marked osteopenia, well-defined osteolytic lesions and cortical defects in tubular bones, severe acro-osteolysis, and destruction of epiphyses of the long bones are also reported (Fig. 13.22). This autosomal, recessive condition is reported in chil-

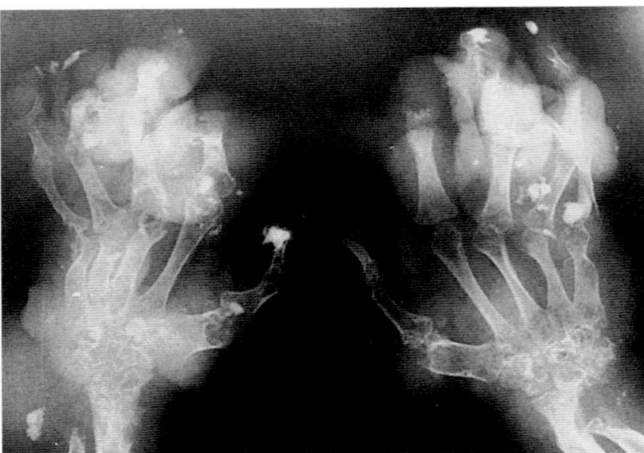

Fig. 13.22. Juvenile hyaline fibromatosis in a 36-year-old woman. Radiograph of the hands. There are multiple, calcified soft tissue nodules and expansile osteolytic lesions in the tubular bones, with marked deformation of the wrists and small joints. Severe acro-osteolysis. (Reproduced from [28], with permission)

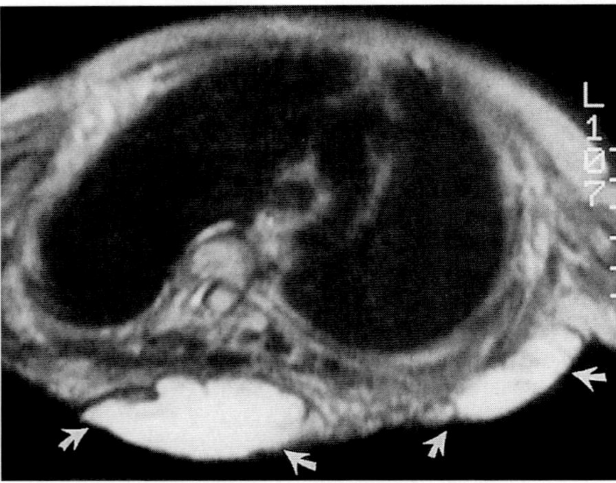

Fig. 13.23. Juvenile hyaline fibromatosis in a 9-year-old girl with multiple palpable nodules throughout the body and severe scoliosis. Axial spin-echo T2-weighted MR image of the trunk Presence of two large subcutaneous masses showing extremely high signal intensity on the T2-weighted image. In this case of juvenile hyaline fibromatosis, the bright signal on the T2-weighted image is consistent with the presence of hyaline matrix. (Reproduced from [38], with permission)

dren of consanguineous parents, and clinical onset occurs between 2 months and 4 years of age. Subcutaneous nodules are slow growing and may reach a large size, producing great deformities. Surgical excision is often followed by tumor recurrence.

Histologically the lesion is characterized by the presence of hyaline substance in the tumoral connective tissue. Diagnosis is confirmed by electron-microscopic examination [28]. On MR images the lesions are bright on T2-weighted images, most likely reflecting the hyaline matrix which is characteristic of the lesions (Fig. 13.23). MRI may be a significant diagnostic aid, as other fibro-

matosis syndromes have nodules that are of low signal on T2-weighted images [38].

13.4.5 Fibromatosis Colli

Fibromatosis colli is a peculiar growth of the sternocleidomastoid muscle that appears within the 1st weeks of life and is often associated with torticollis. It occurs in 0.4% of newborns. There is a marked male predominance. It remains unclear whether the fibroblastic proliferation is reparative or neoplastic. Although there is a history of breech or complicated delivery in more than 4% of the cases, microscopic appearance of the lesion differs from that of proven cases of organizing hematoma, and there is also very little demonstrable hemosiderin within it. Vascular impairment as the result of prolonged venous stasis or ischemia during labor is another possible cause. Nevertheless there is a clear association with other musculoskeletal developmental abnormalities that are associated with abnormal intrauterine positioning, including forefoot anomalies and congenital hip dislocation [20].

Clinically the lesion manifests between the 2nd and 4th week of life as a firm mass of 2–3 cm diameter lying within the lower portion of the sternocleidomastoid muscle. Initially it grows rapidly, but after a few weeks or months, growth comes to a halt. Later it begins to regress and may disappear after a period of 1 or 2 years. It never recurs and at no time does it behave aggressively. During the initial growth period, torticollis occurs in 40% of all cases and usually is mild and transient.

Microscopically the sternocleidomastoid muscle is partially replaced by a fibroblastic process of varying cellularity without pleomorphism or mitotic activity. Residual degenerated muscle fibers are intimately mixed with proliferated fibroblasts. Long-standing lesions may show a lower degree of cellularity and a greater amount of stromal collagen [17].

On ultrasound scans, the mass within the belly of the sternocleidomastoid muscle is spindle shaped and may be hyperechoic (50%), isoechoic, or hypoechoic relative to normal muscle. The echotexture may be homogeneous (50%) or heterogeneous (50%). The mass is surrounded by a hypoechoic rim in 90% of cases [1]. Ultrasound is the method of choice for follow-up of fibromatosis colli (Fig. 13.24b) [9]. On CT scans, fibromatosis colli appears as a focal or diffuse isodense enlargement of the sternocleidomastoid muscle with or without mass effect (Fig. 13.24a). On MR images fibromatosis colli may present with a slightly increased SI on T2-weighted images compared with normal muscle (Fig. 13.24c, d) or with a slightly decreased SI on T2-weighted images consistent with the presence of some fibrous tissue [1]. Imaging findings that are not characteristic of fibromatosis colli are: mass extending beyond

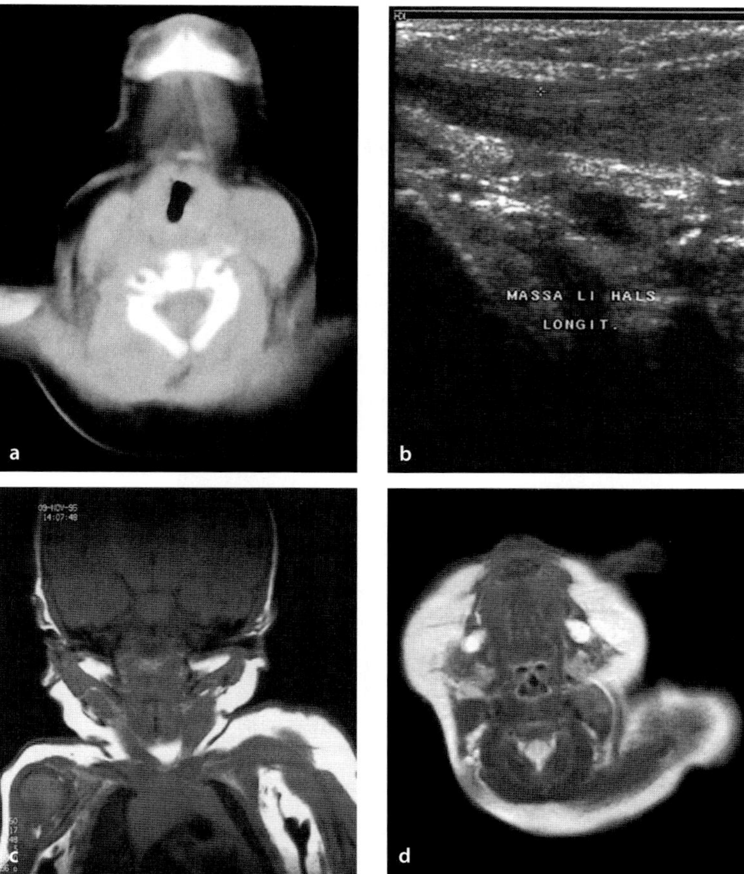

Fig. 13.24a–d. Fibromatosis colli in a 1-day-old boy (**a**) and a 7-week-old girl (**b–d**) presenting clinically with torticollis. **a** CT scan. **b** Ultrasound of the left sternocleidomastoid muscle. **c** Coronal spin-echo T1-weighted MR image. **d** Axial turbo spin-echo T2-weighted MR image. CT scan showing overall enlargement of the left sternocleidomastoid muscle, without obvious change in attenuation (**a**). On ultrasound scans, there is a fusiform mass in the distal part of the muscle. The mass is hyperechoic and lacks muscle fiber structure (**b**). On the T1-weighted image, there is a fusiform enlargement of the left sternocleidomastoid muscle (**c**), while on the T2-weighted image the lesion is less homogeneous and predominantly of high signal intensity (**d**). Characteristic age, location, and shape of a fibroma colli

the margins of the sternocleidomastoid muscle, poor definition of the surrounding fascial planes and/or mass associated with adenopathy, bone involvement, intracranial or intraspinal extension, vascular encasement, and airway compression. If essential clinical and radiological features of fibromatosis colli are present, recognition of this entity by medical imaging can prevent unnecessary diagnostic and therapeutic maneuvers [9].

13.4.6 Infantile (Desmoid-Type) Fibromatosis

Infantile (desmoid-type) fibromatosis represents the infantile variety of musculo-aponeurotic desmoid-type of fibromatosis. Infantile fibromatosis may occur in bone, in soft tissues or in a generalized form (soft tissues, viscera, and bone) Lesions mostly occur in the head and neck region. They appear as nodular, rounded, or oval masses with well-defined margins or as more infiltrative, permeative lesions with indistinct borders extending to encase adjacent neurovascular structures and bone [41]. Most lesions are unifocal at presentation; when multifocal they also show intra-abdominal mesenteric and retroperitoneal spread and ascites. Familial

cases occur, particularly as part of Gardner syndrome [15]. If bony lesions coexist they are purely lytic lesions with an aggressive appearance [86].

Although histologically benign, the lesion tends to gradually infiltrate soft tissues (skin, subcutaneous tissues, muscles, and even tendons, nerves, and blood vessels) and adjacent bone – hence the terms aggressive juvenile fibromatosis, juvenile or infantile fibrosarcoma, congenital fibrosarcoma, desmoplastic fibrosarcoma of infancy, and medullary fibromatosis of infancy [73]. These terms are used for all fibroblastic tumors of infancy that show an abundant number of cells and prominent mitotic activity [86]. Aggressive infantile fibromatosis is usually first detected at birth or within the first 3 months of life. Col [8] has reported on the observation of a fetal tumor on antenatal echography which was diagnosed after birth as aggressive fibromatosis of the trunk. There is no sexual predilection. The condition occurs most frequently in the skeletal muscle or in adjacent aponeuroses of the extremities in the head and neck, shoulder and upper arm, and the thigh. A case of aggressive infantile fibromatosis of the thigh which subsequently metastasized to the lungs has been reported by Shankwiler [73].

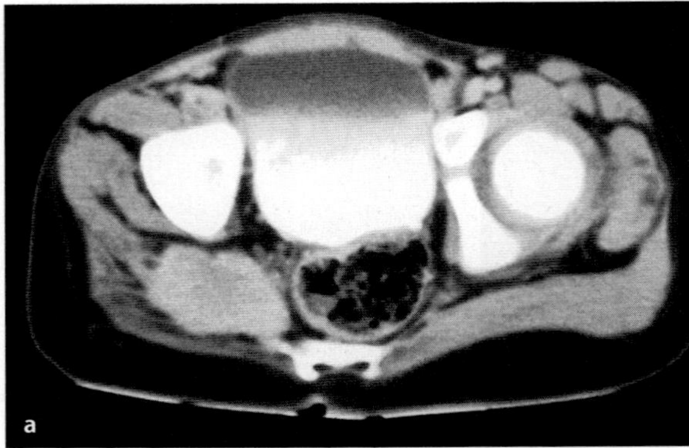

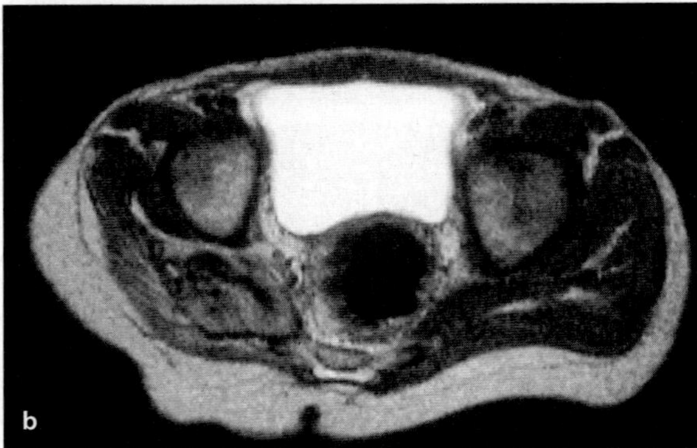

Fig. 13.25 a, b. Infantile fibromatosis in a 2-year-old boy. **a** CT scan. **b** Axial turbo spin-echo T2-weighted MR image. Slowly growing mass in the right gluteal region, with uncharacteristic CT attenuation (**a**). Note the atrophy of adjacent gluteal muscles. On the T2-weighted image, the lesion is of mixed, overall low signal intensity. While the lesion is nonspecific on CT scan, it has a characteristic low signal intensity on the T2-weighted MR image as a consequence of its high collagen content

Microscopically, two patterns can be distinguished that reflect progressive stages in the differentiation of fibroblasts. The immature type is composed of cells which are intermediate in appearance between primitive mesenchymal cells and fibroblasts, and are associated with a dense meshwork of reticulin fibers and considerable amounts of mucoid material. The mature type is composed of more mature fibroblasts associated with varying amounts of collagen. It closely resembles adult musculo-aponeurotic fibromatosis. Aggressive juvenile fibromatosis lesions are hypercellular and composed of pleomorphic, mitotically active, spindle-shaped fibroblasts arranged in a herringbone pattern [73].

Only a few cases of infantile fibromatosis have been reported with uncharacteristic appearance on ultrasound and CT scans, i.e., homogeneous and hypoechoic on ultrasound, and homogeneous, hyper-, or isodense with respect to muscle on precontrast CT scans, enhancing after contrast administration [51]. Extensive ossification within an infantile fibromatosis is a rare finding, which has been described by Fromowitz [26].

The variable MR imaging signal characteristics of infantile desmoid fibromatosis reflect differences in composition, especially cellularity, fibrous tissue content, and the presence of myxomatous degeneration. Most desmoid tumors are heterogeneous soft-tissue lesions of intermediate SI (between those of muscle and fat). Lesions may be hypointense, isointense, or, occasionally, marginally hyperintense with respect to muscle signal on T1-weighted images and of mixed, predominantly high signal (greater than that of muscle but usually less than that of fat) on T2-weighted images. Zones of low SI are often seen on both T1- and T2-weighted images. The difference in T2-weighted SI appears to be determined by the degree of cellularity rather than the amount of collagen present in the lesion (Fig. 13.25). After IV injection of Gd contrast, tumors may show homogeneous, inhomogeneous, or no significant enhancement. No relationship has been shown between the pattern of enhancement and tumor recurrence.

13.5 Intermediate-Grade Fibromyoblastic Tumors

In the new WHO classification, this group contains the extrapleural solitary fibrous tumor, inflammatory myofibroblastic tumor, hemangiopericytoma, and infantile fibrosarcoma.

13.5.1 Solitary Fibrous Tumor

Solitary fibrous tumor is a mesenchymal tumor of probable fibroblastic type which shows a prominent, hemangiopericytoma-like branching vascular pattern. It's an uncommon lesion observed in middle-aged adults without sex predilection. It can be found at any location of which 40% in the subcutaneous tissue. Most solitary fibrous tumors are found at the pleura, face, and meninges. It is mostly a large, well delineated, slowly growing and painless mass. Histopathologically it consists of a mixture of hypocellular and hypercellular areas separated from each other by thick bands of collagen and branching, hemangiopericytoma-like vessels. Malignant solitary fibrous tumors (10–15%) behave aggressively and show histopathological features of hypercellularity, cytological atypia, necrosis, numerous mitoses, and infiltrative growth.

On MR images, solitary fibrous tumors of the extremities have nonspecific features, i.e., inhomogeneous, low to intermediate SI on T1-weighted images and inhomogeneous, intermediate to high SI on T2-weighted images [3] (Fig. 13.26).

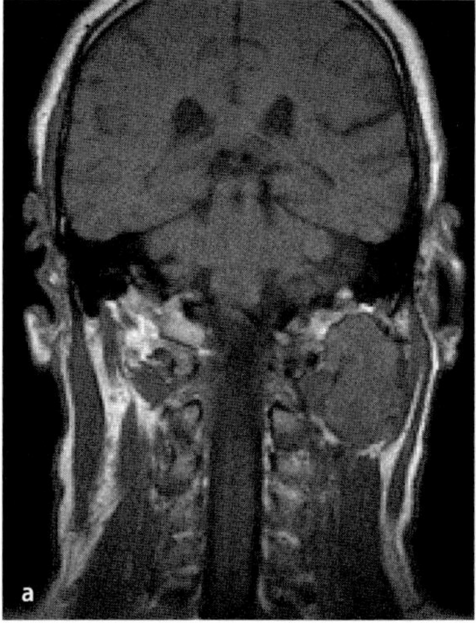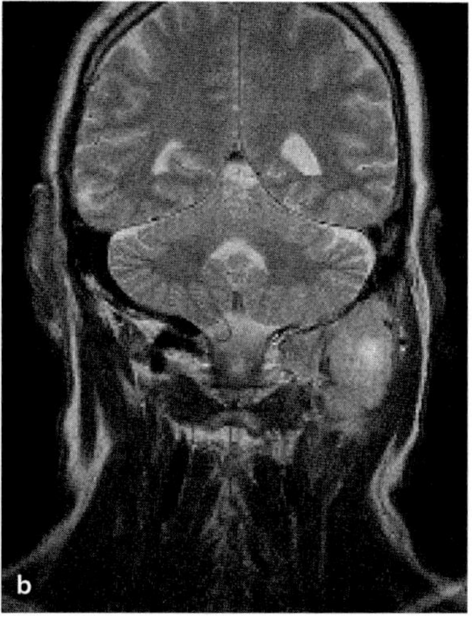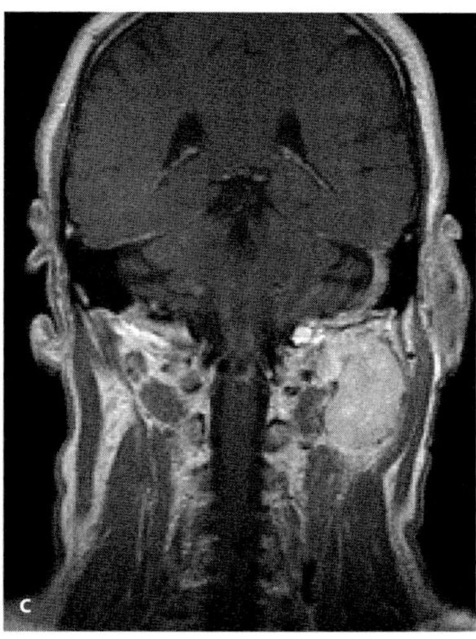

Fig. 13.26 a–c. Solitary fibrous tumor. **a** Coronal spin-echo T1-weighted MR image. **b** Coronal spin-echo T2-weighted MR image. **c** Coronal spin-echo T1-weighted MR image, after gadolinium contrast injection. Mass lesion in between the left sternocleido-mastoid muscle and deep cervical muscles, presenting with low to intermediate SI on both T1- (**a**) and T2-weighted (**b**) MR images and with marked enhancement after contrast administration (**c**)

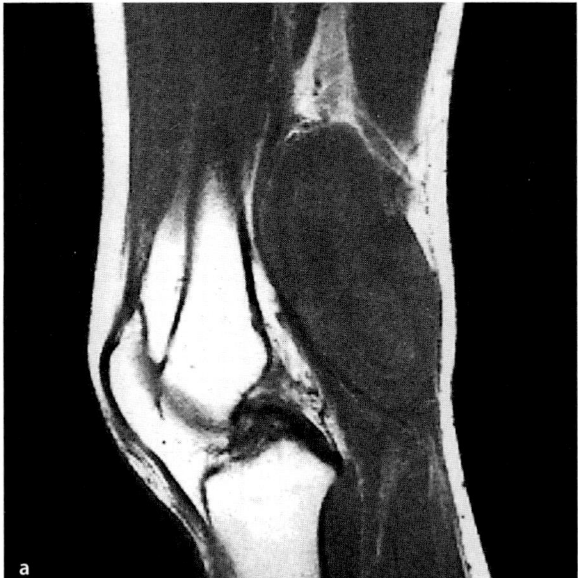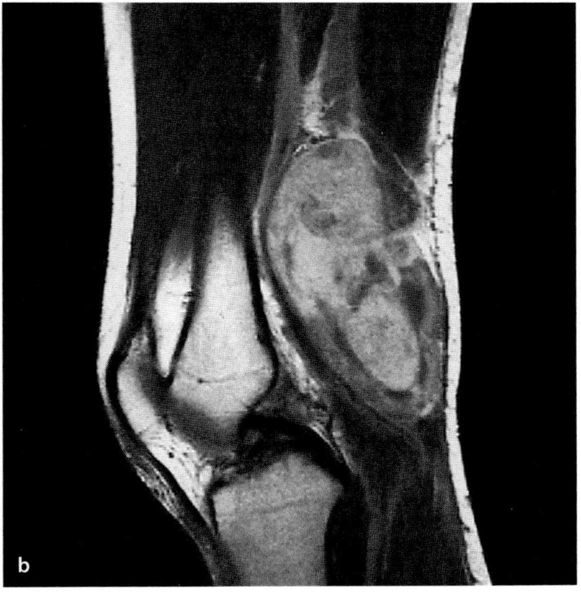

Fig. 13.27 a, b. Hemangiopericytoma of the right popliteal fossa. **a** Sagittal T1-weighted MR image. **b** Sagittal T1-weighted MR image after gadolinium contrast injection. An oval, largely homoge-neous lesion is seen lying superficial to the major vessels. There is no invasion of the subcutis (**a**). After contrast administration, a strong enhancement of the mass is seen (**b**)

13.5.2 Hemangiopericytoma

Hemangiopericytoma is a slow growing tumor of intermediate grade of malignancy that never metastasizes (Fig. 13.27). The term is used to encompass a wide variety of neoplasms which have in common the presence of a thin-walled, branching vascular pattern. They most commonly occur in middle-aged adults, with an apparent female predominance. The pelvis and retroperitoneum are the most frequent locations.

Histopathologically hemangiopericytoma closely resembles solitary fibrous tumor, albeit with the consistent presence of numerous, variably ectatic or compressed, thin-walled branching vessels, often having a staghorn configuration [20].

13.5.3 Inflammatory Myofibroblastic Tumor

It is a distinctive lesion, primarily a visceral and soft tissue tumor of children and young adults, composed of myofibroblastic spindle cells accompanied by an inflammatory infiltrate of plasma cells, lymphocytes and eosinophils. All body parts can be affected and they determine the symptoms of inflammatory myofibroblastic tumor [20]. Lung, mesentery omentum, and orbits are the most common sites.

Findings of a mass lesion are frequently in association with fever, weight loss and pain. Imaging studies reveal a lobulated, solid mass which can be inhomogeneous. Intralesional calcifications are described.

In our own series we have one case of an inflammatory myofibroblastic tumor located in the subcutis with infiltration of the underlying fascia. The lesion is ill defined with nonspecific MR features, i.e., low SI on T1-, and high SI on T2-weighted MR images and peripheral enhancement after contrast administration.

13.5.4 Infantile Fibrosarcoma

Infantile, congenital or juvenile fibrosarcoma is a rare childhood malignancy (3% of all childhood tumors) of mesodermal origin. (Fig. 13.28) For some authors [17], infantile fibrosarcoma is a distinct lesion, while for others [73, 81] it cannot be differentiated from the aggressive infantile type of fibromatosis described above. It usually presents at birth or during the first year of life. Prenatal diagnosis is likely to increase with the advent of routine antenatal ultrasound. There is no sex preponderance. The superficial and deep soft tissues of the extremities, especially distally, are the most common sites, accounting for 61% of cases overall. [20] It tends to show a rapid increase in size and distant metastasis may occur in 8% of cases [34]. Infantile cases are often grotesquely large in proportion to the size of the child [20] Adjacent bone may show some deformity with cortical thickening and failure of normal tubulation. Large tumors may cause bone erosion, bowing, remodeling, or destruction. Intratumoral ossification or calcification is rare.

Histologically, infantile fibrosarcoma is an undifferentiated fibroblastic spindle cell tumor of intermediate grade of malignancy, which is densely cellular, often in a herringbone pattern with numerous mitoses and infiltrative margins. Collagen formation is not prominent. Cystic, myxoid, highly vascular, and necrotic tumor components are often seen [34]. Histological description parallels that of an aggressive juvenile fibromatosis (see Sect. 13.4.6). Tumors are isoechoic on US and mild-

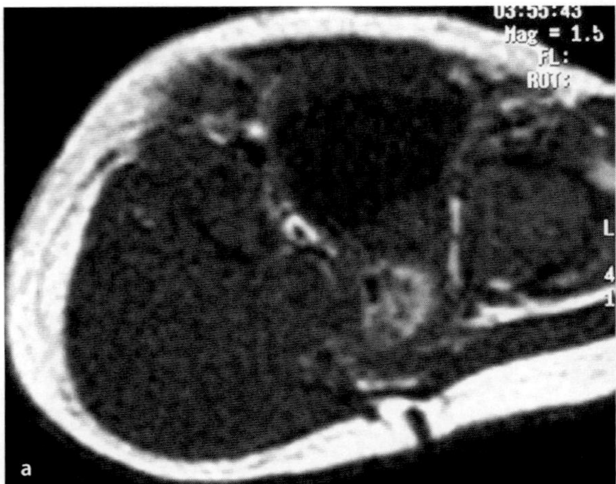

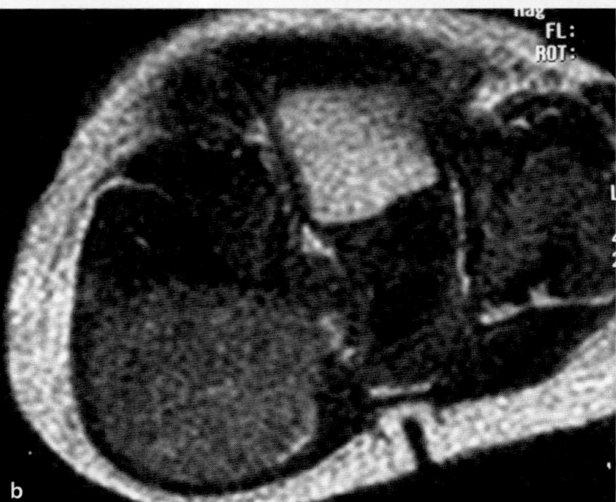

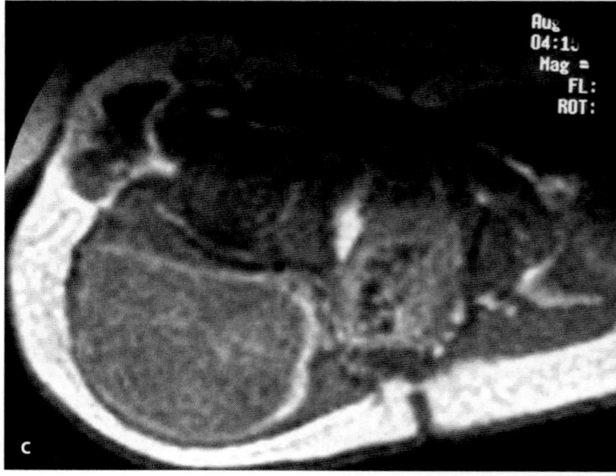

Fig. 13.28 a–c. Infantile fibrosarcoma. **a** Axial spin-echo T1-weighted MR image. **b** Axial turbo- T2-weighted MR image. **c** Axial spin-echo T1-weighted MR image after gadolinium contrast injection. Infantile fibrosarcoma at the right gluteal region presenting with nonspecific MR features, i.e., low SI on T1- (**a**), and intermediate SI on T2-weighted images (**b**). There is moderate enhancement after contrast administration (**c**)

ly hypodense on plain CT. On MR, they appear isointense on T1-weighted images and hyperintense on T2-weighted images. There is an heterogeneous enhancement pattern with low SI areas, both centrally and in the periphery of the lesions [15].

CT is useful in demonstrating the extent of the tumor and the bony involvement, while disruption of soft tissue planes is better shown on MR images. MRI has a role in follow-up and early detection of local tumor recurrence. Use of Gd contrast agents may aid in differentiating between fibrosis and tumor recurrence [81].

13.6 Malignant Fibromyoblastic Tumors

13.6.1 Adult Fibrosarcoma

Adult fibrosarcoma is a malignant tumor composed of fibroblasts with variable collagen production and herring-bone architecture and is capable of recurrence and metastasis [17]. Histologic, immunohistochemical, and ultrastructural examination are important tools for diagnosing fibrosarcoma and for differentiating fibrosarcoma from nodular fasciitis, myxofibrosarcoma, musculoaponeurotic fibromatosis, and other sarcomas. Recognition of these lesions as specific tumors and entities is responsible for the decline in the incidence of fibrosarcoma and for the overdiagnosis of fibrosarcoma in earlier studies.

Clinically, fibrosarcoma presents as a slowly growing, solitary, palpable mass with a diameter of 3–8 cm. It may reach a large size before causing symptoms. The lesion is most common between the ages 30 and 55 years, and the incidence is slightly higher in women. The thigh and the knee region are preferential localizations, followed by the trunk, distal legs, and forearms. Less than 5% present in the head and neck [29]. Deep fibrosarcomas originate from the intramuscular and intermuscular fibrous tissue, fascial envelopes, aponeuroses, and tendons. They may cause periosteal and cortical thickening, and rarely demonstrate intralesional calcifications or ossifications. Superficial or subcutaneous

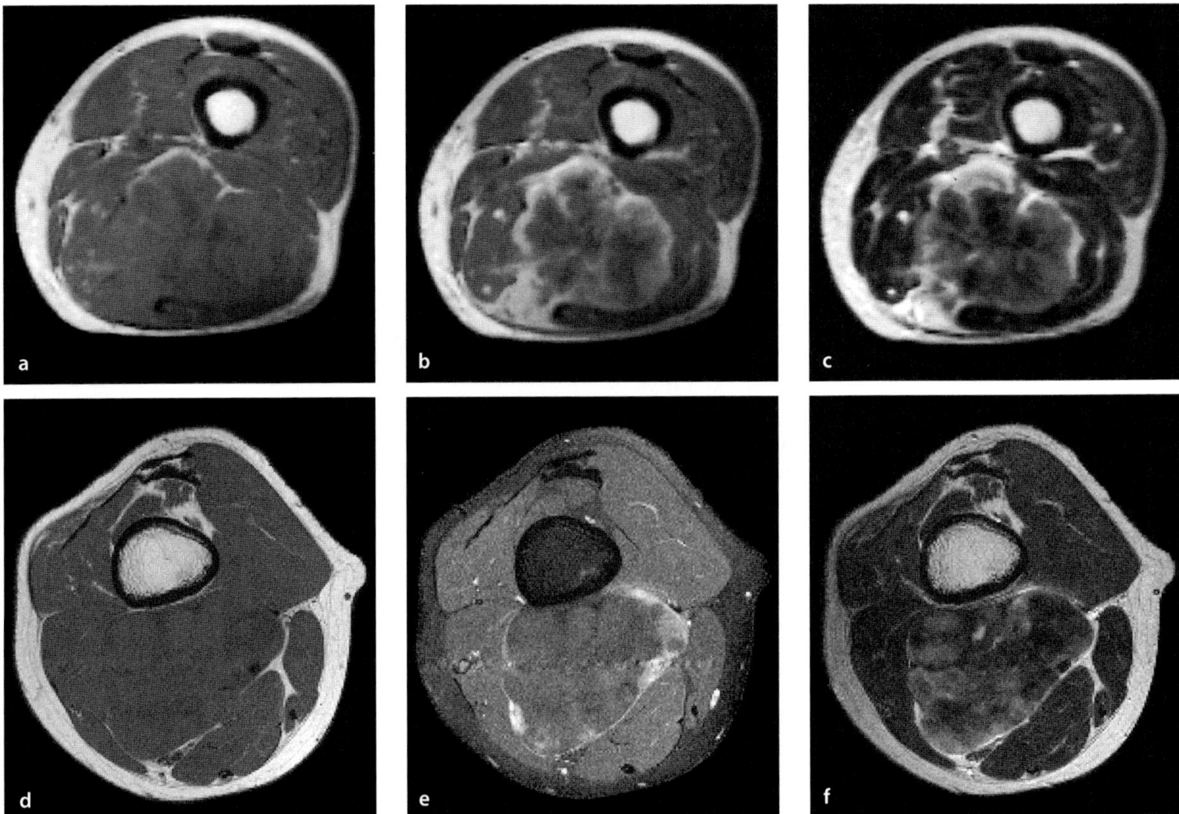

Fig. 13.29a–f. Two cases of Fibrosarcoma (**a–c, d–f**). **a** Axial spin-echo T1-weighted MR images. **b** Axial spin-echo T1-weighted MR images after gadolinium contrast injection. **c** Axial spin-echo T2-weighted MR images. **d** Axial spin-echo T1-weighted MR images. **e** Axial spin-echo T1-weighted MR images after gadolinium contrast injection, with fat suppression. **f** Turbo spin-echo T2-weighted MR images. In both cases lesions are nonhomogeneous and isointense to muscle on T1-weighted MR images (**a, d**), they are nonhomogeneous and of overall low SI on T2-weighted MR images (**b, e**) and enhance in a spoked-wheel pattern after contrast administration (**c, f**). Large size and SIs are compatible with the diagnosis of fibrosarcoma. Good delineation and speckled areas of low SI do not allow differentiation from extra-abdominal desmoids

fibrosarcomas arise in tissues damaged by trauma, scarring, heat (burns), or radiation.

Macroscopically, small fibrosarcomas are well defined, while larger fibrosarcomas tend to be poorly defined, grow in a diffusely invasive manner, and are often multiloculated. Microscopically, fibrosarcomas have a rather uniform or fasciculated growth pattern consisting of spindle-shaped cells separated by interwoven collagen fibers that are arranged in a parallel fashion. Mitotic activity is a condition for diagnosis. Grading of fibrosarcoma (well differentiated versus poorly differentiated) is based on the degree of cellularity, cellular maturity, the amount of collagen produced by the tumor cells, and the presence of necrosis and/or intralesional hemorrhage.

Low-grade fibrosarcoma (well differentiated) is defined by sheets of uniform spindle cells with moderate cellularity arranged in a herringbone pattern, mild nuclear pleomorphism, and only rarely mitoses. A collagenous stroma is usually present. High-grade lesions (poorly differentiated) show greater nuclear pleomorphism, abundant cellularity, frequent mitotic activity, and possible tumor necrosis. Despite the fact that desmoids are characterized more by their localization and that fibrosarcomas are larger in size, differentiation between desmoids (representing more than 70% of tumors of fibrous tissue) and fibrosarcomas (less than 5%) is difficult even on MR images (Figs. 13.29, 13.30). Multicentric presentation of fibrosarcoma is a rare finding which can hardly be differentiated from metastatic fibrosarcoma (Fig. 13.31). The treatment of choice is wide local excision. Simple excision of fibrosarcomas is often followed by local recurrence.

Medical imaging literature about fibrosarcoma is sparse and limited to case reports. In our series of soft tissue tumors, we had nine cases of primary fibrosarcoma and two recurrent fibrosarcomas. The age range of patients was between 16 and 77 years, with a mean age of 47 years. In contrast to results reported in the literature, nine of ten patients were men. Nine lesions were located on the lower limb, from the groin to the sole of the foot. One patient presented with multiple bone and soft tissue localizations. Diameters were between 2 and 27 cm (mean diameter, 12 cm).

All patients underwent MRI. Lesions were either homogeneous or inhomogeneous on both T1- and T2-weighted images. Most lesions showed signal intensities equal to those of muscle on T1-weighted images and low-SI areas on a background of moderate to high SI on T2-weighted images. T1-weighted images after Gd contrast were performed in nine patients. Ninety percent of the lesion showed a marked, peripheral enhancement, with a spoked-wheel appearance in three patients. Nonenhancement of central tumor parts was not a consequence of intratumoral necrosis. In only one case did the nonenhancing central part correspond to an area of

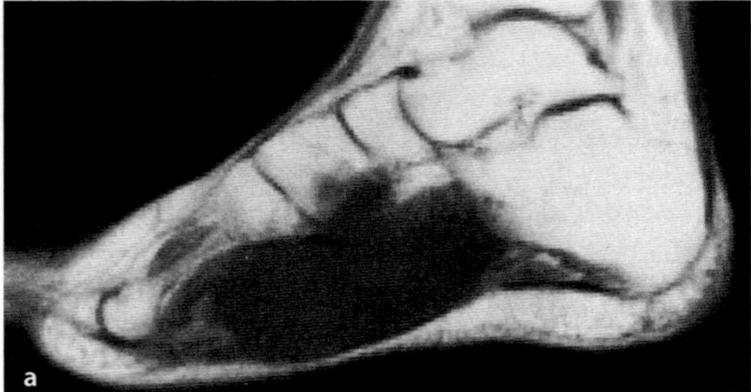

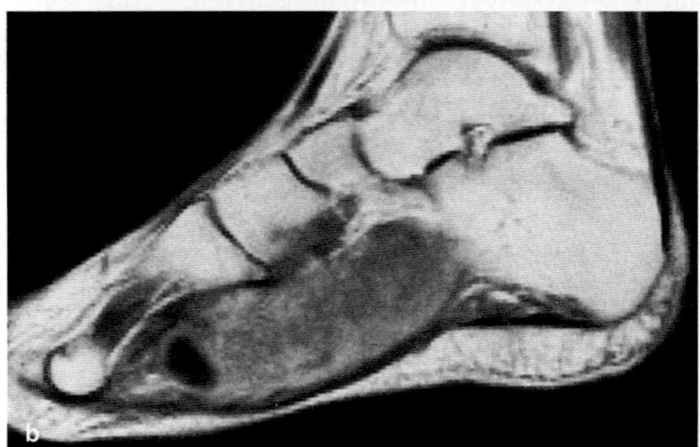

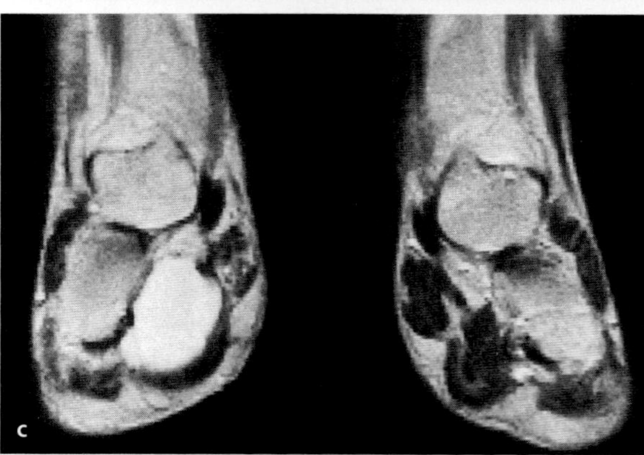

Fig. 13.30 a–c. Fibrosarcoma of the foot in a 34-year-old man. **a** Sagittal spin-echo T1-weighted MR image. **b** Sagittal spin-echo T1-weighted MR image after gadolinium contrast injection. **c** Coronal spin-echo T2-weighted MR image. A large fusiform-mass lesion is present at the foot deep to the plantar aponeurosis, with involvement of the medial cuneiform bone. Overall signal intensity on the T1-weighted image is low (**a**). The lesion shows moderate enhancement, with a nonenhancing (necrotic?) nodule at the distal part (**b**). On the T2-weighted image, the lesion is of homogeneous high signal intensity (**c**). Age, location, and MRI characteristics suggest a malignant tumor but do not allow further histological typing

high SI on T2-weighted images. Osseous involvement was rare, being noted only once in the group of solitary fibrosarcomas. The patient with multicentric fibrosarcoma had numerous osteolytic osseous lesions and two soft tissue nodules at the pelvic girdle (Fig. 13.31).

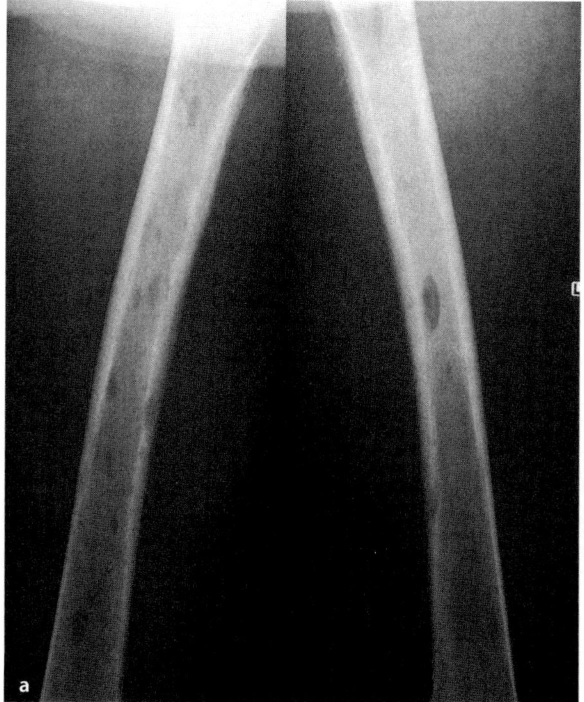

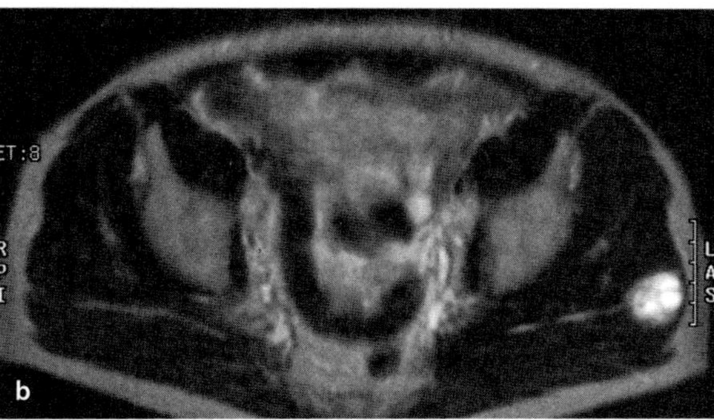

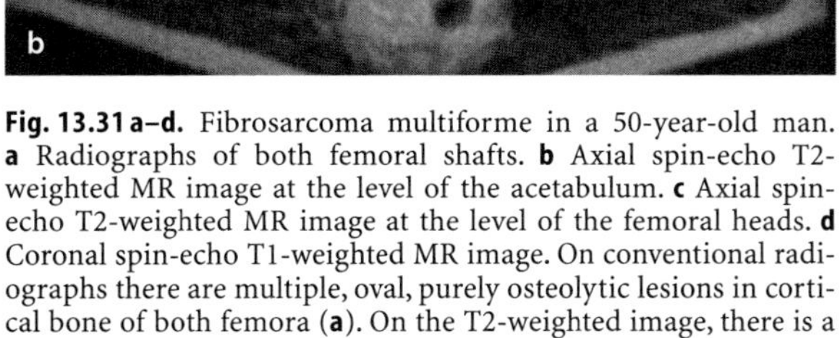

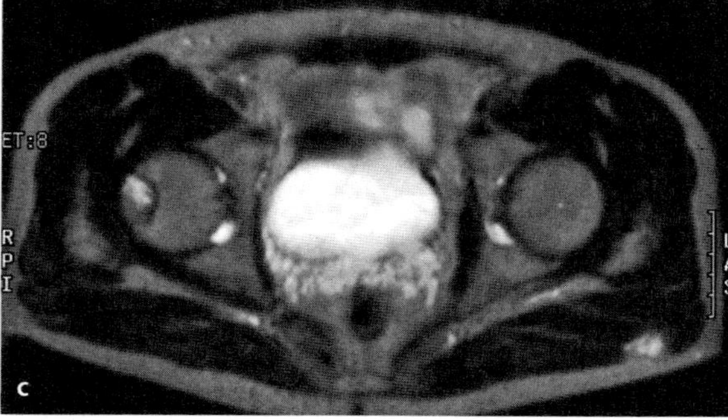

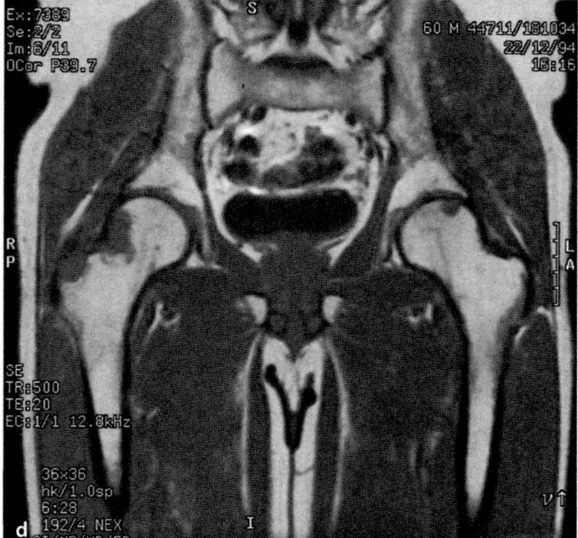

Fig. 13.31 a–d. Fibrosarcoma multiforme in a 50-year-old man. **a** Radiographs of both femoral shafts. **b** Axial spin-echo T2-weighted MR image at the level of the acetabulum. **c** Axial spin-echo T2-weighted MR image at the level of the femoral heads. **d** Coronal spin-echo T1-weighted MR image. On conventional radiographs there are multiple, oval, purely osteolytic lesions in cortical bone of both femora (**a**). On the T2-weighted image, there is a rounded lesion within the left gluteus maximus muscle, consisting of multiple lobules of high signal intensity, separated by septa of intermediate signal intensity (**b**). On the T2-weighted image at the level of the femoral heads, there is an inhomogeneous lesion within the right femoral head, partly of high signal intensity. There is a small, high-intensity soft tissue lesion in the gluteus maximus muscle on the left side (**c**). On the coronal view, there are multiple lesions of intermediate signal intensity at both femoral heads and right greater trochanter (**d**). Coexistence of bone and soft tissue lesions is a rare finding in fibrosarcoma. Differentiation from metastatic fibrosarcoma remains difficult even histologically

13.6.2 Myxofibrosarcoma

Myxofibrosarcoma (MFS), formerly known as myxoid malignant fibrous histiocytoma, is a malignant fibrous lesion that preferentially affects adults (mean age 66 years). It exhibits a slight male predominance. The majority of patients present with a slowly enlarging and painless mass. Most lesions (80%) arise in the extremities, and less frequently in the trunk, retroperitoneum, head and neck, pelvis, and penis. Seventy percent of the masses are located in the subcutis; they commonly have very infiltrative margins [59]. A MFS lesion is defined as low grade if 30% or more is of myxoid component, 20% or less is solid area and only focal, 10% or less is tumor necrosis [35]. Low-grade MFS occur more frequently in a superficial location [62].

Histopathologically, a nodular growth pattern is seen. The myxoid matrix contains elongated, curvilinear, thin-walled capillaries, and fusiform, round or stellate cells with slightly eosinophilic cytoplasm. Low-grade lesions have a hypocellular, mainly myxoid

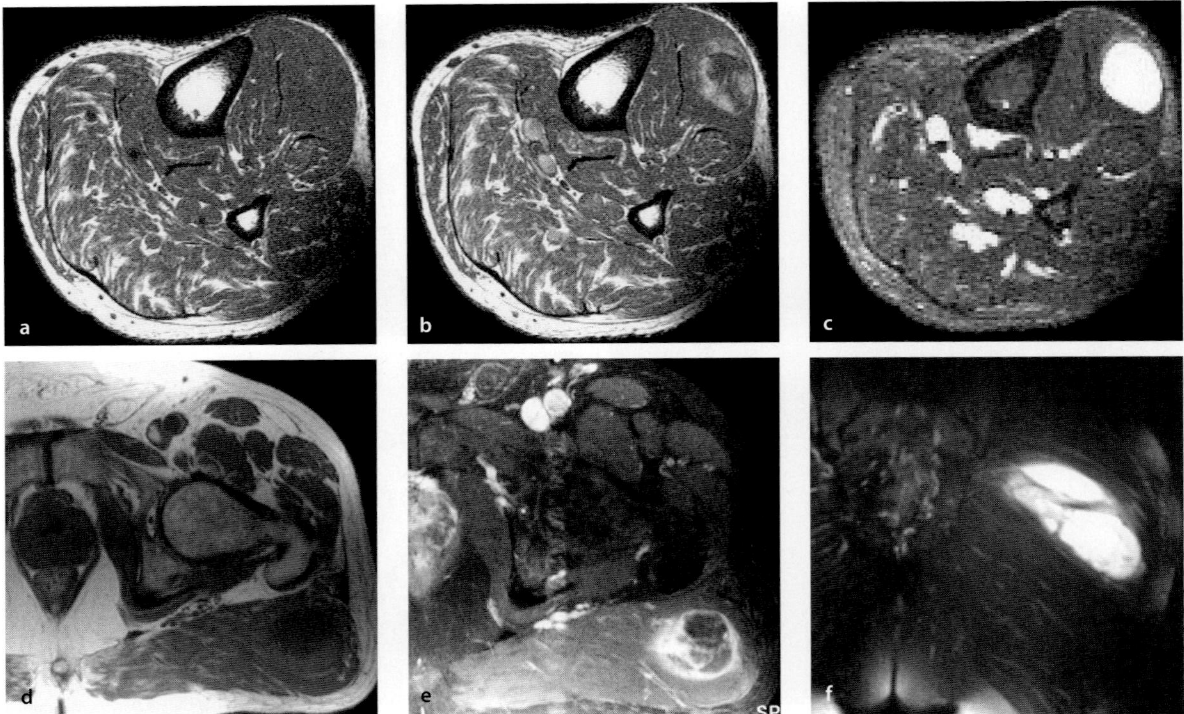

Fig. 13.32 a–f. Two cases of myxofibrosarcoma. **a** Axial spin-echo T1-weighted MR image. **b** Axial spin-echo T1-weighted MR image after gadolinium contrast injection. **c** Axial short-tau inversion recovery MR image. **d** Axial spin-echo T1-weighted MR image. **e** Axial spin-echo T1-weighted MR image after gadolinium contrast injection with fat suppression. **f** Coronal spin-echo T2-weighted MR image: a first one at the left lower leg (**a–c**), a second one at the left gluteal region (**d–f**). Both lesions are of low SI on T1-weighted MR images (**a, d**), show septal and peripheral enhancement after contrast administration (**b, e**) and are of very high SI on T2-weighted MR images (**c, f**) due to abundant myxoid components

aspect, whereas, in high-grade myxofibrosarcoma, high mitotic activity, pleomorphism, and intratumoral necrosis is seen [59].

Mentzel et al. describe local recurrences in 54% of their cases (follow-up of 5–300 months) and metastases in 17%. Neither the depth of the primary lesion nor the histological grade influences the incidence of local recurrence. However, because only intermediate- and high-grade neoplasms metastasize, it is important to recognize low-grade myxofibrosarcoma, because incorrect initial diagnosis and treatment may result in local recurrence, with progression to a higher-grade lesion that has the capability to metastasize [27, 59].

Imaging findings are sparsely reported. On ultrasound scans, a well-circumscribed hypoechoic mass is seen. On T1-weighted MR images, the lesion is homogeneous and has intermediate SI [70]. T2-weighted images reflect the myxoid content of low- and intermediate-grade myxofibrosarcoma, the myxoid content being inversely proportional to the cellularity and the grade of the tumor. High-grade myxofibrosarcoma is not easily distinguished from other adult pleomorphic sarcomas as well histopathologically as on imaging [39] (Fig. 13.32).

Low-grade myxofibrosarcoma may not be confused with low-malignancy fibromyxoid sarcoma, another myxoid mesenchymal sarcoma with fibroblastic differentiation, which has – in contrast to low-grade myxofibrosarcoma – an indolent but ultimately malignant clinical course [57, 58].

13.6.3 Fibromyxoid Sarcoma

Low-grade fibromyxoid sarcoma is a slow-growing, rare neoplasm that preferentially affects young and middle-aged adults (median age 45 years) (Fig. 13.33). Very occasionally it affects children. Most lesions arise from the deep soft tissues at the lower limb or thoracic wall, and less frequently the groin, buttock, axilla, and retroperitoneum [18]. The majority of cases occur in a subfascial location. They are often large at the time of diagnosis.

Histopathologically, the lesion is characterized by intermingled fibrous and myxoid areas, a whorled growth pattern, and bland fibroblastic spindle cells. Cellularity is low and mitotic figures are uncommon.

In contrast to low-grade myxofibrosarcoma, low-grade fibromyxoid sarcoma has an aggressive clinical

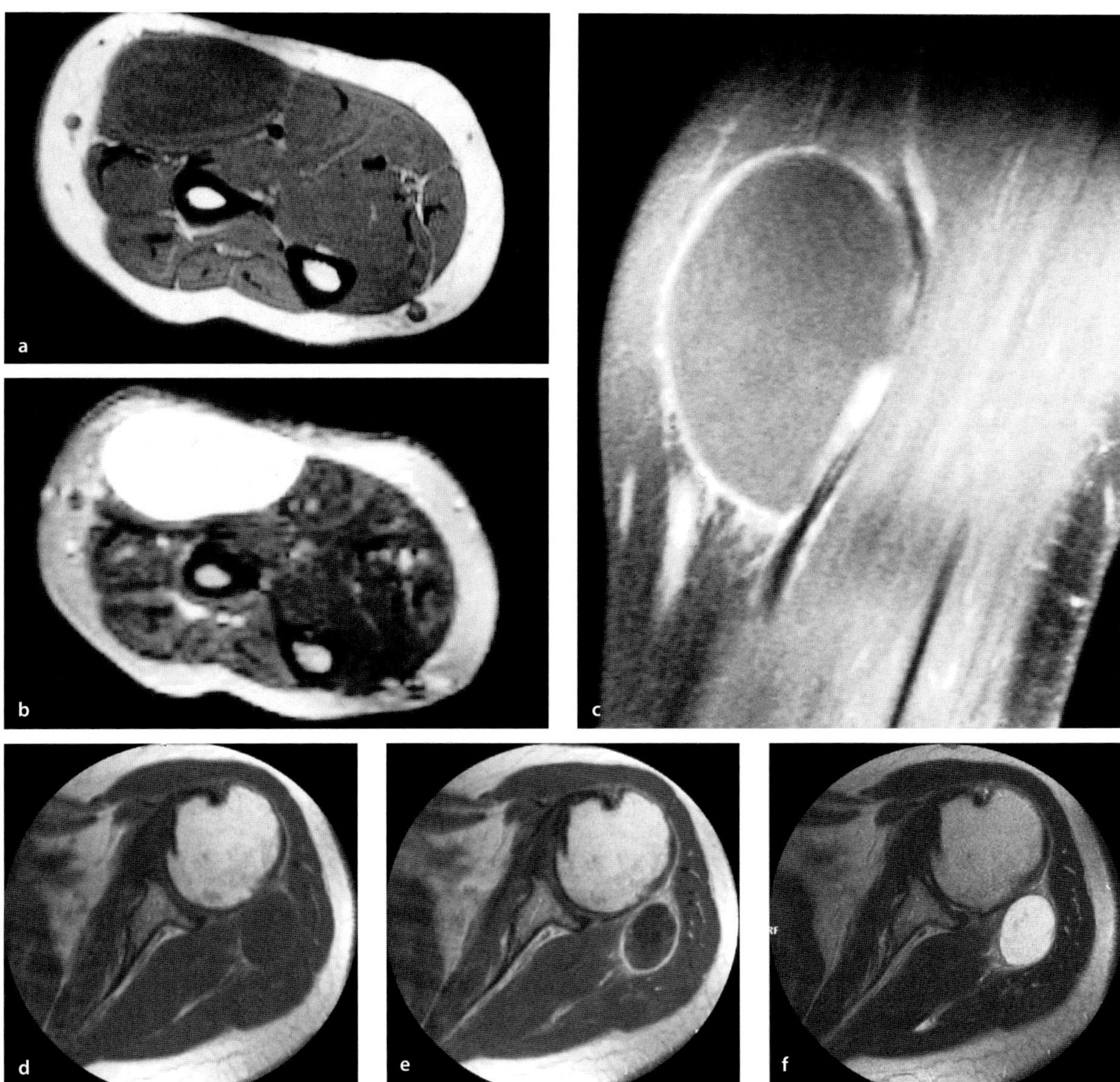

Fig. 13.33 a–f. Two cases of fibromyxoid sarcoma (**a–c, d–f**). **a** Axial spin-echo T1-weighted MR image. **b** Axial spin-echo T2-weighted MR image. **c** Sagittal spin-echo T1-weighted MR image after gadolinium contrast injection with fat suppression. **d** Axial spin-echo T1-weighted MR image. **e** Axial spin-echo T1-weighted MR image after gadolinium contrast injection. **f** Axial spin-echo T2-weighted MR image. Both have similar MRI features. Both lesions are of very low SI on T1-weighted MR image (**a, d**), of very high SI on T2-weighted MR image (**b, c**) and show only minimal capsular enhancement after contrast administration (**c, f**). MR findings reflect the high content of myxoid tissue of both tumors

course characterized by multiple recurrences and with the potential for metastasis to lungs and occasionally to bone. However, recent series show recurrences, metastases, and death from disease in only 9%, 6%, and 2% of patients, respectively. [21, 31].

Imaging features of low-grade fibromyxoid sarcoma are sparsely reported. Koh has reported on two patients with intralesional nodules, one with a large, ovoid mass within the thigh, some of these nodules showing a target-like appearance. A second lesion was dumbbell-shaped with invasive features. There was no intralesional hemorrhage or necrosis.[43].Two high-grade fibromyxoid sarcomas in our series showed a pseudocystic appearance on MR images, i.e., low SI on T1-, high SI on T2-, and only faint, capsular enhancement on Gd contrast T1-weighted images.(Fig. 13.33).

13.7 Strategy

Because they frequently have a characteristic localization and age at presentation (childhood or midlife), tumors of fibrous tissue are diagnosed clinically and not by means of medical imaging. Clinical suspicion may be confirmed by ultrasound, which otherwise has only limited value in diagnostic workup except for demonstration or intratumoral calcifications. Conventional radiography or, even better, CT may confirm the presence of calcifications and show concomitant osseous involvement as a rare finding.

After a lesion has been detected clinically and/or on ultrasound, further evaluation by MRI is mandatory. MRI is able to demonstrate the exact localization, extent, and margins of the lesion. Intratumoral areas of low SI on T2-weighted images that do not enhance on T1-weighted images after Gd contrast administration represent fibrous components of mature tumors of fibrous tissue. Areas of high SI on T2-weighted images that enhance on T1-weighted images after Gd contrast administration represent nonfibrous components of immature tumors of fibrous tissue. Intratumoral necrosis is a rare finding even in fibrosarcoma.

MRI also shows the natural evolution of tumors of fibrous tissue, which have high SI in the initial stages and low SI on T2-weighted images in later stages, paralleling the histological evolution from hypercellular in the initial to more collagenous in the mature, later stage. Staging by MRI helps the physician to choose adequate therapy, leading to a decrease in tumor recurrence because of incomplete surgery.

The purposes of imaging of fibrous tumors in children described by Eich et al. [15] are:
1. Confirmation of a clinically suspected mass
2. Characterization of the mass with regard to location, extension, structure, and margins
3. Determination of either unifocal or multifocal disease, or metastases
4. Observation of additional features as part of a systemic disorder (e.g., Gardner syndrome, hyaline fibromatosis)
5. Formulation of a tentative diagnosis
6. Assistance for biopsy or excision
7. Follow-up for documentation of regression, progression, recurrence, or secondary spread.

Things to remember:
1. Tumors of connective tissue are common.
2. Histopathological and imaging features are related to age of the lesions.
3. Benign tumors mostly have a characteristic location (giant cell tumor of the tendon sheath, elastofibroma, palmar and plantar fibromatosis, nuchal fibroma, abdominal desmoid, etc.).
4. Desmoid tumors present with low-SI components also on T2-weighted MR images; they are aggressive lesions, which frequently recur after surgical resection.
5. Fibromatosis colli is seen within the sternocleidomastoid muscle in newborns.
6. Hemangiopericytoma moves from the vascular to the connective tissue tumors.
7. Myxofibrosarcoma replaces malignant fibrous histiocytoma in the new WHO classification.

References

1. Ablin DS, Jain K, Howell L, West DC (1998) Ultrasound and MR imaging of fibromatosis colli. Pediatr Radiol 28:230–233
2. Ackman J, Whitman G, Chew F (1994) Aggressive fibromatosis. Am J Roentgenol 163:544
3. Akisue T, Matsumoto K, Kizaki T, Fujita I, Yamamoto T, Yoshiya S, Kurosaka M (2003) Solitary fibrous tumor in the extremity: case report and review of the literature. Clin Orthop 411:236–244
4. Allen RA, Woolner LB, Ghormley RK (1995) Soft tissue tumors of the sole with special reference to plantar fibromatosis. J Bone Joint Surg 37:14–26
5. Casillas J, Sais G, Greve J, Iparraguirre M, Morillo G (1991) Imaging of intra- and extraabdominal desmoid tumors. Radiographics 11:959–968
6. Chateil JF, Brun M, Lebail B, Perel Y, Casteu JF, Diard F (1995) Infantile myofibromatosis. Skeletal Radiol 24:629–632
7. Cintora E, Del Cura J, Ruiz J, Grau M, Ereno C (1993) Case report 807. Skeletal Radiol 22:533–535
8. Col JY, Vannier JP, Chabrolle JP, Brottier C (1995) Fibromatosis found during prenatal ultrasonography. J Gynecol Obstet Biol Reprod 24:52–60
9. Crawford S, Harnsberger H, Johnson L et al (1988) Fibromatosis colli of infancy: CT and sonographic findings. AJR Am J Roentgenol 151:1183–1184
10. De Schepper A, Degryse H (1990) Imaging findings in a patient with Pentazocine-induced myopathy. AJR Am J Roentgenol 154:343–344
11. De Schepper A, Degryse H, Ramon F, Van Marck (1992) Extraabdominal desmoid tumors. J Belge Radiol 75:91–98
12. Devaney D, Livesley P, Shaw D (1995) Elastofibroma dorsi: MRI diagnosis in a young girl. Pediatr Radiol 25:282–285
13. Dong P, Seeger L, Eckardt J, Mirra J (1994) Juxtacortical aggressive fibromatosis of the forearm. Skeletal Radiol 23:560–563
14. Duda S, Bittner R, Laniado M, Lobeck H, Langer M (1989) Bildgebende Diagnostik der agressiven Fibromatosen und MRT-pathologischen Korrelation. Fortschr Röntgenstr 151:57–62

15. Eich GF, Hoeffel JC, Tschäppeler H, Gassner I, Nilli UV (1998) Fibrous tumors in children: imaging features of a heterogeneous group of disorders. Pediatr Radiol 28:500–509

16. Einstein D, Tagliabue J, Desai R (1991) Abdominal desmoids: CT findings in 25 patients. AJR Am J Roentgenol 157:275–279

17. Enzinger F, Weiss S (1995) Soft tissue tumors, 3rd edn. Mosby, St Louis, pp 165–292

18. Evans HL (1993) Low-grade fibromyxoid sarcoma. A report of 12 cases. Am J Surg pathol 17:595–600

19. Feld R, Burk L, Mc Cue P, Mitchell D, Lackman R, Rifkin M (1990) MRI of aggressive fibromatosis: frequent appearance of high signal intensity on T2-weighted images. Magn Reson Imaging 8:583–588

20. Fletcher DM, Krishnan Unni K, Mertens F (2002) World Health Organization classification of tumours. pathology and genetics of tumours of soft tissue and bone. IARC, Lyon, pp 47–106

21. Folpe AL, Lane KL, Pauli G, Weiss JT (2000) Low-grade fibromyxoid sarcoma and hyalizing spindle cell tumor with giant rosettes: a clinicopathological study of 73 cases supporting their identity and assessing the impact of high-grade areas. Am J Surg Pathol 24:1353–1360

22. Fornage B (1995) Musculoskeletal ultrasound. Churchill Livingstone, New York

23. Fox MG, Kransdorf MJ, Bancroft LW, Peterson JJ, Flemming DJ (2003) MR imaging of fibroma of the tendon sheath. AJR Am J Roentgenol 180:1449–1453

24. Francis R, Dorovini-Zis K, Glazer G, Lloyd R, Amendola M, Martel W (1986) The fibromatoses: CT-pathologic correlation. AJR Am J Roentgenol 147:1063–1066

25. Frei S, Lange S de, Fechner R (1991) Nodular fasciitis of the elbow. Skeletal Radiol 20:468–471

26. Fromowitz F, Hurst L, Nathan J, Badalamente M (1987) Infantile fibromatosis with extensive calcification. Am J Surg Pathol 11:66–75

27. Fukunaga M, Fukunaga N (1997) Low-grade myxofibrosarcoma: progression in recurrence. Pathol Int 47:161–165

28. Gallego M, Millan J, Gil-Martin R, Cespedes M, Pulpeiro R, Salamanca J (1987) Juvenile hyalin fibromatosis: radiographic and pathological findings of a new case. J Med Imaging 1:251–257

29. Gartlan MG, Hoffman HT, Haller JR, Dolan KD (1993) Fibrosarcoma of the posterior neck. Ann Otol Rhinol Laryngol 102:820–822

30. Gielen JL, De Schepper AM, Vanhoenacker F, Parizel PM, Wang XL, Sciot R, Weyler J (2004) Accuracy of MRI in characterization of soft tissue tumors and tumor-like lesions. A prospective study in 548 patients. Eur Radiol 14(12):2320–2330

31. Goodlad JR, Mentzel R, Fletcher CD (1995) Low-grade fibromyxoid sarcoma: clinicopathological analysis of eleven new cases in support of a distinct entity. Histopathology 26:229–237

32. Hartman TE, Berquist T, Fetsch JF (1992) MR imaging of extraabdominal desmoids: differentiation from other neoplasms. AJR Am J Roentgenol 158:581–585

33. Hawnaur J, Jenkins J, Isherwood (1990) Magnetic resonance imaging of musculoaponeurotic fibromatosis. Skeletal Radiol 19:509–514

34. Hayward PG, Orgill DP, Mulliken JB, Perez-Atayde AR (1995) Congenital fibrosarcoma masquerading as lymphatic malformation: report of two cases. J Pediatr Surg 30:84–88

35. Huang HY, Lal P, Qin J, Brennan MF, Antonescu CR (2004) Low-grade myxofibrosarcoma: a clinicopathologic analysis of 49 cases treated at a single institution with simultaneous assessment of the efficacy of 3-tier and 4-tier grading systems. Hum Pathol 35(5):612–621

36. Ichikawa T, Koyama A, Fujimoto H et al (1994) Abdominal wall desmoid mimicking intraabdominal mass: MR features. Magn Reson Imaging 12:541–544

37. Ishii N, Matsui K, Ichiyama S, Takahashi Y, Nakajima H (1989) A case of infantile digital fibromatosis showing spontaneous regression. Br J Dermatol 121:129–133

38. Jabra A, Taylor G (1993) MRI evaluation of superficial soft tissue lesions in children. Pediatr Radiol 23:425–428

39. Kilpatrick SE, Ward WG (1999) Myxofibrosarcoma of soft tissues: cytomorphologic analysis of a series. Diagn Cytopathol 20:6–9

40. Kim E, Kim C, Romero J, Chung W, Isiklar A (1995) Different biologic features of desmoid tumors demonstrated with MR Imaging, RNSA, scientific exhibition, Poster 278 SK, Chicago, 25 Nov-1 Dec

41. Kingston CA, Owens CM, Jeanes A, Malone M (2002) Imaging of desmoid fibromatosis in pediatric patients. AJR Am J Roentgenol 178:191–199

42. Koenigsberg RA, Faro S, Chen X, Marlowe F (1995) Nodular fasciitis as a vascular neck mass. AJNR Am J Neuroradiol 17:567–569

43. Koh SH, Choe HS, Lee IJ, Park HR, Bae SH (2004) Low-grade fibromyxoid sarcoma: ultrasound and magnetic resonance findings in two cases. Skeletal Radiol 8 [Epub ahead of print]

44. Koujok K, Ruiz RE, Hernandez RJ (2004) Myofibromatosis: imaging characteristics. Pediatr Radiol 19 [Epub ahead of print]

45. Kransdorf M, Murphey M (1997) Imaging of soft tissue tumors. Saunders, Philadelphia, pp 143–186

46. Kransdorf M, Jelinek J, Moser R, Utz J, Hudson T, Neal J, Berrey B (1990) Magnetic resonance appearance of fibromatosis. Skeletal Radiol 19:495–499

47. Kransdorf M, Meis J, Montgomery E (1992) Elastofibroma: MR and CT appearance with radiologic-pathologic correlation. AJR Am J Roentgenol 159:575–579

48. Lang P, Suh KJ, Grampp S, Steinbach L, Steiner E, Peterfy C, Tirman P, Schwickert H, Rosenau W, Genant HK (1995) CT and MRI in elastofibroma. A rare benign soft tissue tumor. Radiologe 35:611–615

49. Lee T, Wapner K, Hecht P (1993) Current concepts review: plantar fibromatosis. J Bone Joint Surg [Am] 75:1080–1084

50. Liessi G, Tregnaghi A, Barbazza R, Scapinello A, Muzzio P (1991) Elastofibroma: CT and MR findings. J Belge Radiol 74:37–39

51. Liu P, Thorner P (1992) MRI of fibromatosis: with pathologic correlation. Pediatr Radiol 22:587–589

52. Lourie JA, Lwin KY, Woods C (1992) Fibroma of tendon sheath eroding 3rd metatarsal bone. Skeletal Radiol 21:273–275

53. Loyer E, Shabb N, Mahon T, Eftekhari F (1992) Fibrous hamartoma of infancy: MR-pathologic correlation. J Comput Assist Tomogr 16:311–313

54. Marin ML, Perzin KH, Markowitz AM (1989) Elastofibroma dorsa: benign chest wall tumor. J Thorac Cardiovasc Sur 98:234–238

55. Massengill A, Sundaram M, Kathol M, El-Khoury G, Buchwalter J, Wade T (1993) Elastofibroma dorsi: a radiological diagnosis. Skeletal Radiol 22:121–123

56. Meiss-Kindblom J, Enzinger F (1996) Color atlas of soft tissue tumors. Mosby-Wolfe, St Louis

57. Mentzel T, Katenkamp D, Fletcher CD (1996) Low malignancy myxofibrosarcoma versus low malignancy fibromyxoid sarcoma. Distinct entities with similar names but different clinical course. Pathologe 17:116–121

58. Mentzel T, Calonje E, Wadden C, Camplejohn RS, Beham A, Smith MA, Fletcher CD (1996) Myxofibrosarcoma. Clinicopathologic analysis of 75 cases with emphasis on the low-grade variant. Am J Surg Pathol 20:391–405

59. Meyer C, Kransdorf M, Jelinek J, Moser R (1991) MR and CT appearance of nodular fasciitis. J Comput Assist Tomogr 15:276–279

60. Michal M, Fetsch JF, Hes O, Miettinen M (1999) Nuchal-type fibroma: a clinicopathologic study of 52 cases. Cancer 85:156–163

61. Morrison W, Schweitzer M, Wapner K, Lackman R (1994) Plantar fibromatosis: a benign aggressive neoplasm with a characteristic appearance on MR images. Radiology 193:841–845

62. Oda Y, Takahira T, Kawaguchi K, Yamamoto H, Tamiya S, Matsuda S, Tanaka K, Iwamoto Y, Tsuneyoshi M (2004) Low-grade fibromyxoid sarcoma versus low-grade myxofibrosarcoma in the extremities and trunk. A comparison of clinicopathological and immunohistochemical features. Histopathology 45(1):29

63. Ogose A, Hotta T, Emura I, Higuchi T, Kusano N, Saito H (2000) Collagenous fibroma of the arm: a report of two cases. Skeletal Radiol 29:417–420

64. O'Keefe F, Kim E, Wallace S (1990) Magnetic resonance imaging in aggressive fibromatosis. Clin Radiol 42:170–173

65. Posner MC, Shiu MH, Newsome JL, Hajdu SI, Gaynoe JJ, Brennan MF (1989) The desmoid tumor. Not a benign disease. Arch Surg 124:191–196

66. Pretorius E, Hrubain R, Fishman E (1995) Recurrent fibromatosis in a patient with breast carcinoma. Invest Radiol 30:381–383

67. Pulitzer D, Martin P, Reed R (1989) Fibroma of tendon sheath. Am J Surg Pathol 13:472–479

68. Quinn S, Erickson S, Dee P, Walling A, Hackbarth D, Knudson G, Mosely H (1991) MR Imaging in fibromatosis: results in 26 patients with pathologic correlation. AJR Am J Roentgenol 156:539–542

69. Reed M, Gooding G, Kerley S, Himebaugh-Reed M, Griswold V (1991) Sonography of plantar fibromatosis. J Clin Ultrasound 19:578–582

70. Reuther G, Mutschler W (1988) An unusual location of a myxofibrosarcoma. ROFO Fortschr Geb Rontgenstr Nuklearmed 149:544–545

71. Robbin MR, Murphey MD, Temple HT, Kransdorf MJ, Choi JJ (2001) Imaging of musculoskeletal fibromatosis. Radiographics 21:585–600

72. Samadi DS, McLaughlin RB, Loevner LA, LiVolsi VA, Goldberg AN (2000) Nuchal fibroma: a clinicopathological review. Ann Otol Rhinol Laryngol 109:52–55

73. Shankwiler RA, Athey PA, Lamki N (1989) Aggressive infantile fibromatosis. Clin Imaging 13:127–129

74. Shields CJ, Winter DC, Kirwan WO, Redmond HP (2001) Desmoid tumors. Eur Journal Surg Oncol 27(8):701–706

75. Shimizu S, Hashimoto H, Enjoji M (1984) Nodular fasciitis: an analysis of 250 patients. Pathology 16:161–166

76. Sifumba S, Thomson SR, Madaree R (1993) Desmoids don't die. S Afr Med J 83:536–537

77. Sundaram M, Duffrin H, McGuire MH, Vas W (1988) Synchronous multicentric desmoid tumors (aggressive fibromatosis) of the extremities. Skeletal Radiol 17:16–19

78. Tourne Y, Saragaglia D, Butel J (1991) Les fibromes desmoïdes des parties molles à localisation extraabdominale. Ann Radiol 34:267–272

79. Tung G, Davis L (1993) The role of magnetic resonance imaging in the evaluation of the soft tissue mass. Crit Rev Diagn Imaging 34:239–308

80. Vandevenne JE, De Schepper AM, De Beuckeleer L, Van Marck E, Aparisi F, Bloem JL, Erkorkmaz Z, Brijs S (1997) New concepts in understanding evolution of desmoid tumors: MR imaging of 30 lesions. Eur Radiol 7:1013–1019

81. Vinnicombe S, Hall C (1994) Infantile fibrosarcoma: radiological and clinical features. Skeletal Radiol 23:337–341

82. Wagstaff MJD, Raurell A, Perks AGB (2004) Multicentric extra-abdominal desmoid tumors. Br J Plast Surg 57 (4):362–365

83. Wang X, De Schepper A, Vanhoenacker F, De Raeve H, Gielen J, Aparisi F, Rausin L, Somville J (2002) Nodular fasciitis: correlation of MRI findings and histopathology. Skeletal Radiol 31:155–161

84. Wassenaar W (1994) Infantile myofibromatosis. Rad Doc 94–10

85. Wetzel L, Levine E (1990) Soft tissue tumors of the foot: value of MR imaging for specific diagnosis. AJR Am J Roentgenol 155:1025–1030

86. Wuisman P, Roessner A, Blasius S, Edel G, Vestring R, Winkelmann W (1994) Solitary congenital or infantile (desmoid-type) fibromatosis of the proximal end of the tibia. Skeletal Radiol 23:381–384

87. Yacoe M, Bergman G, Ladd A, Hellman B (1993) Dupuytren's contracture: MR imaging findings and correlation between MR signal intensity and cellularity of the lesions. AJR Am J Roentgenol 160:813–817

88. Yao L, Toranji S, Doberneck S, Eckardt J (1994) Case report 818. Skeletal Radiol 23:217–219

Fibrohistiocytic Tumors

14

L.H.L. De Beuckeleer, F.M. Vanhoenacker

Contents

14.1 Introduction

Fibrohistiocytic tumors and tumor-like conditions have been the subject of controversy in recent decades, which has centered on whether they arise from histiocytic cells that may assume fibroblastic features or from fibroblastic stem cells. This continuing controversy is beyond the scope of the present chapter. Regardless of the pathogenesis of this disease, however, the term "fibrohistiocytic" remains fashionable in imaging literature to indicate a lesion composed of a mixture of cells with histiocytic and fibroblastic appearance.

Fibrohistiocytic masses are divided into three categories according to their degree of malignancy: (1) benign fibrohistiocytic lesions, (2) lesions of intermediate malignancy, and (3) malignant fibrohistiocytic lesions.

Benign fibrohistiocytic lesions consist of various lesions with similar morphology but different pathogenesis and biological behavior; i.e., true neoplasms (fibrous histiocytoma), tumor-like conditions (xanthoma, reticulohistiocytoma), and indeterminate processes (juvenile xanthogranuloma). Since juvenile xanthogranuloma, reticulohistiocytoma, and other superficial soft tissue masses are often confined to the skin, with a rather characteristic gross appearance, they are often detected and characterized by visual inspection or palpation, and usually not imaged. Imaging findings in cutaneous masses have therefore been published only occasionally in radiological literature. Furthermore, the contrast resolution in computed tomography (CT) is insufficient for imaging these small superficial lesions [49]. The development of a dedicated, high-resolution MR surface coil will facilitate MRI of cutaneous and subcutaneous lesions [102]. It has already been reported that MRI is the method of choice for estimating the depth and extent of cutaneous tumors [72, 102]. Fat-suppression techniques, masking high signal intensity (SI) of surrounding fat, may theoretically improve anatomical detail and contrast resolution [102].

Dermatofibrosarcoma protuberans, Bednár tumor, plexiform fibrohistiocytoma, giant cell fibroblastoma, and angiomatoid fibrous histiocytoma are considered as fibrohistiocytic tumors of intermediate malignancy, since they grow in a more infiltrative fashion and more often recur. Their potential to metastasize, however, is low.

Malignant fibrohistiocytic tumors include the atypical fibroxanthoma and malignant fibrous histiocytoma (MFH). The latter accounts for the majority of reports on fibrohistiocytic tumors reported in the radiological literature. However, there is growing evidence indicating that MFH is not a definite fibrohistiocytic neoplasm. As a result, it has been omitted from the 2002 World Health Organization (WHO) classification (see 14.2.3.2 for further details) [36].

14.2 Classification

14.2.1 Benign Fibrohistiocytic Tumors

14.2.1.1 Giant Cell Tumor of Tendon Sheath and Pigmented Villonodular Synovitis

The most significant contribution to the understanding of giant cell tumors was made by Jaffe, Lichtenstein, and Sutro, who regarded the synovium of tendon sheath, bursa, and joint as an anatomical unit that could give rise to a common family of lesions, including the giant cell tumor of tendon sheath (GCTTS), localized and diffuse forms of pigmented (villo)nodular synovitis of joints, and rare examples of extra-articular pigmented villonodular synovitis (PVNS) arising from bursae. The differences in clinical extent and growth are influenced by the anatomical location.

Lesions of the joints tend to expand inward and grow into the joint surface along the path of least resistance.

Tumors of the tendon sheath of necessity grow outward, molded and confined by the shearing forces of the tendon. Localized and diffuse forms of synovial involvement occur, and subclassification has been indicated by adding the appropriate prefix "L" or "D" [7].

The etiology of PVNS and giant cell tumors of the tendon sheath is unknown, but several possibilities have been suggested, including: (1) a neoplastic process, (2) an inflammatory process, (3) localized abnormal lipid metabolism with secondary inflammatory and traumatic changes, and (4) a reactive response to chronic trauma and repeated hemorrhage. Most authors believe that the disease is either a locally aggressive neoplasm or a reactive synovitis [7].

In favor of a neoplastic origin of this pathology are the observation that these lesions are capable of autonomous growth, the high rate of local recurrence [86], and rare cases of metastatic disease [7].

Giant Cell Tumor of Tendon Sheath

Giant cell tumors of the tendon sheath can be divided into two different groups, the localized form (nodular tenosynovitis), and the diffuse form, which probably represents an extra-articular form of PVNS.

■ **Epidemiology.** The *localized form* of giant cell tumor of the tendon sheath may occur at any age, but it is most common between the ages of 30 and 50 years. The sex ratio is skewed toward women [66]. This form involves usually the hand, particularly the flexor tendon sheaths of the first three fingers, where they represent the most common neoplasm of that region. Less common sites include the wrist, foot, or ankle.

The *diffuse form* of giant cell tumor of the tendon sheath affects slightly younger adults, between 20 and 40 years old. The tumor is frequently located around a large joint, with a distribution similar to that of PVNS [66].

■ **Clinical Behavior and Gross Findings.** The *localized forms* develop gradually over a longer period of time and may retain the same size for several years. In their evolution the earliest lesion is a nodular structure that projects into the synovial space of the tendon sheath. Ultimately these tumors grow outward due to the limited space in the synovial cavity and become cauliflower-shaped masses. They are exophytically attached to the tendon sheath [66]. Their contour is smooth and may be lobulated. Although they are fixed to deep structures, the skin is not involved, unless in the distal finger. Lesions in the fingers are usually small, ranging in size up to 4 cm. Tumors in other locations may become larger.

Surgery is curative, although recurrence after resection is not uncommon and may be seen in approximately 7–27% of patients [96]. Malignancy is unusual, but has been described [12].

The *diffuse forms* are growing, soft tissue masses, and are usually larger and more irregular. Some lesions may reach a considerable size and behave aggressively, with a recurrence rate of as high as 40–50% after surgery [66].

■ **Pathology.** Microscopically the tumor consists of a mix of hemosiderin-laden histiocytic mononuclear cells, giant cells, and xanthoma cells. Most tumors are moderately cellular and are composed of sheaths of rounded or polygonal cells, blending with hypocellular regions of collagen bands. Multinucleated giant cells are formed by fusion of the more prevalent mononuclear cells into large cells with up to 60 nuclei. Although mitotic figures can occasionally be detected, they are a focal finding and do not indicate malignancy.

Some diffuse forms are surrounded by one or more layers of synovial cells or contain pseudoglandular spaces or chronic inflammatory infiltrates. Such lesions are rarely seen in the digit group of lesions [96].

■ **Imaging Findings.** *Standard radiographs* may be normal or display a well-circumscribed soft tissue mass in about half of the patients. Erosive lesions in the underlying bone are present in about 20% of patients, while periosteal reaction, calcifications, or cystic changes are extremely unusual [66].

Ultrasound shows a hypoechoic, solid mass with well-defined margins usually located near tendons. Bone erosions due to pressure of the tumor on the cortex may be demonstrated also. The tendon usually exhibits normal shape and echogenicity. Contrary to

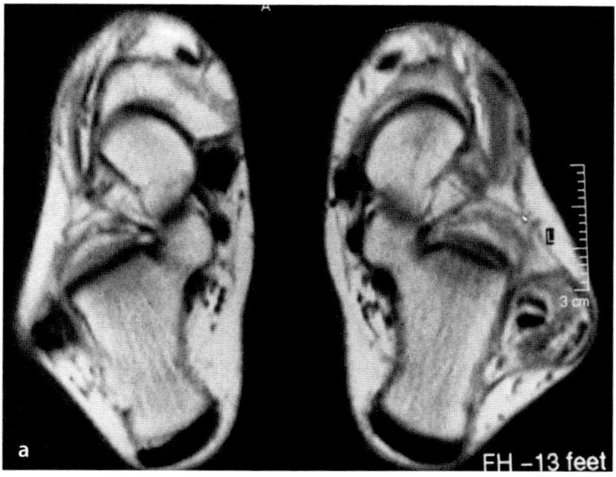
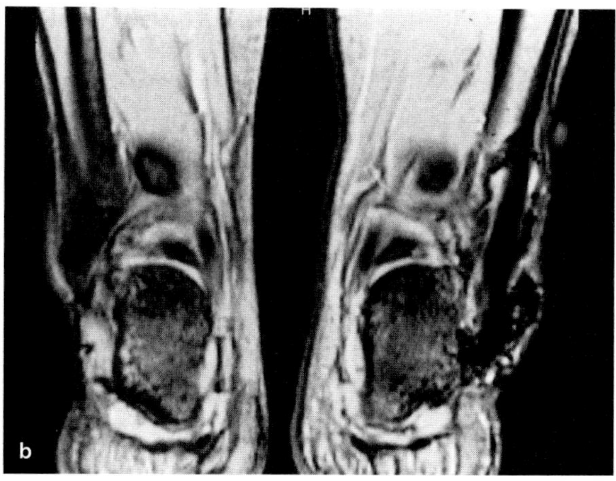

Fig. 14.1 a, b. Localized giant cell tumor of tendon sheath affecting the peroneal tendons. **a** Axial T1-weighted MR image of both ankles. **b** Coronal gradient echo MR image. A soft tissue mass with equal signal intensity compared with muscle is seen around the peroneal tendons. Some low signal-intensity areas are seen at the lateral aspect of the mass (**a**). The low signal intensity of the mass is even more obvious on the gradient-echo MR images. This is due to susceptibility artifacts, caused by hemosiderin. There is also a small amount of fluid in the tendon sheath of the peroneal tendons (**b**). (Case courtesy of Dr. A.M. Davies, Birmingham)

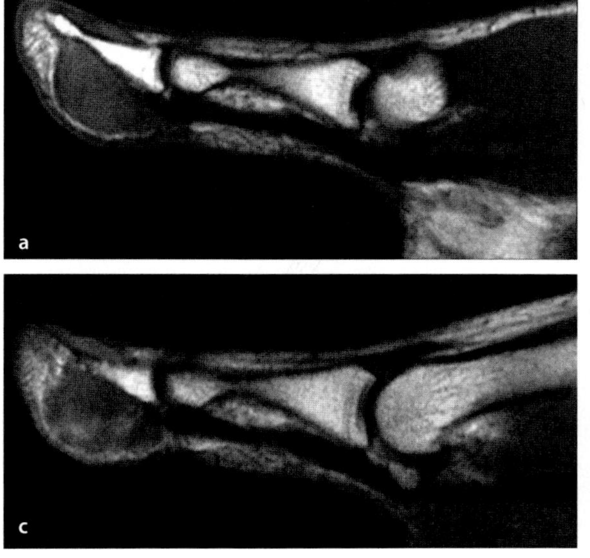
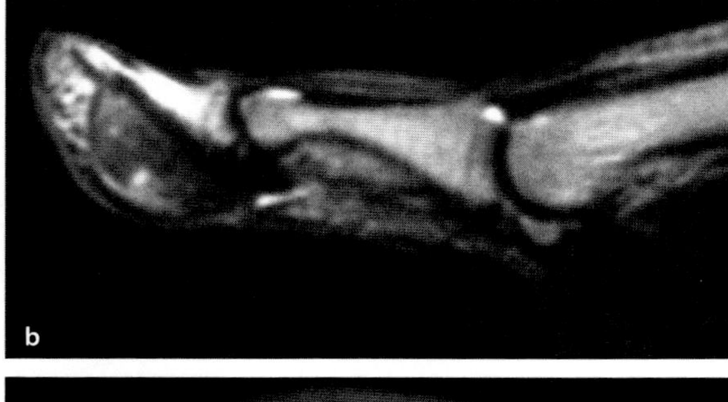
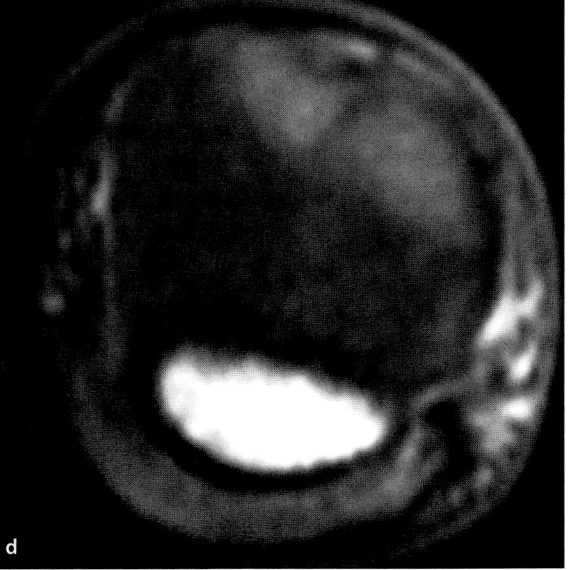

Fig. 14.2 a–d. Giant cell tumor of tendon sheath. **a** Sagittal spin-echo T1-weighted MR image. **b** Sagittal spin-echo T2-weighted MR image. **c** Sagittal spin-echo T1-weighted MR image after gadolinium contrast injection. **d** Axial spin-echo T1-weighted MR image after gadolinium contrast injection. The tumor is located at the volar side of the flexor tendons. It has a typical low signal on T1- and T2-weighted images (**a, b**) and shows moderate enhancement after administration of gadolinium (**c, d**). A soft tissue tumor located on the volar side of a finger is highly suggestive of giant cell tumor of a tendon sheath

ganglia, the giant cell tumor lacks posterior acoustic enhancement, always has internal echoes, and shows Doppler signals [71].

Magnetic resonance images typically show a well-defined mass adjacent to or enveloping a tendon, with a SI similar to or less than that of skeletal muscle on T1-weighted images. On T2-weighted images, the SI of those lesions is predominantly low, with a variable degree of heterogeneity. Strong, homogeneous enhancement is usually seen after contrast administration (Figs. 14.1, 14.2) [20, 66].

Because of their similar signal intensities, old desmoid tumors must be considered in the differential diagnosis of giant-cell tumor of tendon sheath. Old desmoid tumors, which get their low signal on MRI from their low cellularity and high amount of collagenous matrix, may be differentiated on the basis of shape and location [21].

Pigmented Villonodular Synovitis of Joints

The articular counterparts of giant cell tumors of the tendon sheath can also be classified into two forms, depending on their extent of joint involvement. The localized intra-articular form is also known as (pigmented) nodular synovitis, while the diffuse intra-articular form is better known as PVNS.

■ **Epidemiology.** The *diffuse form of intra-articular PVNS* is a rare, monoarticular arthropathy that usually occurs between the ages of 20 and 50 years, with a peak incidence between the third and the fourth decades of life. There is no sex predilection. It usually involves the knee (80%) or the hip, while the ankle, elbow, shoulder, and wrist are less frequent locations (Fig. 14.3) [66].

The *localized form* or *(pigmented) nodular synovitis* is even less frequent than the diffuse intra-articular PVNS. Most lesions are within the knee, particularly in the infrapatellar fat [66].

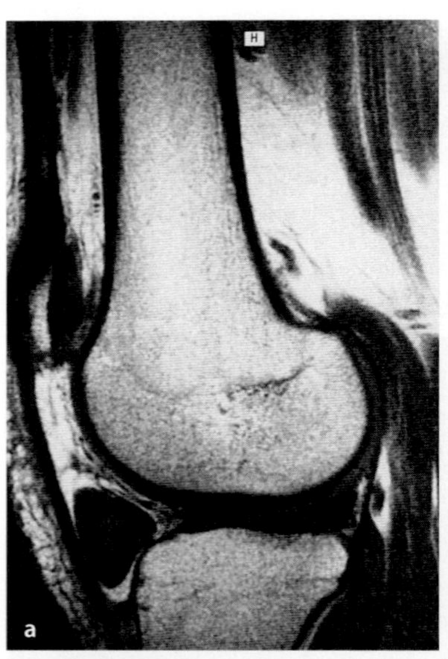
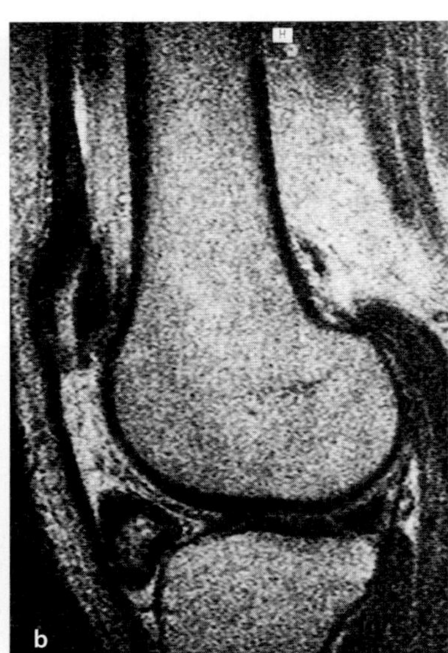
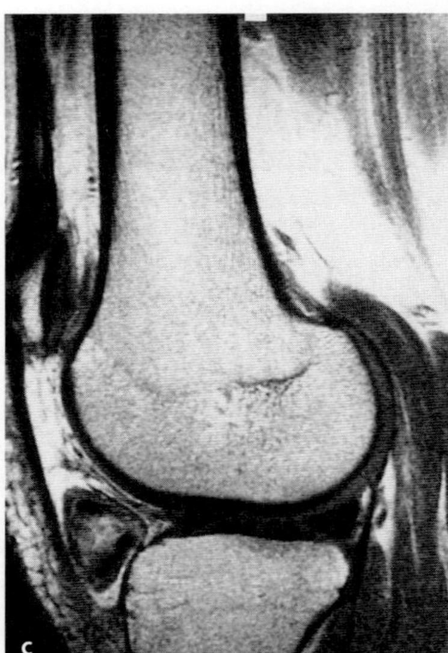
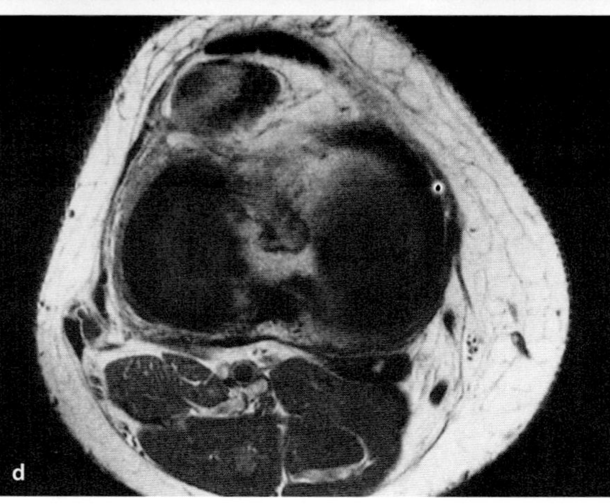

Fig. 14.3 a–d. Localized giant cell tumor of the knee (patellar retinaculum). **a** Sagittal T1-weighted MR image. **b** Sagittal T2-weighted MR image. **c** Sagittal T1-weighted MR image after intravenous gadolinium contrast injection. **d** Axial T1-weighted MR image after intravenous gadolinium contrast injection. On T1-weighted MR images, a sharply demarcated mass in Hoffa's fat pad is seen, which is isointense to muscle at its center and hypointense to muscle at its periphery (**a**). The periphery of the mass is hypointense on T2-weighted images, while its center is slightly hyperintense (**b**). The tumor shows heterogeneous contrast enhancement, especially at the center of the lesion (**c**). The lesion has some linear extension towards the lateral retinaculum, but remains extra-articular (**d**)

■ **Clinical Behavior and Gross Findings.** The *localized form* is characterized by the presence of a nodule, which is usually pedunculated, has a firm consistency, and is yellow to yellow-brown in color. The mass may be lobulated [7]. Patients may not have symptoms or may present with a painless soft tissue mass. Joint effusion is mostly absent.

In the early stages of *diffuse PVNS*, the synovium looks like a tangled red-brown beard. Matting together of the hyperplastic pigmented villi later leads to a spongy orange and brown pad of great complexity. There may also be firm nodules, sessile or pedunculated. Especially in the hip, the adjacent bone may be infiltrated by the pigmented tissue. The clinical picture is characterized by the insidious onset of monoarticular swelling in young adults, stiffness, and progressive pain. Symptoms tend to be continuous, but exacerbations occur from time to time. Aspirated synovial fluid is typically xanthochromic or serosanguinous, but, according to Flandry et al., aspiration is unreliable in establishing the diagnosis [34].

■ **Pathology.** Microscopically the lesions are composed of solid or finger-like masses of hyperplastic synovium with multinucleated giant cells, xanthoma cells, and intra-and extracellular hemosiderin, lying in a fibrous stroma. Long-standing lesions show fibrosis and hyalinization [66]. When the villi become matted together, clefts lined by synovial cells are seen and may give an appearance alarmingly similar to synovial sarcoma.

■ **Imaging Findings.** Conventional *radiographs* may be normal or show only a nonspecific periarticular soft tissue mass (most often in Hoffa's fat pad) in the localized form, while there is usually associated joint effusion in the diffuse form of PVNS. Visible calcifications are extremely unusual [66]. The presence of calcifications should suggest an alternative diagnosis such as synovial osteochondromatosis. Despite the absence of calcification in PVNS, high iron content may be present within the synovium, producing a higher radiodensity than adjacent joint effusion or soft tissue [7]. Associated bone erosions with sclerotic margins may be present on both sides of the affected joints, particularly in joints with a tight capsule, such as the hip (Fig. 14.4) and elbow [66]. These erosive changes are probably due to a pressure phenomenon resulting from entrapment of soft tissue masses between articulating surfaces [78]. These lesions are usually present in nonmarginal locations and may be multiple. If solitary, they may mimic primary osteolytic bone neoplasms [53, 59]. The preservation of the articular space until late in the disease, and the absence of peri-articular osteopenia, is helpful in the differential diagnosis from an inflammatory synovitis.

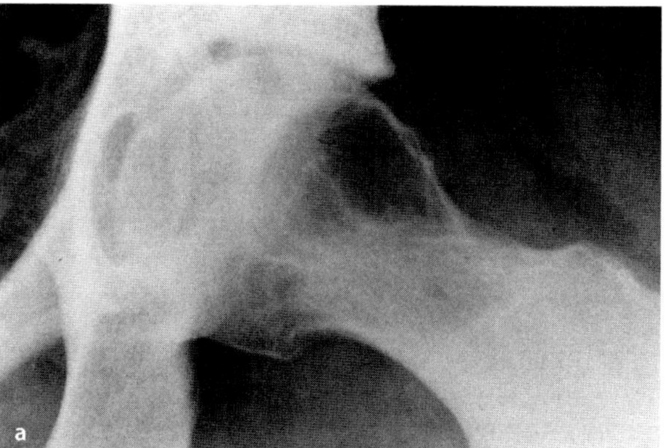

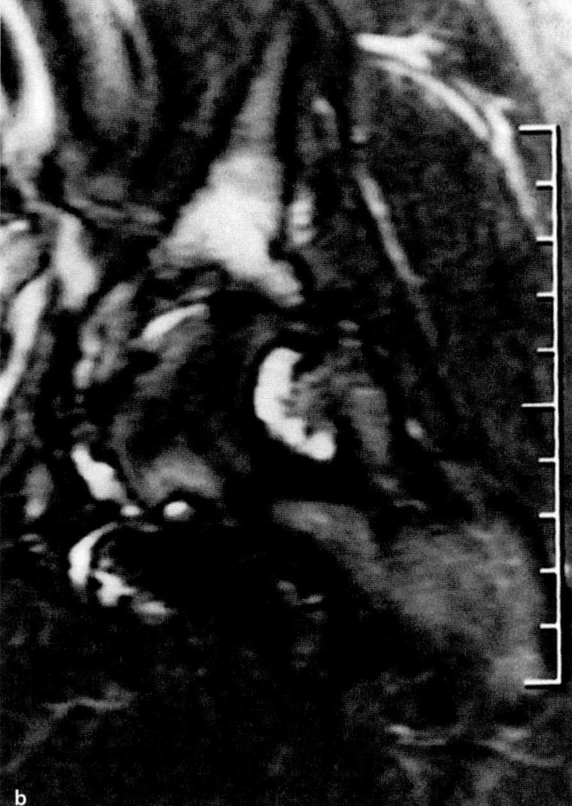

Fig. 14.4 a, b. Pigmented villonodular synovitis (PVNS) of the left hip joint (diffuse form). **a** Radiograph of the hip. **b** Coronal T2-weighted MR image. "Cystic" translucent areas are seen at the superolateral and inferomedial aspects of the left femoral head, owing to pressure erosions along the site of the capsular insertion (**a**). On a T2-weighted MR image, the soft tissue content of the erosive lesions is of a mixed signal intensity. The hypointense components are due to hemosiderin deposits, while the hyperintense components are caused by joint fluid interspersed between the PVNS masses (**b**). (Courtesy of F. Deckers, Wilrijk)

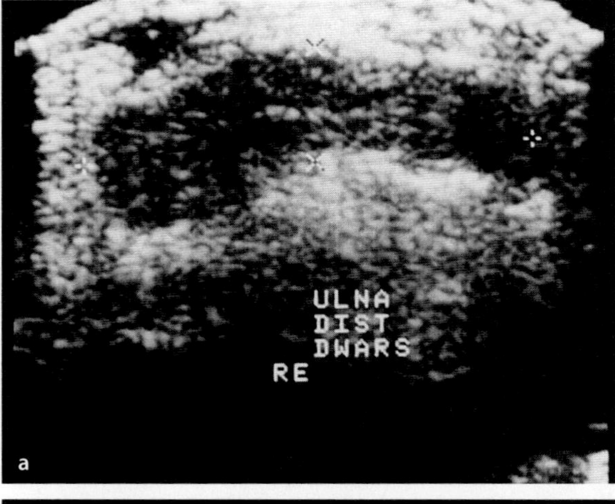

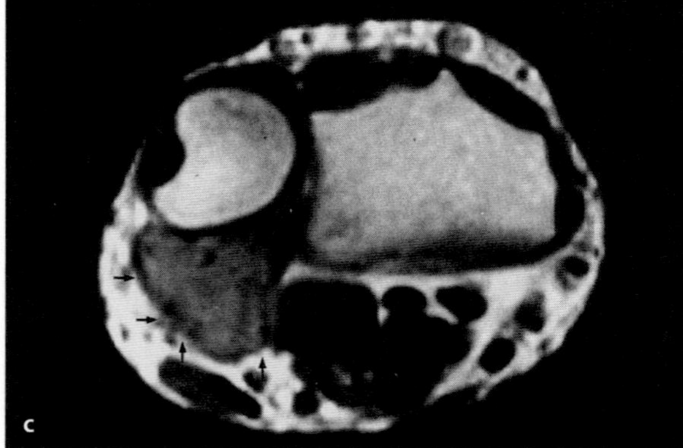

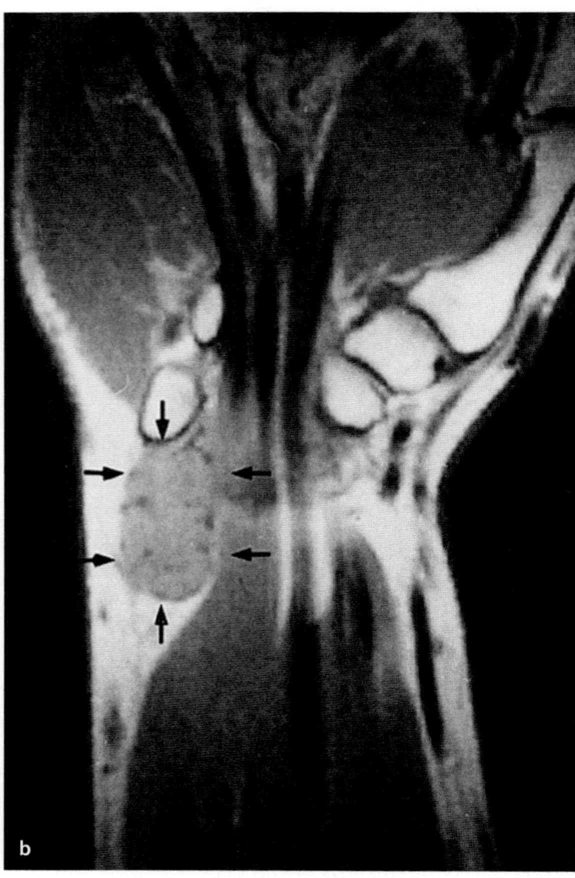

Fig. 14.5a–c. Localized form of pigmented nodular synovitis of the wrist. **a** Axial ultrasound. **b** Coronal T1-weighted MR image. **c** Contrast-enhanced axial T1-weighted MR image. On ultrasound, a hypoechoic mass is seen at the medial aspect of the distal ulna (**a**). On a coronal T1-weighted MR image, the mass (*arrows*) has an in-termediate signal intensity compared with muscle, with some internal low signal-intensity foci due to hemosiderin deposition (**b**). After administration of gadolinium contrast, there is homogeneous contrast enhancement, with sparing of the internal low signal-intensity foci, which represent hemosiderin deposits (**c**)

Bone scintigraphy is rarely performed for the evaluation of PVNS. An increased blood flow and blood pool uptake has been noted in the region of the soft tissue masses on ^{99m}Tc-labeled methylene diphosphonate bone scintigraphy [52]. If erosive bone alterations are present, increased bone uptake is seen on delayed images. Large soft tissue masses may also show subtle areas of increased activity on delayed images.

On thallium (^{201}Tl) scintigraphy, uptake of ^{201}Tl is almost invariable in both PVNS and GCTTS. In PVNS, a diffuse nodular juxta-articular pattern of ^{201}Tl activity is strongly suggestive of PVNS, whereas the increased activity is more focal in GCTTS. Given its tendency to occur in the extremities, GCTTS should be considered in the differential diagnosis of a lesion with ^{201}Tl activity in the hands and feet [68].

Ultrasonography shows a heterogeneous mass lesion (Fig. 14.5a). Sometimes related enlarged or disconnected synovial cysts or bursae with internal septa are noted.

Arthrograms demonstrate an enlarged joint space with multiple, lobulated filling defects (Fig. 14.6). Double-contrast arthrography is better in demonstrating synovial adhesion of the tumoral masses.

CT is able to sharply define lytic bone lesions associated with PVNS. Also associated intraosseous soft-tissue masses extending with a narrow pedicle to the synovium are easily visualized [52]. Joint effusion is atypical, and the tumoral mass itself is also not as characteristic as on MR images. Sometimes a high attenuation tissue is identified within the joint, due to the presence of hemosiderin. The differential diagnosis consists of iron deposition in the joint due to hemophilia or chronic bleeding and calcification. Enhancement after intravenous contrast administration appears to be the rule [7].

On *MR images* the appearance of PVNS as a rule is quite characteristic, due to the presence of hemosiderin within the synovial masses. A heterogeneous, hyperplastic synovial process with significant areas of low SI

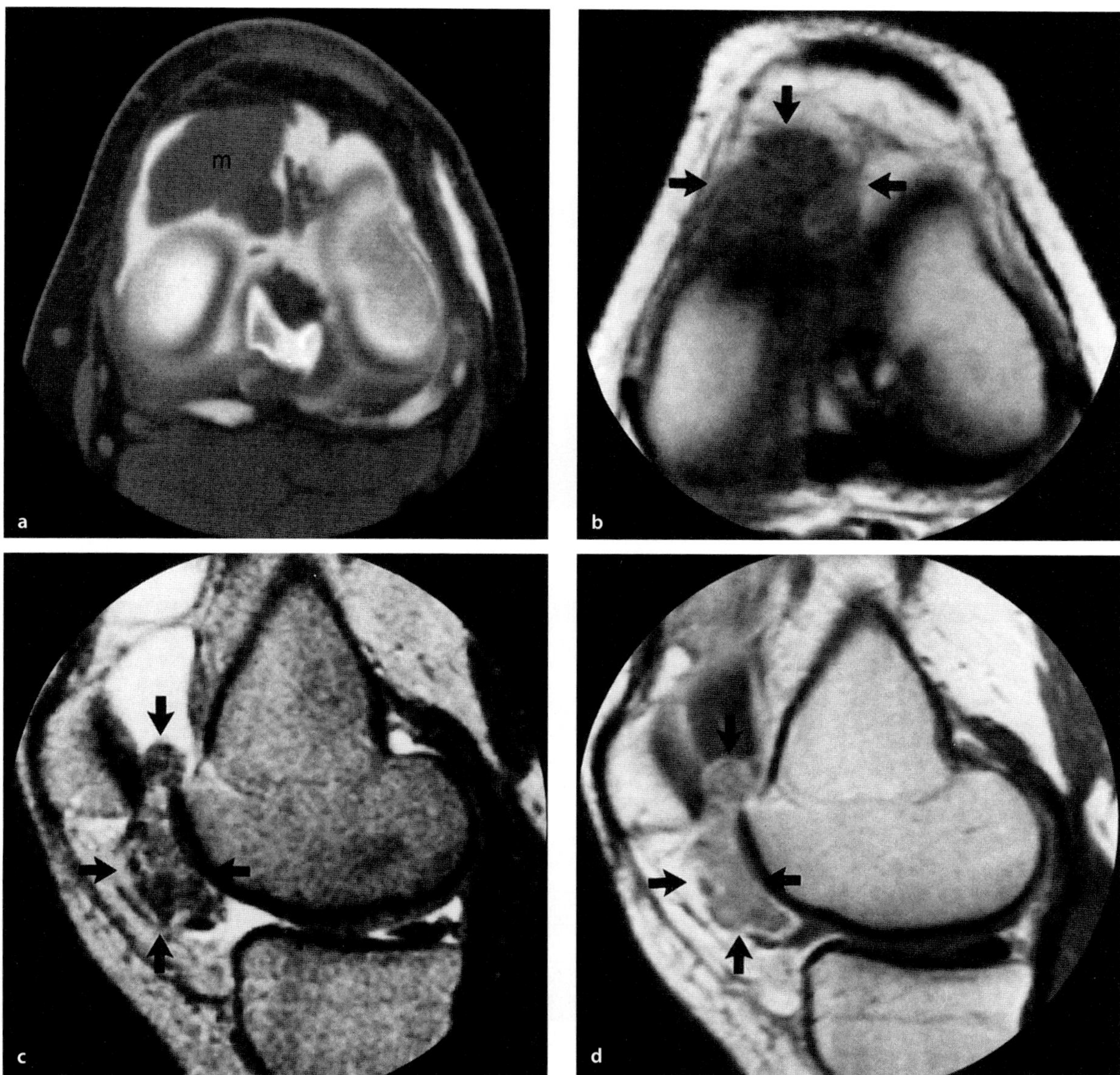

Fig. 14.6a–d. Localized form of pigmented nodular synovitis of the knee. **a** Arthro-CT scan. **b** Axial T1-weighted MR image. **c** Sagittal fast spin-echo (FSE) T2-weighted MR image. **d** Sagittal T1-weighted MR images after intravenous injection of gadolinium contrast. Intra-articular lobulated soft tissue mass (*m*) anteriorly and medially in the knee joint (**a**). The mass (*arrows*) has a predominantly low signal intensity, with some internal, very low signal intensity foci, owing to hemosiderin deposition (**b**). This low signal intensity is even more prominent on T2-weighted images and T2* images, because of the "blooming" artifact caused by hemosiderin deposits: the low signal-intensity mass (*arrows*) is surrounded by the high signal-intensity fluid in the suprapatellar recess (**c**). The mass shows septal contrast enhancement (*arrows* in **d**)

on all sequences, particularly T2-weighted images, is typical (Figs. 14.4–14.10). It is noted in almost 100% of reported cases [7, 52]. The presence of hemosiderin causes local changes in susceptibility and therefore loss of MR signal. This is especially true for gradient-echo sequences and at high field strengths. This decreased SI is most prominent in the periphery of the lesions (the so-called blooming artifact). Occasionally, intralesional areas of high SI on both pulse sequences may be present, due to fat, edema, or inflammation. Joint effusion, appearing as hyperintense areas entrapped between the low signal-intensity areas on T2-weighted images is most common in the knee joint, but much less frequent in other joints (Figs. 14.4, 14.10).

After gadolinium administration, homogeneous or septal enhancement may be observed [66]. The differential diagnosis on MR images includes other causes of chronic hemarthrosis such as chronic trauma, hemophilia, synovial hemangioma, and "burnt out" rheumatoid pannus and amyloid arthropathy. These disorders can be separated on the basis of clinical history, laboratory findings, and enhancement pattern. In hemophilia

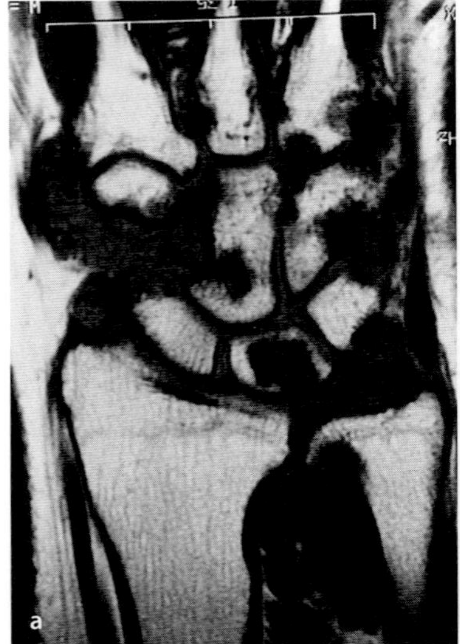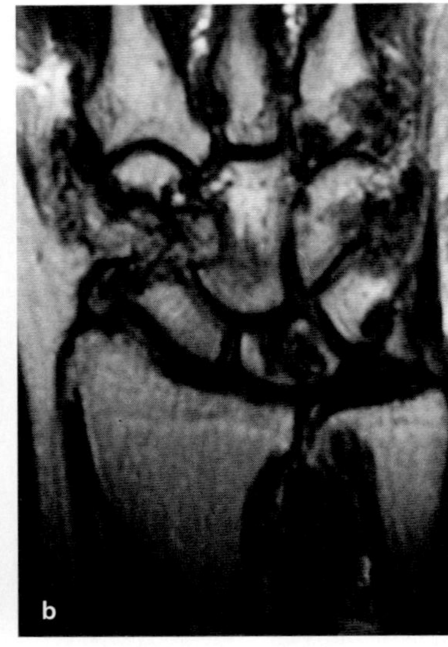

Fig. 14.7a,b. Diffuse intra-articular form of pigmented villonodular synovitis of the wrist. **a** Coronal T1-weighted MR image. **b** Contrast-enhanced coronal T1-weighted MR image. Multiple erosions caused by diffuse PVNS are seen at the carpal bones and the distal radioulnar joint and within the distal radioulnar, radiocarpal, midcarpal, and carpometacarpal joints. Note the low signal intensity of these masses within the several joint spaces (**a**). On coronal T1-weighted MR images after gadolinium contrast injection, there is marked, inhomogeneous contrast enhancement of these intra-articular masses (**b**)

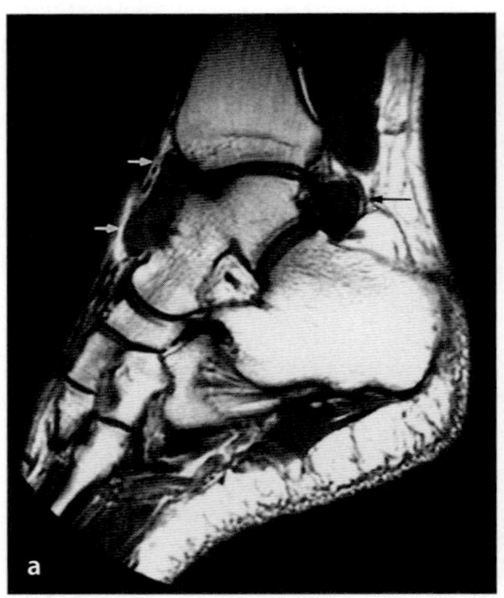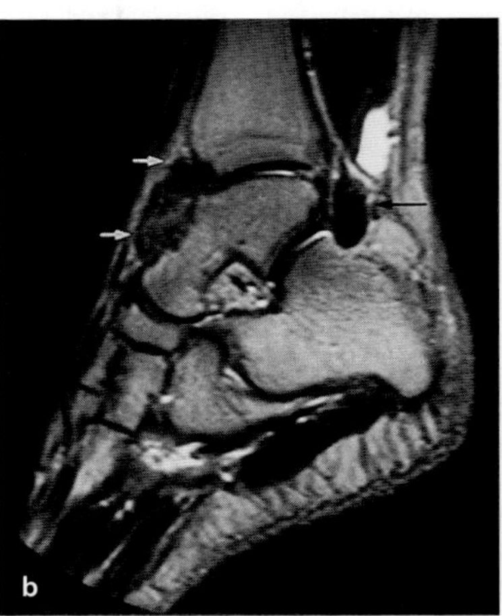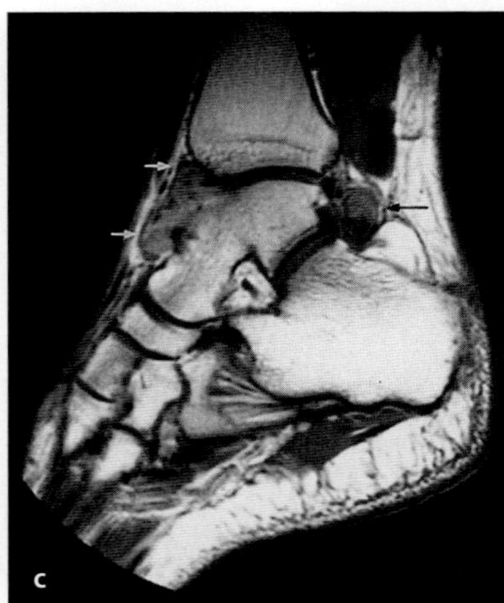

Fig. 14.8a–c. Diffuse intra-articular form of pigmented villonodular synovitis of the ankle. **a** Sagittal T1-weighted MR image. **b** Sagittal FSE T2-weighted MR image. **c** Postcontrast T1-weighted MR image. There is a low signal-intensity mass within the anterior and posterior recess of the tibiotalar joint (*arrows*). The very low signal intensity foci within the anterior recess are due to hemosiderin deposition (**a**). The mass still has low signal intensity on T2-weighted MR images (**b**). There is strong uptake of gadolinium chelates on this postcontrast T1-weighted MR image, with sparing of the low signal-intensity deposits of hemosiderin (**c**)

there are usually diffuse changes in cartilage and bone, including cartilaginous and subchondral erosions, as well as joint-space narrowing. Synovial chondromatosis could potentially simulate PVNS on MR, and in general this is true for all low signal-intensity masses with calcified or ossified components. This should be no problem, since these areas are easily recognized on plain films and CT scans. Tophaceous gout may also mimic PVNS if there is a high concentration of calcium within the tophus [85]. Finally desmoid tumors, benign fibrous histiocytoma, and sclerosing hemangioma could be mistaken for PVNS owing to their low signal on MR images, which is due to their dense fibrous content. The lack of intra-articular changes should alert one to consider another diagnosis besides PVNS.

MRI is the imaging technique of choice to evaluate the possible extra-articular extension and areas of the joint, which are difficult to see arthroscopically. In the knee there is commonly extension of the mass in a Baker's cyst or the tibiofibular joint, while in the hip the iliopsoas bursa may be involved. This information is essential to assist in appropriate surgical planning and to prevent partial surgical resection. The localized form of pigmented nodular synovitis of the joint demonstrates a single mass, but the signal characteristics are similar to those of diffuse PVNS [7].

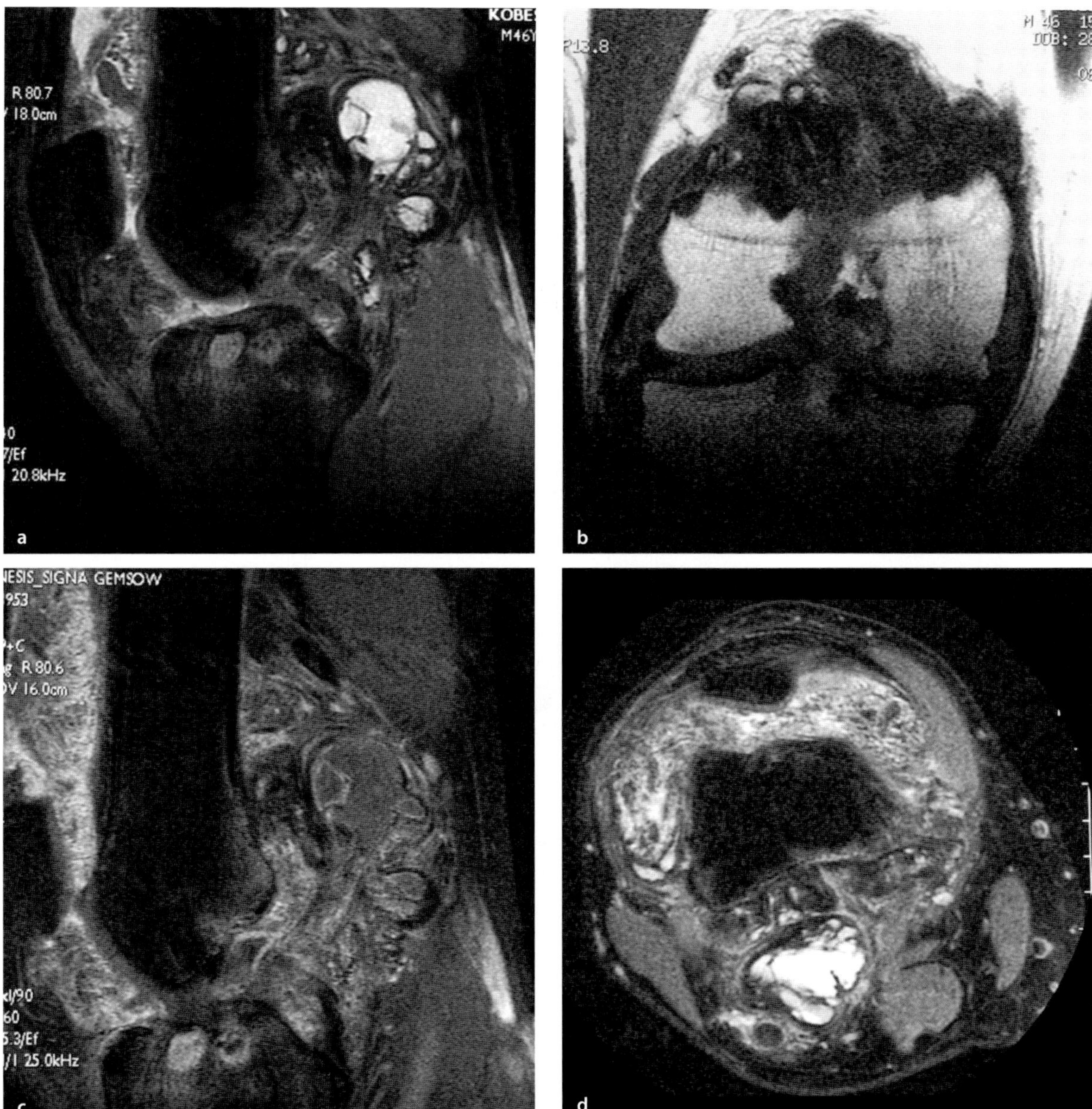

Fig. 14.9 a–d. Diffuse pigmented villonodular synovitis of the knee. **a** Sagittal fat-suppressed, turbo spin-echo T2-weighted MR image. **b** Coronal spin-echo T1-weighted MR image. **c** Sagittal fat-suppressed spin-echo T1-weighted MR image after gadolinium contrast injection. **d** Axial fat-suppressed turbo spin-echo proton density (PD)-weighted MR image. This is an example of the typical MRI presentation of PVNS. The knee is the most frequently affected joint (80%). Heterogeneous, mostly very low signal on both T1- (**b**) and T2-weighted (**a**, **d**) images is the rule in these tumors. This low signal is caused by extreme T2 shortening due to local changes in susceptibility in the vicinity of hemosiderin deposits. These are caused by repetitive bleeding. Remaining portions of synovial membrane show enhancement after gadolinium administration. This results in intra- and peritumoral enhancing curvilinear regions (**c**). In extensive disease, especially in the localized form, erosive bone changes may occur, such as illustrated in the proximal tibia (**a**, **c**)

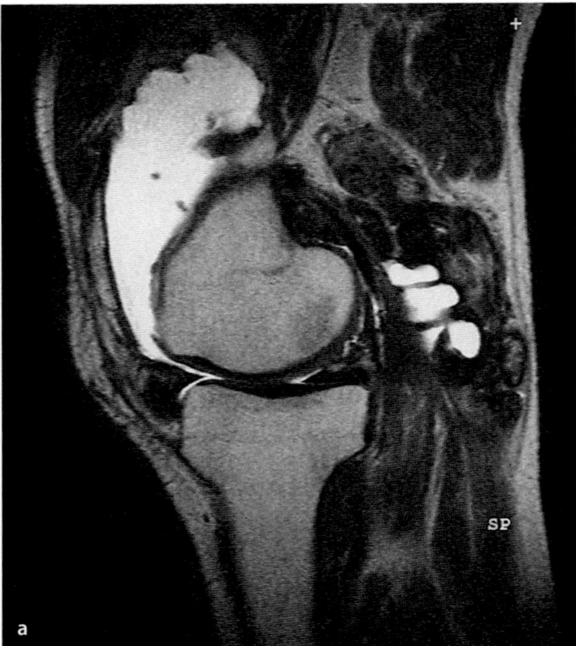
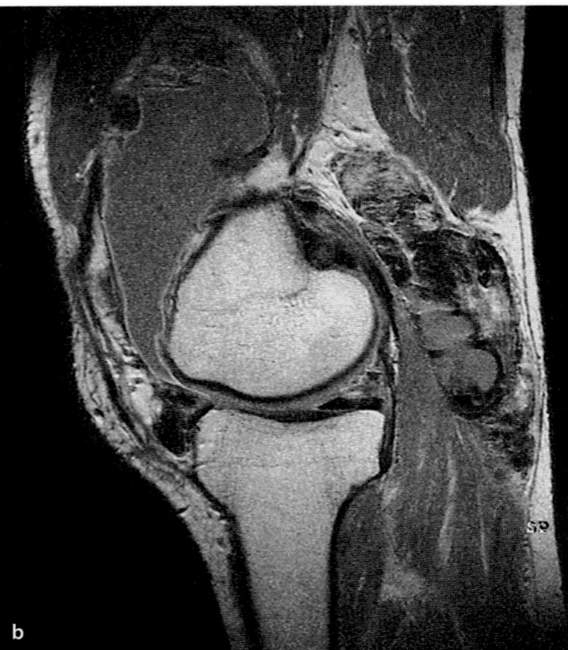

Fig. 14.10a, b. PVNS of the knee and pigmented villonodular bursitis in a 42-year-old man. **a** Sagittal turbo spin-echo T2-weighted MR image. **b** Sagittal spin-echo T1-weighted MR image after gadolinium contrast injection. Tenosynovial giant cell tumor may arise or extend in a bursa, as in this case with involvement of the bursa gastrocnemiosemimembranosa. This is called pigmented villonodular bursitis and can be regarded as a diffuse form of the tumor. Imaging findings, however, are comparable with those found in the localized form, with very low signal on both T1- (**b**) and T2-weighted (**a**) images. After administration of gadolinium, enhancement of the normal synovial lining in the bursa suprapatellaris can be noted (**b**).

■ **Pigmented Villonodular Bursitis.** Sometimes a diffuse synovial giant cell tumor actually arises in a bursa and is known as pigmented villonodular bursitis. The imaging features are similar to PVNS of the joints.

14.2.1.2 Xanthoma

■ **Definition and Clinical Findings.** A xanthoma is a localized reactive proliferation containing lipid-laden histiocytes. It often affects patients with altered serum lipid profiles (familial hypercholesterolemia and type 2 and 3 hyperlipidemia) or with secondary hyperlipidemia (diabetes mellitus, primary biliary cirrhosis, nephrotic syndrome, hypothyroidism). It seldom occurs in normolipemic persons. Xanthoma may be confined to the skin and subcutis but may also involve deep soft tissues such as tendons and synovium.

Cutaneous xanthomas are seen in various types of hyperlipidemia and are divided into eruptive, tuberous, and flat xanthomas and xanthomas of the eyelid, also called xanthelasmas. Their superficial location, gross appearance, and associated clinical and biochemical findings lead to the diagnosis.

In patients with homozygous familial hypercholesterolemia, plane cutaneous xanthoma is often present at birth at sites of trauma such as the knees, buttocks, elbows, and fingers. At these sites, minor trauma or injury may elicit histamine release, resulting in local increased capillary permeability with traverse of serum lipids towards the extravascular compartment, which thus accelerates xanthoma formation [29]. When cutaneous xanthomas occur in normolipemic persons, it is associated in one-half of cases with malignant diseases of the reticuloendothelial system, e.g., myeloma, lymphoma, and malignant histiocytosis.

Tendinous xanthomas are among the first clinical signs of heterozygous familial hypercholesterolemia but are seldom palpable before the age of 30 years [92]. They seldom occur in other forms of hyperlipidemia. Most lesions present as nodular or fusiform, slowly growing, painless masses involving tendons of the extensor surfaces of fingers, wrist, knee, and ankle. Involvement of the Achilles tendon, bilateral in 90% of patients, is a hallmark of this disease [58].

Early detection of familial hypercholesterolemia depends on detection of tendinous xanthomas and is important, because these patients are at high risk for ischemic heart disease and stroke. Since tendon enlargement is only secondary, the ultimate goal of imaging is to assess alterations of the inner tendon structure before they enlarge [25] (Fig. 14.11).

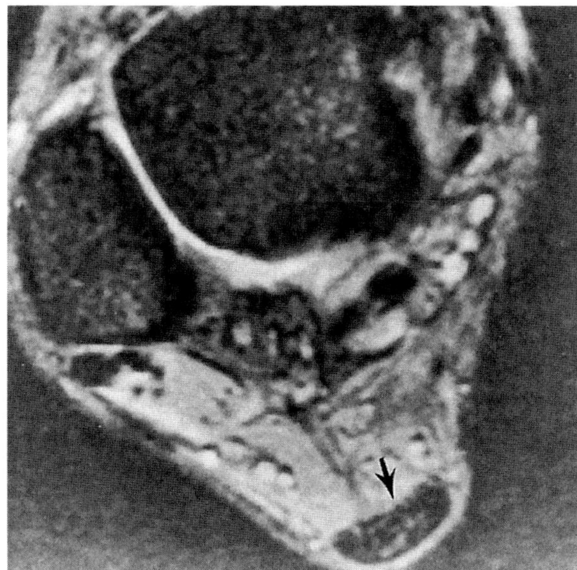

Fig. 14.11. Achilles tendon of a 41-year-old man with familial hypercholesterolemia. Axial gradient T2-weighted MR image shows abnormal signal intensity with diffuse stippled pattern in a normal-sized tendon. This case illustrates that intratendinous xanthomatous alterations are sometimes detected before tendon enlargement occurs. (Reprinted from [25], with permission)

■ **Histological Findings.** On deposition of chylomicron remnants and cholesterol esters in tissue macrophages, swollen foamy histiocytes form. The histological picture is dominated by collagenous fibers, separated by broad sheets of foamy histiocytes which contain cholesterol, cholesterol esters, triglycerides, and phospholipids. Giant cells, some inflammatory cells, extracellular free cholesterol, and cholesterol derivatives are also present. Some cells contain fine granules of hemosiderin. In mature lesions a marked degree of fibrosis may be seen.

■ **Imaging Findings.** In the past, one commonly used physical examination, soft tissue radiography, and CT to assess Achilles tendon size [24, 41, 70, 92]. CT demonstrates the heterogeneous structure of the tendon resulting from cholesterol and cholestanol crystal deposits [47]. Secondary tendon enlargement is easily visualized. Intratendinous abnormalities, however, cannot be detected adequately.

MRI and ultrasound are currently advocated as excellent techniques for the examination of tendons. These modalities provide detailed information about the involved anatomical structures and nature of the pathology [58, 97]. In patients with familial hypercholesterolemia, the Achilles tendons are characterized by overall hypoechogenicity [26]. Older-generation transducers were not able to delineate individual xanthomas; only secondary tendon enlargement could be easily visualized in the laterolateral and sagittal planes. Nowadays, using high-frequency, linear-array transducers, intratendinous xanthomas may be recognized as focal or diffuse hypoechoic nodules [8, 9] (Fig. 14.12b). Normal tendinous fibrillar architecture is disturbed.

The normal appearance of tendons on MR images has been widely discussed [60, 90]. They are homogeneous structures of very low SI on T1- and T2-weighted images. Intratendinous areas of increased SI have been attributed to degenerative, inflammatory, or traumatic changes [87]. However, some scattered spots of slightly increased SI within the tendon body may be seen on T1-weighted images in normal Achilles tendons [87].

MR images of tendinous xanthomas show a diffuse reticulated or speckled signal pattern on T1- and T2-weighted images. The normal tendon fibers are seen as low signal-intensity strands. Intermingled areas of higher SI on T2-weighted images are believed to correspond to xanthomatous deposits, secondary edema, or inflammation [9, 58] (Fig. 14.13). However, the MRI signal pattern is not pathognomonic, and a large overlap in appearance is observed with degenerative and traumatic tendon abnormalities [25]

More accurate demonstration of the heterogeneous aspect of the tendon has been achieved by using fat-suppressed T1-weighted images [9] (Fig. 14.12a). Since liquid cholesterol and cholesterol esters make up to 80% of the xanthoma lipid pool and triglycerides and fatty acids only 6%, the SI of intratendinous xanthomatous areas is not reduced on fat-suppressed T1-weighted images as one might expect at first when thinking of the "lipid content" of xanthomas [9].

Despite the characteristic MR image appearance, state-of-the-art ultrasound has been recommended as the first-choice technique for detecting tendinous xanthomas since it better depicts the number and extent of focal intratendinous lesions [9, 65]. Both imaging modalities provide equal information on anterior-posterior enlargement of the tendon, which is a parameter for success of treatment [92]. In familial hyperlipidemia, the lesions tend to regress upon lipid-lowering therapy. Hence, the thickness and width of the Achilles tendon have been advocated as parameters for assessing disease state and the effect of lipid-lowering treatment [92]. On the other hand, in patients with cerebrotendinous xanthomatosis, a rare, autosomal recessive lipid-storage disease characterized by dementia, ataxia, and early cataract formation, tendinous xanthomas are not affected by conservative treatment. Nevertheless, early detection is important, because the neurological deterioration may be halted when treatment is instituted [4, 13, 47].

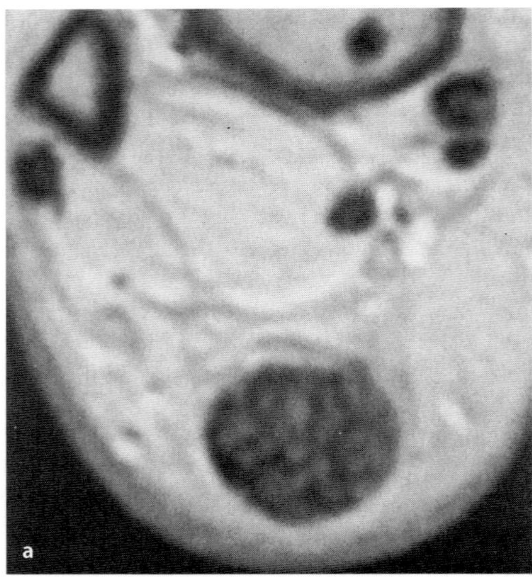
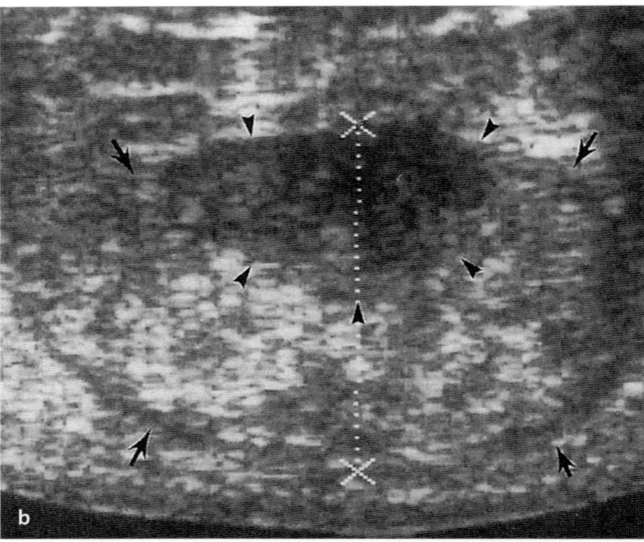

Fig. 14.12 a, b. Achilles tendon xanthoma in a 36-year-old man with familial hypercholesterolemia. **a** Axial fat-suppressed T1-weighted MR image. **b** Axial ultrasound at the same level. Fat-suppressed T1-weighted MR image (**a**) shows marked accentuation of stippled inhomogeneity in comparison with spin-echo T1-weighted image (not shown). On ultrasound a large xanthoma, not de-tected with MRI, is seen as a hypoechoic mass (*arrowheads*) (**b**). Some smaller xanthomas are present in near proximity to the large lesion. This case illustrates the high accuracy of new-generation ultrasound equipment in detecting intratendinous xanthomas. (Reprinted from [9], with permission)

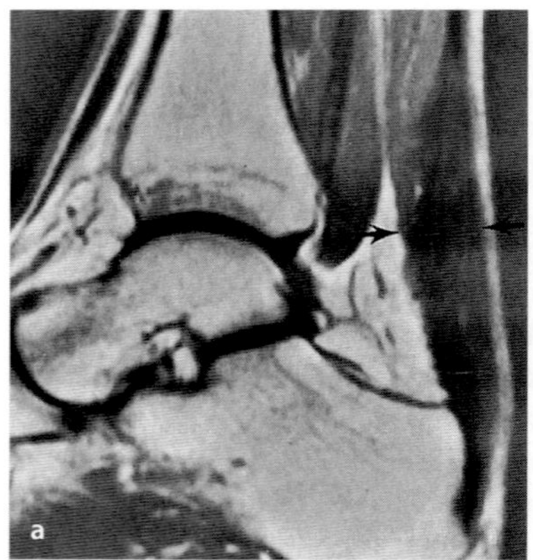
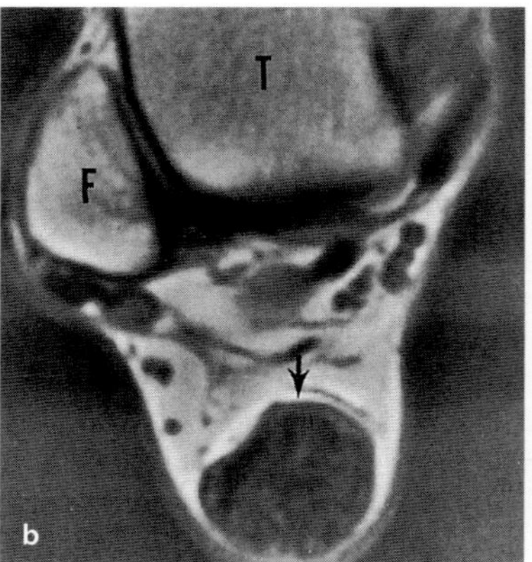
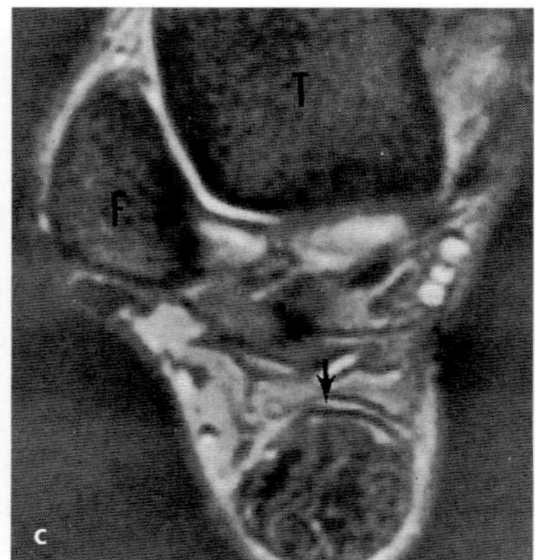

Fig. 14.13 a–c. Achilles tendon xanthoma in a 30-year-old woman with familial hypercholesterolemia. **a** Sagittal spin-echo T1-weighted MR image. **b** Axial spin-echo T1-weighted MR image. **c** Axial gradient-echo T2-weighted MR image. Enlarged tendon with vertical striations of increased signal intensity on T1- and T2-weighted images (**a**, **b**), most probably caused by collagenous strands that are surrounded by high signal-intensity inflammation and bulk of foamy histiocytes. The findings are more obvious on a T2-weighted image (**c**). *F* Fibula, *T* tibia. (Reprinted from [25], with permission)

14.2.1.3 Juvenile Xanthogranuloma

■ **Definition and Clinical Findings.** Juvenile xanthogranuloma, belonging to the non-X histiocytoses, is a predominantly dermatological disorder which affects primarily but not exclusively newborns and young children between 1 month and 2 years of age. Sometimes it is noted at birth. The male-to-female ratio is 1 [42]. It is believed that juvenile xanthogranuloma is a prolifera-tive disorder of dendrocytes, possibly dermal dendrocytes, which shares clinical and pathologic features with Langerhans cell histiocytosis. Therefore, in light of the most recently proposed international classification of histiocytic disorders, both entities are designated together as "dendritic cell-related" histiocytoses [19].

There are both macro- and micronodular forms. The micronodular form is characterized by numerous reddish-yellow to brown macular, papular, or (papulo) nodular skin lesions. They are located principally in the head, neck, mucous membranes, trunk, or the extremities and are considered the main clinical feature [40]. It has been associated with other diseases including juvenile chronic myelogenous leukemia, neurofibromatosis type I, urticaria pigmentosa, insulin-dependent diabetes mellitus, aquagenic pruritus, and possibly cytomegalovirus infection [37]. It has not yet been determined whether this entity is a true neoplasm or a reactive, self-limiting granulomatous process. Nevertheless, most cutaneous and visceral lesions tend to regress spontaneously within several months or a few years [40], lending support to the theory that juvenile xanthogranuloma represents a benign histiocytic proliferation that is likely to be a reactive process [40, 94]. In contradistinction with cutaneous juvenile xanthogranuloma, systemic disease has led to serious complications and even death in some children [37]. In the macronodular form, only one or a few reddish skin lesions are seen. This form may be accompanied by extracutaneous, deeply situated lesions within skeletal muscle or bones, at the eye, lung, peri- and epicardium, liver, colon, oral cavity, brain, kidney, adrenals, spleen, or gonads [40, 42, 44]. In some cases skin lesions are absent. In the literature, one report exists on an intramuscular location of juvenile xanthogranuloma in a 2-month-old boy without other lesions and without overlying skin changes [18]. Systemic involvement, except for the iris and ciliary body, has not been reported to occur in the micronodular form [27]. The risk of spontaneous intraocular hemorrhage with subsequent hyphema and glaucoma exists [69].

■ **Imaging Findings.** Skin biopsy generally affords the correct diagnosis. Hence, few imaging findings have been published, and they are nonspecific. There is one report that described the findings of an intramuscular location of juvenile xanthogranuloma. On ultrasound scans, a hypoechoic solid mass is seen. Upon MR images, the rounded mass has low SI on T1-weighted images, is relatively hyperintense to surrounding tissues on fat-saturated T2-weighted images, and enhances markedly. On T2-weighted images, the lesion is slightly heterogeneous [18, 94]. Other reports are directed solely at the involvement of visceral lesions in cases of macronodular juvenile xanthogranuloma [27, 40, 42, 44].

14.2.1.4 Reticulohistiocytoma

■ **Definition and Clinical Findings.** Reticulohistiocytoma is a rare, probably pseudotumoral condition affecting adults, particularly middle-aged women. The female-to-male ratio is 2:1. There are two forms: localized and cutaneous reticulohistiocytoma, and widespread involvement, as a part of a systemic disease referred to as multicentric reticulohistiocytosis, also known as lipoid dermatoarthritis, lipoid rheumatism, giant cell reticulohistiocytosis, and giant cell histiocytosis [99]. In cutaneous reticulohistiocytoma, red or brown solitary (or rarely multiple) nodules are present in the upper half of the body [29]. These nodules are a few millimeters to a few centimeters in diameter. This lesion tends to regress spontaneously or runs a benign course.

In patients with multicentric reticulohistiocytosis, multiple firm papular or nodular lesions may be seen arising from the dermis. Any part of the body may be involved. However, the dorsum of the hand and fingers, the ear, forehead, scalp, and nasal margins are predilection sites. Larger nodules on forearms, elbows, and knees may clinically be confused with gouty tophi or rheumatoid nodules [11]. Many other tissues or organs such as synovium, bones, skeletal muscle, subcutaneous fat, mucous membranes, liver, lung, lymph nodes, thyroid, and endocardium may contain large amounts of typical histiocytic multinucleated giant cells and periodic acid-Schiff (PAS)-positive histiocytes [11, 29, 101].

The most frequent symptoms are multiple mucocutaneous nodules, constitutional symptoms (such as weight loss, pyrexia, hypertension), erythema, pruritus, and progressive, polyarticular symmetrical arthritis. Virtually any joint may be involved, with interphalangeal joints of hands and feet, knees, wrists, and shoulder being the most commonly affected sites. No periosteal new bone formation is seen. Accompanying periarticular osteopenia is disproportionately mild [11, 43]. In about 60% of cases, the polyarthritis precedes the onset of cutaneous lesions. The articular changes may wax and wane. After some years, in the end stage of the disease, patients are often left with a deforming and disabling arthritis. The etiology has not yet been established, but several authors suggest that it is a reactive inflammatory disorder arising in response to an as yet unidentified stimulus [11].

Metabolic disorders (such as diabetes mellitus, hypothyroidism, Sjögren syndrome, and primary biliary cirrhosis) have been reported in 6–17% of cases of multicentric reticulohistiocytosis. Associated malignancies (mostly adenocarcinoma, lymphoma, or melanoma) may be present in 15–30% [11, 51]. Therefore a careful search for evidence of an underlying malignancy is warranted in every patient with multicentric reticulohistiocytosis [51].

■ **Imaging Findings.** Since the soft tissue lesions which originate within the dermis are very small, imaging features of these papules have not yet been described. There are isolated case reports of extracutaneous soft tissue locations of multicentric reticulohistiocytosis [55]. The findings described are nonspecific, however. Most authors report on the articular changes in multicentric reticulohistiocytosis. On plain film, well-

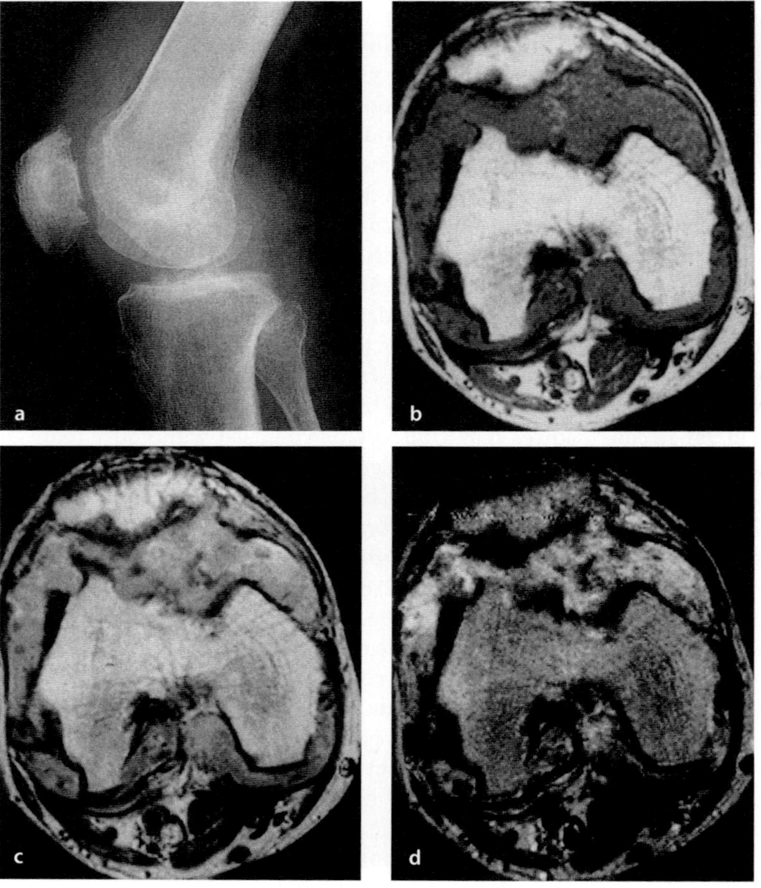

Fig. 14.14 a–d. Multicentric reticulohistiocytosis in a 44-year-old man. **a** Plain film of the right knee. **b** Axial SE T1-weighted image. **c** Axial SE T1-weighed image after intravenous administration of gadolinium contrast. **d** Axial SE T2-weighted image. A soft tissue swelling surrounding the patellofemoral and tibiofemoral joints is seen. Note the presence of well-defined osseous erosions. Extensive synovial proliferation with intermediate SI on SE T1-weighted image are seen (**b**). After intravenous injection of Gd contrast, the synovium enhances markedly (**c**). On T2-weighted image, the synovium has high SI, except for intralesional dots of low SI, corresponding to hemosiderin deposits (**d**). (Reprinted from [99], with permission)

circumscribed marginal erosions without overhanging edges are seen. Symmetrical joint involvement, interphalangeal joint distribution, atlantoaxial subluxation, lack of osteoporosis, lack of ankylosis, and soft tissue nodules are characteristic features [11, 32, 39, 99]. On MR images, severe joint destruction with tumor-like synovial proliferations with intermediate SI on T1-weighted images and high SI on T2-weighted images are seen. Internal low-SI areas correspond with intralesional hemosiderin deposits (Fig. 14.14) [99].

14.2.1.5 Benign Fibrous Histiocytoma

■ **Definition and Clinical Findings.** Benign fibrous histiocytoma is a fibrohistiocytic tumor arising in the skin or the deeper soft tissues. It is one of the most common benign soft tissue tumors of the skin and predominantly affects young adults. Because of its large variety of histological appearances, it is known also as dermatofibroma, sclerosing hemangioma, nodular subepidermal fibrosis, fibrous xanthoma, and histiocytoma cutis [10].

Cutaneous fibrous histiocytoma presents as a painless, slowly growing, flat or pedunculated lesion with reddish or black overlying skin. Multiple lesions are seen in 30% of cases [29]. Deep-seated lesions are larger (2–12 cm), affect middle-aged patients, and are yellowish or white masses. The true incidence is unknown, since deep-seated lesions are often asymptomatic and not biopsied.

Deep benign fibrous histiocytoma is found in subcutaneous tissue, skeletal muscle, and in the abdominal cavity. Sites of predilection are the lower limb and head and neck region [67].

A special clinicopathological variant, the aneurysmal ("angiomatoid") fibrous histiocytoma, is characterized by large, blood-filled cystic spaces without endothelial lining, combined with a storiform proliferation of histiocyte-like and fibroblast-like cells in a capillary-rich stroma, and diffuse hemosiderin deposits. The lesion may clinically be misinterpreted as a high-grade malignancy, since it may be painful and show rapid growth. Intralesional hemorrhage accounts for this growth and may explain the imaging findings (Figs. 14.17d–e; see Imaging Findings, below) [74, 91].

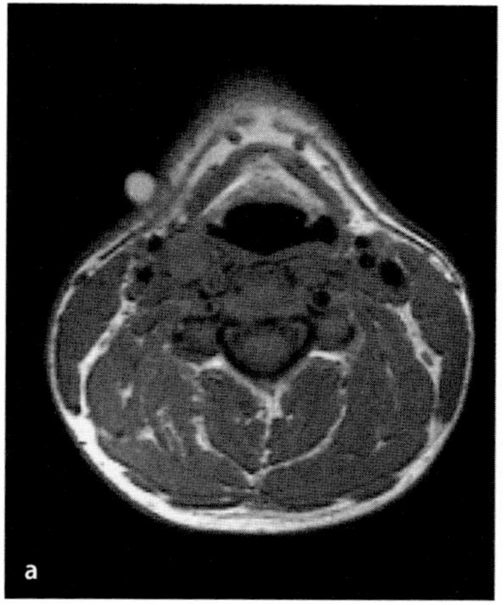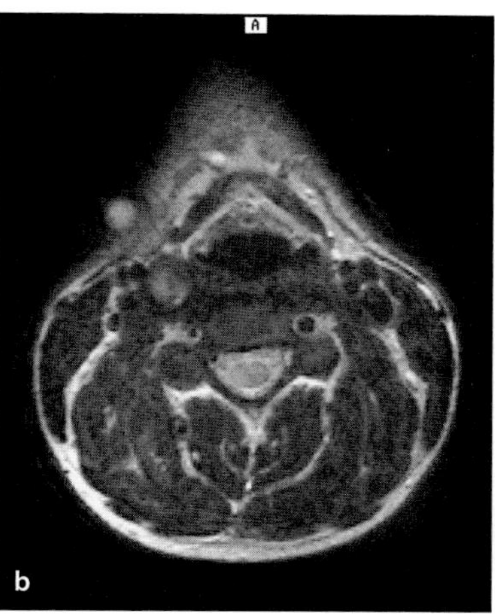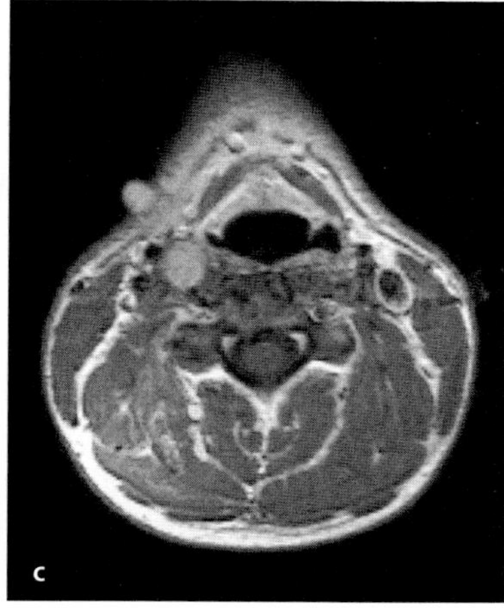

Fig. 14.15 a–c. Deep-seated benign fibrous histiocytoma in the anterior neck triangle of a 25-year-old man. **a** Axial spin-echo T1-weighted MR image. **b** Axial turbo spin-echo T2-weighted MR image. **c** Axial spin-echo T1-weighted MR image after gadolinium contrast injection. Small, well-circumscribed nodular mass show- ing lateral displacement of the adjacent carotid artery. On the T1-weighted image, the lesion has intermediate signal intensity (**a**). On the T2-weighted image, homogeneous low signal intensity is noted (**b**). Strong homogeneous enhancement is seen on gadolinium-enhanced T1-weighted image (**c**)

Fig. 14.16 a–d. Deep benign fibrous histiocytoma in the popliteal fossa of the right knee in a 28-year-old woman. **a** Contrast-enhanced CT scan. **b** Axial turbo spin-echo (TSE) PD-weighted image. **c** Sagittal SE T1-weighted image. **d** Sagittal SE T1-weighted image after intravenous injection of Gd contrast. A huge, well-delineated mass with marked peripheral enhancement and central low-density areas is seen (**a**). On T2-weighted images the mass has intermediate SI (**b**). On T1-weighted image, the mass has intermediate SI (**c**), and shows strong, peripheral enhancement (**d**). (Reprinted from [67], with permission)

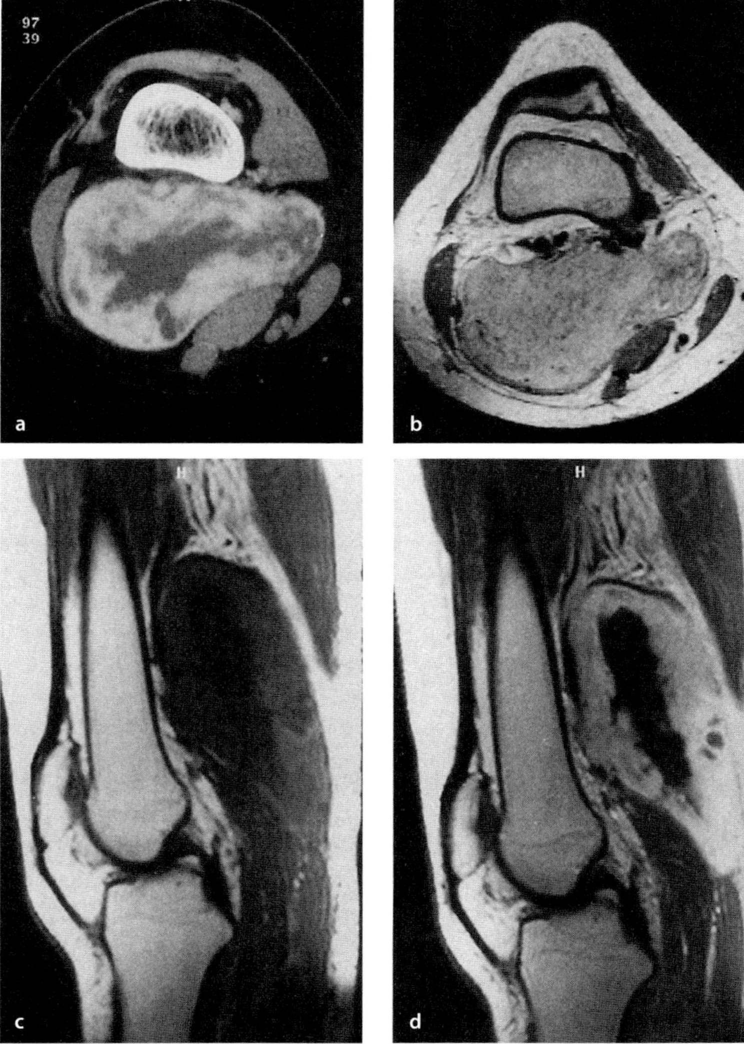

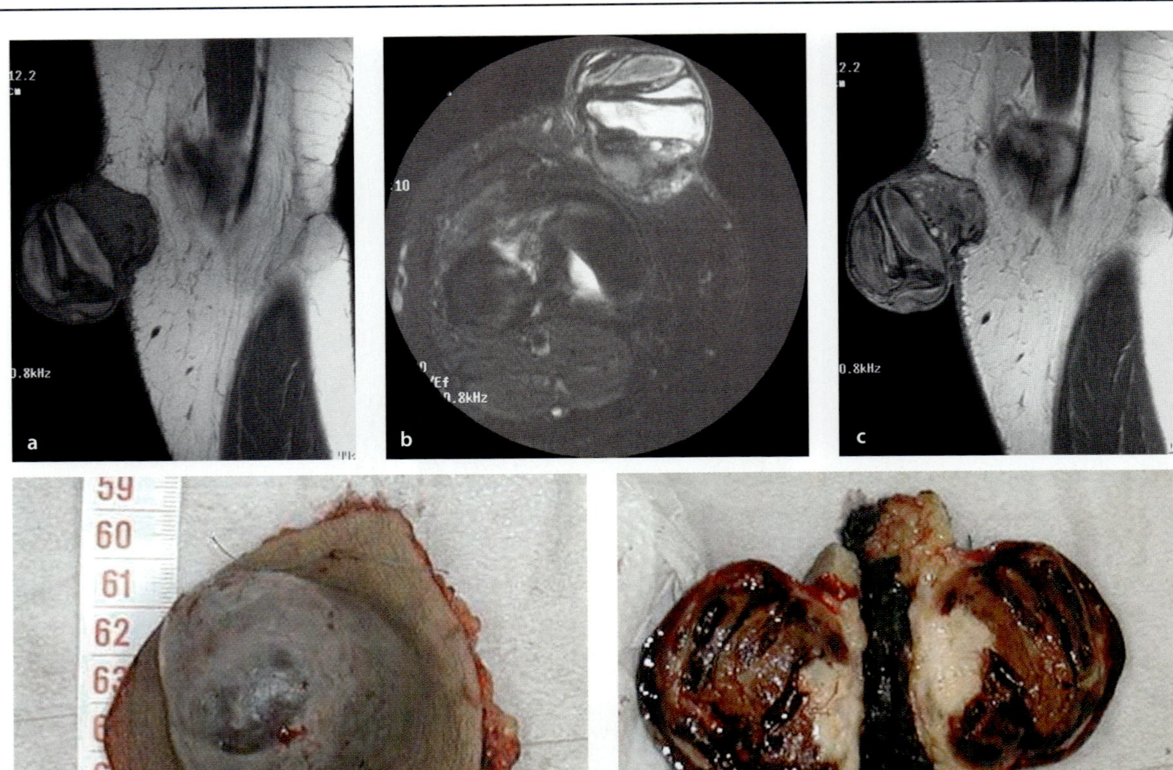

Fig. 14.17 a–e. Aneurysmal benign fibrous histiocytoma at the anterior aspect of the right lower leg in a 39-year-old woman. **a** Sagittal T1-weighted MR image. **b** Axial fat-saturated T2-weighted MR image. **c** Sagittal T1-weighted MR image after intravenous administration of gadolinium. **d** Macroscopic resection specimen. **e**. Macroscopic resection specimen, midsagittal cross section. On T1-weighted MR images, the mass is located within the subcutaneous fat and has heterogeneous signal intensity (**a**). Large clefts with peripheral high signal-intensity components, corresponding to hemorrhagic contents, are noted. On fat-saturated T2-weighted images, the mass has intermediate to high SI (**b**). On T1-weighted images after intravenous administration of gadolinium contrast, diffuse enhancement is seen in the nonhemorrhagic parts of the lesion (**c**). In the center of the mass, large vessels are present (*arrow*). A huge, protruding slowly-growing purple mass is seen at the macroscopic resection specimen of the lower leg (**d**). On sagittal cross section of the resected specimen, the large clefts, containing blood and blood degradation products, are well documented (**e**)

In contradistinction to its benign cutaneous counterpart, an "atypical" form of fibrous histiocytoma of the skin has been reported recently [54]. This entity consists of a nodular, plaque-like or polypoid lesion of the dermis, invading the subcutis in 30% of cases. Besides the classic histological features of fibrous histiocytoma, they show also plump, pleomorphic cells with large, bizarre hyperchromatic nuclei. Furthermore, mitotic figures (up to 15 per 10 high-power fields) are found, including atypical mitotic figures. Sometimes, even more worrisome features such as intralesional necrosis or extension to the subcutis are noted and may represent a potential pitfall for overinterpretation as pleomorphic sarcoma. Rarely, distant metastases may occur.

■ **Imaging Findings.** Since cutaneous benign fibrous histiocytoma is a small dermal tumor, usually not larger than a few millimeters, there are no reports on imaging findings in this entity. Imaging features of deep benign fibrous histiocytoma have been reported by Machiels et al. [67]. On ultrasound, a solid hyperechoic mass is seen. CT scan shows a hypo- to isodense mass, with internal cystic and necrotic areas. On MR images, the lesion has nonspecific signal intensities. On T1-weighted images, the lesion has intermediate SI, similar to that of muscle. On T2-weighted images, the mass is inhomogeneous and has intermediate to high SI (Figs. 14.15, 14.16).

Aneurysmal (angiomatoid) fibrous histiocytoma presents as a protruding, heterogeneous lesion with large internal "clefts" filled with intralesional hemorrhagic deposits (of different age), surrounded by solid tissue components (Fig. 14.17).

14.2.2 Fibrohistiocytic Tumors of Intermediate Malignancy

14.2.2.1 Dermatofibrosarcoma Protuberans

■ **Definition and Clinical Findings.** Dermatofibrosarcoma protuberans is a rare soft tissue tumor with locally aggressive growth potential, occurring early in life (first to fifth decades). Controversy continues about its histogenesis. It accounts for 6% of all soft tissue sarcomas [62]. A slight male preponderance is seen. It is generally located on the trunk, head and neck region, and the extremities [16, 61]. Initially, it presents as a well-defined slowly growing red plaque-like lesion extending from the dermis to invade the epidermis, subcutaneous fat, muscle, fascia, and bone [16]. The lesion may remain unchanged in size for many years before a period of more rapid growth starts. Only at the end stage does the lesion have a typical "protuberant" appearance.

Dermatofibrosarcoma protuberans is very uncommon in childhood, and only a few congenital cases have been reported [1, 73]. Clinically, congenital or childhood cases often have a fibrotic plaque-like aspect, resembling fibrous hamartoma of infancy, solitary infantile myofibromatosis, and infantile fibromatosis [1]. When affecting children, it is seen mostly on the back and hands or feet [83].

On cross section the lesion may have a gelatinous appearance corresponding to myxoid change. Hemorrhage and cystic changes may be present, while intratumoral necrosis is a rare finding [16]. Microscopically it is characterized by spindle-shaped fibroblasts arranged in a distinctive storiform pattern and resembles a benign fibrohistiocytoma [62]. Previous radiotherapy or preceding local trauma are considered to be predisposing factors [2, 5, 75].

Very infrequently a case undergoes fibrosarcomatous change [28, 98]. A tendency to recur, however, exists in up to 50% of patients. In cases of dermatofibrosarcoma protuberans with fibrosarcomatous changes, the recurrence rate reaches approximately 75% [76]. After multiple recurrences the lesion may become more anaplastic. Despite its strong tendency to recur, it is rarely (4.9%) metastatic. Predilection sites for metastases are the regional lymph nodes and lung [5, 28]. Occasionally it may metastasize to unusual sites, including the chest wall, peritoneum, pericardium, retroperitoneum, and soft tissue of the locomotor system [28].

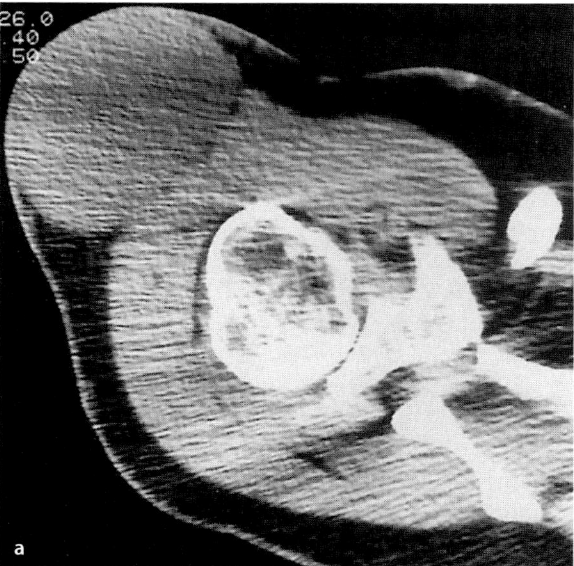

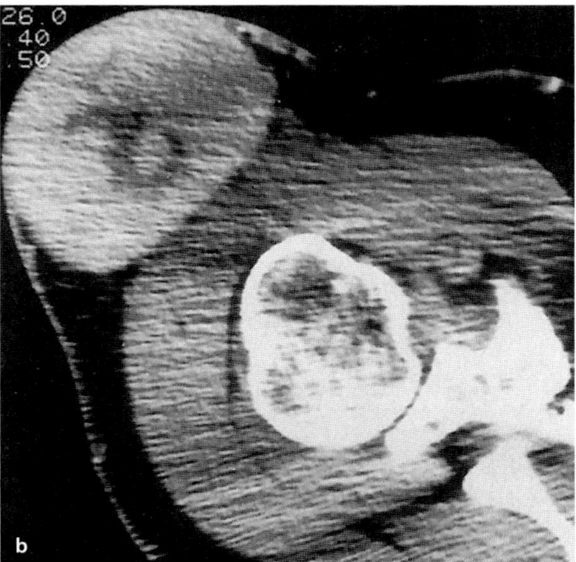

Fig. 14.18a,b. Recurrent dermatofibrosarcoma protuberans of the right shoulder in a 42-year-old man. **a** CT. **b** CT scan after iodinated contrast injection. Presence of a well-circumscribed subcutaneous mass with intermediate density (**a**). After intravenous contrast administration, inhomogeneous enhancement is seen (**b**). (Reprinted from [62], with permission)

■ **Imaging Findings.** On plain radiographs dermatofibrosarcoma protuberans is seen as a nodular subcutaneous mass without calcifications. CT scans show a well-defined, lobular lesion [16, 62]. Tissue attenuation is equal to or slightly higher than that of skeletal muscle (Fig. 14.18a). Bone involvement is not present. After intravenous contrast administration, moderate enhancement is seen (Fig. 14.18b).

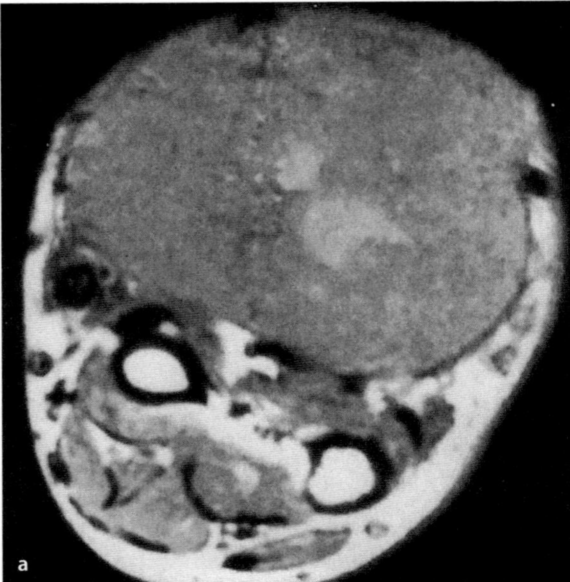

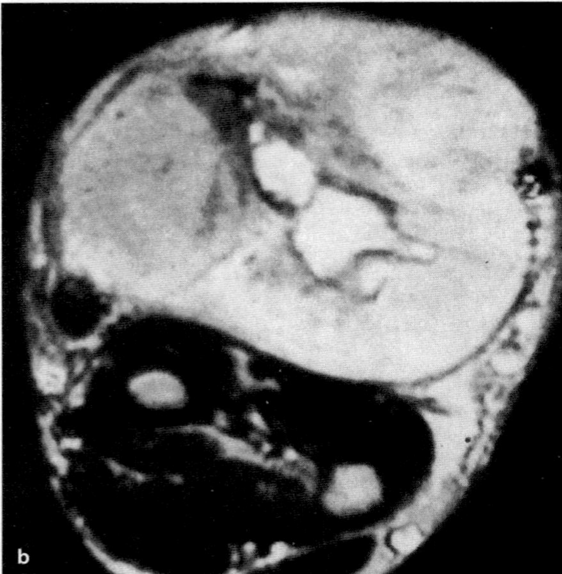

Fig. 14.19a, b. Dermatofibrosarcoma protuberans of the wrist in a 36-year-old man with a mass that had been expanding for 23 years. **a** Axial spin-echo T1-weighted MR image. **b** Axial spin-echo T2-weighted MR image. Large mass in the subcutaneous tissues of the dorsum of the wrist with intermediate signal intensity on T1- (**a**) and high signal intensity on T2-weighted images (**b**). Central focus of increased signal intensity presumably corresponds to focal hemorrhage and/or necrosis. These findings reflect the nonspecific MRI characteristics of dermatofibrosarcoma protuberans. (Reprinted from [62], with permission)

The MRI appearance is nonspecific, showing mostly a low SI on T1-weighted images and a high SI on T2-weighted images [62, 95]. Heterogeneous intratumoral foci of hemorrhage, myxoid change, or necrosis may be present (Fig. 14.19) [62, 76]. Angiography reveals a nonspecific, early-enhancing vascular lesion.

14.2.2.2 Bednár Tumor

■ **Definition and Clinical Findings.** Bednár tumor is a rare, slowly growing cutaneous tumor resembling dermatofibrosarcoma protuberans in clinical appearance and growth behavior [1]. Histologically, however, it is distinguished by the presence of melanin-bearing dendritic cells; therefore, it is also called pigmented dermatofibrosarcoma protuberans. It accounts for 5% of all cases of dermatofibrosarcoma protuberans [31, 62]. Doubt still exists about its exact origin. Some authors propose a neural origin: hence the synonym "storiform neurofibroma." Nevertheless, the lesion has characteristics largely identical to those of dermatofibrosarcoma protuberans [6].

■ **Imaging Findings.** To our knowledge, no reports exist on Bednár tumor's imaging characteristics.

14.2.2.3 Plexiform Fibrohistiocytic Tumor

■ **Definition and Clinical Findings.** Plexiform fibrohistiocytic tumor is a rare, slowly growing tumor of the skin, arising principally in the (upper) extremities of children and adolescents. The male-to-female ratio is 1:3. It frequently recurs (40%) and sometimes (3%) metastasizes to regional lymph nodes [29]. Previous radiation therapy may be a predisposing factor [3]. Histologically it is characterized by its plexiform structure, extensive hemosiderin deposits and numerous multinucleated giant cells and fibroblasts [3]. Some cases present as purely fibroblastic lesions, designated as fibroblastic variant of plexiform fibrohistiocytic tumor [3, 6]. There are no histological features that predict which lesions will metastasize.

■ **Imaging Findings.** To our knowledge only one report exist on imaging findings in plexiform fibrohistiocytic tumor. The lesion has low SI on both T1- and T2-weighted images and shows no contrast enhancement. These imaging features may reflect the high amount of intratumoral collagen [45].

14.2.2.4 Giant Cell Fibroblastoma

■ **Definition and Clinical Findings.** Giant cell fibroblastoma is a nodular (sub)dermal mass arising at the back of the thigh, groins, and chest wall. It affects predominantly infants and children [30]. Macroscopically the lesion presents as a gray to yellow mass.

Recent advances in histological, immunohistochemical, and cytogenetic analysis may show that giant cell fibroblastoma should be considered as the juvenile form of dermatofibrosarcoma protuberans [15, 22]. However, other authors believe that giant cell fibroblastoma is not a definite entity on its own, but might represent rather a host reaction of the connective tissue in association with a locally aggressive or malignant mass [56].

■ **Imaging Findings.** To our knowledge, no imaging reports exist on this entity.

14.2.2.5 Angiomatoid Fibrous Histiocytoma

■ **Definition and Clinical Findings.** The WHO Committee for the Classification of Soft Tissue Tumors recently renamed angiomatoid MFH as "angiomatoid fibrous histiocytoma," because this term better reflects its slow growth potentials and the rarity of metastasis (1%) [30]. Although it has not yet been definitely proven, actual findings support the theory that angiomatoid fibrous histiocytoma will turn out to be a separate entity arising from or being related to myoid cells or lymphoid tissue, which is an argument for its classification in another subdivision in the near future [32, 35, 48, 50].

Angiomatoid fibrous histiocytoma presents as a slowly growing multinodular or multicystic, hemorrhagic (sub)cutaneous mass, characteristically affecting children and adolescents. Clinically, it often resembles a hematoma.

Histologically, it consists of solid masses of histiocytes, irregular blood-filled spaces, intense chronic inflammation, and extensive fibrosis. The histiocytic cells contain hemosiderin and lipids. The most important problem often is marked bleeding [100].

■ **Imaging Findings.** Some case studies describe the presence of multiple fluid-fluid levels, indicative of intralesional hemorrhage [77]. CT scan shows a lobulated, heterogeneous soft tissue mass. On MR images, a heterogeneous cystic-like lesion is seen, with internal fluid-fluid levels (Fig. 14.20). Foci of low SI on T1- and T2-weighted images suggest hemosiderin deposits [64]. On angiography, prominent vascular pooling has been reported [33].

14.2.2.6 Giant Cell Tumor of Soft Tissues

■ **Definition and Clinical Findings.** Giant cell tumor of soft tissues is an extremely rare tumor, which was first described in 1970 by Salm and Sissons, who noted a close resemblance between a subset of giant cell-rich soft tissue tumors and giant cell tumors of bone [6, 89]. Up until 1992, no further reports on this entity were published. In 1992, Nascimento published reports on 10 giant cell tumors of soft tissues that he considered to be soft tissue equivalents of giant cell tumors of bone [79]. In 1999 and 2000, three authors described the findings from another 71 cases [38, 81, 82].

Giant cell tumor of soft tissues is a painless, multinodular or fungating growing mass at the lower limbs (50%), trunk (32%), the upper limbs (14%), and head and neck region (7%). It affects virtually any age group and there is no sex predilection. Most lesions are superficially located. In 30% of cases, extension through the superficial fascia is noted [38, 81, 86].

Microscopically, giant cell tumors of soft tissue is seen as a homogeneously mixed proliferation of spindle and polygonal mononucleate stromal cells and evenly distributed multinucleated osteoclast-like giant cells, arranged in a multinodular architecture, separated by fibroconnective tissue septa. They indeed bear a close resemblance to their bony counterparts, giant cell tumors of bone. In contradistinction to its high-grade counterpart, the cells lack nuclear atypia or pleomorphism and the mitotic rate is low [81]. Foci of intralesional hemorrhage are seen in up to 50% of cases, whereas intratumoral metaplastic bone formation can be found in 40% of lesions, frequently seen as a peripheral shell of woven bone, otherwise as scattered bony structures. Secondary cystic changes and blood-filled lakes are seen in approximately 30% of cases. Intratumoral necrosis is seldom seen. Features typically associated with GCTTS such as dense stromal hyaline, siderophages, and xanthoma cells (see Giant Cell Tumor of Tendon Sheath, above) are nearly always absent.

There is a marked disparity in prognosis and outcome among patients with giant cell tumors of the soft tissues. When treated adequately by complete surgical excision, a benign course is expected in numerous cases. In others, recurrences may occur and metastases may appear within a relatively short interval after local treatment [84]. Since their long-term metastatic risk is not completely defined, the term "giant cell tumor of low malignant potential" is also used for the latter lesions. The term "malignant giant cell tumor of soft parts" or "giant cell MFH" should be restricted to histologically high-grade lesions [38].

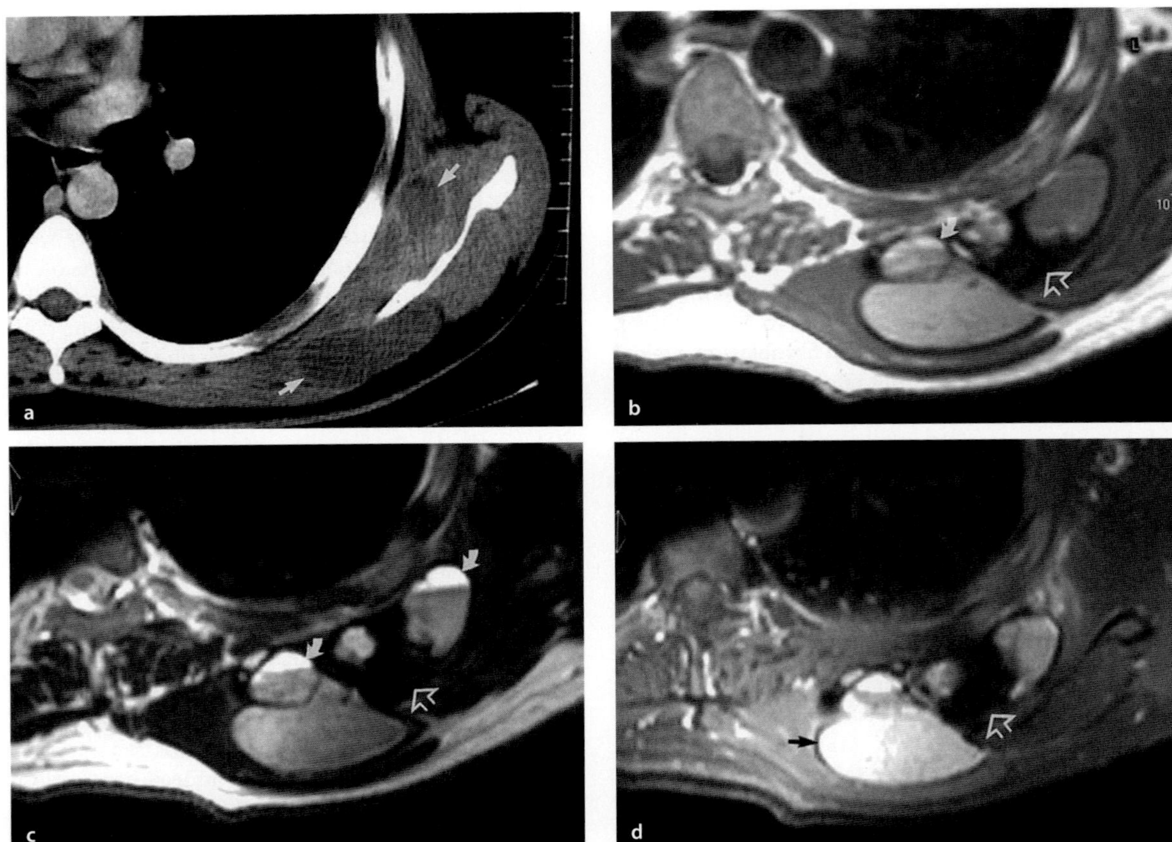

Fig. 14.20a–d. Angiomatoid fibrous histiocytoma of the left scapular region in a 32-year-old man. **a** Contrast-enhanced CT scan. **b** Axial T1-weighted MR image. **c** Axial T2-weighted MR image. **d** Axial fat-saturated T1-weighted MR image after intravenous administration of gadolinium contrast. On contrast-enhanced CT scan, a soft tissue mass with hypodense intralesional components is seen. There is no enhancement of the tumor (**a**). On T1- (**b**) and T2-weighted (**c**) MR images, a heterogeneous, multiloculated mass with intralesional fluid-fluid levels, corresponding to hemorrhage, is noted. A low signal-intensity area (*arrows*) on both T1- and T2-weighted images is indicative of hemosiderin deposits. On fat-saturated T1-weighted images after gadolinium administration, no enhancement is seen. The high signal intensity of the cystic component is an effect of fat suppression. (Reprinted from [64], with permission)

■ **Imaging Findings.** On histological examination, peripheral mineralization is sometimes noted. However, corresponding radiographic or CT findings are not yet reported. On MR images, no specific signs are seen. A heterogeneous mass with intermediate SI on T1-weighted images and high SI on T2-weighted images is seen. Diffuse, heterogeneous enhancement is noted (Fig. 14.21) [23].

14.2.3 Malignant Fibrohistiocytic Tumors

14.2.3.1 Atypical Fibroxanthoma

■ **Definition and Clinical Findings.** Atypical fibroxanthoma is a pleomorphic, solitary, nodular tumor occurring at the sun-exposed parts of the skin in elderly persons and on the extremities or trunk in young adults. Solar, occupational, or therapeutic irradiation may be causative factors. Histologically, it resembles a pleomorphic MFH. In contrast to this entity, it has an excellent prognosis following resection because of its small size and its superficial location. Therefore, it was earlier classified among the benign fibrohistiocytic tumors. However, because of the histological similarity with some forms of MFH, it has to be considered as a malignant fibrohistiocytic tumor. Recurrences are rare, and when a large, deep-seated recurrence does arise, it should be regarded as a MFH and treated accordingly [30].

■ **Imaging Findings.** Because of its superficial location, this lesion is excised or sampled without imaging. To our knowledge, no reports exist on imaging appearance of atypical fibroxanthoma in current radiological literature.

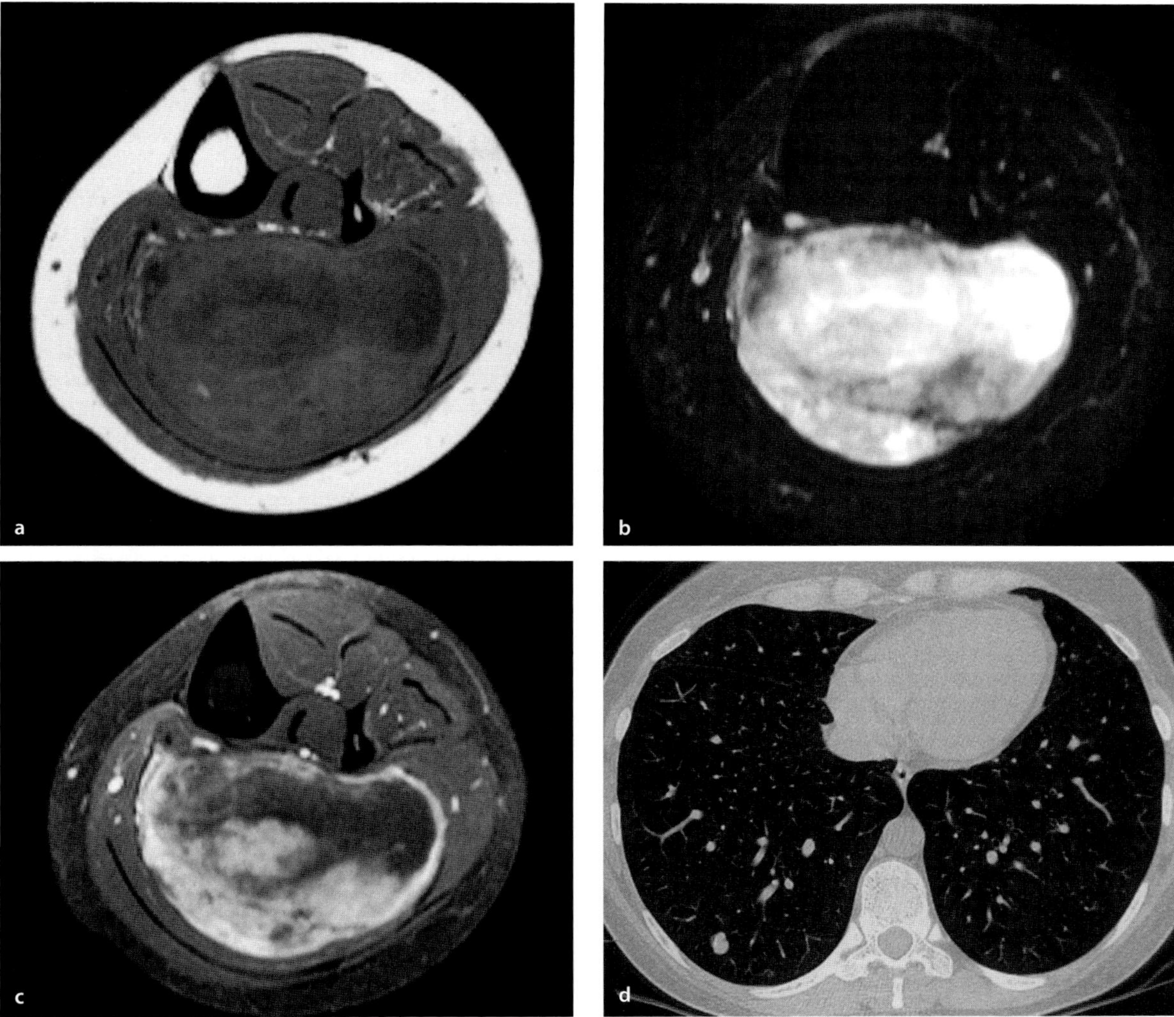

Fig. 14.21 a–d. Giant cell tumor of soft tissues in a 26-year-old man, within the left lateral gastrocnemius region. (Courtesy of J.L. Bloem, Leiden). **a** Axial T1-weighted MR image. **b** Axial fat-saturated T2-weighted MR image. **c** Axial fat-saturated T1-weighted MR image after gadolinium contrast injection. **d** Contrast-enhanced CT scan of the thorax, pulmonary window. On T1- (**a**) and T2-weighted (**b**) MR images, a heterogeneous mass is noted at the posterior aspect of the left lower leg. On fat-saturated T1-weighted images after gadolinium administration (**c**), heterogeneous enhancement is seen. Complete resection of the mass showed low-grade giant cell tumor of soft tissues. After resection, radiation therapy was administered. After a period of 6 years, a local recurrence was found on a follow-up MR study. On CT scan of the thorax (**d**), some metastatic deposits in both lungs were noted

14.2.3.2 Malignant Fibrous Histiocytoma

In the first half of the twentieth century, tumor classification was based on the concept of histogenesis or "cell of origin." The characteristics of the neoplastic cells in culture relative to normal cells defined the cell of origin.

Explanted cells of so-called histiocytic tumors show some of the characteristics of histiocytes in the first days of growth. Afterwards, they exhibit some characteristics of fibroblasts. Therefore, these cells were interpreted as histiocytic in origin, but capable to develop features of fibroblasts (facultative fibroblasts) [88].

The term "malignant fibrous histiocytoma" (MFH) was introduced by Stout and O'Brien and Kaufmann in the early 1960s [57, 77, 80], flourishing throughout the 1970s and 1980s, and the pleomorphic storiform subtype became regarded as the most common soft tissue sarcoma of adulthood. Four other variants (myxoid, inflammatory, giant cell, and angiomatoid) have also been described.

Nowadays, thanks to the recent advances in immunohistochemistry and cytogenetics, molecular biology and pharmacology, many more neoplasms can be identified more accurately. The impact of these new techniques on classification of particular soft tissue sarcomas is illustrated in a large-series retrospective study by Daugaard, in which he revisited histopathological slides and performed immunohistochemical tests (when necessary) on 281 soft tissue sarcomas of the extremities from the period 1972–1994. Initial diagnosis changed in up to 57% of lesions [17]!

Growing evidence has arisen in the last 5 years that formerly classifications of so-called histiocytic neoplasms were incorrect and inappropriate [46]. Recent cytogenetic studies have shown a similar pattern of recurrent genomic imbalances in malignant fibrous histiocytoma and leiomyosarcoma. Also, similar chromosome deletions have been found in both these tumors [63]. Recent developments (new antibodies) in immunohistochemistry are not able to define specific markers or to describe the phenotype of this sarcoma of supposed "fibrohistiocytic" lineage. Furthermore, the immunophenotype overlaps with other malignancies [88]. A substantial number of formerly so-called pleomorphic MFH turns out to be leiomyo-/myogenic sarcomas or dedifferentiated liposarcomas [14].

This has implications on treatment and prognosis, since metastatic potential differs for different subgroups among the neoplasms formerly categorized as pleomorphic MFH (e.g., the metastatic rate of dedifferentiated liposarcomas and high-grade myxofibrosarcomas is about 15–20% and 30–35%, respectively, whereas a much larger amount of leiomyosarcomas does metastasize, resulting in a shorter relapse-free interval and worse long-term prognosis).

As a result of these findings, the term "malignant fibrous histiocytoma" has been partly abandoned in the 2002 WHO classification of soft tissue neoplasms [36]. In this classification, the different types of malignant fibrous histiocytoma are considered to be undifferentiated pleomorphic sarcomas. The storiform-pleomorphic MFH is now designated as undifferentiated high-grade pleomorphic sarcoma. Myxoid MFH has been demonstrated to show fibroblastic differentiation. Furthermore, since it lacks histiocytic differentiation and possesses prominent myxoid areas, this tumor may not be classified as a fibrohistiocytic lesion and should preferentially be renamed as myxofibrosarcoma (see Chap. 13) [48].

Giant cell MFH is now called – in WHO classification terms – undifferentiated pleomorphic sarcoma with giant cells. Inflammatory MFH is reclassified as undifferentiated pleomorphic sarcoma with prominent inflammation.

Notwithstanding these improvements in classification, a large amount of pleomorphic sarcomas with morphological features of MFH cannot become subdivided in one or other category. Ultrastructural features show that these pleomorphic masses consist of an admixture of fibroblastic or myofibroblastic cells, which might in the near future prove to be a distinct clinicopathological entity [93]. Therefore, some authors propose to incorporate these neoplasms into the category of fibrosarcoma, and introduce the terms of storiform-

pleomorphic fibrosarcoma, myxofibrosarcoma, inflammatory pleomorphic fibrosarcoma, and giant cell-rich fibrosarcoma [88].

Because of the developmental race in molecular biology and cytogenetics, the 2002 WHO classification, representing at least a step forward in understanding these soft tissue neoplasms, may soon be outdated. [88].

Things to remember:

1. Giant cell tumors of tendon sheath and pigmented villonodular synovitis are characterized by a typical location (tendon or joint, respectively), a low SI on both pulse sequences, with blooming on gradient echo sequences and a strong enhancement pattern.
2. Xanthomas are highly associated with familial or secondary hyperlipidemia. These patients are at risk of ischemic heart disease and stroke.
3. Imaging features of other benign and malignant fibrohistiocytic tumors are nonspecific.

References

1. Annessi G, Cimitan A, Girolomoni G, Giannetti A (1993) Congenital dermatofibrosarcoma protuberans. Pediatr Dermatol 10:40–42
2. Argiris A, Dardoufas C, Aroni K (1995) Radiotherapy induced soft tissue sarcoma: an unusual case of a dermatofibrosarcoma protuberans. J Clin Oncol 7:59–61
3. August C, Holzhausen HJ, Zornig C, Harms D, Schroder S (1994) Plexiformer Fibrohistiozytischer Tumor. Histologie, Immunohistologie und Ultrastruktur. Pathologe 15:49–53
4. Barkhof F, Verrips A, Wesseling P, et al (2000) Cerebrotendinous xanthomatosis: the spectrum of imaging findings and the correlation with neuropathologic findings. Radiology 217:869–876
5. Bashara ME, Jules KT, Potter GK (1992) Dermatofibrosarcoma protuberans: 4 years after local trauma. J Foot Surg 31:160–165
6. Billings SD, Folpe AL (2004) Cutaneous and subcutaneous fibrohistiocytic tumors of intermediate malignancy: an update. Am J Dermatopathol 26:141–155
7. Bravo SM, Winalski CS, Weissman BN (1996) Pigmented villonodular synovitis. Radiol Clin North Am 34:311–326
8. Bude RO, Adler RS, Bassett DR, Ikeda DM, Rubin JM (1993) Heterozygous familial hypercholesterolemia: detection of xanthomas in the Achilles tendon with US. Radiology 188:567–571
9. Bude RO, Adler RS, Bassett DR (1994) Diagnosis of Achilles tendon xanthoma in patients with heterozygous familial hypercholesterolemia: MR vs sonography. Am J Roentgenol 162:913–917
10. Calonje E, Mentzel T, Fletcher CDM (1994) Cellular benign fibrous histiocytoma: Clinicopathologic analysis of 74 cases of a distinctive variant of cutaneous fibrous histiocytoma with frequent recurrence. Am J Surg Pathol 18:668–676
11. Campbell DA, Edwards NL (1991) Multicentric reticulohistiocytosis: systemic macrophage disorder. Baillieres Clin Rheumatol 5:301–319
12. Carstens HP, Howell RS (1979) Malignant giant cell tumor of tendon sheath. Virchows Arch A Pathol Anat Histol. 382:237–243
13. Chakraverty S, Griffiths PD, Walls TJ, McAllister VL (1995) Cerebrotendinous xanthomatosis in two sisters: case reports and MRI. Clin Radiol 50:117–119

14. Coindre JM, Mariani O, Chibon F, et al (2003) Most malignant fibrous histiocytomas developed in the retroperitoneum are dedifferentiated liposarcomas: a review of 25 cases initially diagnosed as malignant fibrous histiocytoma. Mod Pathol 16:256–262

15. Dal Cin P, Sciot R, De Wever I, et al (1996) Cytogenetic and immunohistochemical evidence that giant cell fibroblastoma is related to dermatofibrosarcoma protuberans. Genes Chromosomes Cancer 15:73–75

16. Daly BD, Currie AR, Choi PCL (1993) Case report: computed tomographic and scintigraphic appearances of dermatofibrosarcoma protuberans. Clin Radiol 48:63–65

17. Daugaard S (2004) Current soft-tissue sarcoma classifications. Eur J Cancer 40:543–548

18. David JK, Anupindi SA, Deshpande V, Jaramillo D (2003) Intramuscular juvenile xanthogranuloma: sonographic and MR findings. Pediatr Radiol 33:203–206

19. De Beuckeleer L, De Schepper A, De Belder F, et al (1997) Magnetic resonance imaging of localized giant cell tumour of the tendon sheath (MRI of localized GCTTS). Eur Radiol 7:198–201

20. Dehner LP (2003) Juvenile xanthogranulomas in the first two decades of life: a clinicopathologic study of 174 cases with cutaneous and extracutaneous manifestations. Am J Surg Pathol. 27:579–593

21. De Schepper AM, Degryse HR, Ramon FA, Van Marck EA (1992) Magnetic Resonance imaging of extraabdominal desmoid tumors. J Belge Radiol 75:91–98

22. Diaz-Cascajo C, Weyers W, Borrego L, et al (1997) Dermatofibrosarcoma protuberans with fibrosarcomatous areas: a clinico-pathologic and immunohistochemic study in four cases. Am J Dermatopathol 19:562–567

23. Dodd LG, Major N, Brigman B (2004) Malignant giant cell tumor of soft parts. Skeletal Radiol 33:295–299

24. Durrington PN, Adams JE, Beastall MD (1982) The assessment of achilles tendon size in primary hypercholesterolaemia by computed tomography. Atherosclerosis 45:345–358

25. Dussault RG, Kaplan PA, Roederer G (1995) MRI of achilles tendon in patients with familial hyperlipidemia: comparison with plain films, physical examination, and patients with traumatic tendon lesions. Am J Roentgenol 164:403–407

26. Ebeling T, Farin P, Pyörälä K (1992) Ultrasonography in the detection of achilles tendon xanthomata in heterozygous familial hypercholesterolemia. Atherosclerosis 97:217–228

27. Eggli KD, Caro P, Quiogue T, Boal DKB (1992) Juvenile xanthogranuloma: non-X histiocytosis with systemic involvement. Pediatr Radiol 22:374–376

28. Eisen RN, Tallini G (1993) Metastatic dermatofibrosarcoma protuberans with fibrosarcomatous change in the absence of local recurrence. A case report of simultaneous occurrence with a malignant giant cell tumor of soft parts. Cancer 72:462–468

29. Enzinger FM, Weiss SW (1995) Benign fibrohistiocytic tumors. In: Enzinger FM, Weiss SW (eds) Soft tissue tumors, 3rd edn. Mosby, St. Louis, pp 293–323

30. Enzinger FM, Weiss SW (1995) Fibrohistiocytic tumors of intermediate malignancy. In: Enzinger FM, Weiss SW (eds) Soft tissue tumors, 3rd edn. Mosby, St. Louis, pp 325–349

31. Enzinger FM, Zhang R (1988) Plexiform fibrohistiocytic tumor presenting in children and young adults. An analysis of 65 cases. Am J Surg Pathol 12:818–826

32. Fanburg-Smith JC, Miettinen (1999) Angiomatoid "malignant" fibrous histiocytoma: a clinicopathologic study of 158 cases and further exploration of the myoid phenotype. Hum Pathol 30:1336–1343

33. Fisher HJ, Lois JF, Gomes AS, Mirra JM, Deutsch L-S (1985) Radiology and pathology of malignant fibrous histiocytomas of the soft tissues: a report of ten cases. Skeletal Radiol 13:202–206

34. Flandry F, Hughston JC, McCann SB, et al (1994) Diagnostic features of diffuse pigmented villonodular synovitis of the knee. Clin Orthop 298:212–220

35. Fletcher CD (1991) Angiomatoid "malignant fibrous histiocytoma": an immunohistochemical study indicative of myoid differentiation. Hum Pathol 22:563–568

36. Fletcher CDM, Unni KK, Mertens F, et al. Eds. (2002) Pathology and genetics of tumours of soft tissue and bone (World Health Organization Classification of Tumours). Lyon, France, IARC Press

37. Freyer DR, Kennedy R, Bostrom BC, Kohut G, Dehner LP (1996) Juvenile xanthogranuloma: forms of systemic disease and their clinical implications. J Pediatr 129:227–237

38. Folpe AL, Morris RJ, Weiss SW (1999) Soft tissue giant cell tumor of low malignant potential: a proposal for the reclassification of malignant giant cell tumor of soft parts. Mod Pathol 12:894–902

39. Friedman PD, Kalisher L (1998) Multicentric reticulohistiocytosis in a child: radiological findings and clinical correlation. Can Assoc Radiol J 49:378–380

40. Garcia-Pena P, Mariscal A, Abellan C, Zuasnabar A, Lucaya J (1992) Juvenile xanthogranuloma with extracutaneous lesions. Pediatr Radiol 22:377–378

41. Gattereau A, Davignon J, Levesque HP (1971) Roentgenological evaluation of Achilles-tendon xanthomatosis. Lancet 2(726):705–706

42. Gilbert TJ, Parker BR (1988) Juvenile xanthogranuloma of the kidney. Pediatr Radiol 18:169–171

43. Gold RH, Bassett LW, Seeger LL (1988) The other arthritides. Roentgenologic features of osteoarthritis, erosive osteoarthritis, ankylosing spondylitis, psoriatic arthritis, Reiter's disease, multicentric reticulohistiocytosis, and progressive systemic sclerosis. Radiol Clin North Am 26:1195 –1212

44. Gupta AK, Bhargava S (1988) Juvenile xanthogranuloma with pulmonary lesions. Pediatr Radiol 18:70

45. Habermann CR, Nicolas V, Steiner P (1995) Magnetic resonance tomography diagnosis of plexiform fibrohistiocytic tumor. Aktuelle Radiol 5:243–245

46. Hatano H, Tokunaga K, Ogose A, Imaizumi S, Hayami T, Yamagiwa H, Hotta T, Endo N, Takahashi HE, Naito M (1999) Origin of histiocyte-like cells and multinucleated giant cells in malignant fibrous histiocytoma: neoplastic or reactive? Pathol Int 49:14–22

47. Hertzanu Y, Berginer J, Berginer VM (1991) Computed tomography of tendinous xanthomata in cerebrotendinous xanthomatosis. Skeletal Radiol 20:99–102

48. Hollowood K, Fletcher CD (1995) Malignant fibrous histiocytoma: morphologic pattern or pathologic entity? Semin Diagn Pathol 12:210–220

49. Hyde JS, Jesmanowicz A, Kneeland JB (1987) Surface coil for MRI of the skin. Magnet Reson Med 5:456–461

50. Jacobs IA, Chevinsky A (2000) Angiomatoid fibrous histiocytoma: a case report and review of the literature. Dermatol Surg 26:491–492

51. Janssen BA, Kencian J, Brooks PM (1992) Close temporal and anatomical relationship between multicentric reticulohistiocytosis and carcinoma of the breast. J Rheumatol 19:322–324

52. Jelinek JS, Kransdorf MJ, Utz JA, et al (1989) Imaging of pigmented villonodular synovitis with emphasis on MRI. Am J Roentgenol 152:337–342

53. Jergesen HE, Mankin HJ, Schiller AL (1978) Diffuse pigmented villonodular synovitis of the knee mimicking primary bone neoplasm. J Bone Joint Surg Am 60:825–829

54. Kaddu S, McMenamin ME, Fletcher CD (2002) Atypical fibrous histiocytoma of the skin: clinicopathologic analysis of 59 cases with evidence of infrequent metastasis. Am J Surg Pathol 26:35–46

55. Kamel H, Gibson G, Cassidy M (1996) Case report: the CT demonstration of soft tissue involvement in multicentric reticulohistiocytosis. Clin Radiol 51:440–441

56. Karabela-Bouropoulou V, Liapi-Avgeri G, Mahera H (1999) Giant cell fibroblastoma: an entity or a reactive phenomenon? Pathol Res Pract. 195:413–419

57. Kauffman SL, Stout AP (1961) Histiocytic tumors (fibrous xanthoma and histiocytoma) in children. Cancer 14:469–482

58. Kenan S, Abdelwahab IF, Klein MJ, Aaron A, Lewis MM (1992) Case report 754. Skeletal Radiol 21:471–473

59. Kindblom LG, Gunterberg G (1978) Pigmented villonodular synovitis involving bone. Case report. J Bone Joint Surg Am 60: 830–832

60. Koblik PD, Freeman DM (1993) Short echo time magnetic resonance imaging of tendon. Invest Radiol 28:1095–1100
61. Koh CK, Ko CB, Bury HPR, Wyatt EH (1995) Dermatofibrosarcoma protuberans. Int J Dermatol 34:256–259
62. Kransdorf MJ, Meis-Kindblom JM (1994) Dermatofibrosarcoma protuberans: radiological appearance. Am J Roentgenol 163:391–394
63. Lagacé R, Aurias A (2002) Requiem pour l'histiocytome fibreux malin? Ann Pathol 22:29–34
64. Li CS, Chan WP, Chen WT, et al (2004) MRI of angiomatoid fibrous histiocytoma. Skeletal Radiol 33:604–608
65. Liem MSL, Gevers Leuven JA, Bloem JL, Schipper J (1992) Magnetic resonance imaging of Achilles tendon xanthomas in familial hypercholesterolemia. Skeletal Radiol 21:453–457
66. Llauger J, Palmer J, Roson N, Cremades R, Bague S (1999) Pigmented villonodular synovitis and giant cell tumors of the tendon sheath: radiological and pathologic features. Am J Roentgenol 172:1087–1091
67. Machiels F, De Maeseneer M, Chaskis C, Bourgain C, Osteaux M (1998) Deep benign fibrous histiocytoma of the knee: CT and MR features with pathologic correlation. Eur Radiol 8:989–991
68. Mackie GC (2003) Pigmented Villonodular Synovitis and Giant Cell Tumor of the Tendon Sheath. Scintigraphic Findings in 10 cases. Clin Nucl Med 28:881–885
69. MacLeod PM (1986) Case report: Juvenile xanthogranuloma of the iris managed with superficial radiotherapy. Clin Radiol 37:295–296
70. March HC, Gilbert PD, Kain TM (1957) Hypercholesterolemic xanthoma of the tendon. Am J Roentgenol 77:109
71. Martinoli C, Bianchi S, Derchi LE (1999) Tendon and nerve sonography. Radiol Clin North Am 37:691–711
72. Mäurer J, Requardt H, Müller F, Steinkamp HJ, Hosten N, Langer R, Felix R (1994) Indikationen zur Applikation einer Hochauflösungsspule in der MR-Tomographie. ROFO Fortschr Röntg 160:353–360
73. McKee PH, Fletcher CDM (1991) Dermatofibrosarcoma protuberans presenting in infancy and childhood. J Cutan Pathol 18:241–246
74. McKenna DB, Kavanagh GM, McLaren KM, Tidman MJ (1999) Aneurysmal fibrous histiocytoma: an unusual variant of cutaneous fibrous histiocytoma. J Eur Acad Dermatol Venereol 12:238–240
75. McLoughlin PM, Girach M, Wood GA (1992) Dermatofibrosarcoma protuberans of the scalp. Br J Oral Maxillofac Surg 30:401–403
76. Miyakawa E, Fujimoto H, Miyakawa K, Nemoto K, Kozawa K, Sugano I, Odani Y, Hirata T, Ogata H, Ohno T (1996) Dermatofibrosarcoma protuberans. CT findings with pathologic correlation in 6 cases. Acta Radiol 37:362–365
77. Murphey MD, Gross TM, Rosenthal HG (1994) Musculoskeletal malignant fibrous histiocytoma: radiologic-pathologic correlation. Radiographics 14:807–826
78. Myers BW, Masi AT (1980) Pigmented villonodular synovitis and tenosynovitis: a clinical epidemiologic study of 166 cases and literature review. Medicine (Baltimore) 59:223–238
79. Nascimento AG (1992) Giant cell tumors of soft parts (abstract). Mod Pathol 68:32A
80. O'Brien JE, Stout AP (1964). Malignant fibrous xanthomas. Cancer 17:1445–1455
81. O'Connell JX, Wehrli BM, Nielsen GP, Rosenberg AE (2000) Giant cell tumors of soft tissue: a clinicopathologic study of 18 benign and malignant tumors. 24:386–395
82. Oliveira AM, Dei Tos AP, Fletcher CD, Nascimento AG (2000) Primary giant cell tumor of soft tissues: a study of 22 cases. Am J Surg Pathol 24:248–256
83. Rabinowitz LG, Luchetti ME, Segura AD, Esterly NB (1994) Acrally occurring dermatofibrosarcoma protuberans in children and adults. J Dermatol Surg Oncol 20:655–659
84. Reilly KE, Stern PJ, Dale JA (1999) Recurrent giant cell tumors of the tendon sheath. J Hand Surg 24:1298–1302
85. Ritchie DA. (1999) MRI of synovial tumours and tumour-like lesions. Br J Radiol 72:212–218
86. Rodriguez-Peralto JL, Lopez-Barea F, Fernandez-Delgado J (2001) Primary giant cell tumor of soft tissues similar to bone giant cell tumor: a case report and literature review. Pathol Int 51:60–63
87. Rollandi GA, Bertolotto M, Perrone R, Garlashi G, Derchi LE (1995) MRI of normal achilles tendon. Eur J Radiol 5:596–598
88. Rosenberg AE (2003) Malignant fibrous histiocytoma: past, present, and future. Skeletal Radiol 32:613–618
89. Salm R, Sissons HA (1972) Giant-cell tumours of soft tissues. J Pathol 107:27–39
90. Schick F, Dammann F, Lutz O, Claussen CD (1995) Adapted techniques for clinical MRI of tendons. Mag Reson Mater Phys Biol Med 3:103–107
91. Sheehan KM, Leader MB, Sexton S, et al (2004) Recurrent aneurysmal fibrous histiocytoma. J Clin Pathol 57:312–313
92. Steinmetz A, Schmitt W, Schuler P, Kleinsorge F, Schneider J, Kaffarnik H (1988) Ultrasonography of Achilles tendons in primary hypercholesterolemia. Comparison with computed tomography. Atherosclerosis 74:231–239
93. Suh Ch, Ordonez NG, Mackay B (2000) Malignant fibrous histiocytoma: an ultrastructural perspective. Ultrastruct Pathol 24:243–250
94. Thomas DB, Sidler AK, Huston BM (1998) Radiological case of the month. Juvenile xanthogranuloma. Arch Pediatr Adolesc Med 152:1029–1030
95. Torreggiani WC, Al-Ismail K, Munk PL, et al (2002) Dermatofibrosarcoma protuberans: MRI features. Am J Roentgenol 179:989–993
96. Ushijima M, Hashimoto H, Tsuneyoshi M, Enjoji M (1986) Giant cell tumor of the tendon sheath (nodular tenosynovitis). A study of 207 cases to compare the large joint group with the common digit group. Cancer 57:875–884
97. Van Holsbeeck M, Introcaso JH (1991) Musculoskeletal ultrasound. Mosby-Year Book, St. Louis
98. Wrotnowski U, Cooper PH, Shmookler BM (1988) Fibrosarcomatous change in dermatofibrosarcoma protuberans. Am J Surg Pathol 12:287–293
99. Yamada T, Kurohori YN, Kashiwazaki S, Fujibayashi M, Ohkawa T (1996) MRI of multicentric reticulohistiocytosis. J Comput Assist Tomogr 20:838–840
100. Yamamoto Y, Arata J, Yonezawa S (1985) Angiomatoid malignant fibrous histiocytoma associated with marked bleeding arising in chronic radiodermatitis. Arch Dermatol 121:275–276
101. Yoshimura Y, Sugihara T, Kishimoto H, Nagaoka S (1987) Multicentric reticulohistiocytosis accompanied by oral and temporomandibular joint manifestations. Br J Oral Maxillofac Surg 45:84–86
102. Zemtsov A, Lorig R, Ng TC, Xue M, Bailin PL, Bergfeld W, Larson K, Yetman R (1991) Magnetic resonance imaging of cutaneous neoplasms: clinicopathologic correlation. J Dermatol Surg Oncol 17:416–422

Lipomatous Tumors

F.M. Vanhoenacker, M.C. Marques, H. Garcia

15

Contents

15.1 Introduction

Histologically adipose tissue is classified into two main types: white fat (lipocytes), widely distributed through the body, and brown fat, which is more common in rodents and hibernating animals. Brown fat is considered an immature form of the white fat and is chiefly found in the interscapular region, neck, mediastinum, axilla, and retroperitoneum [46, 69].

Lipomatous tumors are common mesenchymal lesions that can be both benign or malignant. There is a wide range of histological subtypes, the lipoma being the most frequent of them. Some tumors, including lipoma and some types of liposarcoma, will display typical features which allow a specific diagnosis to be made [85, 86, 144]. In the following discussion, only the subdivisions of lipomatous tumors that arise in the soft tissues of the body are considered.

The role of magnetic resonance imaging (MRI) for the study and evaluation of these common tumors is emphasized throughout this chapter. The superiority of this technique stems from its exquisite sensitivity in displaying minor differences in tissue composition. Many investigators have reported MRI to be diagnostically valuable in distinguishing fat-containing tumors from other tumors, because of its ability for detecting fatty components [21, 75, 89]. On plain radiographs, lipomatous tumors may not be apparent or can be detected as a mass of increased density or of fatty opacity. On ultrasound scans, these tumors can show different patterns of echogenicity: they are mostly isoechoic or hyperechoic, although a hypoechoic pattern may be also encountered [1, 54]. Using computed tomography (CT), diagnosis of a lipomatous tumor can be straightforward when typical low attenuation values are found (–65 to –120 HU). On MR images, the signal intensity (SI) of fatty tumors tends to be equal to that of subcutaneous fat on all pulse sequences, including those obtained with fat suppression: short-tau inversion recovery (STIR) or chemical shift pulse sequences [40, 90, 89, 145, 144, 155] (Fig. 15.1).

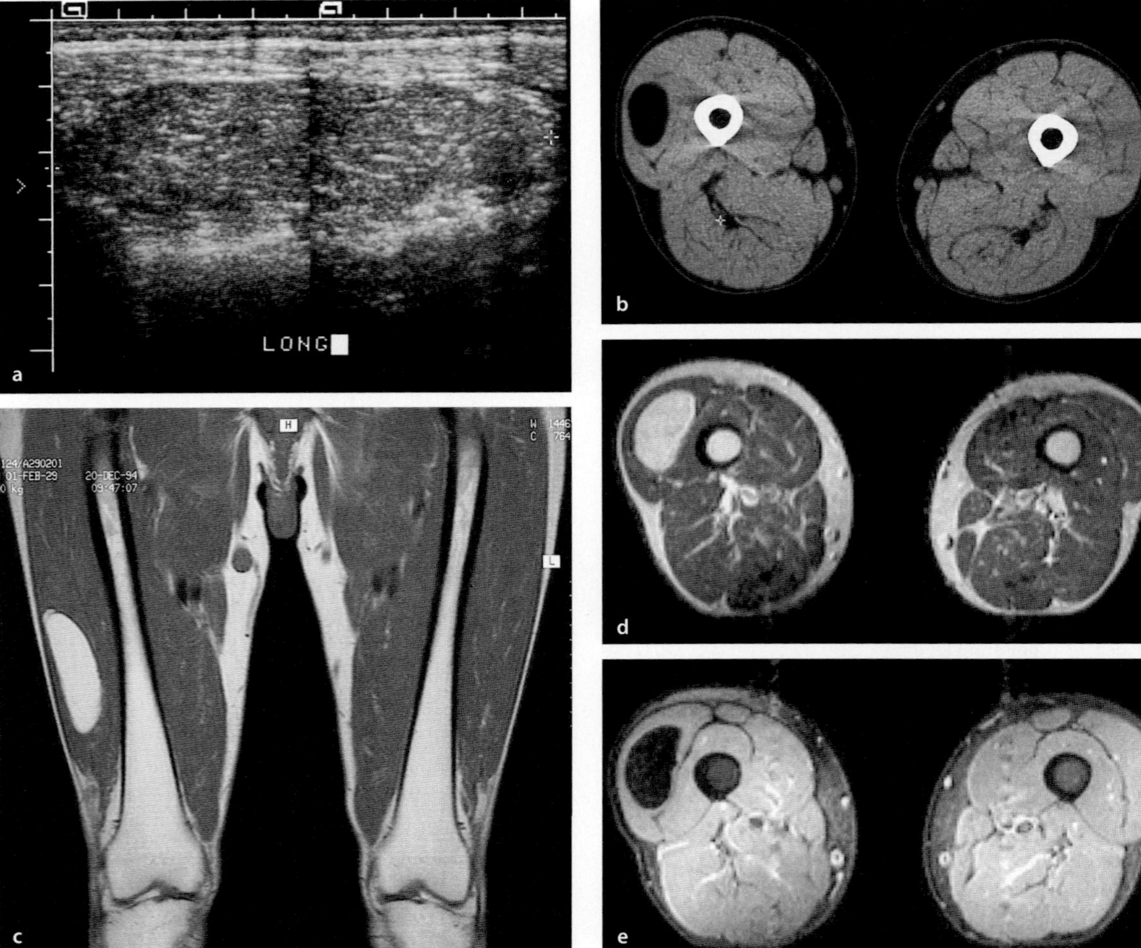

Fig. 15.1a–e. Intramuscular lipoma of the thigh in a 65-year-old man. **a** Ultrasound. **b** CT scan. **c** Coronal SE T1-weighted MR image. **d** Axial SE T2-weighted MR image. **e** Axial fat-suppressed STIR MR image. The ultrasound examination reveals a fusiform, hypoechoic mass, located in the vastus lateralis muscle (**a**). On CT scan a well-defined mass with fat-attenuation values is seen (**b**). The mass is homogeneous on MR and SI is equal to that of subcutaneous fat on different pulse sequences (**c–e**). This case illustrates characteristic shape and imaging findings in a lipoma

15.2 Benign Lipomatous Tumors

The benign lipomatous tumors represent a very common and varied group and, according to the most recent World Health Organization's Committee for the Classification of Soft Tissue Tumors (2002), nine distinct entities are distinguished [26]: lipoma, lipomatosis, lipomatosis of nerve, lipoblastoma/lipoblastomatosis, angiolipoma, myolipoma of soft tissue, chondroid lipoma, spindle cell/pleiomorphic lipoma, and hibernoma. However, this classification does not distinguish true neoplasms, hamartomatous processes, or simple overgrowth of fat, mainly because the differentiation is devoid of any clinical consequences.

15.2.1 Lipoma

Microscopically, lipoma is usually a well-circumscribed, encapsulated mass, composed of mature fat (adipocytes) differing very little from the surrounding fat. Although lipomas are well vascularized, this feature may not be readily apparent owing to vascular compression caused by the distended adipocytes.

Lipoma is the most common mesenchymal tumor and, in a review of 18,677 benign soft tissue tumors, lipoma and lipoma variants were the most common group, representing 16% of all lesions [85]. Lipoma generally affects patients in the fifth to seventh decade of life, more frequently in obese persons. There is no definite sex predilection [42, 72, 85].

Lipomas can be superficially or deeply located (subcutaneous or deep lipomas); they occur most common-

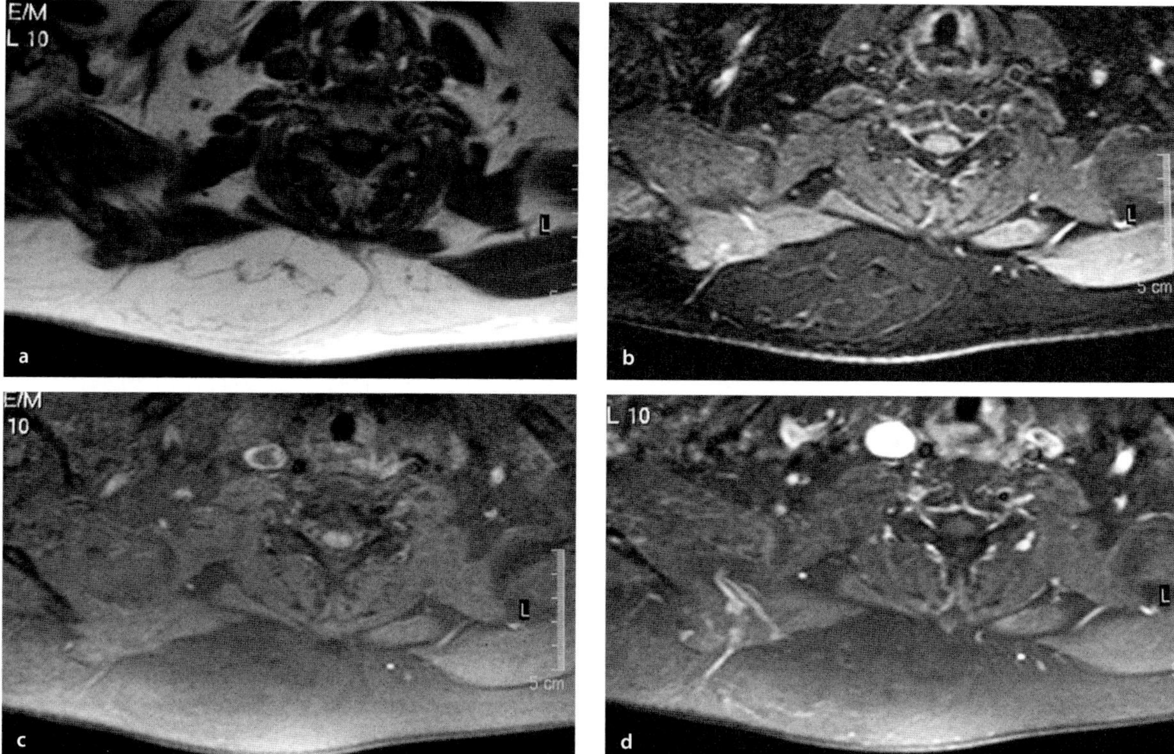

Fig. 15.2 a–d. Subcutaneous lipoma in the back. **a** Axial SE T1-weighted MR image. **b** Axial STIR image. **c** Axial FS SE T1-weighted MR image. **d** Axial FS SE T1-weighted MR image after gadolinium contrast administration. There is a well defined mass within the subcutaneous tissue of the back, with SI similar to that of adjacent subcutaneous fat on all pulse sequences (**a-b-c**). There are multiple septa within the mass, with low SI on T1-weighted images (**a**) and some of them displaying high SI on STIR images (**b**). In some of these septa, faint contrast enhancement is seen (**d**)

ly in the subcutaneous tissue and rarely in the deep soft tissue. Subcutaneous lipomas are most frequently found in the upper back and neck, shoulder, abdomen, and proximal portions of the extremities, while the less common deep lipomas occur most commonly in the chest wall, and subfascial tissues of the hands and feet [87]. Deep lipomas tend to be larger and less circumscribed than the superficial ones [46, 89].

Symptoms depend on the location and size of the tumors. A lipoma typically appears as a slowly growing, painless mass, but rapidly growing lipomas have been reported [117]. Pain is rare, but may occur as a consequence of nerve compression, and, depending on the location and relationship to adjacent structures, other symptoms such as carpal or tarsal tunnel syndrome have been reported [46]. Brady et al. have described recently one case of chronic lower extremity deep vein thrombosis associated with femoral vein compression by a lipoma [16]. Superficial lipoma manifests usually as a small mass, less than 5 cm, rarely exceeding 10 cm [46].

Subcutaneous lipomas are easily diagnosed at clinical examination, without the need for radiographic evaluation. The radiograph may occasionally demonstrate a radiolucent soft tissue mass and rarely osseous deformity by mass effect.

The most frequent sonographic appearance of lipoma is that of an elliptical, compressible and well-defined mass parallel to the skin surface, containing multiple echogenic lines (Fig. 15.1). Ahuja et al. have described the sonographic findings of 25 head and neck lipomas, and they have noted that 76% of all lipomas were hyperechoic, 8% isoechoic, and 16% hypoechoic in comparison with adjacent muscle and without any flow on color Doppler sonography [1].

On CT and MR images, lipomas present as homogeneous, well-circumscribed and encapsulated masses of fatty nature, without enhancement after intravenous contrast administration. The differentiation between the superficial lipoma and the surrounding fat may be difficult due to their similarity on density and SI (Fig. 15.2). Regular, thin septations can be seen both on CT and MR images [40, 56, 72, 91, 88, 145, 152, 156]. The septa appear as low-intensity strands on T1-weighted MR images, which may become hyperintense on T2-weighted MR images, and as soft-tissue density strands on CT scans. The width of these septa can be unmeasurable, with a slight enhancement after intravenous contrast administration, which is more clearly demonstrated on fat-suppressed T1-weighted MR images [71]. An unusual pattern, with diffuse enhancement after intravenous gadolinium administration, has been described by Hosono et al [60]. Lipomas composed of tissue other than adipose tissue may differ from the classic CT or MR imaging appearance (see Variants of Lipoma).

15.2.1.1 Multiple Lipomas

Some patients, especially males, may have multiple lipomas, which are grossly and microscopically similar to other lipomas. They occur predominantly in the back, shoulder, and upper arms, sometimes in a symmetrical distribution [46, 72]. There exists a familiar disorder, referred to as "familial multiple lipoma," which show this typical clinical presentation. Associated hyperlipidemia and hypercholesterolemia have been described in some cases [46, 132].

15.2.2 Variants of Lipoma

Lipomas containing other mesenchymal elements are classified as fibrolipoma, myxolipoma, chondroid lipoma, osteolipoma, myolipoma, or angiolipoma depending on the associated tissue: fibrous connective tissue, mucoid, cartilaginous, bony elements, smooth muscle, or small and thin-walled vessels, respectively. The presence of nonlipomatous areas can alter the MRI appearance of a simple lipoma, making the differential diagnosis with well-differentiated liposarcoma sometimes complicated [58, 59].

Occasionally, lipoma shows no evidence of fat on MR images [40]. These lipomas are usually suggestive of malignancy and may be indistinguishable on CT or MR images from other soft tissue tumors.

In this section, benign lipomatous tumors containing nonlipomatous elements is discussed. Furthermore, the discussion of the variants of lipoma also focuses on those subtypes that differ clinically and histologically from lipoma, such as angiolipoma, lipoblastoma, spindle cell lipoma, and pleomorphic lipoma. Extrarenal angiomyolipoma and extra-adrenal myelolipoma are rare variants, which are not discussed in detail.

15.2.2.1 Fibrolipoma

Fibrous connective tissue is the most common nonlipomatous element found in benign lipomatous tumors, often with the configuration of septa [71]. When lipoma contains connective tissue (fibrolipoma), it may demonstrate some areas of low SI on T1- and T2-weighted images [40, 56].

15.2.2.2 Myxolipoma

If there is myxoid degeneration, lipomas may also display areas of low SI on T1-weighted MR images and high signal on T2-weighted MR images [30, 40, 56].

15.2.2.3 Chondroid Lipoma

This is a rare lipomatous tumor, with a variable background of mature fat with cells resembling lipoblasts and brown fat cells, showing features of both lipoma and hibernoma. It contains myxoid and chondroid material and pathologically mimics myxoid liposarcoma and myxoid chondrosarcoma [46, 64]. Meis et al. have reported 20 patients, with an average age of 36 years (range 14–70 years old), with tumors measuring 1.5–11 cm in size (median, 4 cm) [112]. Chondroid lipoma manifests as a well-circumscribed mass in the subcutis, superficial fascia, or muscles of the extremities and occasionally in the trunk and head and neck [14, 119] and is mostly found in women [112]. The lesion appears as a well-defined mass with prominent fluid-like areas at sonography and CT. Areas of bright echogenicity have been described also [64]. Calcification is usually present on CT scans and radiographs [64, 119]. The presence and nature of the calcifications – which can be irregular and curvilinear – can raise the possibility of either a malignant diagnosis (including synovial sarcoma, malignant peripheral nerve sheath tumor, epithelioid hemangioendothelioma) or a benign diagnosis (e.g., myositis ossificans) [64]. On MR images, a predominant low SI is seen on T1-weighted images, with a only a few strands of high SI identical to fat, either in the periphery or the center of the lesion [119]. These lacy strands of high SI on T1-weighted images are suppressed on STIR images. On T2-weighted MR images, the mass is inhomogeneous and hyperintense, reflecting the largely myxoid consistency of the tumor (Fig. 15.3.). Other features of the mass, such as fine septations and a lobulated margin suggest cartilage matrix [99]. However, chondroid lipoma demonstrates a whole spectrum of cellular and matrix content, which is reflected in variable MR imaging characteristics [14]. Based on the MRI characteristics, chondroid lipoma is difficult to distinguish from myxoid liposarcoma, extraskeletal myxoid chondrosarcoma, and ancient schwannoma [14]. Because MR imaging cannot differentiate absolutely between malignant and benign lesions, biopsy is required to make a final diagnosis [64].

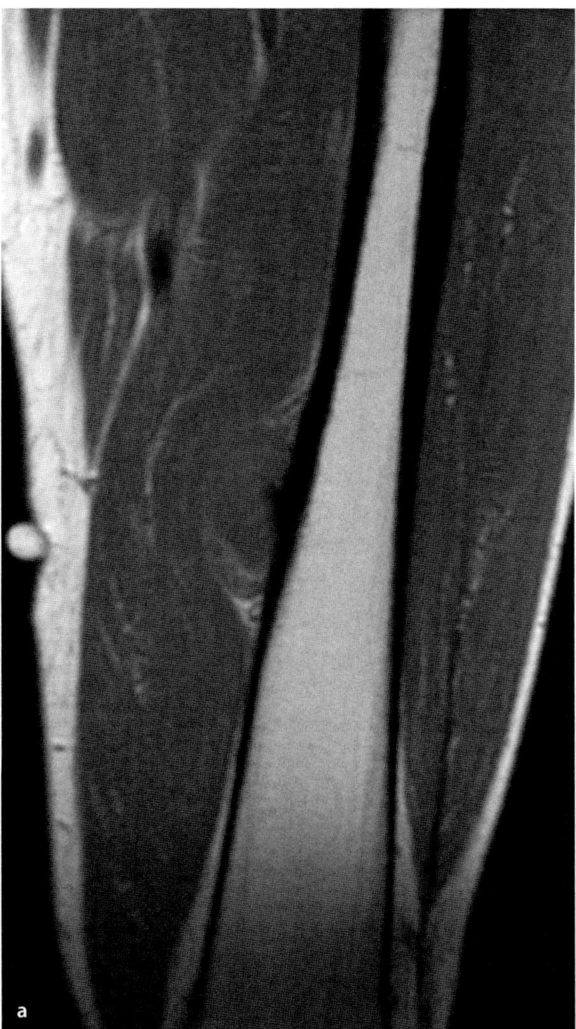
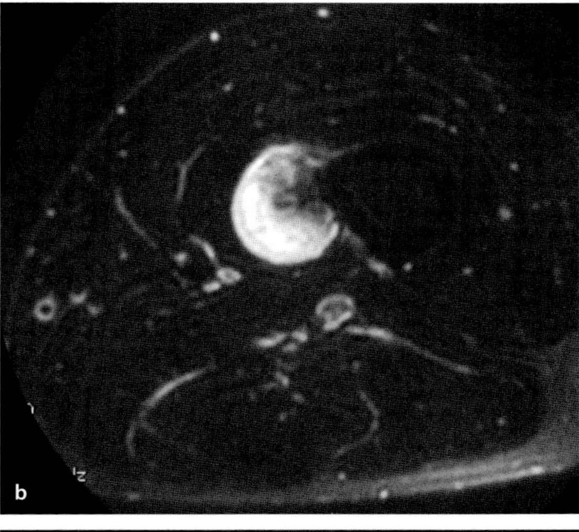
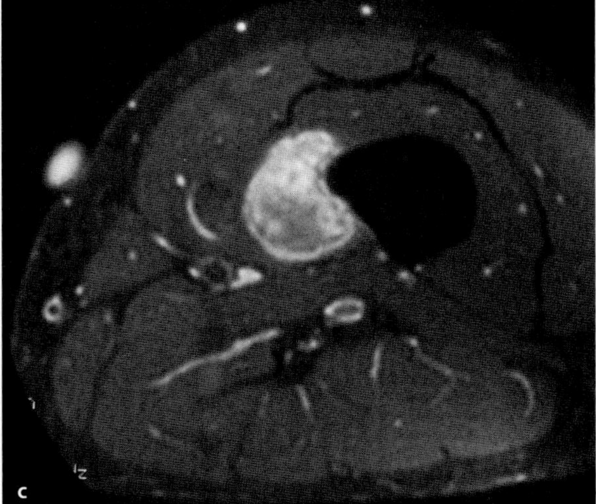

Fig. 15.3 a–c. Chondroid lipoma within the medial aspect of the left vastus intermedius muscle. **a** Coronal SE T1-weighted MR image. **b** Axial FS T2-weighted MR image. **c** Axial FS SE T1-weighted MR image after gadolinium contrast administration. The lesion abuts the cortical bone of the femur and is of predominant low signal intensity seen on T1-weighted images, with only a few strands of high signal intensity identical to fat within the lesion. The external cortex is irregularly delineated (**a**). On FS T2-weighted MR image, these strands are suppressed. The bulk of the tumor is – however – of high SI, reflecting the largely myxoid consistency (**b**). After gadolinium administration, there is a heterogeneous enhancement (**c**)

15.2.2.4 Ossifying Lipoma and Osteolipoma

Osseous metaplasia occurring within a lipoma is referred to as osteolipoma or ossifying lipoma. If the fat component is predominant, the tumor is designated as an ossifying lipoma, whereas the term osteolipoma is used in those lesions without a predominant fat component [98, 128, 129].

The pathogenesis of this rare tumor is still debated. Single or repeated trauma or local ischemia have been suggested as causes of bone formation. According to others, the osseous metaplasia results from blood-borne monocytes entering the tissue and releasing an osteo-inducing factor that results in transformation of fibroblasts into osteoblasts. Ossification from preexisting fibrofatty mesenchymal elements has also been suggested. Most likely, the tumor represents a benign mesenchymoma in which mesenchymal cells differentiate to bone [57, 98].

Within the soft tissues, the tumor may be located at the head and neck area and wrist, although location within the central nervous system at the tuber cinereum, hypothalamic and suprasellar region, and spinal canal has been reported also [98].

Imaging modalities such as standard radiography and CT scan are useful diagnostic tools to demonstrate the ossified components, whereas MR allows further identification of the adipose tissue component. Definitive diagnosis requires pathological examination of the specimen after excision. The patient's prognosis after excision is favorable.

15.2.2.5 Myolipoma

Myolipoma of soft tissue is a rare benign tumor exhibiting features of mature smooth muscle and mature adipose tissue [26]. It is also known as "extrauterine lipoleiomyoma." The lesion is most frequently located in the abdominal cavity, retroperitoneum, and inguinal areas, and more rarely in the subcutis of the trunk and extremities [119]. The majority of the lesions (especially the deeply located abdominal lesions) are large at initial presentation, ranging from 17 to 25 cm in diameter [119].

Due to the presence of nonlipomatous elements within the tumor, imaging does not allow distinction from a well-differentiated liposarcoma. Coarse calcification may be seen in large lesions [119]. On immunohistochemical analysis, smooth muscle components are strongly positive for smooth muscle actin and desmin [119]. Treatment consists of surgical resection. No recurrence or malignant transformation has been described.

15.2.2.6 Angiolipoma

This tumor is composed of mature fat cells and a network of small vessels, containing typical fibrin thrombi. These features allow differentiation from lipoma and from intramuscular hemangioma with prominent fatty elements [46]. It occurs in young adults, being rare in children and in patients older than 50 years.

Angiolipomas have been divided into noninfiltrating and infiltrating types [41]. The most common type is

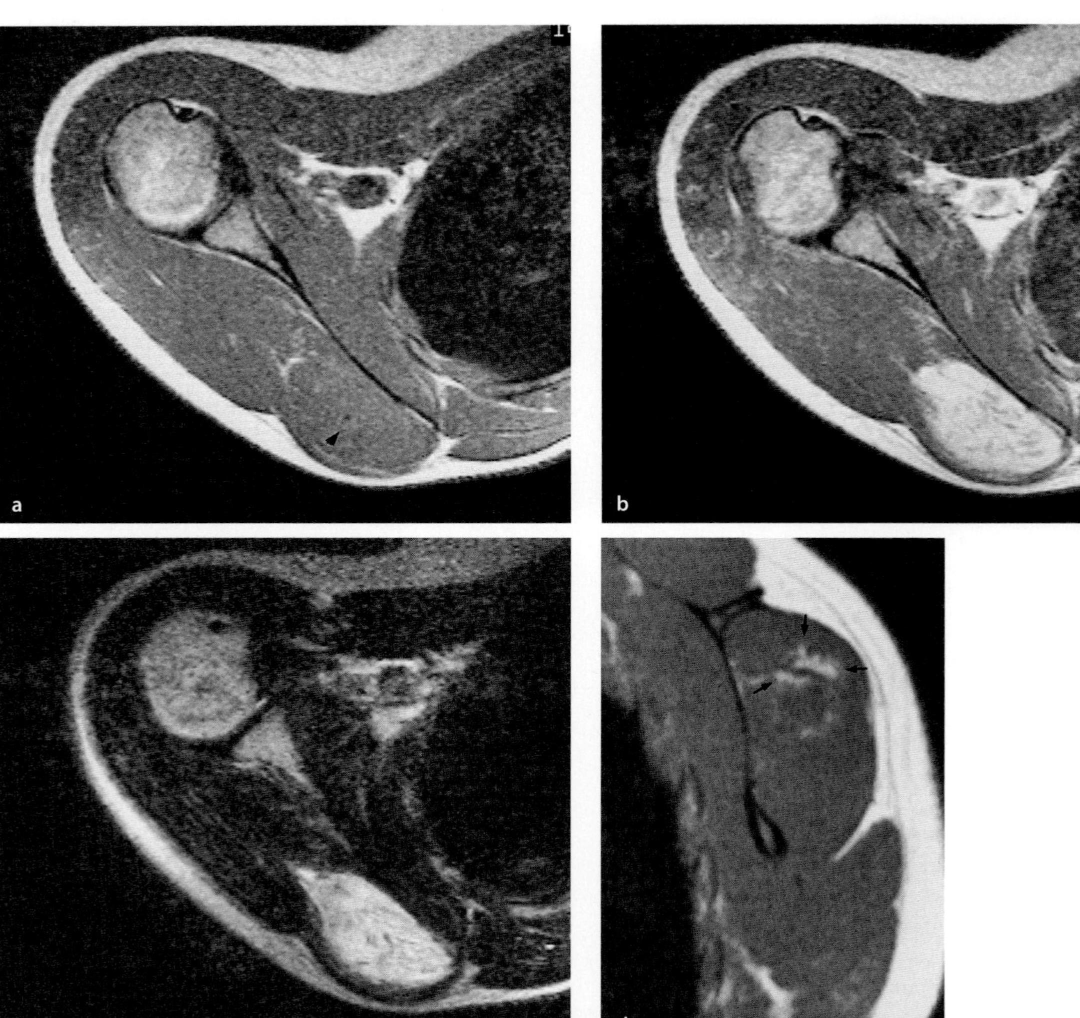

Fig. 15.4a–d. Angiolipoma of right infraspinatus muscle in a 17-year-old girl. **a** Axial SE T1-weighted MR image. **b** Axial SE T1-weighted MR image after Gd-contrast injection. **c** Axial SE T2-weighted MR image. **d** Parasagittal SE T1-weighted MR image. On T1-weighted MR images, there is a mass lesion which is nearly isointense to muscle (**a**). Within the lesion there are tiny fatty components (small arrows) and a few signal voids (arrowhead) (**a, d**). On T2-weighted images, the lesion is of higher SI than fat. There is marked enhancement after gadolinium injection(**b**). MRI does not allow differentiation between intramuscular angioma and angiolipoma. Tiny fatty components can be found in both lesions

the noninfiltrating type, which presents as a small (median size, 2 cm), encapsulated, subcutaneous nodule located in the trunk, upper arm, and particularly the forearm, rarely affecting the face, hands, or feet [46, 91]. Multiplicity of these lesions is frequent [46]. The infiltrating angiolipoma is a rare, locally aggressive, and unencapsulated variant containing foci of angiomatous proliferation [24, 91]. Imaging is only required in the infiltrating variant of this tumor. On plain radiographs this tumor may show as a mass of fat density, with serpiginous densities and punctate calcifications [24]. On CT scans it usually shows as a poorly delineated heterogeneous intramuscular lesion, with attenuation values ranging from those of fat to those of muscle. This variant has a hypervascular pattern on angiography that can be incorrectly diagnosed as a soft tissue sarcoma [24, 72].

On MR images, angiolipoma shows a mixed composition of both fatty and vascular elements. Signal intensities depend on the relative proportion of tumor components. The nonfatty areas exhibit low SI on T1-weighted images, high SI on T2-weighted images and enhance markedly after intravenous injection of gadolinium contrast (Fig. 15.4). The excision of this tumor is rarely radical, due to its poorly circumscribed margins and muscle invasion, and local recurrence is common [24].

15.2.2.7 Lipoblastoma

Lipoblastoma is a well-encapsulated lesion, confined to the subcutis, and is composed of lobules of fat with septations, lipocytes, and lipoblasts (immature fat cells) and poorly differentiated mesenchymal cells in a myxoid stroma with lipoblasts in different stages of development [27, 46]. If it infiltrates the subcutis and adjacent muscles and extends across anatomical planes, it is referred to as lipoblastomatosis. The term "lipoblastoma" was first used in 1926 by Jaffe to describe an embryonic fat cell tumor; whereas the term "lipoblastomatosis" was used in 1958 by Vellios et al. to describe the unencapsulated, diffuse form [74, 150]. Lipoblastoma is approximately twice as common as lipoblastomatosis, which is generally more deeply located [46].

Eighty-eight percent of lipoblastomas occur in patients below 3 years of age, 55% of the cases in patients below 1 year of age, and in some instances they are present at birth [27, 142]. The occurrence of lipoblastoma in patients older than 8 years of age is rare, although it has been documented in some patients of 10–18 years of age [28, 61, 76]. Lipoblastoma affects more often boys than girls [27, 28, 46, 87]. This entity most commonly occurs in the extremities, but lipoblastoma may be apparent in other locations such as the trunk, head, neck, axilla, prevertebral soft tissues, mediastinum, or retroperitoneum [27, 65, 76, 85, 142].

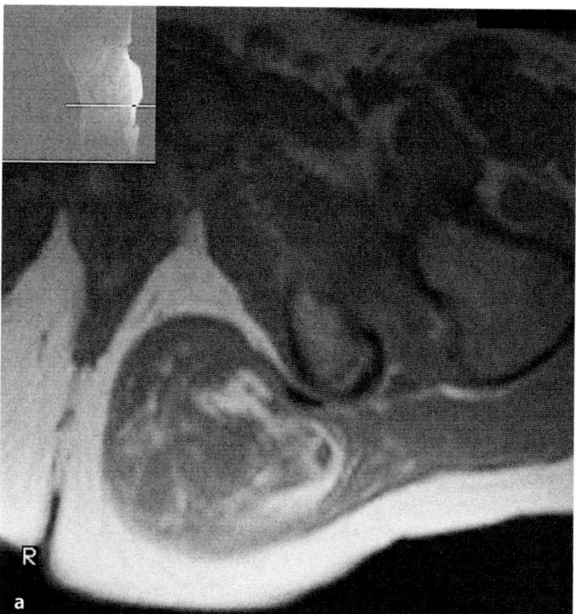

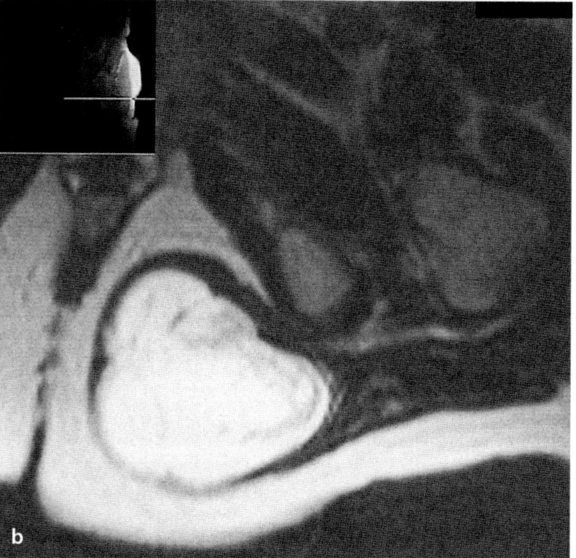

Fig. 15.5 a, b. Lipoblastoma of the buttocks in a 5-year-old boy. **a** Axial SE T1-weighted MR image. **b** Axial TSE T2-weighted MR image. The lesion is located in the medial part of the gluteus maximus muscle protruding into the left ischiorectal fossa. On T1-WI the mass is heterogeneous and ill defined with interspersed areas of high SI (**a**). On T2-WI the lesion is well defined and of overall high SI (**b**). The presence of fatty components is indicative for the lipomatous nature of the tumor. Although MR images do not allow differentiation from liposarcoma, the age of the patient is much in favor of a lipoblastoma

In a review of 25 cases, Collins et al. have reported 11 lipoblastomas and 14 cases of lipoblastomatosis, with 19 cases (79%) occurring in boys; 84% of the patients were less than 5 years old. These lesions measured 1–21 cm in greatest dimension, but 60% measured less

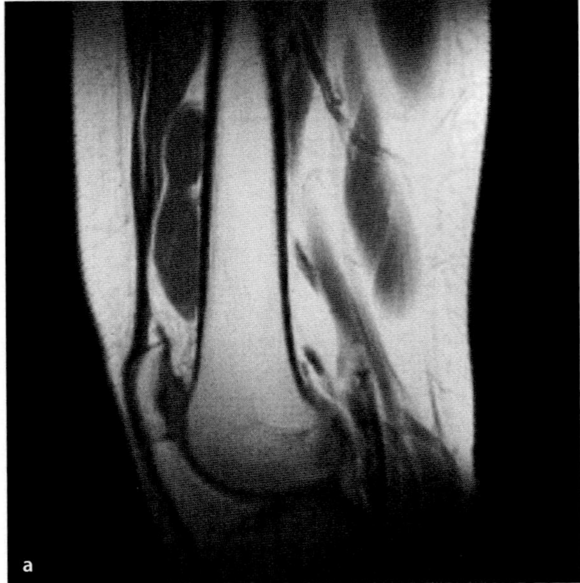

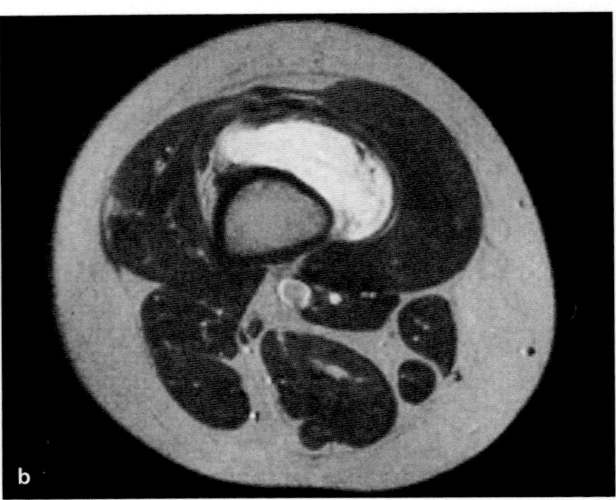

Fig. 15.6 a, b. Lipoblastoma of the thigh in a 30-year-old woman. **a** Sagittal SE T1-weighted MR image. **b** Axial SE T2-weighted MR image. Dumbbell-shaped lesion located between the distal femoral diaphysis and the vastus intermedius muscle. The lesion is isointense to muscle on T1-weighted images (**a**) and has a very high SI on T2-weighted images (**b**). The presence of abundant immature fat cells is probably responsible for the lower SI of the lesion on T1-weighted images. As a consequence such lesions are hardly differentiated from myxoid tumors

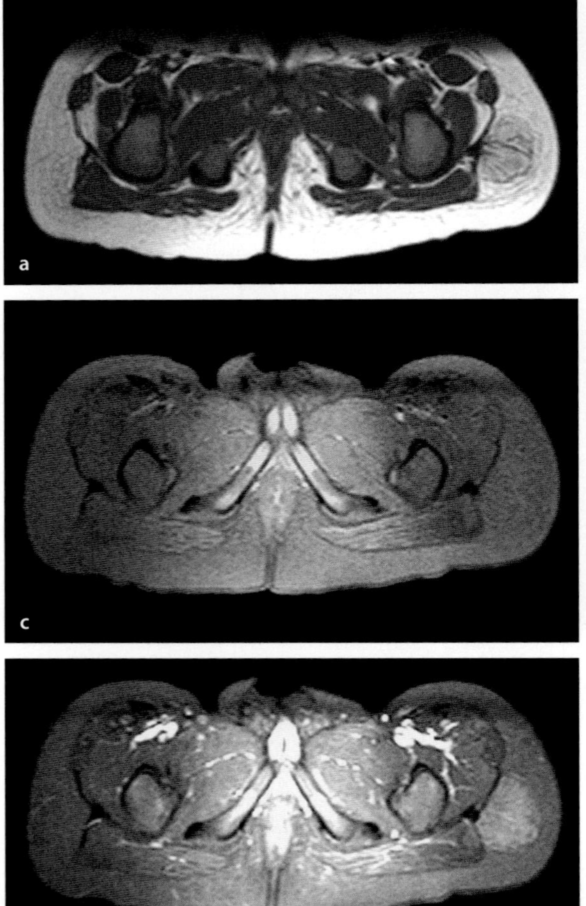

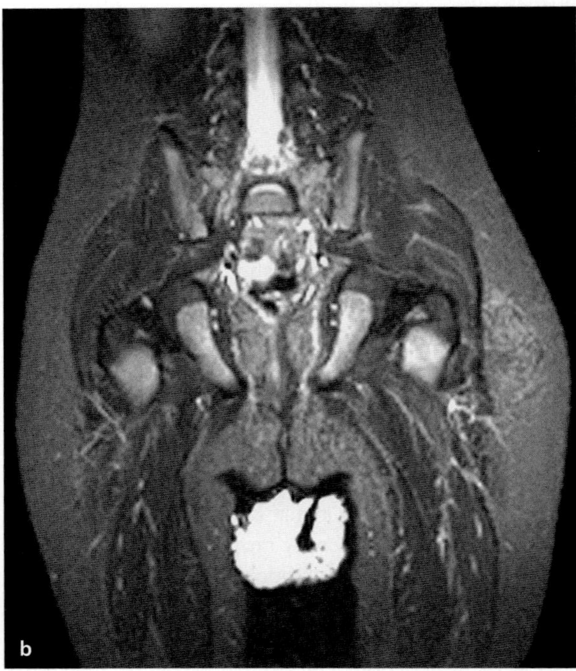

Fig. 15.7 a–d. Lipoblastoma of the buttocks in a 5-year-old boy. **a** Axial SE T1-weighted MR image. **b** Coronal FS TSE T2-weighted MR image. **c** Axial FS SE T1-weighted MR image. **d** Axial FS SE T1-weighted MR image after gadolinium contrast administration. The lesion is located within the left buttocks. On T1-WI the mass is heterogeneous, isointense to subcutaneous tissue and ill defined with interspersed strands of low SI (**a**). These strands are slightly hyperintense on FS T2-WI (**b**) and only a faint contrast enhancement is seen in these nonlipomatous areas (**d**). The presence of fatty components is indicative for the lipomatous nature of the tumor. The age of the patient is an important clue in favor of a lipoblastoma

than 5 cm [28]. The relative number of lipoblastoma and lipoblastomatosis in a series of 114 cases of the Armed Forces Institute of Pathology (AFIP), was 88 well-circumscribed lesions (lipoblastomas) compared with 26 diffuse forms (lipoblastomatosis) [87].

Lipoblastoma usually is a painless, soft tissue mass. The symptoms, although rare, are determined by the size and the location of the tumor. Surgical excision is the treatment of choice and is usually curative in lipoblastoma. Recurrence is rare and affects patients with the diffuse rather than the circumscribed type [28, 46]. Besides recurrence, lipoblastoma may have the capacity to differentiate into mature lesions, such as a lipoma or even fibrolipoma [28, 65, 130].

On sonography images, lipoblastoma manifests as a mass of mixed echogenicity, with highly echogenic regions interspersed with areas of diminished echogenicity [136].

The appearance on CT scans varies according to the amount of the adipose and other soft tissue components [12]. Lipoblastoma usually is seen as a fatty mass with scattered foci of soft tissue density [76, 142].

On MR images lipoblastoma/lipoblastomatosis is mostly bright on T1- and T2-weighted images, but it may be hypointense to subcutaneous fat on T1-weighted images, without the signal characteristics of a fatty tumor [61, 65, 79, 130, 154]. Some hyperintense areas on T2-weighted MR images have been described, consistent with cystic or myxoid areas (Figs. 15.5–15.7). Lipoblastoma does not enhance or shows poor enhancement after intravenous gadolinium administration [61, 154].

The demonstration of a fatty mass on CT or MRI examination in an infant or child should raise the possibility of a lipoblastoma or lipoblastomatosis. Lipoma, lipoma variants, and liposarcoma are uncommon in infants and children. Radiologically and even on microscopic examination lipoblastoma may be misdiagnosed as liposarcoma, especially myxoid liposarcoma [61]. However, in the case of lipoblastoma, the clinical setting is

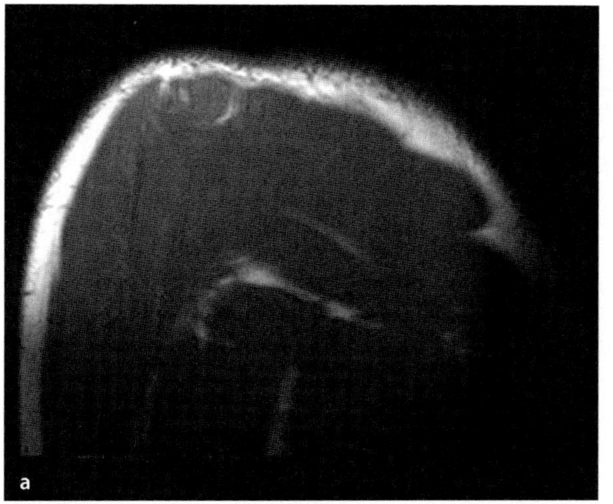

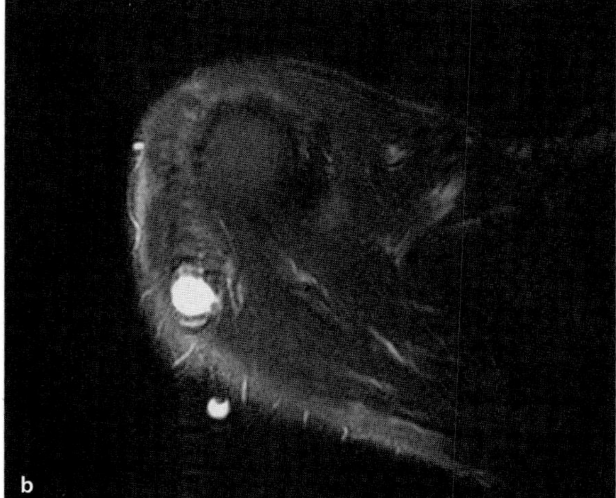

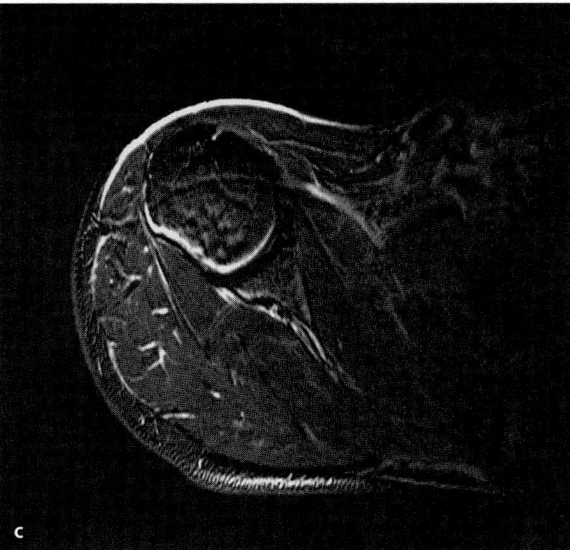

Fig. 15.8 a–c. Spindle cell lipoma within the deltoid muscle. **a** Sagittal SE T1-weighted MR image. **b** Axial FS TSE T2-weighted MR image. **c** Axial subtraction image of FS SE T1-weighted MR images before and after gadolinium contrast administration. The signal intensity of the lesion is predominantly isointense to muscle on T1-weighted images (**a**), whereas T2-weighted images show a high signal intensity (**b**). There is no significant enhancement (**c**)

quite distinct, since lipoblastoma occurs in children, while liposarcoma is very uncommon in this age group [39, 78]. Miller et al., in a review of 149 lipomatous tumors at a children's hospital, has reported 7 lipoblastomas and 2 liposarcomas [114]. The liposarcoma patients were aged 9 and 14 years, and the children with lipoblastoma were younger, but 29% were more than 3 years of age. In a review of more than 2,500 cases of liposarcoma at the AFIP, only two cases of liposarcoma occurred in children below 10 years old [87].

15.2.2.8 Spindle Cell Lipoma and Pleomorphic Lipoma

In these two clinically and pathologically related variants, the mature fat is replaced by collagen-forming spindle cells. Pleomorphic lipoma is considered as a pleomorphic variant of spindle cell lipoma and it is distinguished by the presence of a marked cellular pleomorphism and scattered bizarre giant cells. Histologically the differential diagnosis from liposarcoma may be difficult [46]. Spindle cell and pleomorphic lipomas typically present as a well-circumscribed nodule, confined to the subcutis of the neck or shoulder region in male patients older than 45 years [66]. These lipomas usually manifest as a slow-growing, painless, solitary mass, with an average size between 3 and 5 cm. Although rare, multiple spindle cell lipomas have been described [51, 111]. Fanburg-Smith et al. have reported 7 familial and 11 nonfamilial cases of multiple spindle cell lipomas, all occurring in male patients, and most of them in the sixth to eighth decades of life [51]. These patients had between 2 and more than 220 lesions, on the posterior neck or back and involving also the shoulders.

Pleomorphic and spindle cell lipomas may manifest as inhomogeneous, nonspecific fatty masses with non-lipomatous components that show increased density on CT scans and long relaxation times on both T1- and T2-weighted MR images (Fig. 15.8). A spindle cell lipoma with marked bone erosion of the foot has been documented [17]. Radiologically pleomorphic and spindle cell lipomas are frequently misdiagnosed as liposarcoma [17, 91]. A spindle cell variant of well-differentiated liposarcoma has to be differentiated from a benign spindle cell lipoma [33].

15.2.3 Heterotopic Lipomas

The group of heterotopic lipomas includes lesions that arise or develop in association with tissues other than the adipose tissue.

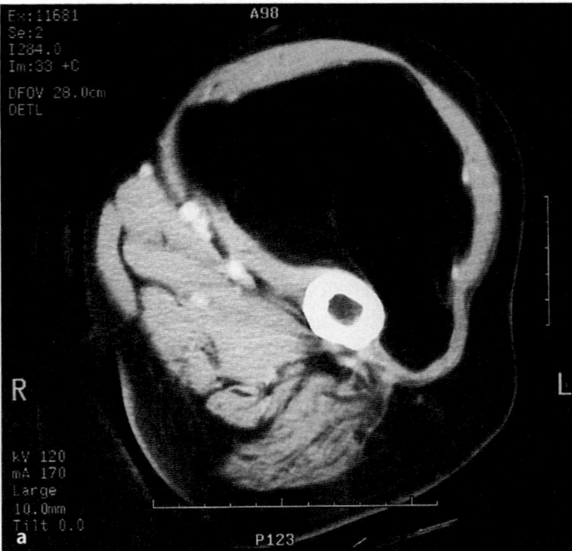

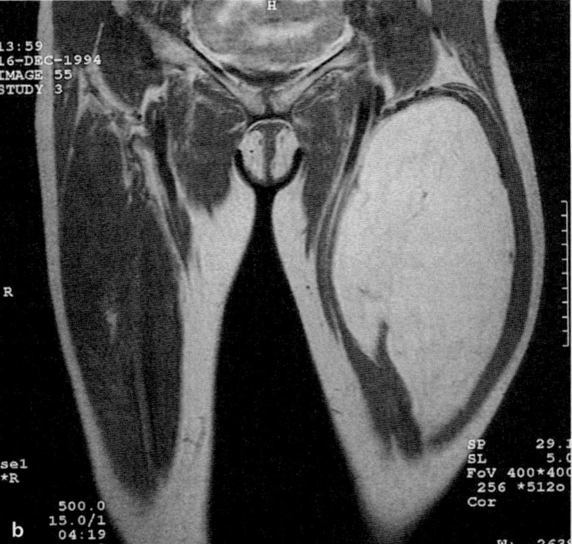

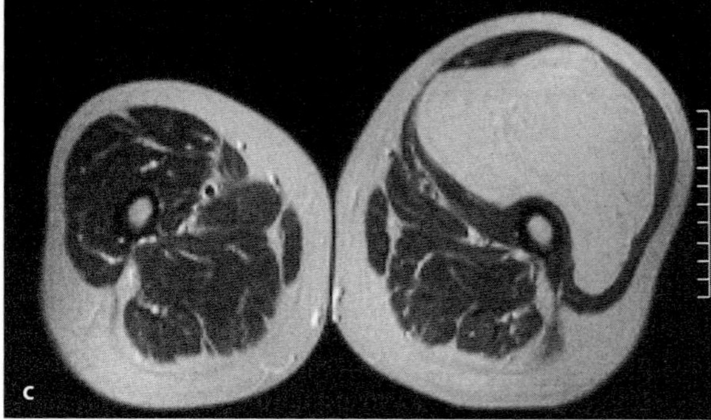

Fig. 15.9 a–c. Intramuscular lipoma of the thigh in a 61-year-old woman. **a** CT scan. **b** Coronal SE-T1-weighted MR image. **c** Axial TSE T2-weighted MR image. Large mass in the quadriceps muscle of the left thigh with low attenuation values on CT (**a**). Note the presence of multiple intratumoral strands of higher density on CT (**a**) and lower SI (**b, c**) on MRI. The signal intensity on different MR sequences equals that of fat (**b, c**)

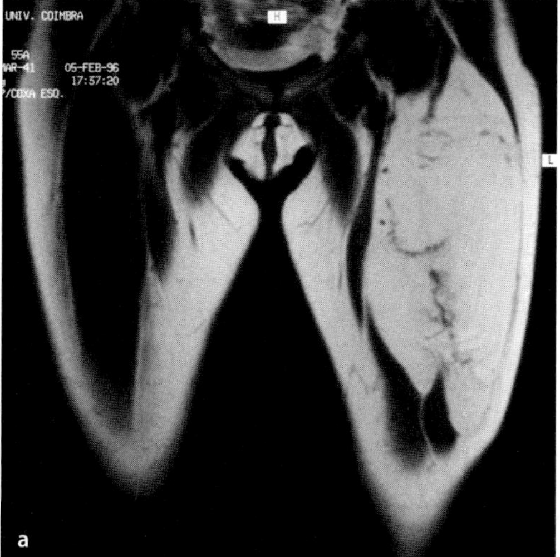
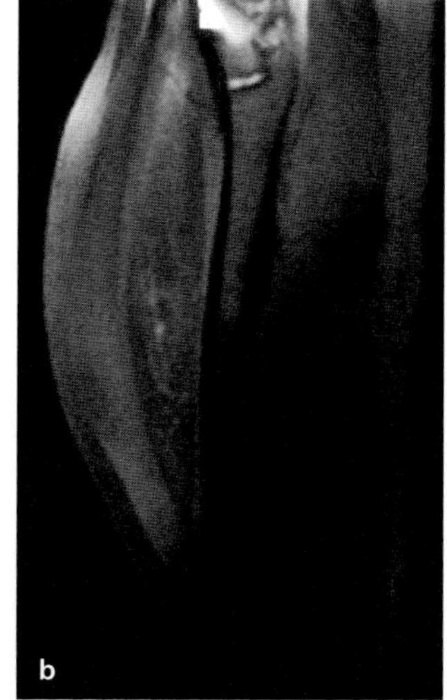
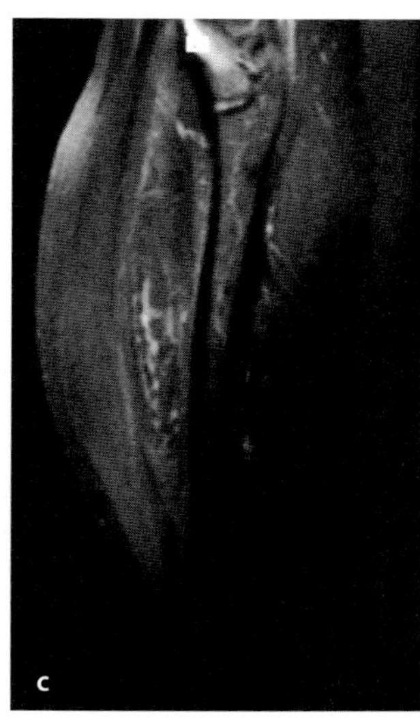

Fig. 15.10a–c. Intramuscular lipoma of the thigh in a 55-year-old woman **a** Coronal SE T1-weighted MR image. **b** Sagittal fat-suppressed SE T1-weighted MR image. **c** Sagittal fat-suppressed SE T1-weighted MR image after Gadolinium contrast injection. On T1-weighted MR image there is a large mass in the quadriceps muscle, with SI identical to that of fat, containing irregularly linear septa of low SI (**a**). On fat-suppressed SE T1-weighted image, there is a reduction in the lesion's SI, according to its fatty nature (**b**). After intravenous gadolinium administration, there is a distinct enhancement of the septa, well-demonstrated on a fat-suppressed SE T1-weighted image (**c**). These characteristics are very frequently seen in well-differentiated liposarcomas, as well, making the differential diagnosis with lipoma extremely difficult

15.2.3.1 Intramuscular and Intermuscular Lipoma

On gross inspection of intramuscular and intermuscular lipomas, fat has replaced the muscle tissue. Microscopically mature lipocytes infiltrate the muscle fibers which may show some degree of atrophy. Widespread invasion of one or more muscles may occur. Intramuscular lipoma has also been referred to as "infiltrating lipoma" due to its frequently infiltrative aspect on histological examination. Intramuscular lipoma is more frequent than the intermuscular variant and it can affect both the muscular and intermuscular tissues [8, 91].

Intramuscular lipoma affects all age groups, mostly occurring in patients over 40 years of age, and, although rare, it has also been reported in children [46, 65]. Most authors have described a male predominance. These lesions tend to involve most commonly the large muscles of the extremities, especially of the thigh, trunk, shoulder, and upper arm [46, 87].

The clinical picture is one of a painless, slow-growing lesion, but occasionally the symptoms may be very different from those of the common subcutaneous variety, and intramuscular lipoma may present as a rapidly growing mass with nerve entrapment [117]. The size of the lipoma varies from a small mass of less than 3 cm to more than 20 cm in diameter [46, 107]. The imaging findings in these heterotopic lipomas are basically the same as in other lipomas [60, 107, 117]. Although most of the intramuscular lipomas are well-defined lesions on CT or MR images, they also may show infiltrative margins, corresponding to the infiltrative type of intramuscular lipoma [20, 65, 91, 107]. On CT and on MR images, some intramuscular lipomas are septate, inhomogeneous masses, with tissue attenuation and interspersed regions of decreased signal on T1- and T2-weighted images, which probably represent either muscle or fibrous tissue within the mass [88, 107, 152, 155] (Fig. 15.9). Matsumoto et al. have reported the MR findings of 17 cases of intramuscular lipoma, 12 being homogeneous and the remaining 5 inhomogeneous with intermingled muscle fibers that were isointense with normal muscle on both T1- and T2-weighted images [107].

The infiltrative nature, which mostly characteristic of malignant tumors, is in favor of benignity, in the case of intramuscular lipoma [107]. These thin or thick linear structures, with low SI on both T1- and T2-weighted images, demonstrate no enhancement in the majority of cases, although faint enhancement may be seen [107] (Fig. 15.10). Intramuscular lipoma most often is a uninodular mass, but binodularity was seen in a minority of cases (2/17) in the series of Matsumoto [107]. Although absence of contrast enhancement and unilobularity are useful signs in the differential diagnosis of intramuscular lipoma from well-differentiated liposarcoma (Table 15.1), these signs are not 100% reliable. This makes the differential diagnosis with well-differentiated liposarcoma difficult, even on histological examination [20, 60, 107].

15.2.3.2 Lipoma of the Tendon Sheath and Joint

This is a very rare lesion that can be seen in two different forms. The first form is a lipomatous mass spreading along the tendon sheaths, usually in the hand or wrist and less frequently in the ankle and foot. Lipoma of tendon sheath usually occurs in young patients, affecting with equal frequency both sexes, and approximately 50% are bilateral [143]. Pain may be referred, and rupture of a tendon has been reported [46]. The lipoma of the tendon sheath manifests as a mass in every way similar to a simple lipoma (Fig. 15.11). The second form is an intra-articular, lipoma-like lesion, consisting of hypertrophic synovial villi distended by fat that replaces the subsynovial tissue. This lesion, called "lipoma arborescens" is more common than the tendon sheath variety.

Lipoma arborescens is of unknown etiology, but it is frequently associated with degenerative joint disease, diabetes mellitus, chronic synovitis, or rheumatoid arthritis and joint trauma. Therefore, lipoma arborescens is usually regarded as a nonspecific reactive and secondary process to traumatic or inflammatory stimuli, involving the synovial membrane [23, 46, 102, 140]. Hallel et al. have suggested renaming this process as "villous lipomatous proliferation of synovial membrane," since "lipoma arborescens" implies a neoplastic connotation [68]. However, according to Vilanova, a minority of lipoma arborescens may appear in joints with no other associated changes, and these lesions could be categorized rather as primary lipoma arborescens [151].

Lipoma arborescens is mainly found in adults, but it has also been documented in children from 9 years old [39, 67, 134, 140]. Some reports have shown that there is a male predominance [104, 139].

The knee is the usual site of involvement, with a predilection for the suprapatellar pouch, although it may also affect the wrist, hip, elbow, and ankle [67, 102, 105, 106, 134]. Bilateral presentation or even multiple joint involvement have been described [6, 105]. Only a few cases of lipoma arborescens of the shoulder have been reported, arising within the subdeltoid bursa in association with rotator cuff tears [31, 94, 122]. The typical clinical presentation is of painless joint swelling over many years, with intermittent effusion and limitation of motion [6]. On plain radiographs lipoma arborescens presents as soft tissue swelling, rarely with radiolucent areas [67, 102, 105]. Lipoma arborescens is displayed as a nonspecific synovially based lesion on ultrasound scans (Fig. 15.12) and at arthrography, the latter showing multiple, irregular filling defects [19, 67, 96, 106]. Dynamic compression during ultrasound demonstrates bending and deformation of the villous projections. CT and MRI demonstrate a frond-like fatty mass, arising from the synovium, associated with joint effusion [6, 23, 31, 52, 67, 105, 106, 122, 134, 140] (Figs. 15.13, 15.14). On MR images, the villous proliferations display a SI of fat on all pulse sequences and a chemical-shift artifact at the interface with the effusion [52, 122, 134]. No enhancement of the villous projections after intravenous contrast administration is noted [23]. A review of eight patients with lipoma arborescens of the knee, by Ryu et al., has demonstrated the presence

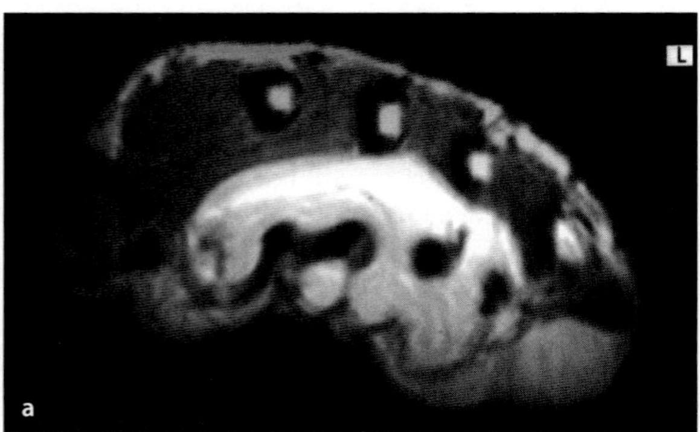

a

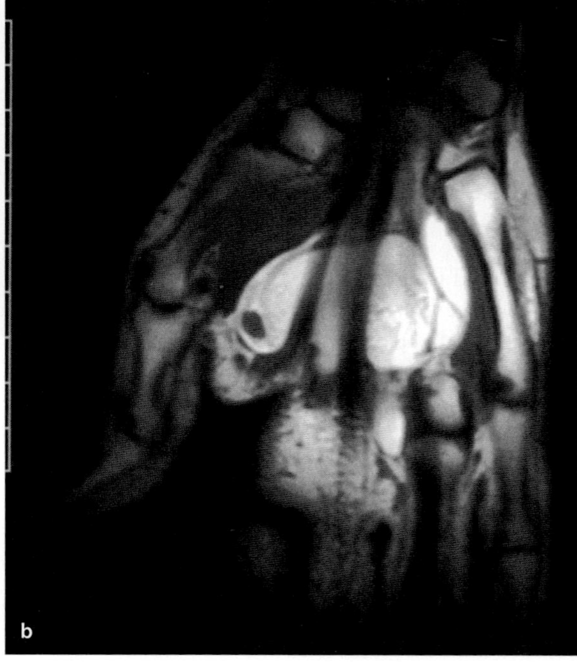

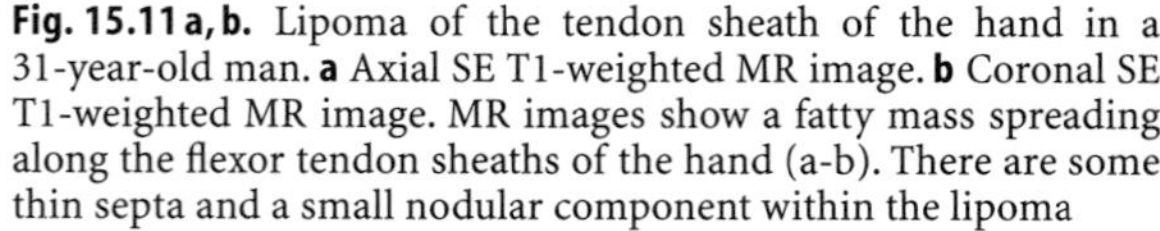

Fig. 15.11 a, b. Lipoma of the tendon sheath of the hand in a 31-year-old man. **a** Axial SE T1-weighted MR image. **b** Coronal SE T1-weighted MR image. MR images show a fatty mass spreading along the flexor tendon sheaths of the hand (a-b). There are some thin septa and a small nodular component within the lipoma

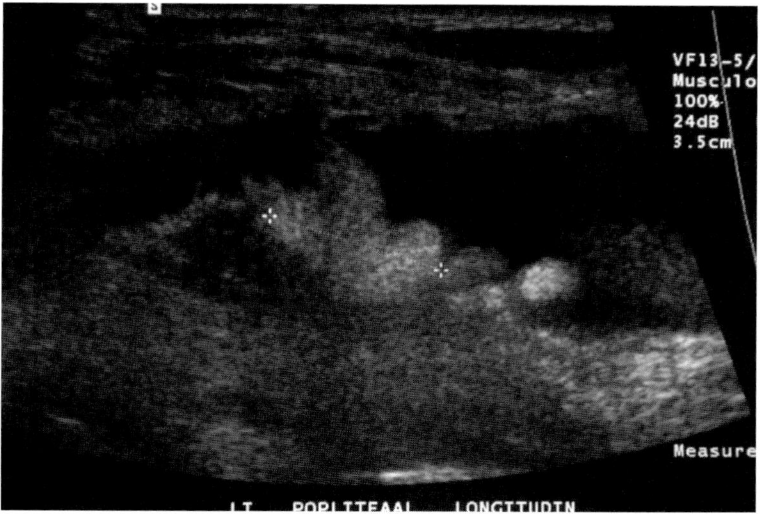

Fig. 15.12. Lipoma arborescens of the knee joint in a 40-year-old woman. Ultrasound of the knee demonstrates a hyperechoic synovially based mass with villous projections protruding within the suprapatellar bursa

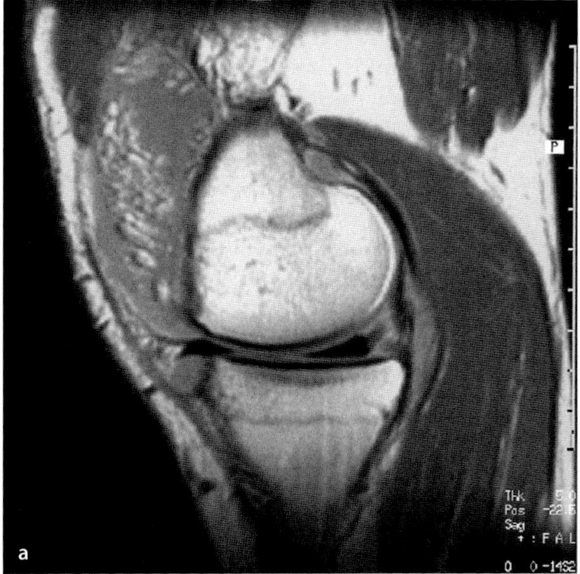

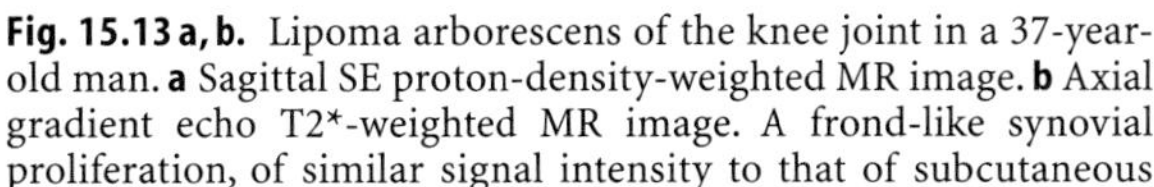

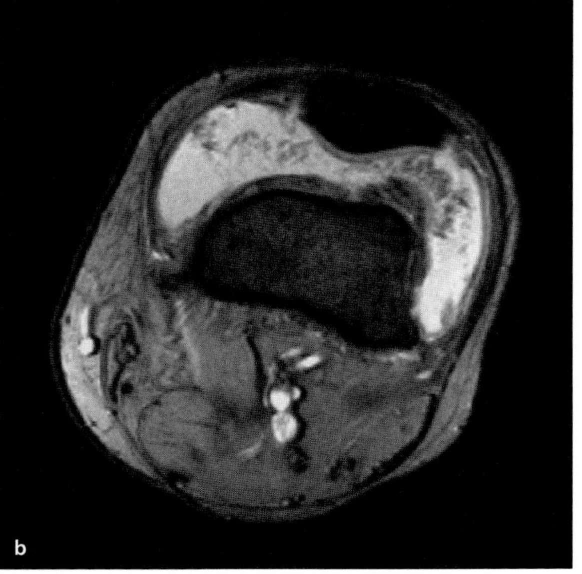

Fig. 15.13 a, b. Lipoma arborescens of the knee joint in a 37-year-old man. **a** Sagittal SE proton-density-weighted MR image. **b** Axial gradient echo T2*-weighted MR image. A frond-like synovial proliferation, of similar signal intensity to that of subcutaneous fat on all pulse sequences. They are located within the suprapatellar pouch, surrounded by a large effusion which is of intermediate SI on proton-density images (**a**) and high SI on T2-weighted images (**b**)

of mass-like subsynovial fat deposits, divided by septa of low SI on both T1- and T2-weighted images, in 38% of cases [134]. They have also found the presence of erosive bone changes at articular margins in three patients (38%), joint effusion in all eight (100%), and a synovial cyst in three (38%). Soler et al. have described the MR characteristics of lipoma arborescens in 13 knee joints and have found three patterns of presentation: multiple villous lipomatous synovial proliferations in 6, isolated, frond-like fatty subsynovial mass in 2, and a mixed pattern in 5 joints [140]. They speculate that the morphological pattern of presentation depends on the duration of the disease, with a longer delay in the group of patients with the mixed form. These lesions affected the suprapatellar bursa but also the posterior joint compartment and one Baker cyst.

The differential diagnosis includes the synovial lipoma, pigmented villonodular synovitis, synovial chondromatosis, plexiform neuroma, and synovial hemangiomatosis due to their identical clinical picture, but the differentiation is readily made by CT and especially by MRI. The recommended treatment for lipoma arborescens is surgical or arthroscopic synovectomy.

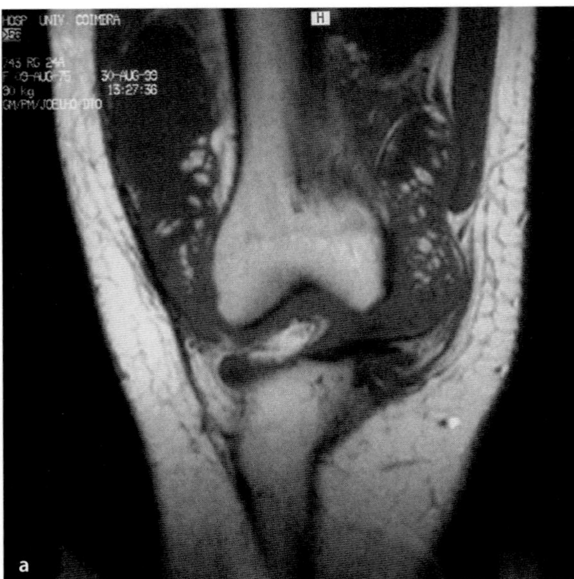

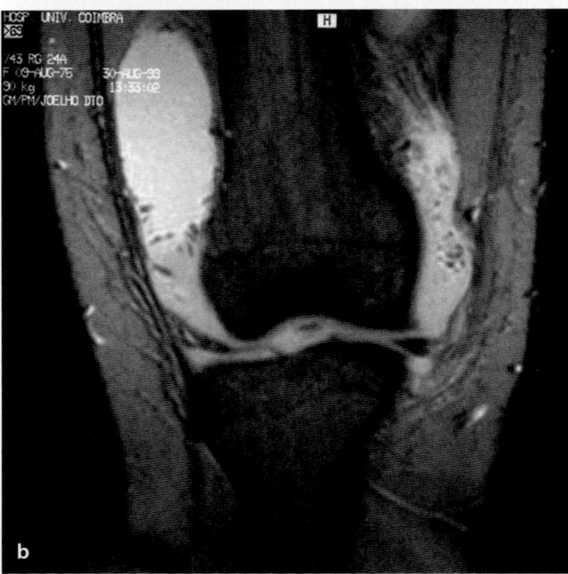

Fig. 15.14 a, b. Lipoma arborescens of the knee joint in a 24-year-old woman. **a** Coronal SE T1-weighted MR image. **b** Coronal gradient echo T2*-weighted MR image. The images demonstrate a large effusion and villous synovial projections, with a frond-like morphology. The signal intensity on T1-weighted image is similar to that of fat (**a**) and there is a decreased signal intensity of synovial proliferation on gradient echo sequence (**b**) as seen with subcutaneous fat

15.2.3.3 Lipomatosis of Nerve

Lipomatosis of nerve has also been designated in the past as fibrolipomatous hamartoma, fibrofatty overgrowth, lipomatous hamartoma, lipofibroma, neurolipoma, intraneural lipoma, fatty infiltration of the nerve, and neural fibrolipoma. In 2002, the WHO adopted the designation of lipomatosis of nerve [26, 119]. The common term "neural fibrolipoma" is, however, still fre-

quently used because it reflects the nature of this entity. It is a very rare tumor, characterized by a proliferation of fatty and fibrous components that surrounds the thickened nerve bundles and infiltrates both the epineurium and the perineurium. No vascular abnormalities are associated with the lesion [46]. Its cause is unknown, but some consider this condition as a congenital lesion, since it is occasionally present at birth, whereas others believe a relationship exists with history of a prior trauma. This tumor affects predominantly children or young adults, although a late presentation at the age of 75 years has been reported recently [22, 49, 103, 139, 153]. According to Enzinger et al., males are affected more frequently than females, although a similar incidence has also been noted [46, 85].

Lipomatosis of nerve occurs chiefly in the volar aspects of the hands, wrist, and forearm and usually involves the median nerve, although occasional involvement of other nerves such as the cubital, radial, ulnar, tibial, superficial peroneal, and sciatic has also been reported [34, 55, 103, 124, 139]. This entity is less common in the lower extremities. A soft tissue mass is frequently present several years before onset of symptoms. Lipomatosis of nerve usually gives rise to pain, paresthesia, or decreased sensation or muscle strength, in the area innervated by the affected nerves [139]. According to some authors, in 27–66% of patients with lipomatosis of nerve there is associated bone overgrowth and macrodactyly of either the fingers or the toes, a condition described as macrodystrophia lipomatosa [3, 46, 139]. Macrodactyly has also been noted in association with neurofibromatosis and vascular lesions or as idiopathic conditions [3]. On plain radiographs, lipomatosis of nerve may manifest by a soft tissue mass or will only be suspected by indirect signs such as the presence of macrodactyly, usually affecting the second and third digits of the hand or foot [15, 89, 139, 149]. There is a soft tissue and osseous hypertrophy, including long, broad and splayed phalanges (Fig. 15.15). Calcifications on plain radiographs due to metaplastic bone formation have been noted [103, 139].

CT and MRI can be used to identify the nervous origin of the tumor due to the presence of tortuous tubular structures, corresponding to enlarged nerve bundles within a predominantly fatty mass (Fig. 15.16). These structures, clearly depicted on MR images, show low SI on both T1- and T2-weighted images according to their fibrous content [15, 22, 32, 34, 49, 103, 124, 153]. According to De Maesseneer et al., the tumor has the tendency to spread along the branches of the nerve, with a significant variation in the distribution of fat along the nerves and their innervated muscle [33]. Marom et al. have reported the MR characteristics in another series of ten patients, in which all tumors consisted of serpiginous low-intensity structures surrounded by fatty tissue [103]. In 80% of the cases, the distribution of fat was

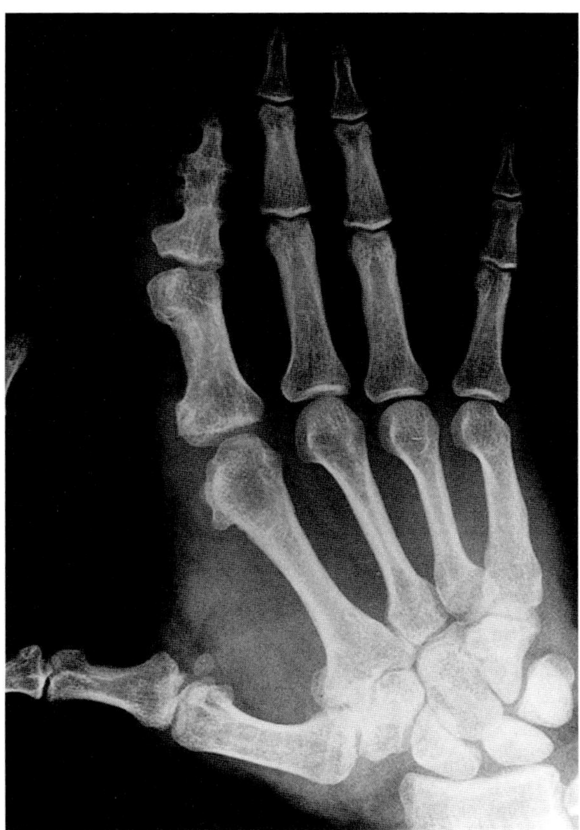

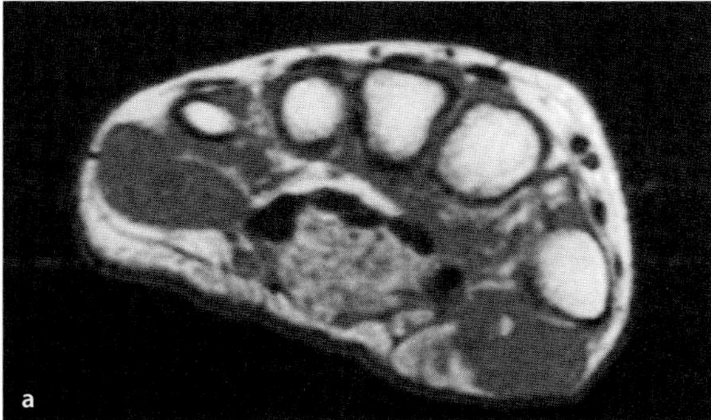

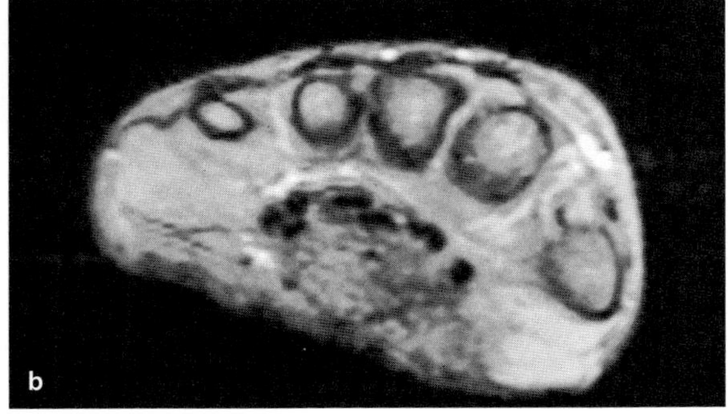

Fig. 15.16a, b. Lipomatosis of nerve of the median nerve at the level of the carpal tunnel in a 40-year-old man. **a** Axial SE T1-weighted MR image. **b** Axial gradient echo T2*-weighted MR image. These MR images reveal a heterogeneous mass within the carpal tunnel. There is a mixed SI of fatty components, fibrous components and neural fascicles (**a, b**). The signal intensity and localization are highly characteristic of a neurofibrolipoma of the median nerve

Fig. 15.15. Macrodystrophia lipomatosa. Posteroanterior radiograph. Osseous and soft tissue enlargement, affecting the second digit

between nerve fibers rather than around them. The contrast between the low-signal nerve fascicles and surrounding high-signal fat results in a "cable-like" appearance of the tumor, when visualized on axial planes on T1-weighted MR images and a "spaghetti-like" appearance on coronal planes [49, 103]. The MR imaging findings of lipomatosis of nerve are very characteristic and, according to Marom et al., they are pathognomonic, allowing a confident diagnosis, and obviating the need for biopsy [103]. Lipomatosis of nerve must be differentiated from a nerve sheath lipoma associated with altered sensibility along the course of some nerves. MRI allows differentiation between these two entities, since lipoma manifests as a focal mass separated from the nerve bundles [9]. Resection of involved neural elements causes considerable sensory and motor deficits, but the symptoms can be relieved by carpal tunnel release [15].

15.2.3.4 Parosteal Lipoma

When affecting the tissue adjacent to the bone, lipoma is referred to as parosteal lipoma [46, 62,119, 131]. Parosteal lipoma constitutes 0.3% of all lipomas and the imaging appearances are characteristic [53, 62]. The gross and histological findings of parosteal lipoma are similar to those of a subcutaneous lipoma, except that the lesion has a broad-based attachment to the subjacent bone [46, 121]. The parosteal lipoma is contiguous with underlying periosteum and some authors have referred to these lesions as "periosteal lipomas." However "parosteal" rather than "periosteal" is the preferred terminology, since fat cells are not found in the periosteum and it indicates contiguity with bone but avoids specifying the tissue of origin [35, 53, 62]. The lesion is often well encapsulated except at the site where it is adherent to the bone. The behavior and morphological and imaging findings of parosteal lipoma are generally identical to those of a subcutaneous lipoma.

The usual age of patients with this lesion is similar to that of those with subcutaneous lipoma, between 40 and 60 years, with a male predominance [62, 118]. The most frequent sites of parosteal lipomas are the arm, forearm, thigh, and calf, adjacent to the diaphysis or diametaphysis of the bone. Other locations have been reported, such as the finger, mandible, shoulder, and adjacent to the upper sacrum and iliac bone [35, 53, 62, 77, 118]. Parosteal lipoma is usually a slow-growing, generally

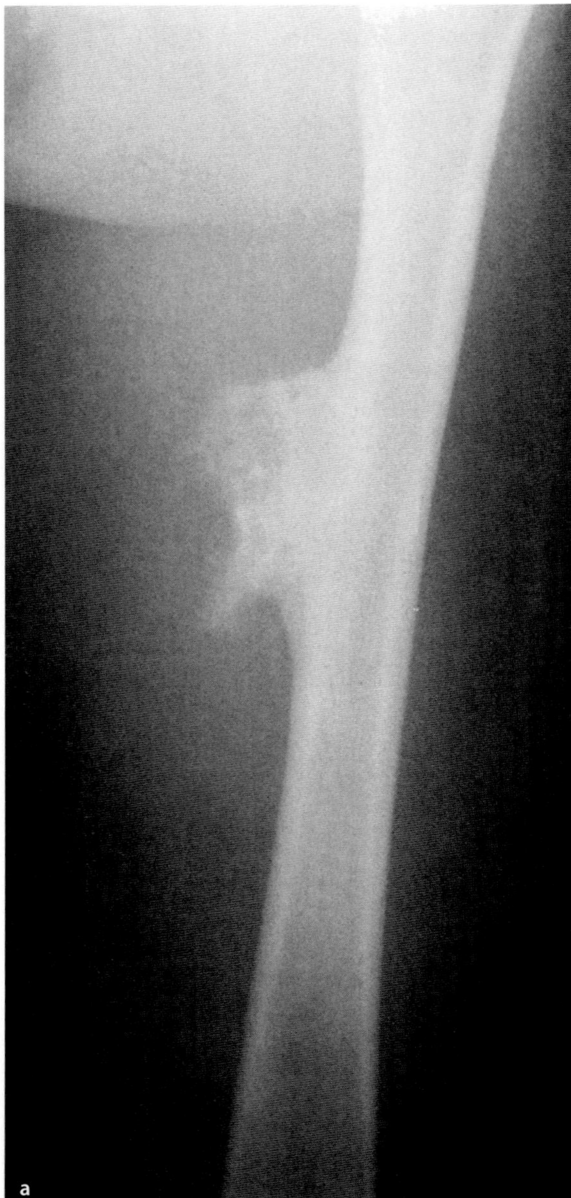

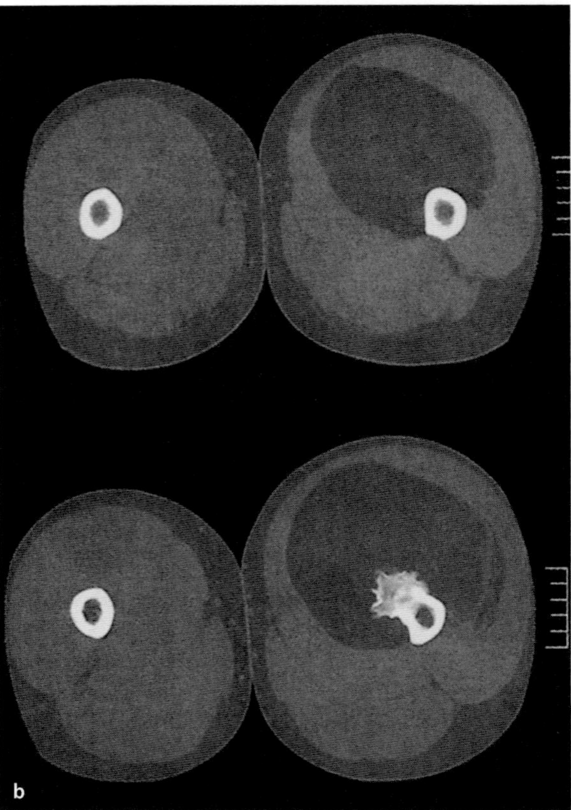

Fig. 15.17 a, b Parosteal lipoma in a 30-year-old man. **a** Radiograph of the left femur. **b** CT of both thighs. The radiograph shows a large soft tissue mass around an exostotic-like lesion at the medial border of the left femur (**a**). There is no continuity between the medullary bone of the femoral shaft and the exostosis. On CT scans, the exostotic lesion at the medial aspect of the left femur is surrounded by a large, well-circumscribed fatty mass (– 80 HU) within or displacing the left quadriceps muscle (**b**). (Case courtesy of D. Frère et al., Brussels)

asymptomatic, large mass, measuring up to 20 cm maximal diameter [53, 131]. Neurological symptoms due to nerve compression have been described in the proximal forearm, with paralysis of the posterior interosseous nerve, but involvement of the radial, sciatic, ulnar, and median nerves has also been reported, resulting in motor and/or sensory disturbances [121].

On plain radiographs this tumor may manifest as a radiolucent lesion in the soft tissues adjacent to cortical bone, with or without osseous change (Fig. 15.17). In parosteal lipoma, occasional osseous changes can be seen at the osseous attachment, such as bowing, bone projections, cortical erosions, periosteal reaction, and intralesional metaplastic bone formation [35, 53, 62, 77, 80, 131]. The most common osseous manifestation is an irregular osseous excrescence into the soft tissue, with variable width at the base [62, 118, 131]. Mild cortical thickening is best evaluated on radiographs, with magnification views, and it may not be demonstrated on MR images [118]. Fleming et al. have described 32 cases of parosteal lipomas and found that 50% were associated with bone changes, but some authors speculate that bony overproduction may be more frequently seen [46, 66, 68]. In a review of eight patients with parosteal lipoma, Murphey et al. have noted osseous reaction in all cases, manifesting as either mild cortical thickening or larger osseous excrescences. Associated muscle atrophy in three cases was caused by nerve impingement and best seen on MR images [118].

CT scans demonstrate a well-marginated mass of fat attenuation, delineating clearly the bony excrescences and the adjacent bony cortex (Fig. 15.17). On MR images the SI of this lipoma is identical to that of subcutaneous fat on all pulse sequences, and the mineralized portion remains of decreased signal on T1- and T2-weighted images. The fatty mass may present various septa as seen in other lipomatous tumors, which appear as low SI on T1-weighted MR images, and may become higher in intensity on long TR images. Large areas of ossification may show marrow components and some cases have been described with hyaline cartilage or small foci of fibrocartilage and endochondral ossification extending into the soft tissue mass, with an osteochondromatous appearance. However, the lack of medullary continuity of the osseous projections, as well as the fatty content of lipoma, argue against the diagnosis of an osteochondroma [62, 77, 80, 118, 131].

15.2.4 Diffuse Lipomatosis

Diffuse lipomatosis represents a diffuse overgrowth of mature adipose tissue histologically similar to simple lipoma. The fatty tissue extensively infiltrates the adjacent structures and contiguous muscles, leading to deformities and limb asymmetry. The distinction between infiltrating lipoma and lipomatosis can be arbitrary at times, and some authors use the two terms interchangeably [89]. However lipomatosis implies a more extensive process with diffuse involvement of the subcutaneous and muscular tissue, while the intramuscular lipoma is always confined to muscle or intermuscular tissue space.

Diffuse lipomatosis is an extremely rare condition that affects most commonly large portions of the trunk or an extremity. Most cases occur during the first 2 years of life, but they also have been reported in adolescents and adults [46]. Lipomatosis may also be associated with osseous hypertrophy and macrodactyly, but, unlike neural fibrolipoma/macrodystrophia lipomatosa, nerves are not involved and the condition is not confined to the extremities.

The radiological findings in lipomatosis include the presence of fatty tissue diffusely distributed within and between the involved muscles (Fig. 15.18). "Infiltrating congenital lipomatosis of the face" is a related entity present at birth or in infancy, consisting of an unencapsulated, infiltrating fatty mass characteristically involving the face. The possibility of association with congenital cytomegalovirus infection has been reported in two cases [38, 125]. MR images depicts an infiltrating fatty mass, and distortion of the facial bones and displacement of the airway by the lesion have been reported [63].

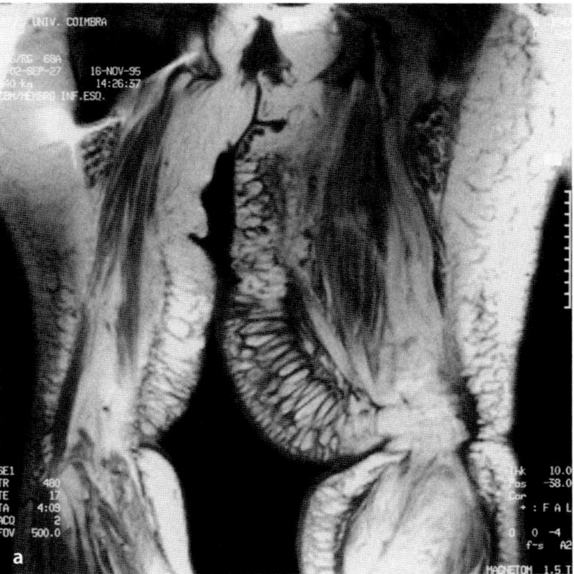

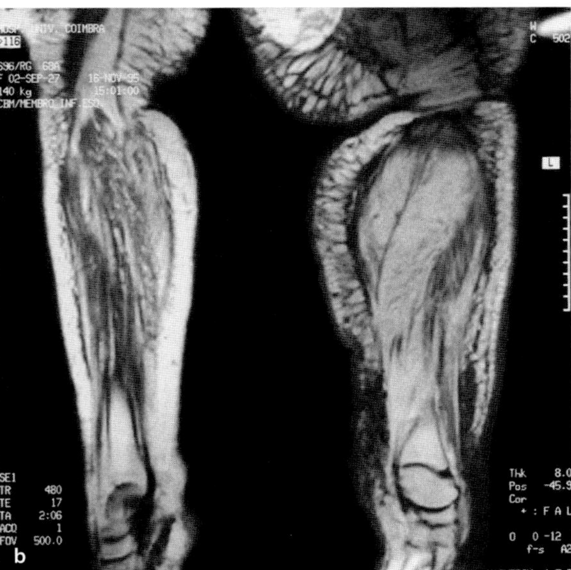

Fig. 15.18 a, b. Diffuse lipomatosis of the thighs and legs in a 66-year-old woman. **a** Coronal SE T1-weighted MR image of the thighs. **b** Coronal SE T1-weighted MR image of the legs. Fat is diffusely distributed within and between the muscles of both thighs (**a**) and legs (**b**) and the subcutaneous fat. Although there is an asymmetry of the size of the limbs, the MR appearances are similar in both sides

15.2.4.1 Multiple Symmetrical Lipomatosis

This rare condition, predominantly affecting middle-aged men, is also known as Madelung disease or Launois-Bensaude syndrome. A familial occurrence has been described. The exact cause is unknown, although a hyperplastic mechanism has been considered [42, 44, 103]. Symmetrical lipomatosis is usually associated with excessive alcohol intake, liver disease, diabetes,

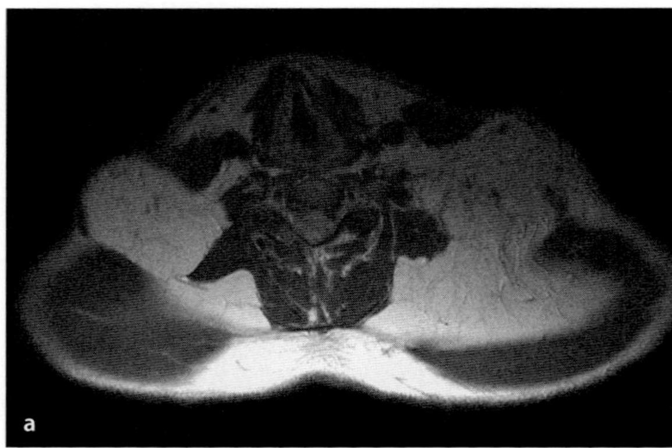

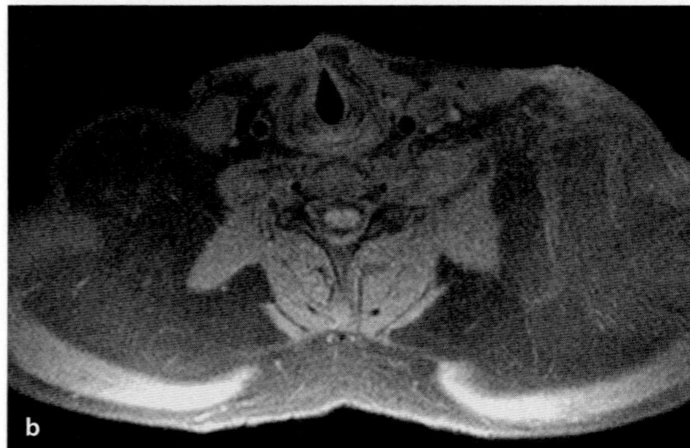

Fig. 15.19a,b. Madelung disease in a 53-year-old man with a history of alcohol abuse. **a** Axial SE T1-weighted MR image of the neck. **b** Axial FS SE T1-weighted MR image of the neck. Symmetric fatty deposits under trapezius and sternocleidomastoid muscles and anteriorly in the neck

hyperlipidemia, hyperuricemia, malignant tumors of the upper airway, and neuropathy [43, 135, 138]. Occurrence is usually sporadic, but some investigators believe an underlying hereditary factor may be present in the form of a mitochondrial dysfunction that disturbs the lipid metabolism [135, 159].

Patients with symmetrical lipomatosis present with massive symmetrical deposition of mature fat in the neck, but also the cheeks, breast, upper arm, axilla, chest, abdominal wall, and groin may be involved [43, 44, 46, 138]. The fatty accumulation progresses frequently over many years and is painless. These fatty masses are unencapsulated, so they are poorly circumscribed with involvement of the subcutaneous fat and deep tissues, mostly posterior relative to the trapezius and sternocleidomastoideus muscles, in the supraclavicular fossa, or between the paraspinal muscles. However, deep fat accumulation may be independent of involvement of adjacent subcutaneous fat, which can be atrophic. This suggests a local formation of fatty masses, rather than penetration of lipomatous tissue by subcutaneous fat [43, 44]. This preferential involvement of compartments distinguishes this disease from obesity. When symmetrical lipomatosis involves the deep soft

tissues of the neck and mediastinum, it may cause dysphagia, hoarseness, severe respiratory insufficiency by extrinsic compression of the trachea, and signs of vascular compression (superior vena cava syndrome) [44–46, 104].

On CT and MR images, symmetric accumulation of fatty, unencapsulated, deep or superficial masses have been reported (Fig. 15.19), with calcifications rarely being observed [45, 104]. Surgical debulking is the treatment of choice, but recurrence is common [135].

15.2.4.2 Adiposis Dolorosa (Dercum Disease)

This condition must be differentiated from symmetrical lipomatosis. It consists of diffuse or nodular painful, multiple subcutaneous fatty deposits. Adiposis dolorosa predominates in postmenopausal women and affects predominantly the regions of the pelvic girdle and the thigh. The patients complain of marked asthenia, depression, and psychogenic disturbances [158]. The inheritance is autosomal dominant with variable penetrance [57].

15.2.4.3 Shoulder Girdle Lipomatosis

This syndrome was first described by Enzi et al., involving the scapulohumeral girdle, with fatty infiltration of muscles in six female adult patients [45]. This is a subtype of lipomatosis with different clinical, pathological and radiological findings. It presents unilateral gradual enlargement and deformity of the shoulder and proximal part of the arm, with shoulder girdle muscle weakness, and motor and sensory neuropathy in the involved limb [45, 109]. Enzi et al. have also noted respiratory symptoms due to compression of the upper airway or infiltration of the laryngeal wall by fatty tissue [45]. MR imaging demonstrates diffuse accumulation of fat, within or between the involved muscles, with high SI identical to normal subcutaneous fat, on T1- and T2-weighted images, without cellular or edematous areas [109].

Bannayan-Zonana syndrome is a rare hamartomatous disorder, which affects men in 68% of cases. Inheritance is autosomal dominant with variable expression. This syndrome is characterized by the presence of moderate macrocephaly, multiple hemangiomas, and subcutaneous and visceral lipomas (in up to 76% of cases) [57].

15.2.5 Hibernoma

Hibernoma is a rare benign tumor composed of brown fat, first described by Merkel in 1906 and named by Gery in 1914. Its name is derived from the tumor's histological similarity to the brown glandular fat of hibernating animals [113]. Brown fat, histologically distinct from white adipose tissue, is present in the human fetus and newborn, but gradually decreases through adulthood [10]. Brown fat plays a role in thermogenesis in hibernating animals and in the newborn, and its role is possibly to maintain a normal body weight [95, 137].

Other names for hibernoma are "lipoma of immature adipose tissue," "lipoma of embryonic fat," and "fetal lipoma," due to the resemblance between brown fat and the early stages of development of white fat [46].

Hibernomas are generally well-circumscribed, encapsulated tumors, but infiltration of the surrounding tissues may occur. They show a lobular pattern, with connective tissue septa, and are composed of granular or multivacuolated cells [46, 110]. The stroma is highly vascularized; the mixed form displaying histological features between lipoma and hibernoma is the most frequent.

The peak incidence of hibernoma is in the third or fourth decade, and although it can be seen at any age, the patients with hibernoma are usually younger than those with lipoma [46, 85]. Enzinger et al. have reported a series of 32 cases, in which the median age is 26 years (range 18–52 years) [46]. Kransdorf has reported 41 cases of hibernoma, with a mean age of 32 years [85]. Several studies have reported a slight female predominance [95, 110].

Usual locations are the scapular and interscapular regions, mediastinum, and upper thorax, sites corresponding to the distribution of remaining brown fat. Involvement of the neck, chest wall, retroperitoneum, arm, buttock, inguinal region, and spinal canal has also been reported, as well as some areas devoid of brown fat such as the thigh or the popliteal fossa [2, 4, 7, 10, 25, 29, 46, 110]. Mugel et al. have reported a hibernoma of the thigh extending into the pelvis, through the obturator foramen [115].

Hibernoma usually manifests as a superficial, soft, well-defined, painless and slow-growing mass that, however, may suddenly increase in size. Local pain has been reported and, since hibernoma is a hypervascular mass, the overlying skin is often warm [110]. It ranges from 5 to 10 cm in diameter, but this tumor can extend to 18 cm in the greatest dimension [46, 95, 120].

Radiographs often demonstrate a mass with a radiolucency consistent with a lipomatous tumor, or some increased density of the soft tissues, without osseous involvement [2, 10, 29, 95]. Sonography displays a hyperechoic mass and, on duplex Doppler examination, several large vascular channels may be identified within the mass [29, 95].

On CT scans this condition may present as a well- or ill-defined lipomatous mass, and it may be heterogeneous, due to the presence of septations and other soft tissue components [2, 10, 29, 37, 95, 115]. Hibernoma may show poor or strong contrast enhancement of the

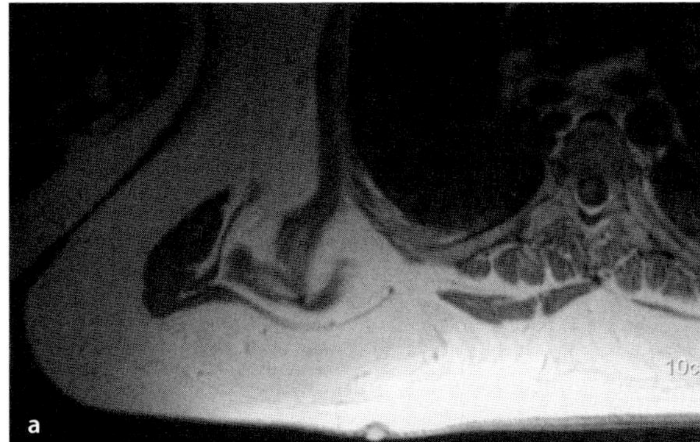

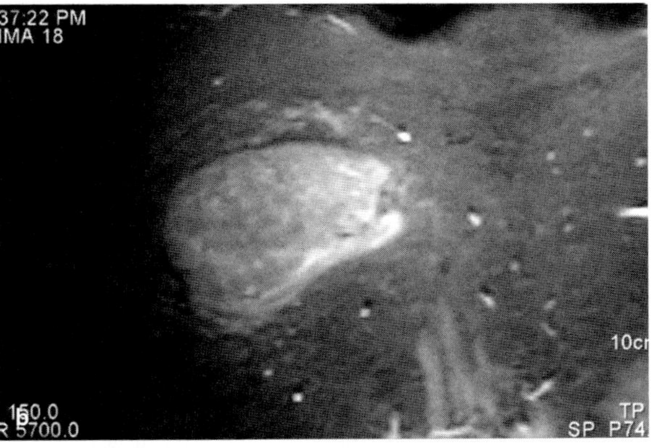

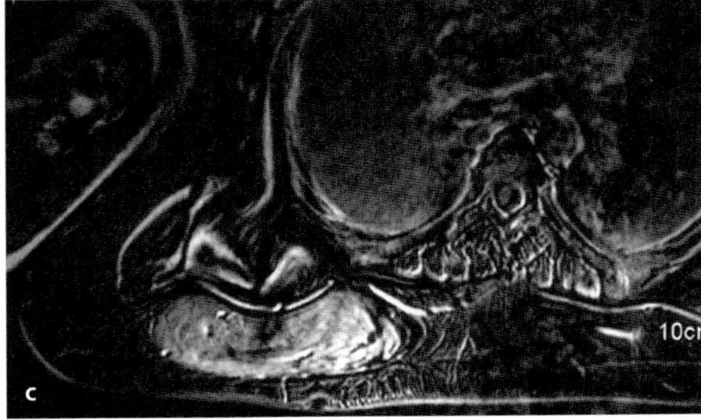

Fig. 15.20a–c. Hibernoma of the right scapular area in a 31-year-old woman. **a** Axial SE T1-weighted MR image. **b** Coronal STIR image. **c** Axial subtraction image of FS SE T1-weighted MR images before and after gadolinium contrast administration. The mass is located deeply within the subcutis of the right dorsal thoracic wall. On T1-weighted images, the signal intensity is slightly lower than subcutaneous fat (**a**). On STIR images, fat-suppression of yellow fat is incomplete, resulting in a relatively higher signal intensity of the mass compared to subcutaneous fat (**b**). After intravenous gadolinium contrast administration, there is marked and diffuse enhancement of the mass (**c**). (Case courtesy of J. Vandevenne, Genk, and reprinted with permission from Daineffe S. et al. 2003 Radiological Documents 21:16)

septa or diffusely within the mass [10, 29, 37, 95]. MR images depict usually a heterogeneous or septated mass, isointense or typically slightly hypointense to subcutaneous fat on T1-weighted MR images (Fig. 15.20), but frequently hyperintense to normal muscle tissue. On T2-weighted MR images, the mass can be nearly isointense to subcutaneous fat, although hypointensity and areas of increased SI have been reported also (7, 13, 29, 37, 95, 115, 137]. Hibernoma demonstrates usually inhomogeneous enhancement after intravenous contrast administration, but absence of enhancement has also been described [29, 95, 115, 137].

Whereas the tumor is almost as intense as fat on T2-weighted images, fat-suppression techniques fail to suppress the fat in the tumor because of the nature and the amount of lipids (Fig. 15.20) [41]. Knowledge of the MR imaging characteristics, particularly hypointensity to subcutaneous fat on T1-weighted images and absence of fat-suppression on STIR or fat-suppressed T2-weighted images may help suggest hibernoma as a potential diagnosis (Fig. 15.20). However, inasmuch as overlap exists in imaging features of hibernomas and a small number of others tumors, a specific diagnosis may not always be possible [78].

Today, angiography has been replaced by MRI in the diagnosis of this tumor, but, when performed, an intense vascular blush can be seen due to high vascularity of the tumor, with absence, however, of neovascularity or arteriovenous shunting [10, 57, 95, 110]. The imaging features make differentiation from liposarcoma almost impossible and therefore surgical resection is usually performed. Definitive diagnosis is usually only made after histopathological examination of the resection specimen. Core needle biopsy has not been recommended in cases of suspected hibernoma owing to the tumor's hypervascularity [2, 29, 59, 78, 95, 110, 120].

Although some reports of malignancy have been described, the existence of malignant hibernoma is still debated, as some cases are considered as variants of round cell liposarcoma [46]. There is no recurrence after complete excision.

15.3 Malignant Lipomatous Tumors

Liposarcoma is the second most common soft tissue sarcoma, accounting for 10–18% of all malignant soft tissue tumors [47, 86]. The tumor originates from mesenchymal cells and differentiates to adipose tissue, the presence of mature fat cells being unnecessary for its development. Liposarcoma can be classified into five histological types: well-differentiated, myxoid, round cell, pleomorphic, and dedifferentiated liposarcoma. In 5–10% of cases, there are mixed forms, which combine two or more histological types [47]. Liposarcoma is preponderant in men (from 55% to 61%), arising in the fifth and sixth decades of life and is extremely rare in infants and children, though some cases have been described [47, 87, 114]. The clinical behavior of liposarcoma varies according to the different histological types and is strongly influenced by its location. Liposarcoma usually manifests as a well-circumscribed, lobulated, and painless mass which may be present for several months or years. The tumor may reach a very large size. Pain or functional disturbance are late complaints.

Liposarcomas are rare in the subcutaneous fat, occurring in deep structures, the majority of them being located in the extremities, particularly in the thigh. The retroperitoneum is the second most common site (15–20%), where liposarcoma may attain a larger size, owing to a later detection [47]. The well-differentiated liposarcoma, as a low-grade malignancy, is in general only locally aggressive, with recurrence if only marginally excised. There is no tendency to metastasize, but it may undergo dedifferentiation to a more aggressive liposarcoma [50, 70, 116]. Retroperitoneal, well-differentiated liposarcomas tend to have a higher recurrence rate than those located in the extremities, probably due to their incomplete excision [47, 48]. The round cell, pleomorphic and dedifferentiated types have a highly malignant behavior, with a strong tendency to recur and metastasize [48]. Recurrence may occur after a long delay (5–10 years) following the initial excision [46]. Metastases are most commonly spread hematogenously, affecting predominantly the lungs and also the visceral organs and bone [47,126]. Myxoid liposarcoma, though of intermediate malignancy grade, may metastasize in 19–34% of the patients, usually to extrapulmonary sites such as serosal surfaces of the pleura, pericardium, diaphragm, and soft tissues of pelvic or chest walls and retroperitoneum [47, 48, 126]. In a study of 95 cases of myxoid and round cell liposarcomas, Kilpatrick et al. have reported the development of metastases in 30 patients (35%). Thirty-one percent died from the disease [82]. They concluded that the presence of spontaneous necrosis, a percentage of more than 25% of round cell differentiation, and age more than 45 years are significantly associated with a poor prognosis. Henricks et al., in a series of 155 dedifferentiated liposarcomas, have described a local recurrence rate of 41%, a metastatic rate of 17%, and a mortality of 28% [70].

Multifocal liposarcoma, although rare, has been reported [47, 81, 93]. A case of multicentric myxoid liposarcoma has been documented by Kemula et al. with three different sizes and location, without pulmonary, hepatic, or osseous metastases [81]. The authors agree with the hypothesis, still debated, that this represents a multicentric rather than metastatic spreading origin.

Because the histological subtype affects both prognosis and surgical planning, an accurate preoperative assessment is essential. The radiological features of a liposarcoma depend on the histological type and tend to reflect its degree of differentiation. Well-differentiated liposarcomas have CT or MRI findings that closely resemble those of subcutaneous fat or a simple lipoma [74, 88, 115]. They are frequently composed of more than 75% of fat, while the other types usually have less than 25%. About 50% of liposarcomas do not have any radiologically detectable fat [36, 75, 88, 100]. This variable fat content accounts for the frequently nonspecific appearance of liposarcoma on CT and MR images [36, 40, 42, 56, 72, 75, 146]. The presence of soft tissue calcification is variable, occurring predominantly in the well-differentiated liposarcomas [75]. The angiographic pattern is nonspecific and cannot be used to distinguish benign from malignant tumors [97].

15.3.1 Well-Differentiated Liposarcoma

Well-differentiated liposarcoma grossly resembles lipoma and consists of variably sized fat cells, but has also scattered lipoblasts, broad fibrous septa, and thick-walled blood vessels. Histologically, there are three major subtypes of well-differentiated liposarcoma: (1) "lipoma-like," (2) inflammatory, and (3) sclerosing [46]. Another variant is the spindle cell liposarcoma, arising in the subcutaneous tissue, mostly around the shoulder girdle or upper limbs. All described cases occurred in adults [34]. The lipoma-like subtype is the most common and it simulates lipoma. The terms "well-differentiated liposarcoma" and "atypical lipoma" have been used interchangeably, but "atypical lipoma" should be reserved to designate the subcutaneous form of well-differentiated liposarcoma, especially of the small size [47, 127]. Well-differentiated liposarcomas tend to be more frequent in the lower extremities, in the retroperitoneum, and trunk [86].

Although the amount of radiologically identifiable fat is variable, a well-differentiated liposarcoma will generally demonstrate at least 75% adipose tissue, although occasionally this will be as little as 25% of the lesion volume [127].

On CT, a well-differentiated liposarcoma may appear as a well-marginated mass, with attenuation values equal to those of simple fat, mimicking a benign lipomatous tumor. However, this type usually has some thickened (more than 2 mm wide) linear or nodular soft tissue septa, which enhance after intravenous administration of contrast material [75]. On MR images, these small, nonlipomatous components are of low SI on T1-weighted images or increased SI on T2-weighted images [5, 20, 40, 75, 89] (Fig. 15.21). The internal septa display a marked enhancement compared with those in lipoma and tend to have irregular width [71] (Fig. 15.22). Although earlier reports state that internal septa enhance only in liposarcoma, while no septal enhancement is seen in lipoma, this has been denied by Hosono, using fat-suppressed T1-weighted sequences after gadolinium

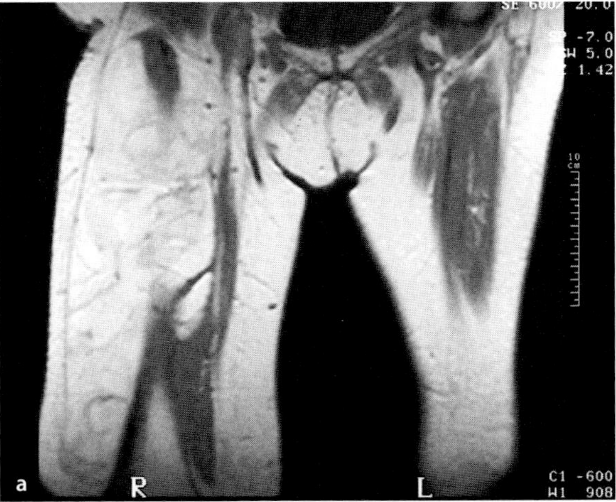
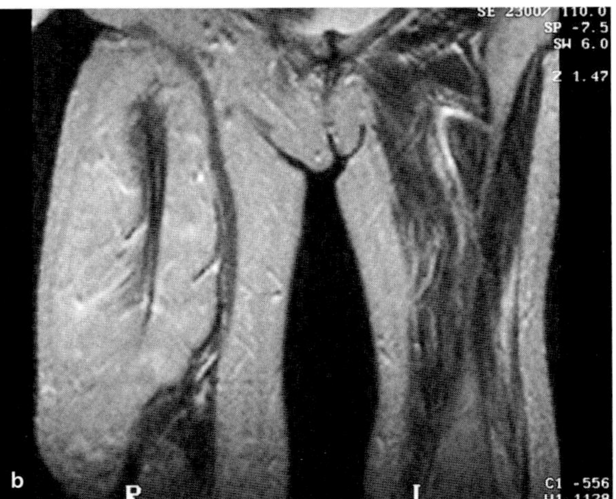

Fig. 15.21 a, b. Well differentiated liposarcoma of the thigh in a 92-year-old female. **a** Coronal SE T1-weighted MR image. **b** Coronal SE T2-weighted MR image. Both images reveal a large mass within the quadriceps muscle. The overall signal intensity equals that of subcutaneous fat, intratumoral strands having low SI on T1- and high SI on T2-weighted images. Intratumoral strands of liposarcoma are more prominent in this case than in the lipoma shown in Fig. 15.9

administration [71]. However, more prominent enhancement is seen in the malignant form. The reason why septa in liposarcoma enhance considerably more than in lipoma is probably due to the presence of malignant cellularity and inflammatory cell infiltration.

On color Doppler examination, these internal septa show increased vascularity [30]. Of all liposarcomas, the well-differentiated type is distinguished from the other variants, due to its predominantly fatty composition [75].

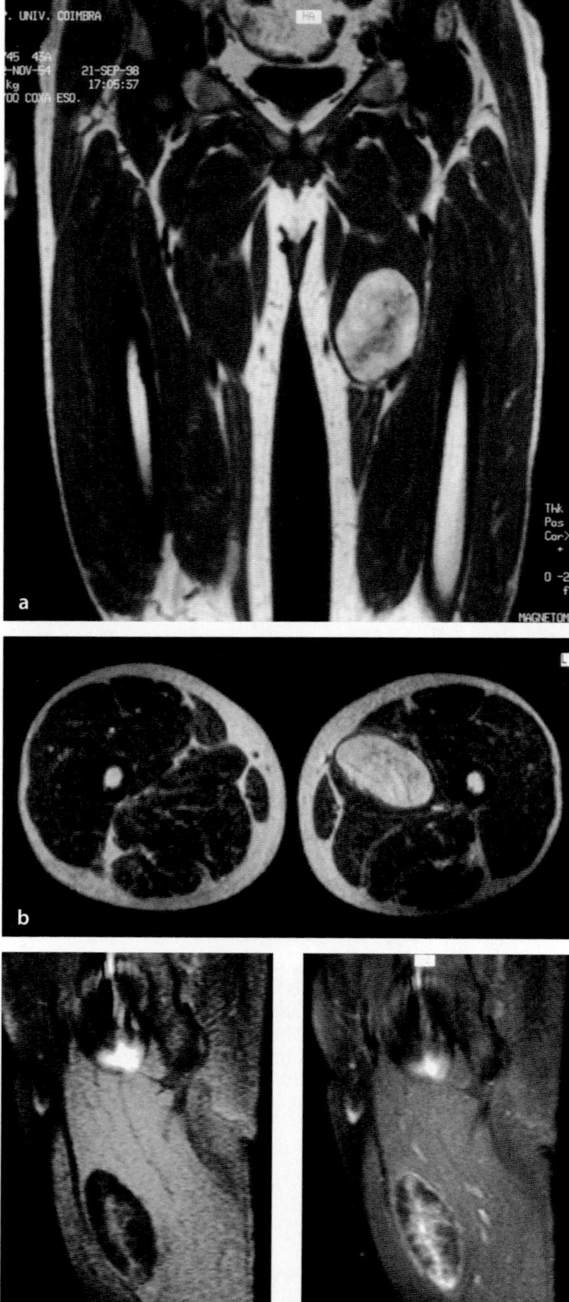

Fig. 15.22 a, d. Well-differentiated liposarcoma, sclerosing subtype of the thigh in a 43-year-old man. **a** Coronal SE T1-weighted MR image. **b** Axial SE T2-weighted MR image. **c** Sagittal fat-suppressed T1-weighted MR image. **d** Sagittal fat-suppressed T1-weighted MR image after Gd-contrast injection. MR displays a very well-defined, heterogeneous fatty mass in the adductor muscles. The central area is of low SI on T1-weighted image (**a**), high SI on T2-weighted image (**b**), and intermediate SI on fat-suppressed image (**c**). The enhancement of this central area is well demonstrated on fat-suppressed image after gadolinium contrast (**d**)

15.3.2 Myxoid Liposarcoma

Myxoid liposarcoma was previously considered as the most common variant of liposarcoma, accounting for 45–55% of all liposarcomas [47, 75]. However, in a review of 1,755 liposarcomas by Kransdorf, this subtype occurred in only 20.5% of the cases, the well-differentiated subtype being the most common (47.5%) [86]. Myxoid liposarcomas are well-differentiated tumors consisting of a plexiform vascular network, and stellate and spindle-shaped mesenchymal cells within a basophilic myxoid matrix or ground substance [47]. Ground substance accounts for 90% of the tumor [146]. Myxoid liposarcoma mostly presents as a painless, slowly growing mass at the lower extremities [50, 75, 86]. Other sites (in decreasing order of frequency) include the buttocks, retroperitoneum, trunk, ankle, proximal limb girdle, head and neck, and wrist. Myxoid liposarcoma occur in the intermuscular fascial planes or deep-seated areas. They are rarely found in the subcutaneous tissue. Liposarcomas may be multicentric, with involvement of two or more anatomical sites. In 10% of patients with primary liposarcoma of the thigh, a second liposarcoma occurs in the retroperitoneum 2 or more years after the removal of the primary tumor [147, 47]. Most patients are aged 18–67 years, with a mean age of 42 years [47].

Very frequently there is no radiological evidence of fat, owing to the small amount of mature fat in this subtype, which usually represents less than 10% of its total volume [75, 146]. Therefore, it may be difficult to establish the correct diagnosis with CT and MRI due to the lack of fat density or intensity.

On CT scans, myxoid liposarcoma manifests as a homogeneous or slightly heterogeneous mass that is less attenuating than the surrounding muscle [116]. On MR images, a spectrum of MR imaging features occurs owing to several factors (Figs. 15.23–15.26). One factor is the fat content of the tumor. Other factors include the amount of myxoid material, the degree of cellularity and avascularity, and the presence of necrosis in the tumor. Most myxoid liposarcomas demonstrate lacy or linear, amorphous hyperintense foci within a hypointense mass on T1-weighted images and behaving like normal fat on all pulse sequences, [146] (Fig. 15.24). These foci are attributed to the presence of minute quantities of detectable fat within the tumor [75, 100, 141, 146]. On T2-weighted images, a high SI is seen, with foci of intermediate SI corresponding to fat. Tumors with increased cellularity and vascularity tend to enhance on contrast-enhanced images, whereas tumor areas with necrosis, hypocellularity, and an accumulation of mucinous material tend not to enhance [5, 75, 146, 147] (Fig. 15.23).

Fig. 15.23 a–c. Myxoid liposarcoma of the thigh in a 83-year-old woman. **a** Sagittal SE T1-weighted MR image. **b** Axial SE T2-weighted MR image. **c** Sagittal fat-suppressed T1-weighted MR image after Gd-contrast injection. A large polylobulated mass is seen in the posterior compartment of the thigh. This mass is almost homogeneous and of very low SI on T1-WI (**a**). On T2-weighted image the lesion is more heterogeneous and strongly hyperintense (**b**). Enhanced fat-suppressed T1-weighted images show a heterogeneous lesion with high SI areas at the periphery and low SI areas more centrally located (**c**). Small streaks of high SI (better visualized on monitor study) on native T1-weighted image in a lesion with overall low SI, the signal on T2-weighted image and the strong enhancement after contrast injection are strongly suggestive of myxoid liposarcoma

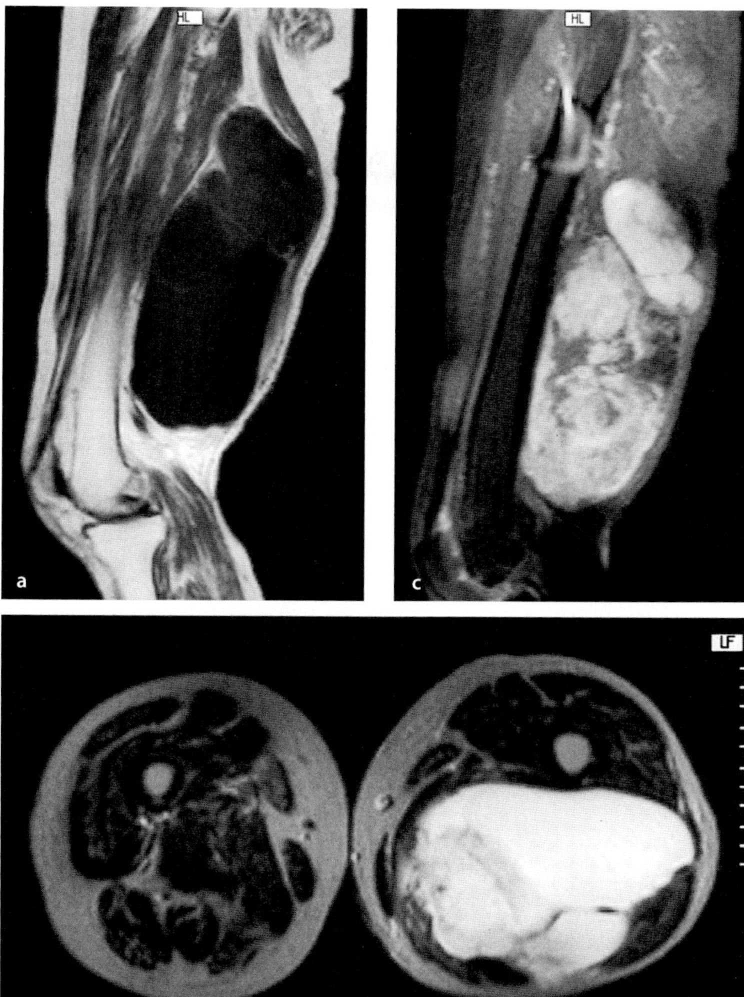

Fig. 15.24 a, b. Myxoid liposarcoma of the thigh in a 83-year-old woman. **a** Coronal spin echo T1-weighted MR image. **b** Coronal spin echo T2-weighted MR image. On the T1-weighted image a poorly delineated heterogeneous mass with small hyperintense foci in the center is found in the adductor muscles (**a**). On the T2-weighted image, the mass is strongly hyperintense, while the fatty foci have decreased signal intensity (**b**). Signal characteristics, presence of minute foci of fatty tissue, and intratumoral septa are indicative of a myxoid type of liposarcoma

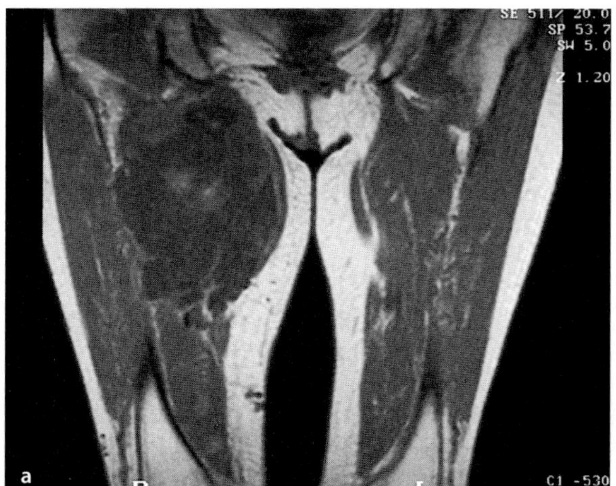
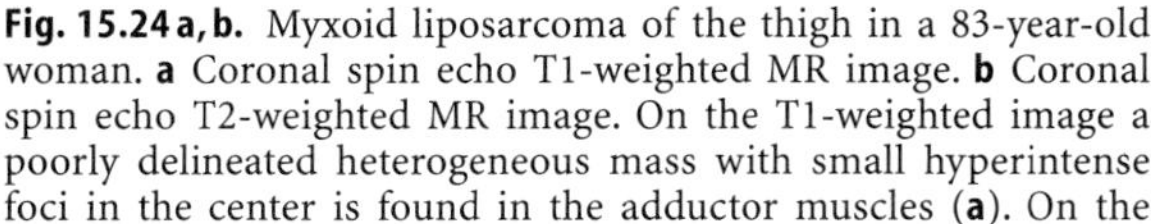
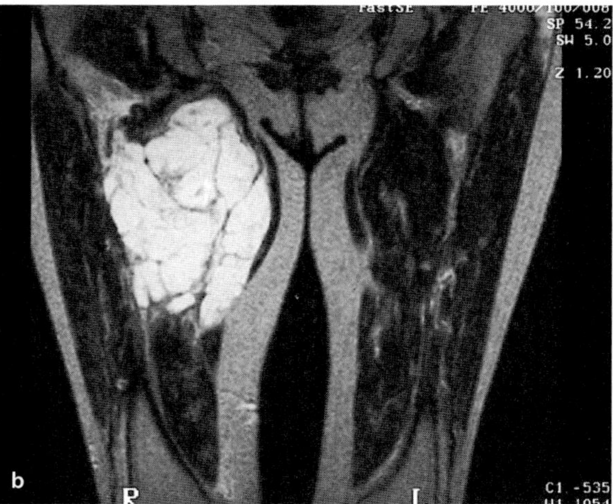

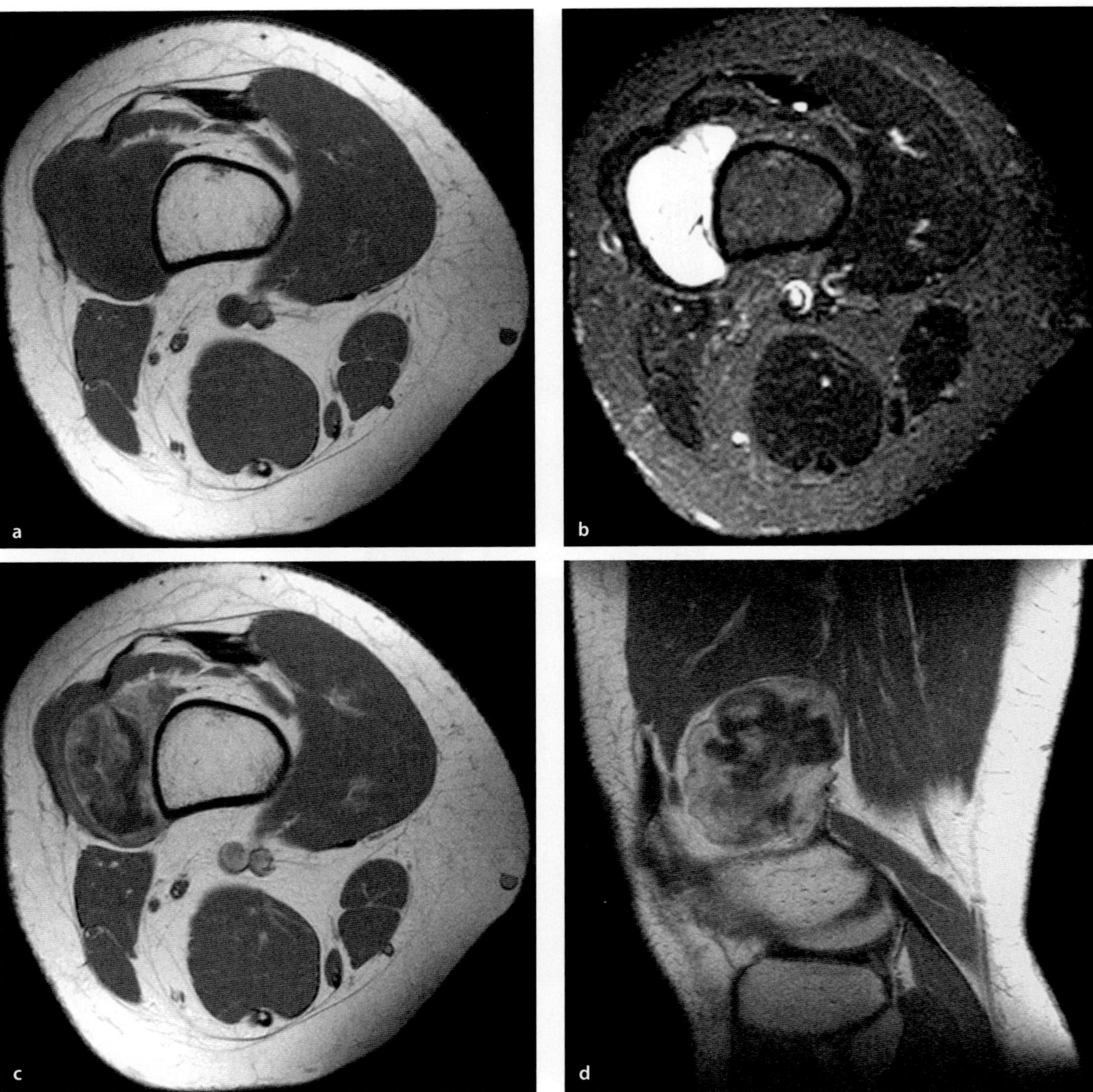

Fig. 15.25 a–d. Myxoid liposarcoma of the thigh with cystic appearance. **a** Axial SE T1-weighted MR image. **b** Axial FS TSE T2-weighted MR image. **c** Axial SE T1-weighted MR image after Gd-contrast injection. **d** Sagittal SE T1-weighted MR image after Gd-contrast injection. A well-delineated oval lesion is seen in the vastus lateralis muscle. The lesion is hypointense to muscle on T1-WI (**a**), homogeneously hyperintense on FS TSE T2-weighted image (**b**) and shows marked heterogeneous enhancement after contrast administration (**c–d**). Although rather nonspecific, a cystic appearance is frequently seen in myxoid liposarcoma. Intravenous gadolinium administration is often necessary to differentiate between true cystic lesions and solid masses

At morphological analysis, the mass is well defined. The lesion is frequently lobulated and may be multilobulated and septated or oval. Edema may be present in the soft tissue surrounding the tumor. There is no evidence of infiltration or invasion into adjacent structures. The lobulated pattern with internal linear septa is best visualized on T2-weighted MR images.

On CT and MR images, a myxoid liposarcoma may occasionally resemble a cyst, due to the lack of fat content, with sharply demarcated margins. On CT scans, it displays attenuation values within the water range. A marked low signal on T1-weighted MR images and a high signal on T2-weighted MR images, due to the predominant myxoid matrix of this tumor, is noted [40, 75,

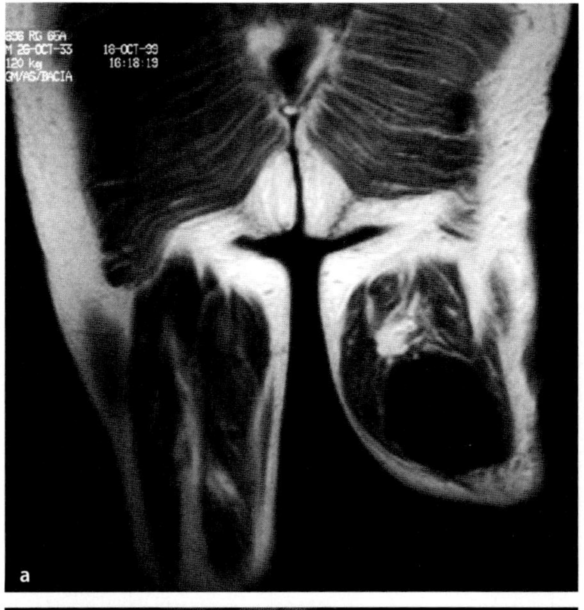

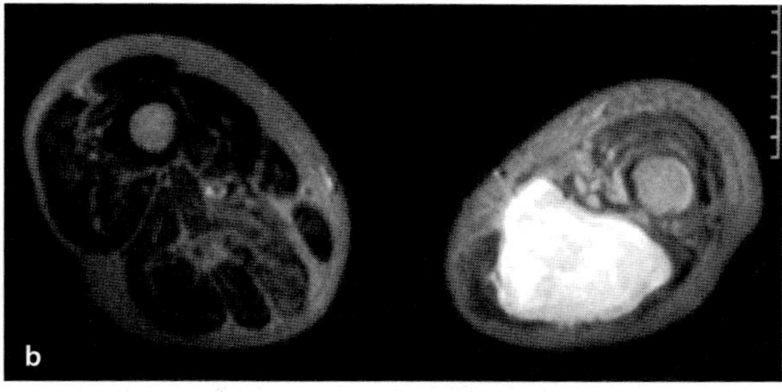

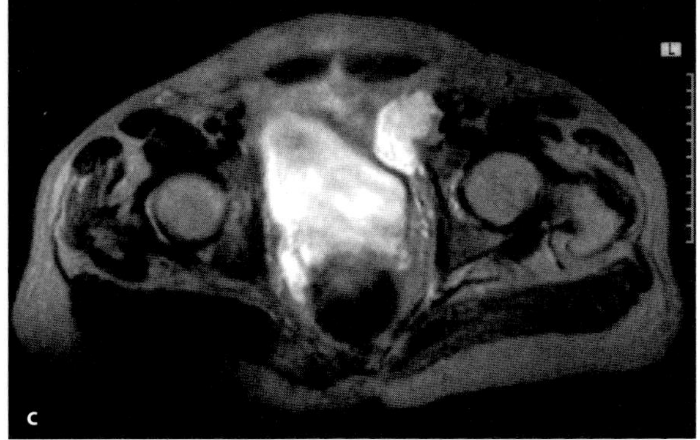

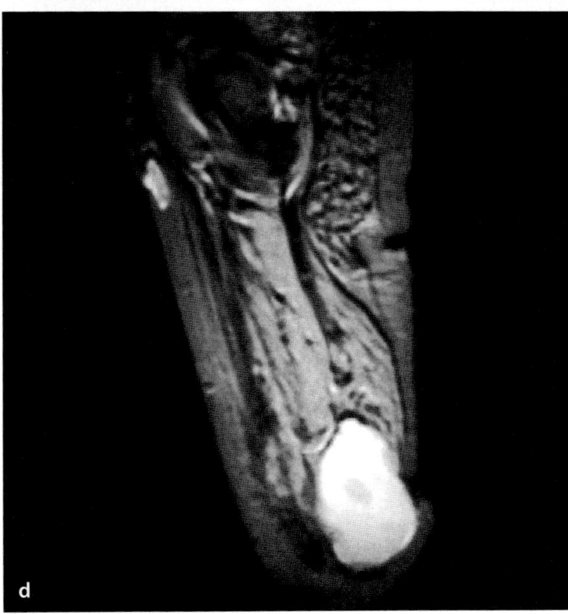

Fig. 15.26 a–d. Postamputation multiple recurrence of myxoid liposarcoma in a 65-year-old man. **a** Coronal SE T1-weighted MR image. **b** Axial SE T2-weighted MR image. **c** Axial SE T2-weighted MR image. **d** Sagittal gradient echo T2*-weighted MR image. On coronal T1-weighted MR image there is a homogeneous mass in the stump with a very low signal intensity, less than the adjacent skeletal muscle (**a**). On T2-weighted MR image this lesion is slightly inhomogeneous and with a marked high signal intensity (**b**). There is another lesion, with the same SI in the pelvis, anterior to the acetabulum and compressing and deviating the bladder (**c**). On sagittal T2*-weighted image, two hyperintense masses are displayed, one in the stump and another in the thigh, in the anterior subcutaneous fat (**d**)

84, 88] (Figs. 15.25, 15.26). The homogeneous or heterogeneous enhancement seen after gadolinium contrast facilitates distinction between myxoid liposarcomas and nonenhancing cystic lesions [101, 147].

Ultrasound is another useful tool in differentiating solid masses from cystic lesions. Myxoid liposarcomas appear complex, hypoechoic masses that do not meet the criteria for a simple cyst at ultrasound [147].

The lesion that is perhaps the most problematic for radiologists to differentiate from the cyst-like form of myxoid liposarcoma is intramuscular myxoma. Although there is an overlap, intramuscular myxoma is far more likely when there is a rind of perilesional fat (rather than intralesional fat), a globular, heterogeneous peripheral and central enhancement pattern, and increased signal in the adjacent muscle on T2-weighted/fluid-sensitive sequences [47, 127].

15.3.3 Round Cell and Pleomorphic Liposarcomas

Round cell liposarcoma represents a poorly differentiated form of myxoid liposarcoma, with proliferation of rounded cells with interspersed lipoblasts. Under the current WHO classification, a round cell liposarcoma would be classified as a myxoid liposarcoma with hypercellular (round cell) component [26]. The pleomorphic variant shows a marked degree of cellular pleomorphism and may contain huge lipoblastic multinucleated cells [47]. Both subtypes are highly aggressive and likely to metastasize.

Most pleomorphic and round cell liposarcomas present as nonspecific, heterogeneous masses with relatively well-circumscribed margins. Both types often do not contain a sufficient amount of fat and therefore exhibit a low SI on T1-weighted images and increased SI on T2-weighted images, as do the majority of other malignant soft tissue tumors [5, 75, 100, 116].There is a marked and heterogeneous enhancement after intravenous contrast administration [5]. Radiologically, these two types are not distinguishable from each other or from other aggressive sarcoma, because they contain little or no fat (Figs. 15.27–15.30).

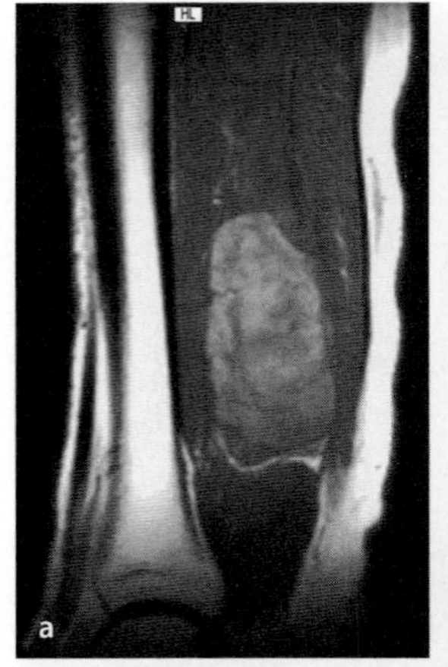
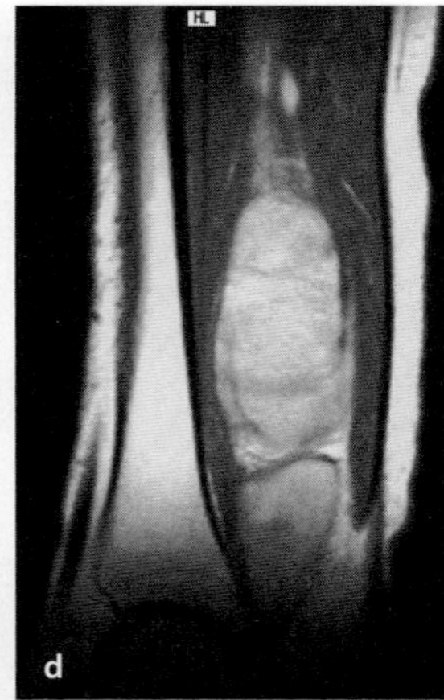
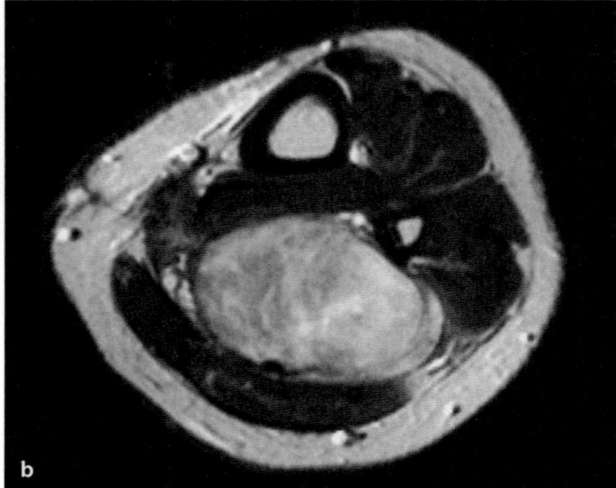
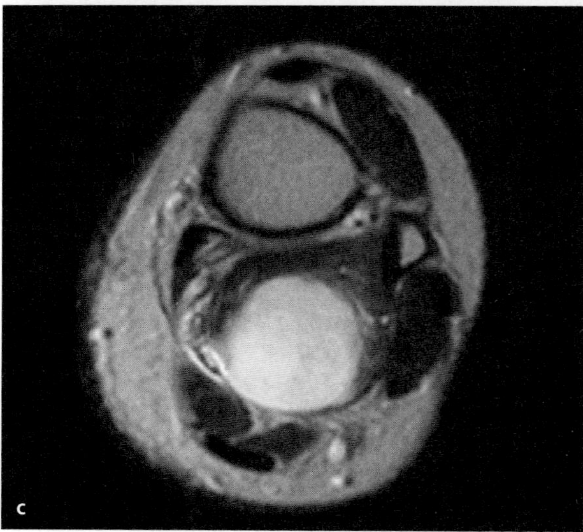

Fig. 15.27 a–d. Round cell liposarcoma of the leg in a 31-year-old man. **a** Sagittal SE T1-weighted MR image. **b, c** Axial SE T2-weighted MR images at different levels. **d** Sagittal SE T1-weighted MR image after Gd-contrast injection. Polylobulated heterogeneous mass within the soleus muscle. The lesion has overall intermediate SI with areas of lower SI on T1-WI (**a**) and areas of high SI on T2-WI (b,c). Enhancement of all components is seen after contrast administration (**d**)

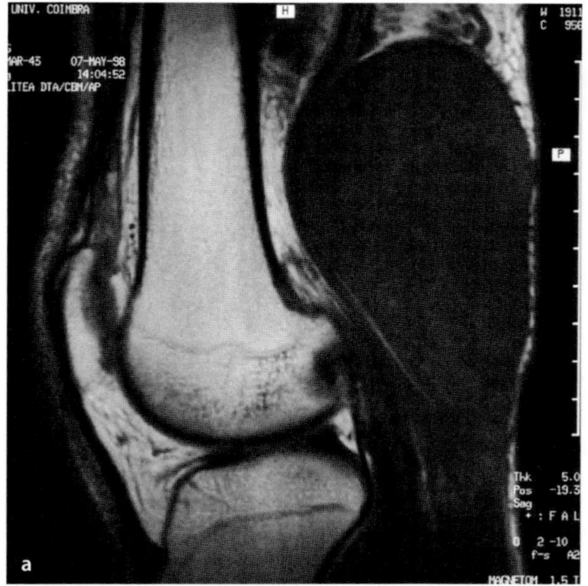
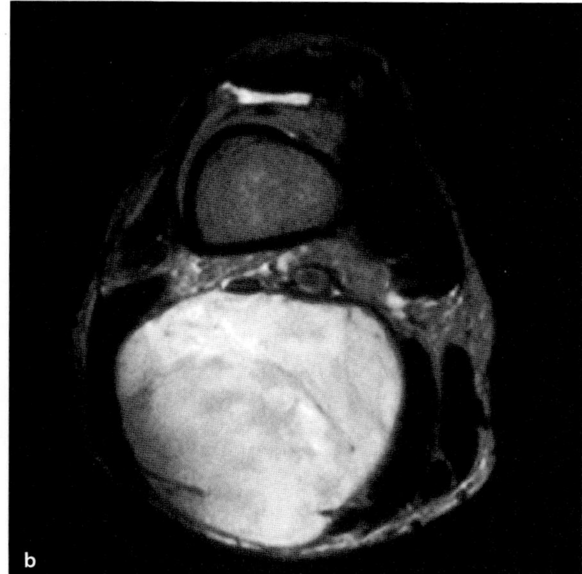
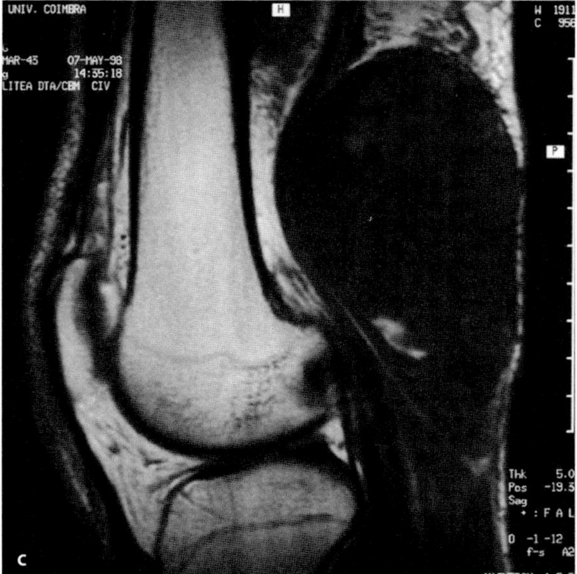

Fig. 15.28 a–c. Round cell liposarcoma in the popliteal fossa in a 53-year-old man. **a** Sagittal SE T1-weighted MR image. **b** Axial SE T2-weighted MR image. **c** Sagittal SE T1-weighted MR image after Gd-contrast injection. The sagittal T1-weighted image shows a large, well-defined, slightly heterogeneous soft tissue mass with SI similar to that of skeletal muscle (**a**). On T2-weighted image the tumor displays high SI (**b**). After intravenous contrast administration despite the high-grade of malignancy of this tumor enhancement is hardly seen, with some discrete hyperintense foci (**c**). The MR appearance is nonspecific for a lipomatous tumor

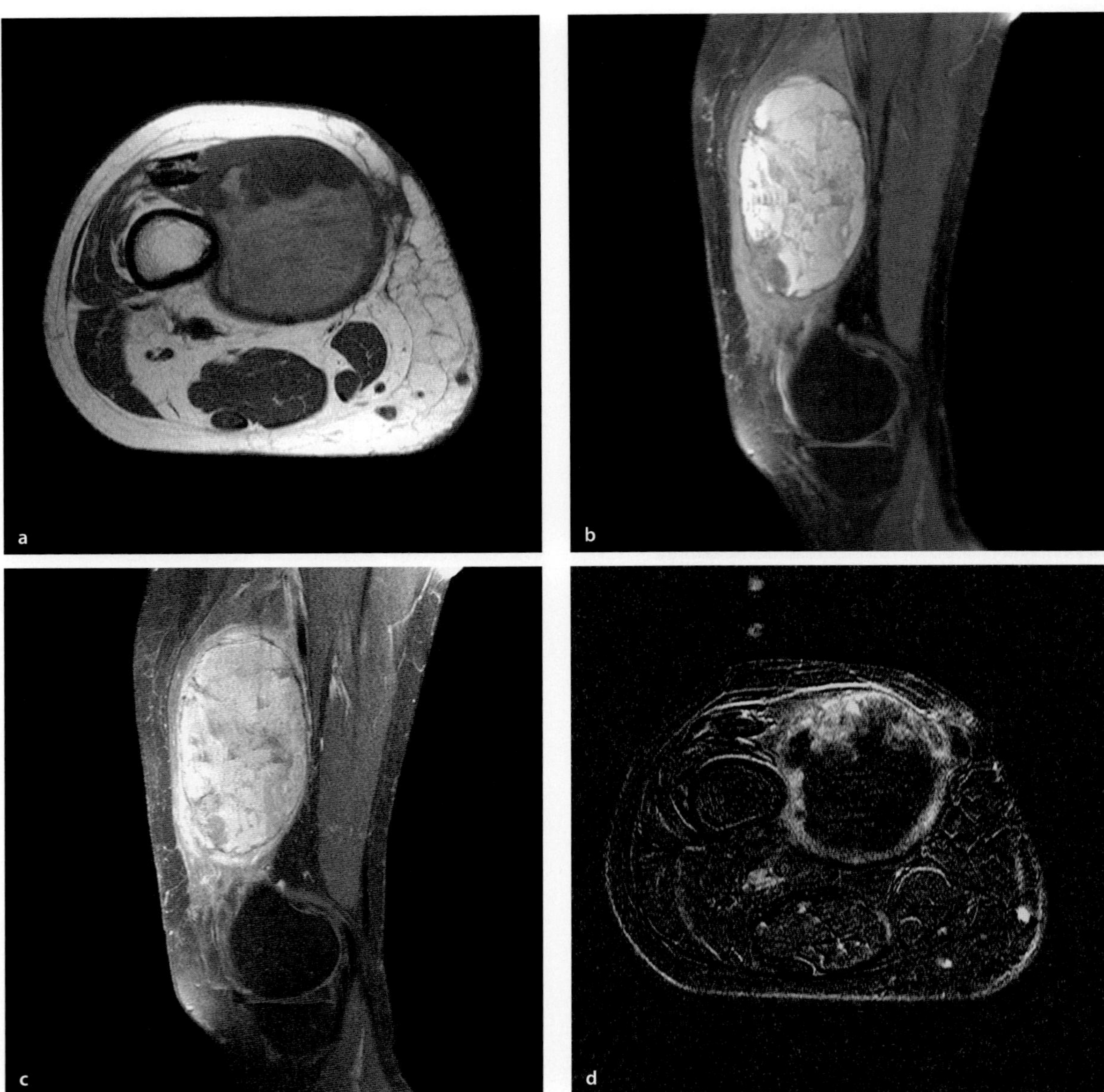

Fig. 15.29 a–d. Pleomorphic liposarcoma of the thigh. **a** Axial SE T1-weighted MR image. **b** Sagittal FS TSE T2-weighted MR image. **c** Sagittal FS SE T1-weighted MR image after gadolinium contrast administration. **d** Axial subtraction image of FS SE T1-weighted MR images before and after gadolinium contrast administration. Most pleomorphic liposarcoma present as nonspecific, heterogeneous masses with relatively well circumscribed margins (**a**). There is usually not a sufficient amount a fat and therefore a low signal intensity is seen on T1-weighted images (**a**) and a high signal intensity on T2-weighted images (**b**). There is a marked and heterogeneous enhancement after intravenous contrast administration (**c–d**)

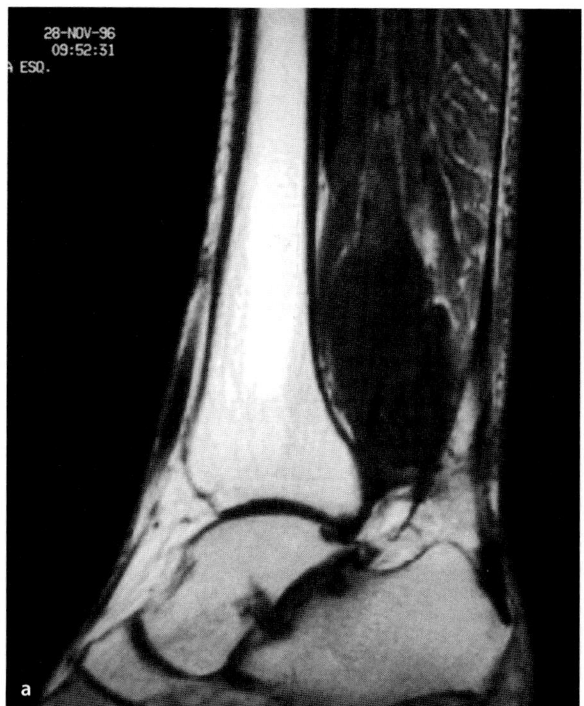
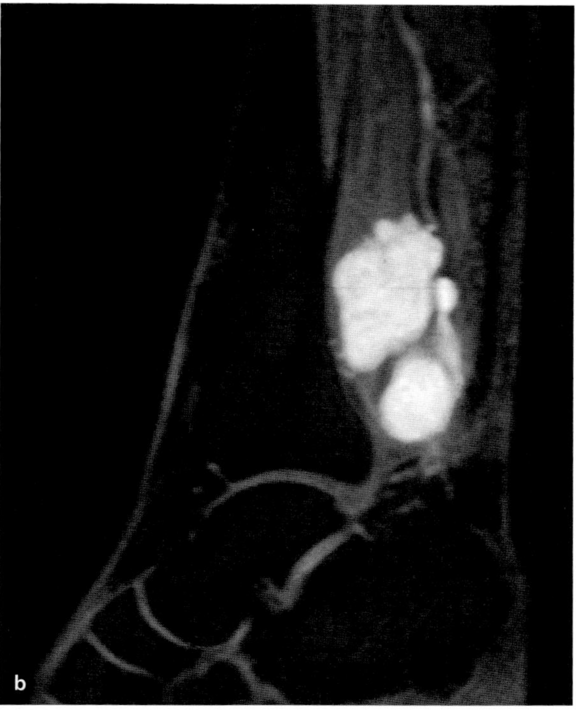

Fig. 15.30 a,b. Mixed liposarcoma (myxoid + round cell types) of the lower leg in a 70-year-old woman. **a** Sagittal SE T1-weighted MR image. **b** Sagittal fat-suppressed SE T1-weighted MR image after Gd-contrast injection. MRI displays a fusiform, near homogeneous mass of low SI on T1-WI, without fatty component (**a**). After Gd-contrast injection the lesion demonstrates a septated appearance and a strong enhancement, well seen with fat-suppression (**b**). These characteristics are nonspecific for a lipomatous tumor, but very suggestive for a sarcoma

15.3.4 Dedifferentiated Liposarcoma

Dedifferentiated liposarcoma is formed by well-differentiated and poorly differentiated nonlipogenic areas. Dedifferentiation can occur into myxofibrosarcoma (formerly known as malignant fibrous histiocytoma, MFH) in more than two-thirds of cases and, occasionally, into fibrosarcoma, leiomyosarcoma, rhabdomyosarcoma, hemangiopericytoma, and even soft tissue osteosarcoma [70, 73, 90, 133, 148]. Dedifferentiation occurs as a late complication (an average interval of 7.7 years) of a preexisting well-differentiated liposarcoma, most commonly of the retroperitoneum, mediastinum, or groin, but can also occur in the extremities and trunk [70, 90, 157]. Dedifferentiation can take place either in the primary tumor as in local recurrences or even metastases, but according to Henricks et al., in a report of 155 cases, the majority of dedifferentiated liposarcoma presented as de novo lesions [70].

Dedifferentiated liposarcoma should be suspected if a nonlipomatous component appears in a previously known, well-differentiated liposarcoma. The tumor retains some of the features of the well-differentiated liposarcoma, while some mass-like areas develop a nonspecific appearance on CT or MR images. These areas display a tissue attenuation greater than fat on CT scans and low SI on T1-weighted images and high SI on T2-weighted images with marked enhancement after intravenous contrast administration [90] (Figs. 15.31, 15.32). Calcification or even ossification may be present [73, 90, 148].

The presence of nonfatty components within a lipomatous tumor should always suggest the possibility of a high grade liposarcoma. However, it is not always possible to distinguish between the dedifferentiated type and other high-grade liposarcomas on the basis of imaging alone.

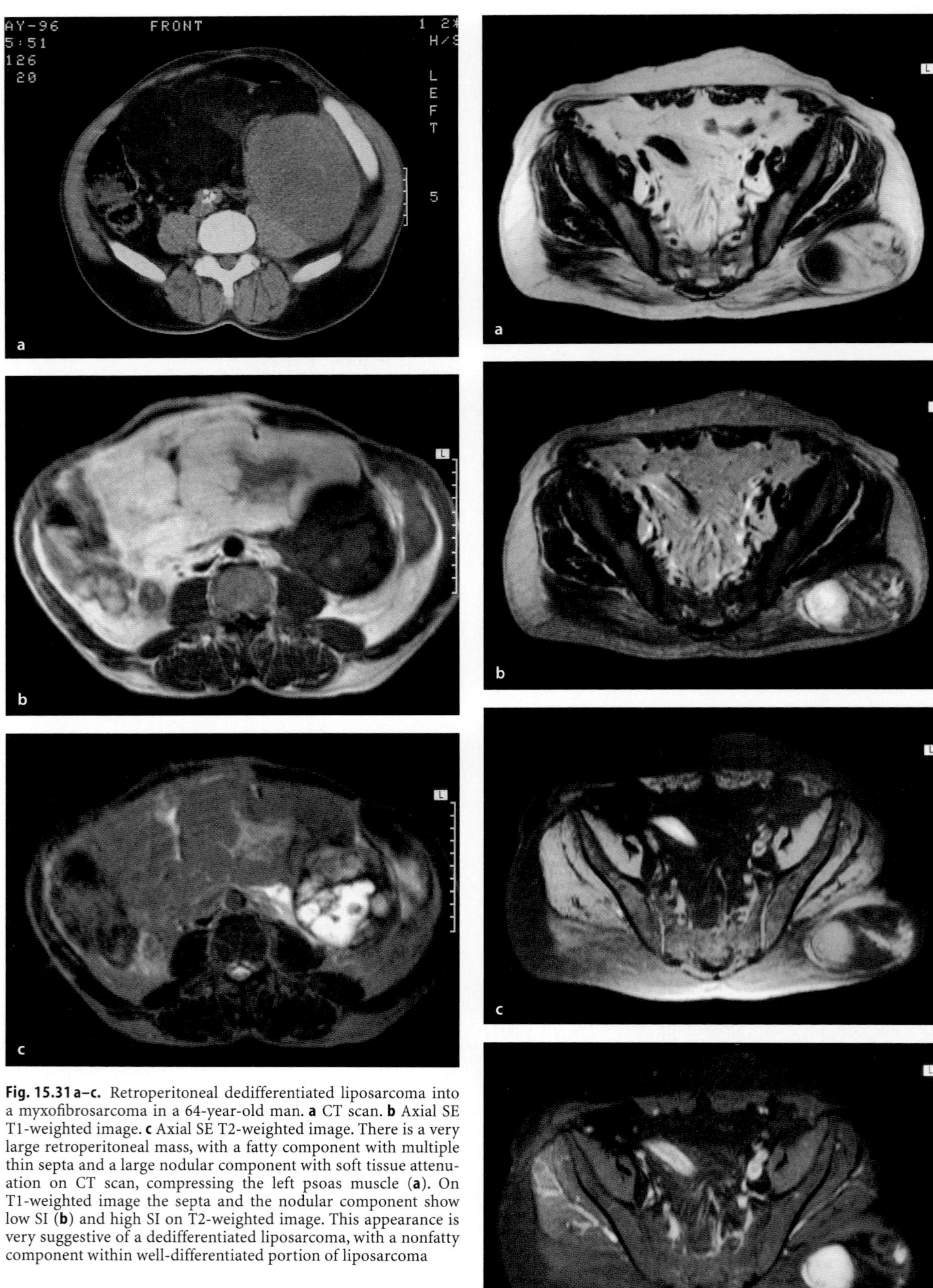

Fig. 15.31 a–c. Retroperitoneal dedifferentiated liposarcoma into a myxofibrosarcoma in a 64-year-old man. **a** CT scan. **b** Axial SE T1-weighted image. **c** Axial SE T2-weighted image. There is a very large retroperitoneal mass, with a fatty component with multiple thin septa and a large nodular component with soft tissue attenuation on CT scan, compressing the left psoas muscle (**a**). On T1-weighted image the septa and the nodular component show low SI (**b**) and high SI on T2-weighted image. This appearance is very suggestive of a dedifferentiated liposarcoma, with a nonfatty component within well-differentiated portion of liposarcoma

Fig. 15.32 a–d. Dedifferentiated liposarcoma, into a myxofibrosarcoma of the buttock, in a 63-year-old man. **a** Axial SE T1-weighted image. **b** Axial SE T2-weighted image. **c, d** Axial fat-suppressed SE T1-weighted MR image before and after Gd-contrast injection. The MR imaging images at the same level, reveal a well-delineated, in the gluteus maximus muscle. On T1-weighted image the mass is predominantly of fatty signal, with some internal septa and a round hypointense component (**a**). On T2-weighted image the nonlipomatous components manifest high signal (**b**) and strong enhancement after contrast administration (**c**)

15.3.5 Mixed-type Liposarcoma

These lipomatous tumors show features of combined myxoid/round cell liposarcoma and well-differentiated liposarcoma/dedifferentiated liposarcoma or of myxoid/round cell liposarcoma and pleomorphic liposarcoma.

15.3.6 Differential Diagnosis of Lipomatous Tumors

Because of differences in treatment, prognosis, and long-term follow-up, it is important to preoperatively distinguish simple lipomas from well-differentiated liposarcomas. In the absence of radiologically identifiable fat, such as in high-grade liposarcoma (pleomorphic and round cell types) imaging is nonspecific. However, recent literature has reported a whole range of useful differentiating features between lipoma and well-differentiating liposarcoma, which are summarized in Table 15.1 [30, 58, 59, 83, 92, 123]. Generally, a lipomatous lesion containing internal septa of more than 2 mm thickness or nonfatty nodular areas without the typical SI of muscle fibers on all pulse sequences should be considered as a liposarcoma till proven otherwise. By using these criteria, MRI is highly sensitive in the detection of well-differentiated liposarcomas and highly specific in the diagnosis of simple lipomas. However, when an extremity or body wall lesion is considered suggestive of well-differentiated liposarcoma, it is more likely (64%) to represent one of many benign lipoma variants, containing nonfatty elements [59]. These tumors include chondroid lipoma, osteolipoma, angiolipoma, hibernoma, lipoleiomyoma, and necrotic lipoma. In these cases, the nonadipose areas represent fat necrosis and associated calcification/ossification, fibrosis, inflammation, and myxoid change [108, 127].

15.4 Other Lesions Containing Fat or Mimicking Its Presence

There are several conditions that may mimic lipomatous tumors of the soft tissues, such as hemangioma, elastofibroma, myxoid or neural tumors [18, 63, 89].

Hemangiomas may contain a variable amount of adipose tissue interspersed between the abnormal vessels. However, its frequently typical appearance on MR images, owing to the presence of the high SI of slow-flowing blood within serpentine or tubular structures, allows the correct diagnosis to be made.

Elastofibroma dorsi, a benign fibrous tissue tumor with fatty elements, usually manifests as a periscapular mass with an intermediate SI and interlaced areas of high SI similar to fat on both T1- and T2-weighted MR images.

Some myxoid and neural tumors may mimic lipomatous tumors owing to their reduced tissue attenuation on CT scans. MRI findings may be utilized as an adjunct to the cytological features to more confidently differentiate intramuscular myxoma [11], myxoid schwannoma, neurofibroma, and ganglion cyst, as well as malignant neoplasms such as myxoid liposarcoma, fibrosarcoma, and myxofibrosarcoma (malignant fibrous histiocytoma) [21].

Table 15.1. Differential diagnostic criteria between lipoma and liposarcoma (modified from [30])

	Lipoma	Intramuscular lipoma	Liposarcoma
Age	adult (mean 52 years)	adult	adult (mean 65 years)
Location	Superficially located (subcutaneous fat) Back, shoulder, neck, arm, thigh, abdomen	Muscle Thigh, shoulder, arm	Muscles/Fascias Muscle/fascia Thigh, retroperitoneum
Size	<5 cm (80%) <10 cm (95%)	frequently >5 cm	exceptionally <5 cm
Margins	Well-defined	Infiltrating or well defined	Usually well defined
Shape	Uninodular	Uninodular (>85%)	Multinodular(>90%)
Septa or nodules	Absent or <2 mm Hypo on FS T2-WI No or weak enhancement	Intermingled muscle fibers Isointense to muscle Enhancement rare	Thick (>2 mm) Hyper on FS T2-WI Strong enhancement

15.5 Conclusions

Because lipomas and low-grade liposarcomas demonstrate identical tumor components and because liposarcomas are frequently mixed tumors, with histological findings of different subtypes, incisional biopsy or incomplete resection may result in substantial sampling error, with important clinical and therapeutic consequences [75]. Imaging on the other hand is capable of evaluating the whole tumoral mass, including all its components. Consequently, imaging plays a significant role in the evaluation of lipomatous soft tissue tumors. In this regard, MRI is superior to other imaging modalities, since it easily demonstrates even minute fatty tumor components and is able to stage soft tissue tumors accurately.

One has to keep in mind that some nonlipomatous tumors may contain fatty components. Fortunately, these tumors have sufficient other characteristics, which permit a more than confident diagnosis by medical imaging. Imaging-guided biopsy should be performed in a mass lesion without MRI characteristics of a benign lipomatous soft tissue tumor and it should always include the nonlipomatous component.

> **Things to remember:**
> 1. The diagnosis of a simple lipoma is usually straightforward on MR images. The use of fat-suppression is an important imaging tool in lesion characterization.
> 2. Lipomas containing other mesenchymal elements than fatty tissue (such as fibrolipoma, myxolipoma, chondroid lipoma, osteolipoma, myolipoma, or angiolipoma) are difficult to distinguish from well-differentiated liposarcomas on MR images.
> 3. Benign intramuscular lipomas may show infiltrative margins.
> 4. Demonstration of a fatty mass in patients below 3 years of age should raise the possibility of a lipoblastoma or lipoblastomatosis.
> 5. Lipomatosis of nerve is frequently associated with soft tissue and osseous hypertrophy.
> 6. The most important imaging parameters for differential diagnosis between a benign lipomatous tumors and a liposarcoma consist of location (superficial versus deep), size, internal composition (presence of thick nonlipomatous septa or nodules), contrast-enhancement pattern and shape of the lesion (uni- versus multinodular).

References

1. Ahuja AT, King AD, Kew J, King W, Metreweli C (1998) Head and neck lipomas: sonographic appearance. Am J Neuroradiol 19(3):505–508
2. Alvine G, Rosenthal H, Murphey M, Huntrakoon M (1996) Hibernoma. Skeletal Radiol 25:493–496
3. Amadio PC, Reiman HM, Dobyns JH (1988) Lipofibromatous hamartoma of nerve. J Hand Surg 13A:67–75
4. Angervall L, Nilsson L, Stener B (1964) Microangiographic and histological studies in two cases of hibernoma. Cancer 17:685
5. Arkun R, Memis A, Akalin T, Ustun EE, Sabah D, Kandiloglu G (1997) Liposarcoma of soft tissue: MRI findings with pathological correlation. Skeletal Radiol 26:167–172
6. Armstrong SJ, Watt I (1989) Lipoma arborescens of the knee. Br J Radiol 62:178–180
7. Atilla S., Eilenberg SS, Brown JJ (1995) Hibernoma: MRI appearance of a rare tumor. Magn Reson Imaging 13:335–337
8. Austin RM, Mack GR, Townsend CM, et al (1980) Infiltrating (intramuscular) lipomas and angiolipomas. Arch Surg 115:281–284
9. Babins DM, Lubahn JD (1994) Palmar lipomas associated with compression of the median nerve. J Bone Joint Surg Am 76:1360–1362
10. Balestreri L, Canzonieri (1998) Case report: axillary hibernoma – radiological and pathological fidings of a rare tumour. Clin Radiol 53:853–855
11. Bancroft LW, Kransdorf MJ, Menke DM, O'Connor MI, Foster WC (2002) Intramuscular myxoma: characteristic MR imaging features. AJR Am J Roentgenol 178:1255–1259
12. Black WC, Burke JW, Feldman PS, Johnson CM, Swanson S (1986) CT appearance of cervical lipoblastoma. J Comput Assist Tomogr 10:696–698
13. Blum A, Henrot P, Sirveaux F et al (2004) Diagnostic des lipomes des parties molles et des liposarcomes cheze l'adulte. In: Laredo JD, Tomeni B, Malghem J et al (eds) Conduite a tenir devant une image osseuse ou des parties molles d'allure tumorale. Sauramps medical, Montpellier, pp 401–416
14. Boets A, Van Mieghem IM, Sciot R, Van Breuseghem I (2004) Chondroid lipoma of the trunk: MRI appearance and pathological correlation. Skeletal Radiol 33:666–669
15. Boren WL, Henry RE, Wintch K (1995) MR diagnosis of fibrolipomatous hamartoma of nerve: association with nerve territory-oriented macrodactyly (macrodystrophia lipomatosa). Skeletal Radiol 24:296–297
16. Brady PS, Spence LD (1999) Chronic lower extremity deep vein thrombosis associated with femoral vein compression by a lipoma. Am J Roentgenol 172:1697–1698
17. Braunschweig IJ, Stein IH, Dodwad MI, Rangwala AF, Lopano A (1992) Case report 751. Spindle all lipoma causing marked bone erosion. Skeletal Radiol 21:414–417
18. Buetow PC, Kransdorf MJ, Moser RP, Jelinek JS, Berrey BH (1990) Radiologic appearance of intramuscular hemangioma with emphasis on MR imaging. Am J Roentgenol 154:563–567
19. Burgan DW (1971) Lipoma arborescens of the knee: another cause of filling defects on a knee arthrogram. Radiology 101:583–584
20. Bush CH, Spanier SS, Gillespy T (1988) Imaging of atypical lipomas of the extremities: a report of three cases. Skeletal Radiol 17:472–475
21. Caraway NP, Staerkel GA, Fanning CV, Varma DG, Pollock RE (1994) Diagnosing intramuscular myxoma by fine-needle aspiration: a multidisciplinary approach. Diagn Cytopathol 11:255–261
22. Cavallaro MC, Taylor JA, Gorman JD, Haghighi P, Resnick D (1993) Imaging findings in a patient with fibrolipomatous hamartoma of the median nerve. Am J Roentgenol 161:837–838
23. Chaljub G, Johnson PR (1996) In vivo MRI characteristics of lipoma arborescens utilizing fat-suppression and contrast administration. J Comput Assist Tomogr 20(1):85–87
24. Chew FS, Hudson TM, Hawkins IF (1980) Radiology of infiltrating angiolipoma. Am J Roentgenol 135:781–787
25. Chitoku S, Kawai S, Watabe Y et al (1998) Intradural spinal hibernoma: case report. Surg Neurol 49:509–512

26. Christopher D, Unni K, Mertens F (2002) Adipocytic tumors. WHO Classification of tumors. Pathology and genetics: tumors of soft tissue and bone. Lyon, France: IARC, pp 19–46
27. Chung EB, Enzinger FM (1973) Benign lipoblastomatosis. An analysis of 35 cases. Cancer 32:482–492
28. Collins MH, Chatten J (1997) Lipoblastoma/lipoblastomatosis: a clinicopathological study of 25 tumors. Am J Surg Pathol 21:1131–1137
29. Cook M, Stern M, Silva RD de (1996) Case report. MRI of a hibernoma. J Comput Assist Tomogr 20(2):333–335
30. Cotten A (2002) L'Imagerie de lipomes et liposarcomes. JBR-BTR 85:14–19
31. Dawson JS, Dowling F, Preston BJ, Neumann L (1995) Case report: lipoma arborescens of the subdeltoid bursa. Br J Radiol 68:197–199
32. Declercq H, De Man R, Van Herck G, Tanghe W, Lateur L (1993) Case report 814. Fibrolipoma of the median nerve. Skeletal Radiol 22:610–613
33. Dei Tos AP, Mentzel T, Newman PL, Fletcher CD (1994) Spindle cell liposarcoma, a hitherto unrecognized variant of liposarcoma. Analysis of six cases. Am J Surg Pathol 18:913–921
34. De Maeseneer M, Jaovisidha S, Lenchik L, Witte D, Schweitzer ME, Sartoris DJ, Resnick D (1997) Fibrolipomatous hamartoma: MR imaging findings. Skeletal Radiol 26:155–160
35. Demos TC, Bruno E, Armin A, Dobozi WR (1984) Parosteal lipoma with enlarging osteochondroma. Am J Roentgenol 143:365–356
36. DeSantos LA, Goldstein HM, Murray JA, Wallace S (1978) Computed tomography in the evaluation of musculoskeletal neoplasms. Radiology 128:89–94
37. Deseran MW, Seeger LL, Doberneck SA, Eckardt JJ (1994) Case report 840. Hibernoma of the right gracilis muscles. Skeletal Radiol 23:301–302
38. Donati L, Candiani P, Grappolini S, Klinger M, Signorini M (1990) Congenital infiltrating lipomatosis of the face related to cytomegalovirus infection. Br J Plast Surg 43:124–126
39. Donnelly LF, Bisset GS III, Passo MH (1994) MRI findings of lipoma arborescens of the knee in a child: case report. Pediatr Radiol 24:258–259
40. Dooms GC, Hricak H, Sollitto RA, Higgins CB (1985) Lipomatous tumors and tumors with fatty component: MR imaging potential and comparison of MR and CT results. Radiology 157:479–483
41. Drevelegas A, Pilavaki M, Chourmouzi D (2004) Lipomatous tumors of soft tissue: MR appearance with histological correlation Eur J Radiol 50:257–267
42. Einarsdottir H, Soderlund V, Larson O, Jenner G, Bauer HCF (1999) MR imaging of lipoma and liposarcoma. Acta Radiol 40(1):64–68
43. Enzi G (1984) Multiple symmetrical lipomatosis: an updated clinical report. Medicine 63:56–64
44. Enzi G, Biondetti PR, Fiore D, Mazzoleni F (1982) Computed tomography of deep fat masses in multiple symmetrical lipomatosis. Radiology 144:121–124
45. Enzi G, Carraro R, Alfieri P, Busetto L, Digito M, Pavan M, Negrin P (1992) Shoulder girdle lipomatosis. Ann Intern Med 117:749–750
46. Enzinger FM, Weiss SW (1995) Benign lipomatous tumors. In: Enzinger FM, Weiss SW (eds) Soft tissue tumors, 3rd edn. Mosby, St Louis, pp 381–430
47. Enzinger FM, Weiss SW (1995) Liposarcoma. In: Enzinger FM, Weiss SW (eds) Soft tissue tumors, 3rd edn. Mosby, St Louis, pp 431–466
48. Enzinger FM, Winslow DJ (1962) Liposarcoma: a study of 103 cases. Virchows Arch [A] 335:367–388
49. Evans HA, Donnelly LF, Johnson ND, Blebea JS, Stern PJ (1997) Fibrolipoma of the median nerve: MRI. Clin Radiol 52:304–307
50. Evans HL (1979) Liposarcoma: a study of 55 cases with reassessment of its classification. Am J Surg Pathol. 3:507–523
51. Fanburg-Smith JC, Devaney KO, Miettinen M, Weiss SW (1998) Multiple spindle cell lipomas: a report of 7 familial and 11 nonfamilial cases. Am J Surg Pathol. 22(1):40–48
52. Feller JF, Rishi M, Hughes EC (1994) Lipoma arborescens of the knee: MR demonstration. Am J Roentgenol 163:162–164
53. Fleming RJ, Alpert M, Garcia A (1962) Parosteal lipoma. Am J Roentgenol 87:1075
54. Fornage BD, Tassin GB (1991) Sonographic appearances of superficial soft tissue lipomas. J Clin Ultrasound 19:215–220
55. Friedlander HL, Rosenberg NJ, Graubard DJ (1969) Intraneural lipoma of the median nerve. J Bone Joint Surg Am 51A: 352–362
56. Friedman AC, Hartman DS, Sherman J, Lautin EM, Goldman M (1981) Computed tomography of abdominal fatty masses. Radiology 139:415–429
57. Fuchs A, Henrot P, IOchum S et al (2002) Tumeurs graisseuses des parties molles des membres et des ceintures de l'adulte. J Radiol 83:1035–1057
58. Galant J, Marti-Bonmati L, Fujimoto R et al (2003) The value of fat-suppressed T2 or STIR sequences in distinguishing lipoma from well-differntiated liposarcoma. 13:337–343
59. Gaskin CM, Helms CA (2004) Lipomas, lipoma variants, and well-differentiated liposarcomas (atypical lipomas): results of MRI evaluations of 126 consecutive fatty masses. AJR Am J Roentgenol 182:733–739
60. Gelineck J, Keller J, Jensen OM, Nielsen OS, Christensen T (1994) Evaluation of lipomatous soft tissue tumors by MR imaging. Acta Radiologica 35(4):367–370
61. Gilbert TJ, Goswitz JJ, Teynor JT, Griffiths HJ (1996) Lipoblastoma of the foot. Skeletal Radiol 25:283–286
62. Goldman AB, DiCarlo EF, Marcove RC (1993) Case report 774. Coincidental parosteal lipoma with osseous excrescence and intramuscular lipoma. Skeletal Radiol 22:138–145
63. Gould ES, Javors BR, Morrison J, Potter H (1989) MR appearance of bilateral periscapular elastofibromas. J Comput Assist Tomogr 13:701–703
64. Green RA, CannonSR, Flanagan AM (2004) Chondroid lipoma: correlation of imaging findings and histopathology of an unusual benign lesion. Skeletal Radiol 33:67–63
65. Ha TV, Kleinman PK, Fraire A, Spevak MR, Nimkin K, Cohen IT, Hirsh M, Walton R (1994) MR imaging of benign fatty tumors in children: report of four cases and review of literature. Skeletal Radiol 23:361–367
66. Haas AF, Fromer Es, Bricca GM (1999) Spindle cell lipoma of the scalp: a case report and review. Dermatol Surg 25(1):68–71
67. Haasbeek JF, Alvillar RE (1999) Childhood lipoma arborescens presenting as bilateral suprapatellar masses. J Rheumatol 26(3):683–686
68. Hallel Tumor, Lew S, Bansal M (1988) Villous lipomatous proliferation of the synovial membrane (lipoma arborescens). J Bone Joint Surg 70A:264–270
69. Heaton JM (1972) The distribution of brown adipose tissue in the human. J Anat 112:35–39
70. Henricks WH, Chu YC, Goldblum JR, Weiss SW (1997) Dedifferentiated liposarcoma: a clinicopathological analysis of 155 cases with a proposal for an expanded definition of dedifferentiation. Am J Surg Pathol 21(3):271–281
71. Hosono M, Kobayashi H, Fujimoto R, Kotoura Y, Tsuboyama T, Matsusue T, Nakamura T, Itoh T, Konishi J (1997) Septum-like structures in lipoma and liposarcoma: MR imaging and pathological correlation. Skeletal Radiol 26:150–154
72. Hunter JC, Johnston WH, Genant HK (1979) Computed tomography evaluation of fatty tumors of the somatic soft tissues: clinical utility and radiographic-pathological correlation. Skeletal Radiol 4:79–91
73. Ippolito V, Brien EW, Menendez LR, Mirra JM (1993) Case report 797. "Dedifferentiated" lipoma-like liposarcoma of soft tissue with focal transformation to high-grade "sclerosing" osteosarcoma. Skeletal Radiol 22:604–608
74. Jaffe RH (1926) Recurrent lipomatous tumors of the groin: liposarcoma and lipoma pseudomyxomatodes. (AMA) Arch Pathol Lab Med 1:381–387
75. Jelinek JS, Kransdorf MJ, Schmookler BM, Aboulafia AJ, Malawer MM (1993) Liposarcoma of the extremities: MR and CT findings in the histological subtypes. Radiology 186:455–459
76. Jimenez JF (1986) Lipoblastoma in infancy and childhood. J Surg Oncol. 32:238–244

77. Jones OG, Habermann ET, Dorfman HD (1989) Case report 553. Parosteal ossifying lipoma of femur. Skeletal Radiol 18:537–540

78. Kallas KM, Vaughan L, Haghighi P, Resnick D (2003) Hibernoma of the left axilla: a case report and review of MR imaging. Skeletal Radiol 32:290–294

79. Katz DS, Merchant N, Beaulieu CF, Blankenberg FG (1996) Clinical image. Lipoblastoma of the thigh: MR appearance. J Comput Assist Tomogr 20(6):1002–1003

80. Kawashima A, Magid D, Fishman EK, Hruban RH, Ney DR (1993) Parosteal ossifying lipoma: CT and MR findings. J Comput Assist Tomogr 17(1):147–150

81. Kemula M, Clerc D, Quillard J, Desmoulins F, Marfeuille M, Bisson M (1999) Liposarcome multicentrique. À propos d'un cas. Rev Méd Interne 20:60–63

82. Kilpatrick SE, Doyon J, Choong PF, Sim FH, Nascimento AG (1996) The clinicopathological spectrum of myxoid and round cell liposarcoma. Cancer 77:1450–1458

83. Kim JY, Park JM, Lim GY, Chun KA, Park YH, Yoo JY (2002) Atypical benign lipomatous tumors in the soft tissue: radiographic and pathological correlation. J Comput Assist Tomogr 29:1063–1068

84. Kim T, Murakami T, Oi H, Tsuda K, Tatsushita M, Tomoda K, Fukuda H, Nakamura H (1996) CT and MR imaging of abdominal liposarcoma. Am J Roentgenol 166:829–833

85. Kransdorf MJ (1995) Benign soft tissue tumors in a large referral population: distribution of specific diagnoses by age, sex and location. Am J Roentgenol 164:395–402

86. Kransdorf MJ (1995) Malignant soft tissue tumors in a large referral population: distribution of diagnoses by age, sex and location. Am J Roentgenol 164:129–134

87. Kransdorf MJ, Murphey MD (1997) Lipomatous tumors. In: Kransdorf MJ, Murphey MD (eds) Imaging of soft tissue tumors. Saunders, Philadelphia, pp 57–101

88. Kransdorf MJ, Jelinek JS, Moser RP, Utz JA, Brower AC, Hudson TM, Berrey BH (1989) Soft-tissue masses: diagnosis using MR imaging. Am J Roentgenol 153:541–547

89. Kransdorf MJ, Moser RP, Meis JM, Meyer CA (1991) Fat-containing soft tissue masses of the extremities. Radiographics 11:81–106

90. Kransdorf MJ, Meis JM, Jelinek JS (1993) Dedifferentiated liposarcoma of the extremities: imaging findings in four patients. Am J Roentgenol 161:127–130

91. Kransdorf MJ, Jelinek JS, Moser RP (1993) Imaging of soft tissue tumors. Radiol Clin North Am 31:359–372

92. Kransdorf MJ, Bancroft LW, Peterson JJ, Murphey MD, Foster WC, Temple HT (2002) Imaging of fatty tumors: distinction of lipoma and well-diiferentiated liposarcoma. Radiology 224:99–104

93. Kulhavy M, Uijs RR, Sur RK, Donde B, Nayler S, Sur M, Giraud A (1997) Symmetrical multifocal liposarcoma. S Afr J Surg 35:68–9

94. Laorr A, Peterfy CG, Tirman PF, Rabassa AE (1995) Lipoma arborescens of the shoulder: magnetic resonance imaging findings. Can Assoc Radiol J 46:311–313

95. Lateur L, Van Ongeval C, Samson I, Van Damme B, Baert AL (1994) Case report 842. Benign hibernoma. Skeletal Radiol 23:306–309

96. Learch TL, Braaton M (2000) Lipoma arborescens: high-resolution ultrasonographic findings. J Ultrasound Med 19:385–389

97. Levine E, Lee KR, Neff JR et al (1979) Comparison of computed tomography and other imaging modalities in the evaluation of musculoskeletal tumors. Radiology 131:431–437

98. Lin YC, Huang CC, Chen HJ (2001) Intraspinal osteolipoma. Case report. J Neurosurg 94:126–128

99. Logan PM, Janzen DL, O'Connell JX, Munk PL, Connell DG (1996) Chondroid lipoma: MRI appearances with clinical and histological correlation. Skeletal Radiol 25:592–595

100. London J, Kim EE, Wallace S, Shirkhoda A, Coan J, Evans H (1989) MR imaging of liposarcomas: correlation of MR features and histology. J Comput Assist Tomogr 13(5):832–835

101. Ma LD, McCarthy EF, Bluemke DA, Frassica FJ (1998) Differentiation of benign from malignant musculoskeletal lesions using MR imaging: pitfalls in MR evaluation of lesions with a cystic appearance. Am J Roentgenol 170:1251–1258

102. Madewell JE, Sweet DE (1988) Tumors and tumor-like lesions in or about joints. In: Resnick D, Niwayama G (eds) Diagnosis of bone and joint disorders, 2nd edn. Saunders, Philadelphia, pp 3889–3943

103. Marom EM, Helms CA (1999) Fibrolipomatous hamartoma: pathognomonic on MR imaging. Skeletal Radiol 28:260–264

104. Martin DS, Sharafuddin M, Boozan J, Sundaram M, Archer C (1995) Multiple symmetric lipomatosis (Madelung's disease). Skeletal Radiol 24:72–73

105. Martín S, Hernández L, Romero J, Lafuente J, Poza AI, Ruiz P, Jimeno M (1998) Diagnostic imaging of lipoma arborescens. Skeletal Radiol 27:325–329

106. Martinez D, Millner PA, Coral A, Newman RJ, Hardy GJ, Path FR, Butt WP (1992) Case report 745. Synovial lipoma arborescens. Skeletal Radiol 21:393–395

107. Matsumoto K, Hukuda S, Ishizawa M, Chano T, Okabe H (1999) MRI findings in intramuscular lipomas. Skeletal Radiol 28:145–152

108. Matsumoto K, Takada M, Okabe H, Ishizawa M (2000) Foci of signal intensities different from fat in well-differentiated liposarcoma and lipoma: correlation between MR and histological findings. Clin Imaging 24:38–43

109. McEachern A, Janzen DL, O' Connell JX (1995) Shoulder girdle lipomatosis. Skeletal Radiol 24:471–473

110. McLane RC, Meyer LC (1978) Axillary hibernoma: review of the literature with report of a case examined angiographically. Radiology 127:673–674

111. Mehregan DR, Mehregan DA, Mehregan AH, Dorman MA, Cohen E (1995) Spindle cell lipomas. A report of two cases: one with multiple lesions. Dermatol Surg 21:796–798

112. Meis JM, Enzinger FM (1993) Chondroid lipoma: a unique tumor simulating liposarcoma and myxoid chondrosarcoma. Am J Surg Pathol 17:1103–1112

113. Merkel H (1906) Uber ein pseudolipom der mamma (Eigenartigr Fettzellentumor). Beitr Path Anat 39:152–157

114. Miller GG, Yanchar NL, Magee JF, Blair GK (1998) Lipoblastoma and liposarcoma in children: an analysis of 9 cases and a review of the literature. Can J Surg 41(6):455–458

115. Mugel T, Ghossain MA, Guinet C, Buy J, Bethoux J, Texier P, Vadrot D (1998) MR and CT findings in a case of hibernoma of the thigh extending into the pelvis. Eur Radiol 8:476–478

116. Munk PL, Lee MJ, Janzen DL, Connell DG, Logan PM, Poon PY, Bainbridge TC (1997) Lipoma and liposarcoma: evaluation using CT and MR imaging. Am J Roentgenol 169:589–594

117. Muren C, Lee M, Juhlin L (1994) CT-diagnosis of deep-seated lipomas with alarming symptoms. Acta Radiol 35:169–171

118. Murphey MD, Johnson DL, Bhatia PS, Neff JR, Rosenthal HG, Walker CW (1994) Parosteal lipoma: MR imaging characteristics. Am J Roentgenol 162:105–110

119. Murphey MD, Carroll JF, Flemming DJ, Pope TL, GannonFH, Kransdorf MJ (2004). From the archives of the AFIP. Benign musculoskeletal lipomatous lesions. Radiographics 24:1433–1466

120. Nigrisoli M, Ruggieri P, Picci P, Pignatti G (1988) Case report 489. Hibernoma of left thigh. Skeletal Radiol 17:432–435

121. Nishida J, Shimamura T, Ehara S, Shiraishi H, Sato T, Abe M (1998) Posterior interosseous nerve palsy caused by parosteal lipoma of proximal radius. Skeletal Radiol 27:375–379

122. Nisolle JF, Blouard E, Baudrez V, Boutsen Y, De Cloedt P, Esselinckx W (1999) Subacromial-subdeltoid lipoma arborescens associated with a rotator cuff tear. Skeletal Radiol 28:283–285

123. Ohguri T, Aoki T, Hisaoka M et al (2003) Differential diagnosis of benign peripheral lipoma from well-diffrentiated liposarcoma. MR imaging: Is comparison of margins and internal characteristics useful? AJR Am J Roentgenol 180:1689–1694

124. Oleaga L, Florencio MR, Ereño C, Grande J, Terrones J, Legorburu A, Grande D (1995) Fibrolipomatous hamartoma of the radial nerve: MR imaging findings. Skeletal Radiol 24:559–561
125. Patel RV, Gondalia MS (1991) Congenital infiltrating lipomatosis of the face. Br J Plast Surg 44:157–158
126. Pearlstone DB, Pisters PW, Bold RJ et al (1999) Patterns of recurrence in extremity liposarcoma: implications for staging and follow-up. Cancer 85:85–92
127. Peterson JJ, Kransdorf MJ, Bancroft LW, O'Connor MI (2003) Malignant fatty tumors: classification, clinical course, imaging appearance and treatment. Skeletal Radiol 32:493–503
128. Plaut GS, Salm R, Truscott DE (1959) Three cases of ossifying lipoma. J Pathol Bacteriol 78:292–295
129. Pudlowski RM, Gilula LA, Kyrialos M (1979) Intraarticular lipoma with osseous metaplasia: a radiographic-pathological correlation. AJR Am J Roentgenol 132:471–473
130. Reiseter T, Nordshus T, Borthne A, Roald B, Naess P, Schistad O (1999) Lipoblastoma: MRI appearances of a rare paediatric soft tissue tumour. Pediatr Radiol 29:542–545
131. Rodriguez-Peralto JL, Lopez-Barea F, Gonzalez-Lopez J, Lamas-Lorenzo M (1994) Case report 821: parosteal ossifying lipoma of femur. Skeletal Radiol 23:67–69
132. Rubinstein A, Goor Y, Gazit E, Cabili S (1989) Non-symmetric subcutaneous lipomatosis associated with familial combined hyperlipidaemia. Br J Dermatol 120:689–694
133. Russell WO, Cohen J, Enzinger FM et al (1977) A clinical and pathological staging system for soft tissue sarcomas. Cancer 40:1562–1570
134. Ryu KN, Jaovisidha S, Schweitzer M, Motta AO, Resnick D (1996) MR imaging of lipoma arborescens of the knee joint. AJR Am J Roentgenol 167:1229–1232
135. Salgado R, Bernaerts A, Op de Beeck B, De Schepper A, P Parizel (2004) Madelung's neck: cross-sectional observations. AJR Am J Roentgenol 182:1344–1345
136. Schultz E, Rosenblatt R, Mitsudo S, Weinberg G (1993) Detection of a deep lipoblastoma by MRI and ultrasound. Pediatr Radiol 23:409–410
137. Seynaeve P, Mortelmans L, Kockx M, Van Hoye M, Mathijs R (1994) Case report 813: Hibernoma of the left thigh. Skeletal Radiol 23:137–138
138. Shugar MA, Gavron JP (1985) Benign symmetrical lipomatosis (Madelung's disease). Otolaryngol Head Neck Surg 93:109–112
139. Silverman TA, Enzinger FM (1985) Fibrolipomatous hamartoma of nerve: a clinicopathological analysis of 26 cases. Am J Surg Pathol 9:7–14
140. Soler T, Rodriguez E, Bargiela A, Da Riba M (1998) Lipoma arborescens of the knee: MR characteristics in 13 joints. J Comput Assist Tomogr 22:605–609
141. Soulie D, Boyer B, Lescop J, Pujol A, Le Friant G, Cordoliani YS (1995) Myxoid liposarcoma. MRI imaging. J Radiol 76:29–36
142. Stringel G, Shandling B, Mancer K, Ein SH (1982) Lipoblastoma in infants and children. J Pediatr Surg 17:277–280
143. Sullivan CR, Dahlin DC, Bryan RS (1956) Lipoma of the tendon sheath. J Bone Joint Surg Am 38A:1275
144. Sundaram M, McGuire MH, Herbold DR, Beshany SE, Fletcher JW (1987) High signal intensity soft tissue masses on T1-weighted pulsing sequences. Skeletal Radiol 16:30–36
145. Sundaram M, McGuire MH, Herbold DR (1988) Magnetic resonance imaging of soft tissue masses: an evaluation of fifty-three histologically proven tumors. Magn Reson Imaging 6:237–248
146. Sundaram M, Baran G, Merenda G, McDonald DJ (1990) Myxoid liposarcoma: magnetic resonance imaging appearances with clinical and histological correlation. Skeletal Radiol 19:359–362
147. Sung M, Kang HS, Suh JS et al (2000) Myxoid liposarcoma: appearance at MR imaging with histological correlation. Radiographics 20:1007–1019
148. Toms AP, White LM, Kandel R, Bell RS (2003) Low-grade liposarcoma with osteosarcomatous dedifferentiation: radiological and histological features. Skeletal Radiol 32:286–289
149. Vanhoenacker FM, De Schepper AM, Gielen JL, Parizel PM (2005) MR imaging in the diagnosis and management of inheritable musculoskeletal disorders. Clin Radiol 60:160–170
150. Vellios F, Baez JM, Schumacker HB (1958) Lipoblastomatosis: a tumor of fetal fat different from hibernoma. Report of a case, with observations of the embryogenesis of human adipose tissue. Am J Pathol 34:1149–1159
151. Vilanova JC, Barcelo J, Villalon M, Aldoma J, Delgado E, Zapater I (2003) MR imaging of lipoma arborescens and the associated lesions. Skeletal Radiol 32:504–509
152. Waligore MP, Stephens DH, Soule EH, McLeod RA(1981). Lipomatous tumors of the abdominal cavity: CT appearance and pathological correlation. AJR Am J Roentgenol 137:539–545
153. Walker CW, Adams BD, Barnes CL, Roloson GJ, FitzRandolph RL (1991) Case report 667: Fibrolipomatous hamartoma of the median nerve. Skeletal Radiol 20:237–239
154. Wang SF, Chang CY, Wu HD (1998) Lipoblastomatosis of the shoulder: unusual MR appearance. Br J Radiol 71:884–885
155. Weekes RG, Berquist TH, Mcleod RA, Zimmer WD (1985) Magnetic resonance imaging of soft tissue tumors: comparison with computed tomography. Magn Reson Imaging 3:345–352
156. Weekes RG, McLeod RA, Reiman HM, Pritchard DJ (1985) CT of soft tissue neoplasms. AJR Am J Roentgenol 144:355–360
157. Weiss SW, Rao VK (1992) Well-differentiated liposarcoma (atypical lipoma) of deep soft tissue of the extremities, retroperitoneum and miscellaneous sites. A follow-up study of 92 cases with analysis of the incidence of "dedifferentiation." Am J Surg Pathol 16:1051–1058
158. Whol MG, Pastor N (1938) Adiposis dolorosa (Dercum's disease). JAMA 110:1261
159. Wu TP, Tsai JG, Chan PH, Lee HC, Wei YH (1994) Mitochondrial respiratory function in multiple symmetrical lipomatosis: report of two cases. J Formos Med Assoc 93:513–518

Tumors and Tumor-like Lesions of Blood Vessels

F. Ramon

16

Contents

16.1 Introduction

Tumors and tumor-like conditions of the vascular system are divided into three categories according to their degree of malignancy: benign vascular lesions, lesions of intermediate malignancy, and malignant vascular tumors. The vast majority of the lesions belong to the benign group. These are found predominantly in younger children and adolescents. They may involve either the skin and subcutis or the deep soft tissues. Classification of these lesions is still the source of much controversy and is based on clinical appearance, pathology, embryology, and endothelial growth characteristics [12, 41, 42]. There are two major classification schemes for vascular tumors. That of Enzinger et al. [12] relies on pathological criteria and includes clinical and radiological features when appropriate. On the other hand, the classification of Mulliken and Glowacki [42] is based on endothelial growth characteristics and distinguishes hemangiomas from vascular malformations. The latter classification shows good correlation with the clinical picture and imaging findings.

Hemangiomas are characterized by a phase of proliferation and a stationary period, followed by involution. Vascular malformations are no real tumors and can be divided into low- or high-flow lesions [65].

Cutaneous and subcutaneous lesions are usually easily diagnosed and present no significant diagnostic problems. On the other hand, hemangiomas or vascular malformations that arise in deep soft tissue must be differentiated from malignant neoplasms. Detailed assessment by medical imaging is necessary for adequate planning of surgery.

On magnetic resonance imaging (MRI) benign vascular lesions have a characteristic configuration, generally allowing a correct diagnosis. MRI is superior to other imaging techniques in defining the extent of these lesions, which is important since some types may involve large segments of the body.

Generally the classification of soft tissue vascular anomalies based on endothelial growth characteristics [66] shows good correlation with MRI appearance of these lesions [37]. Since this classification has been useful clinically [54], recognition of these characteristic MRI features is essential for improving therapeutic outcome in these patients.

Vascular lesions of intermediate malignancy and malignant vascular tumors are far more rare. Hemangioendothelioma is a neoplasm of endothelial cells that can be benign or malignant. Angiosarcoma is an aggressive tumor with high local recurrence rate and risk of distant metastases. Imaging findings have only been sparse, probably due to the tendency of these lesions to involve skin and superficial tissue, in contrast to other soft tissue sarcomas. MRI is used for staging rather than for characterization of these lesions.

16.2 Definition and Classification

16.2.1 Benign Vascular Tumors

In the past it was debated whether vascular tumors are developmental malformations or true tumors. In the nineteenth century vascular lesions were thought to be 'produced by the longing of the mother, for particular things, or her aversion to them'. Expressions such as nevus materneus or stigma metrocelis were in reference to the mother. Because vascular tumors sometimes closely resemble normal vessels, it is difficult to distinguish clearly between neoplasm and malformation on histological examination [41].

The term hemangioma has frequently been used incorrectly, although accurate nomenclature is of utmost importance for correct diagnosis and treatment of these lesions [66].

16.2.1.1 Classification of Mulliken

Some authors have suggested that the clinical presentation provides the necessary perspective for classifying vascular lesions. Mulliken et al. presented a useful scheme for separating cutaneous vascular lesions based on endothelial growth characteristics [42]. Their studies reveal two major types of vascular lesions. One exhibits a rapid growth phase followed by a period of stabilization and finally involution; these show a female

predominance and are usually not present at birth. Because of cellular proliferation and the mass effect, these are called (infantile) hemangiomas (Table 16.1).

The majority of hemangiomas do not need treatment.

On the other hand, many vascular lesions show no cellular proliferation; they usually are not present at birth but grow with the child and have no involution phase. These lesions are called vascular malformations, and they are divided into capillary, venous, arterial and lymphatic types depending on the predominant vessel type [42].

The classification scheme was updated during the 1992 meeting of the International Society for the Study of Vascular Anomalies (ISSVA) [75, 82] (Table 16.2).

The endothelial lining of the vascular malformation group is not proliferative. Although they are stable from a cellular point of view, they can be clinically devastating, specially when there is arteriovenous shunting.

16.2.1.2 Classification of Enzinger

Enzinger et al., however, do not rely on clinical presentation for classification of benign vascular lesions [12]. Some congenital lesions do not become apparent until adult life, depending on their location and growth. In view of this limitation no attempt is made to separate malformations from benign neoplasms. All lesions are called hemangiomas, and hemangioma is defined as 'a benign but nonreactive process in which there is an increase in the number of normal or abnormal-appearing vessels [12]. Hemangiomas may be either of two types: those localized in one area and those involving large segments of the body. The histological classification of vascular tumors proposed by Enzinger et al. [12] is as follows (Table 16.3).

Localized hemangiomas are the more common. They have been classified according to clinical, embryologic, or pathological criteria but no system is entirely satisfactory.

Table 16.1. Differentiating features of hemangiomas and vascular malformations (modified from [65])

Hemangiomas	Vascular malformations
Exhibit cellular proliferation	Comprised of dysplastic vessels
Small or absent at birth	Present at birth
Rapid growth during infancy	Growth proportional to child
Involution during childhood	No regression

Table 16.2. ISSVA classification of vascular anomalies (modified from [76, 83])

Vascular malformations		
Vascular tumor	**Simple**	**Combined**
Hemangioma		
Proliferative phase	Capillary malformation	Arteriovenous fistula, arteriovenous malformation, capillary-venous malformation, capillary-lymphatic-venous malformation (Klippel Trénaunay syndrome)
Involutive phase	Lymphatic malformation	Lymphatic-venous malformation, capillary-arteriovenous malformation (Parkes-Weber syndrome), capillary-lymphatic-arteriovenous malformation
Other tumors	Venous malformation	

A more pertinent issue considering imaging and therapy is classifying vascular malformations as either low-flow or high-flow lesions [84]

Table 16.3. Histological classification of vascular tumors (modified from [12])

Benign vascular tumors
  Localized Hemangioma
    Capillary Hemangioma
    Cavernous Hemangioma
    Venous hemangioma
    Arteriovenous hemangioma
    Epithelioid hemangioma
    Hemangioma of the granulation tissue type
    Deep soft tissue hemangioma
  Angiomatosis

Vascular tumors of intermediate malignancy
  Epithelioid hemangioendothelioma
  Spindle cell hemangioendothelioma
  Malignant endovascular papillary hemangioendothelioma

Malignant vascular tumors
  Angiosarcoma
  Kaposi's sarcoma

Table 16.4. WHO classification of vascular tumors (modified from [68])

Benign
  Hemangiomas of
    Subcutis/deep soft tissue
    Capillary
    Cavernous
    Arteriovenous
    Venous
    Intramuscular
    Synovial
  Epithelioid hemangioma
  Angiomatosis
  Lymphangioma

Intermediate (locally aggressive)
  Kaposiform hemangioendothelioma

Intermediate (rarely metastasizing)
  Retiform hemangioendothelioma
  Papillary intralymphatic angioendothelioma
  Composite hemangioendothelioma
  Kaposi sarcoma

Malignant
  Epithelioid hemangioendothelioma
  Angiosarcoma of soft tissue

They are usually located superficially but may involve deep structures, such as skeletal muscle. Depending on the predominant vessel type, the former are grouped as capillary, cavernous, venous or arteriovenous. Other forms are more rare.

Hemangiomas involving the deep soft tissues are grouped as intramuscular, synovial or intraneural types. Intramuscular hemangioma usually shows an overgrowth of adipose tissue, giving the impression of angiolipoma. Unlike their cutaneous variants, it is not always possible to make a clear distinction between different types of intramuscular hemangiomas. A classification into small-vessel, large-vessel and mixed types with different clinical behavior was proposed by Allen to avoid misinterpretation since some of the small-vessel type lesions show alarming histological features resembling those of a sarcoma [1].

Angiomatosis is a rare condition in which large segments of the body are involved by proliferating vessels. Mostly the extremities are affected. A characteristic feature of this condition is the large amount of mature fat that accompanies the proliferating vessels [12].

The distinction between intramuscular hemangioma and angiomatosis is made better by clinical than pathological criteria.

16.2.1.3 WHO Classification

The classification of the WHO (Table 16.4) closely resembles that of Enzinger. In this classification, no distinction is made between benign vascular neoplasms or vascular malformations. Similarly, it is impossible to reliably distinguish vascular from lymphatic endothelium. Therefore, they classify lymphangioma as a vascular tumor.

16.2.2 Vascular Tumors of Borderline or Intermediate Malignancy

The term hemangioendothelioma is currently used for lesions which are histologically intermediate in appearance between hemangiomas and angiosarcomas.

According to Enzinger, the three types are epithelioid hemangioendothelioma, spindle cell hemangioendothelioma and malignant endovascular papillary hemangioendothelioma. Only the epithelioid subgroup occurs in deep soft tissues, most commonly of the extremities. The other types develop preferentially in the dermis or subcutaneous tissues [13].

The WHO classification differentiates locally aggressive tumors of intermediate malignancy and rarely metastasizing types. Kaposiform hemangioendothelioma is characterized by a 'Kaposi sarcoma like' fascicular spindle cell growth pattern. It most commonly occurs in the retroperitoneum or the skin.

16.2.3 Malignant Vascular Tumors

Angiosarcomas are tumors that can vary from highly differentiated, resembling hemangioma, to those whose anaplasia makes it difficult to distinguish from carcinomas. They are characterized by irregular anastomosing vascular channels lined by atypical endothelial cells.

The terms hemangiosarcoma and lymphangiosarcoma are no longer appropriate [14, 45]. The lesions occur preferentially in the skin or soft tissues of the scalp and face. Kaposi's sarcomas have spindle cell areas containing vascular channels.

The disease is associated with the Human Herpes Virus (HHV-8) infection. It presents as cutaneous lesions in the form of multiple patches. According to the WHO classification Kaposi sarcoma is of intermediate malignancy and epithelioid hemangioendothelioma is malignant.

16.2.4 Glomus Tumor

The glomus tumor is a neoplasm consisting of cells which closely resemble smooth muscle cells of the normal glomus body. The glomus body is an arteriovenous anastomosis that has an important role in thermoregulation. It is located in the subungual region, digits, and palms. The lesion shows both muscle fibers and epithelial-appearing glomus cells [15].

16.2.5 Hemangiopericytoma

Hemangiopericytoma is an uncommon tumor, first described by Stout and Murray, and is composed mainly of pericytes [8, 15, 26, 28, 33, 44, 52, 55, 63]. According to the most recent WHO classification [67], hemangiopericytoma will be discussed in Chap. 13 (Tumors of Fibrous Tissue).

16.3 Incidence and Clinical Behavior

16.3.1 Benign Vascular Tumors

To avoid confusion we follow here a combination of the classification of Enzinger and the WHO [12, 67].

The differentiation of Mulliken and Glowacki between hemangiomas and vascular malformations is only considered when specifically mentioned.

Although hemangiomas are uncommon tumors, they make up about 7% of all benign soft tissue tumors. Most of the lesions, however, are located in the skin or subcutaneous tissues, while only a minority is deeply seated [12].

Capillary hemangiomas form the largest group. Except for cherry angioma they occur predominantly in childhood. Juvenile hemangioma is an immature form of capillary hemangioma with a characteristic clinical evolution. They occur mostly in superficial tissue of head and neck region and arise a few weeks after birth. They grow slowly to reach a maximal size at six months of age and then regress. Some lesions may pose cosmet-

ic problems or threaten vital structures. They are treated by systemic steroid therapy and subsequent surgery. Acquired tufted angioma, verrucous hemangioma, and senile angioma are clinical variants of the same subtype of hemangioma.

Cavernous hemangiomas are less frequent but share age and anatomical distribution with the capillary hemangiomas. However, they are usually larger and less circumscribed and may be locally destructive. The majority require surgical resection.

Superficial arteriovenous and venous types are less common. They are distinguished from the capillary and cavernous counterparts by the presence of thick-walled vessels. Superficially located arteriovenous hemangiomas cause no clinical problems. On the other hand, shunting of blood causing cardiac overload, pain and hypertrophy of the involved extremity are problems associated with deep lesions and require an adequate therapeutic approach.

Epithelioid hemangioma and granulation type hemangioma are unusual vascular tumors.

Epithelioid hemangioma consists of well formed but immature vessels and a prominent inflammatory component. They occur predominantly at the forehead and the digits, and present as a nodular mass which gives the impression of an epidermal cyst.

Compared to superficial hemangiomas, deep-seated lesions are quite uncommon, with a reported frequency of 0.8% of all lesions [44]. However, they deserve specific mention because of their different clinical presentation. Because they present with pain or swelling, it is difficult to make a diagnosis based on physical examination. Some 80–90% of intramuscular hemangiomas occur in the first three decades of life. There is no female predilection, as for superficial hemangiomas. The majority of lesions are located in the lower extremity, especially in the muscles of the thigh. Pain is reported to be more common in tumors involving long, narrow muscles, probably through stretching of the muscle fibers.

Lesions have often been present for many years and it is therefore likely that many examples are congenital.

Physical deformity, cardiac decompensation, or destruction of adjacent vital structures may require surgical intervention. Therapy is aimed at complete excision, with or without prior embolization [10, 63]. Intramuscular hemangiomas are benign, but with a high incidence of local recurrence.

Synovial hemangioma and hemangioma of peripheral nerve are rare. The synovial type almost always involves the knee joint, presenting with pain, swelling and joint effusion. The most common site is the suprapatellar pouch. Because of repetitive bleeding into the joint, a radiographic appearance identical to that of hemophilic arthropathy is seen [12, 28]. Only a small proportion of lesions are correctly diagnosed before surgery (Fig. 16.1).

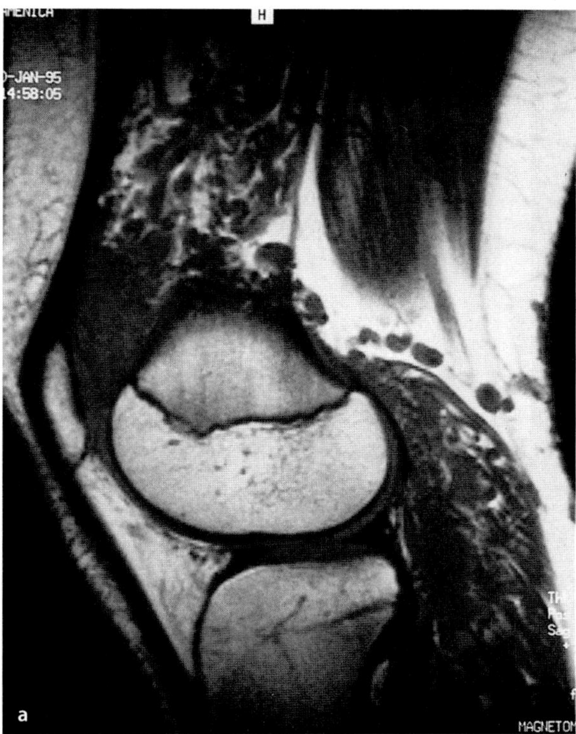

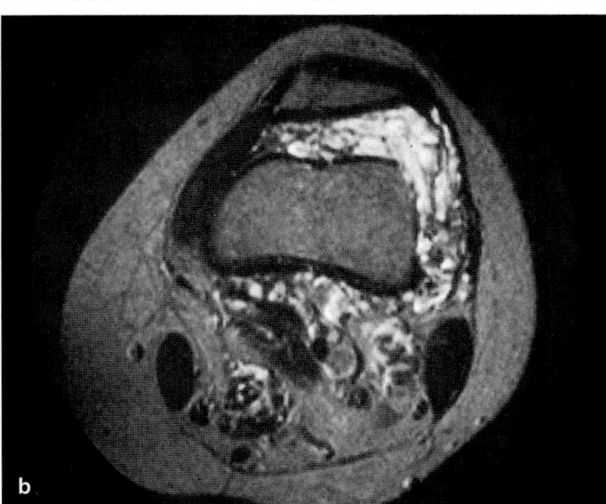

Fig. 16.1a, b. Synovial hemangioma of the knee. **a** Sagittal T1-weighted MR image. **b** Axial T2-weighted MR image. A multilobular inhomogeneous lesion involving both the suprapatellar bursa and the extra-articular fatty tissue and muscles is seen. The lesion is isointense to muscle on T1-weighted images and a large draining or feeding vessel is seen in the popliteal fossa. Axial T2-weighted images show a lesion of high signal intensity. There is no joint effusion

16.3.2 Angiomatous Syndromes

Angiomatous syndromes include Kasabach-Merritt syndrome, Maffucci's syndrome, Klippel-Trénaunay-Weber syndrome, Osler-Weber-Rendu disease, Gorham disease, Proteus syndrome and angiomatosis.

Kasabach-Merritt syndrome was first reported in 1954 [25]. The cardinal features of this syndrome include an enlarging hemangioma, thrombocytopenia and microangiopathic hemolytic anemia with acute or chronic consumptive coagulopathy. The etiology of the coagulopathy is still unknown. Mortality is estimated at approximately 21%. The major cause of death is bleeding. Many therapeutic modalities have been applied, aiming at a twofold objective: to control the bleeding and to reduce the size of the lesion [11, 25, 32, 38]. Maffucci's syndrome is a rare dysplasia characterized by multiple hemangiomas and enchondromas. The vascular tumors are usually noted at birth and are of the cavernous type. According to Silverman et al. [54], the lesions that are termed hemangiomas are in fact vascular malformations. The cartilaginous lesions typically develop after the vascular tumors. The bones are shortened and have multiple exostoses and enchondromas [6, 12] (Fig. 16.2). Malignant sarcomatous degeneration is noted in about 21% of patients.

Klippel-Trénaunay-Weber syndrome consists of cutaneous hemangioma, bone and soft tissue hypertrophy and varicose veins. The syndrome is usually unilateral and involves the lower extremity [68].

Proteus syndrome is a complex hamartomatous disorder defined by local overgrowth (macrodactyly), subcutaneous tumors and various bone, cutaneous and/or vascular anomalies. Vascular anomalies are common and are distributed at random sites of the body. The clinical presentation is highly variable [69, 70].

Angiomatosis is a rare condition in which large segments of the body are involved by proliferating vessels [71]. Principally the extremities are affected. A characteristic feature of this condition is the large amount of mature fat that accompanies the proliferating vessels [12]. The disorder probably starts during intrauterine life when the limb buds form.

Approximately two-thirds of cases develop within the two first decades of life and nearly all are apparent by age 40 years.

It usually presents as a swelling, induration, or discoloration of the affected area with or without limb hypertrophy. Mortality is high because of space occupying effects and consumption coagulopathy [12, 28].

16.3.3 Hemangioendothelioma

Epithelioid hemangioendothelioma of the soft tissues does not occur preferentially in children. All age groups are affected, and there is no sex predilection. Most lesions are solitary. Overall prognosis of this tumor is quite favorable. Only a small proportion does metastasize and cause death. Therapy includes wide local excision without adjuvant chemotherapy or radiotherapy. Regional lymph nodes should be evaluated [30, 41].

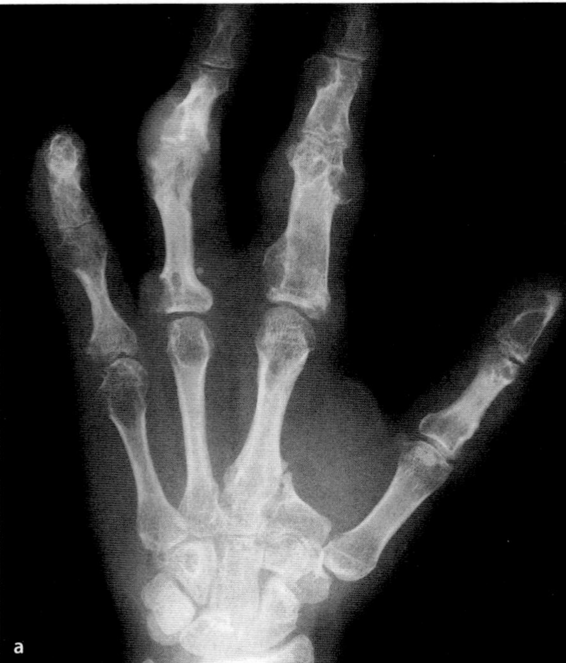

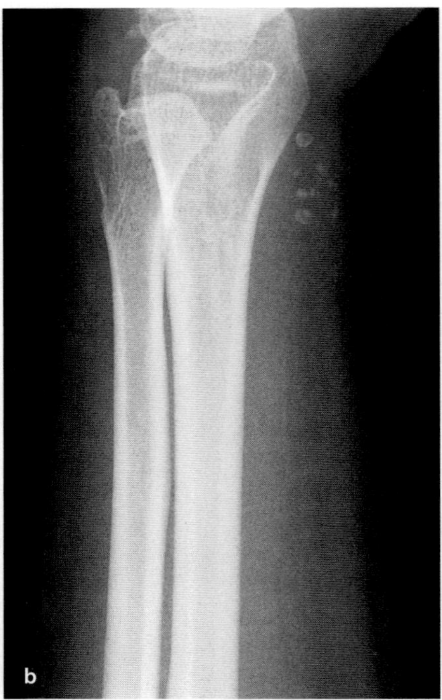

Fig. 16.2a,b. An 18-year-old woman with Maffuci's syndrome. **a** Plain radiograph of the left hand. **b** Plain radiograph (lateral view) of the left wrist. Multiple, expansile, well-defined and predominantly lytic lesions within the phalanges and metacarpals of the left hand are shown. The second digit has previously been amputated. Phleboliths are seen within a soft tissue swelling at the volar aspect of the wrist. The combination of multiple enchondromas and soft tissue hemangiomas is characteristic for Maffuci's syndrome

16.3.4 Angiosarcomas

Angiosarcomas of the deep tissue are one of the rarest forms of soft tissue neoplasms, accounting for less than 1% of all sarcomas. These tumors are evenly distributed throughout all decades and show predilection for the lower extremity and the abdominal cavity, in contrast to the cutaneous forms which are found mostly in head and neck. Chronic lymphedema is the most widely recognized predisposing factor in angiosarcomas. Angiosarcomas are often characterized as enlarging, painful masses lasting for several weeks and are occasionally associated with hemorrhage, anemia or coagulopathy. Epithelioid angiosarcoma is the most frequently observed pattern, but the morphological spectrum is wide [36]. Malignant degeneration in a preexisting benign lesion is probably an unusual event [15].

The paucity of data precludes statements concerning the optimal mode of therapy [5, 45].

16.3.5 Glomus Tumor

Glomus tumors are uncommon, with an equal frequency of occurrence in both sexes. The most common location is the subungual tissue at the tip of the finger. For this location however, there is a striking female predominance. Glomus tumors are also seen at the palm, wrist, forearm, and foot. Multiple lesions may be present, especially during childhood. Glomus tumors cause a radiating pain which is elicited by a change in temperature. Clinical examination usually reveals a characteristic blue-red nodule. Therapy aims at complete excision, still leaving a recurrence rate of 10% [15].

16.3.6 Hemangiopericytoma

As earlier mentioned, hemangiopericytoma (HPC) will be discussed in Chap. 13, which is in line with the most recent WHO classification (2002).

16.4 Imaging

16.4.1 Imaging Studies Other than MRI

Although findings on plain radiography are frequently normal, they are sometimes helpful in diagnosing soft tissue hemangiomas. Plain radiographs reveal the presence of a lesion by displacement or loss of the normal tissue planes. The presence of phleboliths is a specific sign, but unfortunately of low sensitivity.

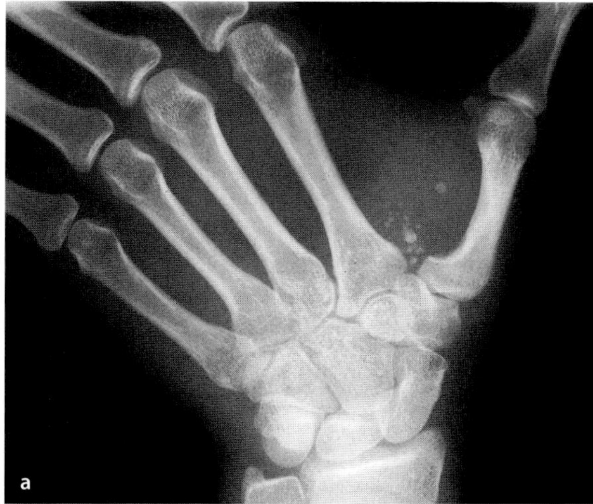

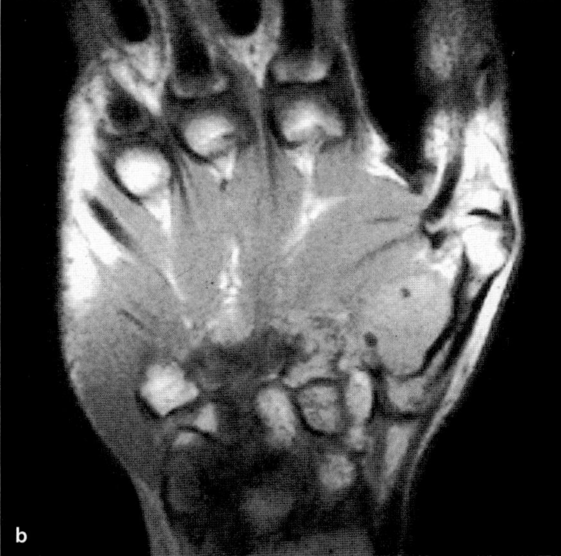

Fig. 16.3 a, b. A 35-year-old man with painless soft tissue mass at the left hand. **a** Radiograph of the left hand. **b** Coronal spin echo T1-weighted MR image. Plain radiography shows an increased density of the soft tissues at the left thenar. Multiple rounded calcifications of varying size are present, corresponding to phleboliths. This finding is characteristic for intramuscular hemangiomas. There is an erosion of the ulnar sided cortex at the base of metacarpal I (**a**). On the MR image the muscles of the thenar are slightly hyperintense due to infiltration by the hemangioma. The rounded spots of low signal intensity correspond to the phleboliths. Pressure erosion of metacarpal I is shown without change in the adjacent bone marrow (**b**)

Phleboliths are found in venous malformations and correspond to calcifications in thrombosis [72].

Lesions that are in close proximity to bone may cause bone erosion or periosteal reaction (Fig. 16.3). Twenty percent of hemangiomas of deep soft tissues cause adjacent bony changes.

The osseous changes can be categorized as periosteal, cortical or medullary. All three categories correlate with

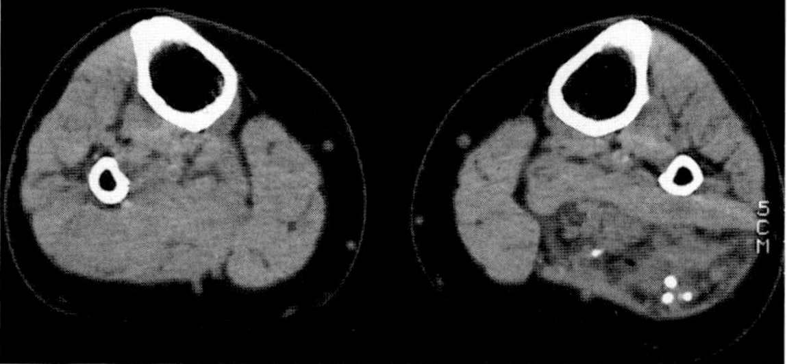

Fig. 16.4. A 47-year-old woman with a swelling of the left calf. Unenhanced CT slice shows an inhomogeneous aspect of the lateral head of the gastrocnemius muscle. The muscle is enlarged and has dispersed internal areas of decreased attenuation. A few rounded phleboliths are seen. There is no involvement of the underlying soleus muscle. Histological examination revealed the presence of a hemangioma. Areas of decreased attenuation correspond to intralesional fat

the proximity of the lesion to bone, whereas medullary changes correspond to size of the hemangioma [73, 74].

Plain film studies are superior to MRI in demonstrating the type and extent of reaction [36]. On the other hand, information about size and extent of the lesion is limited [2, 29, 43, 44, 50, 57].

On computed tomography (CT) benign angiomatous lesions show a mottled low density pattern, partially due to the mixture of fatty, fibrous, and vascular tissue elements. The slow flow and pooling of blood sometimes cause the presence of punctate and curvilinear structures. CT has a greater sensitivity in detecting associated phleboliths (Figs. 16.3 and 16.4) and also clearly shows the relation to adjacent structures in the axial plane. CT may also be useful for exclusion of other soft tissue lesions such as lipomas, which are characterized by a homogeneous low-density attenuation [2, 21, 22, 51].

On angiography the appearance of benign vascular tumors is variable, ranging from small poolings of contrast material over coarse and fine hypervascularity to the presence of large tortuous blood vessels. Angiography has long been the method of choice for defining the lesions extent, vascularity and feeding vessels, allowing distinction from other well-vascularized masses [39, 40].

Angiography of venous malformations, although not indicated, shows contrast pooling in dilated vessels. In arteriovenous malformation, feeding and draining vessels as well as large arteriovenous shunts can be demonstrated [65].

However, underestimation of the extent, false-negative results and inability to define the relationship to adjacent neural structures or fascial planes, have been reported [31, 32]. Moreover, differentiation between hemangiomas and other soft tissue tumors is often not possible. Angiography is, however, still helpful in identification of feeding and draining vessels for planning embolic therapy or preoperative embolization [44, 50].

Excellent palliation has been reported with embolotherapy of symptomatic arteriovenous malformations [11, 64]. The pain is thought to be secondary to perineural congestion.

Subselective embolization using ethanol, coils and particles usually relieves pain [65].

Ultrasound is a very sensitive technique for detecting soft tissue abnormalities, as well as for demonstrating hemangiomas. If phleboliths are present, they are seen as an echogenic focus with acoustic shadowing. Hemangiomas usually present as oval masses with smooth margins. They are heterogeneous and generally hyperechoic. However, there is no ultrasound appearance specific to muscular hemangiomas [7, 58].

Reports on the use of color Doppler are sparse and usually do not deal with vascular lesions in particular. In some hemangiomas no Doppler signal is noted because of low flow. On the other hand, a characteristic low resistance flow pattern can be noted in high flow vascular malformations [75].

Doppler sonography can also be used for follow-up of AVM after therapy [65].

High vessel density and high peak arterial Doppler shift can be used to distinguish hemangiomas from other soft tissue masses [9].

However, literature findings are contradictory [75]. Paltiel et al. have even tried to distinguish hemangioma from vascular malformation on the basis of mean venous peak velocity and mean resistive index [9, 37, 47, 59].

Only one report in the literature mentions the role of positron emission tomography in the evaluation of hemangioma. PET is promising for differentiating benign hemangiomas from other soft tissue tumors [76].

On plain radiographs a glomus tumor is seen as a soft tissue mass usually at the dorsal surface of the finger. A characteristic bone erosion, possibly with sclerotic margin is sometimes noticed [15, 44]. Ultrasound reveals a hypoechoic lesion but is not sensitive [17].

It is not possible to differentiate between hemangioendothelioma and angiosarcoma on the basis of plain radiography [16].

Reports on CT and ultrasound findings in malignant vascular tumors are sparse and usually non-specific [16, 18]. CT show a heterogeneous mass which becomes sharply delineated owing to marked contrast enhancement. Angiosarcoma following chronic lymphedema is characterized by fibrous thickening, increased fat attenuation, and fluid collections surrounding the muscles [27, 50].

16.4.2 Imaging Findings on MRI

MRI is considered the modality of choice in evaluating soft tissue masses, and hemangioma is no exception to this rule [2, 4, 21, 24, 44, 46, 48, 50, 53, 60, 73, 74].

Deeply located and intramuscular hemangiomas usually have no specific clinical signs, unlike their cutaneous variants, and detection is usually delayed [12, 44]. Medical imaging is indispensable for preoperative assessment and is carried out preferentially by MRI.

The descriptions in the literature can be divided into two groups: those that use the term hemangioma and do not distinguish between different subtypes [4, 24, 46, 56]. On the other hand we share the opinion of some authors who believe that MRI can be used to differentiate slow and high flow vascular malformations and hemangiomas, which is of major therapeutic importance [3, 37, 49].

If benign angiomatous lesions are grouped under the term hemangiomas, high signal intensity on T2-weighted images is the most characteristic MRI finding of these lesions [56]. The signal intensity is indeed higher than that of subcutaneous fat. Increased T2-weighting demonstrates increased brightening of the hemangioma and usually improved delineation of the edge and extent of the lesion [46] (Fig. 16.5). On T1-weighted images the signal intensity of the lesions is usually intermediate between that of muscle and fat. Histological comparison shows that slow flow within dilated venous channels, pooling of blood in cavernous spaces, thrombosis, and the presence of fatty elements are responsible for the higher signal intensity on T1- and T2- weighted images (Fig. 16.6). Capillary hemangiomas and small hemangiomas may not present with high signal intensity on T1-weighted images [2].

Except for small lesions (diameter less than 2 cm) and some located in the extremities [4, 73, 77] all hemangiomas are inhomogeneous on both T1- and T2-weighted images. On T2-weighted images punctate or reticular low signal intensity areas may be present corresponding to fibrous tissue, fast flow within blood vessels, or calcified or ossified foci. The presence of those areas is an important feature in the differential diagnosis between hemangiomas and lipomas or intramuscular hematomas [2, 49, 54, 56, 73, 74].

High flow in vessels or fibrous tissue or calcifications can be differentiated using gradient echo sequences with gradient-moment nulling [37].

Hemangiomas are generally composed of multiple lobules of high signal intensity with a 'bunch of grapes' appearance (Fig. 16.7).

Fig. 16.5 a, b. High signal intensity of hemangioma on T2 weighted images: **a** subcutaneous hemangioma of the wrist. Coronal T2-weighted image with fat suppression shows a multilobular mass which involves the subcutaneous fat. The lesion is hyperintense and inhomogeneous due to internal septations; **b** capillary hemangioma of the neck in a two-years old boy. Axial T2-weighted image shows an inhomogeneous septate mass which is sharply delineated and is hyperintense to subcutaneous fat. There is no invasion of the underlying muscle

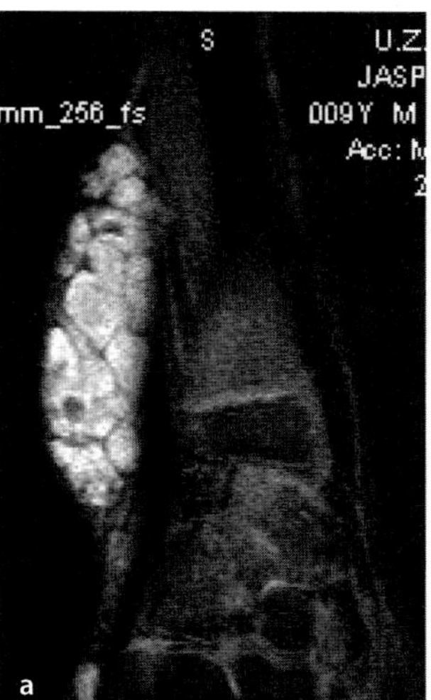

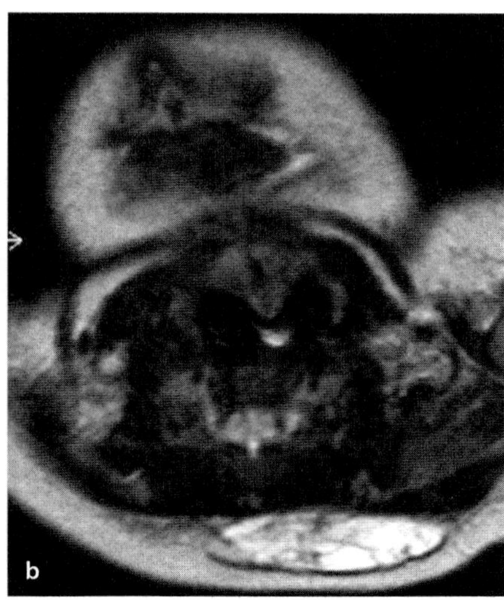

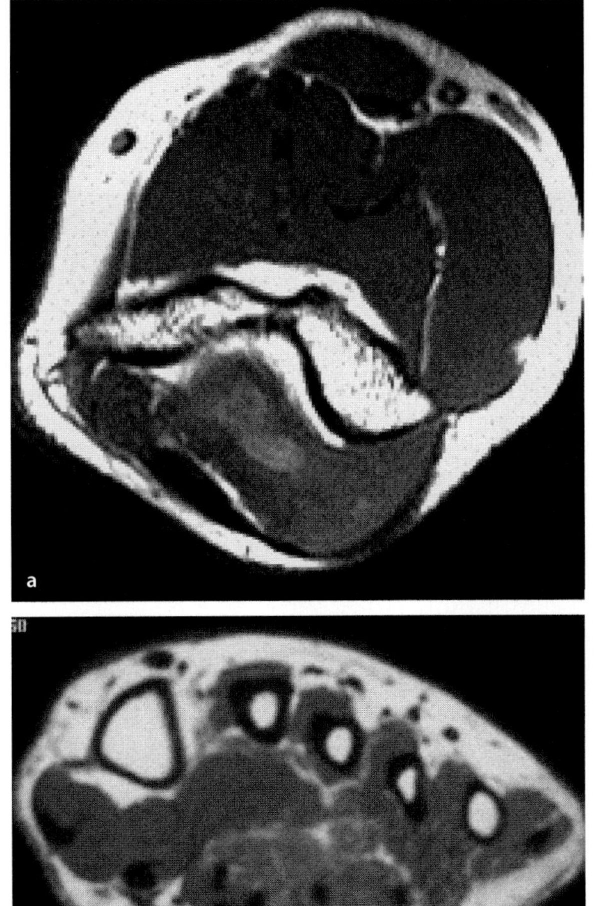

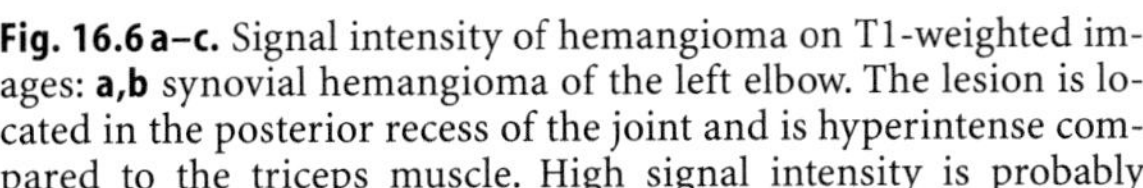

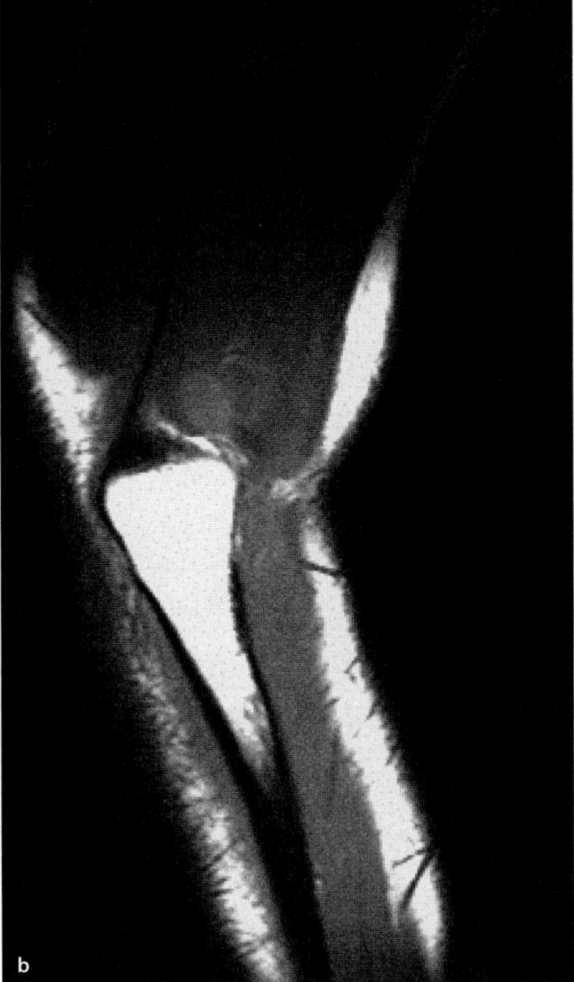

Fig. 16.6 a–c. Signal intensity of hemangioma on T1-weighted images: **a,b** synovial hemangioma of the left elbow. The lesion is located in the posterior recess of the joint and is hyperintense compared to the triceps muscle. High signal intensity is probably caused by stagnant blood; **c** the signal intensity of the flexor digitorum muscles is minimally increased due to the presence of intramuscular hemangioma. Note also the presence of peripheral fatty components

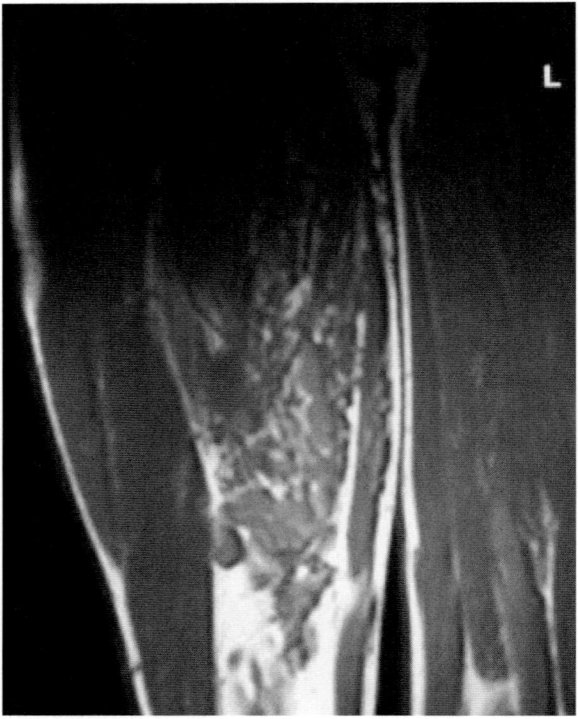

Fig. 16.7. Coronal T1-weighted image of the right thigh shows an intramuscular mass which involves the hamstring muscles. The lesion is composed of multiple nodular components which make it resemble 'a bunch of grapes'

This is probably due to cavernous or cystic vascular spaces containing stagnant blood [4]. It is also within these spaces that fluid-fluid levels can be notes. These fluid-fluid levels are mostly seen in cavernous hemangiomas and are caused by hemorrhage. On T2-weighted images a high signal intensity 'supernatant' corresponding to serous fluid overlies a low signal intensity lower layer. Fluid-fluid levels are not appreciated as easily on T1-weighted images, but they are nevertheless present. On T1-weighted images the signal intensity of the higher layer is low, and that of the lower layer is high (Fig. 16.8).

As noted above, hemangiomas are generally inhomogeneous on T1-weighted image. The lesions are predominantly isointense with muscle, with internal serpiginous high signal intensity strands. These strands correspond to enlarged vessels and generally are orient-

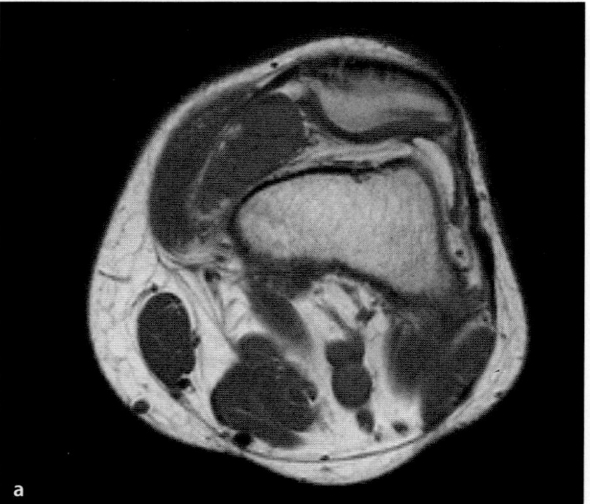

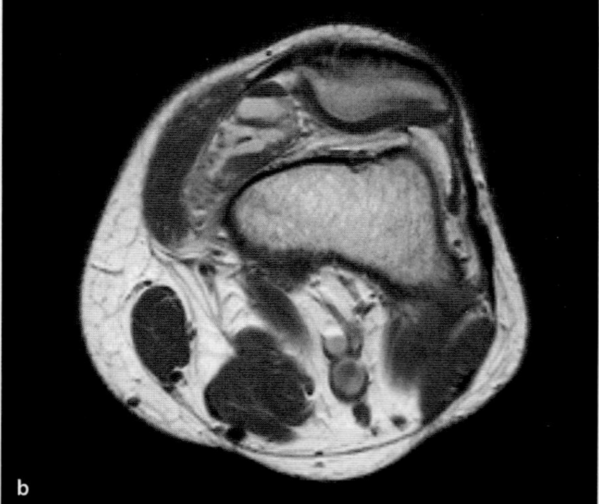

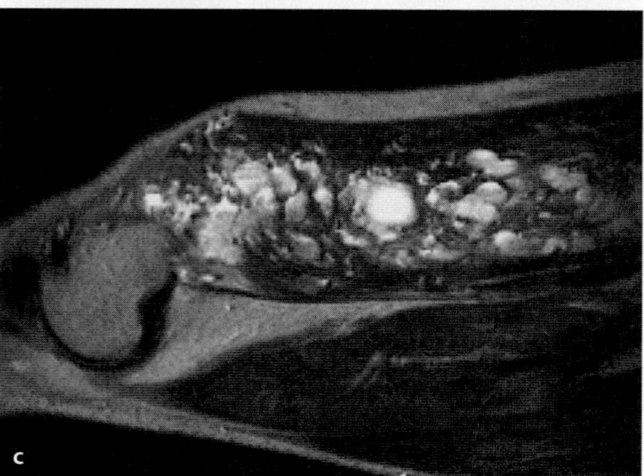

Fig. 16.8. a Axial T1-weighted MR image. b Axial T1-weighted MR image after gadolinium contrast injection. c Sagittal T2-weighted MR image. A fluid–fluid level is seen on axial T1-weighted images. The supernate is slightly hypointense compared with the lower layer due to its serous composition (a). The fluid–fluid level becomes clearer after administration of gadolinium due to the sedimentation of gadolinium to the lower part of the lesion, the same phenomenon as is noted within the bladder after intravenous administration of gadolinium chelates (b). On T2-weighted images there is increased contrast between the hyperintense serous upper layer and the lower layer, which is hypointense due to the sedimentation of erythrocytes (c)

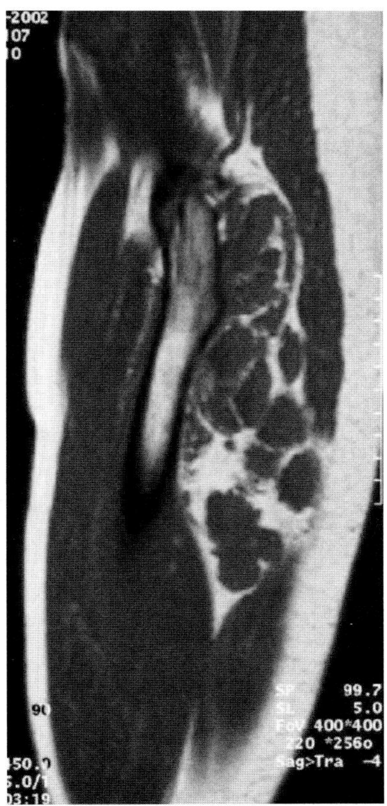

Fig. 16.9. Intramuscular hemangioma in a 40-years-old man. On sagittal T1-weighted images, the signal intensity of the lesion is inhomogeneous. There are central nodular components that are isointense to muscle. The peripheral parts are mainly composed of fatty tissue and are hyperintense to muscle

ed parallel to the muscle fibers [21, 56]. In some hemangiomas peripheral high signal intensity areas are noted on T1-weighted images, corresponding to fat within the lesions (Fig. 16.9).

A frequent finding is hypertrophy or atrophy of the muscle or the subcutaneous fat involved by the hemangiomas (Fig. 16.10). Hypertrophy of the limb in angiomatosis is also known.

The classification of Mulliken differentiates hemangiomas, venous malformations and arteriovenous malformations.

Slow flow vascular malformations include venous, capillary, cavernous and mixed types. The appearance on MRI depends on the composition. Venous portions show large spaces with internal linear or serpentine structures of low or high signal intensity depending on the pulse sequence and blood flow velocity [78, 79].

In addition they are oriented along the long axis of the limb, follow neurovascular distributions, and are sometimes multifocal (Fig. 16.11). Usually there is an enlargement of the neighboring subcutaneous fat. The combination of all findings suggests a congenital tissue dysplasia.

On the other hand, high flow arteriovenous malformations have signal voids on all pulse sequences. Although the lesions can be associated with surrounding edema or fibrofatty stroma, no focal soft tissue mass is found [37, 49] (Fig. 16.12).

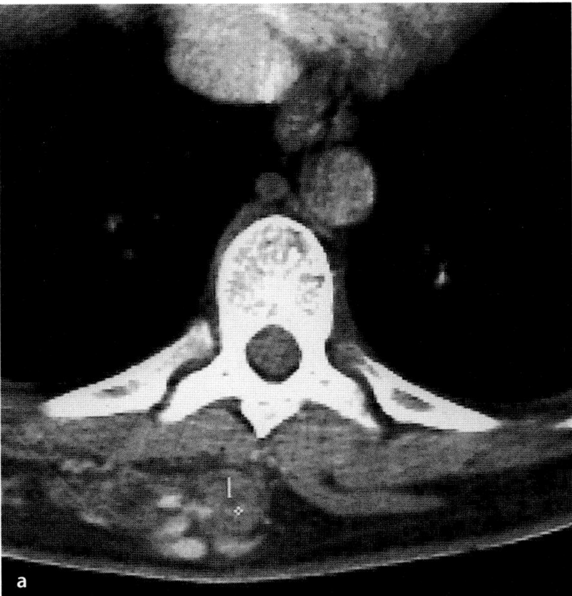

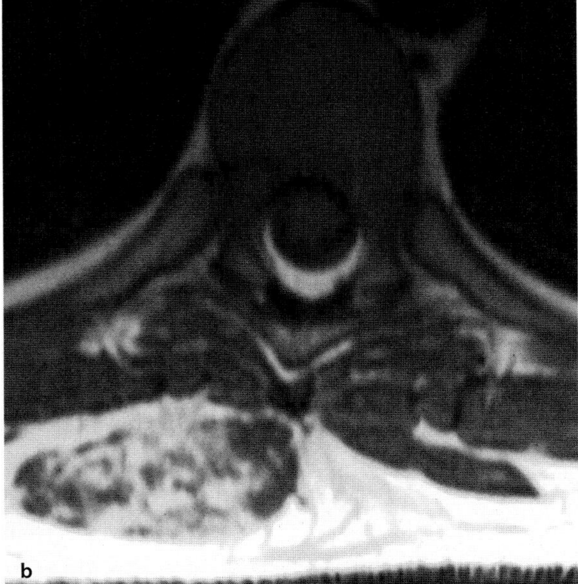

Fig. 16.10 a, b. A 55-year-old woman complaining of interscapular pain. **a** CT after iodinated contrast injection. **b** Axial spin echo T1-weighted MR image. There is a marked hypertrophy of the right trapezoid muscle compared to the contralateral side. Central and peripheral enhancing areas are noted, corresponding to enlarged vessels (**a**). In addition to the hypertrophy, signal intensity of the right trapezoid muscle is inhomogeneous and increased, nearly isointense to subcutaneous fat. The increase is caused by slow flow in enlarged veins (**b**). The presence of enlarged veins and the hypertrophy of the muscle are characteristic for hemangioma

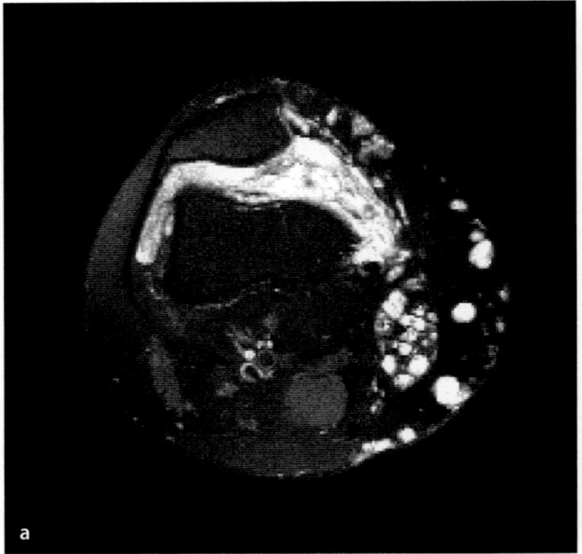

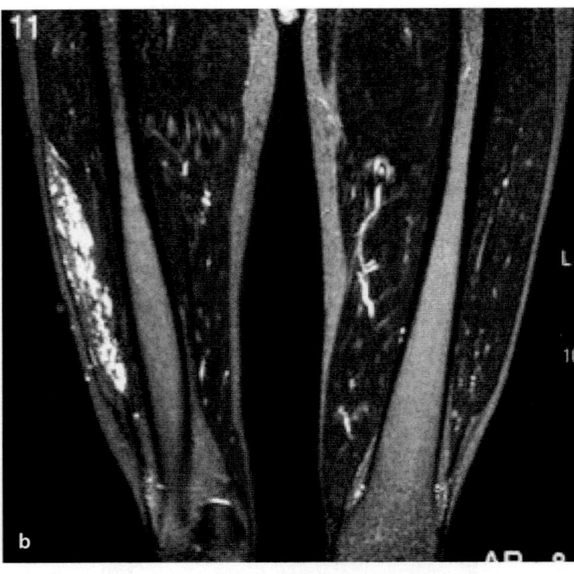

Fig. 16.11a,b. Venous hemangiomas: **a** axial T2-weighted image with fat saturation shows the involvement of multiple compartments of the knee region by the lesion. There are hyperintense nodular and serpentine areas in the subcutis, the semimembranous muscle and within the joint, in the anterior fat pad. High signal intensity is caused by slow flowing blood in dilated venous channels; **b** coronal inversion recovery T2-weighted image in another patient shows pooled blood within saccular dilated blood vessels. There is extension along the long axis of the involved leg

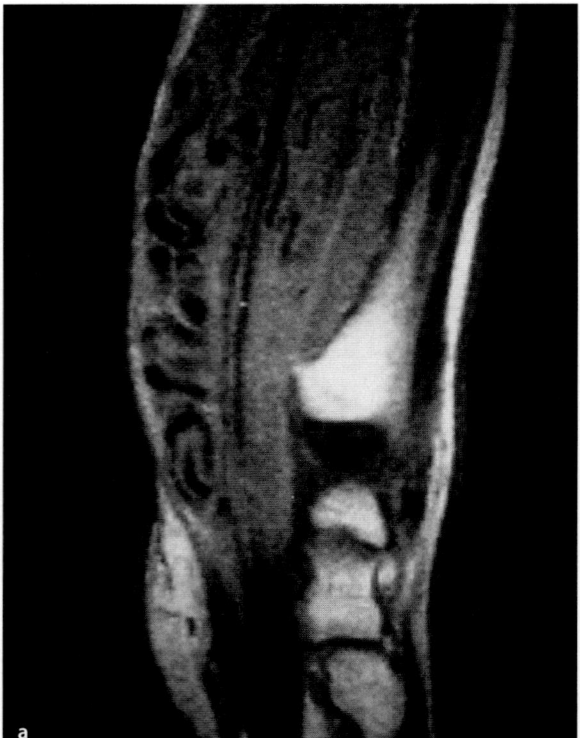

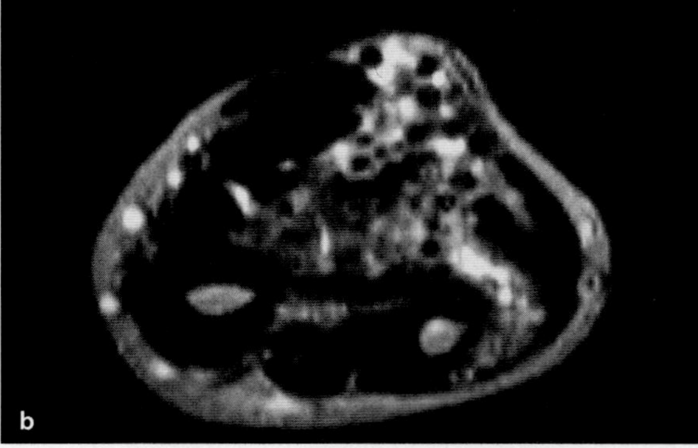

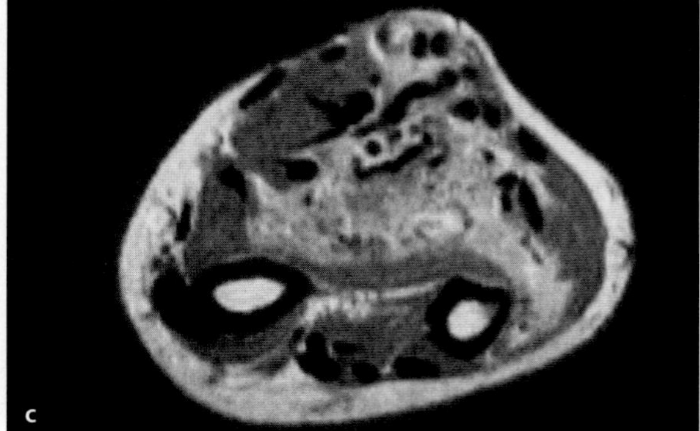

Fig. 16.12a–c. High-flow arteriovenous malformation in the flexor muscles of the forearm. **a** Sagittal T1-weighted MR image. **b** Axial T2-weighted MR image. **c** Axial T1-weighted MR image after gadolinium contrast injection. Multiple serpiginous areas of signal void are present within the flexor muscles of the fingers. These muscles are nearly isointense on T1-weighted images (**a**). On T2-weighted images the involved muscles are slightly hyperintense, with internal areas of signal void. High signal intensity areas correspond to the matrix of vascular malformation, while signal void is caused by high flow in dilated vessels (**b**). After administration of Gd contrast, there is only enhancement of the solid part of the mass (**c**). (From H. Van Moer, with permission)

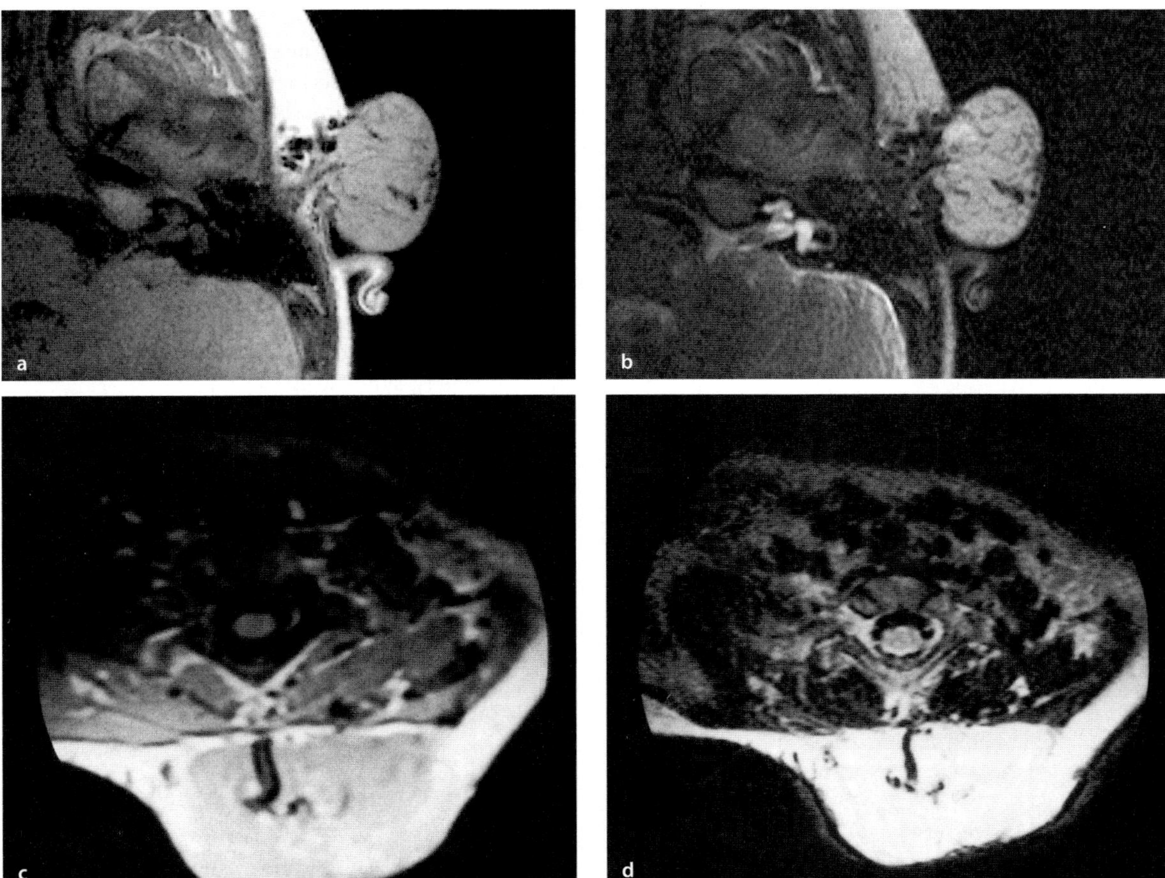

Fig. 16.13 a–d. Hemangiomas of infancy. **a, b** Axial T1- and T2-weighted MR images in a 2-year-old girl. **c, d** Axial T1- and T2-weighted MR images in a 17-month-old girl. A preauricular mass that is isointense on the T1-weighted image and hyperintense on the T2-weighted image is seen (**a, b**). Enlarged feeding vessels are seen within the subcutis anterior to the lesion and peripherally within the lesion. The same findings are noted on axial T1- and T2-weighted images of the neck in the other patient (**c, d**). A horizontal snakelike area of signal void is seen on both images. The presence of enlarged feeding or draining vessels is typical for hemangiomas of infancy and is not seen in venous malformations

Infantile hemangiomas display the features described above: a lobulated mass that is hyperintense on T2-WI and isointense to muscle on T1-WI. They have prominent feeding or draining vessels which are identified as central or peripheral high flow channels (Fig. 16.13).

T1-weighted images after the administration of gadolinium show a moderate to strong enhancement of the vascular lesions. The pattern of enhancement varies with the interval between imaging and the time of injection, depending on the rate of inflow of contrast into the blood-filled spaces [56]. Degree of enhancement varies with flow velocities of blood in the vessels of the hemangioma. Therefore more pronounced enhancement occurs in the low signal intensity parts on native scans, and the lesions become more homogeneous. The contrast-to-noise ratio between hemangiomas and surrounding tissues, however, remains lower than on T2-weighted images (Fig. 16.14).

Conventional MR imaging generally does not allow to making a distinction between different types of venous malformations.

However, Verstraete et al. maintain that dynamic contrast-enhanced MRI and 'first pass' images enable the differentiation between cavernous and capillary hemangiomas and between low flow and high flow vascular malformations [62] (Fig. 16.15; see Chap. 6).

Low slope values are usually found in cavernous types due to low perfusion, while capillary types show high perfusion and high slope values. The first-pass images show good correlation with angiographic findings.

More recent studies confirm that dynamic contrast enhanced MRI provides images that are comparable to conventional angiography. In addition time-intensity curves allow to distinguishing venous malformations from mixed capillary-venous and arteriovenous malformations [80, 81].

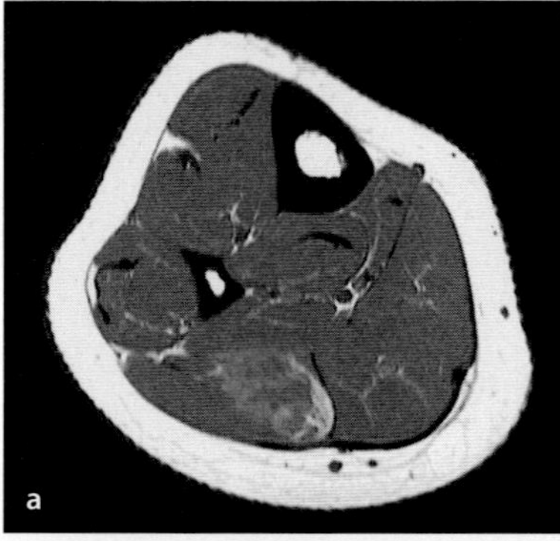

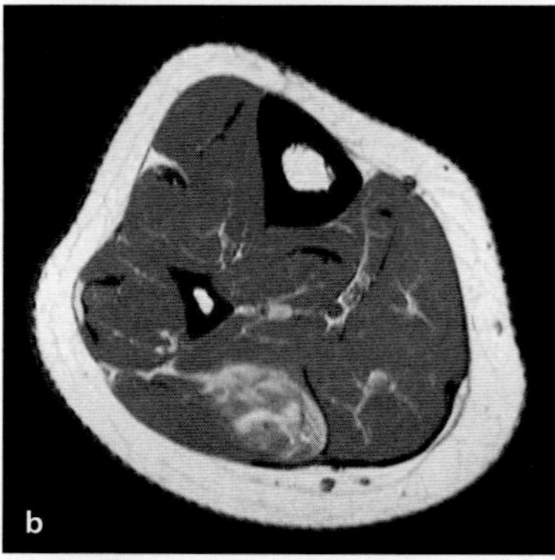

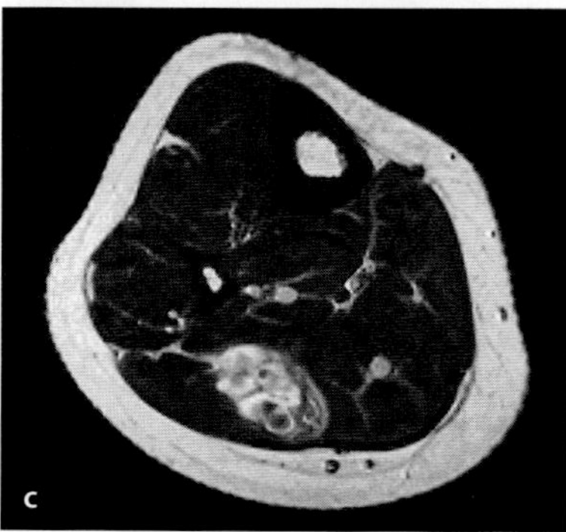

Teo et al. retrospectively reviewed the records of patients with soft tissue hemangiomas and compared them with those having malignant masses. No single MR feature was diagnostic, but analysis of morphology, and signal intensity on native and enhanced images allowed differentiation. The combination of high signal intensity on T2-weighted images, high contrast enhancement, and lobulated, septate morphology was typical for hemangioma [60].

Synovial hemangiomas present with similar features as intramuscular types, except for the high frequency of pressure erosions of adjacent cortical bone and the low signal intensity synovial lining [20, 33, 56] (Figs. 16.2 and 16.16). The appearance of angiomatosis on MRI is identical to that of solitary angiomatous lesions. MRI is ideally suited for defining the extent of soft tissue involvement [40] (Fig. 16.17).

On MRI a glomus tumor is seen as a homogeneous hyperintense lesion on T2-weighted images. Definition of extent is superior to that on other techniques [59].

MRI characteristics of hemangioendothelioma and angiosarcoma may be non specific (Fig. 16.18). Some authors mention the presence of prominent serpentine vessels suggestive for the diagnosis.

Fig. 16.14a–c. A 27-year-old man presenting with a painful swelling of the right calf. **a** Axial T1-weighted MR image. **b** Axial T1-weighted MR image after gadolinium contrast injection. **c** Axial T2-weighted MR image. An ill-defined, inhomogeneous mass within the lateral head of the gastrocnemius muscle is seen. The mass has a hyperintense medial border. The lateral part is nearly isointense to muscle (**a**). After contrast administration homogenization of signal intensity takes place due to a higher degree of enhancement of the low signal intensity parts on native T1-weighted images (**b**). The exact extent of the lesion, however, is still better appreciated on T2-weighted images (**c**)

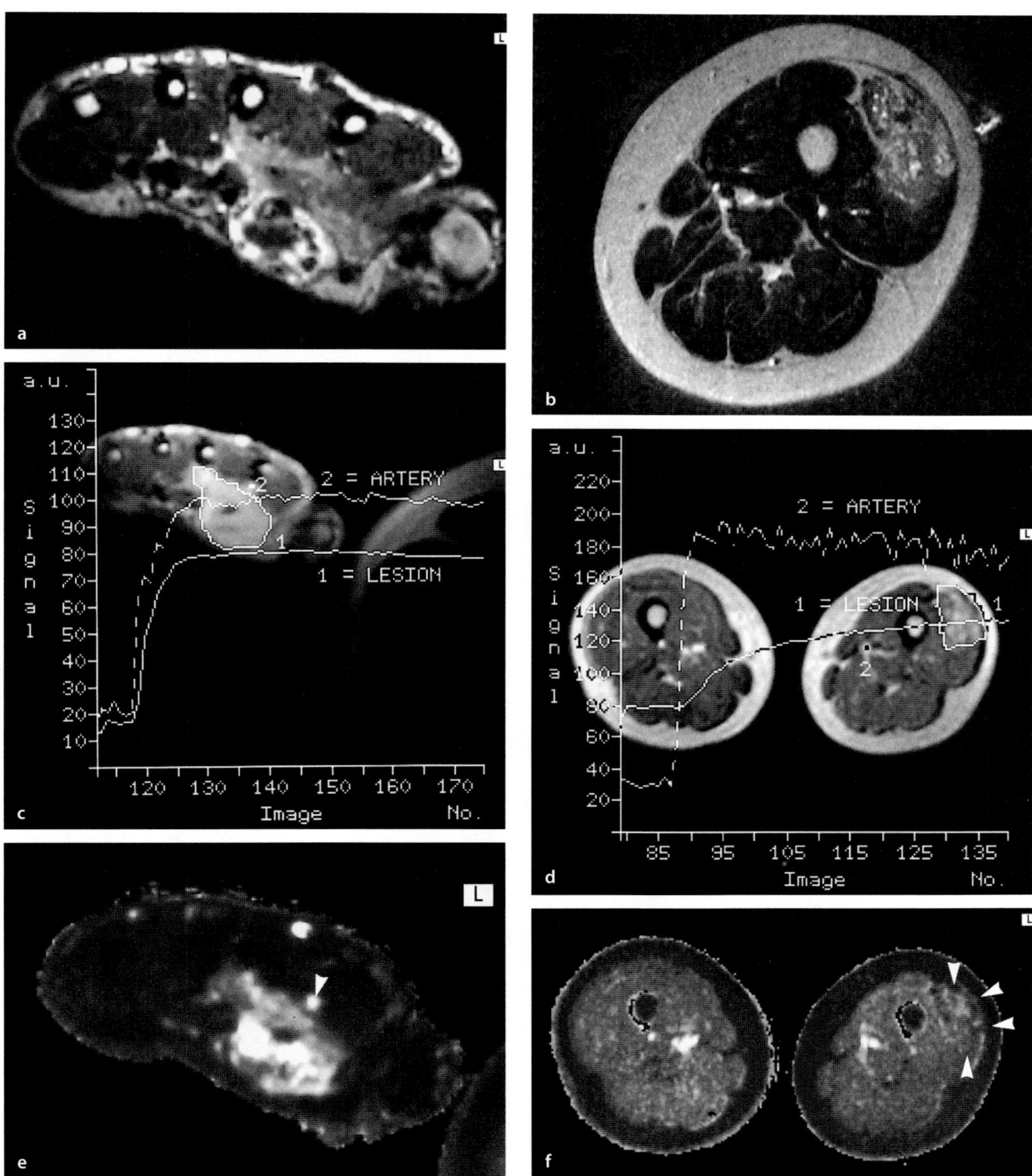

Fig. 13.15 a–f. Differentiation of high-flow from low-flow hemangioma with dynamic MRI. **a** Axial T2-weighted image in a 34-year-old man. **b** Axial T2-weighted MR image in a 19-year-old girl. **c, d** Time–intensity curves. **e, f** First-pass MR images (turbo-FLASH; TR/TE/TI/flip angle: 9 ms/4 ms/200 ms/8°). Axial T2-weighted MR images show a soft tissue lesion of the right hand with low, intermediate, or high signal intensity, corresponding to an arteriovenous hemangioma (**a**) and to a cavernous heman-gioma within the vastus lateralis muscle which displays intermediate to high signal intensity (**b**). On the time–intensity curve, the arteriovenous hemangioma has a high first-pass enhancement that parallels the arterial curve, indicating high perfusion, whereas the cavernous hemangioma has a slow perfusion (**c, d**). On first-pass images the arteriovenous hemangioma appears as bright as the feeding artery (**e**, *arrowhead*), whereas the cavernous hemangioma appears dark, due to slow perfusion (**f**, *arrowheads*)

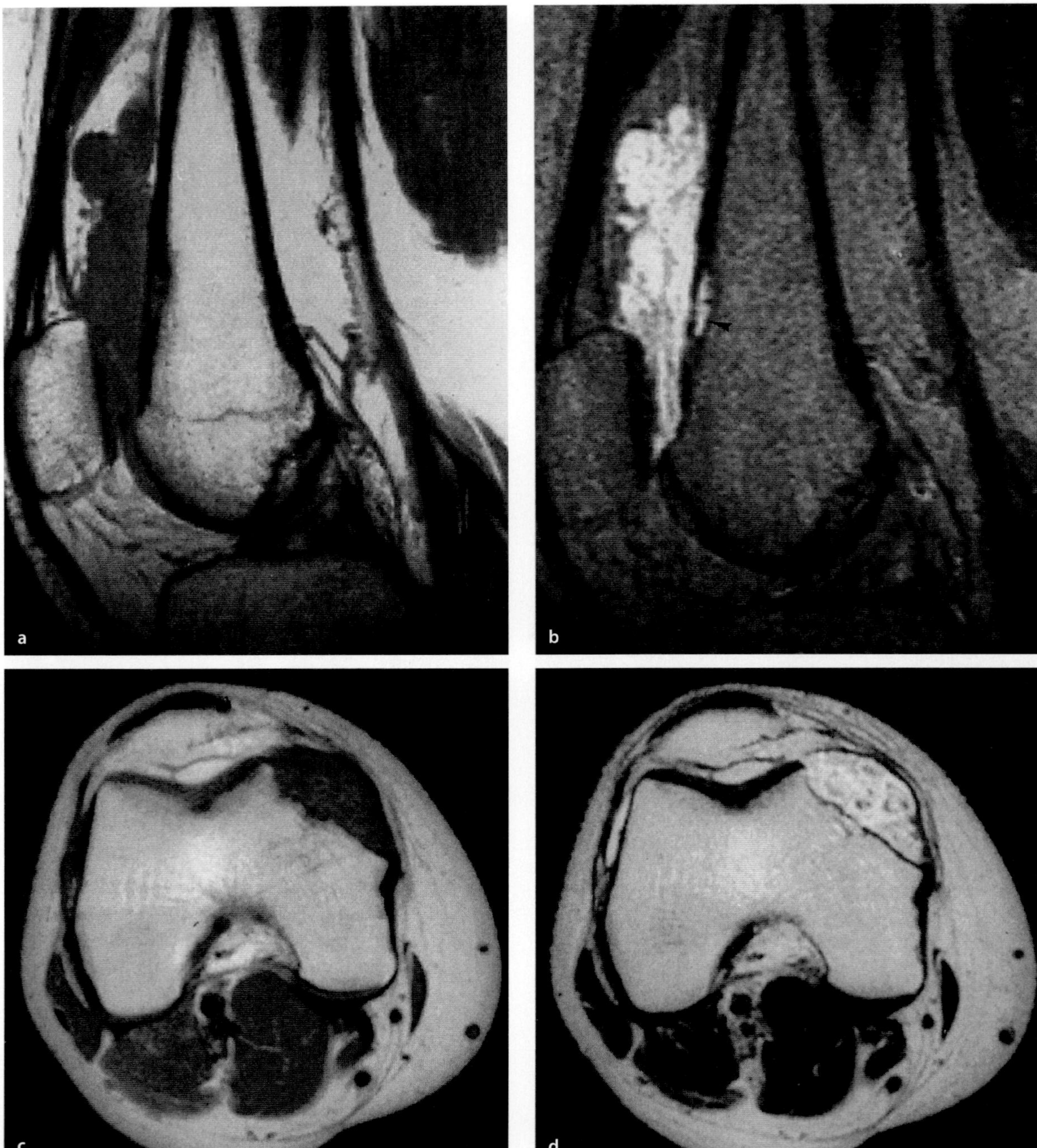

Fig. 16.16 a–d. Synovial hemangioma. **a** Sagittal T1-weighted MR image. **b** Sagittal T2-weighted MR image. **c** Axial T1-weighted MR image. **d** Axial T2-weighted MR image. A well-defined homogeneous lesion with lobulated contours is seen within the suprapatellar bursa. The lesion is isointense to muscle on T1-weighted images (**a, c**) and hyperintense to fat on T2-weighted images (**b, d**) with small linear and punctate areas of low signal intensity. The axial slices reveal erosion of the anterior cortex of the distal femur with adjacent changes within the medullary fat, probably corresponding to bone marrow edema. (Reprinted from [33], with permission)

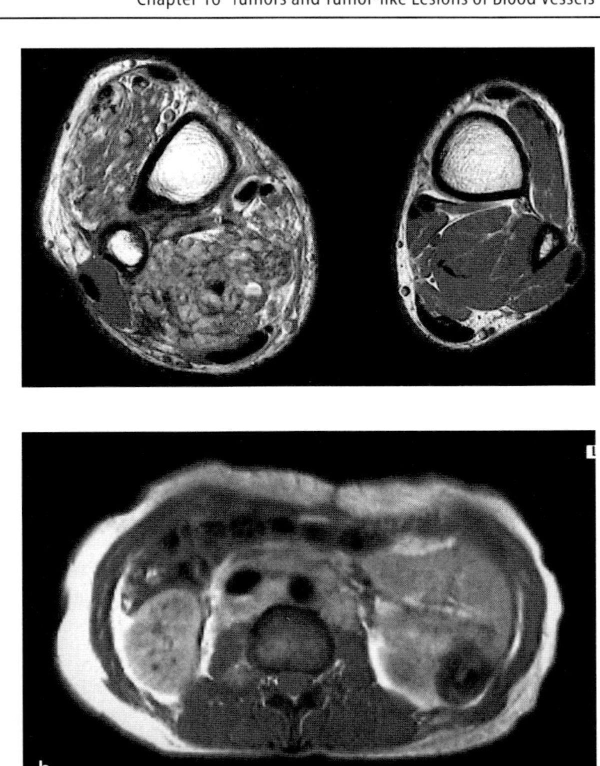

Fig. 16.17. Angiomatosis of the right lower limb. Axial T1-weighted image after gadolinium contrast injection shows the extension of the angiomatous lesion involving the subcutaneous tissues and all muscles with exception of the peroneal muscles, which display normal signal intensity. Note also the obvious hypertrophy of the right lower limb

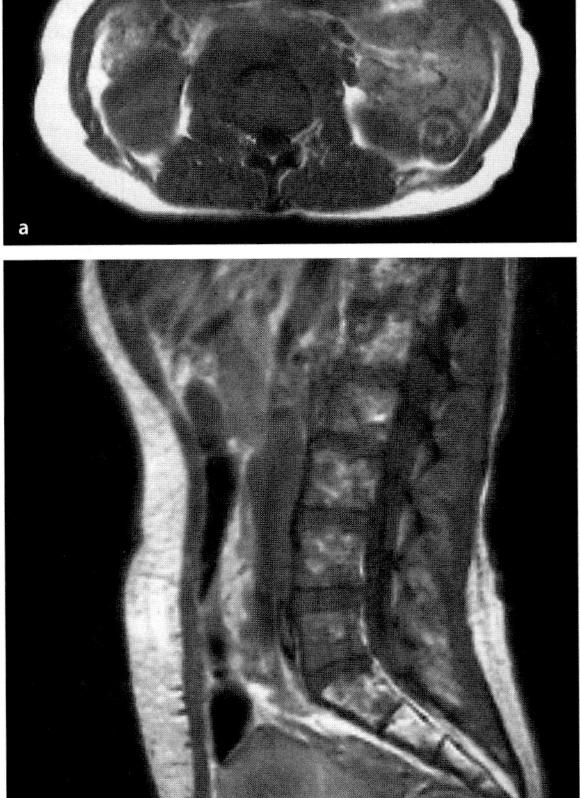

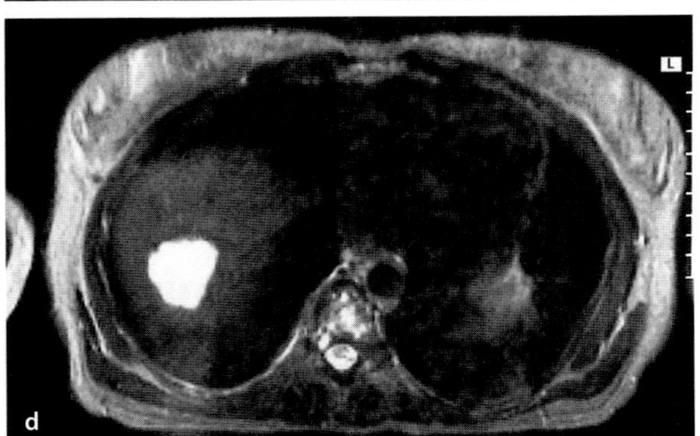

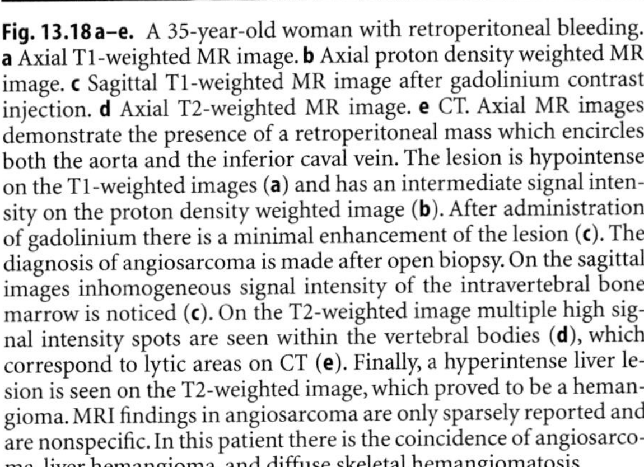

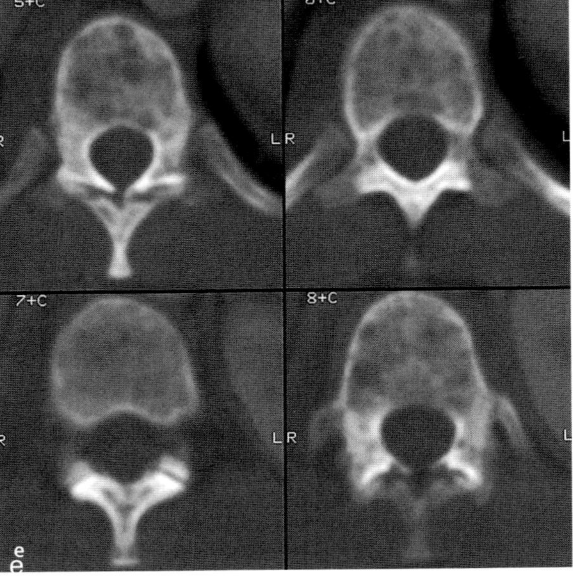

Fig. 13.18a–e. A 35-year-old woman with retroperitoneal bleeding. **a** Axial T1-weighted MR image. **b** Axial proton density weighted MR image. **c** Sagittal T1-weighted MR image after gadolinium contrast injection. **d** Axial T2-weighted MR image. **e** CT. Axial MR images demonstrate the presence of a retroperitoneal mass which encircles both the aorta and the inferior caval vein. The lesion is hypointense on the T1-weighted images (**a**) and has an intermediate signal intensity on the proton density weighted image (**b**). After administration of gadolinium there is a minimal enhancement of the lesion (**c**). The diagnosis of angiosarcoma is made after open biopsy. On the sagittal images inhomogeneous signal intensity of the intravertebral bone marrow is noticed (**c**). On the T2-weighted image multiple high signal intensity spots are seen within the vertebral bodies (**d**), which correspond to lytic areas on CT (**e**). Finally, a hyperintense liver lesion is seen on the T2-weighted image, which proved to be a hemangioma. MRI findings in angiosarcoma are only sparsely reported and are nonspecific. In this patient there is the coincidence of angiosarcoma, liver hemangioma, and diffuse skeletal hemangiomatosis

16.4.3 Imaging Strategy

Cutaneous and subcutaneous vascular tumors usually present with characteristic clinical features. For this reason diagnosis usually poses no problems. Surgical excision can be performed without preoperative radiological assessment [44]. However, if extension to or involvement of the underlying tissues is suspected, MRI has a definite role in the evaluation.

Because patients with deep-seated vascular tumors present with a mass or pain, it is difficult to make a diagnosis based on clinical examination. Nonspecific complaints lead to delayed detection and misdiagnosis. A majority of patients undergo surgery without a definite evaluation of the extent of the lesion or preoperative tissue diagnosis. A high recurrence rate due to incomplete resection is reported.

The choice of imaging techniques is dictated by the availability of equipment and patient-related considerations. When a deep hemangioma is suspected, imaging should start with plain radiography. Characteristic phleboliths and bone erosion can be depicted. Plain radiographs are ideally followed by MRI. MRI can provide characteristic features such as high signal intensity on T2-weighted images and curvilinear or serpentine inhomogeneities on all pulse sequences. Patterns of signal intensity and morphology may allow a presumptive diagnosis of hemangioma even in patients in whom vascular lesions are not suspected. The use of T1-weighted sequences is essential in evaluating hemangiomas since most other lesions have low signal intensity on T1-weighted images.

However, one must be aware of certain pitfalls. Myxoid tumors can show the same reticular high and low signal intensity and the infiltrative appearance of angiomatosis.

Other intramuscular tumors complicated by intralesional hemorrhage or intramuscular hematoma have the same signal intensity as hemangiomas but lack the presence of enlarged vessels. Tumors that infiltrate the subcutaneous fat or are primarily fatty may also resemble hemangiomas [19].

Differentiation of hemangiomas and low flow or high flow vascular malformations is also preferentially done by MRI. Donnely et al. use a combination of axial T1-weighted, fat sat T2-weighted and gradient echo MR images with the addition of coronal or sagittal spin echo T2 weighted images. Differentiation of the lesions is essential for providing appropriate monitoring and therapy. Other authors believe that the combination of conventional MR characteristics with dynamic contrast enhanced features can be used for this purpose [78, 80, 81].

Several reports have shown the superiority of MRI over CT and angiography in delineating the extent of vascular lesions. The multiplanar format permits a complete assessment of size, location, extent and topographic relationship. Since about one third of all lesions, especially venous malformations, are multifocal, this is best achieved by slices oriented parallel to the limb axis. The precision of CT in defining the craniocaudal extent or the extent of lesions without a fatty margin is markedly inferior, due to similar attenuation of hemangioma and muscle. The better differentiation between vascular lesions and the surrounding tissues on T2-weighted images allows a precise definition of the size and the extent [23, 35].

MRI is also superior to evaluate the involvement of vital structures such as neurovascular bundles. Such information is vital to planning surgery or imaging-guided procedures [65].

The extent of venous angiomas is best demonstrated on short inversion time inversion recovery images. Slow-flowing blood is responsible for marked hyperintensity on these short inversion time inversion recovery images, permitting excellent depiction of topography [53]. T1-weighted images may not be useful in cases of subcutaneous hemangiomas because it is difficult to differentiate normal subcutaneous fat from that belonging to the tumor. The only major limitation of MRI compared with plain radiography and CT is the lower sensitivity to identify phleboliths. Large phleboliths can be seen as areas of low signal intensity on T1- and T2- weighted images. However, this is a nonspecific finding, since this cannot be differentiated from fibrous tissue.

Concerning vascular tumors of intermediate malignancy and malignant vascular tumors, no specific literature findings concerning imaging strategy have been published. However, we recommend that imaging starts with plain radiography to demonstrate the presence of calcifications or ossifications. Plain radiographs are followed by MRI because of its superiority in staging of soft tumors [5, 64]. The administration of gadolinium contrast is indispensable since it is essential for the demonstration of intratumoral necrosis, which is a very specific sign indicating malignancy [61]. It is also essential for postoperative assessment in differentiation of postoperative fibrosis and tumor recurrence.

Things to remember:
1. The majority of vascular tumors are benign and are located in the skin or subcutis. They are classified as hemangiomas, which show cellular proliferation, and vascular malformations, which represent a dysplasia rather than a tumor.
2. Hemangiomas can involve large segments of the body, when they are a part of angiomatous syndromes or angiomatosis. However, they are usually small and clinically insignificant.

3. When a deep hemangioma is suspected, plain radiography is performed to demonstrate phleboliths, followed by MRI; T1-weighted images show characteristic high signal intensity, and T2-weighted images show high signal intensity with curvilinear or serpentine inhomogeneities.
4. Diagnosis of vascular malformations is done preferentially by MRI. MRI can be used to differentiate slow and high flow vascular malformations and hemangiomas using both conventional and dynamic contrast enhanced sequences.

References

1. Allen PW, Enzinger FM (1982) Hemangioma of skeletal muscle: an analysis of 89 cases. Cancer 31:8–26
2. Buetow PC, Kransdorf MJ, Moser RP, Jelinek JS, Berrey BH (1990) Radiologic appearance of intramuscular hemangioma with emphasis on MR imaging. AJR Am J Roentgenol 154:653–567
3. Cohen EK, Kressel HY, Perosio T, Lawrence Burk D, Dalinka MK, Kanal E, Schiebler ML, Fallon MD (1988) MR imaging of soft tissue hemangiomas: correlation with pathologic findings. AJR Am J Roentgenol 154:1079–1081
4. Cohen J, Weinreb J, Redman H (1986) Arteriovenous malformations of the extremities: MR imaging. Radiology 158:555–559
5. Coldwell DM, Baron RL, Charnsangavej C (1989) Angiosarcoma: diagnosis and clinical course. Acta Radiol 32:631–631
6. Collins PS, Han W, Williams LR, Rich N, Lee JF, Villavicencio JL (1992) Maffucci's syndrome [hemangiomatosis osteolytica]: a report of four cases. J Vasc Surg 16: 544–551
7. Derchi LE, Balconi G, De Flavii L, Oliva A, Rosso F (1989) Sonographic appearances of hemangiomas of skeletal muscle. J Ultrasound Med 8:263–267
8. De Schepper A, Ramon F, Degryse H (1992) Statistical analysis of MR parameters predicting malignancy in 155 soft tissue tumors. Rofo Fortschr Geb Rontgenstr Neuen Bildgeb Verfahr 155:587–593
9. Dubois J, Patriquin HB, Garel L, Powell J, Filiatrault D, David M, Grignon A (1998) Soft tissue hemangiomas in children and infants: diagnosis using doppler ultrasonography. AJR Am J Roentgenol 171:247–252
10. Ehara S, Sone M, Tamakowa Y, Nishida J, Abe M, Hachiya J (1994) Fluid-fluid levels in cavernous hemangioma of soft tissue. Skeletal Radiol 26:107–109
11. Enjolras O, Riche MC, Merland JJ, Escande JP (1990) Management of alarming hemangiomas in infancy: a review of 26 cases. Pediatrics 85: 551–558
12. Enzinger FM, Weiss SW (1995) Benign tumors and tumorlike lesions of blood vessels. In: Enzinger FM, Weiss SW (eds) Soft tissue tumors, 3 rd edn. Mosby, St Louis, pp 579–626
13. Enzinger FM, Weiss SW (1995) Hemangioendothelioma: vascular tumors of intermediate malignancy. In: Enzinger FM, Weiss SW (eds) Soft tissue tumors, 3 rd edn. Mosby, St Louis, pp 631–654
14. Enzinger FM, Weiss SW (1995) Malignant vascular tumors. In: Enzinger FM, Weiss SW (eds) Soft tissue tumors, 3 rd edn. Mosby, St Louis, pp 655–677
15. Enzinger FM, Weiss SW (1995) Perivascular tumors. In: Enzinger FM, Weiss SW (eds) Soft tissue tumors, 3 rd edn. Mosby, St Louis, pp 701–755
16. Flickinger FW, Corey-Wright J (1994) Angiosarcoma of the extremity: preoperative evaluation with CT, MR imaging, ultrasonography and angiography. South Med J 87: 926–931
17. Fornage BD (1988) Glomus tumor in the fingers: diagnosis with US. Radiology 167:183–185
18. Grant EG, Growal S, Sarosi TE, Birts FT, Holm HH, Schellinger D (1982) Sonographic findings in four cases of hemangiopericytoma. Radiology 154:547–551
19. Greenspan A, MC Gahan JP, Vogelsang P, Szabo RM (1992) Imaging strategies in the evaluation of soft-tissue hemangiomas of the extremities: correlation of the findings of plain radiography, angiography, CT, MR imaging, and ultrasonography in 12 histologically proven cases. Skeletal Radiol 21:11–18
20. Greenspan A, Azouz EM, Matheus J II, Decarie JC (1995) Synovial hemangioma: imaging features in eight histologically proven cases, review of the literature, and differential diagnosis. Skeletal Radiol 24:583–590
21. Hawnaur JM, Whitehouse RW, Jenkins JP, Isherwood I (1990) Musculoskeletal hemangiomas: comparison of MR imaging with CT. Skeletal Radiol 21:261–268
22. Hill JH, Mafee MF, Chow JM, Applebaum EL (1985) Dynamic computerized tomography in the assessment of hemangioma. Am J Otolaryngol 6:26–31
23. Jabra AA, Taylor GA (1993) MR imaging evaluation of superficial soft tissue lesions in children. Pediatr Radiol 26:546–551
24. Kaplan PA, Williams SM (1987) Mucocutaneous and peripheral soft tissue hemangiomas: MR imaging. Radiology 163:163–166
25. Kasabach HH, Merritt KK (1954) Capillary hemangioma with extensive purpura: report of a case. Am J Dis Child 59:1063–1070
26. Kato N, Kato S, Ueno H (1990) Hemangiopericytoma: characteristic features observed by magnetic resonance imaging and angiography. J Dermatol 17:701–706
27. Kazeroni E, Hessler C (1991) CT appearance of angiosarcoma associated with chronic lymphedema. AJR Am J Roentgenol 156:554–555
28. Kneeland JB, Middleton WD, Matlaub HS (1987) High resolution MR imaging of glomus tumor. J Comput Assist Tomogr 11:551–552
29. Kransdorf MJ, Jelinek JS, Moser RP (1993) Imaging of soft tissue tumors. Radiol Clin North Am 31:552–559
30. Lai FM, Allen PW, Yuen PM, Leung PC (1991) Locally metastasizing vascular tumor: spindle cell, epithelioid, or unclassified hemangioendothelioma. Am J Clin Pathol 96:660–663
31. Larsen EC, Zinkham WH, Eggleston JC, Zitelli BJ (1987) Kasabach-Merritt syndrome: therapeutic considerations. Pediatrics 79:971–980
32. Llauger J, Monill JM, Palmer J, Clotet M (1995) Synoval hemangioma of the knee: MR imaging findings in two cases. Skeletal Radiol 24: 579–581
33. Levin D, Gordon D, McSweeney J (1976) Arteriography of peripheral hemangiomas. Radiology 121:626–632
34. Lorigan JG, David CL, Evans HL, Wallace S (1989) The clinical and radiologic manifestations of hemangiopericytoma. AJR Am J Roentgenol 155:545–549
35. McCarville MB, Kaste SC, Pappo AS (1999) Soft tissue malignancies in infancy. AJR Am J Roentgenol 173:973–977
36. Meis-Kindblom JM, Kindblom LG (1998) Angiosarcoma of soft tissue: a study of 80 cases. Am J Surg Pathol 22:683–697
37. Meyer JS, Hoffer FA, Barnes PD, Mulliken JB (1991) Biological classification of Soft-Tissue vascular anomalies: MR correlation. AJR Am J Roentgenol 157:559–564
38. Milikow E, Ash T (1970) Hemangiomatosis, localized growth disturbance and intravascular coagulation disorder presenting with an unusual arthritis resembling hemophilia. Radiology 97:547–548
39. Mitty HA (1993) Musculoskeletal neoplasms: role of angiography in diagnosis and intervention. Semin Interv Radiol 10: 313–317
40. Montgomery SP, Guillot AP, Barth RA (1990) MR imaging of disseminated neonatal hemangiomatosis: case report. Pediatr Radiol 21:214–215
41. Mulliken JB, Glowacki J (1982) Hemangiomas and vascular malformations in infants and children: a classification based on endothelial characteristics. Plast Reconstr Surg 69: 541–552

42. Mulliken JB, Zetter BR, Folkman J (1982) In vitro characteristics of endothelium from hemangiomas and vascular malformations. Surgery 92:548–553
43. Munk PL, Helms CA (1999) Deep soft tissue hemangiomas. Skeletal Radiol 28:57–58
44. Murphey MD, Fairbairn KJ, Parman LM, Baxter KG, Pasa B, Smith WS (1995) Musculoskeletal angiomatous lesions: radiologic–pathologic correlation. Radiographics 15:893–917
45. Naka N, Ohsawa M, Tomita Y, Kanno H, Uchida A, Aozasa K (1995) Angiosarcoma in Japan: a review of 99 cases. Cancer 75:989–996
46. Nelson MC, Stull MA, Teitelbaum GP, Patt RH, Lack EE, Bogumill GP, Freedman MR (1990) Magnetic resonance imaging of peripheral soft tissue hemangiomas. Skeletal Radiol 21:542–557
47. Paltiel HJ, Burrows PE, Kozakewich HP, Zurakowski D, Mulliken JB (2000) Soft tissue vascular anomalies: utility of US for diagnosis. Radiology 214:747–754
48. Peiss VJ, Füzesi L, Bohndorf K, Neuerburg J, Urhahn R, Günther RW (1993) MR-Morphologie von Hemangiomen und Lymphangiomen der peripheren Weichteile – Korrelation mit Angiographie und Histologie. Rofo Fortschr Geb Rontgenstr Neuen Bildgeb Verfahr 158:543–550
49. Rak KM, Yakes WF, Ray RL, Dreisbach WF, Parker SH, Luethke JM, Stavros AT, Slater DD, Burke BJ (1992) MR Imaging of symptomatic peripheral vascular malformations. AJR Am J Roentgenol 159:107–112
50. Ramon F, Degryse H, De Schepper A (1992) Vascular soft tissue tumors: medical imaging. J Belge Radiol 75:323–330
51. Rauch RF, Silverman PM, Korobkin M, Dunnick NR, Moore AV, Wertman D, Martinez S (1984) Computed tomography of benign angiomatous lesions of the extremities. J Comput Assist Tomogr 8:1154–1155
52. Rodriguez-Galindo C, Ramsey K, Jenkins JJ, Poquette CA, Kaste SC, Merchant TE, Rao BN, Pratt CB, Pappo AS (2000) Hemangiopericytoma in children and infants. Cancer 88:198–204
53. Saks AM, Paterson FC, Irvine AT, Ayers BA, Burnand KG (1995) Improved MR venography: use of fast short inversion time inversion recovery technique in evaluation of venous angiomas. Radiology 214: 908–911
54. Silverman RA (1991) Hemangiomas and vascular malformations. Pediatr Dermatol 54:811–854
55. Stout AP, Murray MR (1942) Hemangiopericytoma: a vascular tumor featuring Zimmerman's pericytes. Am Surg 116:26–30
56. Suh JS, Hwang G, Hahn SB (1994) Soft tissue hemangiomas: MR manifestations in 26 patients. Skeletal Radiol 26:621–626
57. Sung MS, Kang HS, Lee HG (1998) Regional bone changes in deep soft tissue hemangiomas: radiographic and MR features. Skeletal Radiol 27:205–210
58. Taylor GA, Perlman EJ, Scherer LR, Gearhart JP, Leventhal BG, Wiley J (1991) Vascularity of tumors in children: evaluation with color-doppler imaging. AJR Am J Roentgenol 157:1267–1311
59. Taylor KJW, Ramos I, Carter D, Morse SS, Snower D, Fortune K (1988) Correlation of Doppler US tumor signals with neovascular morphologic features. Radiology 166:57–62
60. Teo EHJ, Strause PJ, Hernandez RJ (2000) MR Imaging differentiation of Soft Tissue Hemangiomas from malignant soft tissue masses. AJR Am J Roentgenol 174:1623–1628
61. Tung GA, Davis LM (1993) The role of magnetic resonance imaging in the evaluation of the soft tissue mass. Crit Rev Diagn Imaging 54:269–329
62. Verstraete KL, De Deene Y, Roels H, Dierick A, Uyttendaele D, Kunnen M (1994) Dynamic contrast-enhanced MR Imaging of benign and malignant musculoskeletal lesions: parametric 'first-pass' images depict tissue vascularization and perfusion. Radiology 212:854–855
63. Yagmai I (1978) Angiographic features of soft tissue and osseous hemangiopericytomas. Radiology 155:655–659
64. Yakes WF, Luethke JM, Parker SH, Stavros AT, Rak KM, Hopper KD, Dreisbach JN, Griffin DJ, Seibert CE, Carter TE, Guilliband JD (1990) Ethanol embolization of vascular malformations. Radiographics 10:787–796
65. Donnelly LF, Adams DM, Bissett GS III (2000) Vascular malformations and hemangiomas: a practical approach in a multidisciplinary clinic. Am J Roentgenol 174:597–608
66. Vilanova JC, Barcelo J, Villalon M (2004) MR and MR angiography characterization of soft tissue vascular malformations. Curr Probl Diagn Radiol 33:161–170
67. Christopher D, Unni K, Mertens F (2002) Vascular tumours. WHO Classification of tumors. Pathology and genetics: tumors of soft tissue and bone. IARC, Lyon, France, pp 155–177
68. Ziyeh S, Spreer J, Rossler J, Strecker R, Hochmuth A, Schumacher M, Klisch J (2004) Parkes Weber or Klippel- Trénaunay syndrome? Non invasive diagnosis with MR projection angiography. Eur Radiol 14(11):2025–2029
69. Hoeger PH, Martinez A, Maerker J, Harper JI (2004) Vascular anomalies in Proteus syndrome. Clin Exp Dermat 29:222–230
70. Vanhoenacker FM, De Beuckeleer LH, Deprettere A, De Moor A, De Schepper AM (2000) Proteus syndrome: MRI characteristics of plantar cerebriform hyperplasia. Skeletal Radiol 29(2):101–103
71. Vanhoenacker FM, De Schepper AM, De Raeve H, Berneman Z (2003) Cystic angiomatosis with splenic involvement: unusual MRI findings. Eur Radiol 13:Suppl 4:L35–39
72. Bisdorff A, Jomaah N, Bousson V, Capot R, Laredo JD, Enjolras O (2004) Imagerie des anomalies vasculaires des parties molles. In: Laredo JD, Tomeni B, Malghem J et al. (eds) Conduite a tenir devant une image osseuse ou des parties molles d'allure tumorale. Sauramps Medical, Montpellier, pp 417–427
73. Ly JQ, Sanders TG (2003) Hemangioma of the chest wall. Radiology 229:726–729
74. Ly JQ, Sanders TG, Mulloy JP, Soares GM, Beall DP, Parsons TW, Slabaugh MA (2003) Osseous change adjacent to soft tissue hemangiomas of the extremities: correlation with lesion size and proximity to bone. Am J Roentgenol 180:1695–1700
75. Dubois J, Garel L, David M, Powell J (2002) Vascular soft tissue tumors in infancy: distinguishing features on doppler sonography. Am J Roentgenol 178:1541–1545
76. Hatayama K, Watanabe H, Ahmed AR, Yanagawa T, Shinozaki T, Oriuchi N, Aoki J, Takeuchi K, Endo K, Takagishi K (2003) Evaluation of hemangioma by positron emission tomography: role in a multimodality approach. J Comput Assist Tomogr 27(1):70–77
77. Theumann NH, Bittoun J, Goettmann S, Le Viet D, Chevrot A, Drapé JL (2001) Hemangiomas of the fingers: MR imaging evaluation. Radiology 218:841–847
78. Vilanova JC, Barcelo J, Smirniotopoulos JG, Pérez-Andrés R, Villalon M, Miro J, Martin F, Capellades J, Ros PR (2004) Hemangioma from head to toe: MR imaging with pathologic correlation. Radiographics 24:367–385
79. Kern S, Niemeyer C, Darge K, Merz C, Laubenberger J, Uhl M (2000) Differentiation of vascular birthmarks by MR imaging. An investigation of hemangiomas, venous and lymphatic malformations. Acta Radiol 41(5):453–457
80. Herborn CU, Goyen M, Lauenstein TC, Debatin JF, Ruehm SG, Kröger K (2003) Comprehensive time-resolved MRI of peripheral vascular malformations. Am J Roentgenol 181:729–735
81. Van Rijswijk CS, van der Linden E, van der Woude HJ, van Baalen JM, Bloem JL (2002) Value of dynamic contrast-enhanced MR imaging in diagnosing and classifying peripheral vascular malformations. Am J Roentgenol 178:1181–1187
82. Dubois J, Soulez G, Oliva VL, Berthiaume MJ, Lapierre C, Therasse E (2001) Soft-tissue venous malformations in adult patients: imaging and therapeutic issues. Radiographics 21:1519–1531
83. Fishman SJ, Mulliken JB (1993) Hemangiomas and vascular malformations of infancy and childhood. Pediatr Clin North Am 40(6):1177–1200

Lymphatic Tumors

L. van den Hauwe, F. Ramon

17

Contents

17.1 Introduction

At the Workshop on Vascular Anomalies in Rome in June 1996, the Mulliken and Glowacki classification was accepted for various cutaneous vascular lesions. This classification is based upon clinical, histological and cytological features [9, 10, 30]. According to Enzinger, lymphatic tumors can be classified into benign and malignant lesions [14]. As compared with tumors arising from blood vessels, soft tissue tumors of lymphatic origin are rare; benign lesions include the solitary lymphangioma, lymphangiomatosis, lymphangiomyoma and lymphangiomyomatosis. There is growing evidence to suggest that the majority of these lesions represent hamartomas or developmental lymphangiectasias rather than true neoplasms [11, 40].

Although three types of lymphangioma have been described – capillary, cavernous and cystic – they all belong to a single group of lesions [40, 50]. They can affect any part of the body, their presentation depending on the surroundings, but a strong predilection for the neck and axilla has been noted [23].

When bones, soft tissues and visceral organs are involved in a diffuse or multifocal manner, the term 'lymphangiomatosis' is used. Like angiomatosis, this extremely rare disease is most often seen in children [14, 46]. Clinically and histopathologically, there is considerable overlap between these two entities [18]. Lymph-

angiomyoma and its more widespread form, which is called lymphangiomyomatosis, are characterized by a proliferation of smooth muscle in the lymphatic structures of the mediastinum, retroperitoneum and the lung. These benign lesions affect only women. The term lymphangiopericytoma has been abandoned [14].

The collective term of 'angiosarcoma' has been suggested instead of lymphangiosarcoma, as these malignant tumors not only are composed of groups of endothelium-lined empty spaces suggesting lymphatics, but also contain areas resembling hemangiosarcoma [11, 12]. They are seen exclusively in patients with long-standing lymph stasis such as is seen after radical mastectomy (postmastectomy lymphangiosarcoma) or in chronic lymphedema of the lower extremities [12]. They are discussed in Chap. 16.

17.2 Lymphangioma

17.2.1 Classification and Clinical Behavior

Histologically, three types of lymphangioma have traditionally been described based on the size of the lymphatic channels. Capillary lymphangioma or simple lymphangioma ('lymphangioma simplex') is composed of small, capillary-sized endothelium-lined lymphatics, whereas cavernous lymphangioma is made up of larger lymphatic channels with adventitial coats. Cystic lymphangiomas or hygromas are multilocular masses, constituted of large macroscopic lymphatic spaces that possess investitures of collagen and smooth muscle [12]. Some authors have added a fourth entity to this classification system, which is called vasculolymphatic malformation [19, 50]. Although these classification systems are widely used, there are arguments for considering the group of lymphangiomas as a single clinical entity. The distinction between cavernous and cystic lymphangioma is not always clear-cut and is often arbitrary. Moreover, cystic and cavernous components of lymphangioma often coexist in the same lesion, suggesting that cystic lymphangioma can arise out of a long-standing cavernous lymphangioma in which the cavernous

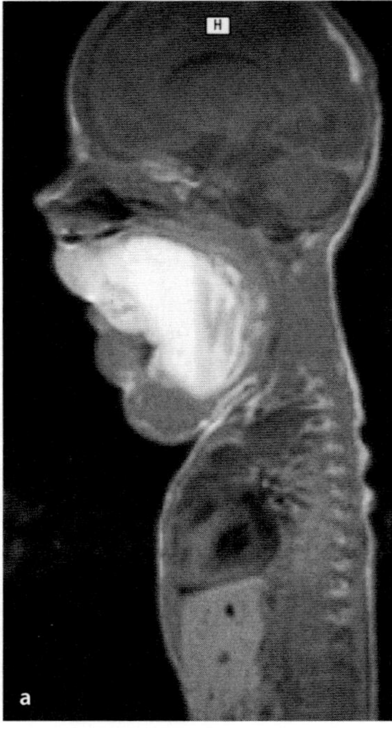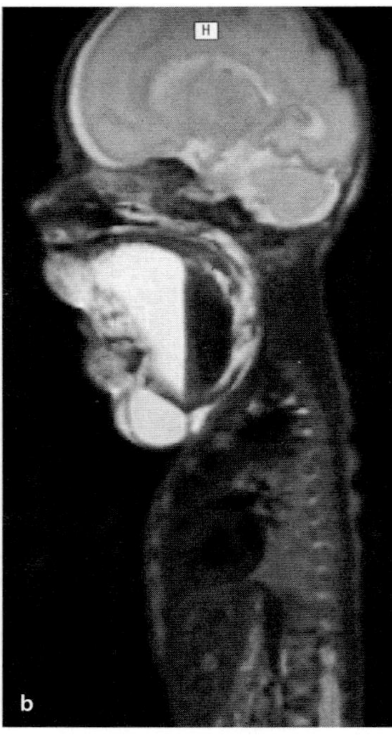

Fig. 17.1 a, b. Cystic lymphangioma of the neck in a 6-day-old premature baby boy. **a** Sagittal SE T1-weighted MR image. **b** Sagittal TSE T2-weighted MR image. A heterogeneous multilocular cystic mass is detected in the region of the neck, extending into the floor of the mouth and oral cavity (**a**). The cystic aspect of the lesion is best demonstrated on the T2-weighted (**b**). Owing to a hemorrhage, most of the cystic components demonstrate high SI on the T1-weighted image with presence of fluid-fluid levels (**a, b**). Low SI of the dependent parts of the cystic components is indicative of the presence of hemosiderin

spaces have progressively widened to form cystic spaces [1]. It has been suggested by Bill and Sumner that the classically described histological differences are the reflection of their anatomical location [3]. This means that the morphology of the lesion is dictated by the histological composition of the surrounding tissues. This theory may explain why cystic lymphangiomas most frequently arise in the neck and axilla (Figs. 17.1, 17.2), where loose connective tissue allows for the expansion of the endothelium lined lymphatic channels. Conversely, cavernous lymphangiomas are encountered in the mouth, lips, cheek, tongue or other areas where dense connective tissue and muscle prevent expansion (Fig. 17.3) [6]. In the tougher dermal and epidermal elements, expansion is further limited, resulting in the formation of a capillary lymphangioma (e. g., lymphangioma circumscriptum) (Fig. 17.4) [50].

There has been a lot of discussion about the exact etiology of these lesions, including whether they are true neoplasms or represent developmental malformations. The 'neoplastic' aspect of these malformations has been made responsible for the local aggressive potential of some lesions [18]. Although lymphangiomas can arise on a obstructive basis after trauma, surgery, radiation or infection, it is now widely believed by most authors that lymphangiomas are congenital lymphatic malformations that are the result of noncommunication between sequestered lymphoid tissue and the peripheral lymphatic system [4, 12, 15, 16, 31, 40, 44, 50].

Three major theories have been proposed to explain this concept [48, 50]. Failure of the primordial lymphatic sacs to drain into the veins will result in enlargement of the isolated lymphatic channels. This may result in the formation of lymphangiomas, especially the more voluminous central cystic hygromas [48]. A second theory may help to explain the characteristics of the more peripherally located lesions, such as capillary and cavernous lymphangiomas, and makes it easier to understand them. When abnormal sequestration of lymphatic tissue occurs early in embryologic life, failure to join the normally developed central lymphatic channels will result in lymphatic malformations [41, 50]. Another theory explains the branching and permeative growth pattern into the surrounding anatomical structures seen in some cavernous lymphangiomas [25]. Aberrant buds of lymphatic material lose their connections with the lymphatic primordia and may give rise to lymph-filled cysts. These cysts keep their ability to branch and grow and do so in an uncontrolled, disorderly manner.

Compared with hemangiomas, lymphatic malformations are a rare finding. There is no clear sexual predilection. About 50–65 % of these lesions are found at birth, and as many as 90 % may be noticed within the first 2 years of life. Cystic lymphangioma or cystic hygroma of the head, neck and axilla is the most frequently encountered and best-known entity (Fig. 17.1). A cervical lobulated, fluctuating mass in the supraclavicular fossa, the posterior triangle or the axillary region, not attached to the skin but fixed to the deep tissues of the neck is seen in these patients [8, 40]. The mass is usually made up of a conglomerate of cysts and sheets of tissue, extending in various directions and separating nerves, vessels and fascial planes. A clear or straw-colored serous fluid can be aspirated out of the cystic com-

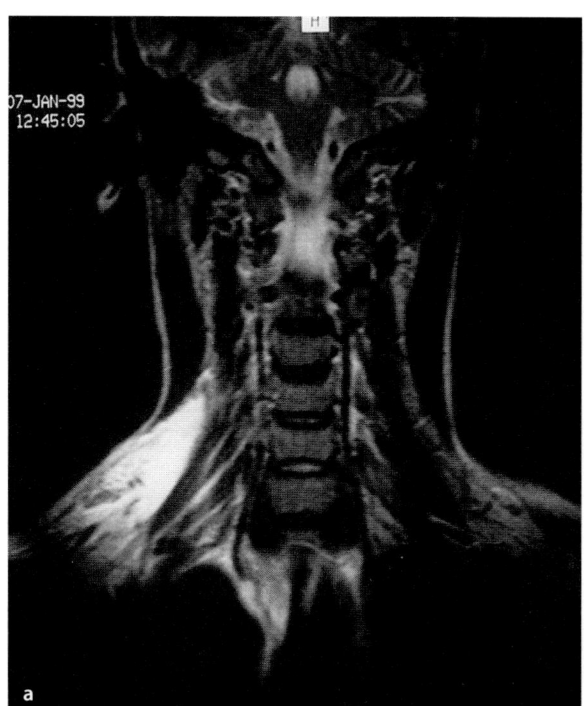

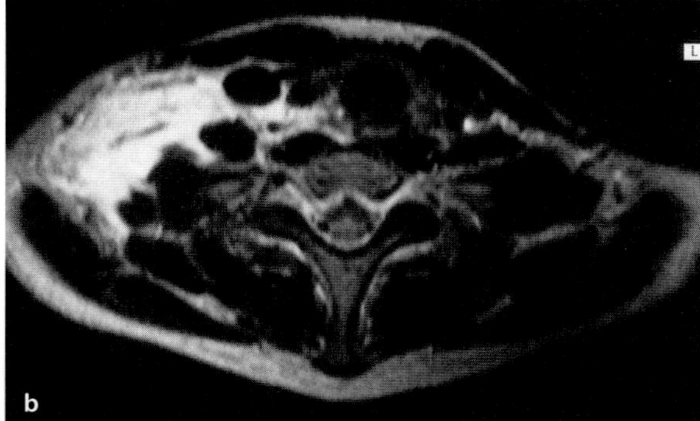

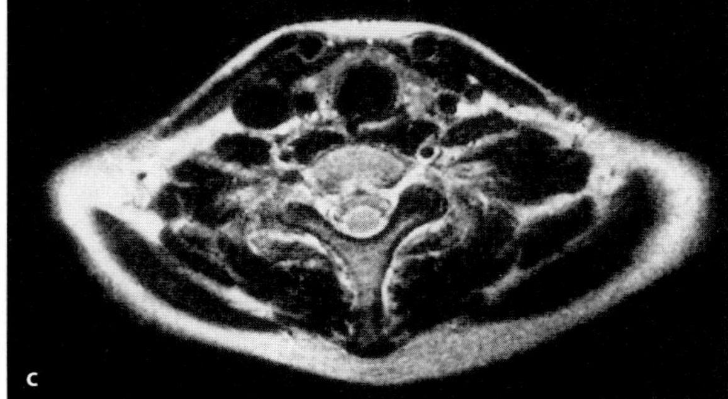

Fig. 17.2 a–c. Fluctuating characteristics of lymphangioma arising in the anterior cervical triangle. **a** Coronal TSE T2-weighted MR image. **b** Axial TSE T2-weighted MR image. **c** Axial TSE T2-weighted MR image at the same level, 6 weeks later. A heterogeneous infiltrating mass is noted, separating vessels, nerves and fascial planes. Note the shift of the trachea (**b**) compared with the control examination 6 weeks later (**c**). Spontaneous involution occurred. There was no history of local infection or trauma

ponents of the mass. When cystic hygromas arise in the anterior cervical triangle – the submandibular area, floor of the mouth, base of tongue or epiglottis – airway obstruction and feeding problems can arise [8]. Also, second branchial cleft cysts arise anterolaterally in the neck, displacing the sternocleidomastoid muscle posterolaterally and the carotid artery posteromedially. Based on their unilocular aspect and their clinical presentation, they can be differentiated quite easily from lymphangioma in most cases [26]. Sudden enlargement is indicative for superinfection of the lesion, which is frequently encountered after trauma or respiratory tract infection (Fig. 17.2) [8]. Cystic hygromas are often isolated malformations, and in this case the remainder of the lymphatic system is normal. In cases of generalized disease with an abnormally developed peripheral lymphatic system, an association with hydrops fetalis and Turner's syndrome is found [5, 50]. In recent years, fetal cystic hygroma has also been described in association with other congenital malformation syndromes, such as Noonan's syndrome, fetal alcohol syndrome, distichiasis–lymphedema syndrome, familial pterygium colli, and several chromosomal aneuploidies [5, 48]. In these cases where a hygroma is detected during fetal life, careful sonographic examination of the entire fetus, determination of the fetal karyotype and an evaluation of the family history are indicated [5]. Sometimes these unicystic or multicystic masses extend from the neck into the mediastinum, but primary mediastinal cystic hygroma can occur. In adults, the radiological diagnosis of these lesions is much more difficult. They are not infrequently an incidental finding on imaging and are generally asymptomatic [36, 39]. Recurrent tumors following incomplete resection during childhood may present in this manner [36]. Sporadically, lesions arise at other sites in the body that are served by the lymphatic system, such as the chest wall (Fig. 17.5), the abdominal wall (Fig. 17.6), the retroperitoneum (Fig. 17.7) and the mesentery [2]. Parenchymal organs, including the lung, gastrointestinal tract, spleen, and liver, can also be involved [13]. The vast majority of lymphangiomas affecting the musculoskeletal system are soft tissue lesions, whereas osseous locations are a rare finding [22, 28]. In Maffucci's syndrome both lymphangiomas and hemangiomas are found.

Lymphangiomas are seldom life-threatening; serious medical problems can, however, arise depending on the size, location and type of the lesion, and these require a surgical approach, which is the treatment of choice. In this context, resection of well-circumscribed cystic lymphangiomas has a higher success rate than resection of cavernous lymphangiomas, arising in and infiltrating the muscle fibers of the tongue or cheek. Inadequate tumor removal almost invariably results in a higher rate

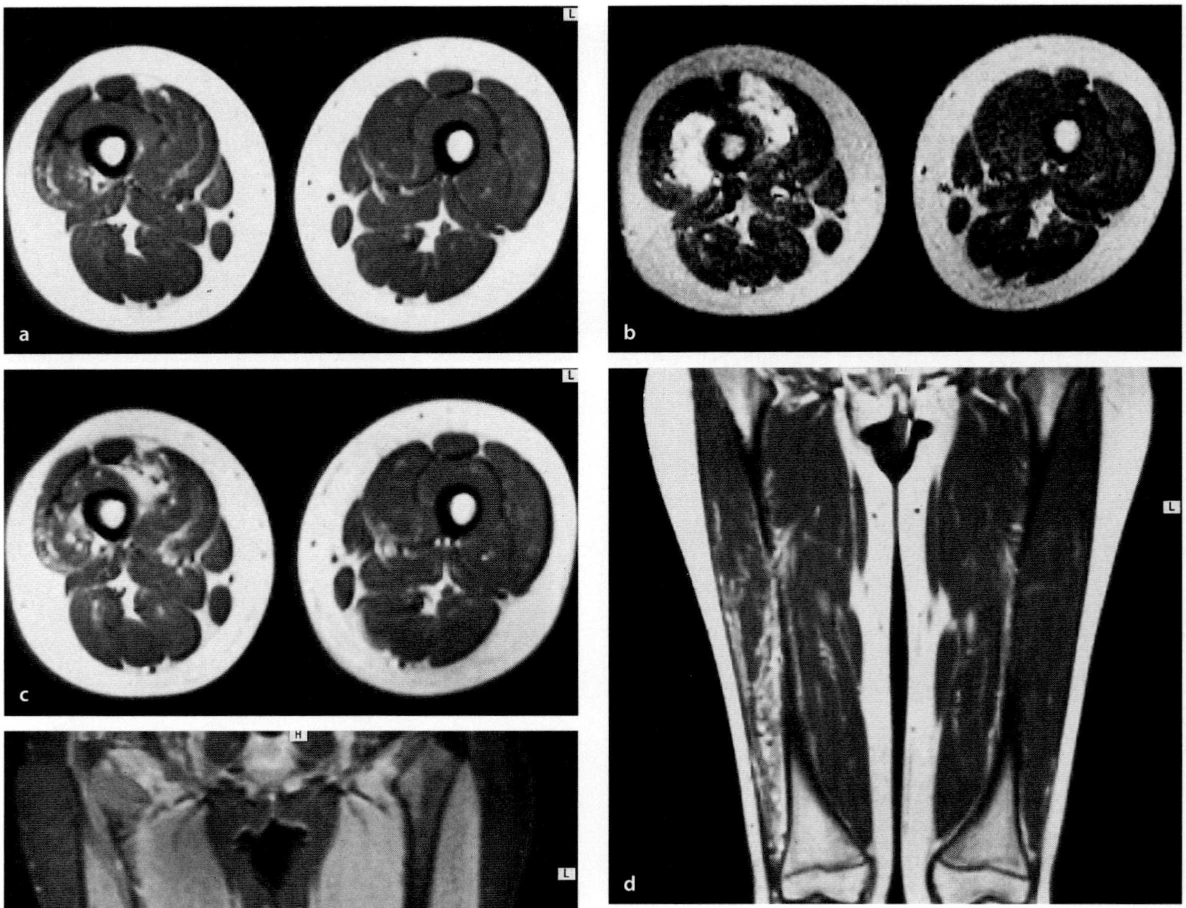

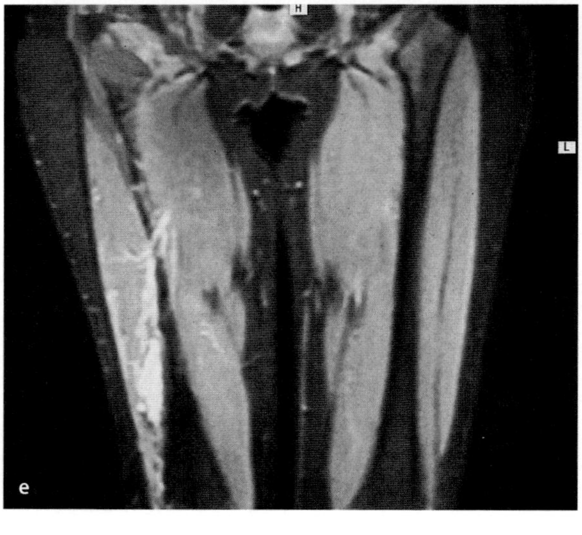

Fig. 17.3 a–e. Intramuscular cavernous lymphangioma in the right vastus lateralis muscle in a 12-year-old boy complaining of pain. **a** Axial SE T1-weighted MR image. **b** Axial SE T2-weighted MR image. **c** Axial SE T1-weighted MR image after Gd-contrast injection. **d** Coronal SE T1-weighted MR image after Gd-contrast injection. **e** Coronal fat suppressed MR image. On a T1-weighted image (**a**) SI is equal to that of muscle. On T2-WI (**b**) the mass has a higher SI than the surrounding muscles. After gadolinium-injection (**c, d**) a more heterogeneous uptake of contrast medium is seen. Note the serpiginous characteristics of the lesion, indicative for a lymphangioma

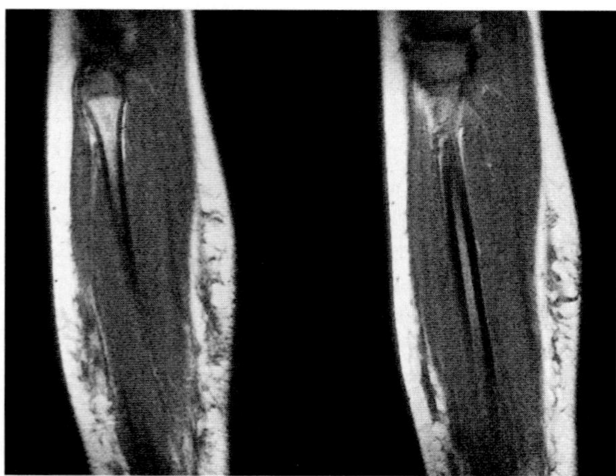

Fig. 17.4. Capillary lymphangioma of the right lower limb in a 6-year-old girl. Sagittal SE T1-weighted MR images. Disappearance of the normal high SI of the fat on both T1- and T2-weighted images by a cluster composed of small, capillary-sized endothelium-lined lymphatics. The tougher dermal and epidermal elements prevent expansion of the lymphatics resulting in the formation of a capillary lymphangioma

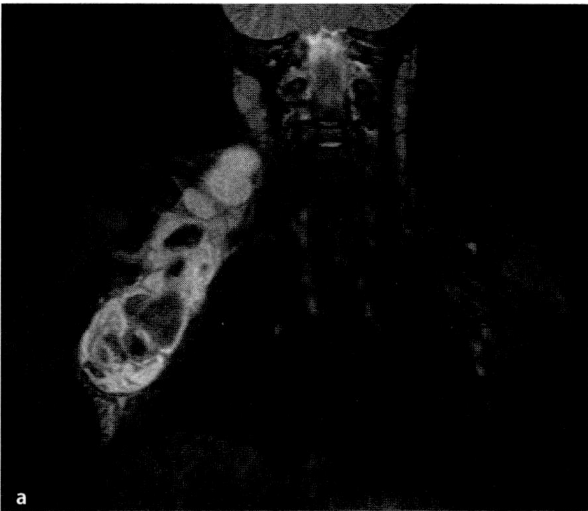

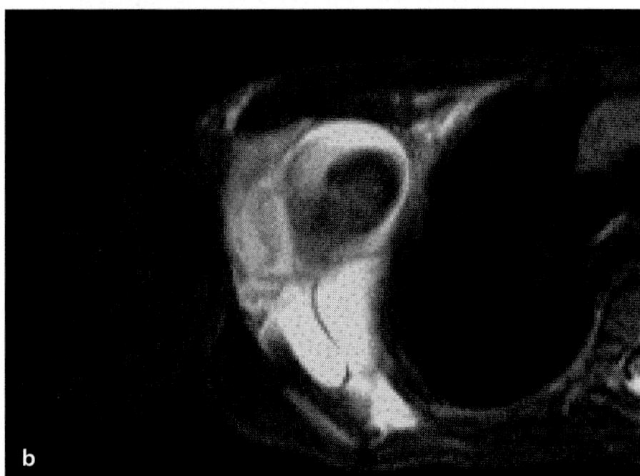

Fig. 17.5 a, b. Swelling at the right axilla in a three-year-old boy that appeared after aspiration-puncture by the general physician: **a** coronal fat suppressed TSE T2-weighted image (STIR); **b** axial STIR-image. Huge heterogeneous mass in the right axilla extending cranially to the supraclavicular fossa and caudally in the thoracic wall. The lesion has a polylobular appearance. Low SI areas correspond probably with hemorrhagic foci

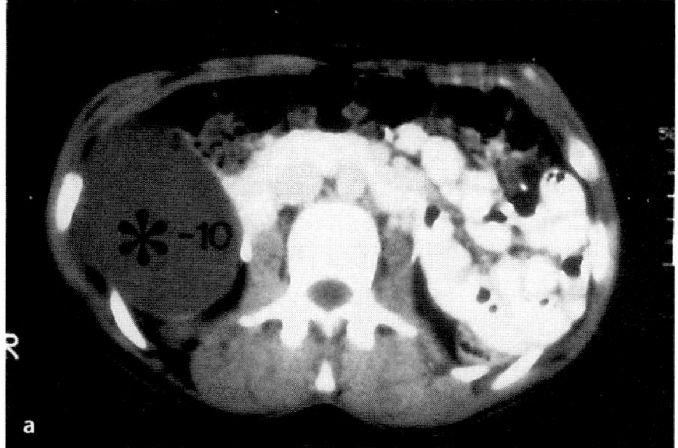

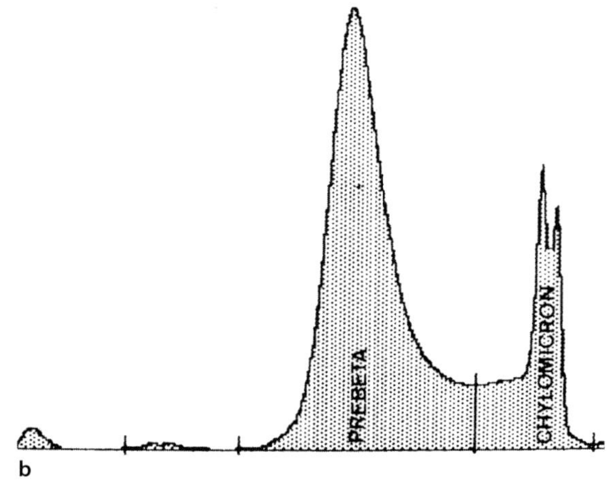

Fig. 17.7 a, b. Cystic retroperitoneal lymphangioma of the upper right abdomen in a 43-year-old woman, presenting with complaints of constipation and intermittent upper right flank pain. **a** CT scan after iodine contrast injection. **b** Electrophoretic analysis of the sample. A large retroperitoneal cystic tumor with negative attenuation value can be seen in Morrison's space, extending in the parietocolic wall and the retropancreatic space (**a**). More than 400 ml of yellow pale fatty fluid was obtained by percutaneous aspiration of the lesion. Lipids electrophoretic analysis (**b**) revealed a high content of pre-beta lipoproteins and chylomicrons, indicating the presence of lymph fluid. (Courtesy of V. Poncelet, Centre Hospitalier de Sainte-Ode, Belgium)

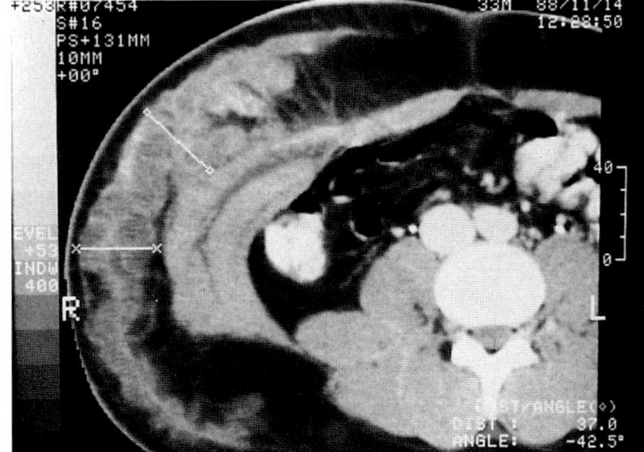

Fig. 17.6. Cavernous lymphangioma of the abdominal wall in a 47-year-old man. Frank swelling with discoloration of the overlying skin was noted. Axial enhanced CT scan. The normal density of the fatty tissue of the right abdominal wall has been replaced by a heterogeneous mass. Multiple cystic structures and internal contrast-enhancing septations can be discerned

of local recurrences and such complications as nerve palsies [8, 40]. Recently, percutaneous sclerotherapy of unresectable lymphangiomas has been described as safe and effective for palliative treatment in these patients [29]. Superinfection, which can arise from traumatic events or therapeutic aspiration, can also occur and be an indication for radical surgical extirpation [12]. For all these reasons, the role of medical imaging is to reveal the exact location and full extent of the lesion, as this may determine the therapeutic approach to be adopted in the particular patient [7].

Lymphangiomatosis is characterized by abnormal lymph tissue at multiple sites, involving every tissue type, except for nervous tissue [47]. Like angiomatosis, this extremely rare disease is most often seen in children [14, 46] (Fig. 17.8). Clinically and histopathologically, there is considerable overlap between these two entities [18]. In patients with visceral involvement differential diagnoses include: lymphoma, leukemic infiltration, metastatic disease, and plain cysts [27]. 'Spinal involvement consists of replacement of bone with lymph tissue, resulting in direct neural compression or bony instability [47]. Gomez et al. recently described a variant form of lymphangiomatosis with limited involvement, predominantly involving the soft tissues of the limbs and bones [18]. Clinical behavior, pathological features, and outcome of the disease are different from those seen in other patients with lymphangiomatosis. On clinical examination, a fluctuant and sponge-like swelling of the limb – either focal or diffuse – is noted.

Overlying skin changes with hyperplasia, vesicle formation and pigmentation changes are noted. On palpation, the accumulated fluid can be moved within the swollen area. Differential diagnosis against angiomatosis of the soft tissues is based on clinical grounds when a contiguous large segment of the body is affected.

17.2.2 Imaging Findings

17.2.2.1 Ultrasonography

Since cystic hygromas are usually located superficially, they can easily be examined with high-resolution ultrasonography (US) [38]. As expected from their cystic nature, they will typically appear as a multiloculated sonolucent mass in the posterior triangle of the neck (Fig. 17.9) [48]. A more heterogeneous appearance is seen when internal septations of variable thickness and/or solid echogenic components of varying size arising from the cyst wall or septa are demonstrated (Fig. 17.15) [38]. An increasing number of lesions are detected on prenatal ultrasonography. Three-dimensional US and MRI may help in assessing the extent of the lesion [35]. When the diagnosis of lymphangioma is made in utero amniocentesis and follow-up examination are mandatory, as these lesions often show tendency to grow with an increase in size of the afflicted area, and diffuse skin edema may develop [48]. Also, any associated anomalies should be ruled out, as these lymphangiomas can be seen in a variety of congenital syn-

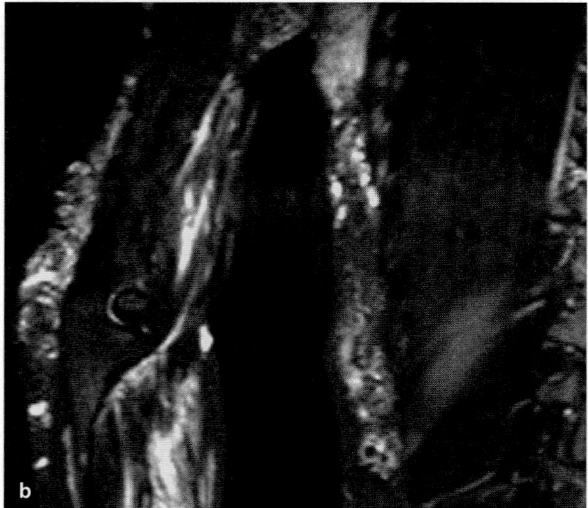

Fig. 17.8 a, b. Lymphangiomatosis in a ten-year-old boy with a prenatal ultrasound diagnosis of swelling at the right upper arm and hemithorax: **a** axial SE T1-weighted image; **b** coronal fat suppressed TSE T2-weighted image (STIR). Large ill-defined mass lesion at the extensor compartment of the forearm, extending proximally and over the axilla to the right thoracic wall. The extensive involvement of different compartments (muscles, subcutis and cutis) by moniliform and serpiginous structures is superbly demonstrated on STIR images

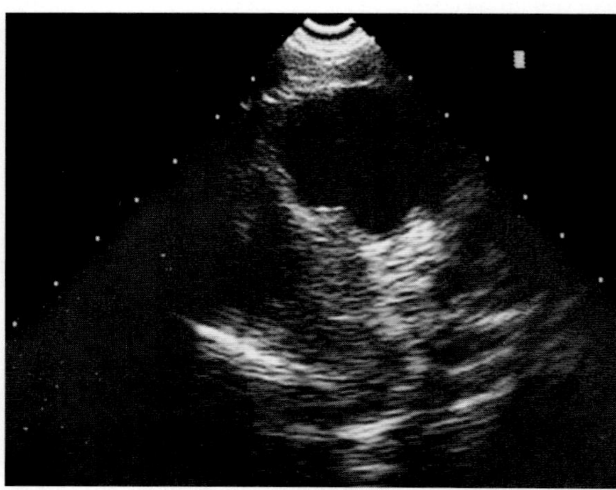

Fig. 17.9. Cystic hygroma of the neck in a newborn patient. Longitudinal sonogram shows an inhomogeneous multilocular mass lesion. Multiple anechogenic cystic components are separated by solid components of mixed echogenicity indicating the internal septations of the lesion

Fig. 17.10 a, b. Cystic lymphangioma in a 17-year-old male patient who presented with a fluctuating mass lesion in the right anterior right neck. **a** Axial enhanced CT-scan. **b** Sagittal reformatted image. Multilocular nonenhancing, cystic mass in the submandibular space, deep to the sternocleidomastoid muscle and slightly pushing the carotid artery medially can be seen on the axial image (**a**). Extension of the lesion into the mediastinum can be excluded on the sagittal reformatted images (**b**)

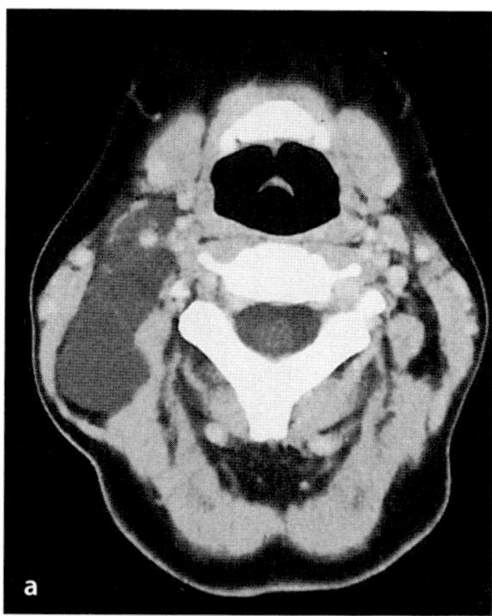
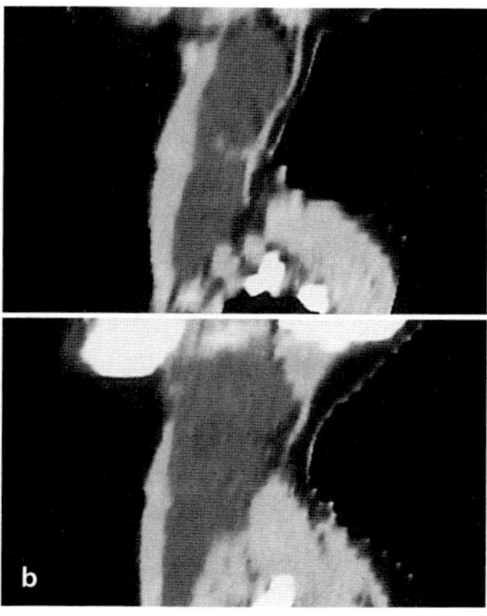

dromes (e. g., Turner's syndrome, Noonan's syndrome, fetal alcohol syndrome, familial pterygium colli, Down's syndrome,...) [5, 48, 50]. Based on the findings of prenatal US and clinical examination, Schuster et al. introduced a classification for lymphangioma colli, to predict the expected morbidity and prognosis with surgical treatment [37].

Other cystic masses arising in the neck are branchial cleft cysts or thyroglossal duct cysts. However, these lesions have a typical location and tend to be unilocular. Differential diagnosis should be made against atypical manifestation forms of abscesses, resolving hematomas and necrotic lymph nodes [38].

17.2.2.2 Computed Tomography

Findings on CT are highly variable; a uniformly cystic mass or a more heterogeneous aspect of the lesion, including both cystic and solid components can be seen (Fig. 17.10). After intravenous administration of contrast agent, no definite enhancement of the lesion can be discerned [36]. CT might hold a minor advantage over MRI in differentiating lymphangiomas from hemangiomas, since the latter group may show the presence of calcified phleboliths in the lesion [26].

17.2.2.3 Magnetic Resonance Imaging

As in other abnormalities seen throughout of the body, MRI has the benefits of multiplanar acquisitions and the lack of ionizing radiation. The strength of MRI in the evaluation of such soft tissue lesions as lymphangiomas and hemangiomas lies in its capability to demonstrate the full extent of the lesion (Fig. 17.11) [7, 26, 49]. This can be most easily achieved on T2-weighted images, where the mass has a higher signal intensity (SI) than the surrounding muscles (Fig. 17.3 a) [40]. However, SI are nonspecific and are similar to those of hemangiomas [26, 34]. For the evaluation of lymphangiomas located in the subcutaneous fat, STIR-sequences are strongly recommended (Fig. 17.3 e). With the use of SE T1-weighted imaging with fat-suppression lymphangiomas may be differentiated from hemangiomas, possibly obviating the use of gadolinium. Hemangiomas will have a high SI, whereas lymphangiomas may have a low SI [17]. Larger series however are necessary to validate this finding. On T1-weighted images, SI is equal to or slightly lower than that of muscle (Fig. 17.3 b), unless complicated by hemorrhage (Fig. 17.1), infection or prior surgery [26]. As already mentioned before, hemangiomas may show the presence of phleboliths which can be visualized on MRI using gradient echo techniques. Flow voids arising from feeding arteries or draining veins can be seen in high-flow hemangiomas and allow rejection of the diagnosis of lymphangioma. Gadolinium injection may offer some help in differentiation between hemangiomas and lymphangiomas, as hemangiomas show a homogeneous enhancement whereas lymphangiomas have a more heterogeneous uptake of contrast medium (Fig. 17.3 c, d) [33]. Although dynamic contrast-enhanced MR-imaging may help to differentiate slow flow lesions (lymphangiomas) from high flow lesions (hemangiomas, fistula), time constraints may prohibit the routine use of this sequence in the work-out of both these benign lesions [43]. More studies are needed to demonstrate the role of magnetic resonance angiography (MRA) and magnetic resonance lymphography in the work-up of lymphatic tumors [46, 24]. Magnetic resonance lymphography with superparamagnetic injection of iron oxide is currently still in an experimental phase, but may prove its validity in the future [1, 20, 42].

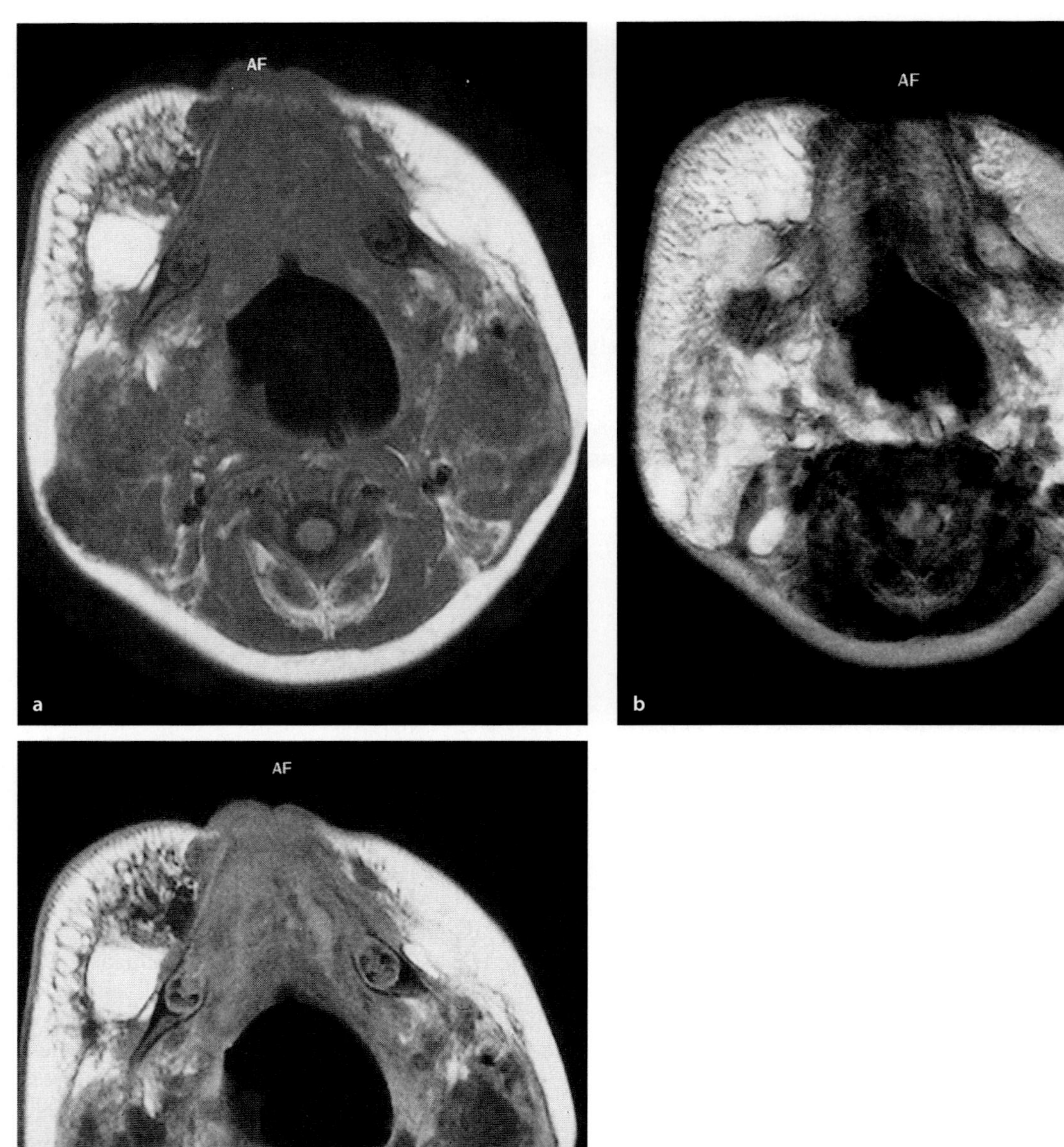

Fig. 17.11 a–c. Lymphangiomatosis with involvement of the head and neck region in a 2-month-old baby-girl. **a** Axial SE T1-weighted MR image. **b** Axial TSE T2-weighted MR image. **c** Axial SE T1-weighted MR image after Gd-contrast injection. Diffuse involvement of the neck bilaterally with extension into the deep spaces of the neck. Involvement of the parotid glands which are difficult to individualize

17.2.2.4 Lymphography

In the work-up of mediastinal or retroperitoneal lesions, the aim of lymphography was to demonstrate the presence of abnormally dilated and cystic lymphatic channels [32, 45]. However, now that CT and MRI are widely available, we believe lymphography is no longer indicated for the diagnosis of lymphangioma.

17.3 Lymphangiomyoma and Lymphangiomyomatosis

Lymphangiomyomatosis is a rare, progressive disease, only afflicting young women of childbearing age (Fig. 17.10). Despite its aggressive nature, lymphangiomyomatosis is not a true neoplastic process, because of its highly organized structure lacking any cellular disarray, cell atypia or mitotic activity. Abnormal smooth muscle proliferation and subsequent gradual obliteration of small airways, lymphatics and vascular structures may result in dyspnea, recurrent pneumothorax, chylous effusion and hemophtisis. Plain chest radiography and CT of the thorax may demonstrate pleural effusion, multiple granular opacities and both mediastinal masses and adenopathies. Pulmonary involvement, which is responsible for most of the morbidity and mortality, is an indicator of a poor prognosis [21]. However, recent findings suggest a favorable prognosis in patients with localized disease, treated with progestational agents [13]. Since patients with tuberous sclerosis may have similar lesions affecting lungs and lymph nodes, speculation has been expressed as to whether lymphangiomyomatosis is a forme fruste of this disease [14].

Things to remember:
1. Tumors of lymphatic origin are rare, and are usually detected early in childhood.
2. Lymphangiomas have been reported in every type of tissue except for neural tissue.
3. An increasing number of lesions are detected on prenatal ultrasonography and fetal MRI.
4. MRI is the imaging method of choice to demonstrate the full extent of the lesion, especially on fat suppressed images.
5. SI of lymphangioma are non-specific and are similar to those of hemangioma. The absence of flow voids and the lack of significant enhancement after Gd-contrast injection are in favor for the diagnosis of lymphangioma.

References

1. Anzai Y, Blackwell K, McLachlan S, Fu YS, Abemayor E, Lufkin RB (1993) Initial clinical experience with an iron-based MR imaging contrast agent for lymphnodes. Radiology 189 (P):108
2. Arts M, De Schepper A, Bracke P, Kockx M (1994) Unusual presentation of a retroperitoneal lymphangiectatic cyst: a case report. Eur Radiol 4:262–264
3. Bill AA, Sumner DS (1965) A unified concept of lymphangioma and cystic hygroma. Surg Gynecol Obstet 120:79–86
4. Blumenthal EZ, Gottehrer NP, Dollberg M, Halevy J (1994) A giant tuberculous lymphangioma extending from the mediastinum to the inguinal region. Chest 105:1279–1280
5. Chervenak FA, Isaacson G, Blakemore KJ, Breg WR, Hobbins JC, Berkowitz RL, Tortora M, Mayden K, Mahoney MJ (1984) Fetal cystic hygroma. N Engl J Med 309:822–825
6. Chisin R, Fabian R, Weber AL, Ragozzino M, Brady TJ, Goodman M (1988) MR Imaging of a lymphangioma involving the masseter muscle. J Comput Assist Tomogr 12:690–692
7. Dubois J, Garel L (1999) Imaging and therapeutic approach of hemangiomas and vascular malformations in the pediatric age group. Pediatr Radiol 29:879–893
8. Emery PJ, Bailey CM, Evans JNG (1984) Cystic hygroma of the head and neck: a review of 37 cases. J Laryngol Otol 98:613–619
9. Enjolras O (1997) Classification and management of the various superficial vascular anomalies: hemangiomas and vascular malformations. J Dermatol 24: 701–710
10. Enjolras O, Mulliken JB (1997) Vascular tumors and vascular malformations. Adv Dermatol 13:375–423
11. Enzinger FM, Weiss SW (1995) Malignant vascular tumors. In: Enzinger FM, Weiss SW (eds) Soft tissue tumors, 3rd edn. St Louis, Mosby, pp 641–677
12. Enzinger FM, Weiss SW (1995) Tumors of lymph vessels. In: Enzinger FM, Weiss SW (eds) Soft tissue tumors 3rd edn. Mosby, St Louis, pp 679–700
13. Enzinger FM, Weiss SW (1996) Lymphatic tumors. In: Meis-Kindblom JM, Enzinger FM (eds) Color atlas of soft tissue tumors. St Louis, Mosby, pp 174–178
14. Enzinger FM, Lattes R, Torloni R (1969) Histological typing of soft tissue tumors. World Health Organization, Geneva
15. Fisher D, Hiller N (1994) Giant tuberculous cystic lymphangioma of posterior mediastinum, retroperitoneum and groin. Clin Radiol 49:215–216
16. Fisher I, Orkin M (1970) Acquired lymphangioma (lymphangiectasis). Arch Dermatol 101:230
17. Gielen JL, De Schepper AM, Parizel PM, Wang XL, Vanhoenacker F (2003) Additional value of magnetic resonance with spin echo T1-weighted imaging with fat suppression in characterization of soft tissue tumors. J Comput Assist Tomogr 27:434–441
18. Gomez CS, Calonje E, Ferrar DW, Browse NL, Fletcher CDM (1995) Lymphangiomatosis of the limbs: clinicopathologic analysis of a series with good prognosis. Am J Surg Pathol 19:125–133
19. Harms SE, Greenway G (1992) Musculoskeletal tumors. In: Stark DD, Bradley WG Jr (eds) Magnetic resonance imaging 2 nd edn. Mosby, St. Louis, pp 2107–2222
20. Heautot JF, Weissleder R, Schaffer B, Brady TJ (1993) Intraarterial MR lymphography: technique to improve accumulation of contrast agents in lymph nodes. Radiology 189 (P):246
21. Johnson SF, Davey DD, Cibull ML, Schwartz RW, Strodel WE (1993) Lymphangioleiomyomatosis. Am Surg 59:395–399
22. Jumbelic M, Feuerstein IM, Dorfman HD (1984) Solitary intraosseous lymphangioma. J Bone Joint Surg [Am] 66:1479–1481
23. Kransdorf MJ (1995) Benign soft-tissue tumors in a large referral population: distribution of specific diagnoses by age, sex, and location. AJR Am J Roentgenol 164:395–402

24. Laor T, Hoffer FA, Burrows PE, Kozakewich HP (1998) MR lymphangiography in infants, children, and young adults. AJR Am J Roentgenol 171:1111–1117

25. Lee K (1980) Surgery of cysts and tumours of the neck. In: Paparella M, Shunrick D (eds) Otolaryngology. Saunders, Philadelphia, p 2987

26. Mancuso AA, Dillon WP (1989) The neck. Radiol Clin North Am 27:407–434

27. Melzer G, Kullnig P, Fluckiger F, Beham A (1991) CT image of diffuse visceral lymphangiomatosis. Fortschr Rontgenstr 155: 282–283

28. Méndez JA, Hochmuth A, Boetefuer IC, Schumacher M (2002) Radiologic appearance of a rare primary vertebral lymphangioma. Am J Neuroadiol 23:1665–1668

29. Molitch HI, Unger EC, Witte CL, van Sonnenberg E (1995) Percutaneous sclerotherapy of lymphangiomas. Radiology 194: 343–347

30. Mulliken JB, Glowacki J (1982) Hemangiomas and vascular malformations in infants and children: a classification based on endothelial characteristics. Plast Reconstr Surg 69:412–422

31. Nosan DK, Martin DS, Stith JA (1995) Lymphangioma presenting as a delayed posttraumatic expanding neck mass. Am J Otolaryngol Head Neck Med Surg 16:186–189

32. Peh WCG, Ngan H (1993) Lymphography – still useful in the diagnosis of lymphangiomatosis. Br J Radiol 66:28–31

33. Peiss J, Fuzesi L, Bohndorf K, Neuerburg J, Urhahn R, Gunther RW (1993) MR morphology of haemangiomas and lymphangiomas of the peripheral soft parts – correlation with angiography and histology. Fortschr Rontgenstr 158:463–470

34. Ramon F (1992) Vascular soft tissue tumors: medical imaging. J Belge Radiol [BTR] 75:303–310

35. Ruano R, Aubry JP, Simon I, Grebille AG, Sonigo P, Dumez Y, Dommergues M (2003) Prenatal diagnosis of a large axillary cystic lymphangioma by three-dimensional ultrasonography and magnetic resonance imaging. J Ultrasound Med 22:419–423

36. Schuster T, Grantzow R, Nicolai T (2003) Lymphangioma colli – a new classification contributing to prognosis. Eur J Pediatr Surg 13:97–102

37. Shaffer K, Rosado-de-Christenson ML, Patz EF Jr, Young S, Farver CF (1994) Thoracic lymphangioma in adults: CT and MR imaging features. AJR Am J Roentgenol 162:283–289

38. Sheth S, Nussbaum AR, Hutchins GM, Sanders RC (1987) Cystic hygromas in children: sonographic-pathologic correlation. Radiology 162:821–824

39. Shin MS, Berland LL, Ho KJ (1985) Mediastinal cystic hygromas: CT characteristics and pathogenetic consideration. J Comput Assist Tomogr 9:297–301

40. Siegel MJ, Glazer HS, St Amour TE, Rosenthal DD (1989) Lymphangiomas in children: MR imaging. Radiology 170:467–470

41. Smith DW (1982) Recognizable patterns of human malformation: genetic, embryologic, and clinical aspects, 3rd edn. Saunders, Philadelphia, pp 472–473

42. Sophocleous S, Ehrenheim C, Hamann A, Hundeshagen H (1994) Cavernous lymphangioma of the pelvic area – MR tomographic and lymphoscintigraphic findings. Fortschr Rontgenstr 160:574–576

43. Rijswijk, van, CS, Geirnaerdt MJ, Hogendoorn PC, Taminiau AH, van Coevorden F, Zwinderman AH, Pope TL, Bloem JL (2004) Soft-tissue tumors: value of static and dynamic gadopentetate dimeglumine-enhanced MR imaging in prediction of malignancy. Radiology 233:493–502

44. Vanel D, Shapeero LG, De Baere T, Gilles R, Tardivon A, Genin J, Guinebretière JM (1994) MR Imaging in the follow-up of malignant and aggressive soft-tissue tumors: results of 511 examinations. Radiology 190:263–268

45. Viamonte M, Jr, Rüttimann AL (1980) Atlas of lymphography. Thieme, Stuttgart, pp 164–172

46. Vogl TJ, Hammerstingl R, Schnell B, Klein Ch, Hauser M, Pfluger T, Lissner J (1992) Magnetic resonance tomography and magnetic resonance angiography of lymphangiomatosis. Fortschr Rontgenstr 157:414–419

47. Watkins RG IV, Reynolds RAK, McComb JG, Tolo VT (2003) Lymphangiomatosis of the spine. Two cases requiring surgical intervention. Spine 28:E45–E50

48. Weingast GR, Hopper KD, Gottesfeld SA, Manco-Johnson ML (1988) Congenital lymphangiectsia with fetal cystic hygroma: report of two cases with coexistent Down's syndrome. J Clin Ultrasound 16:663–668

49. Wunderbaldinger P, Paya K, Partik B, Turetschek K, Hormann M, Horcher E, Bankier AA (2000) CT and MR imaging of generalized cystic lymphangiomatosis in pediatric patients. AJR Am J Roentgenol 174:827–832

50. Zadvinskis DP, Benson MT, Kerr HH, Mancuso AA, Cacciarelli AA, Madrazo BL, Mafee MF, Dalen K (1992) Congenital malformations of the cervicothoracic lymphatic system: embryology and pathogenesis. Radiographics 12:1175–1189

Tumors of Muscular Origin

18

P.C. Seynaeve, P.J.L. De Visschere, L.L. Mortelmans,
A.M. De Schepper

Contents

18.1 Introduction

Generally speaking, tumors of muscular origin are not common. The radiological literature is limited mainly to case reports [17, 27, 38, 55, 59], and even when series of soft tissue tumors are reported, the number of muscular lesions remains low [33, 49]. In two fundamental papers based on lesions seen by the Armed Forces Institute of Pathology over a 10-year period, Kransdorf reported 311 benign tumors of muscular origin (leiomyomas) out of a total of 18,677 benign soft tissue tumors, or 1.7% [32]. Among the 12,370 malignant soft tissue tumors, there were 1,039 leiomyosarcomas (8.4%) and 239 rhabdomyosarcomas (1.9%).

The recently concluded Multicentric European Study on Magnetic Resonance Imaging of Soft Tissue Tumors observed 26 tumors of muscular origin out of a total of almost 800 randomly reported cases [14]. Although muscle tumors have been well described and classified histologically, imaging techniques have remained of limited value in specifying the tissue diagnosis of these masses. However, the newer imaging modalities – computed tomography (CT) and, especially, magnetic resonance imaging (MRI) – have brought some progress in this field.

18.2 Classification, Incidence, and Clinical Behavior

Since imaging techniques lack specificity, it is not possible to classify tumors by their radiological appearance. For this reason we will classify the muscular tumors on the basis of histology according to the WHO classification of soft tissue tumors:

- Smooth muscle tumors
  - A. Benign tumors
    1. Angioleiomyoma
    2. Deep leiomyoma
    3. Genital leiomyoma
  - B. Malignant tumors
    Leiomyosarcoma (excluding skin)
- Skeletal muscle tumors
  - A. Benign tumors
    Rhabdomyoma
    a) Adult rhabdomyoma
    b) Fetal rhabdomyoma
    c) Genital rhabdomyoma
  - B. Malignant tumors
    Rhabdomyosarcoma
    a) Embryonal rhabdomyosarcoma, spindle cell rhabdomyosarcoma, botryoid rhabdomyosarcoma, anaplastic rhabdomyosarcoma
    b) Alveolar rhabdomyosarcoma, solid rhabdomyosarcoma, anaplastic rhabdomyosarcoma
    c) Pleomorphic rhabdomyosarcoma

18.2.1 Tumors of Smooth Muscle

18.2.1.1 Benign Smooth Muscle Tumors

Superficial or cutaneous leiomyomas must be divided into two entities: leiomyomas derived from the arrectores pilorum muscle complex and genital leiomyomas [19].

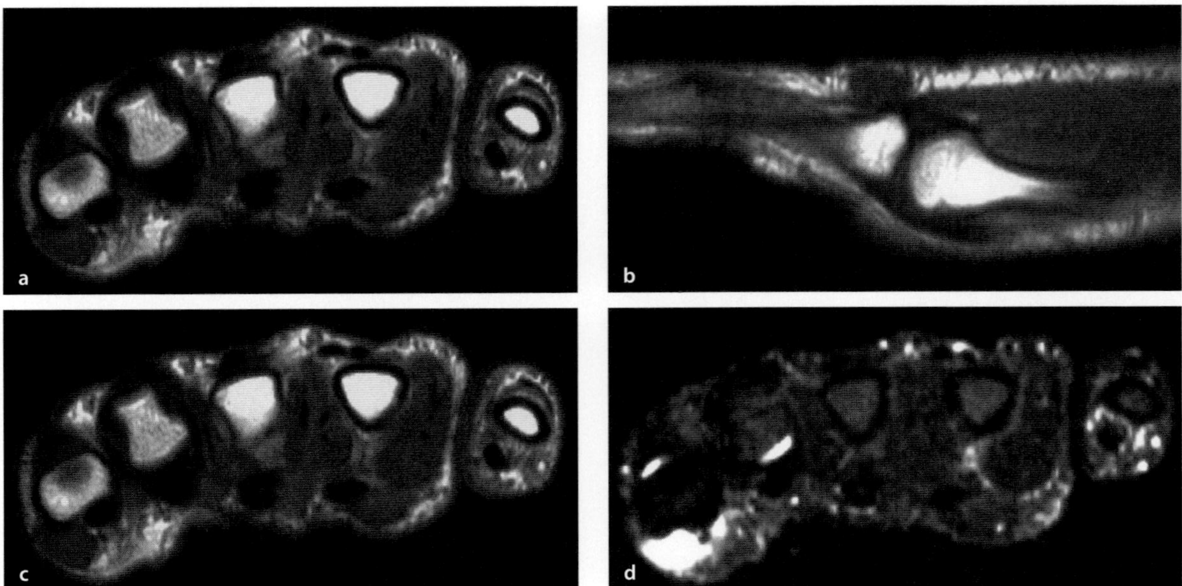

Fig. 18.1 a–d. Angiomyoma in a 46-year-old man with a long standing swelling in the left hand, recently increased in volume. **a** Axial spin-echo T1-weighted MR image. **b** Sagittal spin-echo T1-weighted MR image. **c** Axial spin-echo T1-weighted MR image after gadolinium contrast injection. **d** Axial STIR MR sequence. At the ulnopalmar aspect of the fifth MCP joint, a small, nodular, well-defined mass lesion is seen, with signal intensity equal to ad-jacent normal muscle on T1-weighted MR images (**a, b**). After gadolinium contrast injection, the lesion shows no obvious enhancement (**c**), but on STIR MR sequence there is a very high signal intensity (**d**). Illustration of an angiomyoma with nonenhancement on T1-weighted MR images after gadolinium contrast injection and very high signal intensity on STIR MR sequence

The arrectores pilorum leiomyomas lie within the dermal connective tissue. Most lesions consist of a central zone of smooth muscle cells and blend with the surrounding dermal collagen and adjacent pilar muscle. These leiomyomas are solitary or multiple painful nodules with a diameter of 1–2 cm. These small papules can eventually coalesce to a fine linear pattern in the same dermatome. They may be associated with dermatitis herpetiformis, HLA B8, premature uterine leiomyomas, increased erythropoietin activity, and multiple endocrine adenomatosis type 1. They arise most frequently in the extensor surfaces of the extremities.

Angioleiomyoma, angiomyoma, or vascular leiomyomas are histologically divided into three subtypes: solid, cavernous, and venous. All of these subtypes contain nodular conglomerates of smooth muscle cells and thick-walled vessels (Fig. 18.1).

These are rare; they account for about 5% of all benign soft tissue tumors. These tumors develop most frequently in women in the fourth to sixth decades. Most of the solid histological subtype tumors occur in the lower leg as slowly growing solitary masses of several years' duration. Pain is a prominent feature in about 50% of all reported cases.

Intravenous leiomyomatosis consists of benign smooth muscle tissue nodules that grow in the veins of the myometrium and occasionally extend into uterine and hypogastric veins. The pathogenesis remains un-clear. Whether these lesions develop as a result of vessel invasion by one or several endometrial tumors, or whether they are formed by a proliferation of smooth muscle cells within the vessel wall is still debated. The lesions develop mainly in promenopausal women. Clinically they present as abnormal vaginal bleeding and pelvic pain. In about 50% of these patients, the uterus is enlarged. In certain cases cardiac symptoms may occur or even predominate owing to the presence of tumor in the vena cava or the heart.

Deep leiomyomas histologically have a rich vascularization, which may mimic soft tissue sarcoma. The presence of stippled, plaque-like, or larger mulberry calcifications similar to those in uterine leiomyomas has been described in deep-seated soft tissue leiomyomas, especially in childhood [18, 36, 38]. Deep leiomyomas are less frequent than subcutaneous leiomyomas. Deep leiomyomas can occur in the deep parts of the extremities . They affect both sexes equally, whereas leiomyomas of the retroperitoneum or abdominal cavity occur almost exclusively in women.

In our series (databank of soft tissue tumor of the University Hospital Antwerp), only one histologically proven leiomyoma of the deep flexor compartment of the arm was found (Fig. 18.1).

Leiomyomatosis peritonealis disseminata is another rare entity and is characterized by multiple smooth muscle nodules situated subperitoneally throughout the abdominal cavity. It is not accompanied by any parenchymal disease within the abdominal organs and does not extend extra-abdominally. Leiomyomatosis peritonealis disseminata only occurs in women of childbearing age, is frequently associated with pregnancy or oral contraceptives, and tends to be frequent in Afro-Americans.

Genital leiomyomas are histologically heterogeneous lesions that frequently contain cells with myxoid and epithelioid changes. Genital leiomyomas are small, painless lesions usually less than 2 cm in size that appear in the areola of the nipple, scrotum, labia, penis, and vulva.

18.2.1.2 Malignant Smooth Muscle Tumors

Leiomyosarcomas account for between 5 and 10 % of all soft tissue tumors. They occur typically in adult life, although recently an association of Epstein Barr virus with leiomyosarcomas in young people with AIDS and after organ transplantation has been reported by several groups [37, 40, 45].

All leiomyosarcomas have the same histological characteristics. They are, however, divided into three different subgroups because of their clinical and biological differences [20].

Cutaneous and subcutaneous leiomyosarcomas must be differentiated. The smaller cutaneous lesions are ill-defined tumors with tumor strands blending in with the surrounding collagen and arrectores pilorum muscles. Patients present with cutaneous discoloration, umbilication, and ulceration. The subcutaneous lesions are well circumscribed and form a pseudocapsule. These grow faster and result only in skin elevation.

Cutaneous and subcutaneous leiomyosarcomas account for 2–3 % of all superficial soft tissue sarcomas. They are most common in men in the fifth to seventh decades. Pain is a prominent feature in both tumors. As these tumors are mostly solitary, multiplicity is always suggestive of metastasis from another site. Whereas cutaneous leiomyosarcomas metastasize in 10 % of cases, or less, subcutaneous lesions metastasize in 30–40 % of cases. They differ from the retroperitoneal leiomyosarcomas in their lack of regressive and degenerative changes which is probably related to their smaller size.

Leiomyosarcomas of the deep soft tissues are most frequent in the retroperitoneum and in the abdominal cavity. More than 60 % of this subgroup occur in women, usually after menopause. Symptoms are vague and nonspecific. Less frequently, these tumors can be found in the deep soft tissues of the extremities, affecting both sexes equally.

Vascular leiomyosarcomas are polypoid or nodular masses that are firmly attached to the vessel wall and spread along its surface. In veins the extension to the adjacent tissues is a relatively early event, while in arteries (pulmonary artery) the tunica elastica is usually preserved and invasion of other organs is absent. Vascular leiomyosarcoma is a rare tumor. The inferior vena cava seems to be its primary site and accounts for 50 % of recorded cases, while the greater saphenous vein accounts for 25 % and the bulk of the rest arise from the femoral, internal jugular, and iliac veins in declining order of frequency [29, 30, 60]. Tumor recurrence is not affected by tumor grade, size, or adjuvant therapy [16], the prognosis depending rather on location and surgical accessibility.

In 10 % of cases, metastatic disease, usually in the lung or liver, is already present at the time of diagnosis [31]. Epitheloid or myxoid change and the presence of granular eosinophilic cytoplasm cells in leiomyosarcomas are rare. These tumors are classified as epitheloid, myxoid, or granular cell leiomyosarcomas [22].

18.2.2 Tumors of Striated Muscle

18.2.2.1 Benign Striated Muscle Tumors

In general, benign soft tissue tumors are much more frequent than their malignant counterparts. The opposite is true for striated muscle tumors, where benign lesions account for no more than 2 % of all striated muscle tumors.

Adult rhabdomyoma is a hamartomatous process that is usually solitary and well defined or coarsely lobulated. It shows a gray-yellow to red-brown color on macroscopic inspection and contains large, round polygonal cells intersected by fibrous strands [21].

It presents as a painless, round or polypoid mass in the neck, which seems to arise from the branchial musculature of the third and fourth clefts. Clinically it may cause hoarseness or progressive difficulties in swallowing. Most cases occur in adults over 40 years old and are solitary tumors. However, multifocality has been described in about 20 % but is restricted to the neck (Fig. 18.2).

Fetal rhabdomyoma is a superficial tumor often with a mucoid glistening surface, usually polypoid or pedunculated and less than 5 cm in size. Both myxoid and cellular differentiated subtypes can be found. It is even rarer than the adult subtype and occurs in the head and neck regions of both children and adults. The median age is 4 years (3–58 years), with a 2.4:1 male predominance. The classic fetal rhabdomyoma has a predilection for the postauricular soft tissue. Some may be related to neuromuscular hamartoma (benign Triton tumor).

Genital rhabdomyomas form a group of polypoid or cauliflower-like masses covered by epithelium. These tumors consist of centrally scattered muscle fibers and a matrix of collagen and mucoid material. They present

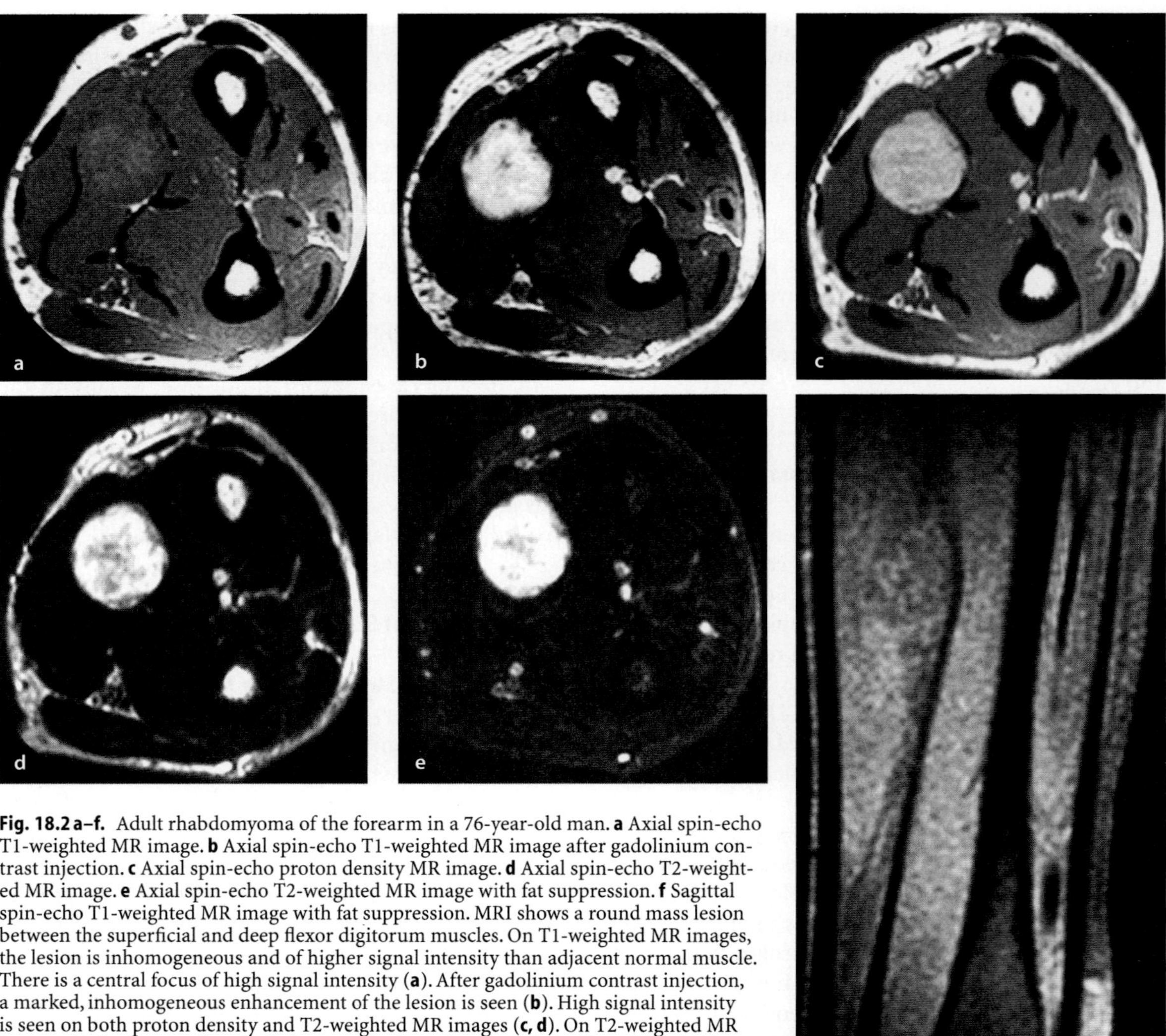

Fig. 18.2 a–f. Adult rhabdomyoma of the forearm in a 76-year-old man. **a** Axial spin-echo T1-weighted MR image. **b** Axial spin-echo T1-weighted MR image after gadolinium contrast injection. **c** Axial spin-echo proton density MR image. **d** Axial spin-echo T2-weighted MR image. **e** Axial spin-echo T2-weighted MR image with fat suppression. **f** Sagittal spin-echo T1-weighted MR image with fat suppression. MRI shows a round mass lesion between the superficial and deep flexor digitorum muscles. On T1-weighted MR images, the lesion is inhomogeneous and of higher signal intensity than adjacent normal muscle. There is a central focus of high signal intensity (**a**). After gadolinium contrast injection, a marked, inhomogeneous enhancement of the lesion is seen (**b**). High signal intensity is seen on both proton density and T2-weighted MR images (**c, d**). On T2-weighted MR image with fat suppression, the lesion remains hyperintense (**e**). On T1-weighted MR image with fat suppression, fatty components can be excluded (**f**)

as slow-growing polypoid or cyst-like masses in the vagina or the vulva of young and middle-aged women. The median age is 42 years (range 30–48 years). A similar lesion has been described in the prostate of a 19-year-old male patient [21, 44].

Rhabdomyomatous mesenchymal hamartomas are subcutaneous lesions composed of poorly oriented skeletal muscle bundles blended with islands of fat, fibrous tissue, and proliferated nerves. They occur in the orbital and periorbital regions of infants and young children.

18.2.2.2 Malignant Striated Muscle Tumors

Rhabdomyosarcoma is frequent in persons under 45 years of age. In children it is actually the most common soft tissue tumor. According to the Armed Forces

Institutes of Pathology, fewer than 15% of rhabdomyosarcomas occur in the extremities, with an equal distribution between upper and lower extremities [61].

Histologically, this group contains several different types of tumors, depending on the cellularity. The WHO classification modifies slightly the previously accepted classification of Horn and Enterline (1958). The malignant striated muscle tumors are subdivided in an embryonal, alveolar, and pleomorphic rhabdomyosarcoma subgroup [28].

The *embryonal group* contains the spindle cell, botryoid, and anaplastic rhabdomyosarcoma subtypes. These subtypes range from poorly differentiated tumors that correspond histologically to the appearance of developing muscle in an early gestational stage to well-differentiated tumors that resemble mature fetal muscle. *Spindle cell rhabdomyosarcoma* is a subtype of this group of tumors and is characterized by the parallel orientation

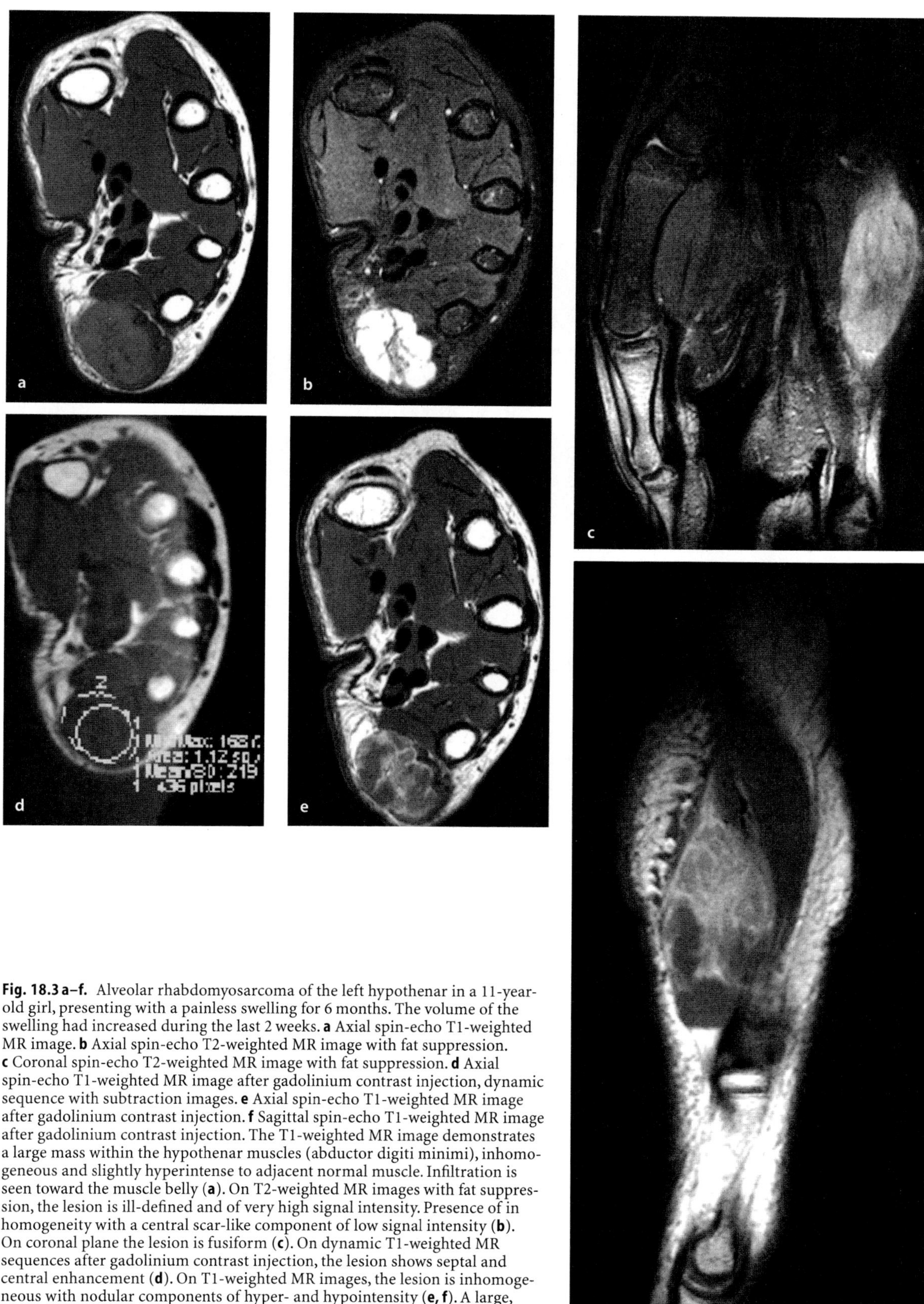

Fig. 18.3 a–f. Alveolar rhabdomyosarcoma of the left hypothenar in a 11-year-old girl, presenting with a painless swelling for 6 months. The volume of the swelling had increased during the last 2 weeks. **a** Axial spin-echo T1-weighted MR image. **b** Axial spin-echo T2-weighted MR image with fat suppression. **c** Coronal spin-echo T2-weighted MR image with fat suppression. **d** Axial spin-echo T1-weighted MR image after gadolinium contrast injection, dynamic sequence with subtraction images. **e** Axial spin-echo T1-weighted MR image after gadolinium contrast injection. **f** Sagittal spin-echo T1-weighted MR image after gadolinium contrast injection. The T1-weighted MR image demonstrates a large mass within the hypothenar muscles (abductor digiti minimi), inhomogeneous and slightly hyperintense to adjacent normal muscle. Infiltration is seen toward the muscle belly (**a**). On T2-weighted MR images with fat suppression, the lesion is ill-defined and of very high signal intensity. Presence of in homogeneity with a central scar-like component of low signal intensity (**b**). On coronal plane the lesion is fusiform (**c**). On dynamic T1-weighted MR sequences after gadolinium contrast injection, the lesion shows septal and central enhancement (**d**). On T1-weighted MR images, the lesion is inhomogeneous with nodular components of hyper- and hypointensity (**e, f**). A large, illdefined mass with inhomogeneous appearance on all MR sequences, arising from the hypothenar in a child

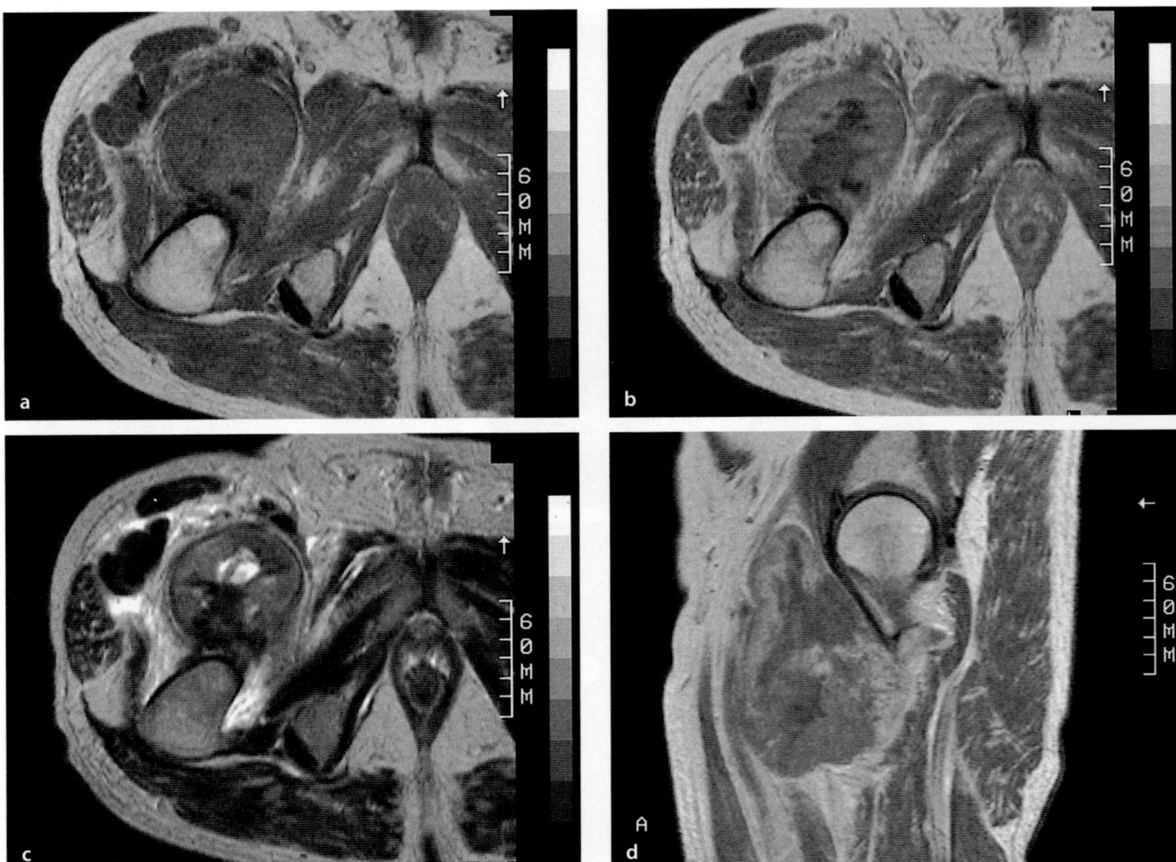

Fig. 18.4 a–d. Pleomorphic rhabdomyosarcoma of the right thigh in a 63-year-old man. **a** Axial spin-echo T1-weighted MR image. **b** Axial spin-echo T2-weighted MR image. **c** Axial spin-echo T1-weighted MR image after gadolinium contrast injection. **d** Sagittal spin-echo T1-weighted MR image after gadolinium contrast injection. The T1-weighted MR image shows a rounded, well-circumscribed mass with mixed signal intensities (**a**). The mass is even more inhomogeneous on T2-weighted MR image, with the presence of a central fluid collection anterior to an area of low signal intensity (**b**). There is no enhancement of both these areas after gadolinium contrast injection (**c, d**). A malignant tumor is suggested by the inhomogeneous appearance in all sequences, location, and volume of the lesion. The pleomorphic subtype is characterized by areas of necrosis alternating with areas of marked enhancement and areas of ring-like enhancement around low signal-intensity areas

of cells having some resemblance to leiomyosarcoma. Recognition of this subtype is important because of its good prognosis.

Embryonal rhabdomyosarcoma accounts for 50–60% of all rhabdomyosarcomas (3 million US children less than 15 years of age). It principally affects children up to the age of 15 years and occurs mainly in the head and neck region, the orbits, the genitourinary system, the retroperitoneum, and the extremities.

Botryoid rhabdomyosarcoma is a variant with a polypoid (grape-like) growth pattern and consists mainly of mucoid matrix with some sparse cells [46]. This myxoma-like tumor is often covered by hyperplastic or squama-like epithelium. It accounts for 5–10% of all rhabdomyosarcomas and occurs principally in mucosa-lined hollow viscera such as the vagina and bladder.

The *anaplastic rhabdomyosarcoma* is histologically defined by the presence of enlarged, atypical cells with hyperchromatic nuclei. Focal anaplastic features can be seen in all subtypes, but in the anaplastic subtype diffuse anaplasia with the presence of clone-like clusters of anaplastic cells are predominant.

Alveolar rhabdomyosarcoma (solid and anaplastic) is composed of individual cellular aggregates that are separated and surrounded by frameworks of dense, fibrous septa that contain dilated vascular channels. It is the second most frequent type and accounts for 20% of all malignant striated muscle tumors. Adolescents and young adults between 10 and 25 years of age are most frequently affected. It can be found in the same locations as the embryonal rhabdomyosarcoma, although it tends to occur more often as a deep-seated mass in the extremities. Alveolar rhabdomyosarcomas has a worse prognosis than other rhabdomyosarcomas (Fig. 18.3).

Pleomorphic rhabdomyosarcoma is histologically difficult to differentiate from other pleomorphic soft tissue tumors. It contains loosely arranged, larger pleomorphic cells. Cross-striations that are found in other subtypes are rare in this group. It accounts for 5% of all rhabdomyosarcomas and occurs mainly in patients over 40 years of age. Its predilection site is the thigh (Fig. 18.4).

Clinically, rhabdomyosarcomas are rapidly growing masses which tend to cause pain and nerve compression symptoms when they reach a large volume. These tumors appear to involve bone more frequently than other soft tissue sarcomas, apart from synovial sarcoma. In a series published by Simmons and Tucker, bone invasion in association with the primary tumor was seen in more than 20% of cases. Remarkably only flat bones were invaded. Bone destruction was permeative and only exceptionally well defined. Sclerosis was an unexpected finding in association with such an aggressive tumor [52].

18.3 Imaging

18.3.1 Imaging Studies Other Than MRI

18.3.1.1 Plain Radiography

Although plain radiography cannot be expected to provide specific information about the nature of a soft tissue lesion, it remains useful to start the evaluation of any soft tissue tumor with plain radiographs [6, 29]. Apart from giving some idea about the size and location of the mass, this reveals the presence of calcifications within the lesion and shows any coexisting bone involvement [34, 50]. For best results, a low-kilovoltage technique should be used to provide maximum density differentiation between tissues [9, 46].

18.3.1.2 Ultrasound

Ultrasound, as a cheap and readily available technique, is of use in the general workup of soft tissue masses providing information about size and internal characteristics [5, 57, 68, 69].

Its main use for establishing a precise diagnosis lies in guiding percutaneous biopsy [3, 10, 33]. Color Doppler techniques are useful in assessing vascularity but offer no help in the diagnosis of muscular tumors.

18.3.1.3 Angiography

■ **Angiography.** Both conventional cut-film and digital subtraction angiography can be used for preoperative vascular mapping and to establish access for intra-arterial chemotherapy [17, 34]. Angiographic findings in soft tissue tumors are entirely nonspecific, and the use of angiography is therefore limited nowadays. This certainly applies to tumors of muscular origin.

■ **Lymphangiography.** Bipedal lymphography has been described as useful only in detecting metastatic lesions arising from muscular tumors in the lower trunk or in the lower extremities [4], but is today replaced by CT.

18.3.1.4 Scintigraphy

Both technetium and gallium were once proposed as useful radiopharmaceuticals, the former for detecting the presence and delineating the extent of a soft tissue tumor, and the latter for demonstrating malignancy. However, a lack of specificity was later established. The main role of scintigraphy lies in detecting skeletal metastases [34, 51, 53, 55].

18.3.1.5 Computed Tomography

Before the advent of MRI, CT was the only imaging modality able to evaluate soft tissue tumor extent and medullary involvement [3, 35]. Its role is now restricted to the detection of calcifications, bone involvement, and intratumoral gas [48, 63].

In a series of 14 tumors reported on by McLeod, leiomyosarcomas were usually large, with frequent necrotic or cystic changes. Calcifications were not seen. Necrotic metastases were observed in several cases [41]. Although the CT appearance remains nonspecific, the presence of necrotic metastases can be suggestive of the diagnosis.

In a series of 73 tumors of the thigh by Rich, there were only 4 rhabdomyosarcomas; in all 4 of these cases, the presence of asymmetrical thickening was noted on CT scans [52].

18.3.2 MRI Findings

The value of MRI in grading and characterization of soft tissue tumors has been the subject of a large number of publications, some of them controversial [1, 2, 6–8, 11–15, 23, 33, 39, 43, 47, 56, 58, 62–67], and has been largely dealt with in Chap. 11.

In the uterus, leiomyomas appear as sharply marginated, homogeneous areas of lower signal intensity on T2-weighted images than the surrounding myometrium; inhomogeneity is indicative for complicated or vascular fibroids [54]. This does not seem to be the case in other locations. In the bladder three leiomyomas presenting as an inhomogeneous mass with overall high signal and dot-like foci of low signal on T2-weighted images have been published [42].

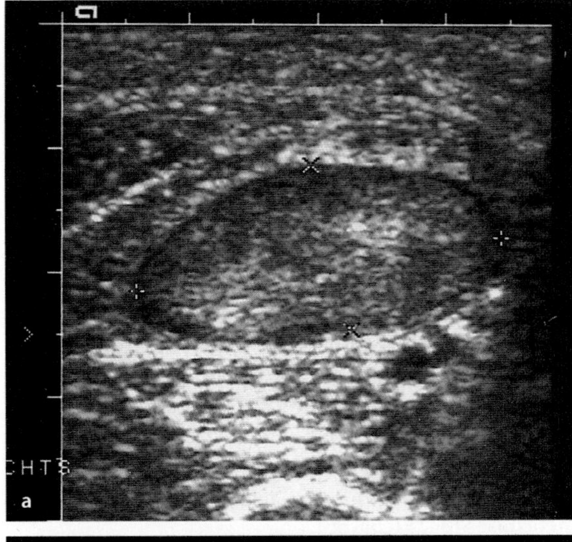

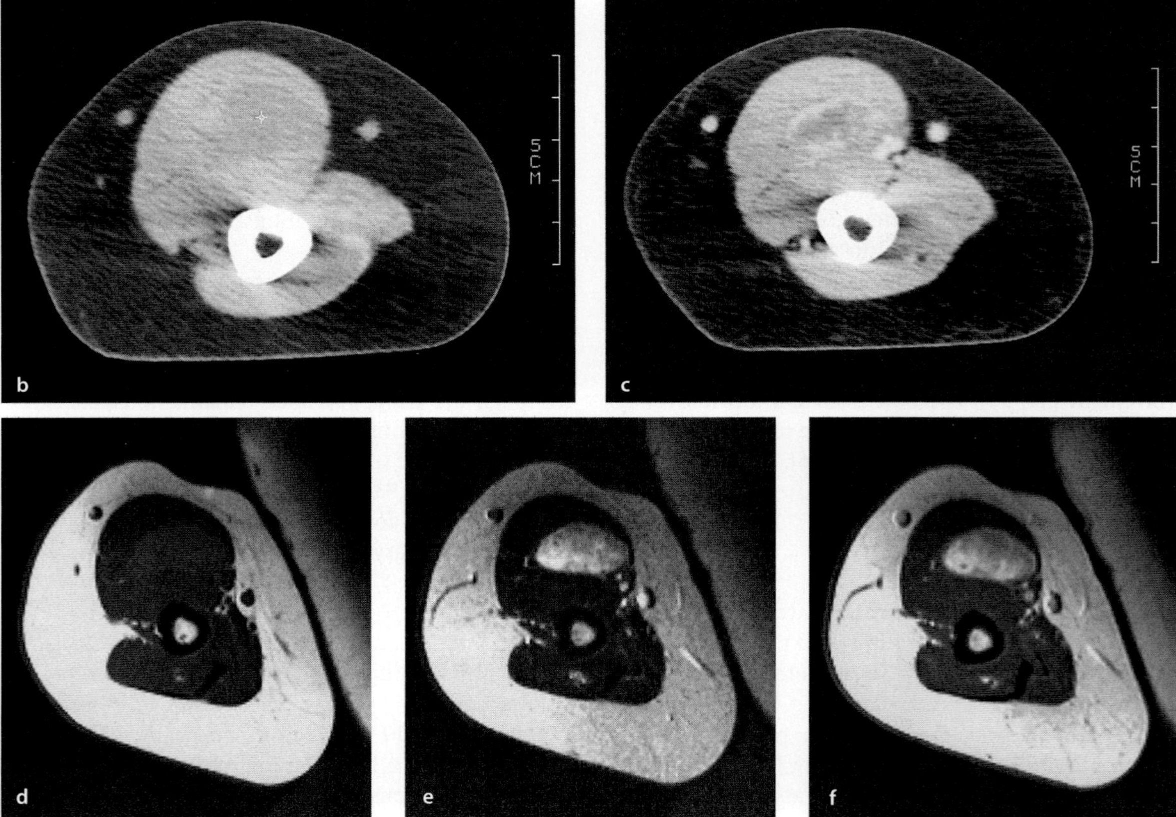

Fig. 18.5 a–f. Leiomyoma of the flexor compartment of the right arm in a 56-year-old woman. **a** Ultrasound, axial plane. **b** Plain CT. **c** CT scan after iodinated contrast injection. **d** Axial spin-echo T1-weighted MR image. **e** Axial spin-echo T2-weighted MR image. **f** Axial spin-echo T1-weighted MR image after gadolinium contrast injection. Ultrasound shows a well-circumscribed, oval and slightly hypoechoic mass within the biceps muscle (**a**). The lesion is of low attenuation on plain CT (**b**) and is enhanced peripherally after contrast injection (**c**). On MRI the well-defined lesion is hyperintense to muscle on T1-weighted MR images (**d**) and shows an inhomogeneous, stippled high signal on T2-weighted images (**e**), and an inhomogeneous enhancement after gadolinium contrast injection (**f**). Nonspecific MR findings of a well-circumscribed, benign intramuscular tumor

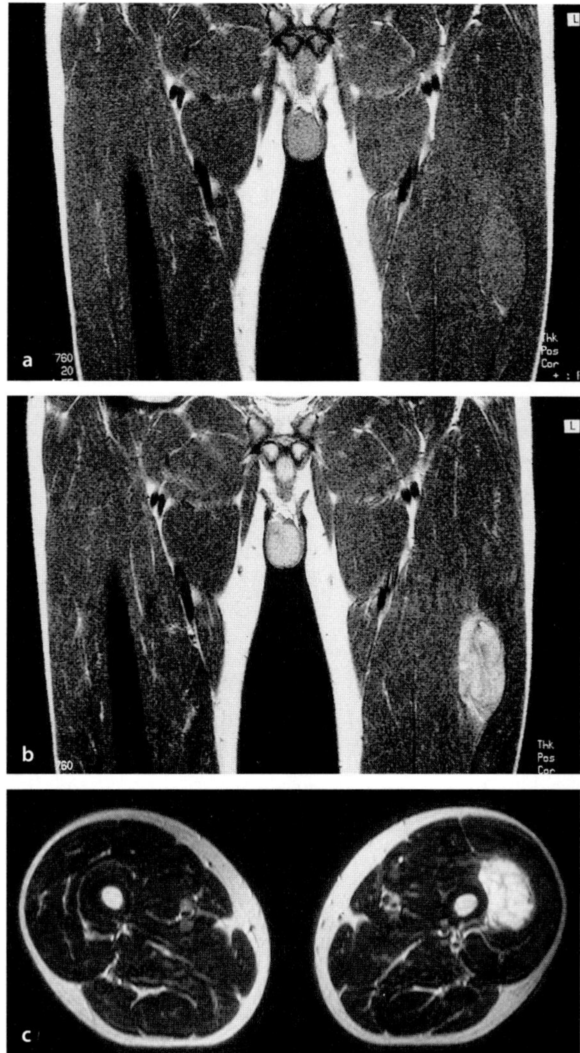

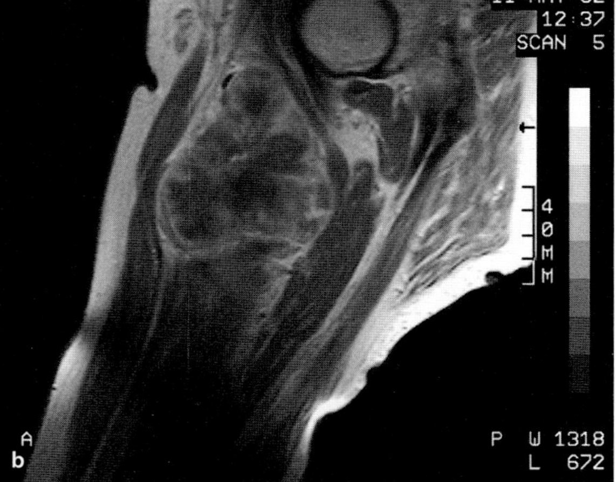

Fig. 18.6a–c. Low-grade leiomyosarcoma of the vastus intermedius muscle in a 33-year-old man presenting with pain and swelling of the left thigh. **a** Coronal spin-echo T1-weighted MR image. **b** Coronal spin-echo T1-weighted MR image after gadolinium contrast injection. **c** Axial spin-echo T2-weighted MR image. Presence of a fusiform soft tissue mass deep in the left thigh hyperintense relative to adjacent normal muscle on T1-weighted images (**a**). After gadolinium contrast injection, there is marked enhancement of the lesion (**b**). On T2-weighted images, the lesion is inhomogeneous and of high signal intensity (**c**). There are numerous feeding vessels indicating a highly vascular lesion. Although the lesion exhibits imaging features similar to those of an alveolar soft tissue sarcoma (Fig. 23.19–23.21), histological diagnosis revealed a low-grade leiomyosarcoma illustrating the difficulty in MR pattern recognition versus histological diagnosis

Fig. 18.7 a, b. Leiomyosarcoma of the thigh in a 88-year-old woman. **a** Sagittal spin-echo T1-weighted MR image. **b** Sagittal spin-echo T1-weighted MR image after gadolinium contrast injection. MRI shows a large and lobulated mass displacing the adjacent muscles. On T1-weighted images the lesion is iso- to hyperintense (**a**). After gadolinium contrast injection, a thick and irregular rim enhancement is seen surrounding areas of central necrosis (**b**). Inhomogeneity of a mass on T1-weighted images and peripheral enhancement are in favor of a malignant tumor

In our series of 26 muscular tumors, only one lesion proved to be a leiomyoma. It was found in the deep soft tissues of the upper arm (Fig. 18.5).

Leiomyosarcomas mostly present with aspecific MR features, i.e., spindle-shaped masses with a long T1 and a long T2 relaxation time (Fig. 18.6). Overall low signal intensity or low signal intensity components allow a more specific diagnosis [62]. In our own series, leiomyosarcomas mostly appeared as large masses with central necrosis and a peripheral rim-like enhancement after gadolinium contrast administration (Fig. 18.7). Bone involvement is seen in 10% of cases (Figs. 18.8, 18.9) [25, 26].

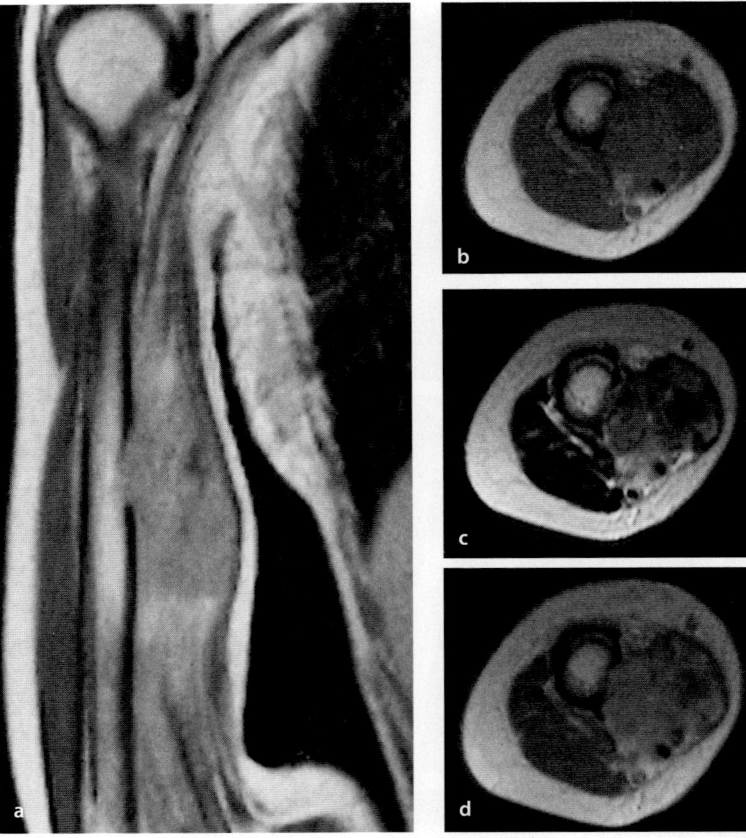

Fig. 18.8 a–d. Leiomyosarcoma of the right arm in a 36-year-old woman. **a** Coronal spin-echo T1-weighted MR image. **b** Axial spin-echo T1-weighted MR image. **c** Axial T2-weighted MR image. **d** Axial spin-echo T1-weighted MR image after gadolinium contrast injection. A spindle-shaped mass is seen, lying along the long axis of the limb and invading the humerus (**a**). The lesion is inhomogeneous and of intermediate signal intensity on the T1-weighted MR images (**a, b**). The tissue inhomogeneity is accentuated on the T2-weighted MR image, which shows mixed signal intensities (**c**). After gadolinium contrast injection, there is inhomogeneous enhancement (**d**). An aggressive muscle tumor with bone involvement

In cases of vascular leiomyosarcomas, differential diagnosis with thrombus is rather straightforward, since tumor expands the vessel to a diameter several times the original, while thrombus never expands the diameter to more than twice the original one. In thrombosis T1 and T2 is generally increased, with a clear delineation of the vessel wall [59].

One case of a myxoid leiomyosarcoma showed high signal intensity on T2-weighted images and a marked enhancement after gadolinium contrast injection, more pronounced at the center of the lesion (Fig. 18.10).

Rhabdomyosarcomas also have rather nonspecific MR features, and they are seldom located in the extremities. Embryonal rhabdomyosarcomas show a more homogeneous low signal intensity on both T1- and T2-weighted images and no obvious intratumoral necrosis (Figs. 18.11, 18.12).

Embryonal subtypes can cause bowing of tubular bones in children, falsely mimicking a slowly growing tumoral process [62]. Alveolar rhabdomyosarcomas are characterized by multiple areas of tumoral necrosis (Figs. 18.12, 18.13, 18.14), while pleomorphic rhabdomyosarcomas have areas of necrosis alternating with areas of marked ring-like enhancement around areas of low signal intensity (Figs. 18.15).

Recent advances in MRI technology allow higher-resolution imaging in shorter acquisition times but no significant progress is seen regarding tissue diagnosis [24]. Dynamic contrast-enhanced MRI (parametric imaging) may help in: (1) defining areas of tumor viability prior to biopsy, (2) determining response to chemotherapy, and (3) evaluating tumor recurrence following surgery [68].

Things to remember:
1. Smooth vessel tumors have no specific imaging features except for vascular leiomyosarcoma, which mostly occurs within the inferior vena cava.
2. Benign striated muscle tumors are extremely rare.
3. Rhabdomyosarcoma is the most common soft tissue tumor in children, the embryonal subtype being by far the most frequent.
4. Leiomyosarcoma mostly present as large, spindle-shaped masses with variable signal intensities, central necrosis, and peripheral contrast enhancement.

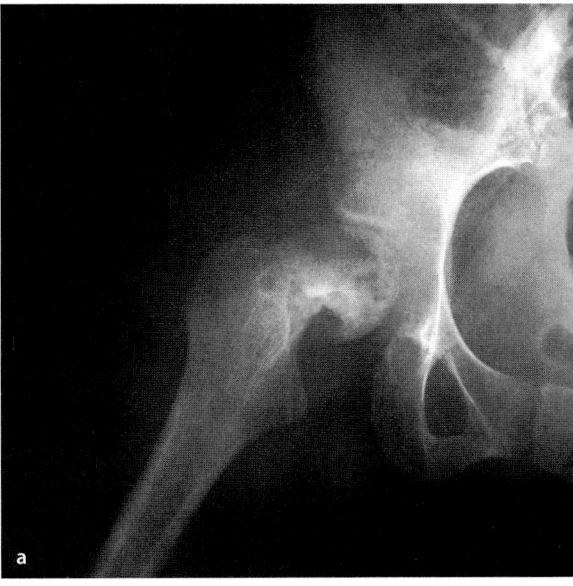
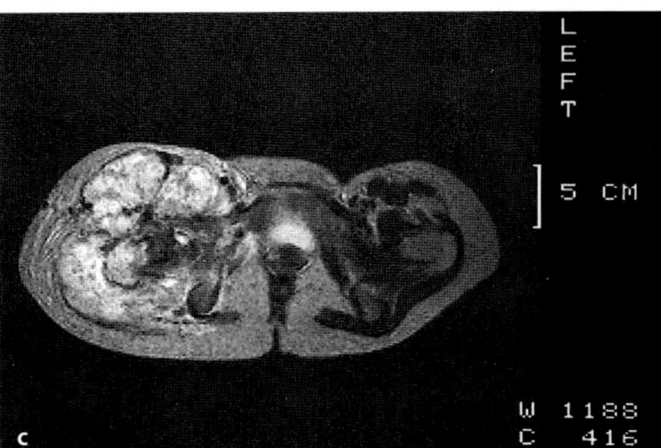
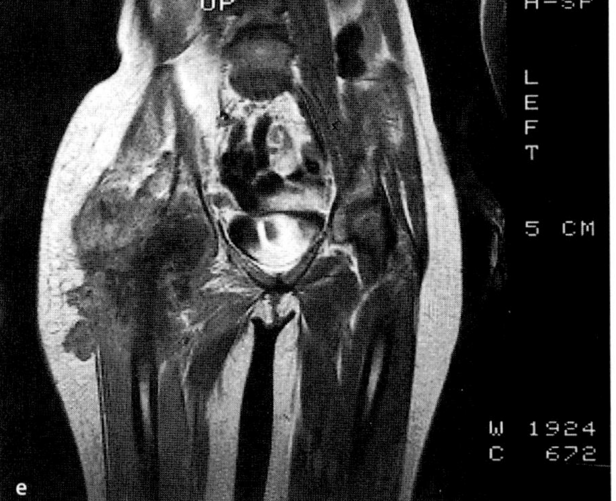
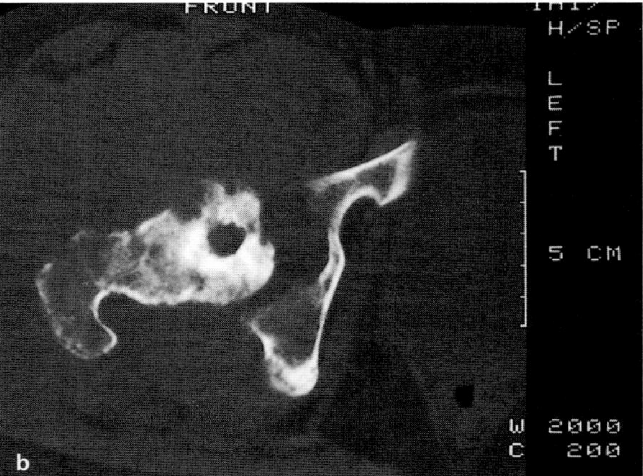
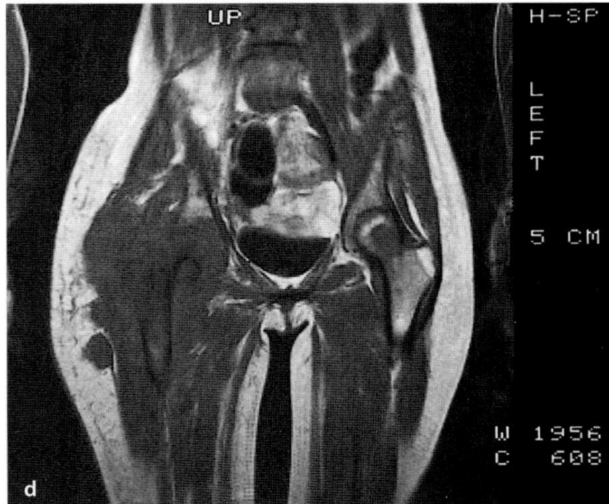

Fig. 18.9 a–e Leiomyosarcoma of the right thigh in a 26-year-old woman. **a** Plain radiograph. **b** Plain CT. **c** Axial spin-echo T2-weighted MR image. **d** Coronal spin-echo T1-weighted MR image. **e** Coronal spin-echo T1-weighted MR image after gadolinium contrast injection. Plain radiography demonstrates an indistinct soft tissue swelling with extensive mottled bone involvement and a pathological fracture of the femoral neck (**a**). CT confirms these areas of bone erosion and patchy sclerosis (**b**). The soft tissue mass surrounds the hip and extends toward the midline. It presents as a very hyperintense mass on T2-weighted MR image (**c**), while the T1-weighted MR image shows an infiltrating tumor (**d**) with essentially peripheral enhancement after gadolinium contrast injection (**e**). Aggressive muscle tumor with extracompartmental (bone and subcutis) extension

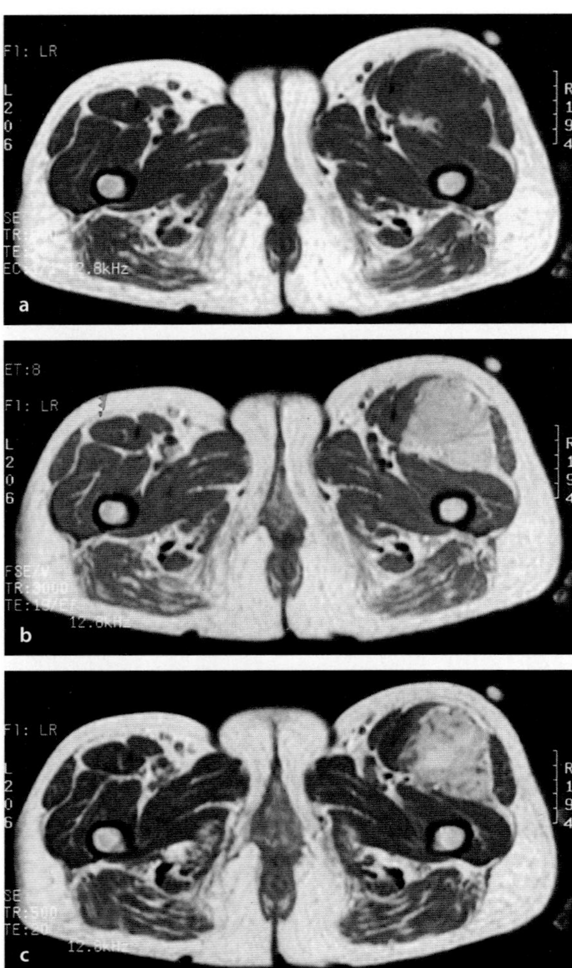

Fig. 18.10 a–c. Myxoid leiomyosarcoma of the anterior left thigh in a 63-year-old woman. **a** Axial spin-echo T1-weighted MR image. **b** Axial spin-echo T2-weighted MR image. **c** Axial spin-echo T1-weighted image after gadolinium contrast injection. MR shows a lobulated mass that is isointense to muscle on T1-weighted MR image (**a**) with mixed but mainly high signal intensity on the T2-weighted MR image (**b**) and inhomogeneous enhancement after gadolinium contrast injection (**c**). Contrast enhancement seems to decrease from the center to the periphery of the mass. Nonspecific mass with overwhelming myxoid components

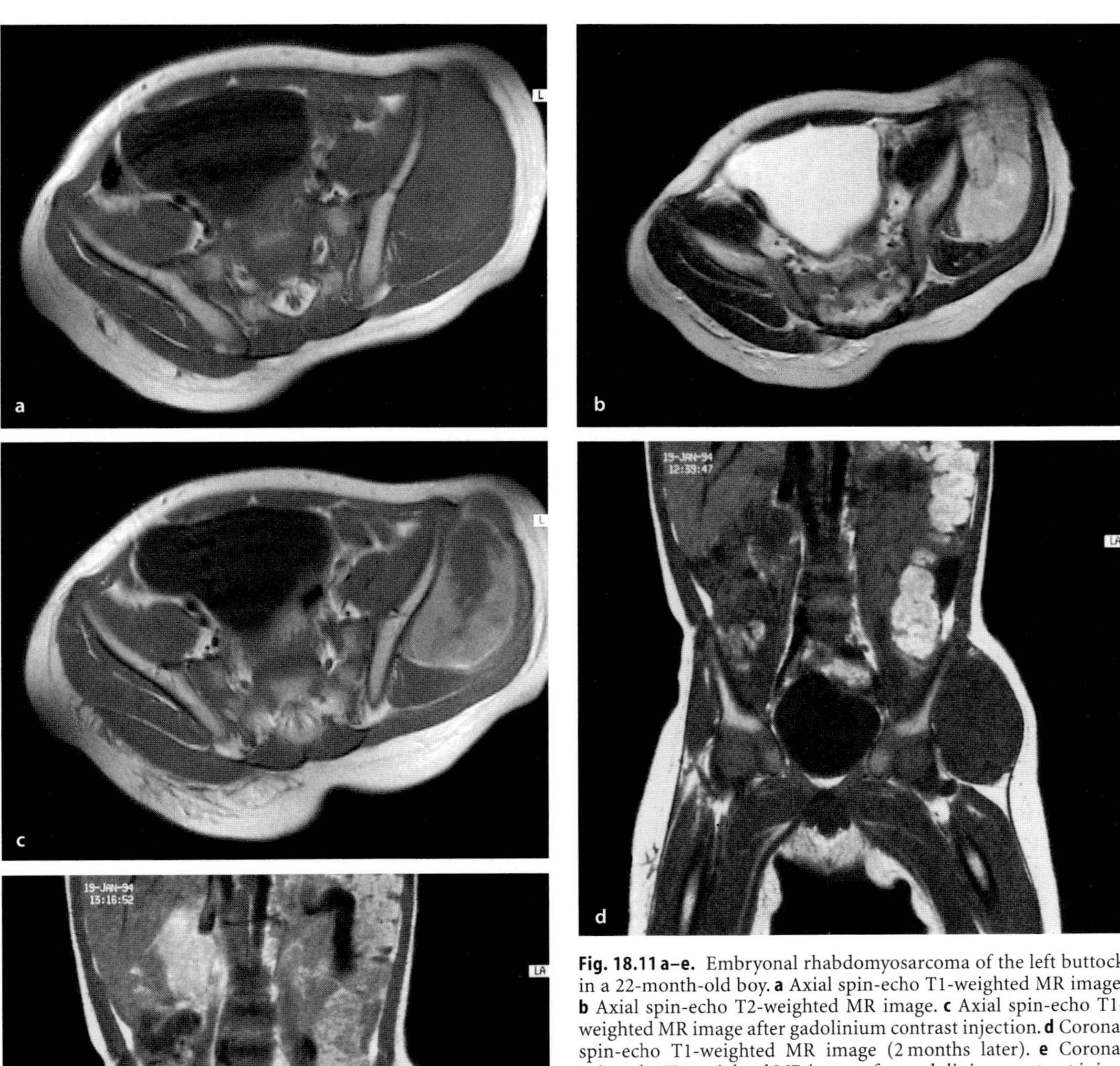

Fig. 18.11 a–e. Embryonal rhabdomyosarcoma of the left buttock in a 22-month-old boy. **a** Axial spin-echo T1-weighted MR image. **b** Axial spin-echo T2-weighted MR image. **c** Axial spin-echo T1-weighted MR image after gadolinium contrast injection. **d** Coronal spin-echo T1-weighted MR image (2 months later). **e** Coronal spin-echo T1-weighted MR image after gadolinium contrast injection (at the same time as **d**). On T1-weighted MR image, the lesion demonstrates a hypo- to isointensity compared with the adjacent muscle (**a**), while there is high signal on T2-weighted MR image with some internal strands of low signal intensity (**b**). After gadolinium contrast injection, there is evident enhancement of some parts of the tumor, but large areas do not enhance at all (**c**). No necrosis is seen. Comparable signal patterns are seen on a follow-up MRI study with a plain T1-weighted MR image (**d**) and a T1-weighted MR image after gadolinium contrast injection (**e**). A large tumor with malignant imaging findings arising from a gluteal muscle in a young child without distinct areas of necrosis. This embryonal subtype of rhabdomyosarcoma shows a marked, slightly inhomogeneous enhancement without extensive necrosis

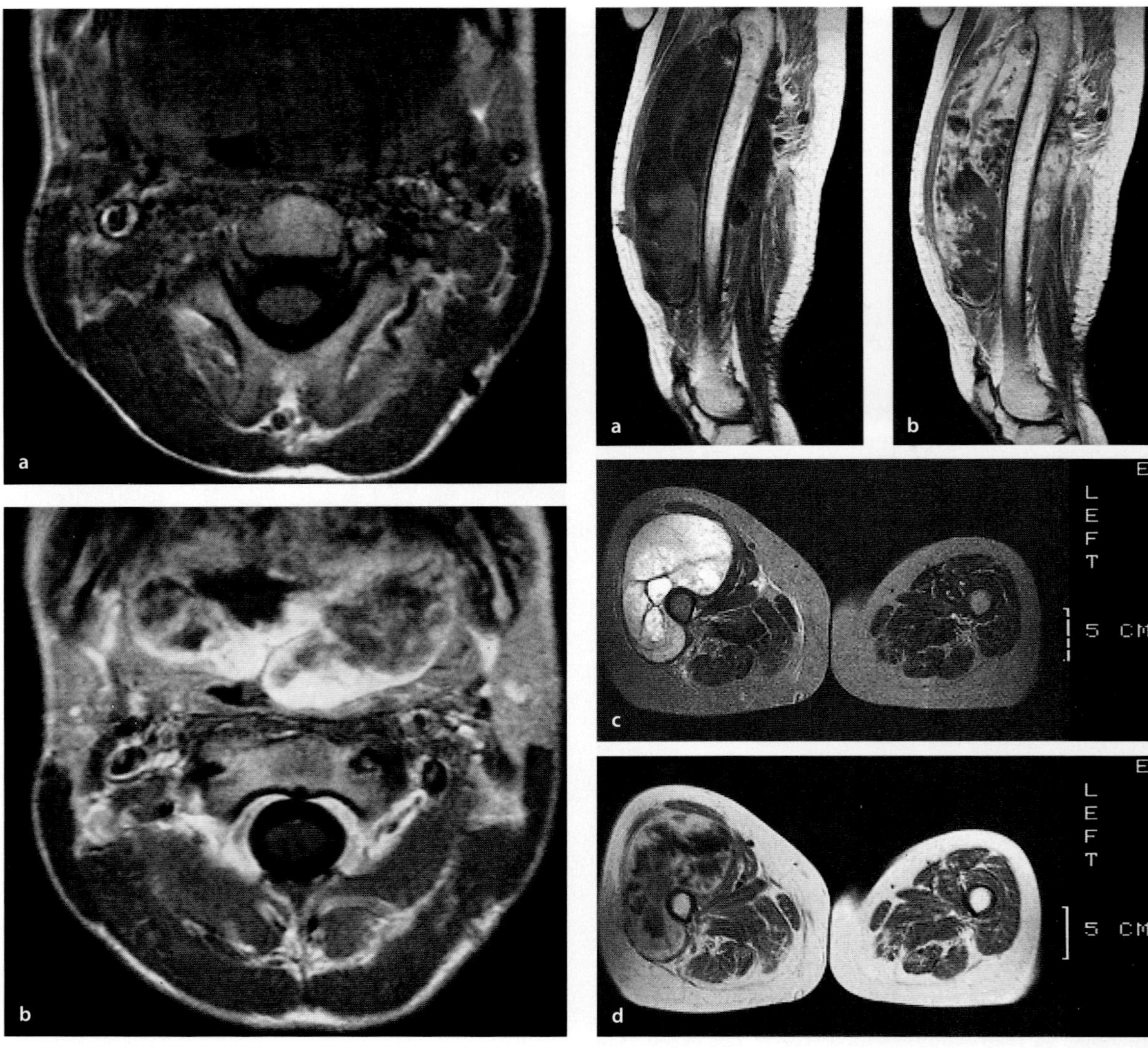

Fig. 18.12 a, b. Embryonal rhabdomyosarcoma of the tongue in a 15-year-old boy, 14 years after treatment for a rhabdomyosarcoma at the same location. **a** Axial spin-echo T1-weighted MR image. **b** Axial spin-echo T1-weighted MR image after gadolinium contrast injection. Huge mass at the tongue base, hardly to differentiate from the intrinsic tongue musculature on a T1-weighted MR image (**a**). After gadolinium contrast injection, there is marked inhomogeneous enhancement of the lesion (**b**)

Fig. 18.13 a–d. Alveolar rhabdomyosarcoma of the right thigh in a 71-year-old woman. **a** Sagittal spin-echo T1-weighted MR image. **b** Sagittal spin-echo T1-weighted MR image after gadolinium contrast injection. **c** Axial spin-echo T2-weighted MR image. **d** Axial spin-echo T1-weighted MR image after gadolinium contrast injection. A voluminous mass with very inhomogeneous signal characteristics is seen on T1-weighted MR images. There are hypointense areas suggestive of central necrosis (**a**). After gadolinium contrast injection, only peripheral enhancement is seen (**b, d**). Higher signal intensity is seen on proton density and T2-weighted MR images especially in the necrotic areas (**c**). Location, large size, inhomogeneous signal intensity on T1-weighted MR images, high signal intensity on T2-weighted MR images, and mostly peripheral enhancement after gadolinium injection are in favor of a malignant muscular tumor. The alveolar subtype is characterized by multiple areas of necrosis

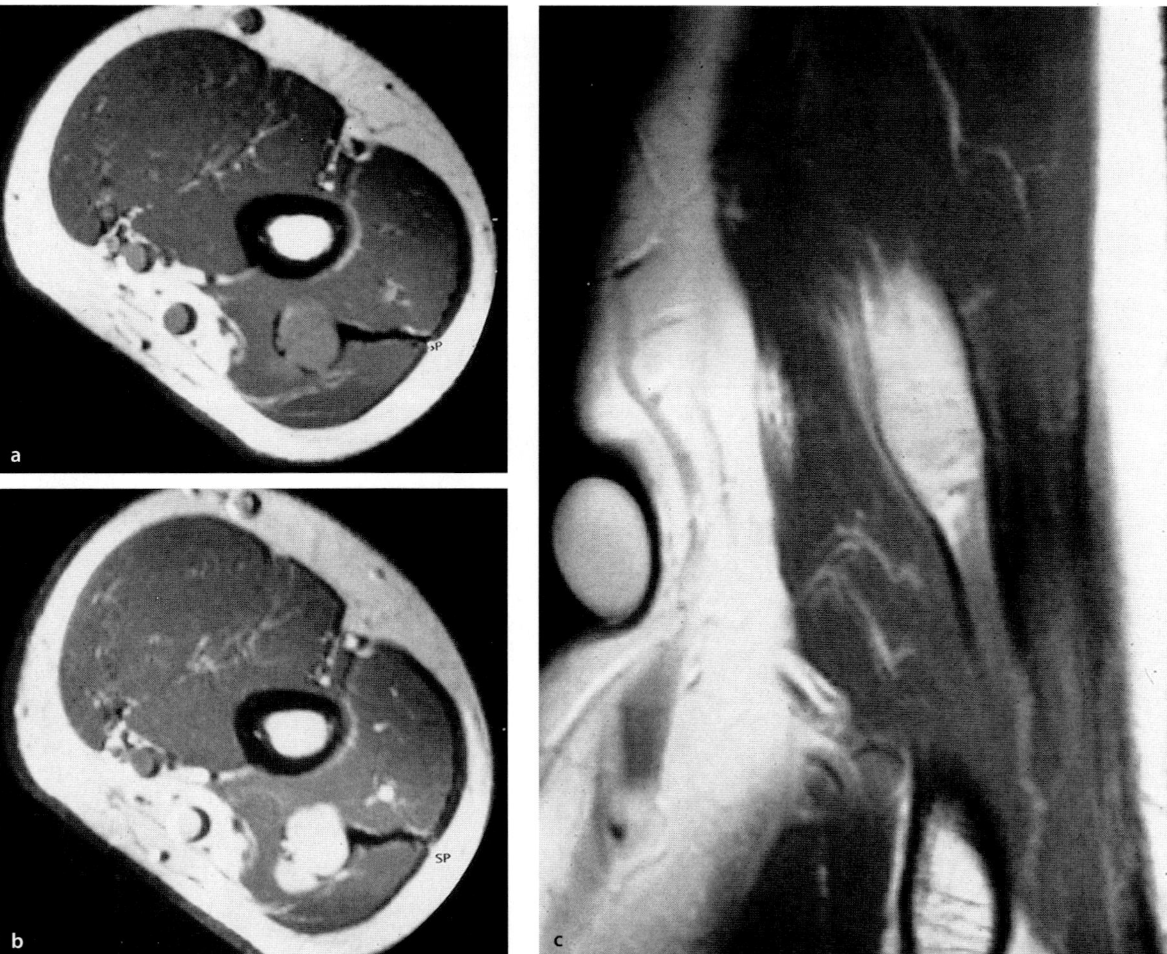

Fig. 18.14a–c. Alveolar rhabdomyosarcoma of the upper arm in a 50-year-old man. **a** Axial T1-weighted MR image. **b, c** Axial (**b**) and sagittal (**c**) T1-weighted MR image after gadolinium contrast injection. Collar button-shaped mass within the triceps muscle of the upper arm, hyperintense to adjacent normal muscle on T1-weighted MR images (**a**) and strongly enhancing after gadolinium contrast injection (**b**). On sagittal plane the lesion has a fusiform shape with ill-defined margins proximally and distally (**c**). Histological examination after biopsy and resection revealed an alveolar rhabdomyosarcoma. This case illustrates the variable morphology and signal-intensity characteristics of rhabdomyosarcomas

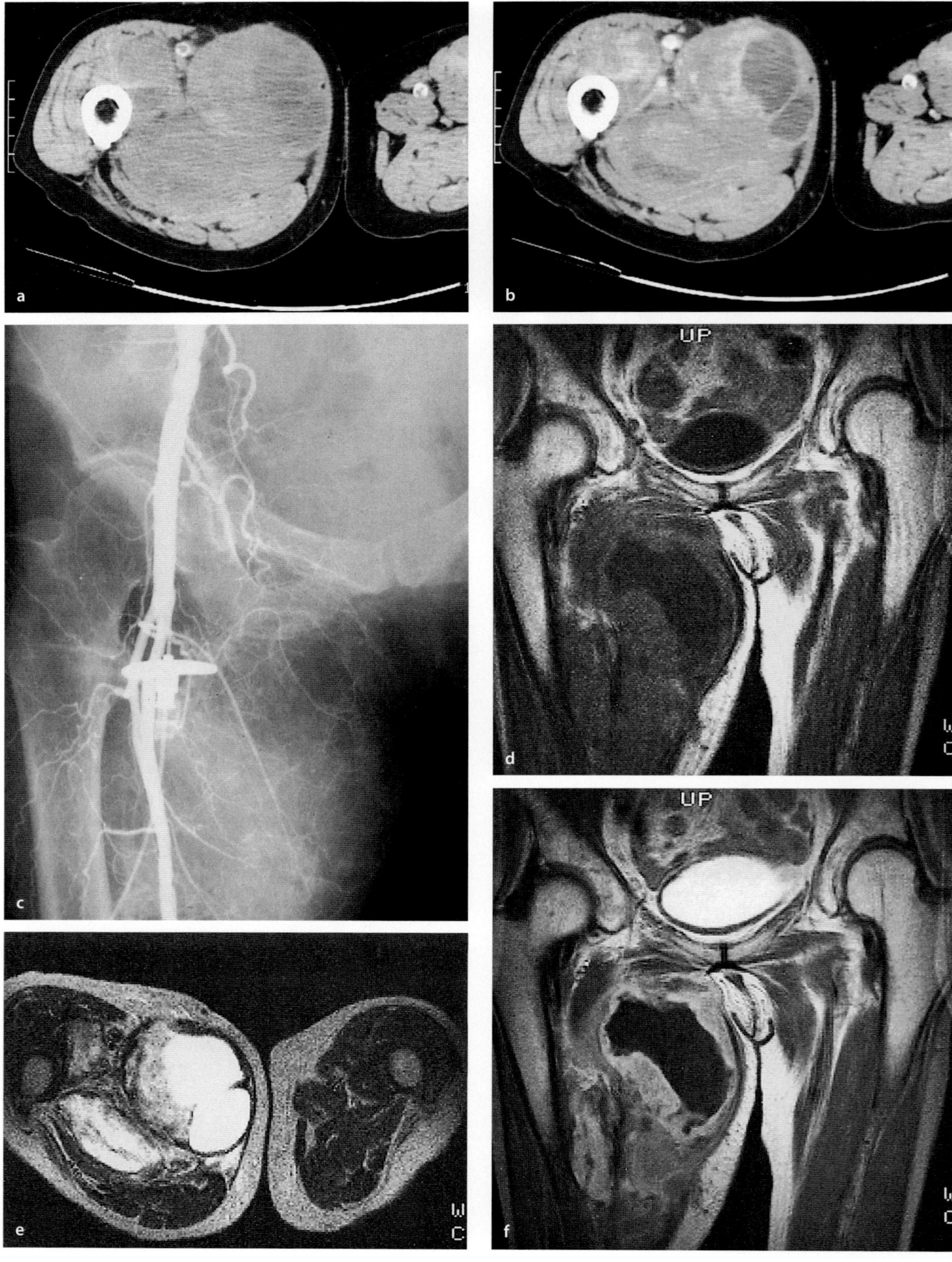

Fig. 18.15a–f. Rhabdomyosarcoma of the adductor region of the right thigh in a 78-year-old woman. **a** Plain CT. **b** CT after iodinated contrast injection. **c** Arteriography with direct retrograde femoral artery injection. **d** Coronal spin-echo T1-weighted MR image. **e** Axial spin-echo T2-weighted MR image. **f** Coronal spin-echo T1-weighted MR image after gadolinium contrast injection. CT shows a large and lobulated soft tissue mass with central hypodensities (**a**). There is a marked enhancement after iodinated contrast injection: rim-like enhancement is seen surrounding areas of necrosis (**b**). Arteriography reveals the presence of neovascularity and of a tumoral blush (**c**). On MR images there is a mass with multiple central hypointensities on T1-weighted MR images (**d**), which become hyperintense on T2-weighted MR images (**e**). After gadolinium contrast injection, strong enhancement at the periphery is seen around the intralesional necrotic areas (**f**). This case of a highly malignant tumor presents with large areas of intratumoral necrosis and neovascularity on angiography

References

1. Armstrong SJ, Wakeley CJ, Goddard PR, Watt I (1992) Review of the use of MR imaging in soft tissue lesions. Clin Radiol 46:311–317
2. Beltran J (1990) MRI musculoskeletal system. Lippincott, Philadelphia, pp 10.4–10.5
3. Berger PE, Kuhn JP (1978) Computed tomography of tumors of the musculoskeletal system in children. Radiology 127:171–175
4. Bergiron C, Markovits P, Benjafaar M, Piekarski JD, Garel L (1979) Lymphography in childhood rhabdomyosarcomas. Radiology 133:627–630
5. Bernardino ME, Jing BS, Thomas JL, Lindell MM Jr, Zornoza JI (1981) The extremity soft-tissue lesions: a comparative study of ultrasound, computed tomography and xeroradiography. Radiology 139:53–59
6. Berquist TH (1990) MRI of the musculoskeletal system, 2nd edn. Raven, New York, pp 447–458
7. Bloem JL (1992) Imaging of soft tissue tumors. J Belge Radiol 75:265–273
8. Bondetti PR, Ehman RL (1992) Soft tissue sarcomas: use of textural patterns in skeletal muscle as a diagnostic feature in postoperative MR imaging. Radiology 183:845–848
9. Cavanagh RC (1973) Tumors of the soft tissues. Semin Roentgenol 8:73–89
10. Christensen RA, Van Sonnenberg E, Casola G, Wittich GR (1988) Ultrasound in the musculoskeletal system. Radiol Clin North Am 26:145–156
11. Crim JR, Seeger LL, Yao L, Chandnani V (1992) Diagnosis of soft tissue masses with MR imaging: can benign masses be differentiated from malignant ones? Radiology 185:581–586
12. Daldrup H, Shames DM, Wendland M, Okuhata Y, Link TM, Rosenau W, Lu Y, Brash RC (1998) Correlation of dynamic contrast-enhanced magnetic resonance imaging with histologic tumor grade: comparison of macromolecular and small molecular contrast media. Pediatr Radiol 28:67–78
13. De Schepper AM, Ramon FA, Degryse HR (1992) Magnetic resonance imaging of soft tissue tumors. J Belge Radiol 75:286–296
14. De Schepper AM, Ramon F, De Beuckeleer L (1995) MRI of soft tissue tumors. In: Baert AL, Grenier P, Willi UV (eds) Syllabus categorical course ECR 95, musculoskeletal imaging: an update. Springer, Berlin Heidelberg New York, pp 155–164
15. Devos V, De Schepper A, Degryse H, Ramon F (1992) Diagnostic imaging of muscular tumors. J Belge Radiol 75:327–334
16. Dzsinich C, Gloviczki P, Van Heerden JA (1992) Primary venous leiomyosarcoma: a rare but lethal disease. J Vasc Surg 15:595–603
17. Ekelund L, Rydholm A (1983) The value of angiography in soft tissue leiomyosarcomas of the extremities. Skeletal Radiol 9:201–204
18. Enzinger FM, Weiss SW (1995) Radiologic evaluation of soft tissue tumors. In: Enzinger MM, Weiss SW (eds) Soft tissue tumors, 3rd edn. Mosby, St Louis, pp 7–8
19. Enzinger MM, Weiss SW (1995) Benign tumors of smooth muscle. In: Enzinger MM, Weiss SW (eds) Soft tissue tumors, 3rd edn. Mosby, St Louis, pp 467–490
20. Enzinger MM, Weiss SW (1995) Leiomyosarcoma. In: Enzinger MM, Weiss SW (eds) Soft tissue tumors, 3rd edn. Mosby, St Louis, pp 491–510
21. Enzinger MM, Weiss SW (1995) Rhabdomyoma. In: Enzinger MM, Weiss SW (eds) Soft tissue tumors, 3rd edn. Mosby, St Louis, pp 523–538
22. Enzinger MM, Weiss SW (1995) Rhabdomyosarcoma. In: Enzinger MM, Weiss SW (eds) Soft tissue tumors, 3rd edn. Mosby, St Louis, pp 539–578
23. Fletcher BG, Hanna SL, Fairclough DL, Gronemeyer SA (1992) Pediatric musculoskeletal tumors: use of dynamic, contrast enhanced MR imaging to monitor response to chemotherapy. Radiology 184:243–248
24. Fujimoto H, Murakami K, Ichikawa T, Matsubara T, Tsumurai Y, Masuda S, Terauchi M, Ozawa K, Nosaka K, Arizimu N (1993) MRI of soft tissue lesions: opposed phase T2* weighted gradient echo images. J Comput Assist Tomogr 17:418–424
25. Geussens E, Vanhoenacker P, Brijs S, Van Aelst F (1995) Leiomyosarcoma. J Belge Radiol 78:228–229
26. Hartman DS, Hayes WS, Choyke PL, Tibbets GP (1992) Leiomyosarcoma of the retroperitoneum and inferior vena cava: radiologic-pathologic correlation. Radiographics 12:1203–1220
27. Herlin K, Willén H, Rydholm A (1990) Deep seated soft tissue leiomyomas. Report of four cases. Skeletal Radiol 19:363–365
28. Horn RC, Enterline HT (1958) Rhabdomyosarcoma: a clinicopathological study of 29 cases. Cancer 11:181
29. Kevorkian J, Cento DP (1973) Leiomyosarcoma of large arteries and veins. Surgery 73:390–400
30. Killoran TP, Wells WA, Barth RJ, Goodwin DW (2003) Leiomyosarcoma of the popliteal vein. Skeletal Radiol 32(3):174–178
31. Kransdorf MJ (1995) Malignant soft tissue tumors in a large referral population distribution of specific diagnoses by age, sex and location. AJR Am J Roentgenol 164:129–134
32. Kransdorf MJ (1995) Benign soft tissue tumors in a large referral population distribution of specific diagnoses by age, sex and location. AJR Am J Roentgenol 164:395–402
33. Kransdorf MJ, Jelinek JS, Moser RP Jr, Utz JA, Brower AC, Hudson TM, Berrey BH (1989) Soft tissue masses: diagnosis using MR imaging. AJR Am J Roentgenol 153:541–547
34. Kransdorf MJ, Jelinek JS, Moser RP (1993) Imaging of soft tissue tumors. Radiol Clin North Am 31:359–372
35. Lateur L, Ramon F (1992) CT of soft tissue tumors. J Belge Radiol 75:281–285
36. Ledesma-Medina J, Oh KS, Girdany BR (1980) Calcification in childhood leiomyoma. Radiology 135:339–341
37. Lee ES, Locker J, Nalesnik M, Reyes J, Jaffe R, Alashari M, Nour B, Tzakis A, Dickman PS (1995) The association of Epstein Barr virus with smooth muscle tumors occurring after organ transplantation. N Engl J Med 332:19–25
38. Lubbers PR, Chandra R, Markle BM, Downey EF Jr, Malawer M (1987) Calcified leiomyoma of the soft tissues of the right buttock (case report 421). Skeletal Radiol 16:252–256
39. Ma LD, Frassica FJ, Scott WW, Fishman EK, Zerhouni EA (1995) Differentiation of benign and malignant musculoskeletal tumors: potential pitfalls with MR imaging. Radiographics 15:349–366
40. McClain KL, Leach CT, Jenson HB, Joshi VV, Pollock BH, Parmley RT, Di Carlo FJ, Chadwick EG, Murphy SB (1995) Association of Epstein Barr virus with leiomyosarcomas in young people with AIDS. N Engl J Med 332:12–18
41. McLeod AJ, Zornoza J, Chirkhoda A (1984) Leiomyosarcoma: computed tomography findings. Radiology 152:133–136
42. Menahem MM, Slywotsky C (1992) Urinary bladder leiomyoma: MRI findings. Urol Radiol 14:197–199
43. Mirowitz SA, Totty WG, Lee JKT (1992) Characterization of musculoskeletal masses using dynamic Gd DTPA enhanced spin echo MRI. J Comput Assist Tomogr 16:120–125
44. Morra MN, Manson AJ, Gavrel GJ (1992) Rhabdomyoma of the prostate. Urology 39:271–273
45. Mueller BV, Butler KM, Higham MC, Husson RN, Montrella KA, Pizzo PA (1994) Smooth muscle tumors in children with HIV. Pediatrics 90:460–463
46. Nelson GL, Staple TW, Ewans RG (1973) Soft tissue radiographic techniques. Semin Roentgenol 8:19–24
47. Olson PN, Everson LI, Griffiths HJ (1994) Staging of musculoskeletal tumors. Radiol Clin North Am 32:151–162
48. Petrasnick JP, Turner DA, Charters JR, Gitelis S, Zacharias CE (1986) Soft tissue masses of the locomotor system. Radiology 160:125–133
49. Petterson H, Gillespy T III, Hamlin DJ, Enneking WF, Springfield DS, Andrew ER, Spanier S, Slone R (1987) Primary musculoskeletal tumors: examination with MR imaging compared with conventional modalities. Radiology 164:237–241
50. Petterson H, Springfield DS, Enneking WF (1987) Radiologic management of musculoskeletal tumors. Springer, Berlin Heidelberg, pp 19–38
51. Resnick D, Niwayama G (1995) Soft tissues. In: Resnick D, Niwayama G (eds) Diagnosis of bone and joint disorders, 3rd edn. Saunders, Philadelphia, pp 4491–4622

52. Rich PJ, King W III (1982) Benign cortical hyperostosis underlying soft tissue tumors of the thigh. AJR Am J Roentgenol 138:419–422
53. Schwartz HS, Jones CK (1992) The efficacy of gallium scintigraphy in detecting malignant soft tissue neoplasms. Ann Surg 215:78–82
54. Scoutt LM, McCarthy SM (1992) Female pelvis. In: Stark DD, Bradley WG Jr (eds) Magnetic resonance imaging, 2nd edn. Mosby-Yearbook, St Louis, pp 1958–1963
55. Shapeero LG, Couanet D, Vanel D, Ackerman LV, Terrier Lacombe MJ, Flamant F, Contesso G, Lumbroso J (1993) Bone metastases as the presenting manifestation of rhabdomyosarcoma in childhood. Skeletal Radiol 22:433–438
56. Shinkwin MA, Lenkinski RE, Daly JM, Zlatin MB, Frank TS, Holland GA, Kressel HY (1991) Integrated magnetic resonance imaging and phosphorus spectroscopy of soft tissue tumors. Cancer 67:1849–1858
57. Simmons M, Tucker AK (1978) The radiology of bone changes in rhabdomyosarcoma. Clin Radiol 29:47–52
58. Sintzoff SA Jr, Gillard I, Van Gansbeke D, Gevenois PA, Salmon I, Struyven J (1992) Ultrasound evaluation of soft tissue tumors. J Belge Radiol 75:276–280
59. Sostman HD, Prescott DM, Dewhirts MW, Dodge RK, Thrall DE, Page RL, Tucker JA, Harrelson JM, Reece G, Leopold KA, Olesson JR, Charles HC (1994) MR Imaging and spectroscopy for prognostic evaluation in soft tissue sarcomas. Radiology 190:269–275
60. Stellard D, Sundaram M, Johnson FE, Janney C (1992) Leiomyosarcoma of great saphenous vein (case report 747). Skeletal Radiol 21:399–401
61. Stout AP, Lattes R (1966) Tumors of the soft tissues. (Atlas of tumor pathology) American Forces Institute of Pathology, Washington DC
62. Sundaram M, McLeod RA (1990) MR Imaging of tumor and tumor like lesions of the bone and soft tissue. AJR Am J Roentgenol 155:817–824
63. Suzuki Y, Ehara S, Shiraishi H, Nishida J, Murooka G, Tamakawa Y (1997) Embryonal rhabdomyosarcoma of foot with expansive growth between metatarsals. Skeletal Radiol 26:128–130
64. Totty WG, Murphy WA, Lee JKT (1986) Soft tissue tumors: MR imaging. Radiology 160:135–141
65. Vanel D, Lacombe MJ, Couanet D, Kalifa C, Spielmann M, Genin J (1987) Musculoskeletal tumors: follow-up with MR imaging after treatment with surgery and radiotherapy. Radiology 164:243–245
66. Vanel D, Shapeero LG, Gilles R, Genin J, Contesso G (1992) Imaging in the follow-up of soft tissue tumors. J Belge Radiol 75:274–275
67. Vanel D, Shapeero LG, De Baere T, Gilles R, Tardivon A, Genin J, Guinebretière JM (1994) MR imaging in the follow up of malignant and aggressive soft tissue tumors: results of 511 examinations. Radiology 190:263–268
68. Verstraete KL, De Deene Y, Roels H, Dierick A, Uyttendaele D, Kunnen MC (1994) Benign and malignant musculoskeletal lesions: dynamic contrast enhanced MR imaging – parametric "first-pass" images depict tissue vascularisation and perfusion. Radiology 192:835–843
69. Vincent LM (1988) Ultrasound of soft tissue abnormalities of the extremities. Radiol Clin North Am 26:131–144

Synovial Tumors

19

F.M. Vanhoenacker, J.W.M. Van Goethem,
J.E. Vandevenne, M. Shahabpour

Contents

19.1 Introduction

The synovial membrane is derived from embryonic mesenchyme and lines nonarticular areas in synovial joints, bursae and tendon sheaths. Cells of the synovial membrane regulate the exchange of substances between blood and synovial fluid, and they synthesize hyaluronate, which is a major component of the synovial fluid [1]. There are considerable differences in the appearance of the synovial membrane, depending on local mechanical factors and the nature of the underlying tissue. For instance, in high-pressure joints the synovium is flat and acellular whereas in low-pressure joints it resembles cuboidal or columnar epithelium [5].

Traditionally, discussion of synovial tumors in radiological textbooks includes benign cystic synovial tumors, as well as giant cell tumors, PVNS and synovial sarcoma.

However, according to the latest World Health Organization Classification of Tumors, PVNS and giant cell tumors are classified as fibrohistiocytic tumors [3]. Therefore, these tumors are discussed more appropriately in Chap. 14.

Synovial sarcoma has been known for longer time as a misnomer, as it is not derived from true synovial cells. Actually, synovial sarcoma is regarded as a malignant tumor of uncertain differentiation [3]. It will be discussed in Chap. 23.

19.2 Benign Synovial Tumors

19.2.1 Benign Cystic Lesions

There exist several types of cystic para-articular soft tissue lesions, like synovial cysts, ganglion(cysts), and bursae. As there is much controversy in the radiological literature about the nomenclature and classification of para-articular cystic lesions, we will first propose a logical classification, related to their possible pathogenesis, before discussing their appearance on imaging.

19.2.1.1 Classification and Pathogenesis

Cystic lesions can be divided into four categories, mainly based upon the combination of two criteria (Table 19.1) [15, 8]:
1. The anatomical location and *relationship with the adjacent joint*, e.g., a communicating stalk with the joint. This communication can be visualized by imaging or can be surgically proven.
2. The *histological composition* of the cyst wall and the contents.

■ **(Arthro)synovial Cyst.** The term synovial cyst describes a continuation or herniation of the synovial membrane through the joint capsule. In the French literature, the term "arthrosynovial" cyst is preferred, which refers to their intimate relationship with the adjacent joint. Indeed, there is always a communication with the adjacent joint, and the histological composition is identical to that of the joint cavity. It consists of a collec-

Table 19.1. Classification of para-articular cystic lesions

	Communication with joint	Wall composition	Cell lining	Contents
(Arthro)synovial cyst	Present	Continuous mesothelial lining	"True" synovial cells	Mucinous fluid
Ganglion (cyst)	May be present	Discontinuous mesothelial lining	Flattened pseudo-synovial cells	Mucinous fluid
Bursitis de novo	Absent	Fibrous wall	No mesothelial lining	Fibrinoid necrosis
Bursa (permanent)	Absent	Continuous mesothelial lining	"True" synovial cells	Mucoid fluid

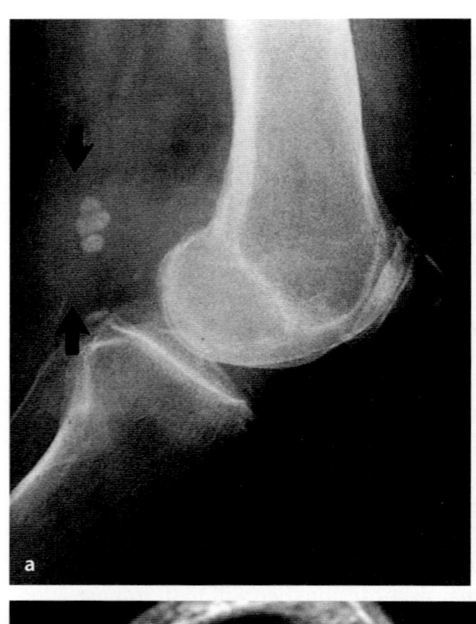

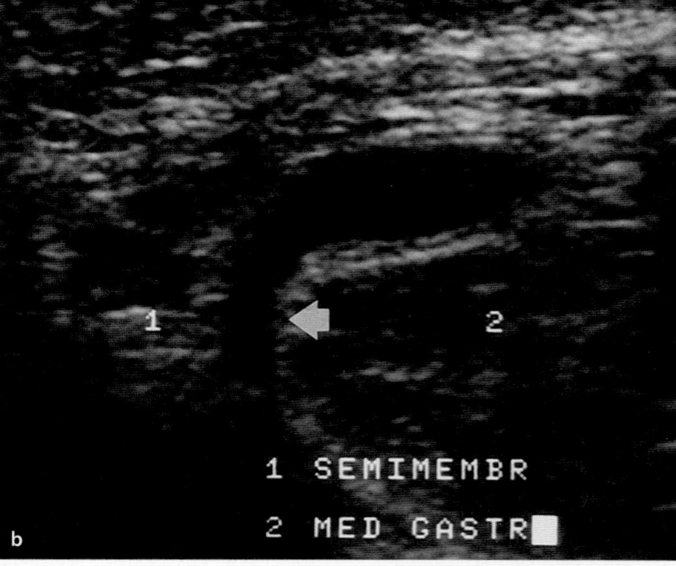

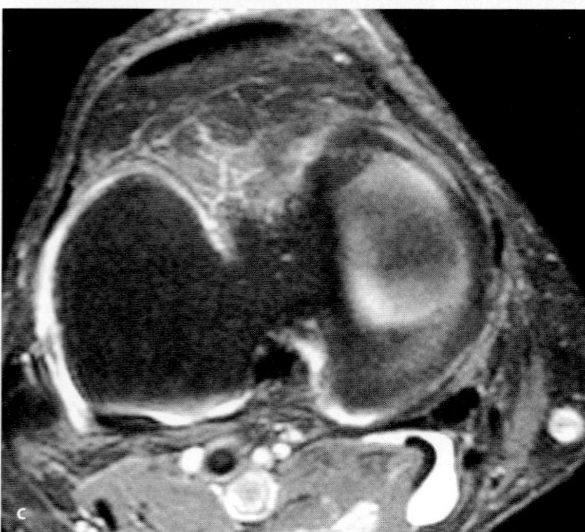

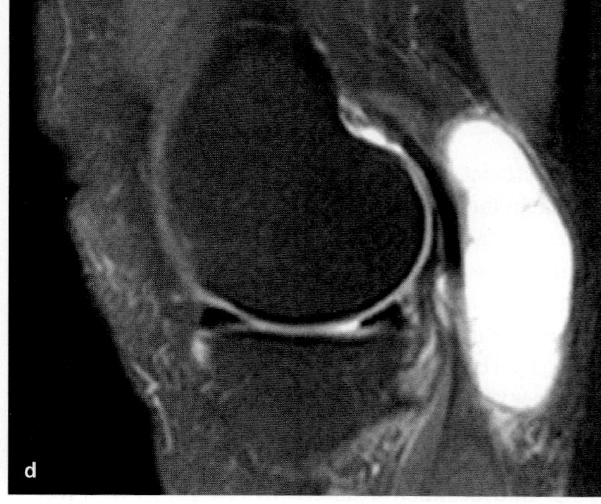

Fig. 19.1 a–d. Synovial cyst – Baker's cyst in different patients: **a** lateral radiograph of the left knee; **b** axial ultrasound of the popliteal fossa; **c** axial fat suppressed turbo spin echo T2-weighted MR image; **d** sagittal fat suppressed turbo spin echo T2-weighted MR image. Soft tissue mass in the popliteal fossa, with internal secondary osteochondromatosis, due to longstanding degenerative joint disease (a). Anechoic structure (b) with a communicating stalk (arrow) towards the knee joint between the semimembranosus tendon (1) and the medial gastrocnemius muscle (2). This typical extension towards the joint is also well appreciated on the axial fat suppressed TSE T2 MR Images (c). Due to its fluid content, the lesion is of high signal intensity on T2-weighted images (c,d). Baker's cyst is a very common synovial cyst located in the popliteal fossa. It represents a distended bursa gastrocnemio-semimembranosa and is as other synovial cysts lined by a normal synovial membrane. It may be the result of increased intra-articular pressure in cases of substantial joint effusion. In the knee joint these effusions are often associated with meniscal tears, rheumatoid disease, osteochondral lesions or degenerative disease

tion of synovial fluid, lined by a continuous layer of "true" synovial cells. The prototype is the Baker's cyst, which results from an extrusion of synovial fluid through a breach between the gastrocnemius muscle and semimembranosus tendon at the popliteal fossa (Fig. 19.1). Other examples can be seen near other joints (spine, shoulder, elbow, hip, hand, foot, and ankle), but are less frequent. They are usually associated with joint diseases, like osteoarthrosis, inflammatory and post-traumatic joint diseases. The elevated intraarticular pressure, due to an accumulation of joint fluid, causes herniation of joint fluid and synovium through a "locus minoris resistentiae" within the joint capsule.

■ **Ganglion (Cyst).** Ganglia also contain mucinous fluid, but their wall consists of a (discontinuous) layer of flattened pseudosynovial cells, surrounded by connective tissue (pseudocapsule) [8, 10, 15, 16].

A communication with the adjacent joint is not always present.

There remains much controversy in the literature concerning the pathogenesis of ganglion cysts. Several theories have been proposed, including displacement of synovial tissue during embryogenesis, proliferation of pluripotential mesenchymal cells, degeneration of connective tissues after trauma, and migration of synovial fluid into the cyst (synovial herniation theory) [9].

Based upon the similar appearance on imaging and surgery and on the similar wall composition of synovial cysts and ganglion cysts, we believe that the synovial herniation hypothesis is the most satisfactory. According to this theory, both synovial cysts and ganglion cysts are formed by a herniation of synovium through a breach in the adjacent articulation. Both types of paraarticular cysts are believed to be variants of the same disease spectrum. At one end of the spectrum, we have the pure (arthro)synovial cysts, which represent an extension of the joint cavity outside the joint, caused by a herniation through a "locus minoris resistentiae" within the joint capsule. This explains why the histological composition of those cysts is exactly a copy of that of the adjacent joint, and why the cellular lining consists of a continuous layer of "true" synovial cells. As those cysts grow and may extend further away from the joint into the soft tissues, they may undergo degenerative changes. First, the cellular lining may become discontinuous and individual cells may flatten, as they may be subject to fluctuations in intracystic pressure. This results in paraarticular cysts, in which the wall composition consists of a discontinuous layer of pseudosynovial cells. Ultimately, the original communication with the joint may be obliterated. Therefore, at the other end of the disease spectrum, a ganglion cyst may represent an advanced degenerative stage of a synovial cyst, in which the continuous synovial lining and the communication with the joint may be lost during the process of degeneration (Fig. 19.2).

The following arguments support the "synovial" theory in their pathogenesis:
1. The *similar histological composition* of synovial and ganglion cysts: both the contents (mucinous fluid), and the cellular lining are very similar (continuous layer of true synovial cells in arthrosynovial cysts vs a discontinuous lining of flattened pseudosynovial cells in ganglion cysts).
2. The *morphology* of some ganglion cysts, e.g. their course along capsular arteries or capsular nerve branches, may explain a peculiar form. This is especially true for adventitial cystic disease and perineural cysts, which can be considered as variants of ganglion cysts [7, 12, 17] (Fig. 19.3).

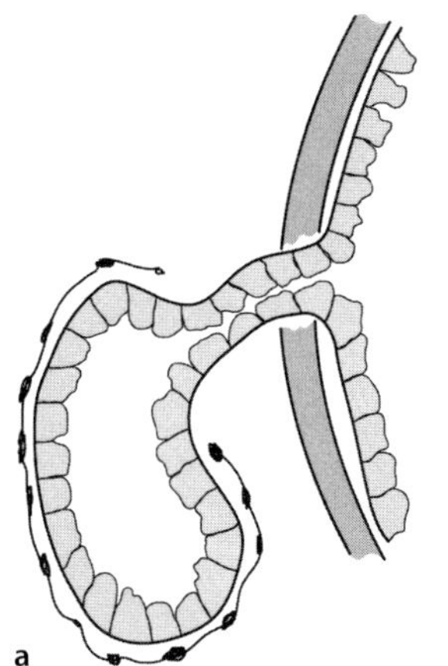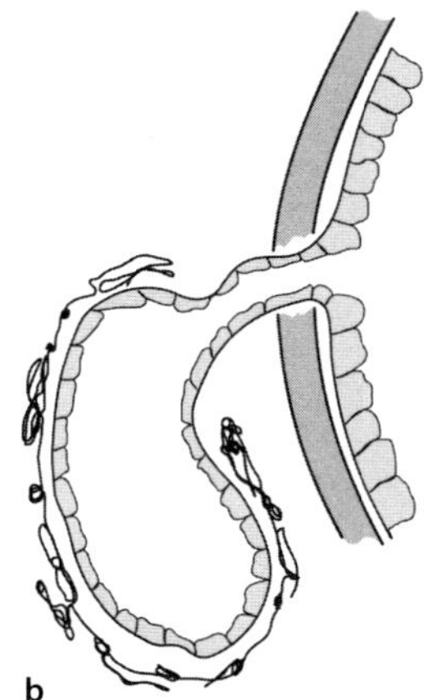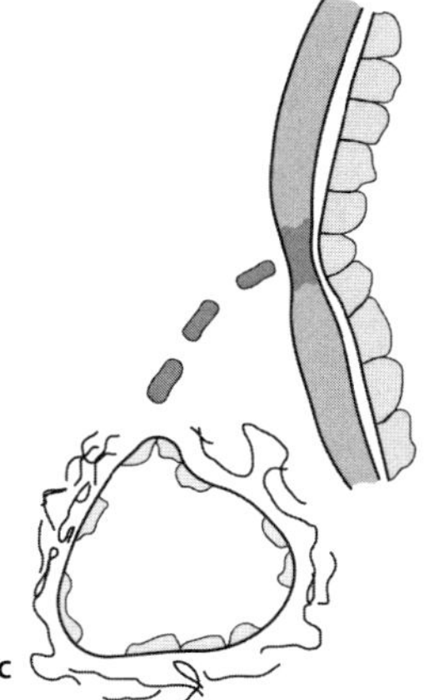

Fig. 19.2 a–c. Pathogenesis according to the "synovial herniation hypothesis" of: **a** (arthro)synovial cyst: this lesion originates from a herniation of the synovial membrane through the joint capsule. The histological composition is identical to the joint cavity, and the cellular lining consists of true synovial cells; **b,c** ganglion cyst: during the process of degeneration, the cellular lining may change, and become discontinuous. Ultimately, the original communication with the joint may be obliterated

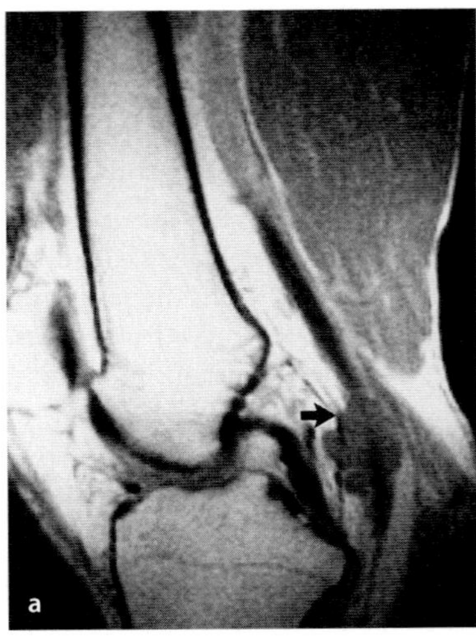
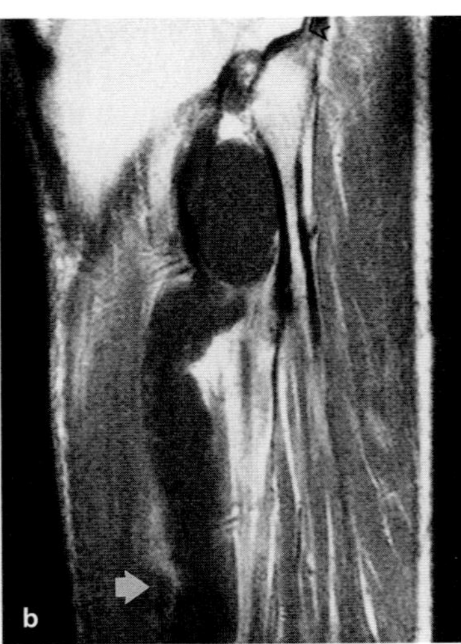

Fig. 19.3. a Adventitial cystic disease. **b** Perineural ganglion cysts. Both may result from dissection of fluid around articular branches of arteries, veins or nerves. a shows a sagittal T1-weighted image of the knee joint, b a sagittal T1-weighted MR image. In adventitial cystic disease, the popliteal artery is encased and focally narrowed by a polylobular hypointense structure (*arrow*), corresponding surgically to a cyst in the adventitia of the vessel wall (a). A ganglion cyst of the proximal tibiofibular joint consists of a moniliform hypointense structure along the course of the articular branch of the deep peroneal nerve (*white arrow*), running to the proximal tibiofibular joint (*open arrow*)

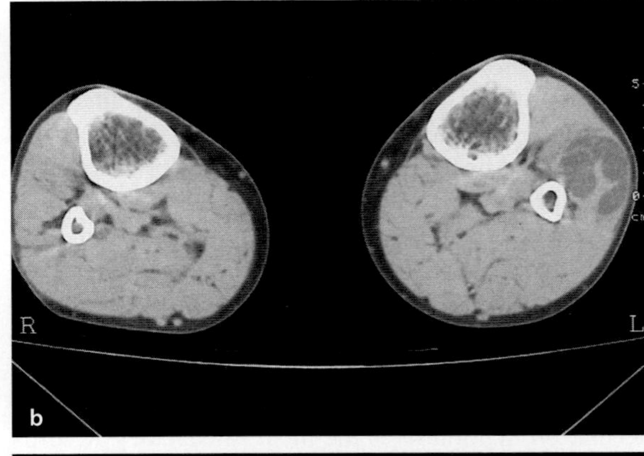
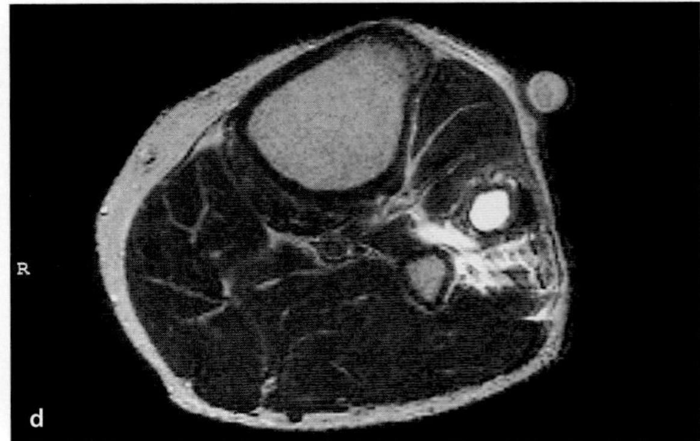
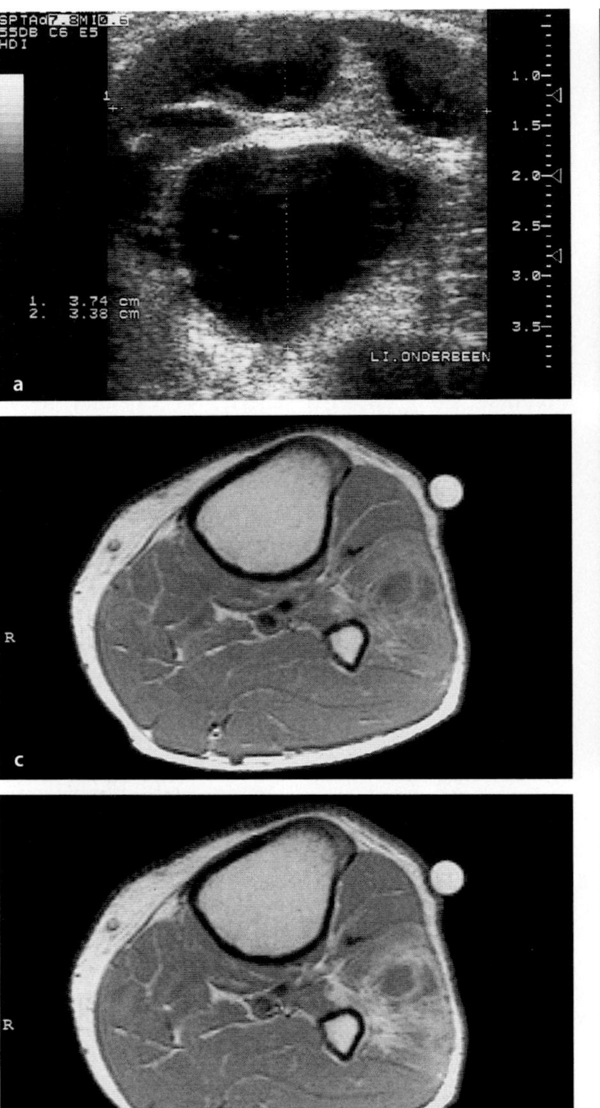

Fig. 19.4a–e. Ruptured ganglion cyst in the lower leg of a 54-year-old man: **a** ultrasound; **b** CT after iodinated contrast injection; **c** axial spin echo T1-weighted MR image; **d** axial turbo spin echo T2-weighted MR image; **e** axial spin echo T1-weighted MR image after gadolinium contrast injection. Ultrasound clearly shows a multiloculated cystic lesion in the lower leg (a). The image corresponds perfectly with the findings on nonenhanced CT (b). The lesion is clearly delineated with sharp borders. The adjacent fibular bone is not eroded. The MRI examination (c–e) was performed two weeks later. The cyst is ruptured, and there is fluid in the inter- and intramuscular fat planes (d). There is no evidence of hemorrhage (c). After gadolinium injection (e) enhancement is seen in the periphery of the lesion as a result of local inflammatory changes. This may lead to confusion in the differential diagnosis against other inflammatory soft tissue changes

3. *Functional arguments*
- When the para-articular cyst is directly injected or after arthrography of the adjacent joint, there is often a delayed opacification of the joint or cyst respectively [8, 9].
- The fluctuating volume of some cysts, sometimes complicated by rupture (Fig. 19.4), argues for a communication with the adjacent joint, which acts as a reservoir of synovial fluid [8, 15].

Ganglion cysts may be located anywhere around the joints. A para-articular location in fat layers (Fig. 19.5) or muscle (Fig. 19.6) is most frequently seen. Dissection of fluid around arteries or veins or nerves results in adventitial cystic disease or peri- or intraneural cysts [7, 12, 17]. A meniscal cyst (Fig. 19.7) can also be considered as a particular form of a ganglion cyst, in which synovial fluid is extruded through a horizontal meniscal tear, resulting in an encapsulated mass around the meniscus [13]. Other para-articular locations like in the subperiosteal area of the diaphyses of the long bones (periosteal ganglion) are rare [5, 9], while intraosseous ganglia are frequent.

Examples of intra-articular locations are paralabral cyst (Figs. 19.8 and 19.9) (shoulder and hip) and cruciate ligament cysts (Fig. 19.10) [2].

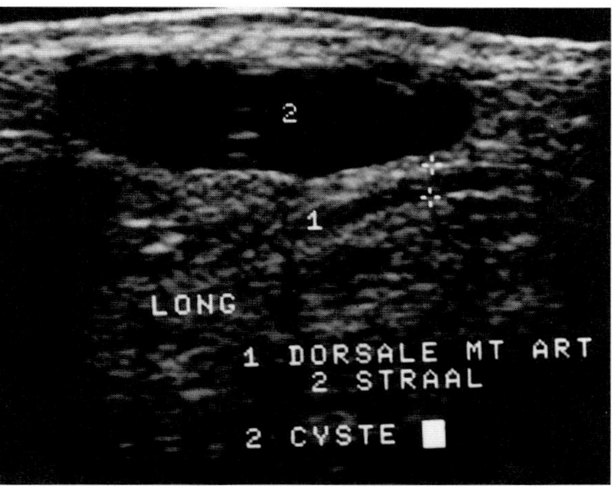

Fig. 19.5. Ganglion cyst in the subcutaneous fat of the dorsum of the foot, presenting as an ovoid, well demarcated anechoic lesion at the metatarsophalangeal joint. There is no obvious communication with the underlying joint

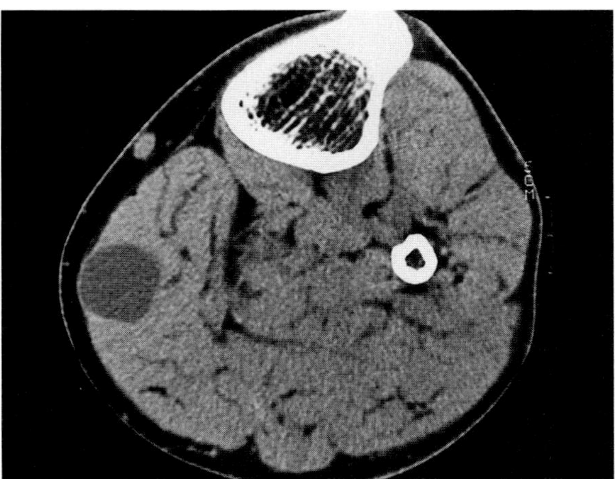

Fig. 19.6. Intramuscular ganglion cyst. CT-scan of the left lower leg shows a sharply demarcated low density lesion within the medial gastrocnemius muscle

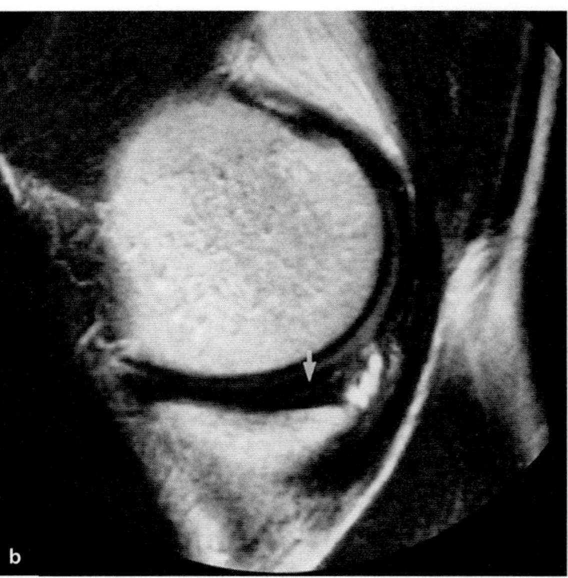

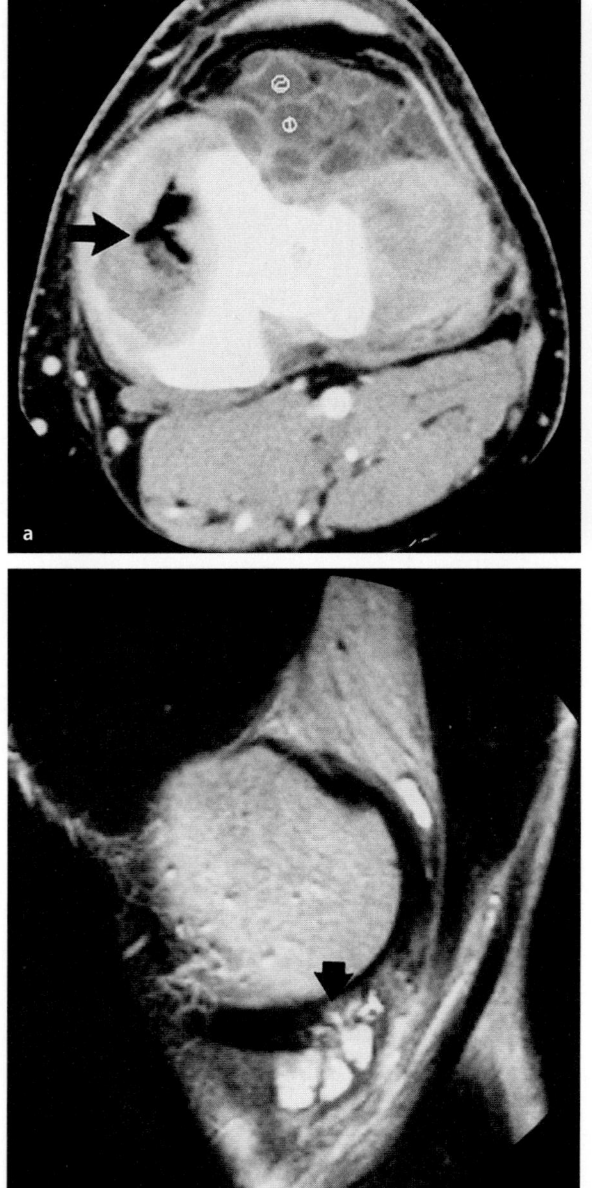

Fig. 19.7 a–c. Meniscal cyst: **a** CT-scan of the knee; **b, c** sagittal TSE T2-weighted MR images. Multicystic lesion within the Hoffa's fat pad (a), associated with an air-containing tear within the medial meniscus (*arrow*). An oblique tear within the meniscus (b), communicating with a multicystic structure at the dorsomedial aspect of the medial meniscus (c) is better appreciated on the corresponding MR images

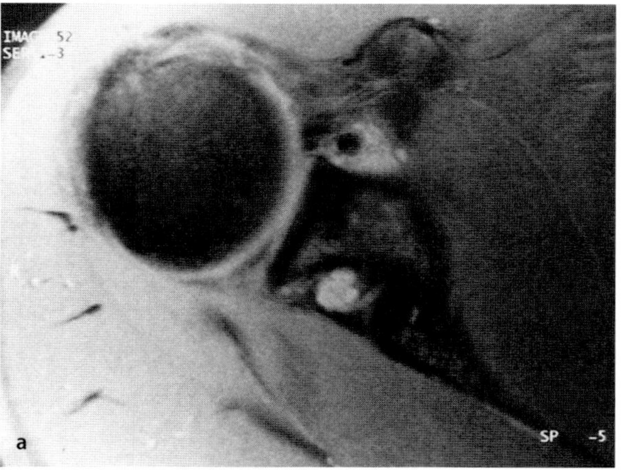

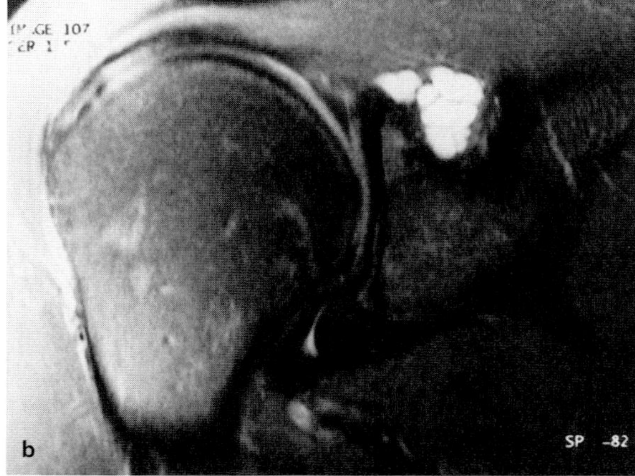

Fig. 19.8 a, b. Ganglion cyst in the spinoglenoid notch of the shoulder (paralabral cyst): **a** axial T2*-weighted image; **b** coronal T2-weighted image with spectral fat saturation. A hyperintense structure with some internal low signal intensity septations is seen in the spinoglenoid notch of the scapula.

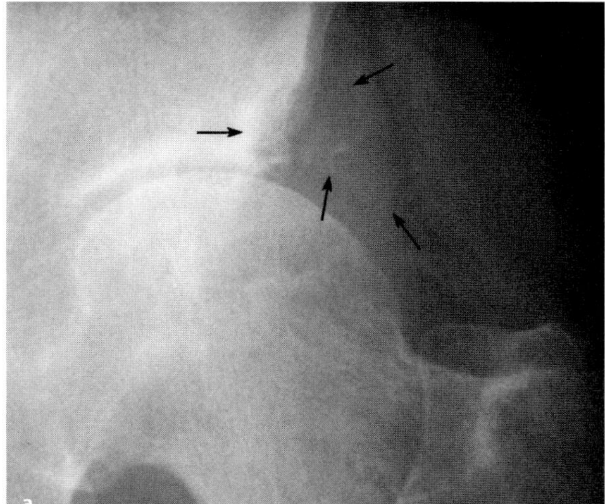

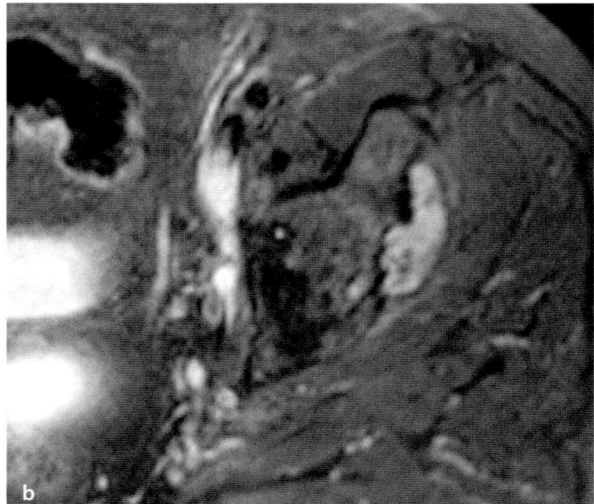

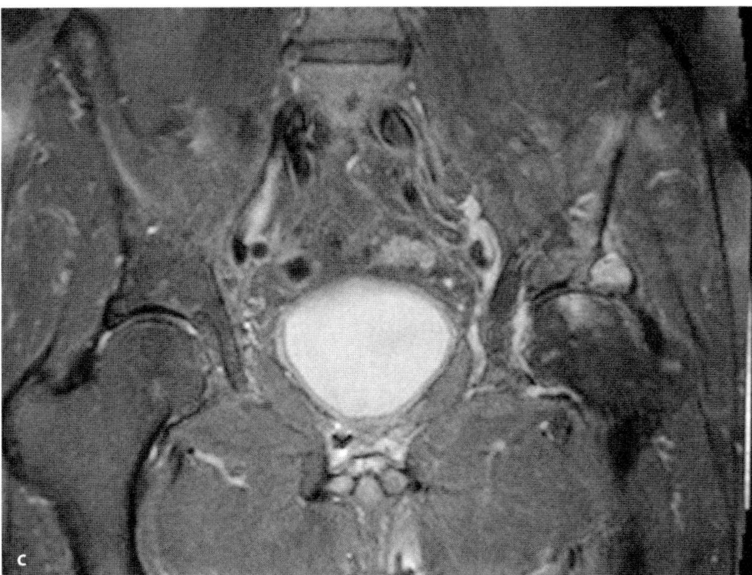

Fig. 19.9 a–c. Paralabral cyst of the left hip: **a** standard radiograph; **b** axial fat suppressed TSE T2-weighted MR image; **c** coronal fat suppressed TSE T2-weighted MR image. The standard radiography (a) reveals the presence of a sclerotic defined erosion at the superolateral aspect of the left acetabulum (*arrows*). On axial and coronal FS TSE T2-weighted MR images, there is a multicystic structure within the acetabular labrum, extending at the lateral aspect of the left acetabulum, causing pressure erosion (b,c). Note also the presence of internal bone debris on the standard radiographs (a), which appears as *hypointense dot-like structures* within the labral cyst on the FS TSE T2-weighted MR images. There is bone marrow edema at the lateral aspect of the left femoral head, as well as in the acetabulum, due to pre-existing osteoarthrosis of the hip

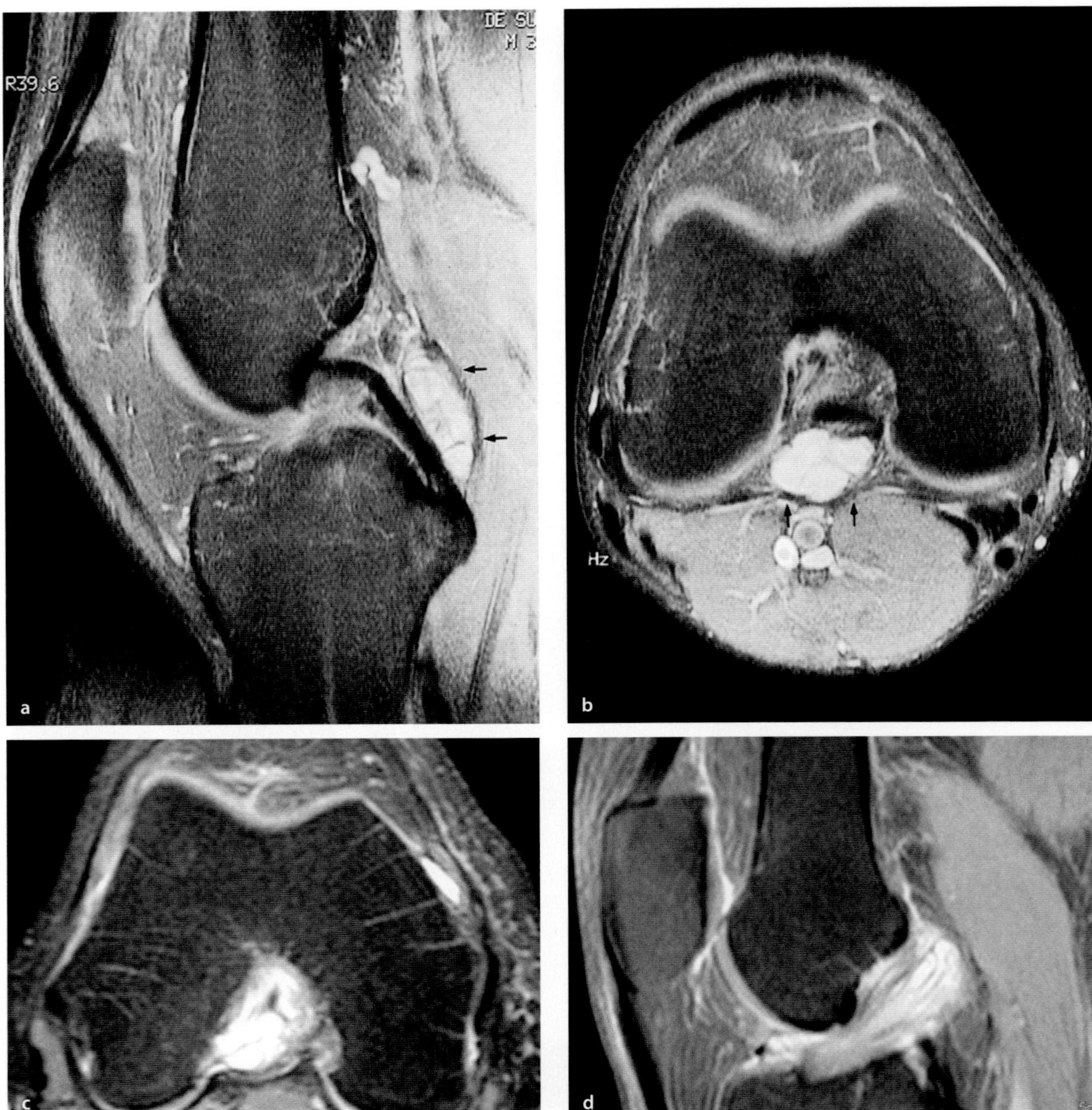

Fig. 19.10 a–d. Cysts of: **a, b** the posterior; **c, d** the anterior cruciate ligaments in two different patients. a is a sagittal fat suppressed T2-weighted MR image, b an axial fat suppressed T2-weighted MR image, c an axial fat suppressed TSE T2-weighted MR image and d a sagittal fat suppressed TSE T2-weighted MR image. A high signal intensity lesion with internal septations (a,b) is seen at the posterior border of the posterior cruciate ligament in the first patient (*arrows*). The fibers of the anterior cruciate ligament are interspersed by linear areas of high signal intensity on T2-weighted MR images in the second patient (c,d). Anterior cruciate ligament (ACL) cysts may be difficult to distinguish from partial tears of the ACL

Fig. 19.11 a–c. Adventitious bursa due to chronic friction at the first metatarsophalangeal joint: **a** clinical picture; **b** radiograph; **c** ultrasound of the first metatarsophalangeal joint. Soft tissue swelling at the medial side (a,b) of a hallux valgus deformity (*arrows*). On ultrasound, a well demarcated hypoechoic structure is seen at the medial aspect of the first metatarsal head

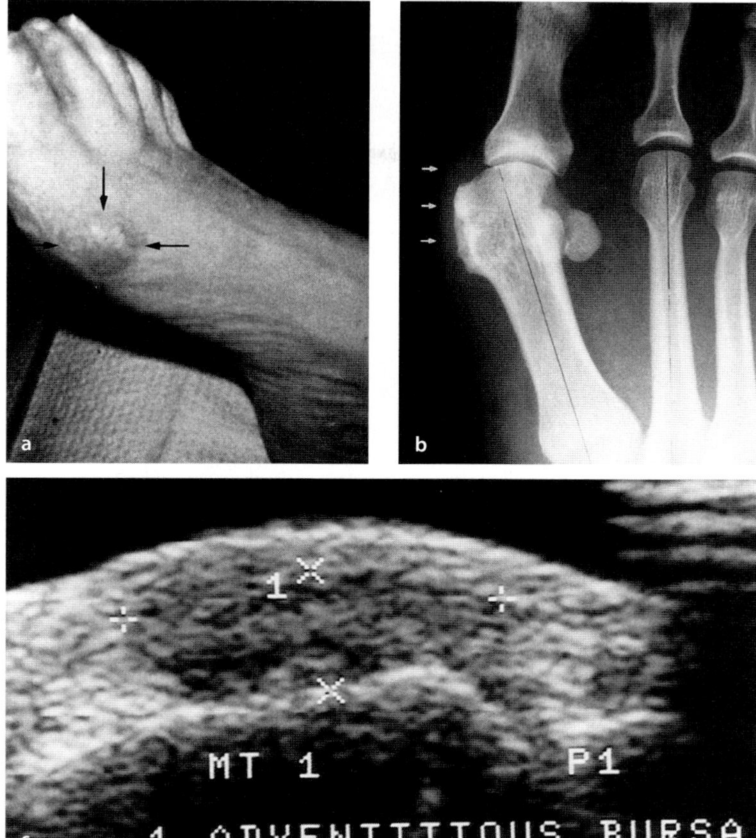

■ **Bursa De Novo (Adventitious Bursa).** Inflammation of connective tissue in areas subject to chronic frictional irritation may result in fibrinoid necrosis, with formation of a bursa de novo or an adventitious bursa. This consists of a cystic structure filled with cellular debris, extracellular fluid, altered ground substance, and inflammatory exudate [14]. The most common example is a bursitis de novo at the medial side of the first metatarsophalangeal joint, due to chronic friction over a hallux valgus (Fig. 19.11).

■ **Bursa.** Bursae are synovial lined structures, which are found in an anatomically predisposed topography. They contain a small amount of lubricating, mucinous fluid and their function is to avoid friction between two adjacent structures. Bursitis is an inflammation of a bursa, usually due to chronic mechanical friction, but may be caused by an infectious or rheumatoid disease as well. Bursitis results in abnormal accumulation of fluid within those bursae (Figs. 19.11–19.15).

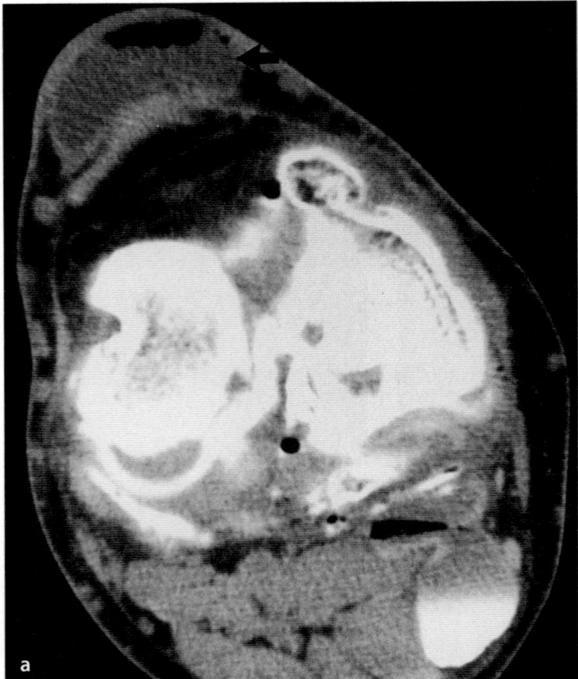

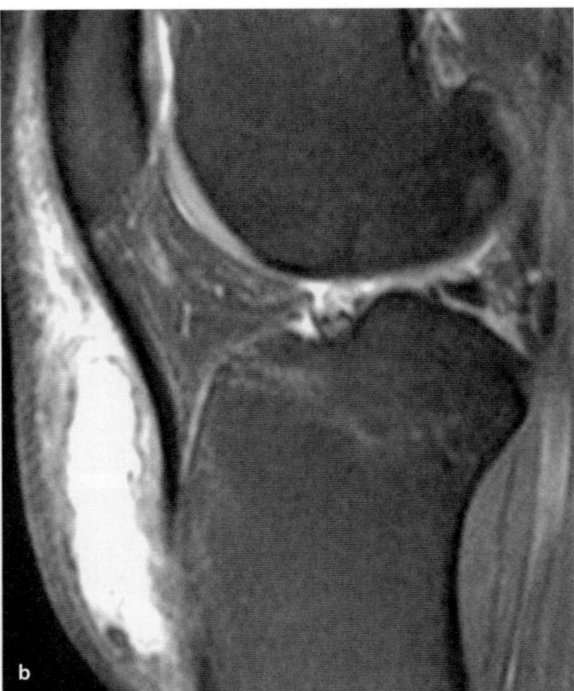

Fig. 19.12a, b. Chronic frictional infrapatellar bursitis in two different patients: **a** axial CT scan; **b** sagittal fat suppressed turbo spin echo T2-weighted MR image. In the first patient, a well delineated hypodense structure at the ventral aspect of the patellar tendon (*arrow*). The internal air is due to a previous puncture (*a*). In the second patient, an ill defined high signal intensity structure is seen anteriorly to the distal patellar tendon. The irregular delineation may be explained by repetitive friction

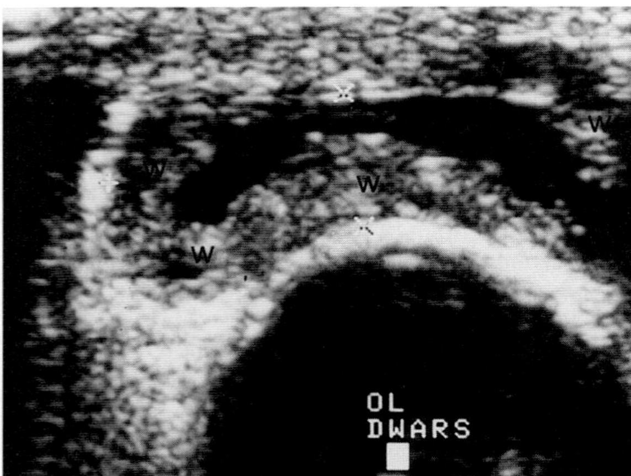

Fig. 19.13. Chronic frictional bursitis olecrani. Axial ultrasound at the dorsal aspect of the olecranon process of the elbow reveals an oval structure with a thickened hypoechoic wall (w) and an anechoic center.

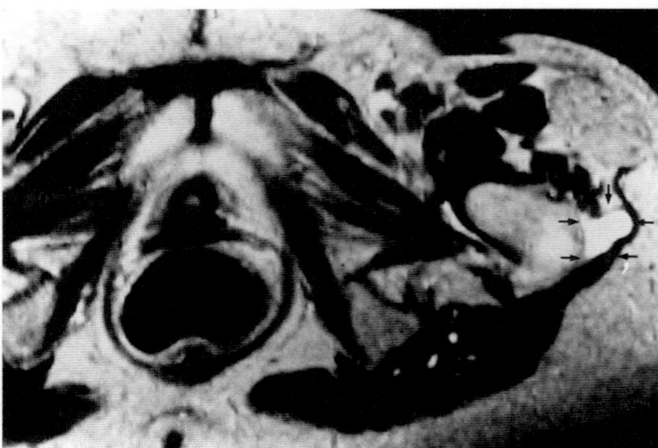

Fig. 19.14. Chronic bursitis (*arrows*) at the greater trochanter, presenting as a hyperintense structure on an axial T2-weighted image. Note the associated bone marrow edema in the greater trochanter

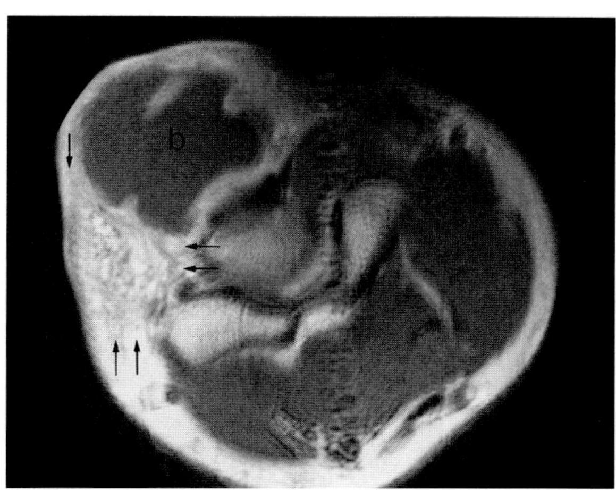

Fig. 19.15. Infectious bursitis olecrani. Axial T1-weighted image after intravenous gadolinium contrast administration: the bursa olecrani (b) is distended with peripheral rim enhancement. There is associated infiltration of the subcutaneous fat (*small arrows*)

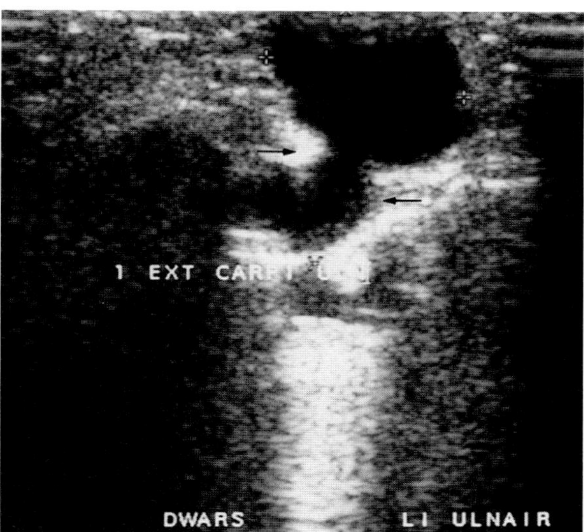

Fig. 19.16. (Arthro)synovial cyst of the wrist. For superficial joints, like the wrist, ultrasound represents an efficient tool for demonstrating the cystic nature, as well as the communication with the underlying joint (arrows). This can be much more difficult for deeply located joints

19.2.1.2 Clinical Manifestations

Clinically, these cysts present as palpable soft tissue masses. Symptoms, including local pain or limitation of joint mobility, are usually due to mass effect on the surrounding tissues [13], but small cysts are usually asymptomatic. Pseudo-thrombophlebitis is a well known complication, due to rupture of a Baker's cyst.

19.2.1.3 Imaging

The role of imaging is to define the cystic nature of those lesions, and to demonstrate a possible communication with the joint (Figs. 19.16 and 19.17). This is important for the surgeon because the resection of the communicating stalk with the joint is essential to avoid postsurgical recurrence of the cyst.

■ **Conventional Radiography.** Standard radiography is nonspecific and may reveal an ill-defined or rounded, noncalcified soft tissue mass. Radiographs may also demonstrate signs of associated degenerative joint disease, bone erosion (Fig. 19.9), calcification, gas, or calcified loose bodies in a communicating cyst (Fig. 19.1) [13].

■ **Ultrasound.** On US, synovial cysts and ganglion cysts appear as anechoic masses (Fig. 19.5), and may have a visible communication with a joint (Fig. 19.16) or

tendon sheath [18]. The lesion may be multiseptate and may contain some fine internal septations. US is an accurate technique to define the cystic nature in superficial cysts around the wrist and the hand, but it has limited ability to visualize deeper lying structures and their relationship with the adjacent joint. Furthermore, cysts containing debris or hyperplastic synovium may simulate solid mass lesions on ultrasound examinations [13].

A normal bursa is not visualized on ultrasound, or is seen only as a thin hypoechoic space or sac in a typical anatomic location. When a bursa is distended, it appears as a hypoechoic structure with well-defined margins and contents of variable echogenicity. The internal appearance varies according to the pathology. In a simple bursitis, there may be just anechoic fluid, with or without septa. In chronic bursitis due to impingement or overuse, more frequently there is bursal wall thickening (Fig. 19.13), with internal debris of variable echogenicity. The echogenic contents may even mimic a solid mass [18]. This is especially true for a bursitis de novo (Fig. 19.11).

■ **CT-scan.** Due to its low soft-tissue contrast, CT is of limited value in assessing soft-tissue lesions. Para-articular cysts are of lower attenuation than muscle (Fig. 19.6) and of higher attenuation than fat. Rim enhancement is seen after intravenous contrast administration [13]. A possible communication with the joint is sometimes difficult to define on axial images.

■ **Arthrography/Direct Cyst Puncture.** Arthrography can be useful to demonstrate the communication of the cyst with the joint cavity. However, cysts may fail to fill when the communication is very narrow or when the cyst is filled with highly viscous fluid [13]. Joint communication can sometimes be demonstrated on delayed images (2 h after the injection) [9].

■ **MRI.** MR imaging demonstrates the exact location and extent of the cystic lesions, and its relationship to the joint and surrounding structures (Figs. 19.1, 19.3, 19.4, 19.7–19.10, 19.12, 19.14, 19.15, 19.17). It is very accurate in depicting associated joint disorders, such as meniscal tears (associated with meniscal cysts) (Fig. 19.7), labral tears (in case of a paralabral cyst) (Figs. 19.8, Fig. 19.9), ligamentous abnormalities or inflammatory changes [13]. Maximum Intensity Projections (MIP) of 3D acquisitions with fat saturation may be helpful to demonstrate the stalk communicating with the adjacent joint.

The diagnosis of a cystic mass is usually straightforward by analysis of the signal intensities of the lesion. They are typically hypo- or isointense to muscle on T1-weighted images, especially if they contain protein-rich gelatinous substances, and homogeneously hyperintense on T2-weighted images. However, there are some pitfalls. Atypical cyst content due to debris or hemorrhage may alter the imaging appearance of the cysts. Chronic inflammation may cause marked thickening of the synovial membrane, and, therefore mimic a solid soft-tissue mass. A cruciate ligament ganglion may demonstrate the same signal intensity as a cruciate ligament tear and may simulate a false-positive diagnosis of cruciate ligament tear [13].

Cystic lesions are well circumscribed, but may be lobulated, or multicystic with internal septa. Ruptured cysts, due to an elevated pressure are irregularly delineated, and must be differentiated from other soft tissue tumors and hemorrhagic or inflammatory lesions.

After gadolinium contrast administration, subtle rim enhancement of the peripheral fibrovascular tissue in the cyst wall is seen, but there is never central enhancement like in other well delineated soft tissue lesions with high signal intensity on T2-weighted images, such as myxoma, myxoid liposarcoma, hemangioma, synovial sarcoma and mucinosis [3, 16].

19.2.2 Giant Cell Tumors and PVNS

According to the most recent WHO classification, these tumors will be discussed in Chap. 14.

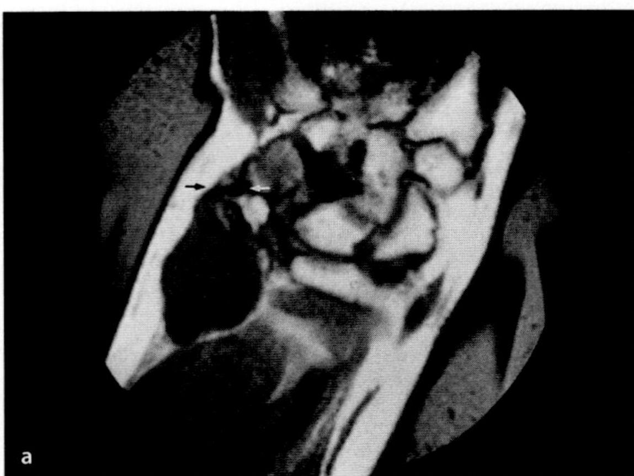

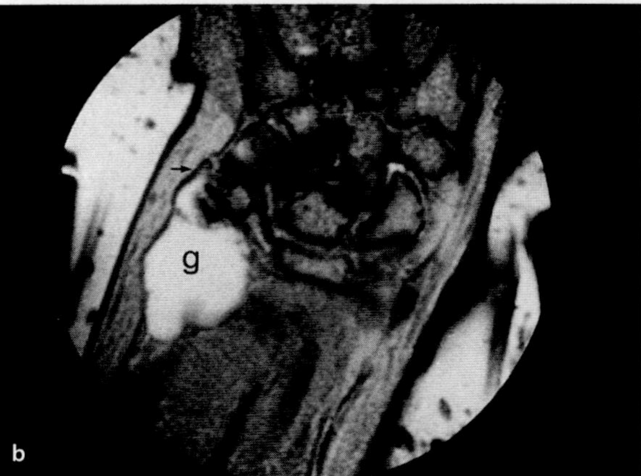

Fig. 19.17 a, b. Uncomplicated ganglion cyst (g) of the wrist in a 59-year-old man: **a** coronal spin echo T1- weighted MR image; **b** coronal turbo spin echo T2-weighted MR image. Ganglion cysts rarely communicate with the adjacent tendon sheath or joints (*arrows*). In this case of a ganglion cyst (g) at the volar aspect of the wrist and forearm there is no associated increase in intra-articular fluid (b). The signal characteristics of ganglion cysts are usually comparable with those of synovial cysts: bright on T2-weighted image (b) and dark on T1-weighted image (a)

19.2.3 Other Synovial Tumors and Tumor-like Lesions

19.2.3.1 Synovial Chondromatosis and Synovial Chondrosarcoma

Synovial chondromatosis is characterized by metaplasia of the subsynovial connective tissue with subsequent cartilage formation. In rare cases there is malignant degeneration into synovial chondrosarcoma. These entities are discussed in Chap. 21.

19.2.3.2 Synovial Hemangioma

Synovial hemangioma is a separate localization of a hemangiomatous tumor. However since it is a vascular and not a synovial tumor by histological criteria this entity is discussed in Chap. 16.

19.2.3.3 Synovial Osteochondroma

Synovial osteochondroma is a very rare cartilaginous tumor that is not connected to bone. It occurs almost exclusively near the joints in hand and feet. It is discussed in detail in Chap. 21.

19.2.3.4 Lipoma Arborescens

This rare tumor will be discussed in the chapter of lipomatous tumors (Chap. 15).

19.3 Malignant Tumors Around the Joints

19.3.1 Synovial Sarcoma

As discussed earlier in the introduction of this chapter, synovial sarcoma is a misnomer. According to the most recent WHO classification (2002), this tumor will be discussed in Chap. 23 (Lesions of Uncertain Differentiation).

19.3.2 Metastatic Spread of Cancer

The metastatic spread of cancer to the joint and synovium is one of the rarest manifestations of malignant diseases, and involvement of more than one joint is exceptional. It is more commonly seen in patients with leukemia and other hematologic malignancies and is rarely reported in those with solid tumors [11]. MRI shows a combination of bone and joint involvement, with nonspecific signal behavior. The diagnosis can be confirmed by joint cytology and/or synovial biopsy.

Synovial involvement of a lymphoma will be discussed in the chapter of soft tissue lymphoma (Chap. 26).

Things to remember:
1. Cystic soft tissue lesions can be divided into four groups (synovial cyst, ganglion cyst, bursa de novo and permanent bursa), based upon the combination of their anatomical location and histological composition.
2. The diagnosis of a cystic lesion is usually straightforward on ultrasound and/or MR imaging. If there is any doubt, however, on the true cystic nature of the lesion, gadolinium contrast administration should be performed to exclude a pseudo-cystic benign or malignant tumor.

References

1. Barland P, Novokoff AB, Hamerman D (1962) Electron microscopy of the human synovial membrane. J Cell Biol 14:207
2. Bui-Mansfield LT, Youngberg RA (1997) Intraarticular ganglia of the knee: prevalence, presentation, etiology, and management. Am J Roentgenol 168:123–127
3. Fletcher CDM, Unni KK, Mertens F (2002) Pathology and genetics of tumours of soft tissue and bone (World Health Organization Classification of Tumours). IARC Press, Lyon, France
4. Kim MG, Kim BH, Choi JA et al. (2001) Intraarticular ganglion cysts of the knee: clinical and MR imaging features. Eur Radiol 11:834–840
5. Kobayashi H, Kotoura Y, Hosono M, Tsuboyama T, Sakahara H, Konishi J (1996) Periosteal ganglion of the tibia. Skelet Radiol 25:381–383
6. Lever JD, Ford EHR (1958) Histological, histochemical and electron microscopic observations on synovial membrane. Anat Rec 132:525
7. Levien LJ, Benn CA (1998) Adventitial cystic disease: a unifying hypothesis. J Vasc Surg 28:193–205
8. Malghem J, Lebon C, Vandeberg B, Maldague B, Lecouvet F (2004) Les kystes mucoides atypiques. In: Laredo JD, Tomeni B, Malghem J et al. (eds) Conduite a tenir devant une image osseuse ou des parties molles d'allure tumorale. Sauramps Medical, Montpellier, pp363–376
9. Malghem J, Vande berg BC, Lebon C, Lecouvet FE, Maldague BE (1998) Ganglion cysts of the knee: articular communication revealed by delayed radiography and CT after arthrography. Am J Roentgenol 170:1579–1583
10. McCarthy CL, McNally EG (2004) The MRI appearance of cystic lesions around the knee Skelet Radiol 33:187–209
11. Metyas SK, Lum CA, Raza AS, Vaysburd M, Forrestier DM, Quismorio FP (2003) Inflammatory arthritis secondary to metastatic gastric cancer. J Rheumatol 30:2713–2715
12. Nucci F, Artico M, Santoro A, Bardella L, Delfini R, Bosco S, Palma L (1990) Intraneural synovial cyst of the peroneal nerve: report of two cases and review of the literature. Neurosurg 26:339–344

13. Steiner E, Steinbach LS, Schnarkowski P, Tirman PF, Genant HK (1996) Ganglia and cysts around joints. Radiol Clin North Am 34:395–425
14. Van Holsbeeck M, Introcaso JH (2001) Sonography of bursae. In: Van Holsbeeck M, Introcaso JH (eds) Musculoskeletal ultrasound, 2nd edn. Mosby, St Louis, pp 131–169
15. Vandevenne JE, Vanhoenacker F, Hauben E, De Schepper AM (1997) Nosologie des kystes para-articulaires. In: Bard H, Drapé JL, Goutallier D, Laredo JD (eds) Le genou traumatique et dégeneratif. Sauramps Médical, Montpellier, pp 293–303
16. Vanhoenacker FM, Van de Perre S, De Vuyst D, De Schepper AM (2003) Proceeding of the meeting of The KBVR-SRBR Osteo-articular section Brussels, June 21, 2003. Cystic lesions around the knee. JBR-BTR 86:302–304
17. Vanhoenacker FM, Vandevenne JE, De Schepper AM, De Leersnijder J (2000) Letter to the editor. Regarding "Adventitial cystic disease: a unifying hypothesis". J Vasc Surg 31:621–622
18. Wang SC, Chhem RK, Cardinal E, Cho KH (1999) Joint sonography. Radiol Clin North Am 37:653–668

Tumors of Peripheral Nerves

Paul M. Parizel, Catherine Geniets

20

20.1 Introduction

Tumors of peripheral nerves most commonly originate from the nerve sheath. In this chapter, they will be referred to as peripheral nerve sheath tumors (PNST). Arthur Purdy Stout (1885–1967) was a pioneer in the development of our current understanding of the histogenesis of these tumors. He was the first to identify the Schwann cell as the major contributor to the formation of benign as well as malignant neoplasms of the nerve sheath [106].

Benign nerve sheath tumors are subdivided into two separate morphological groups with different histopathological characteristics: schwannoma (also known as neurilemoma or neurinoma) and neurofibroma [30]. Intraneural ganglion is also considered to be a tumor of nerve origin. For a discussion on this tumor we refer to Chap. 1, Sect. 3.2.1.

Malignant nerve sheath tumors are known under a confusing multitude of names including malignant schwannoma, malignant neurilemoma, nerve sheath fibrosarcoma, neurogenic sarcoma, and neurofibrosarcoma. In this chapter we will use the generic and widely accepted term malignant peripheral nerve sheath tumor (MPNST).

20.2 Schwannomas

20.2.1 Epidemiology

Schwannomas represent approximately 5% of benign soft-tissue neoplasms. They can occur at all ages, though they are uncommon in children. While literature data indicate that they are most prevalent between the ages of 20 and 50 [29, 75], our own findings appear to indicate a bimodal age distribution with peak incidences in the third and seventh decades. Men and women are equally affected [30, 106]. The majority of schwannomas arise sporadically in patients without a genetic predisposition. However, histologically identical tumors also occur in patients with neurofibromatosis type 2 (NF2), or schwannomatosis [51, 46]. Schwannomas associated with NF tend to occur in younger patients.

20.2.2 Topography

Schwannomas most commonly involve the major nerve trunks of the head, neck and limbs; the flexor surfaces of the extremities are more frequently affected, especially near the elbow, wrist and knee [30, 75, 98]. Consequently, the most common topographical locations of schwannomas include: the spinal roots and cervical plexus, the vagus, peroneal and ulnar nerves. Deeply situated schwannomas are predominantly found in the posterior mediastinum and the retroperitoneum [29, 75]. Relatively few schwannomas appear on the trunk, which contrasts with the distribution of neurofibromas in neurofibromatosis type 1 (NF-1). Other sites of involvement include the scalp and the hands; the feet are usually spared. Less frequently, schwannomas have been recorded in the tongue, palate and larynx. Although the stomach is also held to be a site, confusion here may occur with the common leiomyoma [98]. Solitary schwannomas of the viscera are exceptional in the absence of NF-1 but have been reported in the heart and in the lung [32, 101]. In this chapter, we will focus our discussion on peripheral schwannomas.

20.2.3 Histology

20.2.3.1 General Histologic Features of Schwannomas

Schwannomas are benign, slowly growing neoplasms. They originate in a nerve and are composed exclusively of Schwann cells in a collagenous matrix [46, 75]. In general, they are firm, circumscribed and encapsulated. Unlike a neurofibroma, which incorporates axons, the schwannoma displaces normal elements of the nerve to one side [25]. This implies that surgical excision can usually spare the parent nerve because the schwannoma is separable from the underlying nerve fibers. Small schwannomas tend to be spheroid, whereas larger tumors can be ovoid, sausage-shaped, or irregularly lobulated [98]. Macroscopically, the cut surface is relatively homogeneous, tan or grey, with irregular yellow areas and cysts, particularly in large tumors. Sometimes, only a nodule of tumor remains in what is otherwise a fibrous-walled cyst, filled with watery fluid. Less often schwannomas can be (partially) hemorrhagic [46].

According to the morphology and spatial arrangement of tumor cells, two types of tissue are distinguished: Antoni A and B tissue [3, 75].

In the *Antoni A type* tissue, the texture is composed of compactly arranged spindle-shaped cells, with long oval or rod-shaped nuclei, that are frequently oriented with their long axes parallel to one another, creating a pattern of palisades [46]. The cytoplasm is uniformly pale. A characteristic feature, seen in sections stained with hematoxylin-eosin [46], is the alignment of nuclei in rows, separated by clear hyaline bands along the longitudinally cut bundles. These areas are often called Verocay bodies [98]. Commonly, but not invariably, a part of, or all of a schwannoma has a less cellular *Antoni B type pattern* [46]. It has a looser texture and the tumor cells are more polymorphic, with indefinite outlines and separated by a finely honeycombed eosinophilic matrix in which reticulin fibers are relatively sparse and unevenly distributed. Mucinous and microcystic changes occur more often in the type B tissue. When confluent, they presumably result in the production of intratumoral cysts [107].

In some schwannomas, tumor nuclei, especially in the Antoni B areas, may become enlarged and hyperchromatic, and assume a bizarre appearance. This development is sometimes described as *"ancient schwannoma"* and may also be reflected in the connective tissue of the tumor. The fibrous stroma becomes more abundant and consists of dense bands of hyalinized collagen. This change does not denote a malignant transformation, but refers to long standing lesions with advanced degeneration exhibiting calcification, hyalinization, relative loss of Antoni A areas, and cystic avitation. [98]. Therefore ancient schwannomas must be considered as a degenerative schwannoma subtype. [58].

Vessels in schwannomas are usually prominent [46], and are liable to spontaneous thrombosis with consequent necrosis, and sometimes hemorrhage, in the adjacent areas [98]. The rich vascular supply of schwannomas is reflected in the often intense enhancement of these tumors on imaging studies.

The histologic features of schwannomas can account for their occasional inhomogeneous appearance on computed tomography (CT) or magnetic resonance imaging (MRI) examinations and can be summarized as follows:

1. Areas of decreased cellularity (Antoni B) adjacent to areas of increased cellularity (Antoni A)
2. Cystic degeneration due to vascular thrombosis and subsequent necrosis
3. Xanthomatous regions, containing aggregates of lipid-laden (foam) cells [47, 98]

Calcifications are seen less frequently in schwannomas than in neurofibromas [13].

20.2.3.2 Special Histologic Types of Schwannomas

Histologically, several variants of benign schwannoma can be distinguished.

Cellular schwannomas have a predominantly cellular growth but no Verocay bodies, and are almost exclusively composed of Antoni A areas [75]. They appear circumscribed, if not encapsulated [30]. They typically occur in women and middle-aged people [34], and are more frequently found in deep structures, e.g. the retroperitoneum and posterior mediastinum [30]. They can cause erosion of bone and recur locally. Despite the increased cellularity, there is no basis for malignant behavior of a cellular schwannoma [70, 75, 115].

(Psammomatous) Melanotic schwannoma is characterized by a strong melanocytic -differentiation of the Schwann cells. Like classic schwannomas [81, 90, 92], they are usually diffusely and strongly reactive for S-100 protein and not infrequently reactive for Leu-7 and MBP [115]. Schwann cells and melanocytes share a common precursor stem cell derived from the neural crest, hence this differentiation [17, 83]. Melanotic schwannomas have a predilection for spinal nerve roots, and commonly arise near the midline [30]. It has been suggested that they display malignant behavior with local recurrence after surgery. Although melanotic schwannomas are very rare [74], they merit recognition because of the paramagnetic properties of melanin. CT cannot reliably discriminate these tumors from other neurogenic neoplasms, and is most useful in detecting bone erosion or intratumoral calcifications. MRI shows high signal intensity on T1-weighted MR images, reflecting T1-shortening due to the presence of melanin [68]. Differential diagnosis includes benign and malignant melanotic tumors, pigmented neurofibroma, melanotic medulloblastoma, pigmented neuroblastoma, ganglioneuroblastoma, neurotropic melanoma, and melanotic neuroendocrine carcinomas and carcinoids [76, 77, 96].

Plexiform (multinodular) schwannomas constitute 5% of all schwannomas. The multinodular or plexiform pattern of growth may or may not be apparent macroscopically [30]. Only 4% of all cases of this form reported in the literature occurred in patients with NF-1 [33, 54]; therefore, it is not to be considered associated with NF-1 [26, 33, 75]. Plexiform schwannoma arises in the dermis or subcutaneous tissues, and occurs predominantly in young adults, without sex predilection [33, 63]. Although it can display nuclear pleomorphism and increased cellularity in places, it appears to be a benign lesion [98].

20.2.4 Clinical Presentation

Small schwannomas are usually asymptomatic. Paresthesias, pain or other symptoms can occur when the tumor reaches sufficient size to compress the involved nerve. Pain may radiate along the course of the peripheral nerve, and can be constant and intractable, not influenced by rest or activity. The tumor may be tender to palpation. On physical examination or at surgery, it can be moved from side to side, but not along the long axis of the nerve. Deep schwannomas can become symptomatic because of increasing size and impingement on neighboring structures [46]. Muscle atrophy with fatty replacement can occur in muscle groups located distally to the lesion.

In case of a *melanotic schwannoma*, over 50% of patients develop Carney's syndrome, i.e. myxomas, spotty pigmentation and endocrine overactivity producing Cushing's syndrome [11].

In rare instances, the clinical history may indicate a specific diagnosis, as in the case of *Morton's neuroma*. A Morton's neuroma is a benign reactive perineural sclerosing process, and is *not* a tumor originating from Schwann cells [30, 75]. The term "neuroma" is therefore misleading, and can be considered a misnomer. It is preferable to refer to these lesions as "Morton's fibroma". Morton's fibroma typically originates from the interdigital nerves of the foot, usually in the third and less frequently in the second intermetatarsal space [30, 75, 118]. It has also been reported in the hands [75].

Morton's fibroma is probably due to repeated minor trauma, with compression of the interdigital nerve against the transverse metatarsal ligament [75, 118]. This entrapment hypothesis is favored by the presence of Renaut bodies (densely packed whorls of collagen) which are characteristically found in entrapped peripheral nerves [44, 58]. However, a biomechanical study has shown that in full plantar and dorsal flexion the neurovascular bundle moves parallel to the surrounding structures such as this ligament. There is as yet no definite consensus as to the etiology of Morton's neuroma, and other causes such as ischemia should also be considered [84, 99, 118, 119].

Morton's fibroma is more frequent unilateral than bilateral, and is more common in middle aged women than in men [30, 66] (Fig. 20.1). In early stages, patients may only complain of a mild ache or discomfort in the area of the metatarsal head. A burning sensation or tingling can be experienced. The type of shoe can be a contributory factor in the severity of symptoms. Gradually, the sensations become more specific, often causing constant burning, radiating to the tip of the toes. Patients feel as if a marble were inside the ball of the foot. Diagnosis can be established by the characteristic clinical history and by palpation of the foot sole. Pain is elicited when pressure is exerted between the heads of the metatarsals. It is important to know that Morton's fibroma can elicit pain that is related to another intermetatarsal space [44]. Frequently, Morton's fibroma can be asymptomatic. Small Morton's fibromas may be more commonly asymptomatic. A threshold of 5 mm for the transverse diameter is suggested beyond which the neuroma more commonly produces symptoms [94].

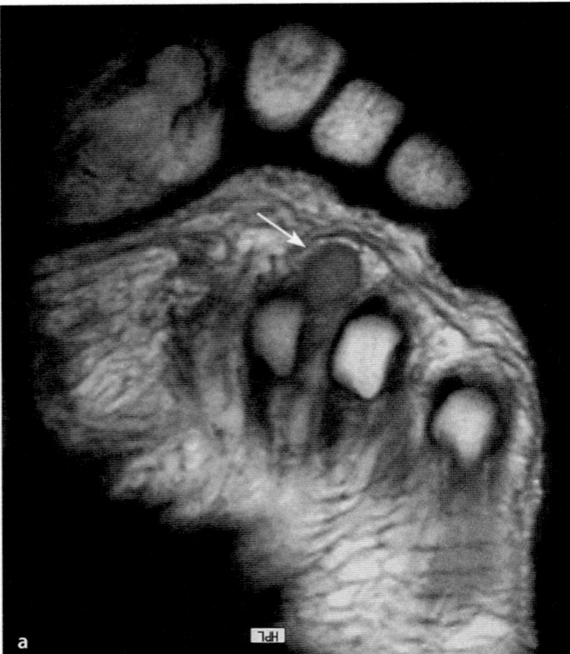

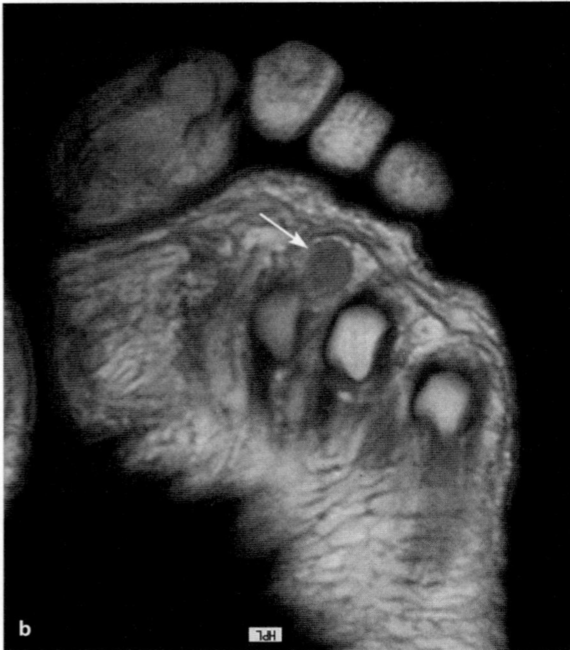

Fig. 20.1 a, b. Morton's neuroma in a 46-year-old woman: **a** oblique coronal precontrast spin echo T1-weighted MR image through the right forefoot; **b** post-contrast spin echo T1-weighted MR image (same location and imaging parameters). There is a sharply delineated ovoid lesion in the third intermetatarsal space, between the heads of the third and fourth metatarsals (*arrow*). The lesion has a maximum diameter of 13 mm and is isointense relative to muscle (**a**). After intravenous contrast injection, the nodular lesion enhances moderately and homogeneously (**b**). At the periphery, there is a hypointense non-enhancing rim. The location and morphology of the tumor are characteristic of Morton's neuroma

The diagnosis of Morton's fibroma on the basis of imaging findings should be made only in the context of the clinical setting [118]. The MR diagnosis of Morton's fibroma is based on three criteria. First, the lesion has to be centered in the region of the neurovascular bundle within the intermetatarsal space, and must be situated on the plantar side of the transverse ligament. Second, the lesion should be well demarcated. This excludes partial volume effects with the adjacent joint capsule to be interpreted as a Morton's fibroma, a frequent problem in hammer toe deformities. Third, the lesion is isointense relative to muscle on T1-WI, and homogeneously or inhomogeneously hypointense relative to fat tissue on T2-WI.

Moreover, MR plays an important role in excluding other pathologies that can mimic Morton's fibroma such as intermetatarsal or subcapitometatarsal bursitis (which occurs dorsal to the transverse metatarsal ligament), osteonecrosis of the metatarsal heads, metatarsophalangeal joint synovitis or dislocation, tendon sheath ganglion, pigmented villonodular synovitis, stress fractures and other disorders associated with metatarsalgia [66, 118].

In most cases, therapy is conservative with perineural infiltrations of a local anesthetic and/or long acting corticosteroids. Surgical excision is only performed when necessary.

Traumatic neuroma is a painful lesion, which is also *not* a tumor of Schwann cell origin. It is a nonneoplastic reactive hyperplasia of nerve tissue and usually occurs at the proximal end of a nerve trunk that has been severed, partially transected, or injured as a result of trauma. The most common location for traumatic neuromas is the lower extremity after amputation, followed by the head and neck, where they have been reported to occur after the extraction of teeth. In contradistinction to a Morton's fibroma, it is neatly circumscribed [80], and it displays mainly proliferative changes, whereas Morton's fibroma shows degenerative changes [30].

20.2.5 Imaging Characteristics

20.2.5.1 Plain Radiography

Peripheral nerve schwannomas are usually not seen on plain radiography, unless the tumor is very large or appears as a round mass with a peripheral sulcus (Fig. 20.2). Some schwannomas exhibit a slightly lower attenuation of the X-ray beam than muscle. Bone erosion (scalloping) can be caused by benign schwannomas, especially the cellular variant [98]. Widening of neural foramina is a frequently encountered sign of schwannomas tracking along the exiting spinal nerves. This can be documented on oblique X-ray films of the spine. Rarely, rib notching can be seen in schwannoma of the intercostal nerves (Fig. 20.3). A posterior mediastinal mass on a chest radiograph, should suggest the possibility of a neurogenic tumor, for they account for 30% of posterior mediastinal mass lesions.

20.2.5.2 Ultrasound

On ultrasound, schwannomas are usually seen as a solid, ovoid, typically hypoechoic mass [9, 13, 36, 40, 50, 52]. Internal cystic cavities provide easier sound-through transmission [9, 13, 36, 39, 50, 52]. Posterior signal reinforcement is seen in 50% of cases [36, 39]. Schwannomas are usually eccentric in relation to the nerve axis. A schwannoma has hyperechoic boundaries. It appears neatly circumscribed from the adjacent structures, which are not infiltrated by the neoplasm. The schwannoma is attached to the band-like structure of the nerve from which it originates. Together, on a longitudinal projection along the axis of the nerve, they can produce an ultrasound image which resembles a spoon. This spoon-like aspect can be considered as pathognomonic for this nerve sheath tumor [39]. The nerve of origin retains its normal echoic qualities [36].

20.2.5.3 Computed Tomography

On unenhanced CT scans schwannomas are seen as well-circumscribed homogeneous lesions. They are hypo- to isodense relative to muscle [14, 15, 63]. However, an inhomogeneous tumor appearance with low density areas is frequently seen in larger tumors. This is believed to reflect the histologic diversity (see Sect. 20.2.3.1.). As a rule, hyperdense areas do not occur in schwannomas [14, 63].

On contrast-enhanced CT scans, most schwannomas become iso- or hyperdense to muscle. Non-enhancing cystic or necrotic areas are typically found in large schwannomas, and are a valuable element in the differ-

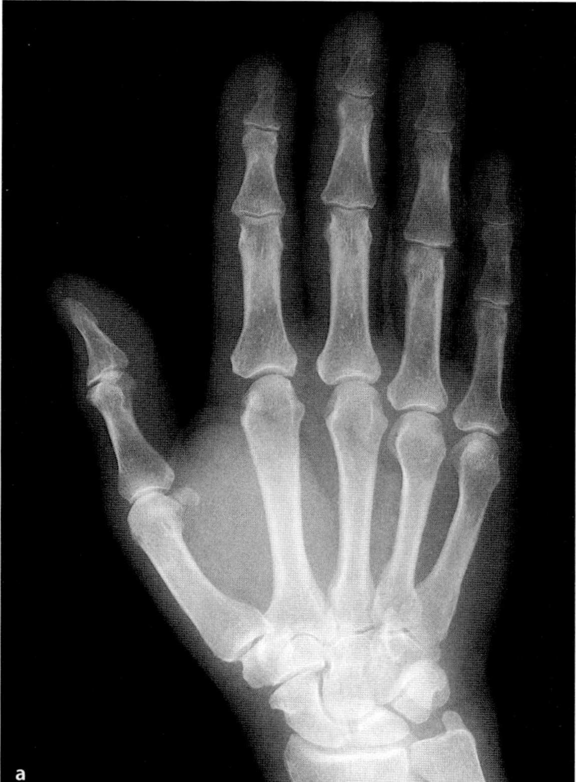

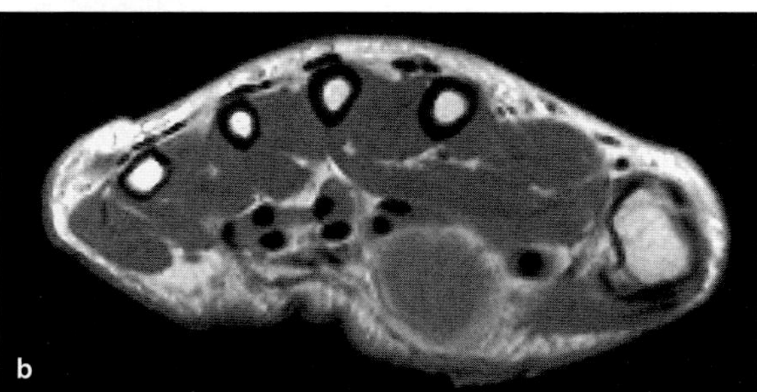

Fig. 20.2 a, b. Schwannoma of the right hand in a 73-year-old man: **a** plain radiograph of the right hand; **b** axial spin echo T1-weighted MR image after gadolinium-contrast injection. A soft tissue mass is seen between the first and second metacarpal of the right hand. The ovoid soft tissue mass is outlined by a translucent rim, possibly representing displaced fatty tissue (**a**). MRI examination confirms the presence of a well circumscribed soft tissue tumor, with minimal peripheral enhancement (**b**). Histology showed a schwannoma

ential diagnosis [14] (Fig. 20.3). They almost never display a uniformly hypodense appearance.

Differential CT diagnosis should include: neurofibromas, malignant peripheral nerve sheath tumors, enlarged lymph nodes [18], synovial cysts, and other soft tissue tumors.

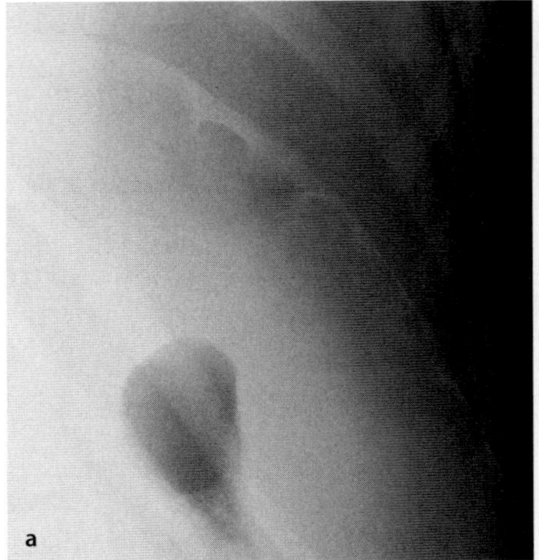

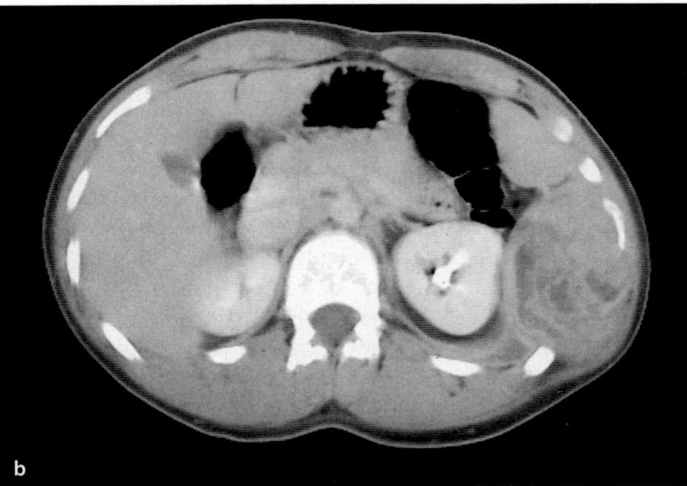

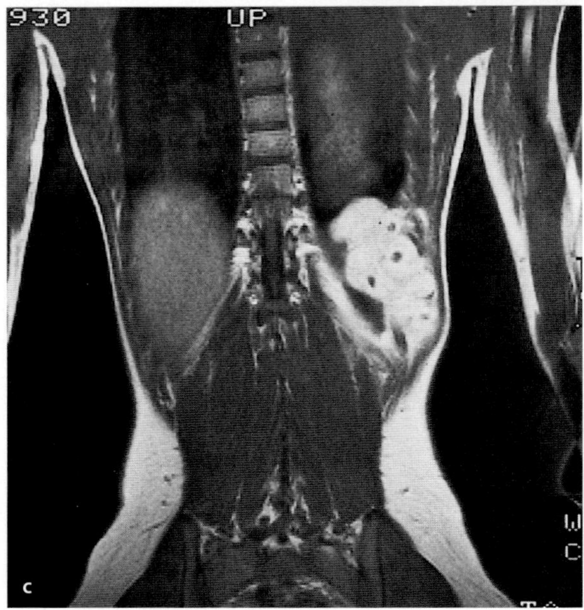

Fig. 20.3 a–c. Schwannoma of the chest wall in a 16-year-old boy: **a** plain radiograph of the rib cage; **b** CT scan after iodinated-contrast injection at the level of the upper abdomen; **c** coronal spin echo T1-weighted MR image after gadolinium-contrast injection. Irregular scalloping (notching) of the inferior border of the left 10th rib and widening of the intercostal space can be seen (**a**). CT displays a large, irregularly enhancing, sharply defined tumor. Within the tumor mass, necrotic or cystic non-enhancing cavities are observed (**b**). MRI examination shows a markedly enhancing tumor subjacent to the 10th rib (**c**). The tumor inhomogeneity can be caused by cystic degeneration, necrosis, xanthomatous change or heterotopic calcifications. At surgery a large tumor mass (23×10×8 cm) was resected. Histology revealed a benign schwannoma

20.2.5.4 Magnetic Resonance Imaging

Prior to performing the MRI examination, it is useful to mark the palpated abnormality by placing a skin marker, which is visible on MRI. For this purpose, a small cod-liver oil (retinol and cholecalciferol) or vitamin E capsule can be used. These markers display a high signal intensity on all pulse sequences. This is especially important in T1-weighted MR images, in which the tumor can be isointense to skeletal muscle (Fig. 20.4).

If the tumor arises at the level of a nerve bifurcation, this can result in a typical forked appearance on parallel scans, or in a bilobed appearance on perpendicular MR or CT images. (Fig. 20.6). Also of importance is the fact that schwannomas grow eccentrically in relation to the nerve of origin (Fig. 20.7), whereas neurofibromas do not (Fig. 20.9).

On nonenhanced T1-weighted MR images, schwannomas have an identical or slightly higher signal intensity than muscle (Figs. 20.4, 20.5 and 20.7). Sometimes they are hardly visible (Fig. 20.6). On proton density-weighted MR images, they are hyperintense to muscle (Fig. 20.6). Signal intensity is markedly increased on T2-weighted MR images (Figs. 20.4–20.6), resulting in a sharp contrast between the hyperintense nerve sheath tumor, medium intensity fat, and lower intensity muscles [8]. Cystic or pseudocystic lesions display a low signal intensity on T1-weighted MR images and a high signal intensity on proton density- and T2-weighted MR images (Fig. 20.8). Solid, highly cellular lesions have an intermediate signal intensity on T1-weighted MR images. In our experience, small schwannomas tend to enhance brightly and uniformly after gadolinium injection, whereas the enhancement pattern in larger lesions

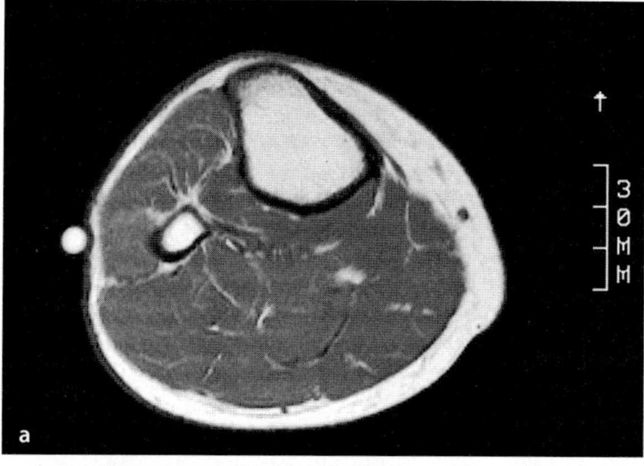

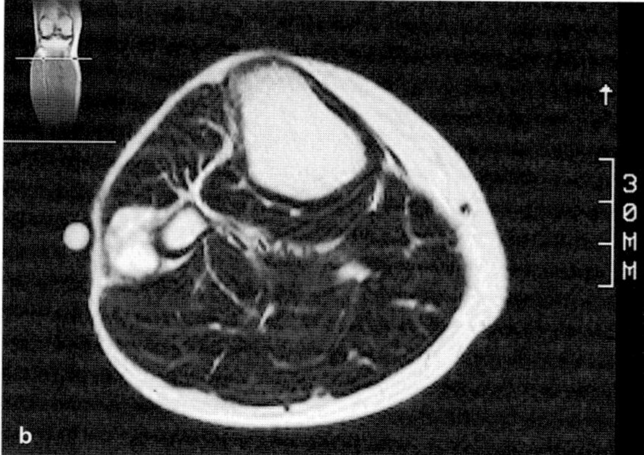

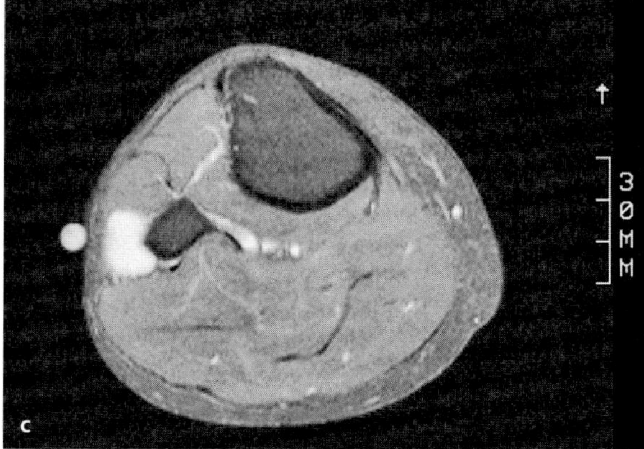

Fig. 20.4a–c. Schwannoma of the right leg in a 62-year-old woman. A cod-liver oil skin marker is used to locate the small soft tissue tumor: **a** axial spin echo T1-weighted MR image through the lower leg, 1.5 cm below the tibial plateau; **b** axial turbo spin echo T2-weighted MR image; **c** axial spin echo T1-weighted MR image after gadolinium-contrast injection with spectral fat saturation. On a T1-weighted scan, the skin marker is of high signal intensity, whereas the tumor is completely isointense to the adjacent muscles (**a**). On a T2-weighted scan, both the skin marker and the tumor display a high signal intensity (**b**). On the fat-saturated post-contrast T1-weighted scan, the tumor enhances intensely and homogeneously (**c**). Note that, even though the subcutaneous fat signal is suppressed on this sequence, the skin marker remains hyperintense (**c**). At histology after surgery, the tumor, located along the course of the fibular nerve, turned out to be a schwannoma

may be more heterogeneous (Figs. 20.2–20.8). It has been suggested that the enhancement pattern of nerve sheath neoplasms could be used to predict benign versus malignant behavior [63] or to differentiate schwannomas from neurofibromas [14]. This hypothesis is still controversial and needs to be confirmed by larger patient series [57].

Nonenhanced and enhanced MR images are superior in depicting intratumoral inhomogeneities, which reflect the histologic nature of the lesion (see Sect. 20.2.3.1). Differential diagnosis must be made with malignant neoplasms, in which inhomogeneities also can occur as a result of hemorrhage or necrosis [16, 63, 67, 113]. As a consequence, tumor heterogeneity is of limited value in predicting the histologic nature of nerve sheath tumors [16, 63, 67].

MR examination is reliable in discriminating between intramuscular and extramuscular tumors, which is of importance for preoperative staging [28].

The detection on MRI of a capsule, visualized as a thin hyperintense rim along the margin of the tumor, has been proposed as a criterion for differentiating schwannomas from neurofibromas [57]. Schwannomas are frequently encapsulated, whereas neurofibromas

usually are not [29]. However, this parameter is not reliable. In one study 30 % of all neurofibromas were found to be encapsulated and 30 % of all schwannomas nonencapsulated [12]. It has been suggested that the relationship between the nerve and the tumor is a more useful differential diagnostic tool [5, 12, 30, 31]. It was reported that in the case of a schwannoma the nerve could be seen along one side of the mass, whereas in a neurofibroma the nerve was either trapped within the tumor, or was obliterated by it and no longer visible [5, 12, 30, 31] (Figs. 20.7 and 20.9). Unfortunately the relationship between nerve and tumor suffers from a high interobserver variability. Some authors have questioned whether the location of a tumor in relationship to the nerve can be determined accurately, unless high resolution thin section images are used [102].

Characteristic MR imaging signs of PNSTs include the split fat sign, fascicular sign and associated muscle atrophy. The *split-fat sign* represents a rim of fat surrounding the tumor, due to the fact that the neurovascular bundle is normally surrounded by fat. The split fat sign is more common in benign PNSTs. The detection on MRI of a split-fat sign can be used as a criterion for differentiating benign from malignant PNSTs [69].

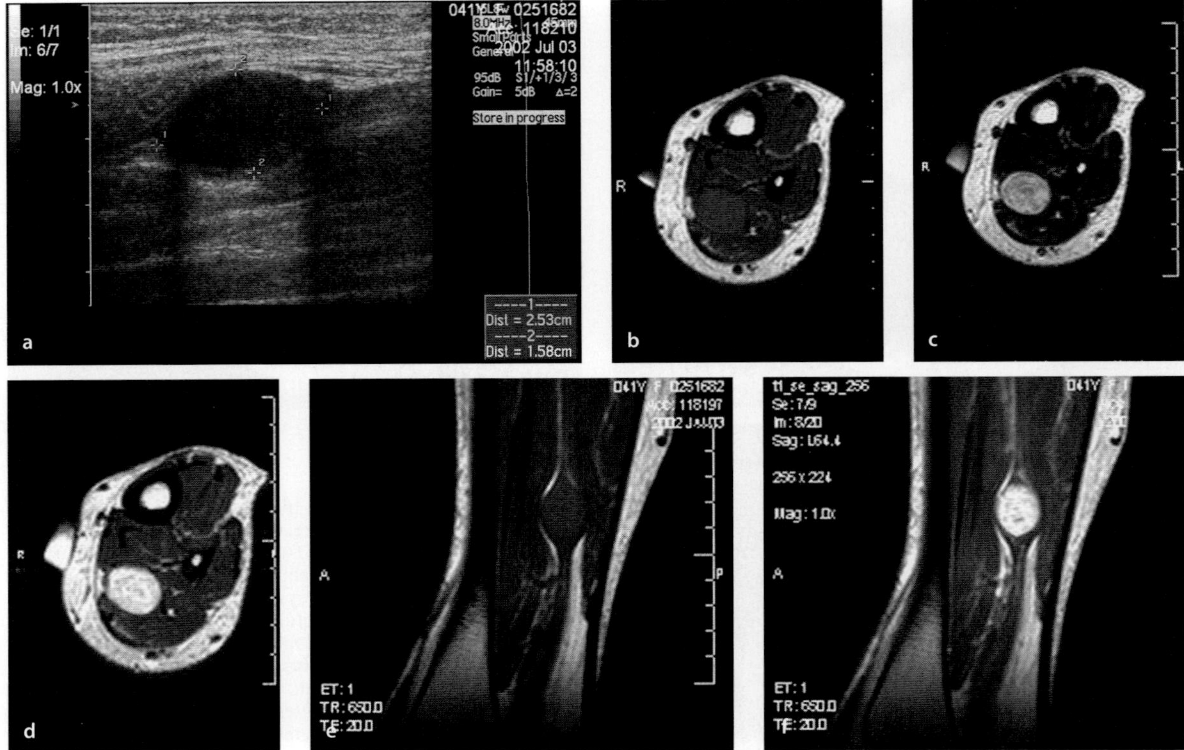

Fig. 20.5a–f. Benign schwannoma at the flexor surface of the left lower leg in a 41-year-old woman: **a** ultrasonography of the left lower leg; **b** axial spin echo T1-weighted MR image; **c** axial spin echo T2-weighted MR image; **d** axial spin echo T1-weighted MR image after gadolinium-contrast injection; **e** coronal spin echo T1-weighted MR image; **f** coronal spin echo T1-weighted MR image after gadolinium-contrast injection. A fusiform, sharply defined, homogeneously hyporeflective tumor is seen, in close relationship to the nerve at the flexor surface of the left lower leg (**a**). Axial T1-weighted image shows a well delineated, homogeneous, hypointense mass, isointense to the adjacent muscles (**b**). On a T2-weighted MR image the tumor has a high signal intensity with fascicular sign (**c**). Axial contrast-enhanced T1-weighted image shows an marked and homogeneous enhancement (**d**). Coronal T1-weighted image shows a well demarcated, fusiform mass with entering and exiting nerve, a split fat sign and an intense enhancement (**e,f**)

The *fascicular sign* represents multiple small ring-like structures (with higher signal intensity peripherally) on T2-weighted images, corresponding to fascicular bundles seen in neurogenic neoplasms [69]. The detection on MRI of the fascicular sign has been proposed as a criterion for differentiating schwannomas from neurofibromas. However, this parameter is not reliable for definitive differentiation [57].

The MR imaging characteristics of neurogenic tumors are not specific, and can be mimicked by other neoplasms. The most common mimickers are myxofibrosarcoma (formerly known as malignant fibrous histiocytoma) and metastases [102].

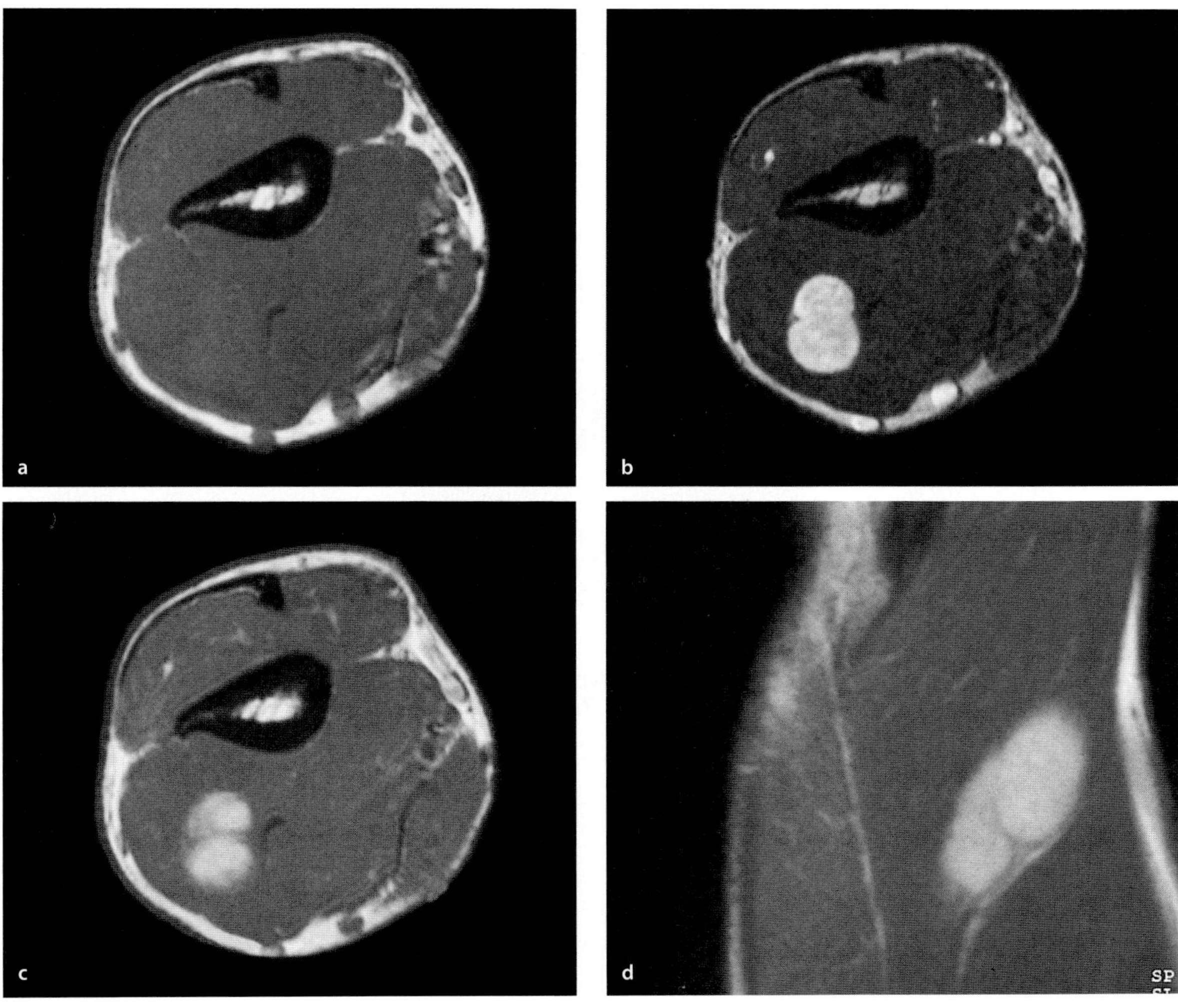

Fig. 20.6 a–d. Bilobed schwannoma of the upper arm in a 31-year-old man: **a** axial spin echo T1-weighted MR image through the right upper arm, 3 cm proximal to the elbow joint; **b** axial turbo spin echo T2-weighted MR image; **c** axial spin echo T1-weighted MR image after gadolinium-contrast injection; **d** sagittal spin echo T1-weighted MR image after gadolinium-contrast injection. On the T1-weighted MR image, the tumor is completely isointense to muscle and nearly indiscernible (**a**). On the T2-weighted MR image (**b**), the tumor is markedly hyperintense to muscle. After gadolinium injection (**c,d**), the tumor enhances homogeneously. Note the bilobed appearance, which is typical for a neurogenic tumor

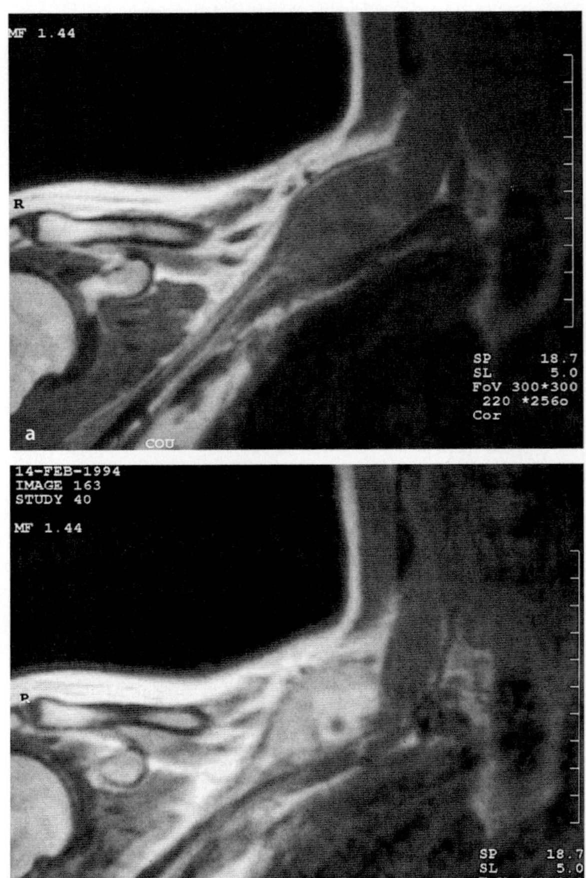

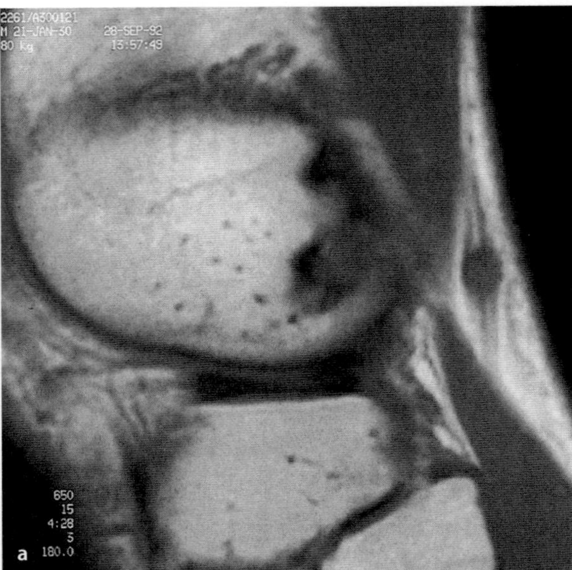

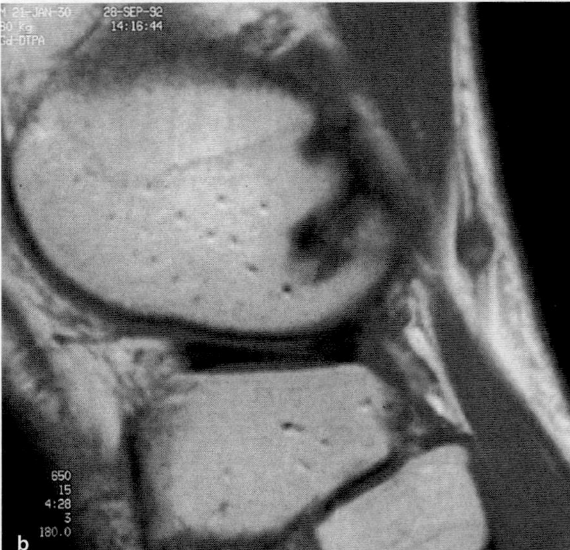

Fig. 20.7 a, b. Solitary schwannoma of the brachial plexus in a 24-year-old woman: **a** coronal spin echo T1-weighted MR image; **b** coronal T1-weighted MR image after gadolinium-contrast injection. A sharply defined, fusiform tumor of intermediate signal intensity is identified in the right brachial plexus (**a**). Note that the tumor is eccentric to the nerve trunk of origin, which is displaced upwards. After gadolinium injection, intense but inhomogeneous tumor enhancement is recognized. The tumor can now easily be discerned from the adjacent scalenus muscle (**b**). At surgery, an oblong, well circumscribed tumor was resected (7×5×3 cm), with slightly tapered edges. Histology established the diagnosis of a benign schwannoma (Antoni type B)

Fig. 20.8 a, b. Peripheral neurofibroma of the popliteal fossa in a 62-year-old man: **a** sagittal spin echo T1-weighted MR image; **b** sagittal spin echo T1-weighted MR image after Gd-contrast injection. There is a rounded lesion within the subcutaneous fat, presenting with homogeneous signal intensity and sharp margins. The lesion has a "bead on a string" appearance, and is situated along the course of the fibular nerve, with entering and exiting the nerve. On the precontrast images, it is isointense to muscle (**a**). After intravenous contrast administration, central enhancement is noted (**b**). The superficial localization in the subcutaneous fat and the relationship with the nerve are suggestive for a peripheral nerve sheath tumor

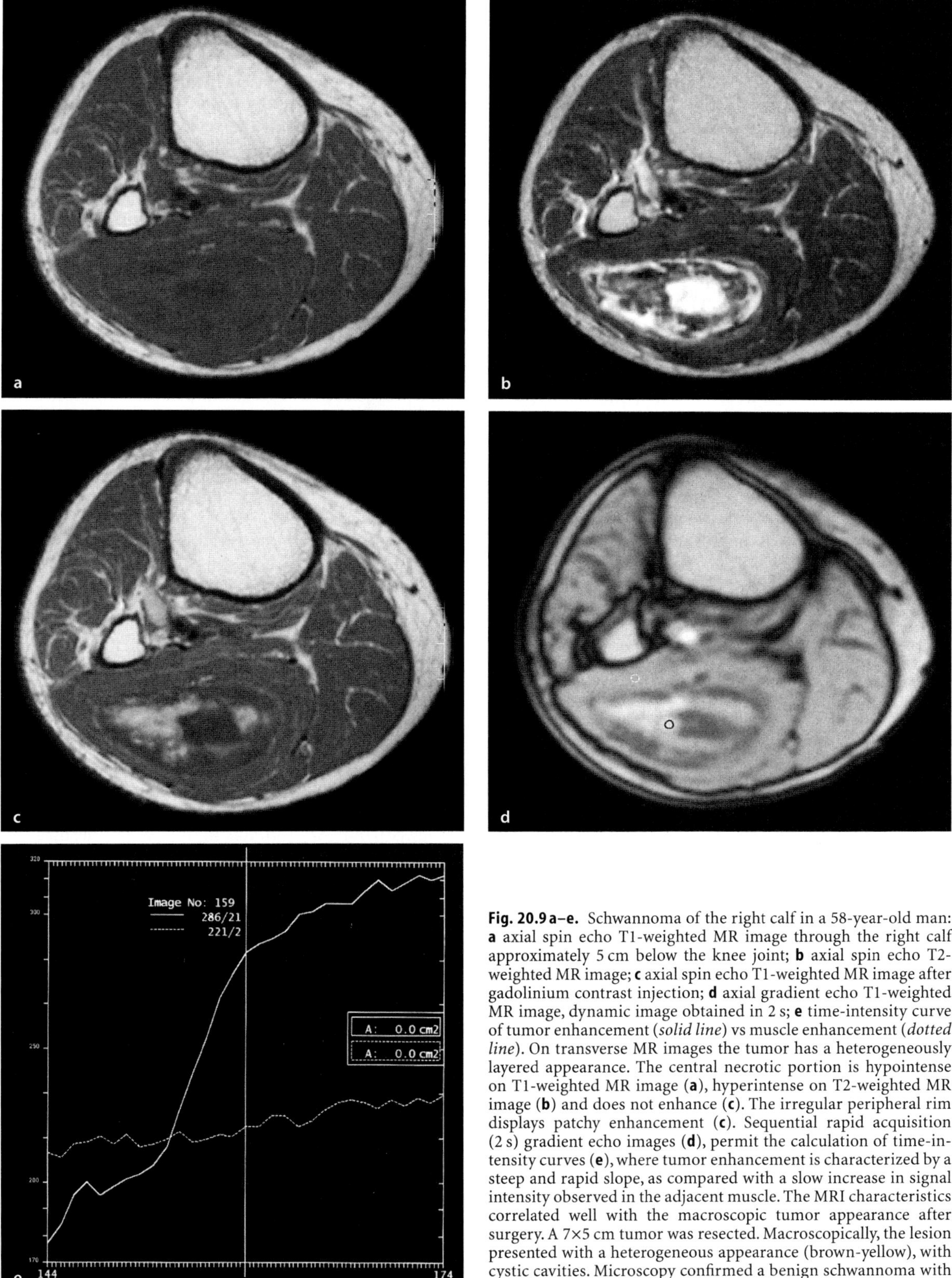

Fig. 20.9 a–e. Schwannoma of the right calf in a 58-year-old man: **a** axial spin echo T1-weighted MR image through the right calf approximately 5 cm below the knee joint; **b** axial spin echo T2-weighted MR image; **c** axial spin echo T1-weighted MR image after gadolinium contrast injection; **d** axial gradient echo T1-weighted MR image, dynamic image obtained in 2 s; **e** time-intensity curve of tumor enhancement (*solid line*) vs muscle enhancement (*dotted line*). On transverse MR images the tumor has a heterogeneously layered appearance. The central necrotic portion is hypointense on T1-weighted MR image (**a**), hyperintense on T2-weighted MR image (**b**) and does not enhance (**c**). The irregular peripheral rim displays patchy enhancement (**c**). Sequential rapid acquisition (2 s) gradient echo images (**d**), permit the calculation of time-intensity curves (**e**), where tumor enhancement is characterized by a steep and rapid slope, as compared with a slow increase in signal intensity observed in the adjacent muscle. The MRI characteristics correlated well with the macroscopic tumor appearance after surgery. A 7×5 cm tumor was resected. Macroscopically, the lesion presented with a heterogeneous appearance (brown-yellow), with cystic cavities. Microscopy confirmed a benign schwannoma with areas of ischemic hemorrhagic necrosis

20.3 Neurofibromas

20.3.1 Epidemiology

There is no obvious predilection for any racial or ethnic group to develop neurofibromas, and these lesions have been described throughout the world [46]. They represent approximately 5% of benign soft-tissue neoplasms. [67].

Three types of neurofibromas are classically described: localized, diffuse, and plexiform.

The *localized neurofibroma* variety is the most common, representing approximately 90% of these lesions, and the vast majority is solitary and not associated with NF-1 [22, 29]. They develop mostly between the ages of 20 and 30. Like schwannomas, they affect both sexes equally [75]. The *diffuse neurofibroma* is an uncommon but distinctive form of neurofibroma, that primarily affects children and young adults. The majority of diffuse neurofibromas are isolated lesions not associated with NF-1. *Plexiform neurofibromas* are essentially pathognomonic of NF-1 (see below), and development of these lesions usually occurs in early childhood. Neurogenic tumors in the setting of NF-1 constitute a special entity, because they are always a local expression of a larger, dispersed disorder [17].

20.3.2 Topography

Most localized, solitary neurofibromas are superficial lesions of cutis or subcutis (Fig. 20.8) [75]. Obviously, neurofibromas can also occur in conjunction with NF-1 [46]. Neurofibromas in NF-1 are relatively frequent on the trunk, which contrasts with the distribution of peripheral nerve schwannomas, which are more frequent in the extremities [98]. The diffuse neurofibromas demonstrate a plaque-like elevation of the skin with thickening of the entire subcutis. Plexiform neurofibromas may involve any or all of the following sites: cranial and spinal nerve roots and ganglia, the major nerves of the neck, trunk and limbs, including the sympathetic system and its ganglia, the subcutaneous branches of the major nerves and the visceral sympathetic plexuses [98]. Below the diaphragm, plexiform neurofibromas are typically located in the retroperitoneal space and paraspinal region [38]. Representative retroperitoneal localizations are (bilateral) parapsoatic and presacral neurofibromas. Less commonly, retroperitoneal neurofibromas are found in the region of the celiac axis and near the origin of the superior mesenteric artery [4].

Involvement of the myenteric plexuses and mesentery of the gastro-intestinal tract by plexiform neurofibromas is rare [38]. Neurofibromas in this location cause pain, intestinal bleeding and obstruction [42]. The regional nerves are enlarged and nodules of varying size are found, especially in Auerbach's plexus. The most common site is the jejunum, followed by the stomach [49].

20.3.3 Histology

Typically, the solitary neurofibroma (Table 20.1) is a benign, slowly growing, and variably encapsulated neoplasm, originating in a nerve [12, 46, 75]. Neurofibromas are intimately associated with the parent nerve, growing in a longitudinal fusiform manner with the nerve "entering and exiting" from the lesion. Surgical resection requires sacrificing the parent nerve because the neurofibroma cannot be separated from the nerve fibers [25].

As opposed to schwannomas, most neurofibromas are solid tumors macroscopically. Areas of cystic degeneration, hypocellularity and xanthomatous material are uncommon. Calcifications and ossification occur more frequently in neurofibromas than in schwannomas [47, 98]. Neural axons traversing the tumor often follow a tortuous course [46]. As in schwannomas, the capacity of neurofibromas for melanogenesis, although rare, has been well documented [2, 6, 21, 46, 74, 87, 89].

Table 20.1. Comparative pathology of schwannoma and neurofibroma

	Schwannoma	Neurofibroma
Cell type	Schwann cells	Schwann cells and fibroblasts
Capsule	Usually encapsulated	Usually nonencapsulated
Extension along nerve bundle	Focal	Infiltrative growth
Tumor shape	Round or fusiform	Fusiform
Tumor topography	Eccentric tumor Displacing tissue along axis nerve	Central Separates tissue
Intratumoral cysts	Common	Rare
Intratumoral necrosis	Common	Rare
Intratumoral hemorrhage	Common	Rare
Malignant degeneration	None	More frequent
Blood supply	Thickened arteries, prominent veins	No thickened arteries, no prominent vessels

Plexiform neurofibroma relates to a diffuse enlargement and distortion of a major nerve trunk. Disorganized growth of nerves is noticed within and occasionally also outside the nerve trunk [75]. Multiple masses are found along the course of nerve bundles or trunks, with irregular cylindrical enlargement of the affected nerves [107]. Fusiform or spherical neurofibromas along their course can produce a moniliform effect, or sometimes give rise to massive growths of a similar character [98].

Many tumors have a central zone composed of tightly packed eosinophilic fibers with a highly cellular component and sparse non-fibrillary stromal substance (such as myxoid material). The peripheral zone is composed of loosely arranged eosinophilic fibers with less cellular components but abundant nonfibrillary stromal material. This histologic pattern is called a zonal distinction [107]. This concept is important to understand because it is presumed to be the histologic correlate of the so-called 'target-appearance' of neurofibromas on CT and MR imaging studies.

20.3.4 Clinical Presentation

Solitary neurofibroma presents as a relatively non-tender mass in the skin or subcutaneous tissue. It is somewhat movable and moderately firm but compressible. An isolated neurofibroma in the skin usually does not exhibit an associated local change in pigmentation of the skin, although hyper- or hypopigmentation is possible. If a solitary neurofibroma occurs along the course of a peripheral nerve, the clinical symptoms are usually related to a space-occupying lesion but can be much the same as those described for schwannoma [46].

The clinical presentation of NF-associated neurofibroma will be discussed below (see Sect. 20.5).

20.3.5 Imaging Characteristics

20.3.5.1 Plain Radiography

The appearance of neurofibromas on plain radiography is similar to that of schwannomas.

20.3.5.2 Ultrasound

Like schwannomas, neurofibromas are hypoechoic (Fig. 20.10) [9, 13, 36, 50, 52]. High frequency ultrasound can visualize the junction between the hypoechoic tumor and the parent nerve [36]. Neurofibromas are often elongated along the nerve axis and lobulated. Nevertheless, there is a considerable overlap between the appearance on ultrasound of schwannomas and neurofibromas [37]. Neurofibromas tend to be less sharply delineated. Like schwannomas, they do not always show distal acoustic enhancement [13, 36, 50].

20.3.5.3 CT

On unenhanced CT scans neurofibromas mostly appear as hypodense lesions, due to the presence of Schwann cells, neural elements and adipocytes. Occasionally, hyperdense areas are found in neurofibromas, and this feature is uncommon in schwannomas. They are believed to result from dense bands of collagen tissue, produced by fibroblasts [63]. On enhanced CT scans, neurofibromas usually show little or no contrast uptake (Fig. 20.10). More than half of neurofibromas remain hypodense after contrast injection [14]. In some cases, ill-defined, cloudy areas of enhancement are found (Fig. 20.11). Retroperitoneal plexiform neurofibromas are usually bilateral and symmetric. They display special imaging characteristics on contrast-enhanced CT. They are mostly homogeneously hypodense, but unusual swirling and serpiginous patterns of increased attenuation superimposed on a low attenuation background have been described [4]. No calcification is identified. Generally, plexiform neurofibromas have well-defined margins, but in some cases, the margins are indistinct, suggesting possible infiltration into the iliopsoas muscle. Such apparent infiltration should not be considered indicative of malignancy [4]. Bilateral parapsoas or presacral masses are characteristic for retroperitoneal plexiform neurofibromas, corresponding to the distribution of the lumbosacral plexus [1]. Nevertheless rare cases of unilateral retroperitoneal plexiform neurofibroma have been reported [20, 88, 95]. This pattern is apparently a less common manifestation of the disease.

The bilaterally symmetric nature of retroperitoneal neurofibromas facilitates differentiation from malignant nerve sheath neoplasms. Some authors have demonstrated that when bilateral lesions are present, asymmetry in axial diameter of more than 2 cm, and asymmetric attenuation pattern are always associated with malignant tumors [4]. When assessing a unilateral retroperitoneal mass, distinction of malignant versus benign behavior is unreliable by imaging criteria [4].

CT findings of multiple soft-tissue nodules within the mesentery, distributed along the course of peripheral nerves, and wall thickening of the affected bowel loops can suggest a diagnosis of plexiform neurofibromatosis in patients with NF-1. In contrast to the solitary mass lesion, there is normal appearing fatty tissue trapped between the small nodules. Differential diagnosis includes: Crohn's disease, ileocecal lymphoma, carcinoid, intraperitoneal seeding of malignancy, mesenteric panniculitis, and tuberculosis [38, 109].

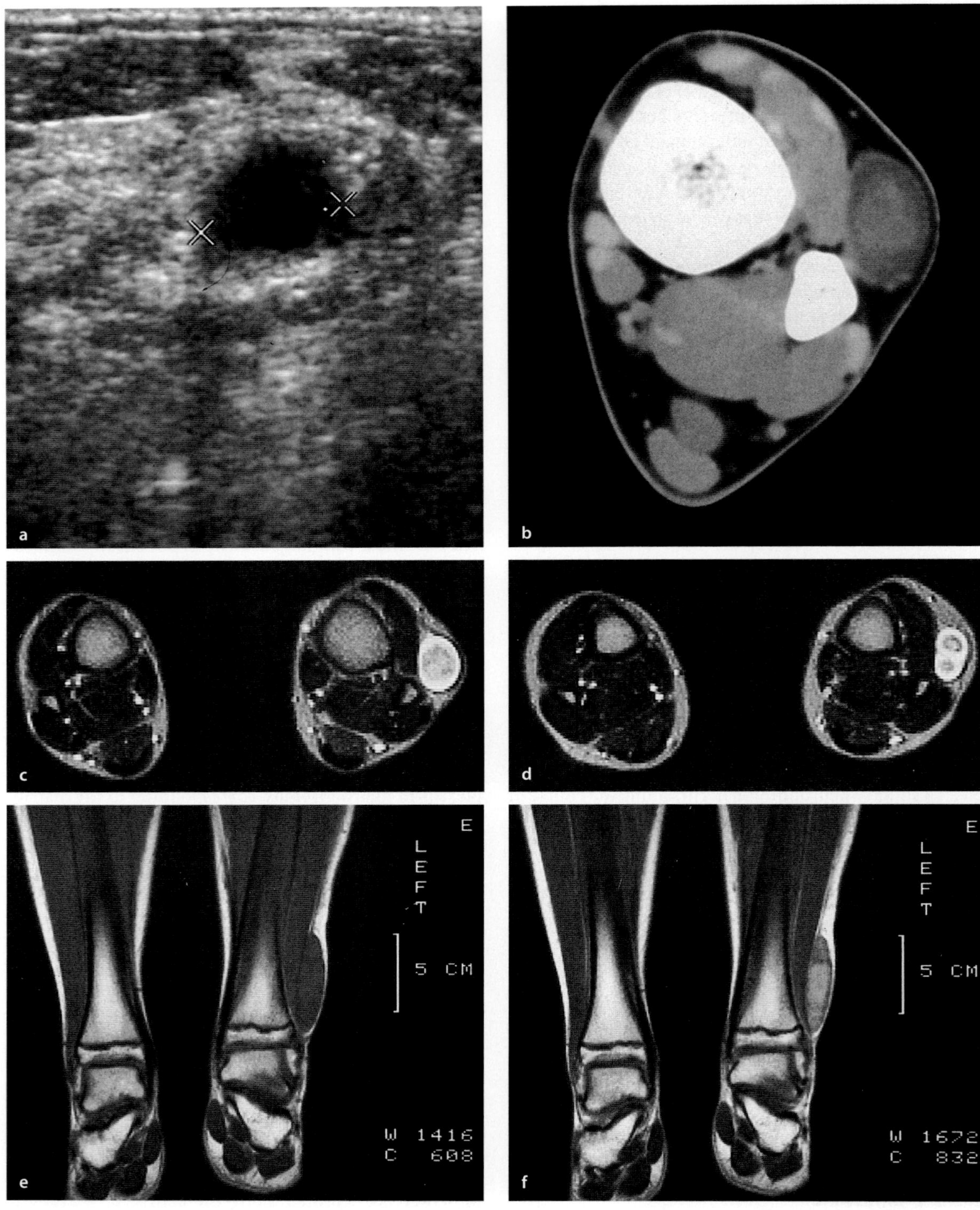

Fig. 20.10 a–f. Neurofibroma of the cutaneous tributary of the left superficial fibular nerve in a 14-year-old boy: **a** axial ultrasound image 8 cm proximal to the left fibular malleolus; **b** CT scan after iodinated-contrast injection, proximal to the left ankle joint; **c** axial spin echo T2-weighted MR image 7 cm proximal to the ankle joints; **d** axial spin echo T2-weighted MR image 3 cm proximal to the ankle joints; **e** coronal spin echo T1-weighted MR image; **f** coronal spin echo T1-weighted MR image after gadolinium-contrast injection. This young man presented with a painful mass above the left lateral malleolus. Ultrasound examination showed a well circumscribed anechoic mass (**a**). Contrast -enhanced CT scan confirmed the mass lesion in the subcutaneous fat next to the extensor digitorum longus muscle. The central part of the lesion shows a slightly higher density than the peripheral rim (target appearance) (**b**). Axial T2-weighted MR image confirms the target appearance, with a central area of moderately high signal intensity surrounded by a rim of extremely high signal intensity. In the inferior part of the lesion, there is a bifurcation (**c, d**). On the T1-weighted MR image, the tumor is isointense relative to muscle (**e**). After gadolinium injection, the central part of the tumor enhances (**f**). Histology revealed a neurofibroma

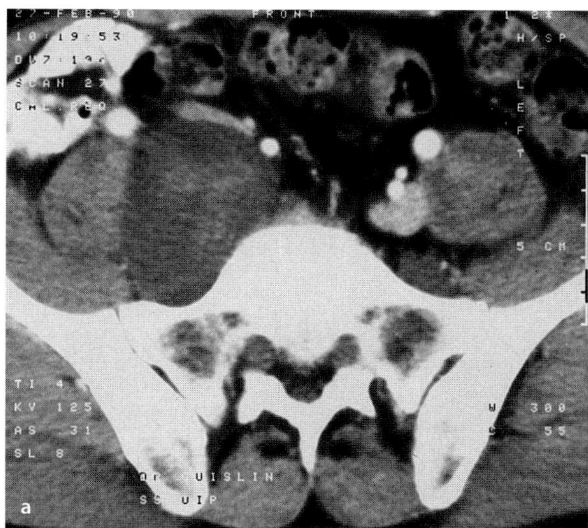
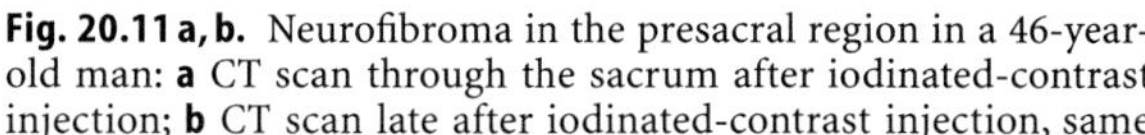
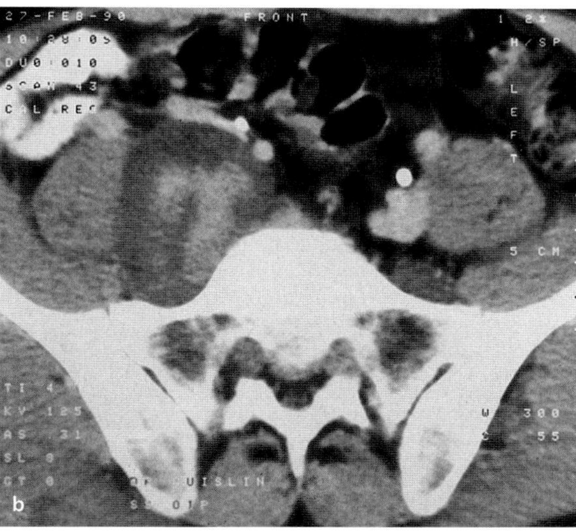

Fig. 20.11a, b. Neurofibroma in the presacral region in a 46-year-old man: **a** CT scan through the sacrum after iodinated-contrast injection; **b** CT scan late after iodinated-contrast injection, same level as (**a**). On the early phase contrast CT, the tumor is predominantly hypodense, relative to muscle tissue (**a**). Late after contrast, ill-defined, cloudy areas of enhancement are seen (**b**)

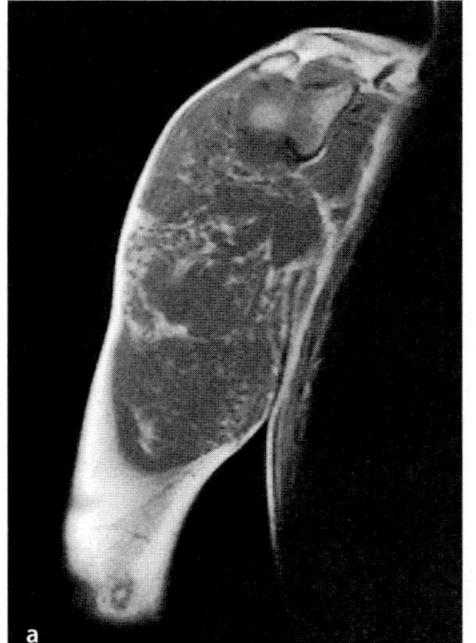
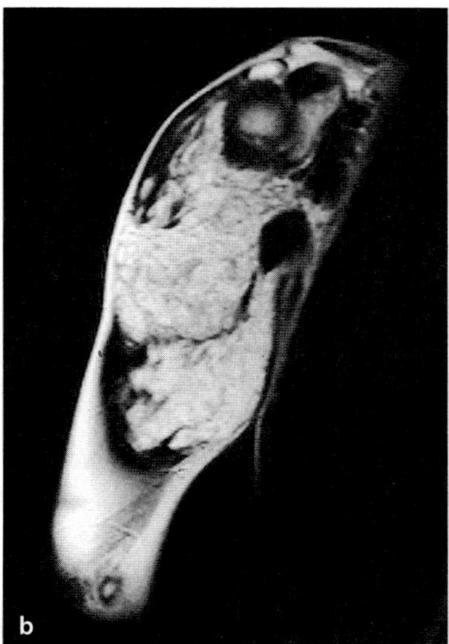
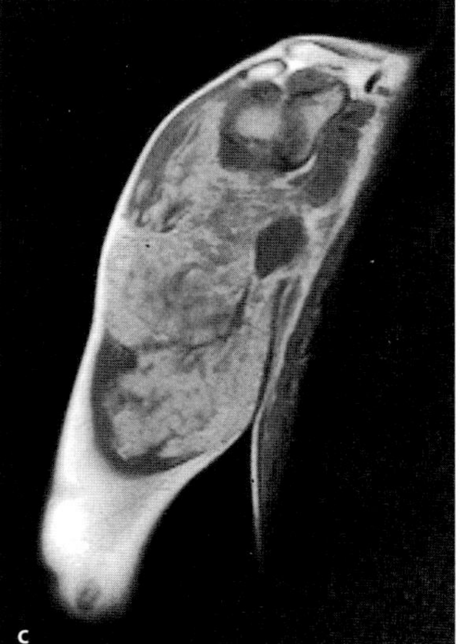
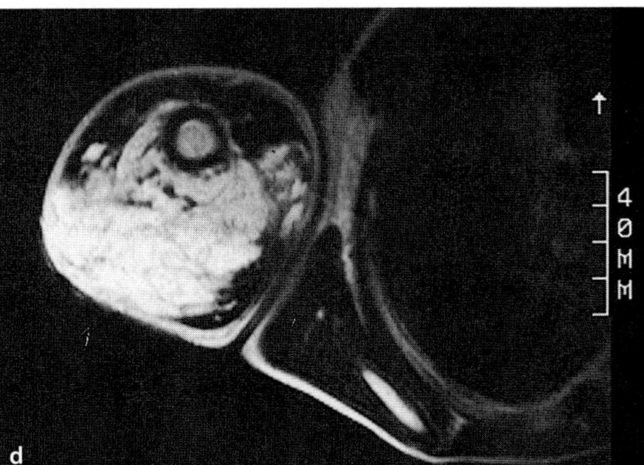

Fig. 20.12a–d. Neurofibroma of the right upper arm in an 11-year-old boy: **a** coronal spin echo T1-weighted MR image through the posterior compartment of the right upper arm; **b** coronal turbo spin echo T2-weighted MR image; **c** coronal spin echo T1-weighted MR image after gadolinium contrast injection; **d** axial turbo spin echo T2-weighted MR image. A large heterogeneous tumor is seen in the posterior muscle group of the right upper arm. On the precontrast T1-weighted MR image, the tumor is isointense with muscle, and is interspersed with fatty tissue (**a**). On the T2-weighted MR images, the lesion is hyperintense throughout (**b, d**). After contrast administration, there is heterogeneous enhancement of the tumor (**c**). The lesion occurred in the clinical setting of NF-1. Note the invasion of multiple muscles by the neoplasm

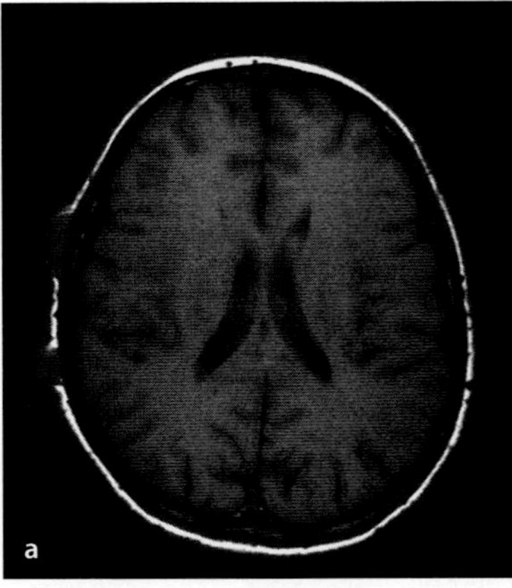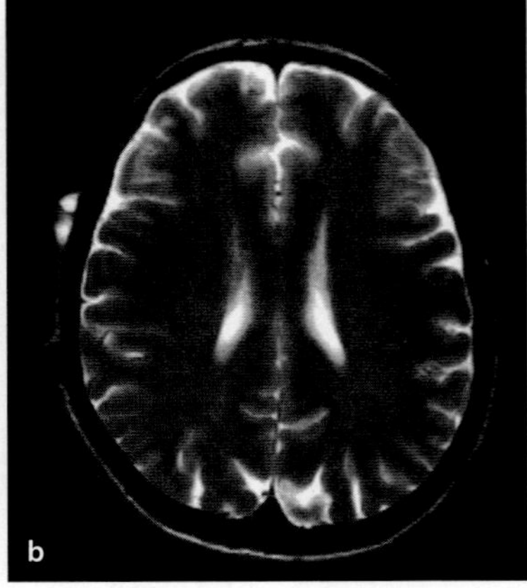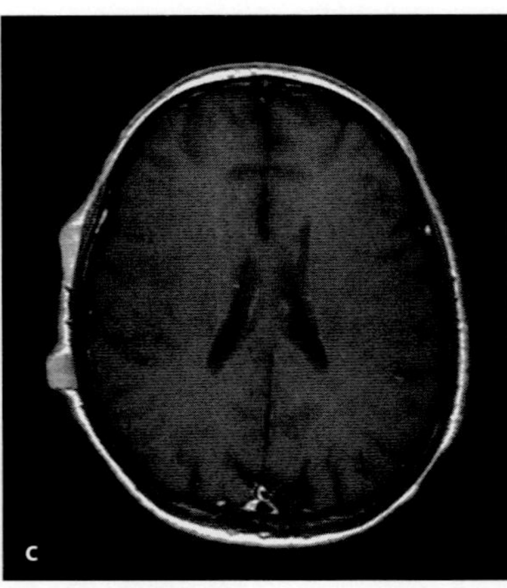

Fig. 20.13 a–c. Subcutaneous neurofibromas in a 41-year-old woman with NF-1: **a** axial spin echo T1-weighted MR image through the brain; **b** axial turbo spin echo T2-weighted MR image (same level); **c** contrast-enhanced axial spin echo T1-weighted MR image (same level). There are two subcutaneous nodules in the right frontal and parietal region (*arrows*). The lesions are sharply demarcated and are hypointense relative to the subcutaneous fatty tissue (**a**). On a T2-weighted scan, the anterior nodule is hyperintense and appears bilobed; the posterior nodule is iso- to hypointense, presumably reflecting fibrous cellular tissue (**b**). After intravenous injection of gadolinium contrast, both lesions enhance, indicating a vascular supply (**c**). Note that the underlying temporalis muscle enhances to a much lesser degree (**c**)

20.3.5.4 MRI

Neurofibromas display an intermediate signal intensity on T1-weighted MR images, i.e. they are isointense or slightly hyperintense to muscle (Figs. 20.9, 20.10 and 20.12). On proton density-weighted images, they are hyperintense to muscle tissue. On T2-weighted scans, neurofibromas are usually hyperintense (Figs. 20.11 and 20.12). This provides a sharp contrast difference between the hyperintense nerve sheath tumor, medium intensity fat, and lower intensity muscles [8]. They can display a salt-and-pepper appearance on T2-weighted images, though this so-called fascicular sign is more common in schwannomas [57, 103]. Central areas of decreased signal intensity may be due to condensations of relatively fibrous cellular tissue (decreased amount of intercellular water) (Fig. 20.12b). Cystic or pseudocystic transformation is less common in neurofibromas than in schwannomas. After intravenous injection of gadolinium, the enhancement pattern is variable. In our experience, approximately two-thirds enhance inhomogeneously (Fig. 20.11), while one-third enhance brightly and uniformly. A dumbbell-shape is characteristic for spinal nerve root neurofibromas, which may enlarge the neuroforamen. Another typical feature is a fusiform shape oriented longitudinally in the nerve distribution.

■ **Target-appearance.** Neurofibromas can display a "target-appearance". On T2-weighted MR images, the target appearance is characterized by a peripheral rim of increased signal intensity, while the central part of the tumor is less hyperintense (Fig. 20.10). This pattern corresponds to a distinctive zonal histologic appearance that can be found in neurofibromas [107]. The high signal-intensity in the peripheral zone may be related to more myxoid tissue with high water content. The central area of lower signal intensity is probably related to the amount of dense collagen and fibrillary tissue which causes T2 shortening [107]. The target appearance on T2-weighted scans is suggestive of neurofibroma ($p<0.05$), though it can also occur in schwannomas (58% in neurofibromas vs 15% in schwannomas) [57]. On Gd-enhanced studies, the target appearance is reflected by the more intense central enhancement. Central enhancement is equally suggestive of neurofibroma, since this finding is much less common in schwannomas (75 vs 8%) [57]. The combination of both findings, i.e. target appearance on T2-weighted scans and central enhancement pattern is useful in differentiating neurofibromas from schwannomas (63 vs 3%) [57, 95].

Some of the more peripheral neurofibromas have a mixed signal intensity. The target-pattern may not be seen in very small lesions. Likewise, it can be absent in large tumors and lesions with cystic, hemorrhagic, or necrotic degeneration, though these features are relatively uncommon in neurofibromas (Fig. 20.14). Prior surgical intervention or malignant change can also disturb the zonal architecture [107, 111].

The target appearance can also occur in schwannomas, be it much less frequently. As a rule, MPNST do not exhibit such a target pattern on MRI.

In conclusion, the target pattern is an indication of the benign character of the lesion, and exhibits a high specificity for benign peripheral nerve sheath tumors.

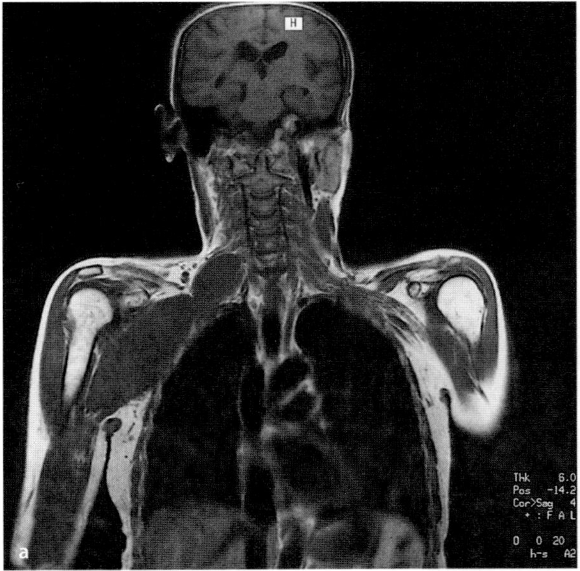

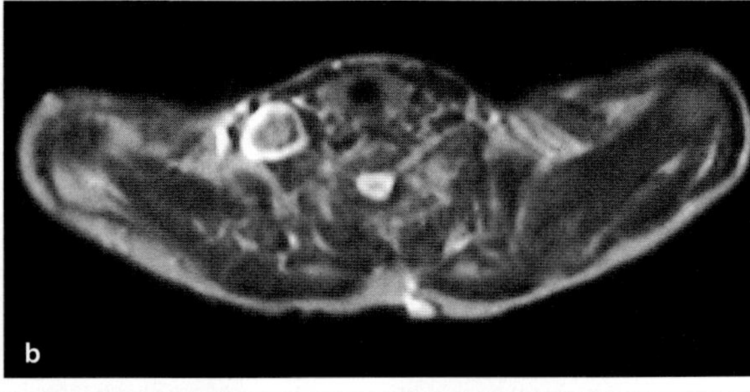

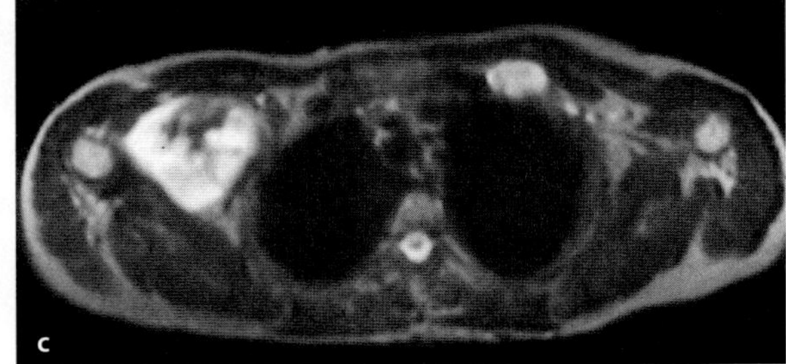

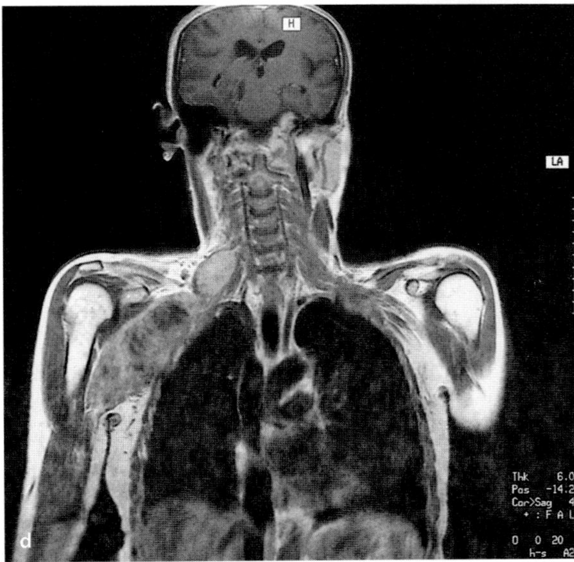

Fig. 20.14 a–d. Neurofibroma of the right axilla in a 33-year-old woman with NF-1: **a** coronal spin echo T1-weighted MR image through the thorax; **b** axial spin echo T2-weighted MR image through the supraclavicular fossa; **c** axial spin echo T2-weighted MR image through the axilla; **d** coronal spin echo T1-weighted MR image after gadolinium contrast injection. A large, bilobed tumor extends along the nerves of the right brachial plexus. There is a small tumor nodule in the supraclavicular fossa and a large fusiform mass extending into the right axilla (**a**). On the T2-weighted MR images, the small nodule in the supraclavicular fossa shows a typical target appearance with peripheral hyperintense rim, whereas the large lesion in the right axilla shows a much more heterogeneous internal architecture. Note the presence of a third lesion in the anterior chest wall on the left (**b, c**). After intravenous gadolinium contrast administration, there is predominantly central enhancement of the small supraclavicular tumor, and heterogeneous enhancement of the right axillary tumor (**d**). The lesions occurred in the clinical setting of NF-1

Unfortunately it has a low sensitivity, and it does not reliably allow differentiation between a schwannoma and a neurofibroma. It should be kept in mind that, even for the pathologist, it is sometimes difficult to distinguish a neurofibroma from a schwannoma. Thus it is not surprising that MR signal intensity patterns may be similar in these lesions [111].

According to some authors, tumor capsule and relationship of the tumor with the nerve can be used as a criterion to differentiate between neurofibromas and schwannomas. For this we refer to Sect. 20.2.5.4.

20.4 Malignant Peripheral Nerve Sheath Tumors

20.4.1 Epidemiology

MPNST (Fig. 20.15) represent about 6 % of all malignant soft tissue tumors [62]. In sporadic cases of MPNST, the sex ratio is approximately equal, whereas in the setting of NF-1, MPNST are four times more frequent in men than in women [75]. The mean age of incidence of MPNST is 42 years, with 80 % of all cases occurring between ages 17 and 70 [62]. In up to 50 % of MPNST, an association with NF-1 is found [24, 43, 46, 75, 104]. On the other hand only a small fraction of patients with NF-1 (approximately 5 %) develop MPNST.

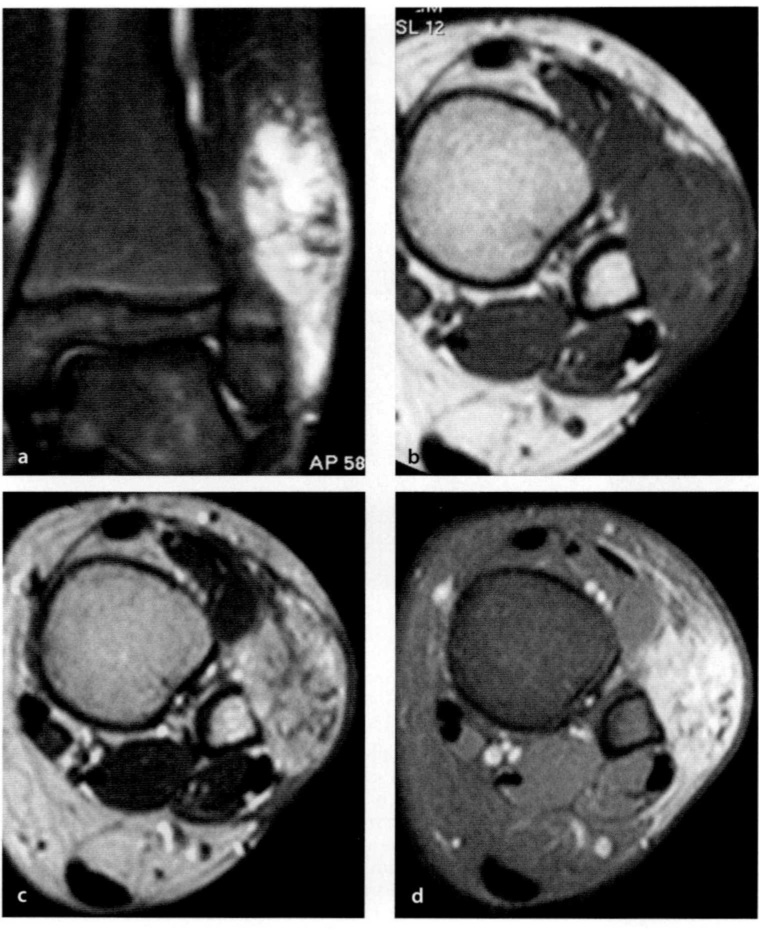

Fig. 20.15 a–d. Fast growing MPNST of left ankle in a middle aged man: **a** coronal STIR T2-weighted MR image; **b** axial T1-weighted MR image; **c** axial contrast-enhanced T1-weighted MR image; **d** axial fat-suppressed contrast-enhanced T1-weighted MR image. There is a large, fusiform, ill defined soft tissue mass at the left ankle, with some perilesional edema (**a**). The tumor is heterogeneous and hypointense with cortical bone invasion at the distal fibula (**b**). The contrast enhanced MR images show an inhomogeneous enhancement with ill-defined tumor margins maybe due to perilesional lymphangitis (**c, d**). Histology showed a MPNST originating from the peroneal nerve

MPNST can develop as a possible delayed sequel of radiation therapy. One study showed 11 % of all MPNST to be post-radiation sarcomas [24]. The mean latency period ranges from 5 to 40 years [23, 24, 35]. The simultaneous presence of NF-1 does not seem to be an influencing factor [24].

20.4.2 Topography

MPNST have a propensity to occur in the proximal limbs and trunks [75]. They typically affect the large nerves of the neck, and proximal extremities (including the sciatic nerve, brachial plexus and sacral plexus), as well as the retroperitoneum, mediastinum and viscera [87] (Fig. 20.15). In a landmark review study on malignant soft tissue tumors, 775 malignant schwannomas were registered with the following distribution according to their anatomic location: lower extremity (25 %), trunk (17 %), upper extremity (12 %), head and neck region (11 %), proximal limb girdle (9 %), retroperitoneum (8 %), hips and buttocks (8 %), foot and ankle (4 %), hand and wrist (3 %), other (7 %) [65]. Primary intraosseous origin of malignant peripheral nerve sheath tumors is exceedingly rare, particularly involving a long bone; such lesions most commonly arise from the mandible [108].

However, tumor topography must not be used as a differential diagnostic criterion, since many other malignant soft tissue tumors, and notably myxofibrosarcoma, display a similar pattern of anatomic distribution. MPNST complicating NF-1 usually arise from one of the large peripheral nerves. Those originating from the intracranial nerves are quite exceptional [98].

20.4.3 Histology

By definition, a malignant nerve sheath tumor is a malignant neoplasm of nerve sheath origin that locally infiltrates and also metastasizes. It can develop in an unaltered nerve or in a neurofibroma. Many of the malignant tumors arising from, or in association with neurofibromas in NF-1, are indistinguishable from fibrosarcomas of soft tissue [46]. It is estimated that between 5 and 13 % of neurofibromas in NF-1 eventually become malignant. Conversely, malignant transformation of schwannomas is extremely rare [87].

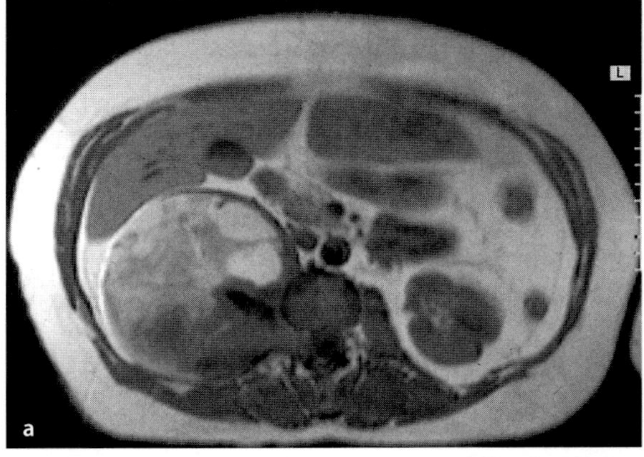

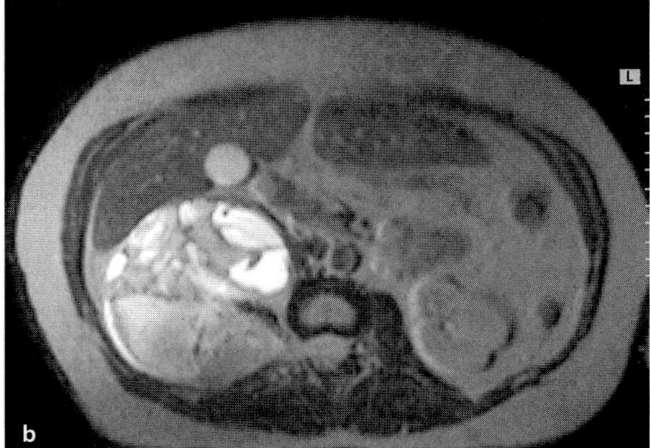

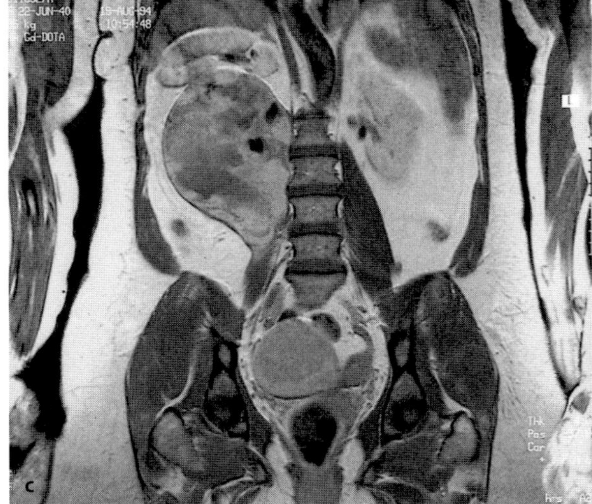

Fig. 20.16 a–c. Parapsoas MPNST in a 54-year-old woman; **a** axial spin echo T1-weighted MR image; **b** axial spin echo T2-weighted MR image; **c** coronal T1-weighted MR image after gadolinium contrast injection. This large, solitary tumor appears to arise from the right intervertebral foramen at L1-L2 (**a, b**). The tumor is markedly heterogeneous with different signal intensity components. Dark areas correspond to calcifications. After contrast (**c**), enhancement is heterogeneous. Note the relationship with the right psoas muscle, and the upward displacement of the right kidney. Histology showed a MPNST with heterologous elements (ossification)

MPNST are microscopically well circumscribed to multinodular masses with fascicles resembling fibrosarcoma. The alternation of sharply demarcated hypercellular and hypocellular zones causes a marbled appearance. Areas of tumor necrosis are common. Divergent differentiation is frequently seen leading to heterologous elements such as bone (Fig. 20.15), cartilage, skeletal muscle (rhabdomyoblastic), and epithelium (glandular or squamous). MPNST with rhabdomyoblastic differentiation are named: "malignant Triton tumor" [7, 19, 24, 31, 80, 112]. These neoplasms are not infrequently associated with NF-1 [115].

20.4.4 Clinical Presentation

Like other sarcomas, MPNST present as enlarging masses that are usually noted several months before the diagnosis is made. Symptoms rarely antedate the detection of a mass.

Clinical manifestations of sarcomatous degeneration of a neurofibroma are not specific. Though pain can herald malignancy, it is also a very common feature of benign neurofibromas. Therefore the presence of pain cannot be used as an indicator of malignancy [16]. MPNST originating from major nerves can also cause other symptoms of sensory or motor nerve deficit, such as paresthesias and weakness [24].

Sudden enlargement of a pre-existing neurofibroma in the setting of NF-1 should be viewed with great suspicion of malignant transformation and lead to immediate diagnostic imaging. When imaging findings indicate an aggressive lesion, biopsy should be performed to exclude malignant transformation of a neurofibroma [75, 114]. As a general rule, biopsy must not be performed without the benefit of prior imaging studies. The tumor carries a higher mortality when it occurs in patients with NF-1, with a poor five-year survival rate of 15–30%, compared to 75% for the solitary form [29].

The aggressive nature of MPNST is evidenced by their tendency to local recurrence after resection [41, 43]. Metastasis, accounting for most of the disease-associated mortality, usually ensues within two years of initial diagnosis and is most common in the lungs, followed by other sites such as liver, subcutis and bone [41, 43, 75] (Fig. 20.16).

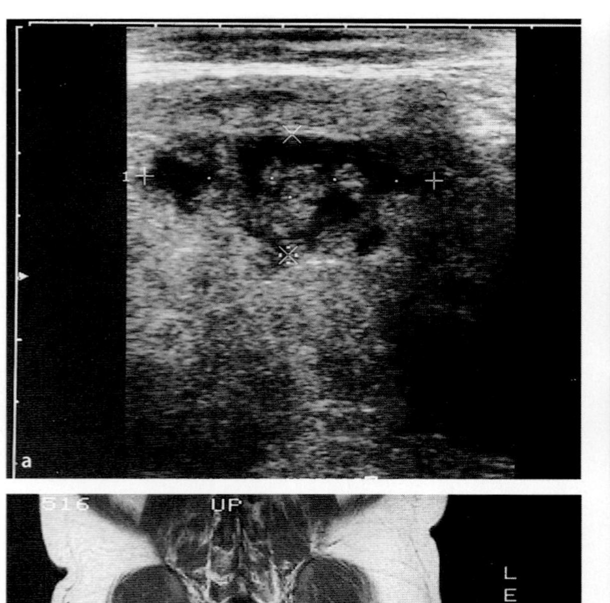
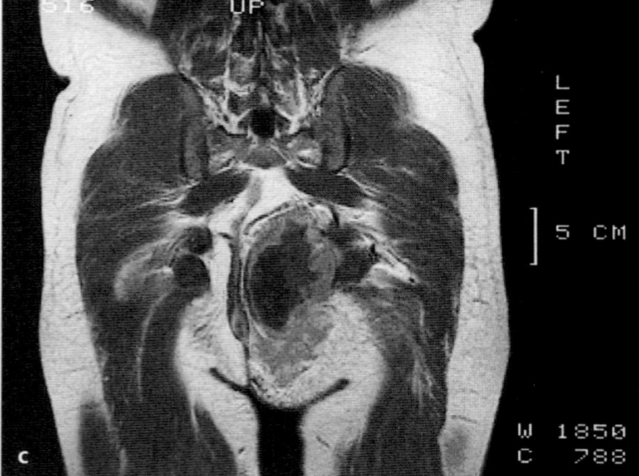
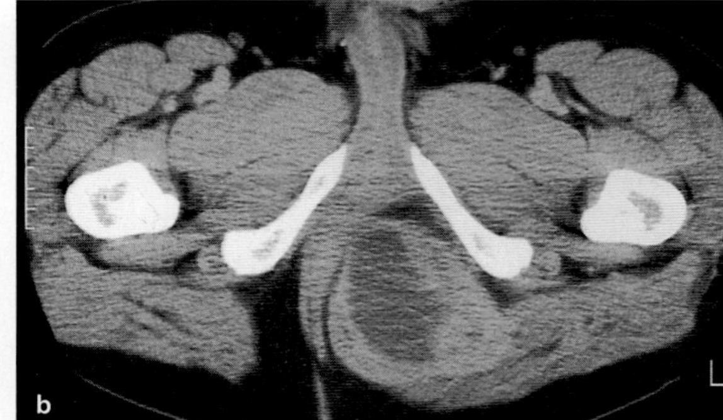
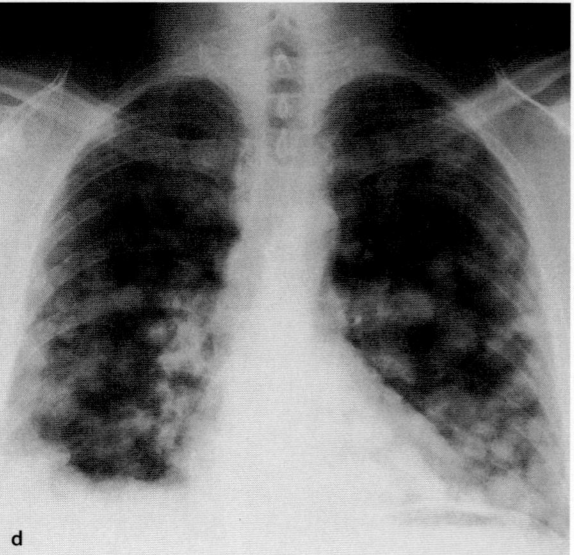

Fig. 20.17 a–d. MPNST in the left ischiorectal fossa in a 45-year-old man: **a** ultrasonography of the left buttock; **b** CT scan of the pelvis after iodinated contrast injection; **c** coronal spin echo T1-weighted MR image after gadolinium contrast injection; **d** chest radiograph, ten months later. A markedly heterogeneous tumor is identified in the left ischiorectal fossa, medial and deep to the gluteus maximus muscle. The lesion contains hypoechoic foci, presumably reflecting necrosis (**a**). This appearance is confirmed by CT scan (**b**). The maximum diameter of the tumor is 7.5 cm. The gadolinium enhanced MR image shows irregular tumor enhancement peripherally, whereas the central necrotic portions do not enhance (**c**). Chest radiograph ten months later, shows multiple lung metastases ("lâcher des ballons") (**d**)

20.4.5 Imaging Characteristics

20.4.5.1 Plain Radiography

Radiological findings of bone erosion and destruction do not necessarily imply that the tumor is malignant, as they can also occur with benign nerve sheath tumors [61, 98]. However, when osseous changes are seen in a patient with NF-1, immediate further investigation is needed because of the known propensity of these patients to develop MPNST [43].

20.4.5.2 CT and MRI

MPNSTs share common imaging findings with other neurogenic tumors: fusiform shape, longitudinal orientation along the parent nerve. CT and MRI offer little help in demonstrating the malignant nature of peripheral nerve sheath tumors [17]. On T1-weighted images, MPNST are isointense or slightly hyperintense compared to muscle. On proton density-weighted images, MPNST tend to be hyperintense to muscle tissue, whereas on T2-weighted images, the signal intensity is markedly increased [8]. The internal structure of the tumor can be heterogeneous and irregular, corresponding pathologically to areas of necrosis [8]. Criteria that can be of help in establishing the diagnosis of MPNST include [16, 63, 78, 113]:

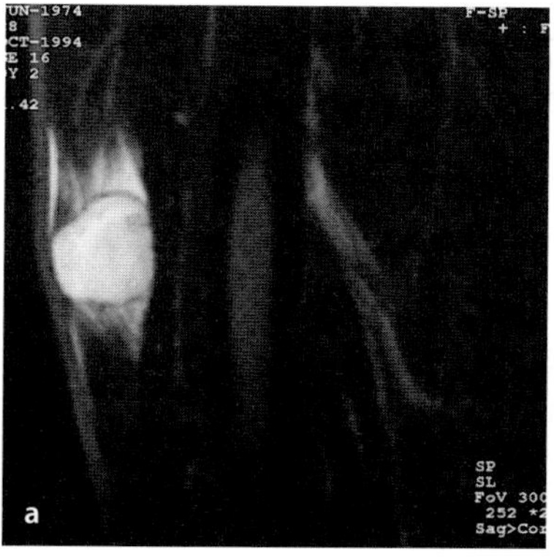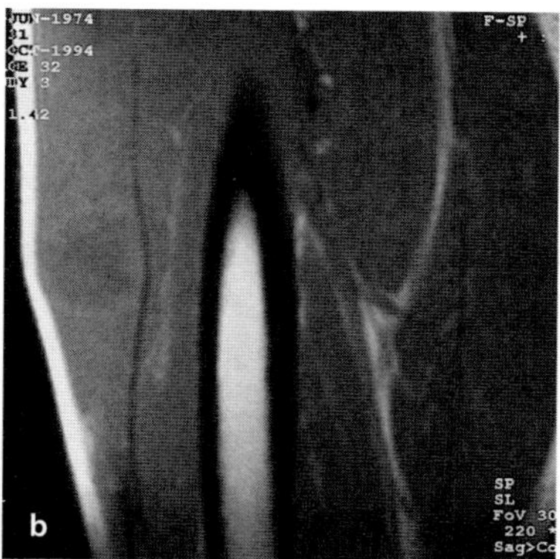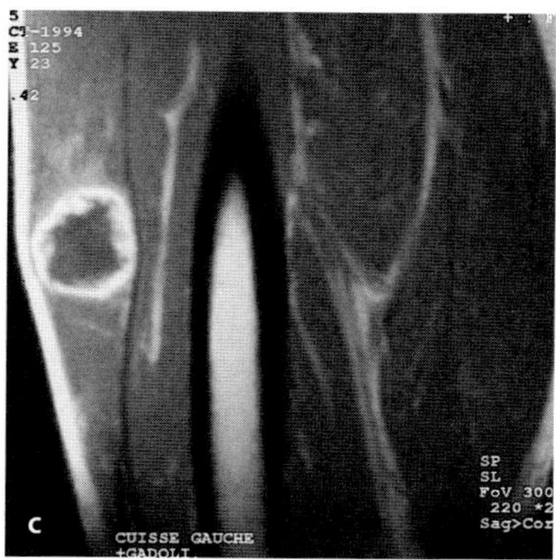

Fig. 20.18 a–c. MPNST in a 20-year-old man: **a** sagittal fat-suppressed short tau turbo inversion recovery MR image; **b** sagittal spin echo T1-weighted MR image; **c** sagittal spin echo T1-weighted MR image after gadolinium contrast injection. A nodular tumor is identified in the left rectus femoris muscle. The tumor is encapsulated, but is surrounded by a halo of edema (**a**). Before contrast, the lesion is almost isointense to muscle (**b**). After gadolinium contrast injection, there is enhancement of a peripheral capsule-like structure (**c**), while the central necrotic part of the tumor does not enhance. Note that the tumor is similar in appearance to a benign schwannoma (see Fig. 20.19), except for the perilesional edema, which is unusual in benign tumors

- A large mass (>5 cm) with compression of adjacent structures
- Inhomogeneous tumor architecture, usually resulting from hemorrhage or necrosis (Figs. 11.1, 11.2 and 20.14)
- Ill-defined margins (Fig. 20.14)
- Invasion of fat planes or neighboring structures (Fig. 11.1)
- Perilesional edema (Figs. 20.14 and 20.17)
- Irregular bone destruction (Fig. 20.14)
- Involvement of lymph nodes
- Pleural effusion

Calcification is more commonly associated with malignant lesions, but can also be present in ancient schwannomas (Fig. 20.18).

These criteria are by no means absolute, and many difficulties remain [64]. MPNST and benign peripheral nerve sheath tumors can be astonishingly similar on imaging modalities (compare Figs. 20.17 and 20.19). Benign plexiform neurofibromas can undergo sudden explosions of growth and present as irregular, lobulated, infiltrating mass lesions. Any tumor of greater dimension can undergo necrosis and hemorrhage. Tumors that were seen as homogeneous and circumscribed masses on medical imaging have been found to be MPNST on histology.

As mentioned above (see Sect. 20.3.5.3.), symmetry can be helpful in differentiating retroperitoneal tumors. When bilateral masses are present, asymmetry in axial diameter of more than 2 cm and asymmetric attenuation aspect are reported to be very strongly associated with malignancy [4]. When assessing a unilateral retroperitoneal mass, one cannot reliably determine its benign or malignant character on the basis of imaging characteristics [4] (Figs. 20.15 and 20.20).

The problem is especially difficult when assessing neural masses in patients known to have NF; a considerable number of these patients will develop a MPNST within a latency period of 10 to as many as 20 years [26].

Gadolinium chelates improve the delineation of an ill-defined lesion from the surrounding soft-tissues. However, it should be remembered that an enhancing tumor may become isointense to the surrounding fat. For this reason, T2-weighted MR images are more sensitive than Gd-enhanced T1-weighted images to detect small local recurrences after surgery, unless T1-weighted MR images with spectral fat saturation pulses are employed. In our experience, MRI is a useful tool in differentiating between MPNSTs and other malignant soft tissue tumors.

MRI findings suggestive of MPNST (p<0.05) are: intermuscular location, location on the course of a large nerve, nodular (fusiform) morphology and overall non-homogeneity on T1-weighted images, T2-weighted images and T1-weighted images after Gd-chelate contrast injection. MRI findings in favor of non-MPNST were intramuscular location, ill-delineated appearance of more than 20% of the lesion's circumference and presence of intralesional blood vessels, perilesional edema and lymphangitis. There is no significant difference for degree and pattern of enhancement after Gd-chelate contrast injection, or for presence of bone involvement or cysto-necrotic areas [48].

Primary intraosseous MPNSTs show a lytic osseous lesion with cortical destruction and soft-tissue extension. In general, radiologic findings are nonspecific; however, given an aggressive osseous lesion in the setting of NF, radiologists should consider an intraosseous MPNST [108].

Table 20.2. Imaging characteristics of peripheral nerve sheath tumors

	Schwannoma	Neurofibroma	MPNST
CT characteristics			
– Contrast	Hypodense	Hypodense	Hypodense
+ Contrast	Diffuse enhancement	Central enhancement	Marked peripheral enhancement
MRI characteristics			
T1-weighted	Hypointense	Hypointense	Non-homogeneous, overall hypointense
T2-weighted	Hyperintense	Hyperintense	Non-homogeneous, overall hyperintense
	Target sign (uncommon)	Target sign (common)	No target sign
	Fascicular sign (common)	Fascicular sign (uncommon)	No fascicular sign
Contrast-enhanced T1-weighted	Diffuse enhancement (unless necrosis, cystic areas)	Central enhancement	Marked non-homogeneous enhancement

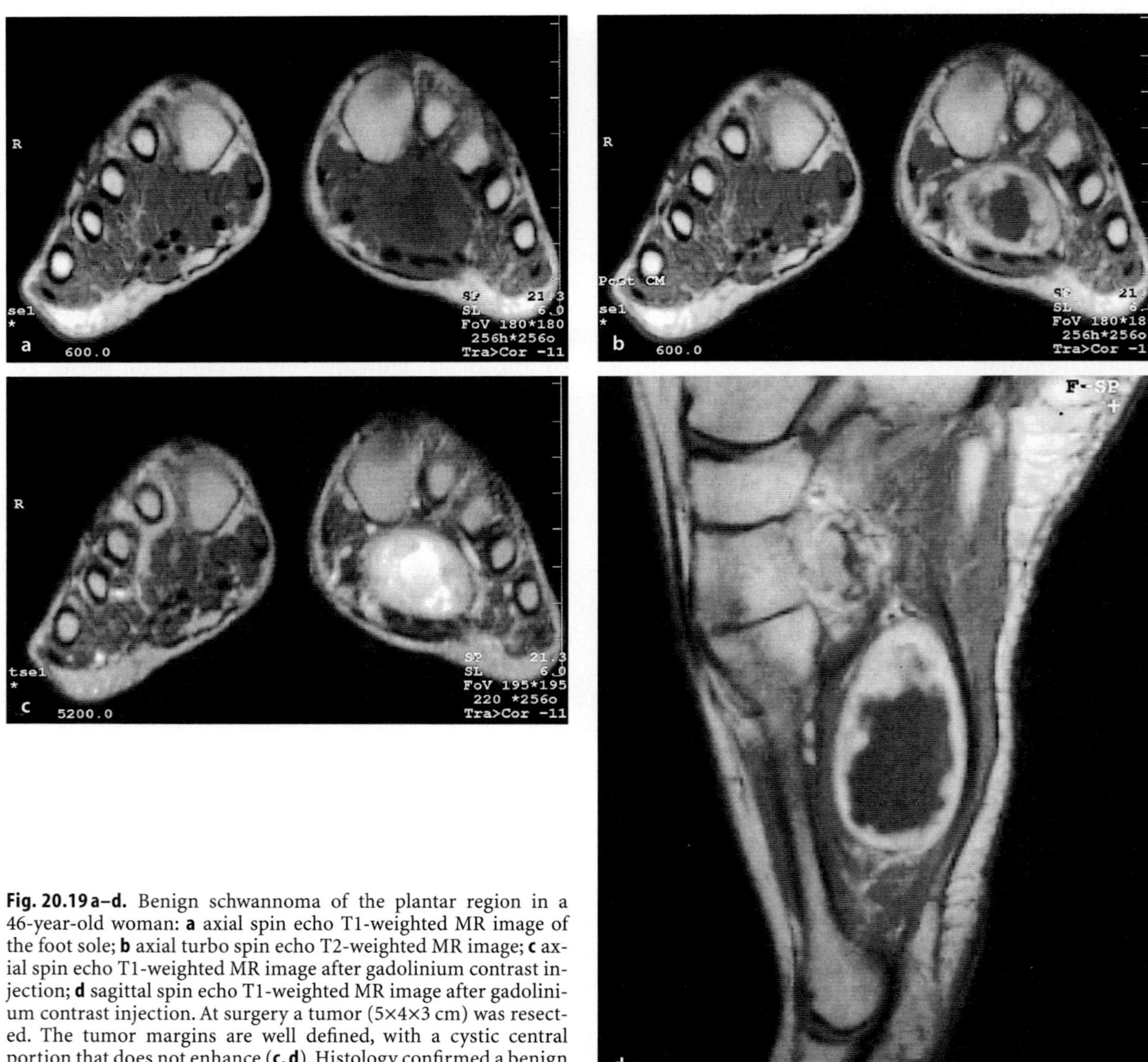

Fig. 20.19a–d. Benign schwannoma of the plantar region in a 46-year-old woman: **a** axial spin echo T1-weighted MR image of the foot sole; **b** axial turbo spin echo T2-weighted MR image; **c** axial spin echo T1-weighted MR image after gadolinium contrast injection; **d** sagittal spin echo T1-weighted MR image after gadolinium contrast injection. At surgery a tumor (5×4×3 cm) was resected. The tumor margins are well defined, with a cystic central portion that does not enhance (**c, d**). Histology confirmed a benign schwannoma

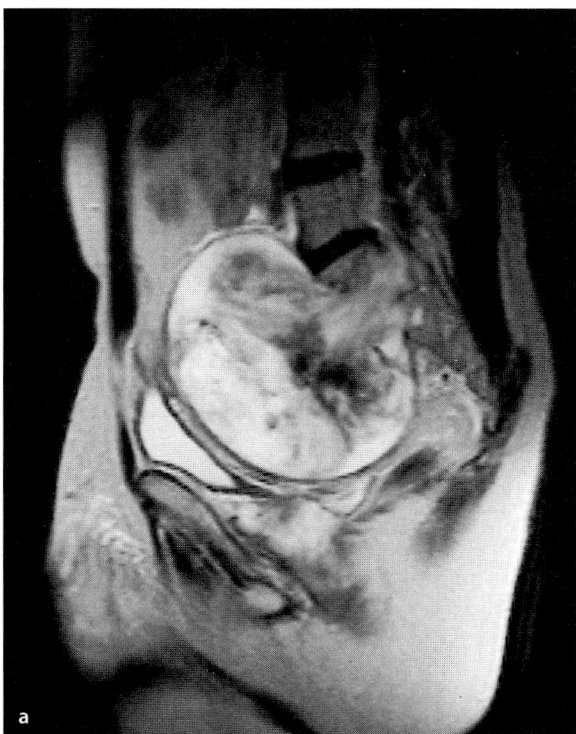
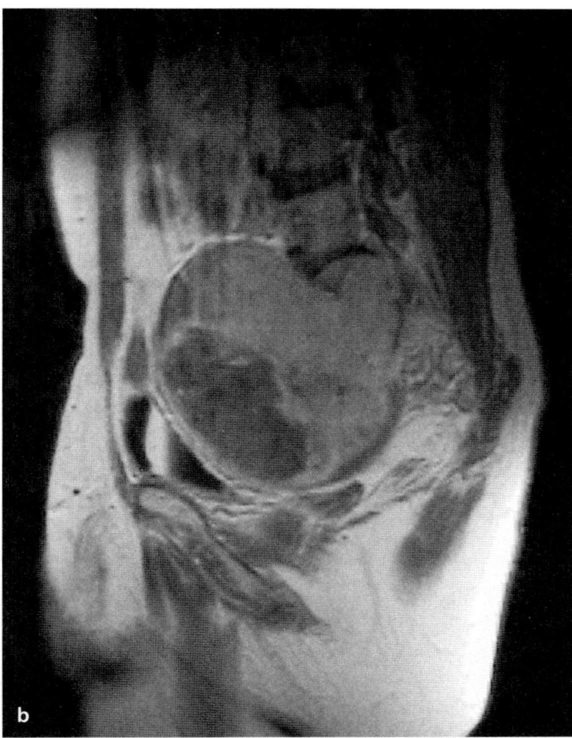

Fig. 20.20 a, b. Presacral MPNST in a 57-year-old man: **a** sagittal turbo spin echo T2-weighted MR image; **b** sagittal spin echo T1-weighted MR image after gadolinium contrast injection. There is a mushroom-shaped tumor with a stalk extending from the right S1–S2 intervertebral foramen into the presacral space (**a**). Tumor architecture and signal intensity are highly heterogeneous (**a**). A large cystic-necrotic portion is seen. After contrast, mild enhancement is seen and the heterogeneity is confirmed (**b**). The tumor flattens the bladder which is displaced inferiorly (**b**). The typical "layering phenomenon" is seen in the bladder [23]

Table 20.2 summarizes the similarities and differences between the different neurogenic tumors with regard to their radiologic presentation.

20.4.5.3 Nuclear Medicine

Differentiation of benign from malignant nerve sheath tumors by conventional preoperative imaging is often unreliable [10]. Benign neurofibromas and MPNST commonly develop in patients with neurofibromatosis. Historically, ^{67}Ga-citrate scanning has been used to evaluate patients with NF-1 and suspected malignant change [45, 67]. Is know that ^{67}Ga-citrate uptake in benign neoplasms, including nerve sheath tumors, is uncommon; conversely, ^{67}Ga-citrate uptake does occur in malignant tumors, including MPNST [45]. Abnormal ^{67}Ga-citrate uptake suggests the possibility of malignancy, and indicates the need for further evaluation by CT or MRI.

Recently, however, FDG-PET has become the predominant non-invasive technique for biological tumor evaluation. Three-dimensional qualitative and quantitative FDG-PET can accurately identify primary and recurrent MPNST [10]. Benign lesions do not demonstrate high FDG uptake. Standard uptake values are significantly higher in MPNST than in benign tumors [10]. Some authors have reported that FDG-PET allows discrimination of benign from malignant neurogenic tumors, with 100% sensitivity and 83% specificity. FDG-PET is particularly useful in patients with neurofibromatosis as it may help to avoid multiple surgical procedures for benign tumors.

Nuclear medicine techniques are known for their high sensitivity, but generally provide poor spatial resolution. Therefore, when a lesion with high FDG uptake is detected, additional cross-sectional imaging with CT and/or MRI is required to provide accurate tumor delineation, and to elucidate the relationship between the malignant tumor and the surrounding structures, for surgical planning. With PET-CT, the best of both worlds can be obtained, with high sensitivity and spatial resolution.

20.5 Association with NF

Any discussion of peripheral nerve sheath tumors would be incomplete without referring to NF, the most common neurocutaneous disease in humans. Schwan-

Table 20.3. Comparison of neurofibromatosis type 1 and 2

	Neurofibromatosis type 1 (NF-1)	Neurofibromatosis type 2 (NF-2)
Pathogenesis	Dysplasia of mesodermal and neuroectodermal tissue, with possibility to diffuse systemic involvement	
Incidence	1:2500 live births	1:50000 live births
Inheritance	Autosomal dominant 50% are new mutations Chromosome 17, variable expression, high penetrance.	Autosomal dominant Chromosome 22
Diagnostic criteria	>1 of following findings: * Café -au -lait spots >5 and >5 mm (>15 mm postpubertal) * One plexiform neurofibroma or >1 neurofibromas of any type * >1 Lisch-nodule * Axillary or inguinal region freckling * Optic nerve glioma * First-degree relative with NF-1 * Characteristic bone lesions *Sphenoid dysplasia* *Thinning of long bone cortex*	Bilateral masses of the eight cranial nerve *or* First degree relative with NF-2 plus either: *Single eight nerve mass *Any of the two following: – *Schwannoma* – *Neurofibroma* – *Meningioma* – *Glioma* – *Juvenile posterior subcapsular lens opacity*
CNS lesions	15–20% – *Optic nerve glioma* – *Astrocytomas* – *Plexiform neurofibromas* – *Neurofibrosarcoma*	Nearly 100% – *CN VIII schwannomas* – *Bilateral multiple schwannomas of other CN*
Associations described	*MEN IIb*: phaeochromocytoma + medullary thyroid carcinoma + multiple neuromas *CHD*: ASD, VSD, IHSS, pulmonary valve stenosis Frequently *schwannomas*	No Lisch nodules, no skeletal dysplasia, no optic pathway glioma, no vascular dysplasia Café-au-lait spots are pale, <5 in number
Cutaneous manifestations	Prominent	Rare

CHD = congenital heart disease; *ASD* = atrial septum defect; *VSD* = ventricular septum defect; *IHSS* = idiopathic hypertrophic subvalvular stenosis (= hypertrophic cardiomyopathy); *MEN* = multiple endocrine neoplasia; *CN* = cranial nerve; *CNS* = central nervous system

nomas, neurofibromas and MPNST can all occur in patients with NF. The term 'neurofibromatosis' covers a heterogeneous group of diseases of neurocutaneous origin [26]. NF is a phakomatosis that displays a wide spectrum of clinical expression with neurocutaneous abnormalities and involvement of multiple organ systems. Although several variants of NF have been reported, to date the National Institutes of Health (NIH) Consensus Development Conference has defined only two clinically and genetically distinct types, namely, NF type 1 (von Recklinghausen's disease, sometimes called peripheral NF), and NF type 2 (bilateral acoustic schwannomas, or central NF) [79, 82]. Because central lesions are often found in NF-1, and because NF-2 can occasionally show peripheral manifestations, the terms "central" and "peripheral" should be avoided. Table 20.3 provides a comparison between NF-1 and NF-2 based on recent literature data [79, 92].

20.5.1 NF and Neurofibroma

All three types of neurofibromas (localized, diffuse, and plexiform) can be associated with NF-1. Only a minority of patients with localized or diffuse neurofibromas are affected by NF-1 [75]. Consequently, localized or diffuse neurofibromas are not specific for NF-1. In the setting of NF-1 they tend to be larger, multiple and more commonly deeply located. Conversely, *plexiform neurofibromas* are the hallmark of NF-1, although as an isolated finding, they are not pathognomonic for this condition [75]. One-third of all patients with NF-1 display plexiform neurofibromas. Plexiform neurofibromas are multiple, tortuous, wormlike masses that arise along the axis of major nerves, resulting in the so-called "bag of worms" appearance [53, 107]. They may involve any or all of the following sites: cranial and spinal nerve roots,

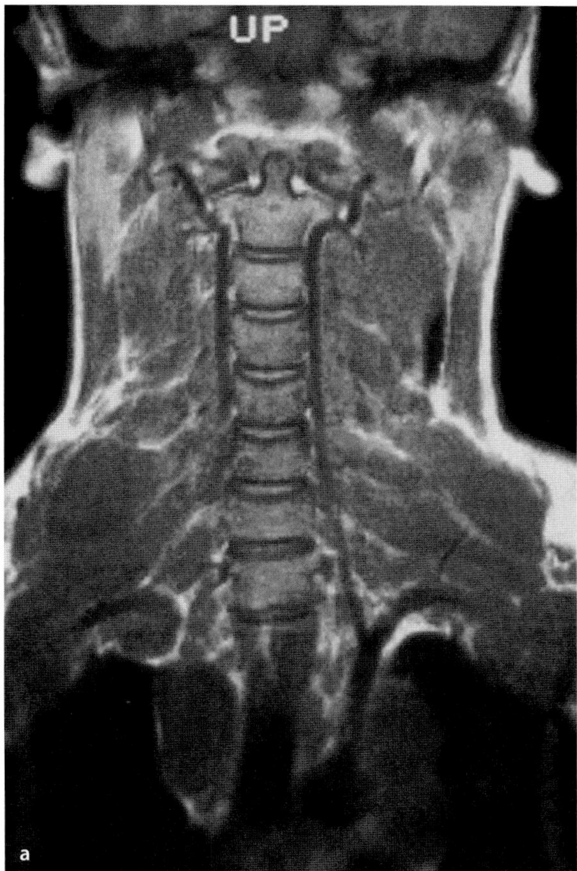

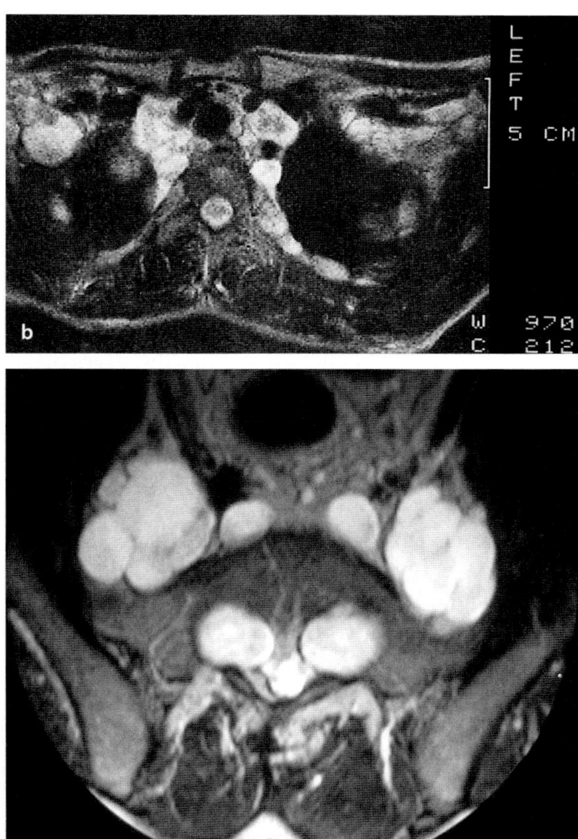

Fig. 20.21 a–c. Plexiform neurofibromas in a 23-year-old woman with NF-1: **a** coronal spin echo T1-weighted MR image through the neck; **b** axial spin echo T2-weighted MR image through the upper mediastinum; **c** axial spin echo T2-weighted MR image through the sacrum. Multiple elongated fusiform or pear-shaped tumors extend along the cervical nerves and the brachial plexus. The tumors are isointense to muscle on the T1-weighted MR image (**a**). They appear sharply marginated and are presumably encapsulated. On the T2-weighted MR image the tumors are hyperintense and somewhat inhomogeneous. At the level of the thoracic inlet, the plexiform tumors extend into the upper mediastinum, and along the chest wall (intercostal nerves) At the level of the sacrum the tumors extend into the presacral space (**b, c**)

and ganglia; the major nerves of the neck, trunk and limbs, including the sympathetic system and its ganglia; the subcutaneous branches of major nerves, and the visceral sympathetic plexuses [98]. They tend to infiltrate and separate the normal nerve fascicles, producing a fusiform appearance (Fig. 20.21) [53, 107]. Plexiform neurofibromas can become extremely large, involving an entire extremity. This causes the condition known as elephantiasis neuromatosa. The entire extremity is enlarged and the overlying skin is loose, redundant, and hyperpigmented, while the underlying bone may be hypertrophied, a phenomenon probably related to the increased vascular supply to the limb [16, 75, 98]. The uncomplimentary term "elephant man" refers not to NF-1, but rather to the Proteus syndrome (cerebriform fibrous proliferation), a prototypic phakomatosis with cutaneous pigmentation, subcutaneous nodules, intracranial tumors and mental retardation [110].

20.5.2 NF and Schwannoma

Association of schwannoma with NF-1 is less common than with NF-2, where acoustic nerve involvement is so frequent that it is the defining diagnostic criterion for the condition [29]. The presence of bilateral acoustic schwannomas has come to imply the diagnosis of NF-2 [75]. In general, NF-2 is a condition that affects the coverings of the central nervous system. It is thus characterized mainly by the presence of multiple schwannomas, meningiomas and ependymomas, though other tumors may also be encountered.

20.5.3 NF and MPNST

Malignant nerve sheath tumors occur frequently in patients with NF, especially NF-1. Although all neurofibromas may undergo malignant degeneration, those arising in the setting of NF-1 [75], and especially plexiform neurofibromas, display the greatest propensity for malignant transformation [98]. In a large survey of the Mayo Clinic patient population, the investigators estimated the incidence of malignant nerve sheath tumors at 4.6% of patients with NF-1, as compared with 0.001% of their general patient population [24]. Other researchers have estimated that between 3 and 13% of patients with NF-1 will develop a MPNST, usually after a long latent period of 10 to 20 years [43, 75, 105]. Given the predisposition for the development of MPNST in patients with NF-1, it is important to thoroughly investigate any new symptoms or signs. The survival rate of patients with MPNST in the setting of NF-1 is significantly lower, with NF-1 apparently an independent adverse prognostic factor [75]. When the diagnosis of MPNST has been established, a combined therapy of aggressive surgery (i.e. mass debulking), and adjuvant radiotherapy should be undertaken. The role of chemotherapy is unclear, but some regimens may be beneficial [114].

20.6 Association with Schwannomatosis

Schwannomatosis is a rare tumor syndrome characterized by the presence of multiple schwannomas arising on cranial, spinal and peripheral nerves, without clinical or radiological evidence of neurofibromatosis (NF) Type 1 or 2 (Fig. 20.22). Molecular and genetic analysis of these patients suggests that schwannomatosis may be a distinct genetic and clinical syndrome [56, 72, 100]. These patients do not develop vestibular tumors. The hallmark of this condition is chronic pain, which can occur in any part of the body, depending on which peripheral nerves are affected. Other clinical neurological findings include paresthesias, sciatica or leg pain, muscle atrophy [51]. Patients with schwannomatosis should undergo regular medical surveillance and genetic counseling is advised.

Table 20.4. Imaging findings suggestive of neurogenic tumors

Fusiform shape
Low attenuation on CT
Entering and exiting nerve
Split-fat sign
Target sign
Fascicular sign
Muscle atrophy

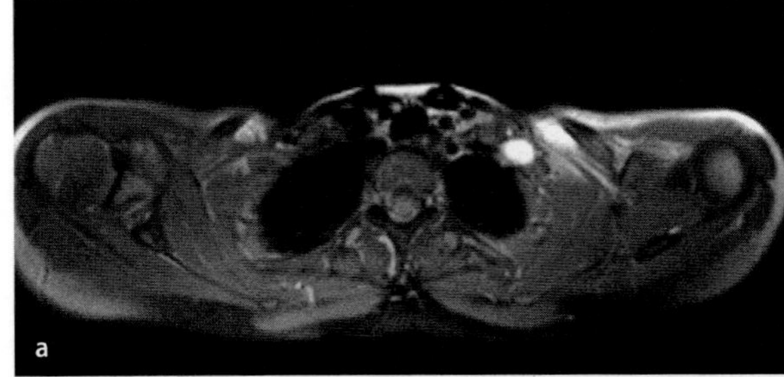
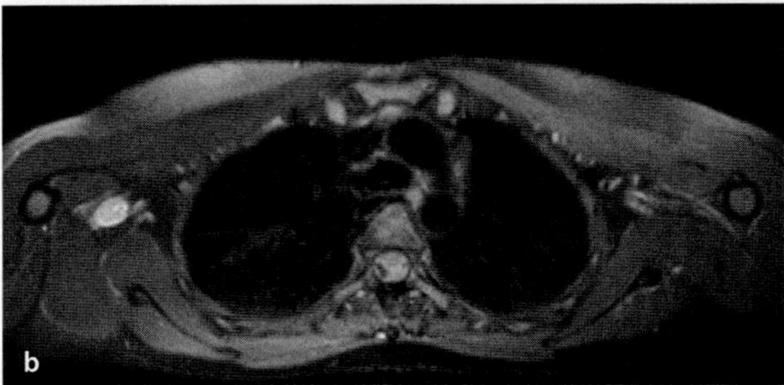
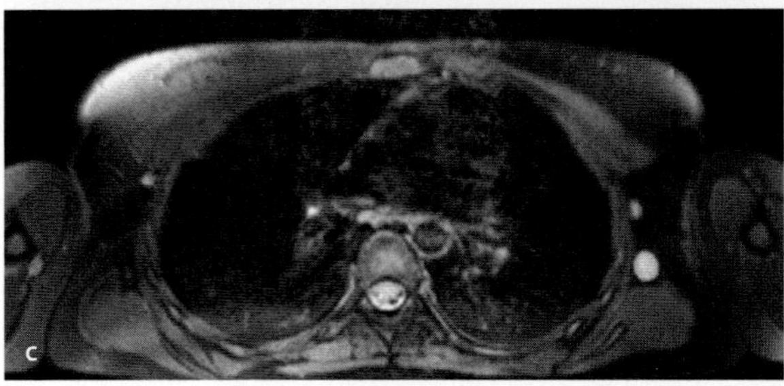

Fig. 20.22 a–c. Schwannomatosis in a midlle aged women with complaints of pain: **a** axial spin echo T2-weighted MR image through the upper mediastinum; **b** Axial spin echo T2-weighted MR image through the upper mediastinum; **c** axial spin echo T2-weighted MR image through the the upper mediastinum. Multiple nodular to fusiform tumors extend along the cervical nerves and the brachial plexus. The tumors are sharply marginated and appear homogeneously hyperintense to muscle on the T2-weighted MR images (**a, b, c**).

Things to remember:
1. Tumors of the peripheral nerves comprise schwannomas, neurofibromas, and malignant peripheral nerve sheath tumors.
2. Benign neurogenic tumors (schwannomas, neurofibromas) are sharply demarcated, round or fusiform lesions, occurring along a peripheral nerve. Other imaging features suggestive for a neurogenic tumor are the finding of an entering/ exiting nerve, the target sign, the fascicular sign, the split fat sign and associated muscle atrophy (Table 20.4).
3. On imaging studies, the differential diagnosis between a schwannoma and a neurofibroma cannot be reliably made. MRI features suggestive of a schwannoma include a fascicular appearance on

T2-weighted images, a thin hyperintense rim on T2-weighted images, and diffuse enhancement. Imaging findings suggestive of neurofibroma include a target sign on T2-weighted images, central enhancement, or a combination of both findings.

4. Criteria that can be of help in establishing the diagnosis of malignant peripheral nerve sheath tumors include a large mass (>5 cm) with mass effect, inhomogeneous tumor architecture (due to areas of necrosis and hemorrhagic foci), ill-defined margins, perilesional edema, heterogeneous enhancement, irregular bone destruction and involvement of lymph nodes.

5. Schwannomas, neurofibromas and MPNST can all occur in patients with neurofibromatosis.

6. Schwannomatosis is a rare tumor syndrome characterized by the presence of multiple schwannomas arising on cranial, spinal and peripheral nerves, without clinical or radiological evidence of neurofibromatosis. These patients do not develop vestibular tumors. The hallmark of this condition is chronic pain.

References

1. Agur AM, Lee MJ (eds) (1991) Grant's atlas of anatomy, 9th edn. Williams and Wilkins, Baltimore, p 138
2. Anderson B, Robertson DM (1979) Melanin containing neurofibroma: case report with evidence of Schwann cell origin in melanin. Can J Neurol Sci 6:139
3. Antoni N (1920) Ueber Rückenmarkstumoren und Neurofibrome. Bergmann, Munich
4. Bass JC, Korobkin M, Francis IR, Ellis JH, Cohan RH (1994) Retroperitoneal plexiform neurofibromas: CT findings. Am J Roentgenol 163:617–620
5. Beggs I (1997) Pictorial review: imaging of peripheral nerve tumors. Clin Radiol 52:8–17
6. Bird CC, Willis RA (1969) The histogenesis of pigmented neurofibromas. J Pathol 97:631
7. Brooks JSJ, Freeman M, Enterline HT (1985) Malignant 'triton' tumors. Natural history and immunohistochemistry of nine new cases with literature review. Cancer 55:2543–2549
8. Burk DL Jr, Brunberg JA, Kanal E, Latchaw RE, Wolf GL (1987) Spinal and paraspinal neurofibromatosis: surface coil MR imaging at 1.5 T. Radiology 162:797–801
9. Cantos-Melian B, Arriaza-Loureda R, Aisa-Varela P (1990) Tibialis posterior nerve schwannoma, mimicking Achilles tendinitis: ultrasonographic diagnosis. J Clin Ultrasound 18:671
10. Cardona S, Schwarzbach M, Hinz U, Dimitrakopoulou-Strauss A, Attigah N, Mechtersheimer G, Lehnert T (2003) Evaluation of F18-deoxyglucose positron emission tomography (FDG-PET) to assess the nature of neurogenic tumours. Eur J Surg Oncol. 29(6):536–541
11. Carney JA (1990) Psammomatous melanotic schwannoma: a distinctive heritable tumor with special associations including cardiac myxoma and the Cushing syndrome. Am J Surg Pathol 14:206–222
12. Cerofolini E, Landi A, DeSantis G, Maiorana A, Canossi G, Romagnoli R (1991) MR of benign peripheral nerve sheath tumors. J Comput Assist Tomogr 15(4):593–597
13. Chinn DH, Filly RA, Callen PW (1982) Unusual ultrasonographic appearance of a solid schwannoma. J Clin Ultrasound 10:243–245
14. Chui MC, Bird BL, Rogers J (1988) Extracranial and extraspinal nerve sheath tumors: computed tomographic evaluation. Neuroradiology 30:47–53
15. Cohen ML, Schwartz AM, Rockoff SD (1986) Benign schwannomas: pathologic basis for CT inhomogeneities. Am J Roentgenol 147:141–143
16. Coleman BG, Arger PH, Dalinka MK, Obringer AC, Raney BR, Meadows AT (1983) CT of sarcomatous degeneration in neurofibromatosis. Am J Roentgenol 140:383–387
17. Coulomb M, Ferretti G, Dal Soglio S, Ranchoup Y, Thony F, Pittet-Barbier L, Blanc F (1995) Tumeurs neurogènes périphériques du thorax chez l'adulte. Feuillets de Radiologie 35(1):1–25
18. Daar AS (1981) Neurilemmoma of femoral nerve-a possible pitfall. Brit J Clin Pract 35:240–241
19. Daimaru YH, Hashimoto H, Enjoji M (1984) Malignant 'triton' tumors: a clinicopathologic and immunohistochemical study of nine cases. Hum Pathol 15:768–778
20. Day DL, Allan BT (1985) Pediatric case of the day. Am J Roentgenol 144:1296–1302
21. Dibble JH (1963) Verocay bodies and pseudo-meissnerian corpuscules. J Pathol Bacteriol 85:425
22. Donner TR, Voorhies RM, Kline DG (1994) Neural sheath tumors of major nerves. J Neurosurg 81(3):362–373
23. Ducatman BS, Scheithauer BW (1983) Postirradiation neurofibrosarcoma. Cancer 51:1028
24. Ducatman BS, Scheithauer BW, Piepgras DG, Reiman HM, Ilstrup DM (1986) Malignant peripheral nerve sheath tumors. A clinicopathologic study of 120 cases. Cancer 57:2006
25. Ellison D, Love S, Chimelli L, Harding BN, Lowe J, Vinters HV (eds) (2004) Peripheral nerve sheath neoplasms. In: Neuropathology, 2nd edn. Mosby, Edinburgh, pp 695–702
26. Elster AD (1992) Radiologic screening in the neurocutaneous syndromes: strategies and controversies. Am J Neuroradiol 13:1078–1082
27. Elster AD, Sobol WT, Hinson WH (1990) Pseudolayering of Gd-DTPA in the urinary bladder. Radiology 174(2):379–381
28. Enneking WF (1986) A system of staging of musculoskeletal neoplasms. Clin Orthop 204:9
29. Enzinger FM, Weiss SW (1983) Benign and malignant tumors of peripheral nerves. In: Enzinger FM, Weiss SW (eds) Soft tissue tumors, 1st edn. Mosby, St Louis, pp 580–656
30. Enzinger FM, Weiss SW (1995) Benign tumors of peripheral nerves. In: Enzinger FM, Weiss SW (eds.) Soft tissue tumors, 3rd edn. Mosby, St. Louis, pp 821–888
31. Enzinger FM, Weiss SW (1995) Malignant tumors of peripheral nerves, In: Enzinger FM, Weiss SW (eds.) Soft tissue tumors, 3rd edn. Mosby, St Louis, pp 889–928
32. Factor S, Turi G, Biempica L (1976) Primary cardiac neurilemoma. Cancer 37:883
33. Fletcher CD, Diavies SE (1986) Benign plexiform (multinodular) schwannoma: a rare tumour unassociated with neurofibromatosis. Histopathology 10(9):971–980
34. Fletcher CDM, Davies SE, McKee PH (1987) Cellular schwannoma: a distinct pseudosarcomatous entity. Histopathology 11:21–35
35. Foley KM, Woodruff JM, Ellis FT, Posner JB (1980) Radiation-induced malignant and atypical peripheral nerve sheath tumors. Ann Neurol 7(4):311–318
36. Fornage BD (1988) Peripheral nerves of the extremities: imaging with US. Radiology 167:179–182
37. Fornage BD (1995) Soft tissue masses In: Fornage BD (ed) Musculoskeletal ultrasound. Churchill Livingstone, Edinburgh, pp 21–42 (Clinics in diagnostic ultrasound volume 30)

38. Fukuya T, Lu CC, Mitros FA (1994) CT findings of plexiform neurofibromatosis involving the ileum and its mesentery. Clin Imaging 18:142–145

39. Genchi V, Moramorco F, Pepe AS, Scarciolla G, Favale E (1993) Schwannoma gigante del nervo mediano: imaging integrato US-TC. Giornale Italiano di Ultrasonologia 4(4):216–219

40. Getachew MM, Whitman GJ, Chew FS (1994) Retroperitoneal schwannoma. Am J Roentgenol 163:1356

41. Ghosh BC, Ghosh L, Huvos AG, Fortner JG (1973) Malignant schwannoma. A clinicopathologic study. Cancer 31:184–190

42. Ghrist TD (1963) Gastrointestinal involvement in neurofibromatosis. Arch Intern Med 112:357–362

43. Guccion JG, Enzinger FM (1979) Malignant schwannomas associated with von Recklinghausen's neurofibromatosis. Virchows Arch Pathol Anat 383:43–57

44. Guiloff RJ, Scadding JW, Klenerman L (1984) Morton's metatarsalgia: clinical, electrophysiological and histological observations. J Bone Joint Surg 66:586–591

45. Hammond JA, Driedger AA (1978) Detection of malignant change in neurofibromatosis (von Recklinghausen's disease) by gallium-67 scanning. Can Med Assoc J 119:352–353

46. Harkin JC, Reed JR (1968) Tumors of the peripheral nervous system. Armed Forces Institute of Pathology, Washington, DC

47. Harkin JC, Reed RJ (1969) Atlas of tumor pathology, second series, fascicle 3. Armed Forces Institute of Pathology, Washington, DC

48. Heyman S, Van Herendael BJ, De Temmerman G, Vanhoenacker F, Bloem GL, De Schepper AM (2005) Value of magnetic resonance imaging in the differentiation between malignant peripheral nerve sheath tumors and non-neurogenic malignant soft tissue tumors. Personal communication. Abstract, ESSR, Oxford

49. Hochberg FH, Dasilva AB, Galdabini J, Richardson EP (1974) Gastrointestinal involvement in von Recklinghausen's neurofibromatosis. Neurology 24:1144–1151

50. Hoddick WK, Callen PW, Filly RA, Mahony BS, Edwards MB (1984) Ultrasound evaluation of benign sciatic nerve sheath tumor. J Ultrasound Med 3:505–507

51. Huang JH, Simon SL, Nagpal S, Nelson PT, Zager EL (2004) Management of patients with schwannomatosis: report of six cases and review of the literature. Surg Neurol 62:353–361

52. Hughes DG, Wilson DJ (1986) Ultrasound appearances of peripheral nerve sheath tumors. Br J Radiol 59:1041–1043

53. Huson SM (1988) Von Recklinghausen neurofibromatosis: a clinical and population study in south-east Wales. Brain 111:1355–1381

54. Iwashita T, Enjoji M (1986) Plexiform neurilemoma: a clinicopathologic and immunohistochemical analysis of 23 tumors from 20 patients. Virchows Arch Pathol Anat 422:305–309

55. Isobe K, Shimizu T, Akahane T, Kato H (2004) Imaging of ancient schwannoma. Am J Roentgenol 183:331–336

56. Jacoby LB, Jones D, Davis K, Kronn D, Short MP, Gusella J, MacCollin M (1997) Molecular analysis of the NF2 tumor-suppressor gene in schwannomatosis. Am J Hum Genet 61:1293–1302

57. Jee WH, Oh SN, McCauley T, Ryu KN, Suh JS, Lee JH, Park JM, Chun KA, Sung MS, Kim K, Lee YS, Kang YK, Ok IY, Kim JM (2004) Extraaxial neurofibromas versus neurilemmomas: discrimination with MRI. Am J Roentgenol 183:629–633

58. Jefferson D, Neary P, Eames RA (1981) Renaut body distribution at sites of human peripheral nerve entrapment. J Neurol Sci 49:19–29

59. Kao GF, Laskin WB, Olsen TG (1989) Solitary cutaneous plexiform neurilemoma (schwannoma): a clinicopathologic, immunohistochemical, and ultrastructural study of 11 cases. Mod Pathol 2:20–26

60. Katsumi K, Ogose A, Hotta T, Hatano H, Kawashima H, Umezu H, Endo N (2003) Plexiform schwannoma of the forearm. Skeletal Radiol 32:719–723

61. Kolbenstvedt A, Skjennald A, Higgins CB (1995) The lungs and mediastinum. In: Petterson H (ed) The NICER Centennial Book 1995: A global textbook of radiology, vol 2, chap 18, p 694

62. Kransdorf MJ (1995) Malignant soft tissue tumors in a large referral population: distribution of diagnosis by age, sex, and location. Am J Roentgenol 164:129–134

63. Kumar AJ, Kuhajda FP, Martinez CR, Fishman EK, Jezic DV, Siegelman SS (1983) Computed tomography of extracranial nerve sheath tumors with pathological correlation. J Comput Assist Tomogr 7:857–865

64. Le Brigand H, Bouquet P, N'Guimbous JF (1977) Enquête sur l'évolution et le pronostic des tumeurs neurogènes endothoraciques de la maladie de Recklinghausen. Ann Chirg 16:195–203

65. Lemaître L, Rémy J, Saint-Michel J (1987) Masses et pseudomasses médiastinales. In: Rémy J (ed), Tomodensitométrie du thorax, Vigot, Paris, pp 47–87

66. Lemont H (1992) Common foot disorders. In: Berkow R, Fletcher AJ (eds) The Merck manual of diagnosis and therapy. Merck and Co, Inc., Rahway NJ, pp 1375–1376

67. Levine E, Huntrakoon M, Wetzel LH (1987) Malignant nerve-sheath neoplasms in neurofibromatosis: distinction from benign tumors by using imaging techniques. Am J Roentgenol 149:1059–1064

68. Liessi G, Barbazza R, Sartori F, Sabbadin P, Scapinello A (1990) CT and MR imaging of melanocytic schwannomas; report of three cases. Eur J Radiol 11(2):138–142

69. Lin J, Martel W (2001) Cross-sectional imaging of peripheral nerve sheath tumors. Am J Roentgenol 176:75-82

70. Lodding P, Kindblom LG, Angerveall L, Stenman G (1990) Cellular schwannoma. A clinicopathologic study of 29 cases. Virchows Arch Pathol 416(3):237–248

71. MacCollin M, Willett C, Heinrich B, Jacoby LB, Acierno JS Jr, Perry A, Louis DN (2003) Familial schwannomatosis: exclusion of the NF2 locus as the germline event. Neurology 24:1968–1974

72. MacCollin M, Woodfin W, Kronn D, Short MP (1996) Schwannomatosis: a clinical and pathologic study. Neurology 46:1072–1079

73. Mallory FB (1920) The type cell of the so-called dural endothelioma. J Med Res 41:349

74. Mandybur TI (1974) Melanotic nerve sheath tumors. J Neurosurg 41:187–192

75. Meis-Kindblom JM, Enzinger FM (1996) Color atlas of soft tissue tumors. Mosby-Wolfe, St. Louis

76. Mennemeyer RP, Hallman KO, Hammar SP, Reisis JE, Tytus JS, Bochus D (1979) Melanotic schwannoma: clinical and ultrastructural studies of three cases with evidence of intracellular melanina synthesis. Am J Surg Pathol 3:3–10

77. Miller RT, Sarikaya H, Sos A (1986) Melanotic schwannoma of the acoustic nerve. Arch Pathol Lab Med 220:153–154

78. Moon W, Im JG, Han M (1993) Malignant schwannomas of the thorax: CT findings. J Comput Assist Tomogr 17:274–276

79. Mulvihill JJ, Parry DM, Sherman JL, Pikus A, Kaiser-Kupfer MI, Eldridge R (1990) NIH Conference on neurofibromatosis 1 (Recklinghausen's disease) and neurofibromatosis 2 (bilateral acoustic schwannoma): an update Ann Intern Med 113:39–52

80. Murphey MD, Smith WS, Smith KE, Kransdorf MJ, Temple HT (1999) From the archives of the AFIP. Imaging of musculoskeletal neurogenic tumors: Radiologic–pathologic correlation. Radiographics 29:1253–1280

81. Nakajima T, Watanabe S, Sato Y, Kameya T, Hirota T, Shimosato Y (1982) An immunoperoxidase study of S-100 protein distribution in normal and neoplastic tissues. Am J Surg Pathol 6:715–727

82. National Institute of Health (NIH) Consensus development conference: neurofibromatosis conference statement (1988) Arch Neurol 45:575–578

83. Nichols DH, Weston JA (1977) Melanogenesis in cultures of peripheral nervous tissue. I. The origin and prospective fate of cells giving rise to melanocytes. Dev Biol 60:217

84. Nissen KI (1948) Plantar digital neuritis: Morton's metatarsalgia. J Bone Joint Surg 30:84–94

85. Ogose A, Hotta T, Morita T, Higuchi T, Umezu H, Imaizumi S, Hatano H, Kawashima H, Gu W, Endo N (2004) Diagnosis of peripheral nerve sheath tumors around the pelvis. J Clin Oncol 34:405–413

86. Ogose A, Hotta T, Morita T, Yamamura S, Hosaka N, Kobayashi H, Hirata Y (1999) Tumors of peripheral nerves: correlation of symptoms, clinical signs, imaging features, and histologic diagnosis. Skeletal Radiol 28:183–188

87. Osborn AG (1994) Miscellaneous tumors, cysts and metastases. In: Diagnostic neuroradiology. Mosby, St-Louis, pp 626–670

88. Paling MR (1984) Plexiform neurofibroma of the pelvis in neurofibromatosis: CT findings. J Comput Assist Tomogr 8:476–478

89. Payan MJ, Gambarelli D, Keller P, Lachard A, Garcin M, Vigouroux C, Toga M (1986) Melanotic neurofibroma: a case report with ultrastructural study. Acta Neuropathol 69:148–152

90. Penneys NS, Mogollon R, Kowalczyk A, Nadjii M, Adachi K (1984) A survey of cutaneous neural lesions for the presence of myelin basic protein. An immunohistochemical study. Arch Dermatol 120:210–213

91. Perentes E, Rubinstein LJ (1985) Immunohistochemical recognition of human nerve sheath tumors by anti-Leu 7 monoclonal antibody. Acta Neuropathol 68:319–324

92. Perentes E, Rubinstein LJ (1987) Recent applications of immunoperoxidase histochemistry in human neuro-oncology. An update. Arch Pathol Lab Med 111:796–812

93. Pilavaki M, Chourmouzi D, Kiziridou A, Skordalaki A, Zarampoukas T, Drevelengas A (2004) Imaging of peripheral nerve sheath tumors with pathologic correlation. Eur J Radiol 52(3):229–239

94. Redd RA, Peters VJ, Emery SF, Branch HM, Rifkin MD (1989) Morton neuroma: sonographic evaluation. Radiology 171:415–417

95. Ros PR, Eshaghi N (1991) Plexiform neurofibroma of the pelvis: CT and MR findings. Magn Reson Imaging 9:463–465

96. Rowlands D, Edwards C, Collins F (1987) Malignant melanotic schwannoma of the bronchus. J Clin Pathol 4:1449–1455

97. Russell DS, Rubenstein LJ (1977) Pathology of tumors of the nervous system, 4th edn. Williams and Wilkins, Baltimore

98. Russell DS, Rubinstein LJ (1989) Tumours of the cranial, spinal and peripheral nerve sheaths. In: Pathology of tumours of the nervous system, 5th edn. Edward Arnold, London, pp 533–589

99. Scotti TM (1957) The lesion of Morton's metatarsalgia (Morton's toe). Arch Pathol 63:91–102

100. Seppala MT, Sainio MA, Haltia MJ, Kinnunen JJ, Setala KH, Jaaskelainen JE (1998) Multiple schwannomas: schwannomatosis or neurofibromatosis type 2? J Neurosurg 89:36–41

101. Silverman JF, Leffers BR, Kay S (1976) Primary pulmonary neurilemoma. Arch Pathol Lab Med 100:644–648

102. Simoens WA, Wuyts FL, De Beuckeleer LH, Vandevenne JE, Bloem LJ, De Schepper AMA (2001) MR features of peripheral nerve sheath tumors: can a calculated index compete with radiologist's experience? Eur Radiol 11(2):250–257

103. Som PM, Braun IF, Shapiro MD, Reede DL, Curtin HD, Zimmerman RA (1987) Tumors of the parapharyngeal space and upper neck: MR imaging characteristics. Radiology 164:823–829

104. Sordillo PP, Helson L, Hajdu SI, Magill GB, Kosloff C, Golbey RB, Beattie EJ (1981) Malignant scwhannoma – clinical characteristics, survival, and response to therapy. Cancer 47:2503–2509

105. Sorensen SA, Mulvihill JJ, Nielsen A (1986) Long-term follow-up of von Recklinghausen neurofibromatosis. Survival and malignant neoplasms. N Engl J Med 314:1010–1015

106. Stout AP (1935) Peripheral manifestation of the specific nerve sheath tumors (neurilemoma). Am J Cancer 24:751–796

107. Suh JS, Abenoza P, Galloway HR, Everson LI, Griffiths HJ (1992) Peripheral (extracranial) nerve tumors: correlation of MR imaging and histologic findings. Radiology 183:341–346

108. Terry DG, Sauser DD, Gordon MD (1998) Intraosseous malignant peripheral nerve sheath tumor in a patient with neurofibromatosis. Skeletal Radiol 27:346–349

109. Vanhoenacker FM, De Backer AI, Op de Beeck B, Maes M, Van Altena R, Van Beckevoort D, Kersemans P, De Schepper AM (2004) Imaging of gastrointestinal and abdominal tuberculosis. Eur Radiol 14:103–115

110. Vanhoenacker FM, De Beuckeleer LH, Deprettere A, De Moor A, De Schepper AM (2000) Proteus syndrome: MRI characteristics of plantar cerebriform hyperplasia. Skeletal Radiol. 2000 29(2):101–103

111. Varma DG, Moulopoulos A, Sara AS, Leeds N, Kumar R, Kim EE, Wallace S (1992) MR Imaging of extracranial nerve sheath tumors. J Comput Assist Tomogr 16(3):448–453

112. Victoria L, McCulloch TM, Callaghan EJ, Bauman NM (1999) Malignant triton tumor of the head and neck: a case report and review of the literature. Head Neck 21:663–670

113. Vogl TJ (1991) Neurogene tumoren. In: Vogl TJ (ed) Kernspintomographie der Kopf-Hals-Region. Springer, Berlin Heidelberg New York, pp 163–165

114. Wanebo JE, Malik JM, Vandenberg SR, Wanebo HJ, Driesen N, Persing JA (1993) Malignant peripheral nerve sheath tumors. A clinicopathological study of 28 cases. Cancer 71(4):1247–1253

115. White W, Shiu MH, Rosenblum MK, Erlandson RA, Woodruff JM (1990) Cellular schwannoma. A Clinicopathologic study of 57 patients and 58 tumors. Cancer 66(6):1266–1275

116. Woodruff JM, Chernik NL, Smith MC (1973) Peripheral nerve tumors with rhabdomyosarcomatous differentiation (malignant "Triton" tumors). Cancer 32:426–439

117. Yimaz MR, Bek S, Bekmezci T, Gokduman C, Solak A (2004) Malignant triton tumor of the lumbar spine. Spine 15(18):399–401

118. Zanetti M, Strehle JK, Zollinger H, Hodler J (1997) Morton neuroma and fluid in the intermetatarsal bursae on MR images of 70 asymptomatic volunteers. Radiology 203:516–520

119. Zollinger H, Jacob HA (1989) Is Morton's disease caused by biomechanical factors? Acta Orthop Belg 55:473–477

Extraskeletal Cartilaginous and Osseous Tumors

21

H.R. Degryse, F. Aparisi

Contents

21.1 Introduction

Except for myositis ossificans, both osseous and cartilaginous tumors of the soft tissues are uncommon. The radiographic and/or magnetic resonance imaging (MRI) appearance of these tumors and tumor-like lesions frequently suggests a specific diagnosis. Even when a specific diagnosis cannot be obtained, knowledge of the various types of lesions is essential to make a relevant differential diagnosis.

21.2 Classification

The most common classification of extraskeletal cartilaginous and osseous tumors is that of the World Health Organization. In the most recent classification only soft tissue chondroma and extraskeletal osteosarcoma are retained under the heading chondro-osseous soft tissue tumors. As the approach in this chapter is from the point of view of the presentation of lesions on various imaging techniques, other conditions, even non-neoplastic, but with similar appearance, will also be considered and discussed.

21.3 Cartilaginous Tumors and Tumor-like Conditions of the Soft Tissues

21.3.1 Benign Lesions

21.3.1.1 Extraskeletal Chondroma (Soft Tissue Chondroma)

■ **Definition.** The term extraskeletal chondroma refers to small, well-defined nodules that are composed of at least focal areas of cartilage and do not have any connection with bone, periosteum nor intra-articular synovium. Two-thirds of the lesions contain mature, viable cartilage, whereas immature chondroblasts are observed in the other one-third of cases [23]. The greatest diameter of the lesion seldom exceeds 3 cm. Most chondromas are ovoid or have a lobular appearance and are sharply delineated. Some of these lesions undergo focal fibrosis (fibrochondroma), ossification (osteochondroma) or myxoid changes (myxochondroma), possibly combined with focal hemorrhage or granuloma formation. Older lesions may contain diffuse calcifications. These predominantly occur at the center of the lesion. Pronounced calcification may obscure its cartilaginous nature and may mimic tumoral calcinosis [14].

■ **Incidence and Clinical Behavior.** Extraskeletal chondromas are rare, representing approximately 1.5% of all benign soft tissue tumors [20]. Almost all extraskeletal chondromas afflict the distal extremities (in up to 96% of cases) [20, 25]. Preferential sites of involvement are the hands (54–64%) especially the fingers – and feet (20–28%) [7, 20, 25]. Trunk, head and neck region are seldom involved. Repeated microtrauma has been stressed as an important provoking factor in the development. This may explain the relative high incidence of soft tissue chondroma in the hands and fingers [20]. The tumors are more common in men and, although they may be seen in patients at any age, are most commonly encountered between 30 and 60 years of age [4, 25, 46]. In the majority of cases the extraskeletal chondroma presents as a slowly growing soft tissue mass, which is occasionally associated with pain or tenderness. On palpation the chondroma is usually firm and mobile. Local surgical resection is the treatment of choice. Despite the benign nature of the lesion, recurrence rates of 15–25% are reported [7, 23, 46]. Malignant transformation has not been reported [14, 46].

■ **Imaging.** On plain radiography and CT, an extraskeletal chondroma presents as a well-demarcated soft tissue mass. Calcifications are observed in 33–77% of cases [11, 20, 46]. The pattern of calcification is most typically that of curvilinear, ring-like densities, outlining the soft tissue lobules. However, these calcifications may also be punctate or mixed punctate and curvilinear [4, 46] (Fig. 21.1). Less commonly, ossification and peripheral rim calcification are observed [20]. Secondary osseous changes of adjacent bone, such as cortical pressure erosions and reactive cortical sclerosis, have been reported [20, 46].

On MRI, soft tissue chondromas appear on T1-weighted images as well-circumscribed masses that are isointense relative to skeletal muscle (Fig. 21.2). On T2-weighted images the hyaline cartilage typically presents with very high signal intensity, greater than that of fat. Mineralized areas cause foci of signal void on all sequences [20] (Fig. 21.3). Diagnosis of chondromas without foci of calcification is more difficult, and these lesions have to be differentiated from other soft tissue masses, especially those of synovial origin. After intravenous injection of gadolinium the majority of chondromas exhibit marked and mostly peripheral contrast enhancement (Figs. 21.3 and 21.4).

Clinical data together with findings on plain radiography, CT and MRI are highly valuable in the differential diagnosis of extraskeletal chondroma. This benign tumor should be differentiated principally from benign intra-articular and juxtacortical calcified lesions, malignant soft tissue tumors containing calcifications, para-articular crystal depositions, myositis ossificans, and soft tissue calcifications [14, 40, 46]. Benign intra-artic-

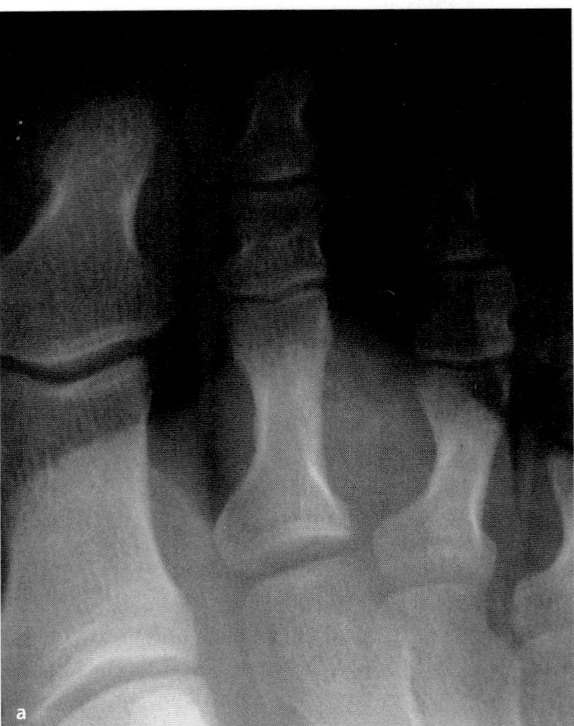
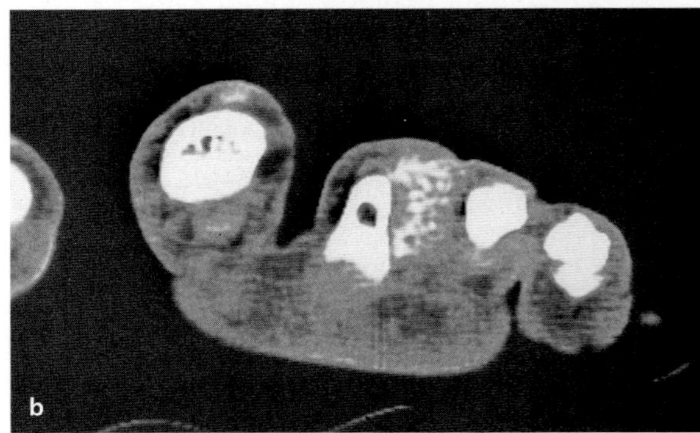

Fig. 21.1 a, b. Extraskeletal chondroma of the foot in a 37-year-old man: **a** plain radiograph; **b** CT. Soft tissue mass with multiple punctate and ring-like calcifications between the second and third toes (**a**). Calcifications are better demonstrated on CT (**b**). Localization in the forefoot and presence of characteristic calcifications are suggestive of extraskeletal chondroma

ular calcified lesions comprise synovial chondromatosis, in which the lesions are often multiple and located within large joints or bursae, the solitary intra-articular chondroma, which is commonly large, and the periosteal chondroma, which shows characteristically severe cortical erosion [40, 46]. Malignant soft tissue tumors containing calcifications more commonly affect other regions of the body, commonly have indistinctive margins, reveal a more irregular pattern of calcification, and usually show bony involvement. In para-articular deposition of crystals occurring in some metabolic dis-

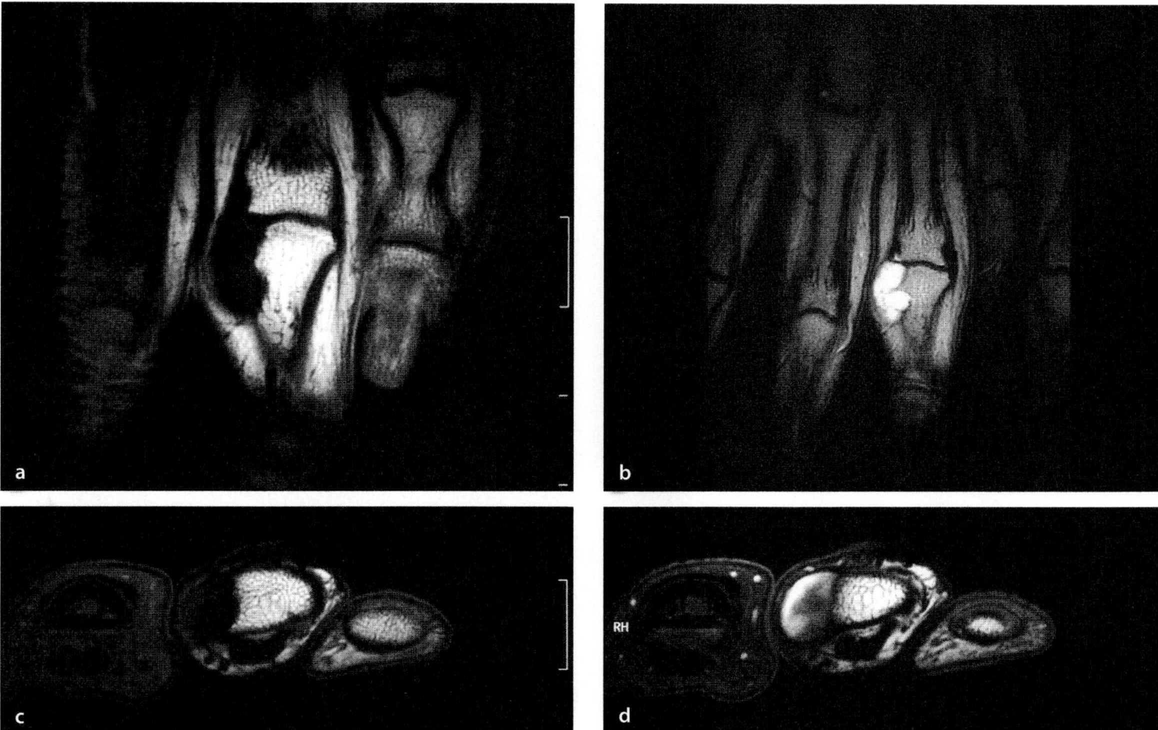

Fig. 21.2 a–d. Soft tissue chondroma of the finger in a young woman: **a** coronal spin echo T1-weighted MR image; **b** coronal spin echo T2-weighted MR image; **c** transverse spin echo T1-weighted MR image; **d** transverse spin echo T1-weighted MR image after gadolinium contrast injection (same level as in **c**). Lobulated soft tissue mass near the radial aspect of the proximal third of the basic phalanx of the fourth finger. On T1-weighted image the mass presents with homogeneous low intensity (**a,c**) T2-weighted image reveals very high signal intensity of the matrix of the lesion, with internal low-intensity linear structures, corresponding to septations separating the cartilaginous lobules (**b**). Gadolinium-enhanced T1-weighted images show pronounced ring-like enhancement at the periphery of the lesion (**d**)

orders, such as gout, the pattern of calcification is more amorphous or multilobulated.

Furthermore, as in soft tissue calcifications occurring in systemic disorders such as scleroderma, the clinical history is generally suggestive of the true nature of the disease. As described in Sect. 21.4.1.1, myositis ossificans seldom occurs in hands and feet, reveals a rapid evolution on serial radiographs, and shows another type of mineralization, which is linear and most dense at the periphery of the lesion.

Clinical and radiologic features that make the diagnosis of extraskeletal chondroma apparent are: the small size of the lesion despite its long history, its characteristic location in a distal extremity, and the nature of its calcifications, as described above. This diagnosis, however, must be confirmed by histopathologic examination.

21.3.1.2 Para-articular Chondroma

■ **Definition.** Para-articular chondroma is a rare tumor, composed of hyaline cartilage with variable endochondral ossification in the central area. The tumors arise from the capsule or the para-articular connective tissue of a large joint (mainly the knee) and are due to cartilaginous metaplasia [19, 32].

■ **Incidence and Clinical Behavior.** As only about 35 cases have been reported in the Anglo-Saxon literature, para-articular chondroma is very rare. The tumor afflicts both males and females, with equal sex distribution, between ages from 12 to 75 years (mean approximately 49 years). The knee is most frequently involved, the tumors being mainly intracapsular, infrapatellar and medial in location. Other locations, such as elbow joint and hip, although much less common, have also been reported [32]. Clinically the tumor manifests as a swelling and by moderate pain, lasting from several months to many years (up to 20 years!) and by limitation of joint movement. The treatment of choice is surgical excision. Local recurrence has been reported, malignant transformation has never been observed.

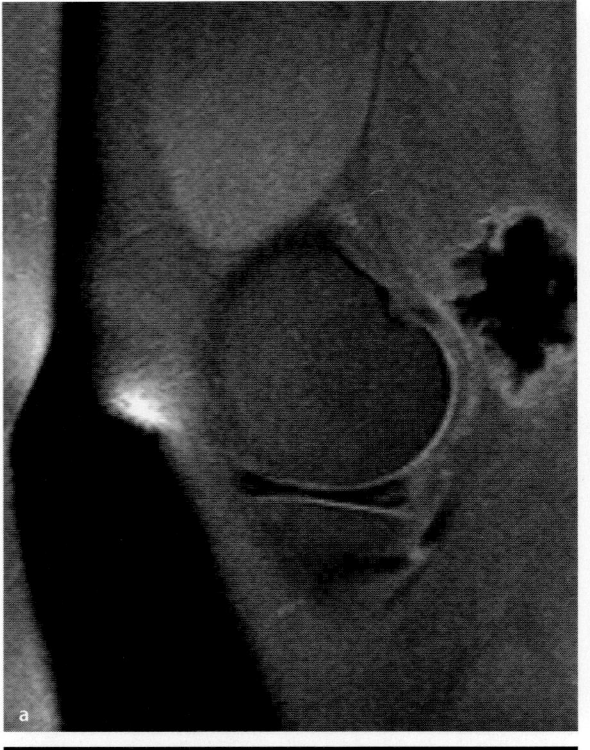
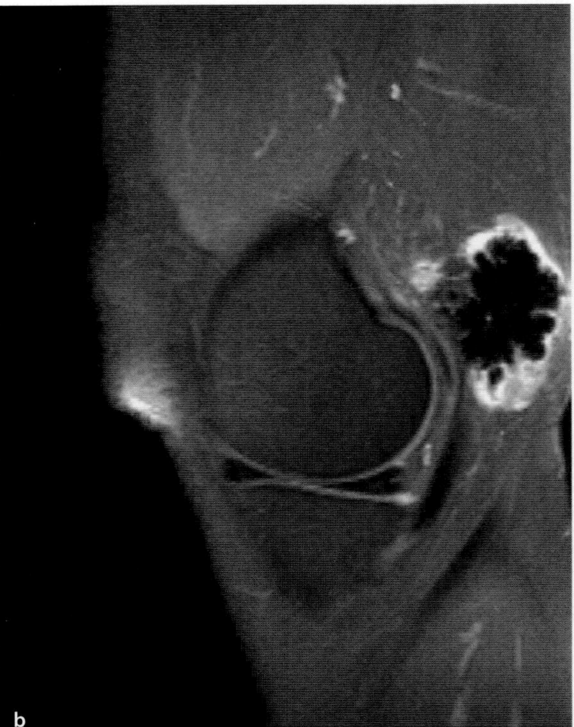
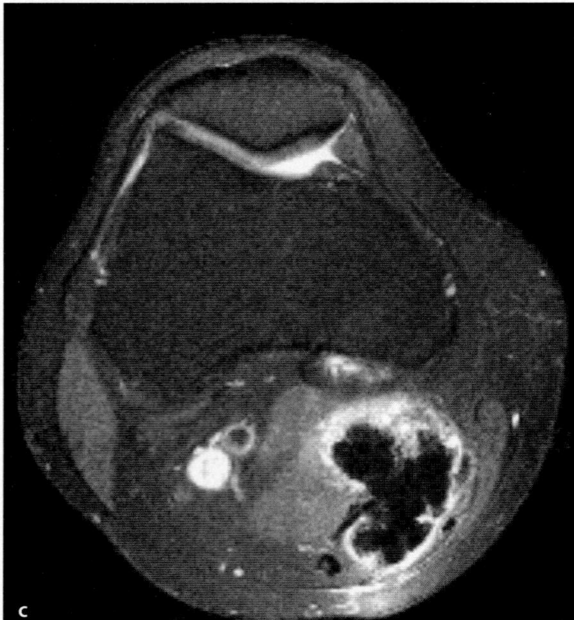

Fig. 21.3 a–c. Extraskeletal osteochondroma at the popliteal fossa:
a sagittal spin echo T1-weighted MR image with fat suppression;
b sagittal spin echo T1-weighted MR image with fat suppression
after gadolinium contrast injection; **c** axial spin echo T2-weighted
MR image with fat suppression. Rounded soft tissue mass at the
popliteal fossa. The central region of signal void corresponds
to extensive calcification, as observed in extraskeletal osteochondroma. The periphery of the lesion is slightly hyperintense to
muscle and fat on fat suppressed T1-weighted images (**a**), markedly hyperintense on fat suppressed T2-weighted images (**c**), and
shows pronounced enhancement following gadolinium contrast
injection (**b**)

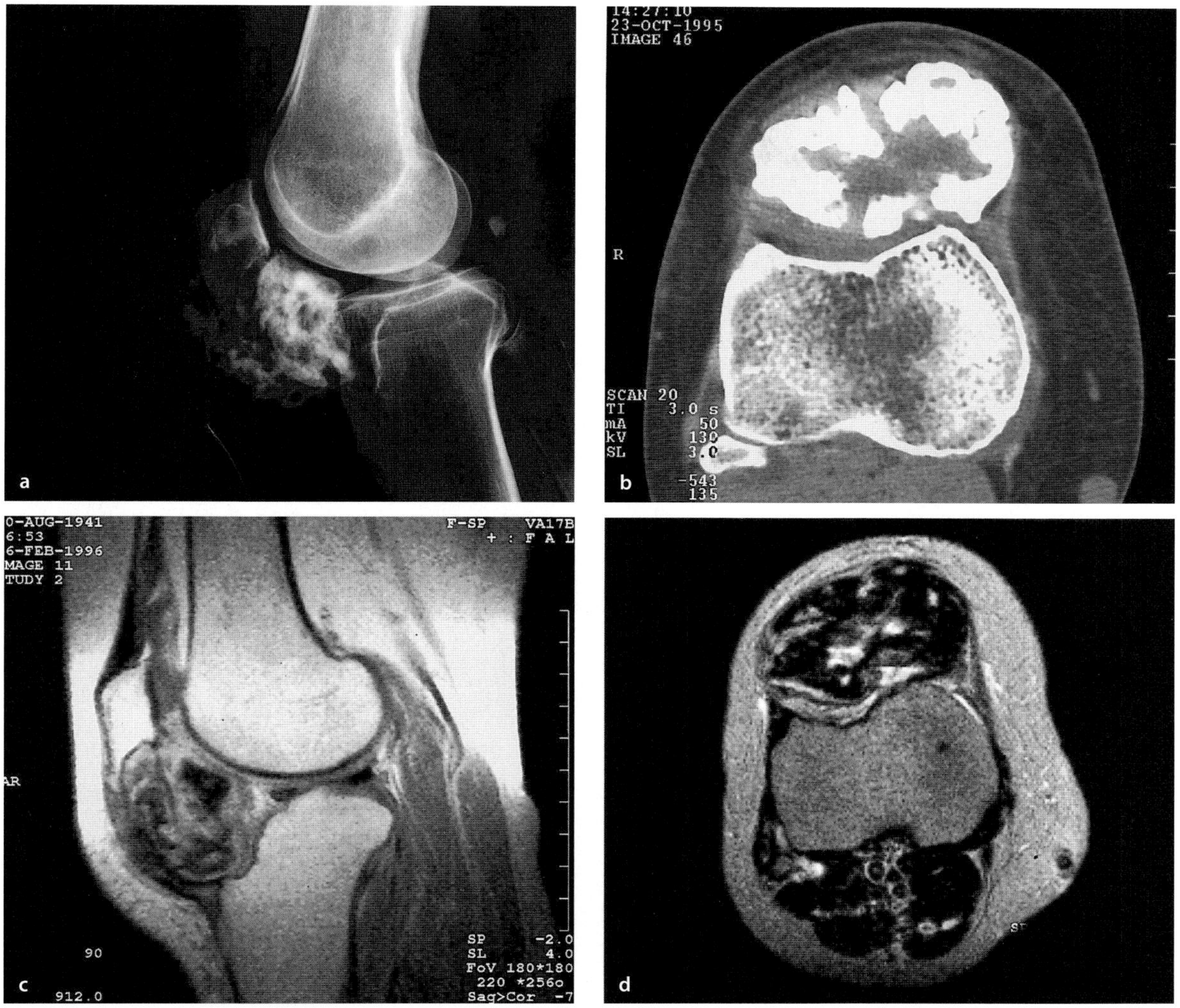

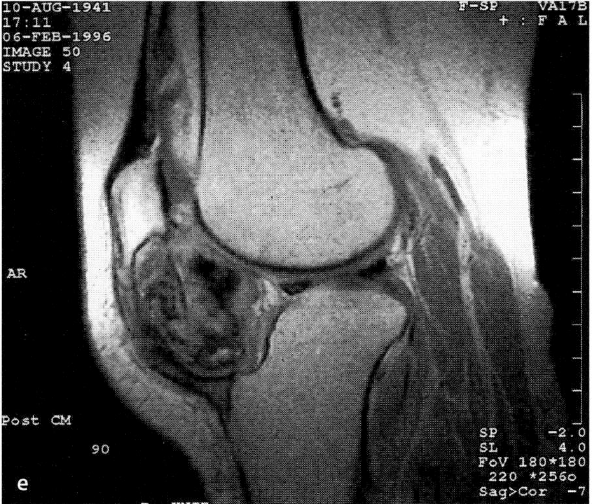

Fig. 21.4a–e. Extraskeletal chondroma (intracapsular type) below the right patella in a 54-year-old woman: **a** plain radiograph; **b** CT at the level of the proximal tibia; **c** sagittal spin echo T1-weighted MR image; **d** axial spin echo T2-weighted MR image at the level of the proximal tibia; **e** sagittal spin echo T1-weighted MR image after gadolinium contrast injection. Presence of a mass below the patella within the infrapatellar fat body. Plain radiograph and CT show a pronounced, dense calcification at the periphery of the mass (**a,b**). On the T1-weighted image, signal intensity is inhomogeneous but predominantly isodense to slightly hyperintense relative to muscle (**c**). No obvious enhancement is observed following gadolinium contrast injection (**e**). Very hyperintense areas are observed in the center of the lesion on T2-weighted image (**d**). On MR images the calcified areas cause large foci of signal void (**c–e**). Although in an unusual location, this case demonstrates well the features of extraskeletal chondroma on various imaging techniques

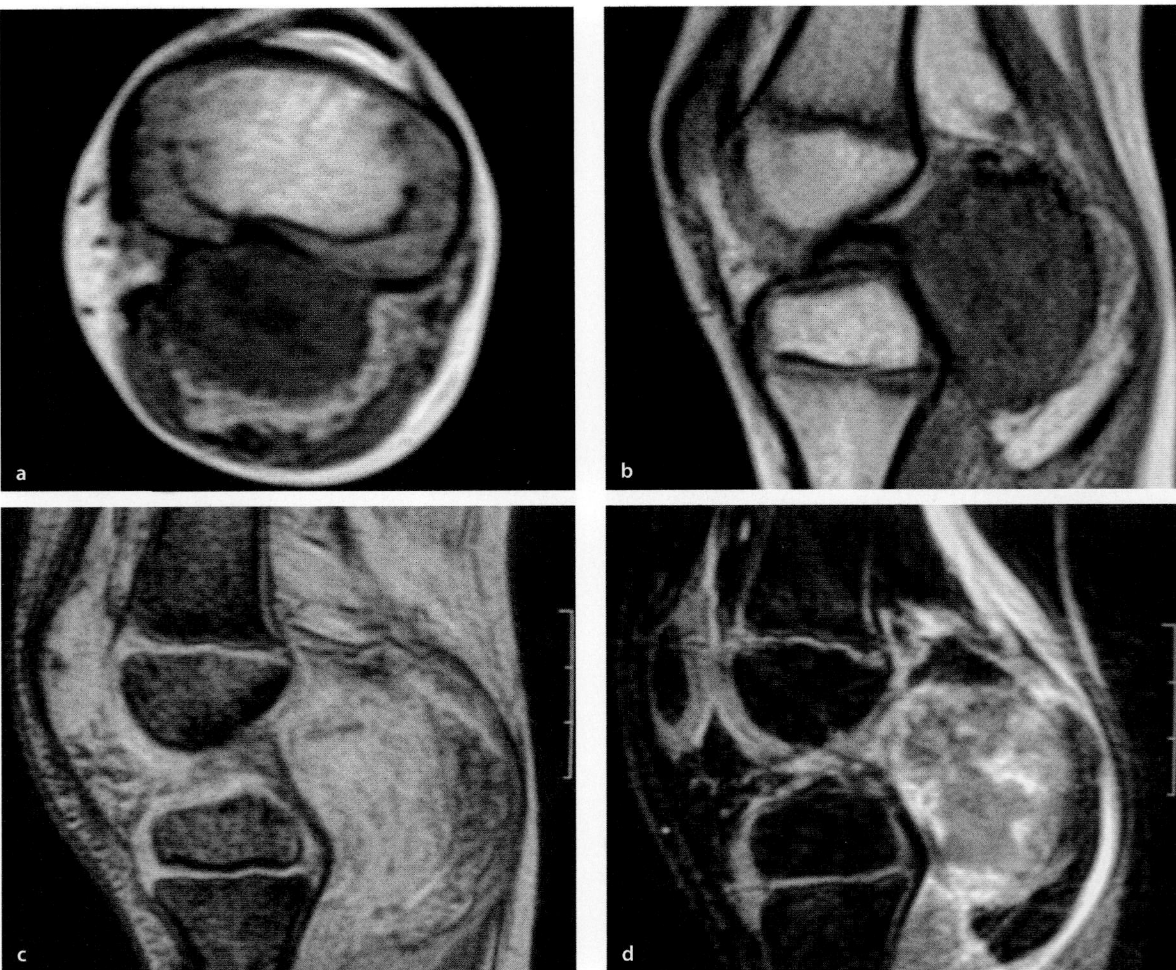

Fig. 21.5 a–d. Extraskeletal chondroma (extracapsular type) in the popliteal fossa of a six-year-old boy: **a** axial spin echo T1-weighted MR image; **b** sagittal spin echo T1-weighted MR image; **c** sagittal gradient recalled echo T2-weighted MR image; **d** sagittal fat-suppressed T1-weighted MR image after gadolinium contrast injection. Soft tissue mass in the popliteal fossa. The lesion is of low signal intensity on the T1-weighted images, and is surrounded by a thin layer of fatty tissue (**a**). The mass appears to be homogeneous and does not contain internal calcifications (**b,c**). Following contrast administration, marked, peripheral enhancement is seen (**d**)

■ **Imaging.** Plain radiographs reveal a soft tissue mass with central high density due to central calcification-ossification. The CT appearance is similar (Fig. 21.5). On MRI para-articular chondroma presents as a mass of relatively low signal, with areas of signal void in the center, corresponding with calcification and ossification [19]. On T2-weighted images, high signal intensity areas are seen within the lesion. After contrast injection peripheral enhancement is observed (Fig. 21.5).

In differential diagnosis other radiological calcified soft tissue masses about the joints must be considered, such as old hematomas, calcifying bursitis, tumoral calcinosis, periosteal chondromas, calcified synovial sarcomas, primary synovial chondromatosis and synovial chondrosarcoma. The differential diagnosis is made on histological basis [19, 32].

21.3.1.3 Synovial Osteochondromatosis

■ **Definition.** Synovial osteochondromatosis is characterized by the formation of numerous metaplastic cartilaginous or osteocartilaginous nodules of small size, attached to the synovial membrane of joint or tendon sheath [14, 43]. This lesion may also occur in a bursa or popliteal cyst. The nodules often detach and form loose bodies in the joint space. Approximately two-thirds of them calcify or ossify.

Rarely, the nodules are extra-articular (Figs. 21.6 and 21.7). Chondrosarcoma arising in synovial chondromatosis has been reported but is uncommon [5].

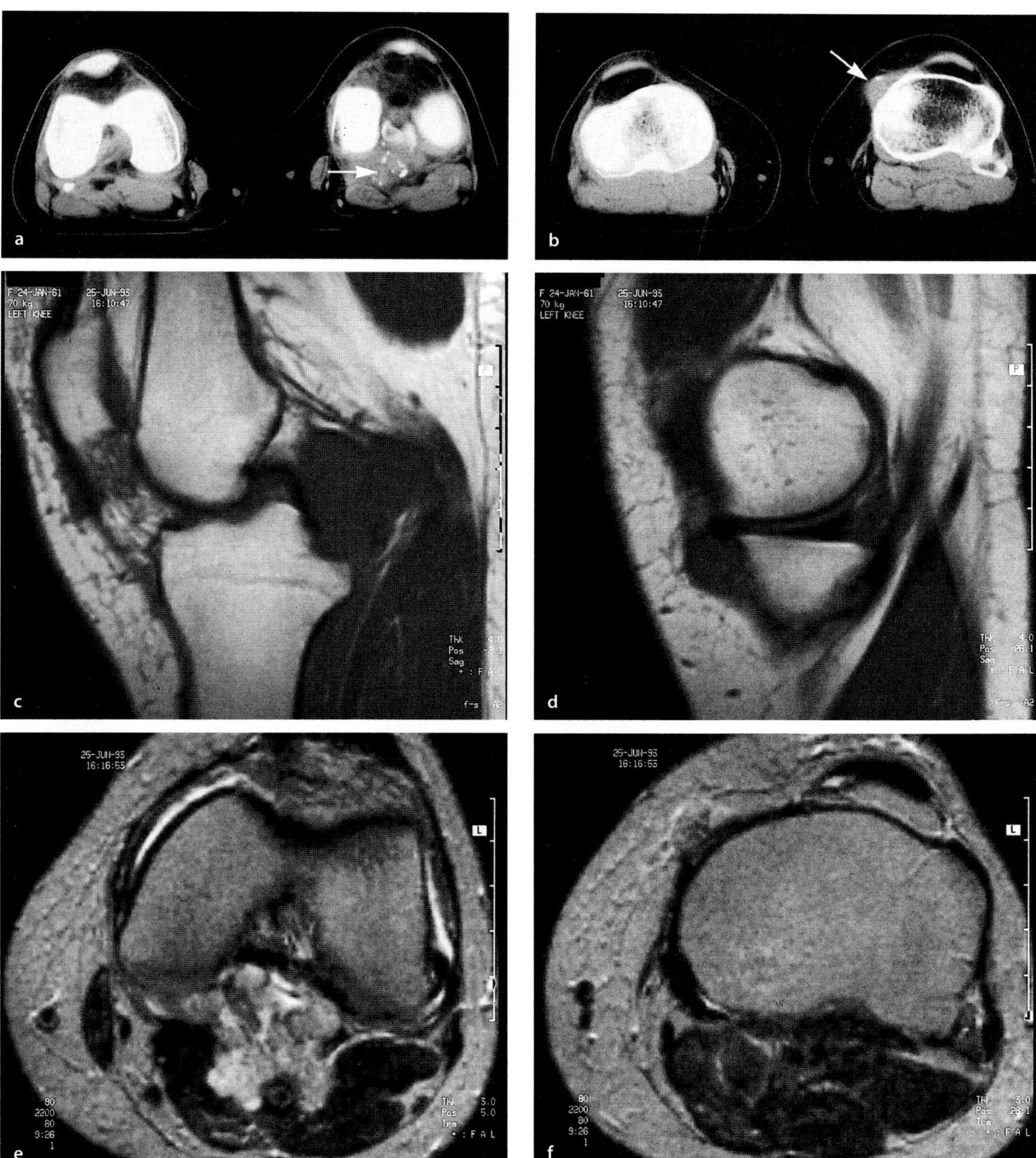

Fig. 21.6a–f. Multifocal synovial chondromatosis of the right knee in a 32-year-old woman: **a** CT at the level of femoral condyles; **b** CT at the level of the proximal tibial epiphysis; **c** sagittal spin echo T1-weighted MR image at the midline; **d** sagittal spin echo T1-weighted MR image at the medial femoral condyle; **e** axial spin echo T2-weighted MR image at the level of the femoral condyles; **f** axial spin echo T2-weighted MR image at the level of the proximal tibial epiphysis. Presence of two small soft tissue masses with punctate intralesional calcifications (**a,b**, *arrows*). Both lesions are lobulated and of intermediate signal intensity on the T1-weighted images (**c,d**). They are adjacent to the anterior horn of the medial meniscus and the posterior cruciate ligament. Both lesions in the popliteal fossa exhibit intermediate signal intensity on the T2-weighted images (**e,f**). Popliteal artery and vein are gently displaced and not invaded by the process (**e**). CT and MRI findings are indicative for a multifocal synovial pathology. Absence of characteristic calcified loose bodies. The polylobular appearance and intermediate signal intensity on T2-weighted images allow differential diagnosis with meniscal cyst

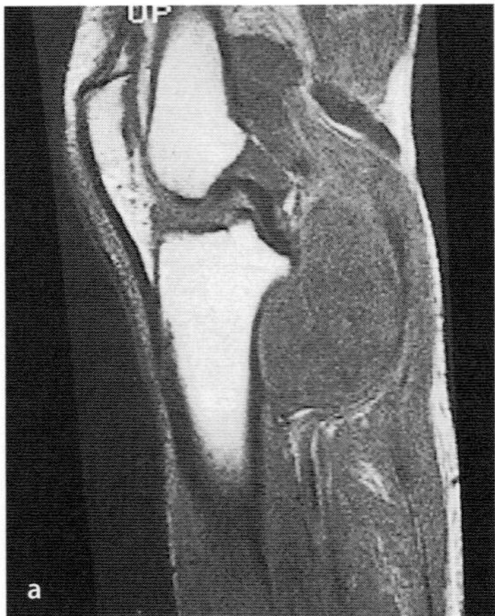

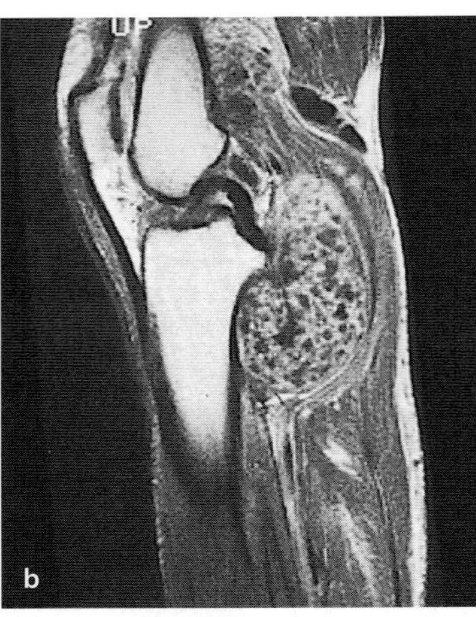

Fig. 21.7 a,b. Multifocal extra-articular synovial chondromatosis of the popliteal fossa in a 68-year-old man: **a** sagittal spin echo T1-weighted MR image; **b** sagittal spin echo T1-weighted MR image after gadolinium contrast injection. There are two rounded masses within the popliteal fossa. They are of low to intermediate signal intensity on the first T1-weighted image (**a**). After contrast injection there is strong enhancement of the synovial tissue without enhancement of multiple small cartilaginous nodules (**b**). On T2-weighted image (not shown) the lesion presents with an overall high signal intensity. Characteristic presentation of an extra-articular synovial chondromatosis without calcification of cartilaginous bodies

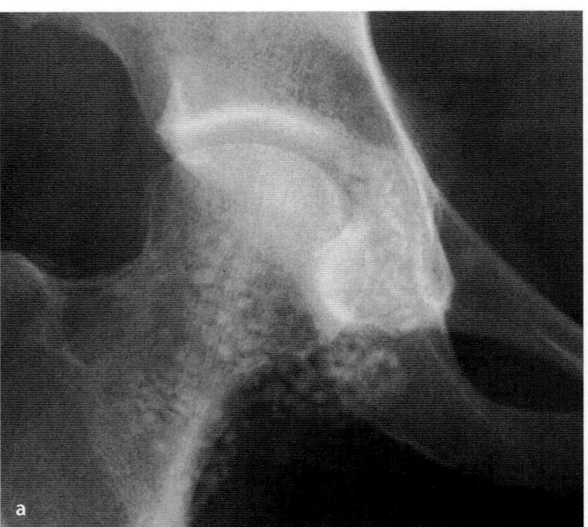

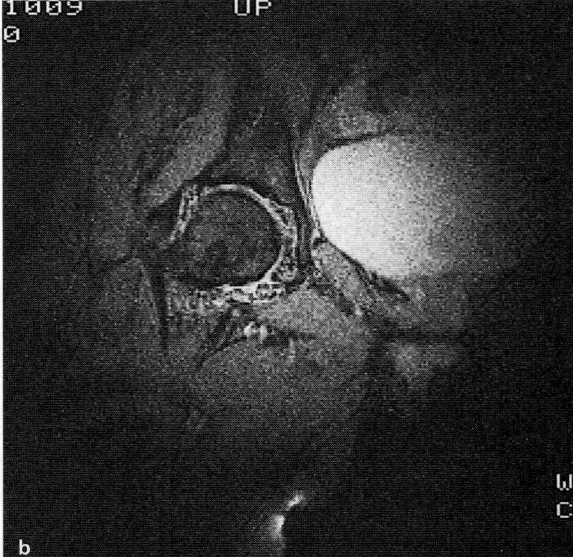

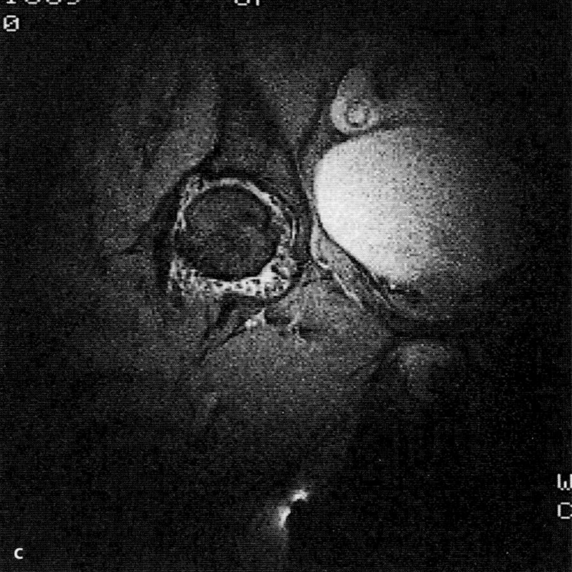

Fig. 21.8 a–c. Intra-articular synovial osteochondromatosis of the right hip joint in a 36-year-old woman: **a** plain radiograph; **b,c** coronal gradient-recalled echo (flash) T2*-weighted MR images. Presence of typical rice grain-like ossified nodules in the region of the right hip joint (**a**). On the T2-weighted images these nodules are seen as ring-like signal voids within the joint fluid. Ossification rather than calcification is suggested on MRI by the presence of a central hyperintense area, with signal intensity of fatty bone marrow, within the largest nodules (**b,c**). This case illustrates characteristic features of ossified intraarticular synovial chondromatosis on plain radiography and MRI

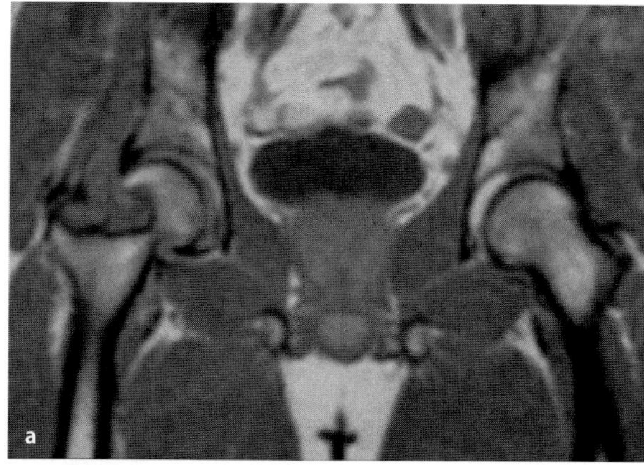

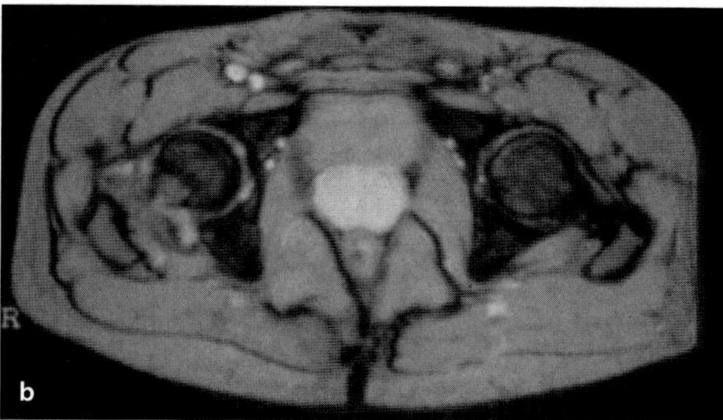

Fig. 21.9 a, b. Synovial chondromatosis of the hip in a 58-year-old woman, with chronic hip pain: **a** coronal spin echo T1-weighted MR image; **b** axial gradient recalled echo T2-weighted MR image. Intra-articular mass lesion with lobulated margins, associated with erosions of adjacent bone. There are no intralesional calcifications

■ **Incidence and Clinical Behavior.** Synovial osteochondromatosis occurs in large joints, such as hip, knee, shoulder or elbow [43]. The clinical history is often characterized by joint pain of several years' duration.

■ **Imaging.** Plain radiography and CT easily demonstrate the calcified or ossified nodules of chondromatosis (Figs. 21.6 and 21.8). Nonmineralized nodules are seen on arthrograms as filling defects outlined by contrast material. Bone scintigraphy shows an uptake of tracer within the nodules [43].

MRI findings are an increased amount of joint fluid and a lobular intra-articular mass. Uncalcified osteochondromas are isointense relative to muscle on T1-weighted images and hypointense relative to synovial fluid. Calcified lesions, occurring in up to 77% of cases, are seen as small, round signal voids. Ossified nodules may demonstrate signal intensities of fatty bone marrow [43]. In joints that have a very tense capsule, such as the hip joint, synovial chondromatosis can cause erosions of bone (Fig. 21.9).

The diagnosis of osteochondromatosis is still mostly made on findings on plain radiography or CT. Conven-

tional arthrography or CT arthrography is recommended if noncalcified nodules must be excluded. In the latter cases, however, high-resolution MRI may become a competitive imaging technique owing to its noninvasive character.

21.3.2 Malignant Lesions

Accounting for approximately 2% of all soft tissue sarcomas, chondrosarcomas in an extraskeletal location are relatively uncommon neoplasms and are far less frequent than those in intraosseous locations. A distinction is made between myxoid, mesenchymal, and well-differentiated types of extraskeletal chondrosarcoma (Figs. 21.10–21.13). A common feature of these neoplasms is that all, except the well-differentiated type, show minimal cartilage formation [20].

21.3.2.1 Extraskeletal Well-Differentiated Chondrosarcoma

■ **Definition.** This is the least common variant of extraskeletal chondrosarcoma. The tumor consists of lobules of well-differentiated hyaline cartilage [20].

■ **Incidence and Clinical Behavior.** Well-differentiated extraskeletal chondrosarcoma is extremely rare, and only very few cases have been mentioned in the literature [20, 25].

■ **Imaging.** In the few cases that have been reported, both plain radiography and CT demonstrated well defined but very densely mineralized soft tissue masses [20]. MRI findings have so far not been reported.

21.3.2.2 Extraskeletal Myxoid Chondrosarcoma (Chordoid Sarcoma)

■ **Definition.** The macroscopic appearance of myxoid chondrosarcoma is that of a soft to firm, well-defined polylobular soft tissue mass with a gelatinous consistency, mostly with a diameter of 4–7 cm. The tumor often contains cystic and hemorrhagic areas. If the hemorrhagic components dominate, the lesion may be mistaken for a hematoma [14, 20]. The term *chordoid sarcoma* refers to the superficial resemblance of this tumor to chordoma [14]. Microscopic examination shows a fibrous capsule surrounding the lesion and fibrous septations that separate the multiple lobules from each other. The lobules consist of strands of chondroblasts that are embedded in an abundant myxoid matrix [20].

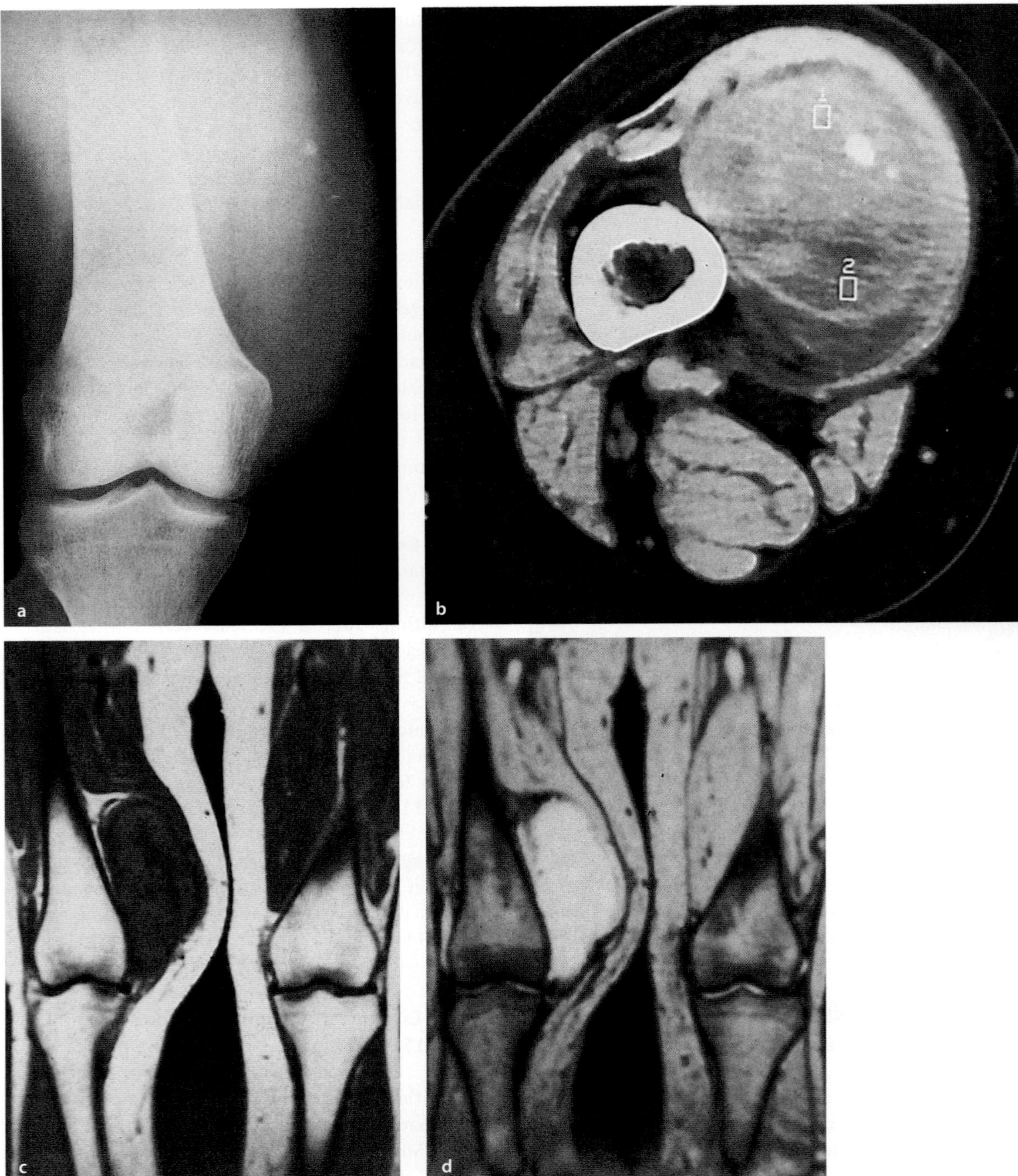

Fig. 21.10 a–d. Low-grade extraskeletal myxoid chondrosarcoma in the left thigh of a 50-year-old woman: **a** plain radiograph; **b** CT at the level of the distal femur; **c** coronal spin echo T1-weighted MR image; **d** coronal gradient-recalled echo T2-weighted MR image. Ill-defined soft tissue mass on the medial aspect of the distal femur. A rounded calcified area is seen in the upper pole of the lesion on the plain radiograph (**a**). CT shows a well-demarcated lesion with a round shape. The presence of sparse calcifications is confirmed. The tumor appears inhomogeneous, with irregularly outlined hypodense areas in its posterior aspect (**b**). On the coronal T1-weighted image the lesion is ovoid. The signal intensity of the tumor predominantly equals that of muscle, although an oblong hypointense area is observed centrally within the lesion (**c**). On the T2-weighted image uniform high signal intensity is observed, higher than that of fat (**d**). The very high signal intensity on T2-weighted image is indicative of the myxoid nature of this extraskeletal chondrosarcoma

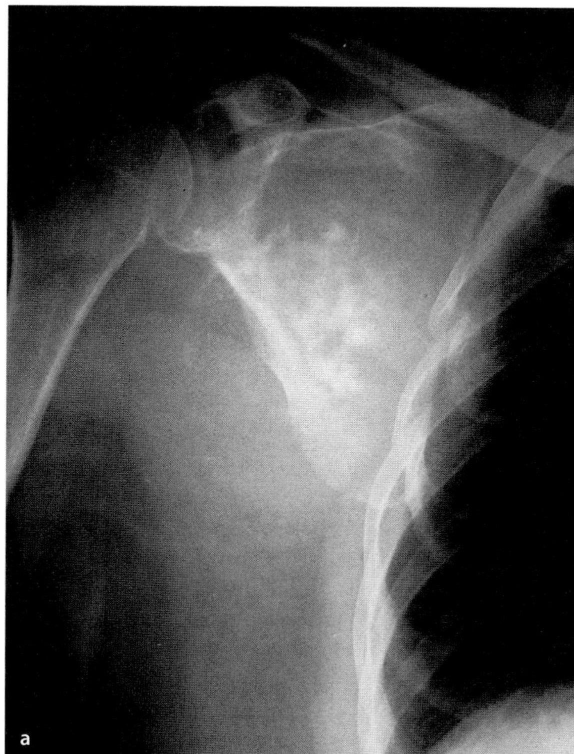

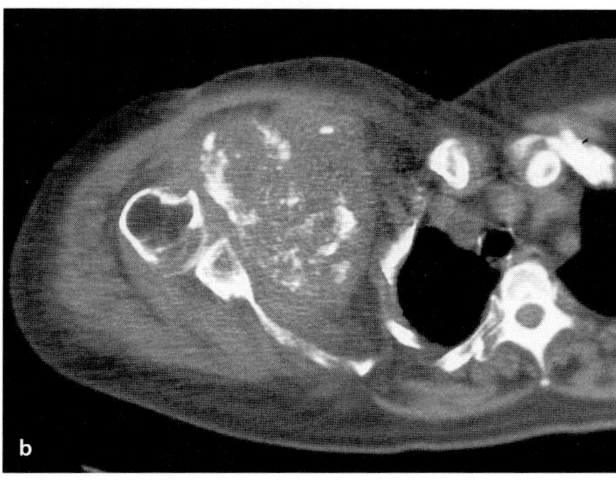

Fig. 21.11 a,b. Extraskeletal mesenchymal chondrosarcoma of the right axilla in a 50-year-old man: **a** plain radiograph; **b** CT. Ill-defined mass with coarse intralesional calcifications located in the subscapular region (**a,b**). Calcifications are commonly seen in the mesenchymal type of extraskeletal chondrosarcoma

■ **Incidence and Clinical Behavior.** The myxoid type of extraskeletal chondrosarcoma is the most common. The tumor afflicts mainly middle-aged adults, with the age of onset being approximately 50 years, but it has been described in patients ranging in age from 4 to 92 years. A higher prevalence is observed in men [14, 20,

24, 25, 29, 34]. Most tumors are located in the proximal extremities and limb girdles, the thigh being most frequently affected. Usually it presents as a slowly growing soft tissue mass, causing pain or tenderness only in about one-third of cases. Extraskeletal myxoid chondrosarcoma is commonly considered to be a low-grade sarcoma, in contrast to its intraosseous counter-part. Reported ten-year survival rates vary from 45 to 75% [20, 25]. Although recent reports suggest that the tumor has a high potential for development of metastases, survival of 5–15 years after the detection of metastases is not uncommon [24, 25, 34]. Metastatic spread commonly occurs, to lungs, followed by lymph nodes, bone, and brain [25]. Unfavorable prognostic factors are large tumor size and advanced age at the time of diagnosis. Local recurrence after surgery is common and often multiple [24, 25].

■ **Imaging.** The only finding on plain radiography and CT is a soft tissue mass that does not contain calcification or bone formation and does not involve adjacent bone. CT shows lobular contours and low attenuation of the tumor [20, 29].

Extraskeletal myxoid chondrosarcoma appears on MRI as a lobulated soft tissue mass (Fig. 21.10). Although the tumor may be well-delineated and homogeneous, in general. its appearance on MRI is that of an inhomogeneous, ill-defined mass. Signal intensity on T1-weighted images is variable and ranges from low, to intermediate, approximately equal to that of skeletal muscle, to high, equal to that of fat. High intensity areas on T1-weighted images are presumed to correspond with hemorrhagic changes within the tumor [29]. On T2-weighted images signal intensity is equal to or, more commonly, greater than that of fat [20, 29, 30, 41]. In cases with predominant myxoid component the lesion may present with very high signal intensity on T2-weighted images, resembling the appearance of cyst or myxoma. In tumors containing hyaline cartilage the appearance of the latter is similar to that of intraosseous chondrosarcoma and consists of homogeneous, high-intensity lobules defined by thin septa of lower signal intensity [9]. After gadolinium injection peripheral enhancement as seen in a chondroid tumor is frequently observed [29].

In view of the better demonstration of various tumor components and tumoral extent, MRI is the preferred imaging technique for both characterization and for staging extraskeletal myxoid chondrosarcoma. Initial plain radiography or CT, however, remains valuable for disclosing calcifications, although these are extremely rare in this tumor, and for determination of integrity of adjacent bone.

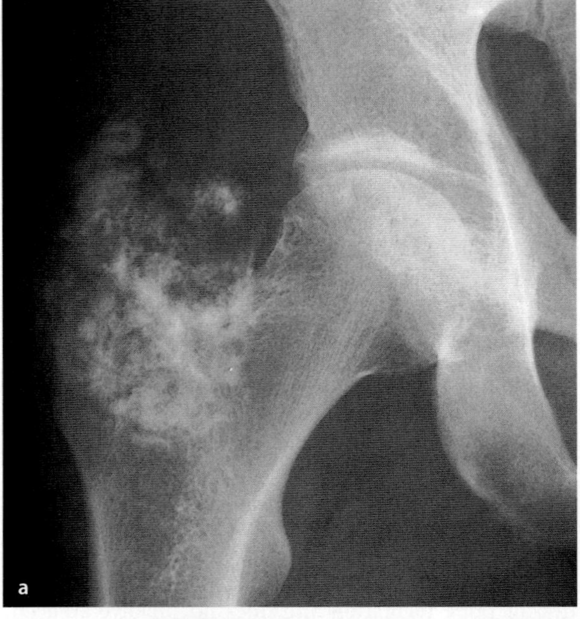

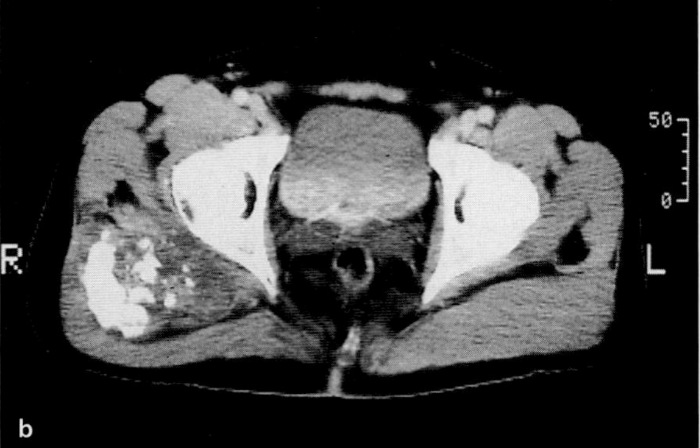

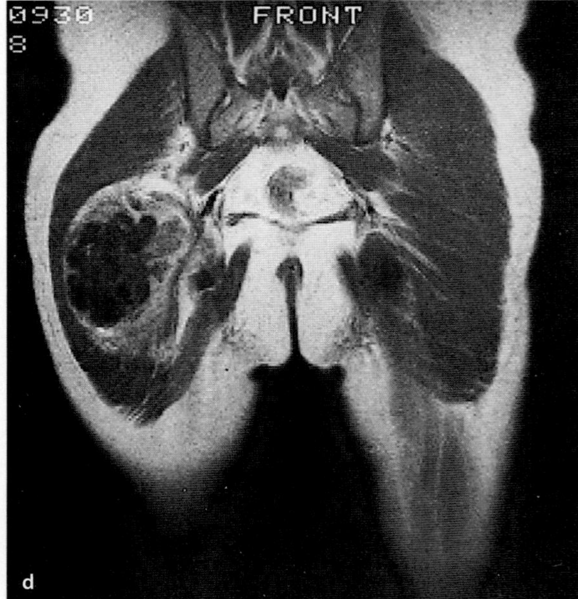

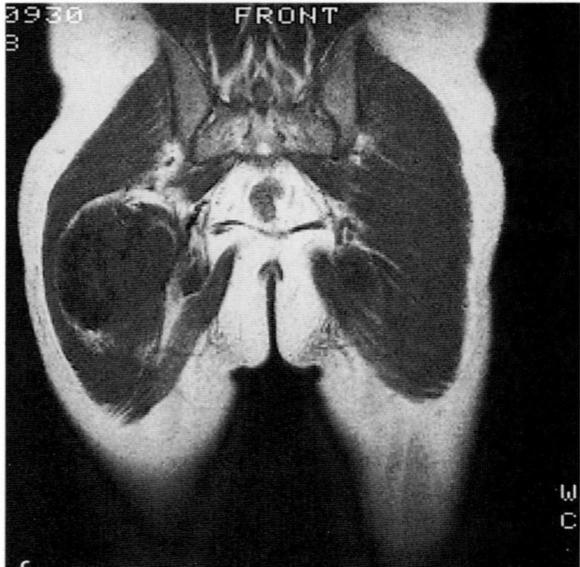

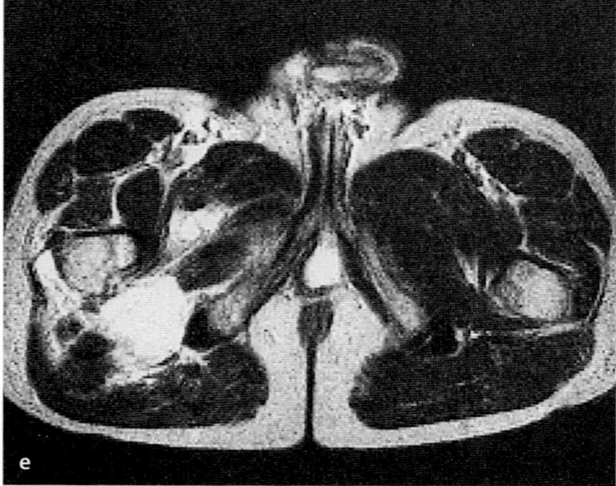

Fig. 21.12 a–e. Extraskeletal mesenchymal chondrosarcoma of the buttock in a 32-year-old man: **a** plain radiograph; **b** CT; **c** coronal spin echo T1-weighted MR image; **d** coronal spin echo T1-weighted MR image after gadolinium contrast injection; **e** axial spin echo T2-weighted MR image. Large calcified mass superior to the trochanter major (**a**). CT reveals a soft tissue component medially and the calcified component laterally within the mass (**b**). On bone window (not shown) there is no obvious osseous involvement. Inhomogeneity of the mass on the T1-weighted image is partially due to intralesional calcifications (**c**). After contrast injection, there is peripheral enhancement with central signal voids due to calcifications (**d**). On T2-weighted image the soft tissue component of the tumor is of extremely high signal intensity (**e**). Findings on plain radiography and CT together with high signal intensity of soft tumor lobules are indicative of a lesion of cartilaginous origin

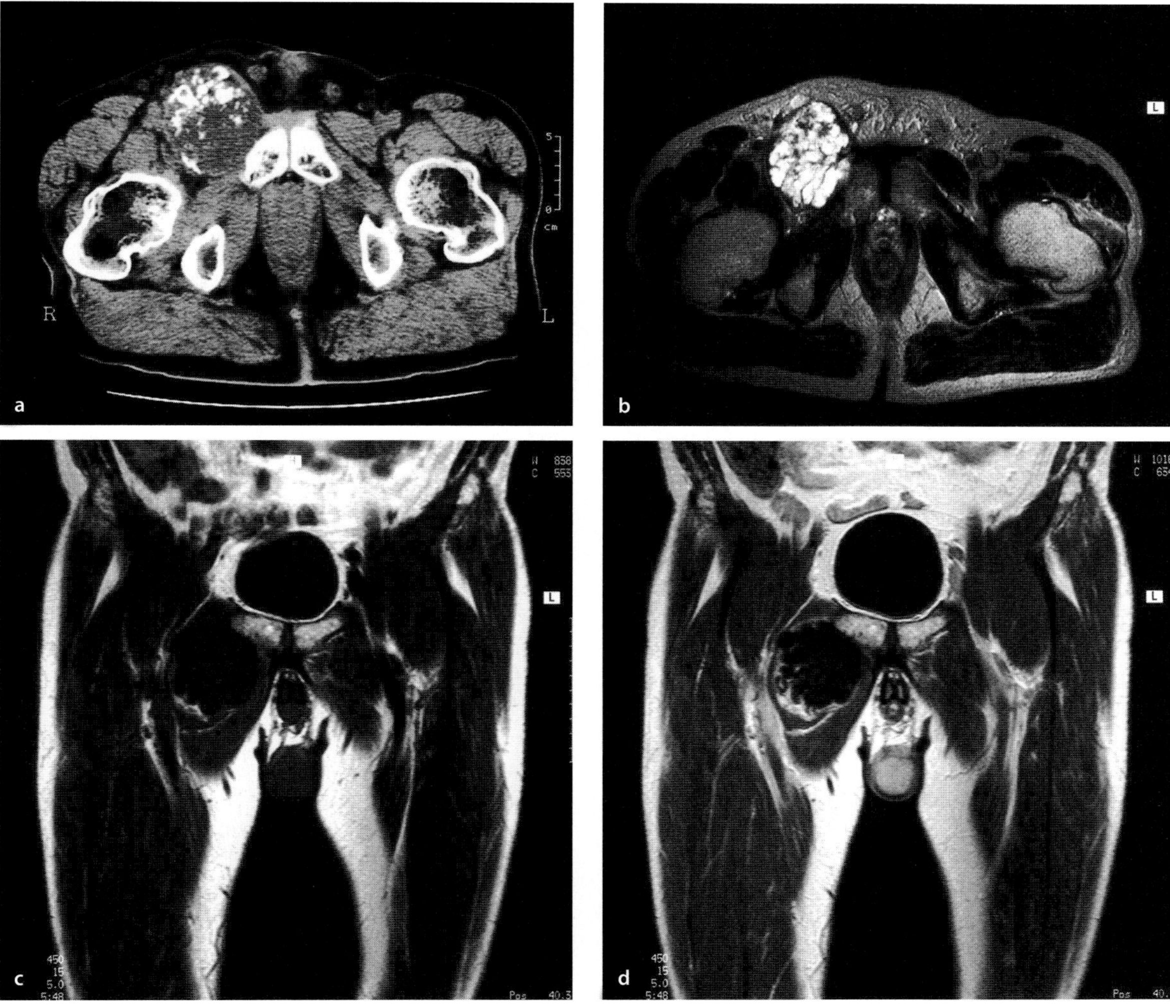

Fig. 21.13 a–d. Extraskeletal mesenchymal low-grade chondrosarcoma of the groin in a 58-year-old man, with known hereditary, multiple exostoses: **a** unenhanced CT; **b** coronal spin echo T1-weighted MR-image; **c** transverse spin echo T2-weighted MR image; **d** coronal spin echo T1-weighted image following administration of gadolinium. CT shows a rounded soft tissue mass at the origin of the right adductor muscles. Numerous calcifications are seen within the mass (**a**). MR images reveal the lobulated shape of the lesion better. On T1-weighted images, the mass has a predominantly very low intensity, and contains only thin strands of discrete higher intensity (**b**). The lobulated architecture of the mass is demonstrated best on the T2-weighted images (**c**). On these images the cartilaginous lobules are markedly hyperintense contrasting with the low-intensity septations and the amorphous areas of signal void and corresponding to the intralesional calcifications. Following administration of gadolinium, pronounced peripheral enhancement is observed (**d**)

21.3.2.3 Extraskeletal Mesenchymal Chondrosarcoma

■ **Definition.** This type of chondrosarcoma presents on macroscopy as a multilobulated mass of variable size. On cross section the tumor shows a mixture of gray-white tissue and foci of cartilage and bone. Small areas of hemorrhage or necrosis may be present but are less prominent than in the myxoid chondrosarcoma. On microscopy the tumor exhibits a proliferation of primitive mesenchymal cells and interspersed small islands of well-differentiated cartilage. Calcification is common but variable [14, 20].

■ **Incidence and Clinical Behavior.** Extraskeletal mesenchymal chondrosarcoma occurs less frequently than the myxoid variant. However, nearly half of all mesenchymal chondrosarcomas are extraskeletal in location, whereas the other 50% are intraosseous [36]. There is no apparent sex predominance [26]. A bimodal age distribution is noted and related to anatomic location. When occurring in the third decade of life, tumors are located mainly in the head or neck, often in the meningeal and periorbital regions. Tumors arising in the fifth decade of life afflict preferentially the thigh [25, 26]. The mesenchymal chondrosarcoma has an aggressive behavior and frequently metastasizes to lungs and lymph nodes. The prognoses is poor, with a ten-year survival rate of nearly 25% [14, 26, 36].

■ **Imaging.** Calcifications within the tumor, which are present in 50–100% of the cases, are well demonstrated by plain radiography and CT (Figs. 21.11–21.13). The degree and type of calcification are variable and range from ring and arcs, flocculent or stippled calcification to dense mineralization [26, 34, 41]. In rare cases the tumor involves underlying bone.

On MRI the extraskeletal mesenchymal chondrosarcoma presents as a lobulated soft tissue mass. Signal intensity of the tumor equals that of muscle on T1-weighted images and is higher than that of fat on T2-weighted images [36]. Following administration of gadolinium complexes, inhomogeneous enhancement is observed, especially at the periphery [36].

Plain radiography and CT are valuable as they demonstrate the calcifications within the tumor and hence point to the histological nature of the tumor. MRI, in contrast, shows only nonspecific findings but is best suited to determining the soft tissue extent of the lesion.

21.4 Osseous Tumors and Tumor-like Conditions of the Soft Tissues

21.4.1 Benign Lesions

21.4.1.1 Myositis Ossificans, Panniculitis Ossificans, Fasciitis Ossificans

■ **Definition.** Myositis ossificans is a generally solitary, benign, self limiting ossifying process occurring in the musculature of the extremities in young men and is related to trauma in about half of all cases [15, 25]. Sometimes it occurs within other tissues, such as subcutaneous fat (panniculitis ossificans) – in one-third of the cases – tendons or fasciae (fasciitis ossificans), and periosteum of the digits (fibro-osseous pseudotumor of the digits) [15, 25].

Most lesions in myositis ossificans measure 3–6 cm in diameter. On cross-section they have a white, soft, and rather gelatinous center and firm, yellow gray periphery with rough, granular surface [15]. Microscopically a zonal pattern is observed. This refers to a progressive degree of cellular maturation from the center to the periphery, maturation being lowest in the center and highest with mature bone formation – at the periphery.

■ **Incidence and Clinical Behavior.** Myositis ossificans is by far the most common bone-forming lesion of the soft tissues. The exact pathogenesis of this disorder is still unclear. A history of preceding mechanical trauma is pre-

sent in about half of all cases [15, 25]. As causative factors in some of the other cases, infection and coagulopathy have been mentioned [15, 25]. Furthermore, the disease may also occur in association with burns, paraplegia, and quadriplegia or with other neuromuscular disorders such as tetanus [1, 25]. Finally, generalized periarticular myositis ossificans as a complication of pharmacologically induced paralysis has been reported [1].

Myositis ossificans commonly affects young, active adults and adolescents, predominantly men (Figs. 21.14–21.18), but occasionally involves persons of other age groups. Pain and tenderness are the first symptoms, followed by a diffuse swelling of soft tissues. This swelling typically becomes more circumscribed and indurated after two to three weeks. Thereafter it progressively changes into a firm hard mass approximately 3–6 cm in diameter, which is well outlined on palpation [15]. Although malignant transformation into extraskeletal osteosarcoma has been suggested in the literature, it has never been proven [15, 27]. Hence, the prognosis of myositis ossificans is generally accepted to be excellent [15].

Principal sites of involvement are the limbs, which are affected in more than 80% of cases. The quadriceps muscle and brachialis muscle are favored sites in the lower and upper extremity, respectively. Areas prone to trauma are more commonly afflicted.

The incidence of panniculitis ossificans differs slightly from that of myositis ossificans in that it prevails in the upper extremities of women [15, 25].

Fibro-osseous pseudotumor of the digits occurs predominantly in the fingers or toes of young adults [25].

■ **Imaging.** Acute myositis ossificans refers to early stages of disease, before ossification is radiologically visible [10, 12]. During these initial stages of disease only a slight increase in soft tissue density is observed radiologically. Angiography at that time may disclose pronounced hypervascularity. In general, calcification develops between four and six weeks after the initial trauma and results in a "mature" lesion. Initially these calcifications present as irregular, floccular radiopacities. Over time lamellar bone forms at the periphery of the lesion and proceeds toward its center [15, 25]. The centrifugal pattern of progressive maturation is well reflected by the CT appearance of the lesion during the active stage of disease: the central immature zone of the lesion appears radiolucent, whereas the outer mature zone shows calcification and ossification (Figs. 21.15 and 21.16). This appearance is referred to in the literature as the "zoning" phenomenon [2]. The appearance of panniculitis ossificans and fibro-osseous pseudotumor of the digits is similar to that of myositis ossificans except that these conditions lack an obvious zoning phenomenon [25, 28]. In the latter case cortical erosion of underlying bone and stippled calcification may be observed [25].

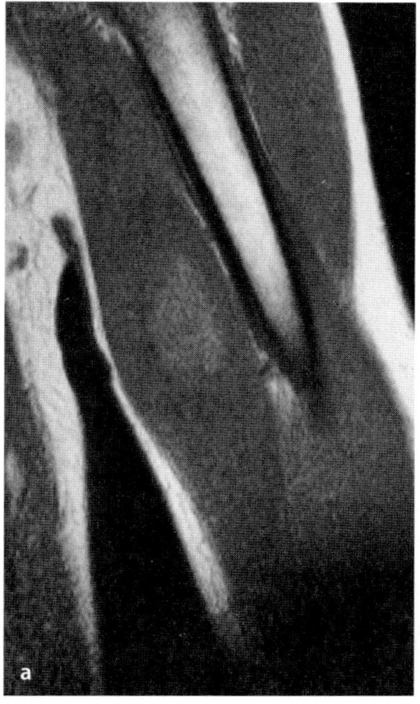
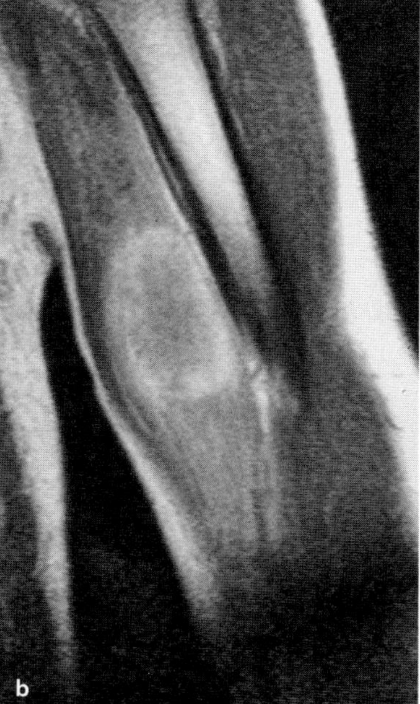
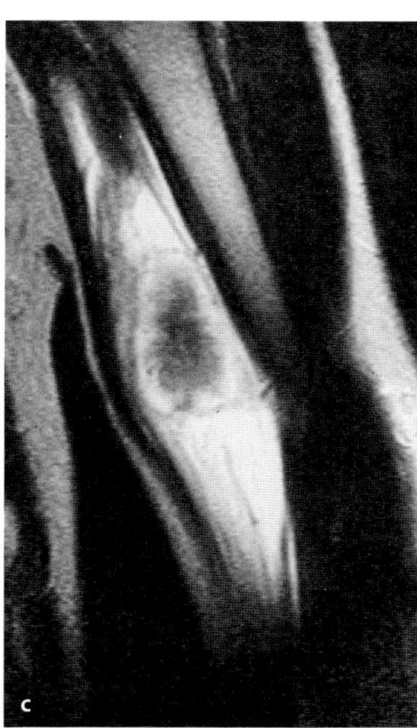

Fig. 21.14 a–c. Myositis ossificans, early stage, in the left upper arm of a seven-year-old boy: **a** coronal T1-weighted MR image; **b** coronal T1-weighted MR image after gadolinium contrast injection; **c** coronal T2-weighted MR image. Ill-defined mass within the biceps muscle. On the T1-weighted image the mass is slightly hyperintense to muscle (**a**). After contrast injection there is a marked peripheral enhancement (**b**). On the T2-weighted image the center of the lesion remains hypointense, while the hyperintense periphery is outlined by a small hypointense rim. Extremely high signal intensity within the whole biceps muscle (**c**). Characteristic appearance of an early stage myositis ossificans. (Biopsy revealed large amounts of osteoid bone, surrounded by numerous osteoblasts)

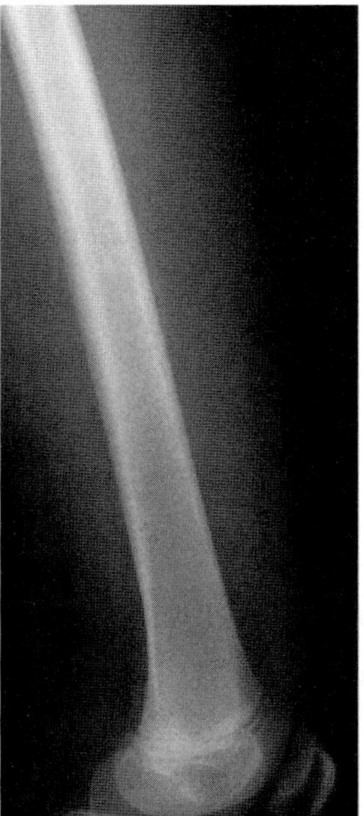
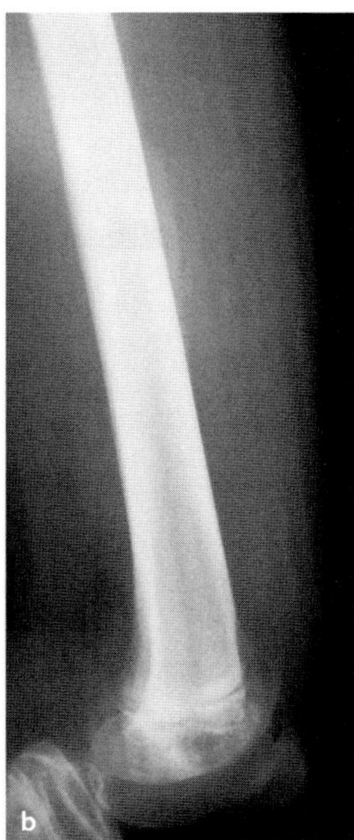
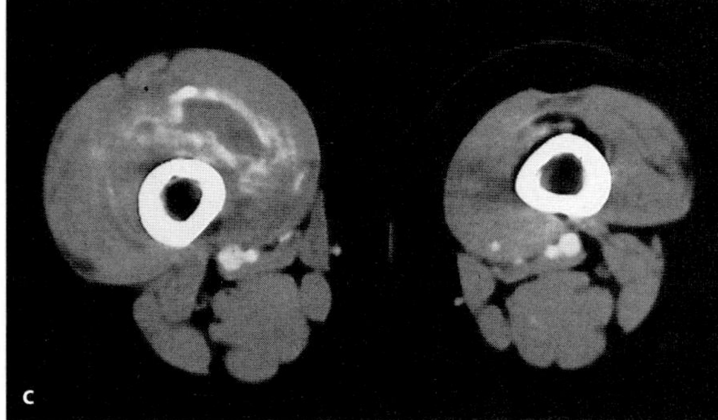

Fig. 21.15 a–c. Myositis ossificans, intermediate stage of the right thigh in a 13-year-old boy: **a** plain radiograph a few days after trauma; **b** plain radiograph five days later; **c** CT. Presence of a faint linear parosteal calcification on the ventral aspect of the right thigh (**a**). Five days later there is extensive calcification within the quadriceps muscle (**b**). On CT there is diffuse swelling of the right thigh with an egg-shell calcification within the vastus intermedius muscle (**c**). The zoning phenomenon is characteristic for an intermediate stage of posttraumatic myositis ossificans

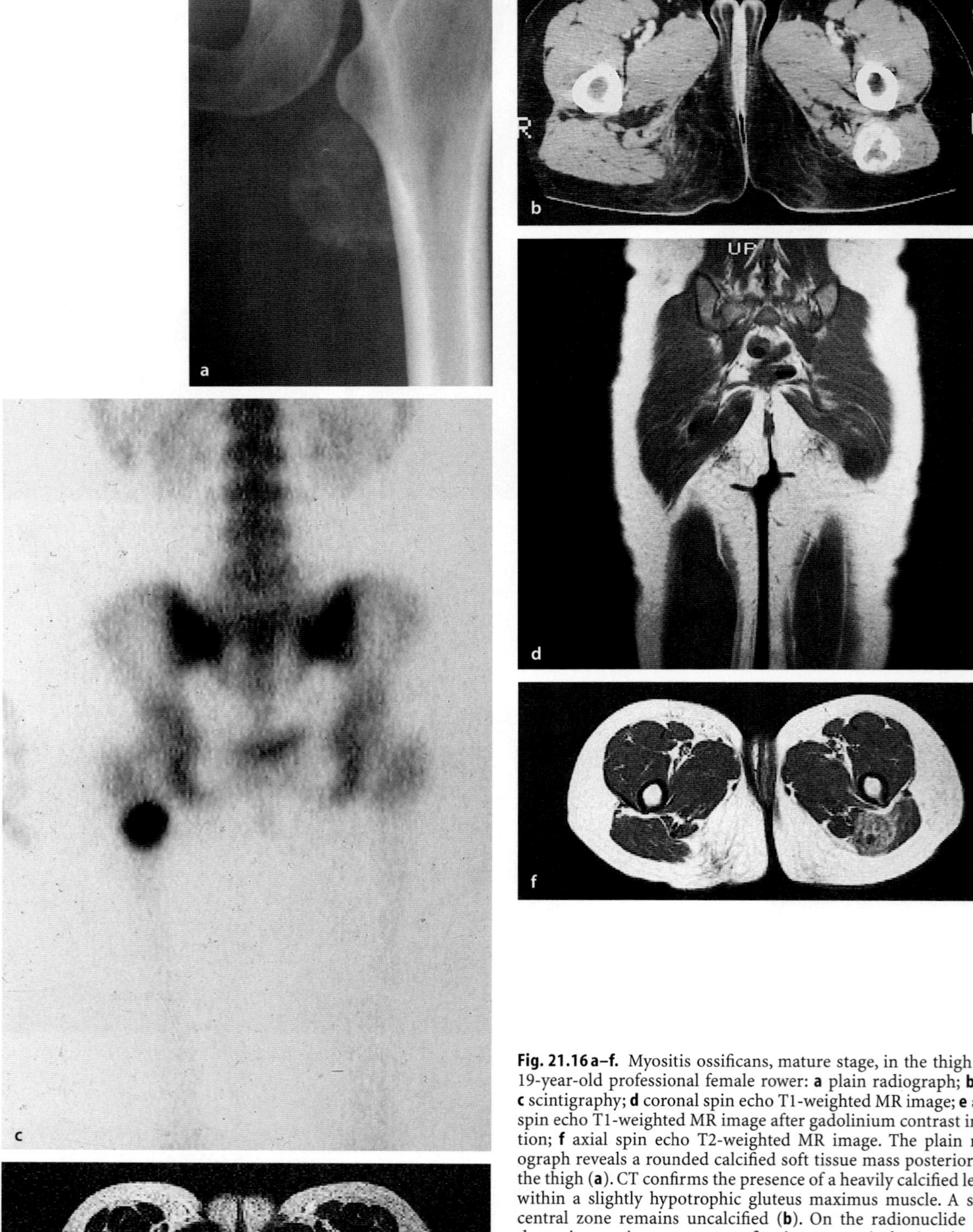

Fig. 21.16a–f. Myositis ossificans, mature stage, in the thigh of a 19-year-old professional female rower: **a** plain radiograph; **b** CT; **c** scintigraphy; **d** coronal spin echo T1-weighted MR image; **e** axial spin echo T1-weighted MR image after gadolinium contrast injection; **f** axial spin echo T2-weighted MR image. The plain radiograph reveals a rounded calcified soft tissue mass posteriorly in the thigh (**a**). CT confirms the presence of a heavily calcified lesion within a slightly hypotrophic gluteus maximus muscle. A small central zone remains uncalcified (**b**). On the radionuclide scan there is an intense tracer fixation posteriorly in the left trochanteric region (**c**). The lesion is hypointense on the T1-weighted image (**d**), hyperintense on the T2-weighted image (**f**), and shows marked enhancement (onion-skin pattern) after contrast injection (**e**). Absence of concomitant mass effect is also obvious on all MR images. History of the patient and imaging findings are in favor of a mature myositis ossificans. Despite the huge calcifications, the lesion still generates high signal intensity on the T2-weighted image

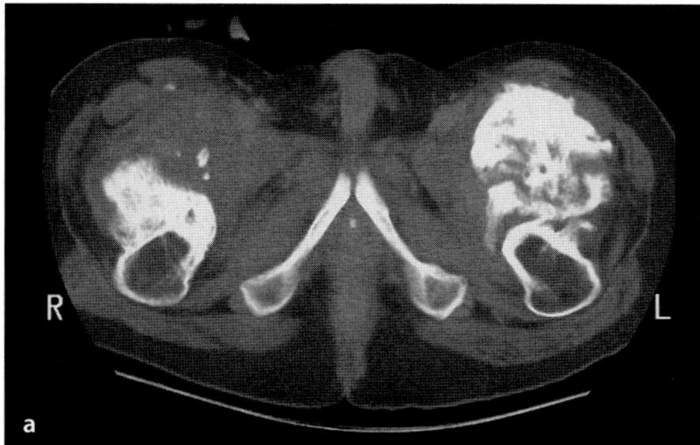

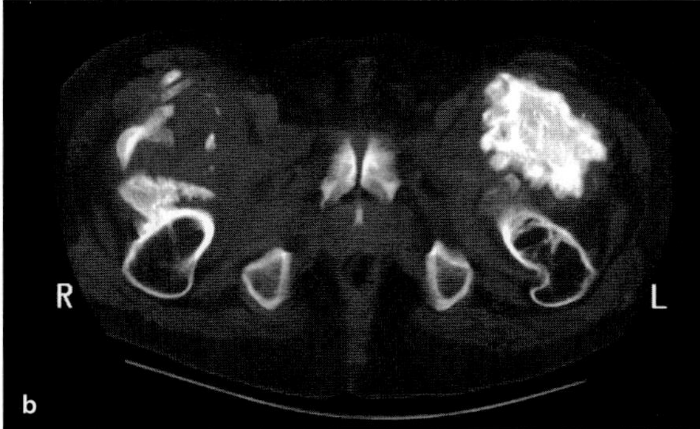

Fig. 21.17 a, b. Posttraumatic myositis ossificans, mature stage, anteriorly in the proximal third of both thighs in a 33-year -old man: **a** CT at the level of the lesser trochanter of the femur (soft tissue window setting); **b** same CT section as in a (bone window setting). Huge, considerably calcified soft tissue masses within both quadriceps muscles, corresponding to the mature stage of myositis ossificans

Three different appearances of myositis ossificans are noted on MRI, corresponding to the stage of maturation [10, 12, 21, 37, 44]. Early stages of myositis ossificans, the so-called acute form, present on MRI as a mass that is isointense or even slightly hyperintense to muscle on T1-weighted images, but hyperintense on T2-weighted images (Fig. 21.14). The lesion is surrounded with variable amounts of edema, appearing hyperintense on T2-weighted image, and a hypointense rim in some cases [10, 12, 21, 37]. Following administration of gadolinium a well-defined rim of enhancement is observed, allowing differentiation between the lesion and primary soft tissue sarcoma, which is enhanced homogeneously [10, 16, 37]. The MRI appearance of the lesions during the intermediate or subacute stage is characterized by isointensity with muscle on T1-weighted images and mild increase of signal intensity on T2-weighted images. These findings are explained by a central fibrous transformation as observed histologically. Occasionally a thin rim of signal void surrounding the lesion may be observed, especially on T2-weighted images, and corresponds to a rim of calcification, although this is better observed on plain radiography and CT [37]. Findings

consistent with hemorrhage and fluid-fluid levels have been reported in some cases [21]. Mature lesions (i.e., the "chronic stage") show more extensive signal voids on all sequences, corresponding to a considerable degree of peripheral calcification and ossification (Fig. 21.16). In this stage lesions demonstrate increased signal intensity in an "onion-skin pattern" on T2-weighted images [37] (Fig. 21.16).

The diagnosis of myositis ossificans commonly relies on findings on plain radiography. Attention must be paid to the presence of a central radiolucent area, as a manifestation of the zoning phenomenon and of a lucent fine separating the lesion from the underlying cortex, which are both better demonstrated on CT. As biopsies, establishing the diagnosis, may have been taken during early stages of the disease, the lesion may continue to grow for some period of time. In these cases repeated plain radiographs CT are useful to document the maturation and to exclude a destructive growth pattern [15, 27] (Figs. 21.17 and 21.18). Plain radiography and CT are superior to MRI in demonstrating calcifications and ossification; however, in the case of early disease – "acute myositis ossificans" – MRI has proven the most accurate imaging technique, although findings are non-specific.

21.4.1.2 Fibrodysplasia Ossificans Progressiva

■ **Definition.** This term refers to a rare, inheritable disorder that is characterized by a progressive ossification of connective tissue and muscle, and by osseous anomalies, particularly short thumbs and great toes [15, 38]. The disease affects primarily connective tissue and is followed by secondary changes in muscle, leading to calcification and ossification of subcutaneous fat, skeletal muscle, tendons, aponeuroses, and ligaments. The first manifestation of the disease is edema, with proliferation of fibroblasts. In a more advanced stage this is followed by deposition of abundant collagen. Finally, this collagenized fibrous tissue calcifies and ossifies. In contrast to myositis ossificans, the ossification takes place in the center of the lesions [15, 17, 38].

■ **Incidence and Clinical Behavior.** The onset of fibrodysplasia ossificans progressiva is typically in the first few years of life, generally before the age of six years and in about half of the cases at the age of two years [15, 38]. The occurrence of the disease is usually sporadic, but it may be inherited in an autosomal dominant way with variable penetrance. A slight male predominance is noted. Symmetric malformations of the digits, especially the thumbs and great toes, are concomitant findings [15, 17, 38].

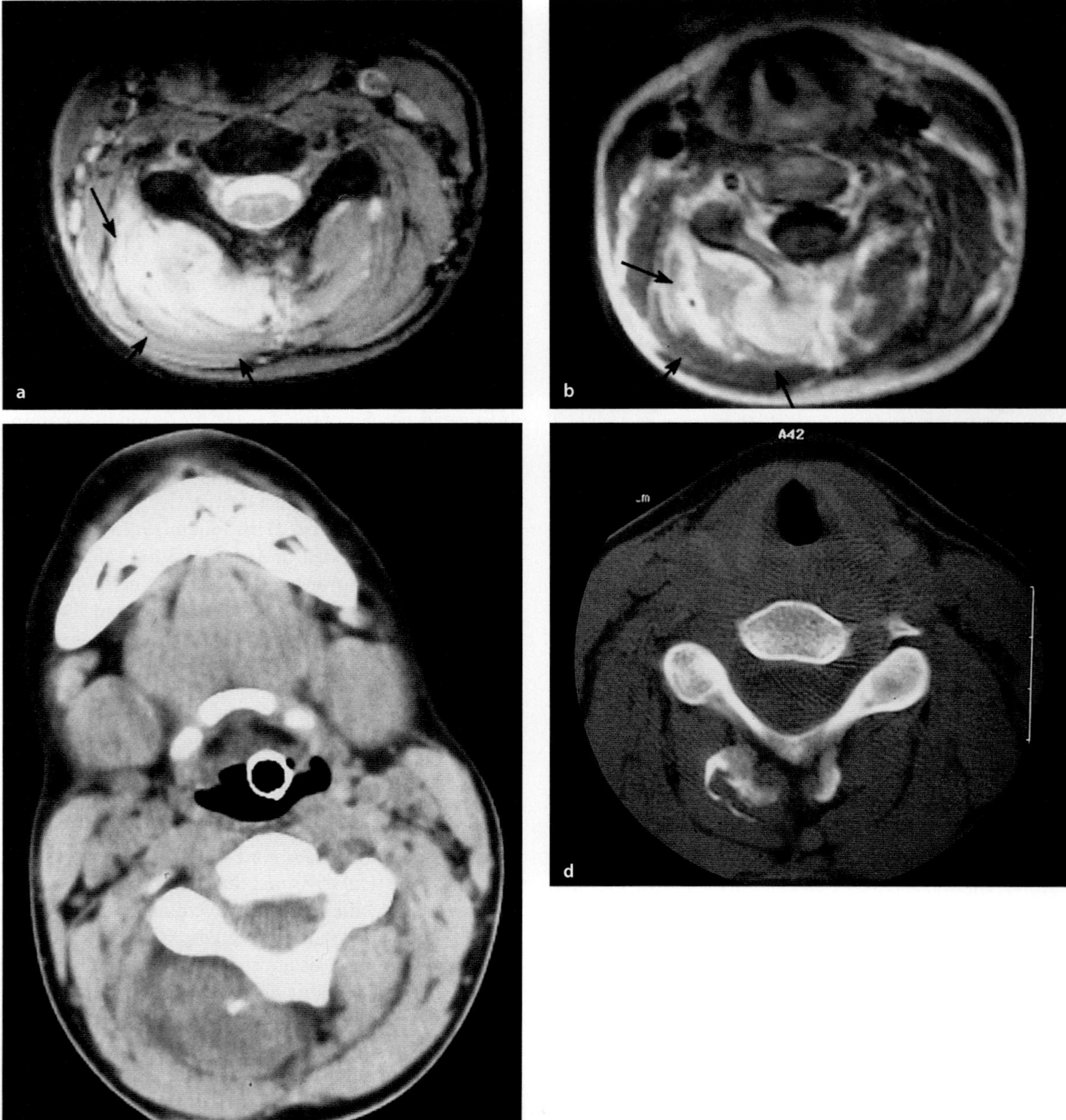

Fig. 21.18a–d. Myositis ossificans evolution from early to mature stage. Myositis ossificans on the neck of a nine-year-old boy who initially presented with torticollis: **a** axial spin echo fat-suppressed T2-weighted MR image; **b** axial spin echo T1-weighted MR image after gadolinium contrast injection; **c** plain CT at the time of initial presentation; **d** plain CT six months later. There is a large soft tissue mass deeply seated in the neck, adjacent to the vertebra. On T1-weighted MR images (not shown) the lesion is of intermediate signal intensity. On T2-weighted images, the lesion is uniformly hyperintense *(arrows)* and outlined by a large area of perilesional edema (**a**). After gadolinium injection, intense enhancement is observed at the lesion *(arrows)*, while only moderate enhancement occurs in the perilesional edematous area (**b**). Plain CT at presentation reveal subtle calcification within the lesion (**c**). Biopsy performed at that time showed foci of inflammation without evidence of malignancy. After six months, the patient became asymptomatic, while on plain CT, a typical zonal calcification is seen (**d**). The images recorded in this case are a good illustration of the evolution from the early to the mature stage in myositis ossificans

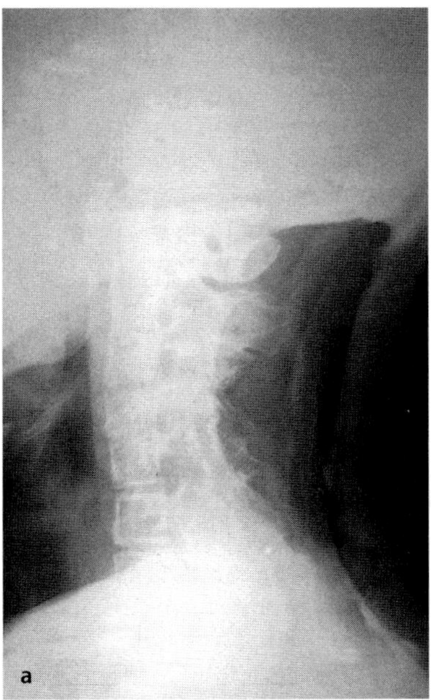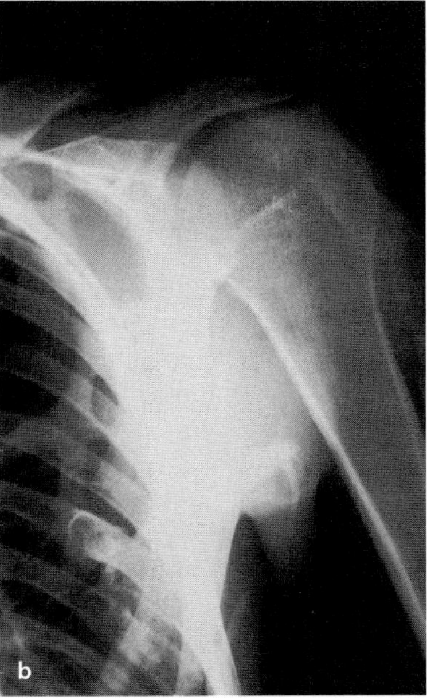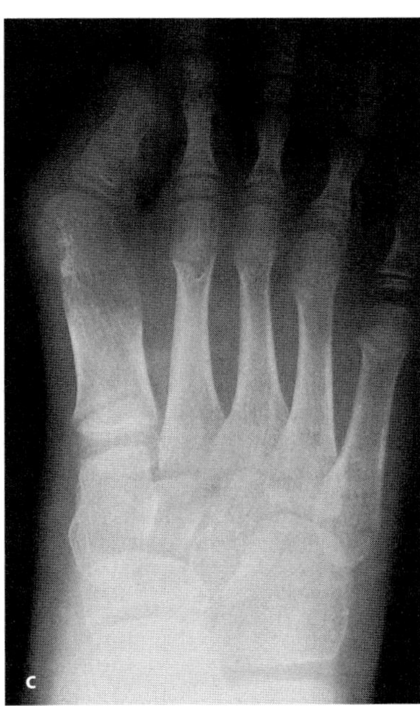

Fig. 21.19 a–c. Fibrodysplasia ossificans progressiva in a 15-year-old boy: **a** plain radiograph of neck; **b** plain radiograph of left shoulder; **c** plain radiograph of right foot. Ossification of ligamentum nuchae, trapezius muscle, and muscles of thoracic wall and shoulder girdle. Concomitant fusion of posterior elements of cervical spine (**a,b**). Microdactyly and valgus deformity of the great toe (**c**). Typical example of a fibrodysplasia ossificans progressiva

Localized soft tissue swellings associated with local heat, edema, mild fever, and often pain are the first symptoms. These nodules commonly arise in the musculature of neck, back, shoulder, and paravertebral regions. This stage is followed over time by resolution of the swelling or by progression to ossification. The latter leads to formation of "bony bridges", which cause impaired function and may be responsible for skeletal contractures and respiratory disturbances [17, 38]. This process generally takes place within several months, occasionally within a few weeks [31]. The course is characteristically one of remission and exacerbation but leads to progressive ossification of muscle and connective tissue. Progression of the disease commonly leads to extensive immobility. Most patients survive to adulthood, but a fatal outcome is commonly observed within a period of 10–15 years. Restrictive pulmonary disease and pneumonia following involvement of the chest wall constitute the major factors of early mortality. The course of the disease may be accelerated by local trauma and surgery [6, 15, 31, 38].

■ **Imaging.** Findings on plain radiography include principally ectopic ossification, short bone abnormalities, and vertebral abnormalities. Secondary signs are epiphyseal changes, calcaneal spurs, high patella, hallux valgus, and cortical thickening along the medial border of the tibia [38]. Ectopic soft tissue ossification usually begins in the neck and paravertebral area and pro-gresses to ossified bony bridges throughout the soft tissues. In some cases ectopic bone from the axial skeleton forms false joints with ectopic bone in the soft tissues of the extremities. This most commonly occurs between the shoulder girdle and paravertebral regions (Figs. 21.19 and 21.20). Nearly all patients have microdactyly of the great toes and/or hallux valgus. Short thumbs, shortening of the middle phalanx of the fifth finger, and short, broad femoral necks are associated findings. Uncommon features are narrowing of the anteroposterior diameter of the cervical and lumbar vertebral bodies, and fusion of the posterior arches in the cervical spine [20, 38]. CT may disclose early soft tissue abnormalities, such as swelling of the muscular fascial planes and edema of muscle and soft tissue ossification, before this is apparent on plain radiography. An interesting observation on CT is that the ossification starts at different sites within the fascia and does not develop as an advancing sheet. This finding is an argument in favor of the hypothesis that the disease begins within the connective tissue [31].

Up to now, MRI findings of fibrodysplasia ossificans progressiva are extremely sparse [6]. In one case with involvement of the chest wall MRI revealed a soft tissue mass with nonspecific prolongation of T1 and T2 relaxation times. On follow-up MRI, performed one year later, the size of the lesion had decreased. In addition, signal intensity of the lesion had decreased on T2-weighted images, and a small area with signal void was observed on

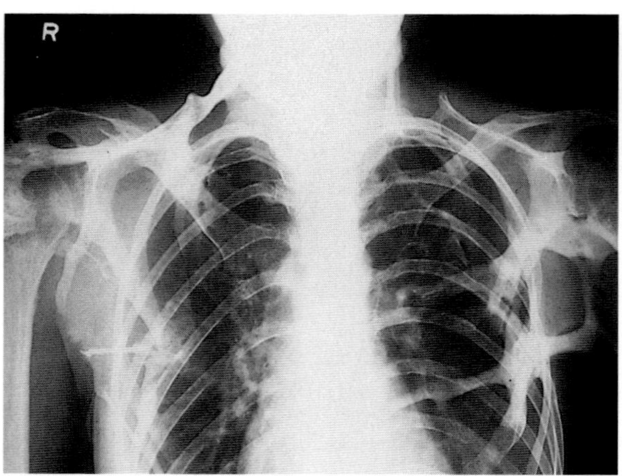

Fig. 21.20. Fibrodysplasia ossificans progressiva in a young man. Plain radiograph of the chest. Multifocal ossification in muscles around thoracic cage and shoulder girdle

all images. The latter was believed to represent calcification, ossification, or dense fibrous tissue. In addition, MRI showed a new area of recent involvement [6].

By demonstrating soft tissue ossification and associated anomalies of bone, plain radiographs are useful in diagnosing and following up patients with fibrodysplasia ossificans progressiva. CT is more sensitive for detecting early lesions and superior for showing the extent of the disease. Therefore, CT is recommended for diagnosis in early and equivocal cases. In addition, CT may be helpful by avoiding the need for biopsy, which has been noted to aggravate the disease. The role of MRI has not yet been defined; it may be useful in detecting early lesions and in determining the extent of the disease. Given the widespread use of MRI in evaluating soft tissue tumors, however, knowledge of the MRI findings in fibrodysplasia ossificans progressiva is recommended.

21.4.1.3 Extraskeletal Osteoma

■ **Definition.** This lesion consists of mature lamellar bone, containing a haversian system and bone marrow with small amounts of cartilage in the periphery, located within the soft tissues. Some authors believe that this lesion represents the end result of posttraumatic ossifying lesions [35].

■ **Incidence and Clinical Behavior.** Extraskeletal osteoma is an extremely rare tumor. Nearly all of these tumors are located in the head, usually in the posterior portion of the tongue. Two cases have been reported with location in the thigh [20, 35]. Symptoms are caused by mass effect of the lesion. When superficially located, the tumor presents as a hard palpable mass. Surgical excision seems to be curative.

■ **Imaging.** Plain radiography and CT show a dense, ossified mass with mature osseous architecture in the soft tissues [35].

Findings of only one MRI report are available. In this case the osteoma presents as a well-circumscribed mass of mixed signal intensity containing signal voids both on T1- and T2-weighted images. The signal intensities are consistent with cortical bone and areas of fatty and hematopoietic marrow [35].

The diagnosis is suggested by the characteristic appearance on plain radiography and CT. MRI does not offer useful supplementary information.

21.4.2 Malignant Lesions

■ **Definition.** Extraskeletal osteosarcoma is a malignant mesenchymal neoplasm that forms osteoid or bone. In some extraskeletal osteosarcomas however also cellular elements from the chondroblastic and fibroblastic cell lines occur. Therefore, although all osteosarcomas contain neoplastic bone, some may also have cartilaginous or fibroblastic components. The neoplasm is located in the soft tissues, unattached to underlying bone or periosteum [8, 15]. Most tumors are deep seated, and they are often fixed to surrounding tissues. Although on gross examination the tumor seems to be encapsulated, microscopically it frequently reveals ill-defined borders and infiltration of adjacent structures. A distinction is made between various subtypes, depending on the relative amounts of tissue constituents. These reflect the subtypes of conventional osteosarcoma of bone and include osteoblastic, chondroblastic, fibroblastic, and occasionally telangiectatic types. The small cell variant is unusual [8, 15, 25].

■ **Incidence and Clinical Behavior.** Soft tissue osteosarcoma is rare and accounts for approximately 1% of all soft tissue sarcomas and nearly 4% of all osteosarcomas [3, 33]. The tumor afflicts adults, with mean age of 50 years at presentation, which is in contrast to its intraosseous counterpart, which is most common in the first two decades of life [3, 8, 20, 44]. Males are affected nearly twice as much as females [28]. More than half of the tumors occur in the lower extremity, in approximately 50% of cases in the thigh. Other common locations are the upper extremity and retroperitoneum. A history of irradiation is found in 4–13% [3, 8, 22]. The role of trauma is still unclear, although a history of trauma is reported in 12–31% of extraskeletal osteosarcoma [3, 8, 13, 15]. The tumor typically presents as a slowly growing soft tissue mass, causing pain and tenderness in 25–50% of cases. Development of local recurrences following surgery and metastatic spread, usually to lungs and lymph nodes, are the rule rather than the ex-

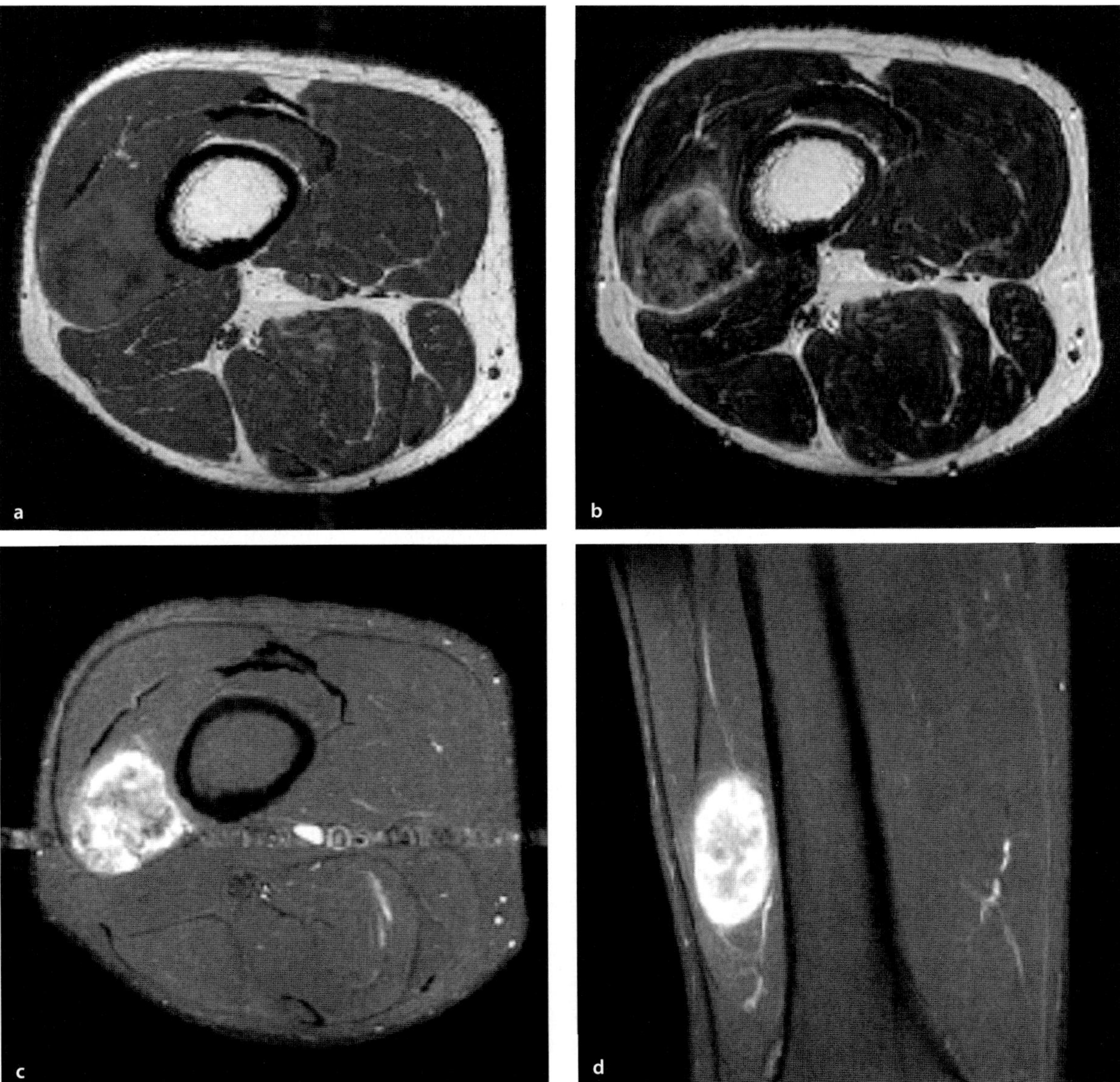

Fig. 21.21 a–d. Extraskeletal osteosarcoma of the thigh in a 48-year-old male (reproduced from [39], with permission): **a** axial spin echo T1-weighted MR image; **b** axial fast spin echo T2-weighted MR image; **c,d** axial (**c**) and coronal (**d**) spin echo T1-weighted MR images with fat suppression after gadolinium contrast injection. Ovoid soft tissue mass, deeply located within the muscle compartment adjacent to the bony structures. The mass re-mains unattached to the underlying bone. Patchy areas of signal void within the center of the lesion on all sequences, consistent with osteoid tissue. The tumor itself appears discretely hyperintense to muscle on T1-weighted images (**a**), hyperintense on T2-weighted images (**b**). Following contrast injection marked enhancement is observed throughout the lesion (**c,d**)

ception and are observed in more than 80–90% of patients [3, 8]. Hence, the overall prognosis is poor, despite radical surgery and adjuvant therapy. Nearly 75% of patients die of the tumor within five years. Tumor size is the major predictor of survival, tumors less than 5 cm in diameter having a relatively better prognosis than those larger than 5 cm. The histological appearance of the tumor does not seem to influence patient outcome [3, 25].

■ **Imaging.** Calcifications within the tumor are observed on plain radiography and CT in about half of all cases [39]. Their appearance depends on the amount of mineralization. Most commonly the calcifications appear as a cloudlike density within the soft tissue. Adjacent bone mostly remains unaffected. CT is superior for detecting small amounts of calcifications and for determination of the degree of mineralization. An important feature on CT is the spatial distribution of the mineralization and calcifications: in extraskeletal osteosarcoma this mineralization is greatest in the center of the lesion and least at the periphery, whereas the opposite is true for myositis ossificans [13, 28]. Furthermore, CT gives good visualization of central necrosis within the tumor. Angiography shows a hypervascularization of the tumor [3].

On T1-weighted MR images the extraskeletal osteosarcoma presents as a well-defined mass with mixed low signal intensity [13, 42, 45] (Fig. 21.21). Tumors in which calcification or osteoid material is not discernible on plain radiography may be hyperintense to muscle on T1-weighted images [42, 45]. Mixed but predominantly high signal intensity is observed on T2-weighted images (Fig. 21.21). Areas of high signal intensity on both T1- and T2-weighted images are consistent with hemorrhage within the tumor. In some tumors large cystic components have been demonstrated [42, 45]. Calcifications present as signal voids on all sequences [13].

Plain radiography remains the initial examination, demonstrating mineralization within the lesion and the absence of involvement of adjacent bone. CT offers valuable additional information by showing the extent of the lesion, distribution of the calcifications within the tumor, and central necrosis more accurately. As noted above, this information is very useful for differential diagnosis. MRI findings are nonspecific, but MRI currently offers the best delineation of the extent of the tumor.

Things to remember:

1. The presence of calcifications or ossifications within a soft tissue mass should suggest the possibility of an extraskeletal cartilaginous or osseous tumor or tumor-like condition.
2. Plain radiography and/or CT remain very powerful tools in the preoperative characterization of these tumors.
3. MRI is useful for evaluation of non calcified lesions, such as early stage osteochondromatosis.
4. The MRI appearance of myositis ossificans is variable, according to the age of the lesion.

References

1. Ackman JB, Rosenthal DI (1995) Generalized periarticular myositis ossificans as a complication of pharmacologically induced paralysis. Skeletal Radiol 24:395–397
2. Amendola MA, Glazer GM, Agha FP, Francis IR, Weatherbee L, Martel W (1983) Myositis ossificans circumscripta: computed tomographic diagnosis. Radiology 149:775–779
3. Bane BL, Evans HL, Ro JY, Carrasco CH, Grignon DJ, Benjamin RS, Ayala AG (1990) Extraskeletal osteosarcoma. Cancer 66: 2762–2770
4. Bansal M, Goldman AB, DiCarlo EF, McCormack R (1993) Soft tissue chondromas: diagnosis and differential diagnosis. Skeletal Radiol 22:309–315
5. Bertoni F, Unni KK, Beabout JW, Sim FH (1991) Chondrosarcomas of the synovium. Cancer 67:155–162
6. Caron KH, DiPietro MA, Aisen AM, Heidelberger KP, Philips WA, Martel W (1990) MR imaging of early fibrodysplasia ossificans progressiva. J Comput Assist Tomogr 14:318–321
7. Chung EB, Enzinger FM (1978) Chondroma of soft parts. Cancer 41:1414–1424
8. Chung EB, Enzinger FM (1987) Extraskeletal osteosarcoma. Cancer 60:1132–1142
9. Cohen EK, Kressel HY, Frank TS et al. (1988) Hyaline cartilage-origin bone and soft-tissue neoplasms: MR appearance and histologic correlation. Radiology 167:477–481
10. Cvitanic O, Sedlak J (1995) Acute myositis ossificans. Skeletal Radiol 24:139–141
11. Dahlin DC, Salvador AH (1974) Cartilaginous tumors of the soft tissues of the hands and feet. Mayo Clin Proc 49:721–726
12. De Smet AA, Noris MA, Fisher DR (1992) Magnetic resonance imaging of myositis ossificans: analysis of seven cases. Skeletal Radiol 21:503–507
13. Doud TM, Moser RP, Giudici MAI, Frauenhofer EE, Maurer RJ (1991) Case report 704: extraskeletal osteosarcoma of the thigh with several suspected skeletal metastases and extensive metastases to the chest. Skeletal Radiol 20:628–632
14. Enzinger FM, Weiss SW (1995) Cartilaginous soft tissue tumors. In: Enzinger FM, Weiss SW (eds) Soft tissue tumors, 3rd edn. Mosby, St Louis, pp 991–1012
15. Enzinger FM, Weiss SW (1995) Osseous soft tissue tumors. In: Enzinger FM, Weiss SW (eds) Soft tissue tumors, 3rd edn. Mosby, St Louis, pp 1013–1038
16. Erlemann R, Reiser MF, Peters PE (1989) Musculoskeletal neoplasms: static and dynamic GdDTPA-enhanced MR imaging. Radiology 171:767–773
17. Gebhardt MC, Parekh SG, Rosenberg AE, Rosenthal DI (1999) Extraskeletal myxoid chondrosarcoma of the knee. Skeletal Radiol 28:354–358
18. Ghrea M, Mathieu G, Apoil A, Soubrane P, Dumontier C, Sautet A (2003) Soft tissue chondroma of the hand: a case report and analysis of diagnostic procedures for extra-osseous cartilaginous lesions of the hand. Revue de Chir Orthopéd et Réparatrice de l'Appareil Moteur 89(3):261–265
19. Gonzalez-Lois C, Garcia-de-la-Torre JP, SantosBriz-Torron A, Vila J, Manrique-Chico J, Martinez-Tello FJ (2001) Intracapsular and para-articular chondroma adjacent to large joints: report of three cases and review of the literature. Skeletal Radiol 30:672–676
20. Kransdorf MJ, Meis JM (1993) From the archives of AFIP. Extraskeletal osseous and cartilaginous tumors of the extremities. Radiographics 13:853–884
21. Kransdorf MJ, Meis JM, Jelinek JS (1991) Myositis ossificans: MR appearance with radiologic-pathologic correlation. Am J Roentgenol 157:1243–1248
22. Laskin WB, Silverman TA, Enzinger FM (1988) Postradiation soft tissue sarcomas: an analysis of 5 cases. Cancer 62:2330–2340
23. Lichtenstein L, Goldman RL (1964) Cartilage tumors in soft tissues, particularly in the hand and foot. Cancer 17:1203–1208
24. Meis JM, Martz KL (1992) Extraskeletal myxoid chondrosarcoma: a clinicopathologic study of 120 cases (abstract). Lab Invest 66:9
25. Meis-Kindblom JM, Enzinger FM (1996) Extraskeletal osseous and cartilaginous tumors. In: Meis-Kindblom JM, Enzinger FM (eds) Color atlas of soft tissue tumors. Mosby-Wolfe, St Louis, pp 259–272
26. Nakashima Y, Unni KK, Shives TC, Swee RG, Dahlin DC (1986) Mesenchymal chondrosarcoma of bone and soft tissue: a review of 111 cases. Cancer 57:2444–2453
27. Nuovo MA, Norman A, Chumas J, Ackerman LV (1992) Myositis ossificans with atypical clinical, radiographic or pathologic findings: a review of 23 cases. Skeletal Radiol 21:87–101
28. Okada K, Ito H, Miyakoshi N, Sageshima M, Nishida J, Itoi E (2003) A low-grade extra-skeletal osteosarcoma. Skeletal Radiol 32:165–169
29. Okamoto S, Hara K, Sumita S, Sato K, Hisaoka M, Aoki T, Hashimoto H (2002) Extraskeletal myxoid chondrosarcoma arising in the finger. 31:296–300

30. Peterson KK, Renfrew DL, Feddersen RM, Buckwalter JA, El-Khoury GY (1991) Magnetic resonance imaging of myxoid containing tumors. Skeletal Radiol 20:245–250

31. Reinig JW, Hill SC, Fang M, Marini J, Zasloff MA (1986) Fibrodysplasia ossificans progressiva: CT appearance. Radiology 159:153–157

32. Rodriguez-Peralto JL, Lopez-Barea F, Gonzalez-Lopez J (1997) Intracapsular chondroma of the knee: un unusual neoplasm. Int J Surg Pathol 5:49–54

33. Sabloff B, Munden RF, Melhem AI, El-Naggar AK, Putnam JB Jr (2003) Extraskeletal osteosarcoma of the pleura. Am J Roentgenol 180:972

34. Saleh G, Evans HL, Ro JY, Ayala AG (1992) Extraskeletal myxoid chondrosarcoma: a clinico-pathologic study of ten patients with long term follow-up. Cancer 70:2827–2830

35. Schweitzer ME, Greenway G, Resnick D, Haghighi P, Snoots WE (1992) Osteoma of soft parts. Skeletal Radiol 21:177–180

36. Shapeero LC, Vanel D, Couanet D, Contesso G, Ackerman LV (1993) Extraskeletal mesenchymal chondrosarcoma. Radiology 186:819–826

37. Shirkhoda A, Armin AR, Bis KG, Makris J, Irwin RB, Shetty AN (1995) MR imaging of myositis ossificans: variable patterns at different stages. J Magn Reson Imaging 5:287–292

38. Thickman D, Bonakdar-pour A, Clancy M, Van Orden J, Steel H (1982) Fibrodysplasia ossificans progressiva. Am J Roentgenol 139:935–941

39. Vanhoenacker FM, Van de Perre S, Van Marck E, Somville J, Gielen J, De Schepper AM (2004) Extraskeletal osteosarcoma: a report of a case with unusual features and histopathological correlation. Eur J Radiol Extra 49:97–102

40. Varma DGK, Kumar R, Carrasco CH, Guo SQ, Richli WR (1991) MR imaging of periosteal chondroma. J Comput Assist Tomogr 15:1008–1010

41. Varma DGK, Ayala AG, Carrasco CH, Guo SQ, Kumar Edeiken J (1992) Chondrosarcoma: MR imaging with pathologic correlation. Radiographics 12:687–704

42. Varma DGK, Ayala AG, Guo SQ, Moulopoulos LA, Kim EE, Charnsangavej C (1993) MRI of extraskeletal sarcoma. J Comput Assist Tomogr 17:414–417

43. Van Slyke MA, Moser RP, Madewell JE (1995) MR imaging of periarticular soft-tissue lesions. MRI Clin North Am 3:651–668

44. Wang XL, Malghem J, Parizel PM, Gielen JL, Vanhoenacker F, De Schepper AM (2003) Pictorial essay. Myositis ossificans circumscripta. JBR-BTR 86(5):278–285

45. Yu JS, Ashman CJ, Dardani M (2000) Extraskeletal osteosarcoma. Am J Roentgenol 175:886–887

46. Zlatkin MB, Lander PH, Begin LR, Hadjipavlou A (1985) Soft-tissue chondromas. Am J Roentgenol 144:1263–1267

Primitive Neuroectodermal Tumors and Related Lesions

22

W. A. Simoens, H. R. Degryse

Contents

22.1 Primitive Neuroectodermal Tumors

22.1.1 Introduction

Primitive neuroectodermal tumors (PNET) form part of the heterogeneous group of small round (blue) cell tumors of childhood and adolescence. This group also contains conventional neuroblastoma, rhabdomyosarcoma, lymphoma, and Ewing's sarcoma [36, 37, 40].

Purely for practical reasons, Dehner introduced the distinction between central PNET (cPNET) and peripheral PNET (pPNET), as he was well aware that little knowledge was available concerning the actual biology of these neoplasms and of their interrelationships [12]. This classification applies knowledge of neuroectodermal derivatives to the PNET. The neuroectoderm generates the brain and spinal cord, on the one hand, and the entire autonomic nervous system, dorsal root ganglia, adrenal medulla, and part of the neuroendocrine system, on the other, among many other derivatives. It must be stressed that this division of the PNET does not have any clinicopathologic or prognostic implications. In this chapter only pPNET will be discussed. Peripheral primitive neuroectodermal tumors constitute a group of uncommon tumors with similar histology, and are aggressive and poorly differentiated neoplasms, occurring mainly in children and young adults.

These tumors originate in the soft tissues or bone, outside the central or sympathetic nervous system, and are composed of undifferentiated, small, round, hyperchromatic tumor cells.

pPNET and Ewing's sarcoma form a special group within the small round (blue) cell tumors. Several common characteristics have been discovered that distinguish them from other small round (blue) cell tumors, namely a unique chromosomal translocation, t(11;22)(q24;12), and the expression of a membrane glycoprotein, known as the MIC2 gene product (see Chap. 7: Genetics and Molecular Biology of Soft Tissue Tumors). In addition to pPNET of soft tissue and Ewing's sarcoma of bone, there are also osseous pPNET and extraskeletal Ewing's sarcoma [4]. It was also noted that extraskeletal Ewing's sarcoma and some atypical forms of Ewing's sarcoma of bone display neuroectodermal features. Because of these shared phenotypical and genotypical characteristics, very typical for Ewing's sarcoma and pPNET, it is now generally accepted that these two neoplasms are related to each other. They are thought to correspond to distinct neural crest lineages or tumors arrested at different stages of development. pPNET is the most differentiated and can be considered the neural variant of Ewing's sarcoma [5, 10, 13, 27, 31].

According to the Ewing's sarcoma/pPNET classification proposed by Schmidt [31], diagnosis of pPNET is reserved to those cases that express at least two different neural markers and/or Homer-Wright rosettes, the others being termed Ewing's sarcoma. This classification has proven to be useful [7].

Due to the identification of the common non-random chromosome rearrangements in Ewing's sarcoma, peripheral primitive neuroectodermal tumor, Askin tumor, and neuroepithelioma, these tumors are now considered entities of the Ewing's sarcoma family of tumors (ESFT).

22.1.2 Incidence and Clinical Behavior

Most pPNET are diagnosed between the ages of 175 and 250 months. Seventy-five percent occur before the age of 30 [15, 24, 31]. Peripheral PNET presenting at birth is uncommon, but reported [14]. Peripheral PNET occurs predominantly in Whites and Hispanics, and rarely occurs in individuals of African or Asian descent [28]. Men are affected more frequently than women [23, 24, 31]. These tumors represent about 1% of all sarcomas.

By definition, pPNET never arise from the sympathetic nervous system. Therefore cases usually occur outside the vertebral axis of the body [15]. They are found most frequently in the thoracopulmonary region, abdomen, pelvis, and lower extremities [22, 31, 35]. They are also reported in the orbit, kidney, stomach [11], retroperitoneum [21], vulva, colon, hand [14], uterus [28], middle ear, diploe and maxilla [2, 22].

The pPNET can give rise to symptoms and signs of neurologic failure [15].

According to Schmidt's classification, prognosis is worse for pPNET than for Ewing's sarcoma [31].

A special entity of pPNET is the Askin tumor. This was first described as a "malignant small cell tumor of the thoracopulmonary region of childhood" [5], but it is now classified as a pPNET of the chest wall [53, 38]. It is found principally in young adults and adolescents [7] but can occur at all ages [29] (Fig. 22.6).

In contrast to the pPNET in general, Askin tumors seem to have a preference for girls [5, 20]. Usually the mass has already achieved a considerable size by the time of diagnosis [8] and is painful in just over half of the cases [30]. Pleural effusion may also occur [5, 8, 17, 19, 25, 32, 34].

pPNET can provoke constitutional symptoms. Fever, anorexia, weight loss, cough, and dyspnea are frequent. In cases of Askin tumor, shoulder pain, Horner's syndrome, cervical lymphadenopathy can also occur [5, 17, 19, 22, 32, 34].

Askin tumors, as with PNET in general, are highly aggressive. One study of 30 cases showed a 2-year survival rate of 38 % and a 6-year survival rate of 14 % [9].

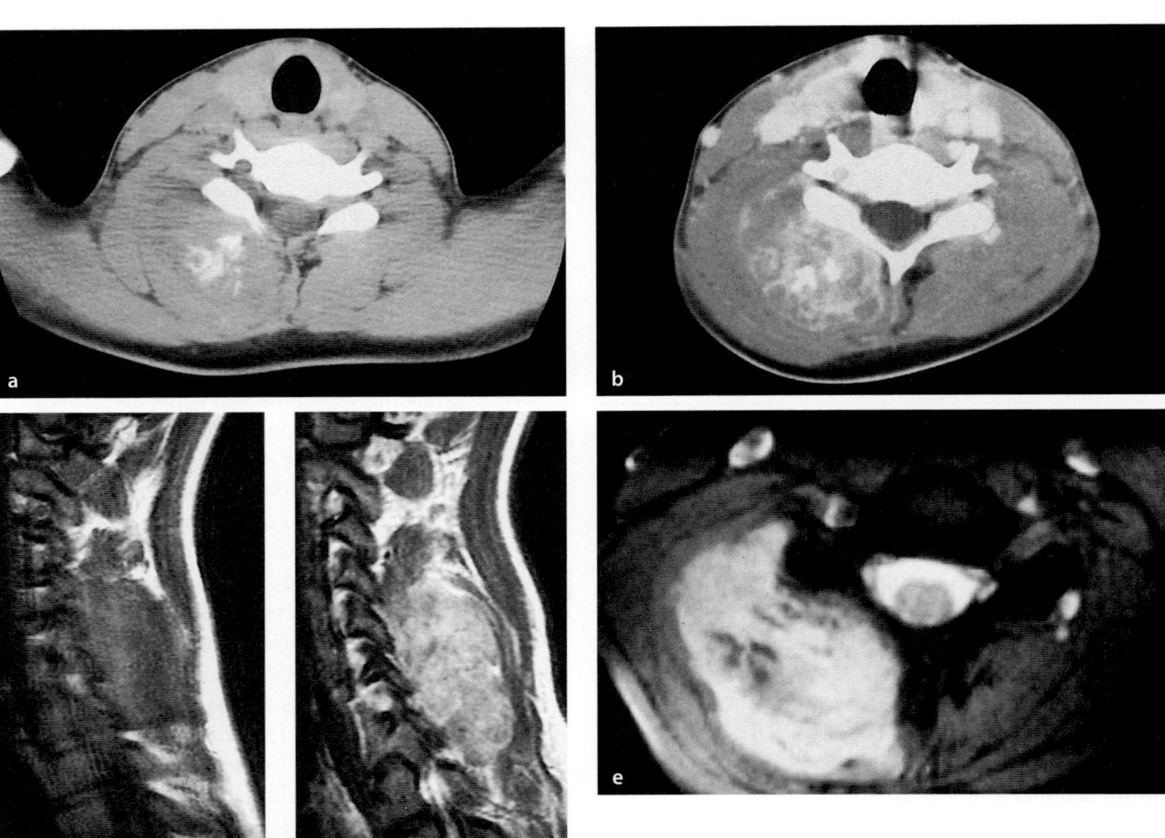

Fig. 22.1 a–e. pPNET of the lower neck in a 12-year-old girl. **a** CT. **b** CT, after iodinated contrast injection. **c** Sagittal spin echo T1-weighted MR image. **d** Sagittal spin echo T1-weighted MR image after gadolinium contrast injection. **e** Axial gradient echo T2-weighted MR image. Large mass within the deep cervical muscles on the right side of the neck. The tumor contains irregular calcifications (**a**). There is marked enhancement after contrast injection (**b**). On the T1-weighted images, the lesion is of low signal intensity and shows considerable enhancement after intravenous administration of gadolinium contrast (**c, d**). On the T2-weighted image, the lesion has a high signal intensity with central signal voids, due to intralesional calcifications. The lesion neighbors the cervical vertebrae, without manifest osseous involvement (**e**)

Relapse is most common at the thorax, where it presents as local chest wall recurrence or disseminated pulmonary metastasis. Metastasis to mediastinal lymph nodes may also occur. The next most common manifestation of relapse is distant skeletal metastasis. Infrequently the disease recurs in liver, adrenals, brain, retroperitoneum, and sympathetic chain. These sites must be considered in follow-up computed tomography (CT) examinations [5, 17, 19, 32, 34].

Esthesioneuroblastoma, also known as olfactory neuroblastoma, has long been considered a member of the pPNET/Ewing's sarcoma family. Although a primitive neural tumor, recent studies raise doubts about the legitimacy of its membership because of the failure to identify the MIC2 gene product [21].

22.1.3 Imaging Characteristics

22.1.3.1 Plain Radiography

Little is known concerning the radiographic presentation of pPNET. On plain radiographs, Askin tumor commonly presents as a mass of the chest wall with soft tissue density. Rib erosion occurs very often [5, 9, 17, 19, 32, 34]. In about 10 % of cases the tumor is seen as a paraspinal or mediastinal mass. In 15 % of cases a usually small, pleural effusion is observed. Rarely, calcifications are present [5, 17, 19, 20, 32, 34].

22.1.3.2 Ultrasound

As in the plain radiograph, ultrasound of Askin tumor reveals only nonspecific features. A complex, solid mass may be revealed, with mixed echogeneity and sometimes with cystic components. When present, a pleural effusion can be seen [30].

22.1.3.3 CT and MRI

On CT, pPNET presents as a large, ill-defined mass with a heterogeneous appearance due to extensive cystic degeneration. As a rule, there is no calcification [22], although our series contains a pPNET with extensive calcification (Fig. 22.1). After the injection of iodinated contrast the tumor has a heterogeneous appearance [22, 30, 39].

On T1-weighted MR images pPNET generally has a signal intensity equal to or greater than that of muscle. Frequently evidence of hemorrhage or necrosis is found. Larger tumors show up as heterogeneous masses, while smaller ones tend to be more homogeneous [16, 22, 39].

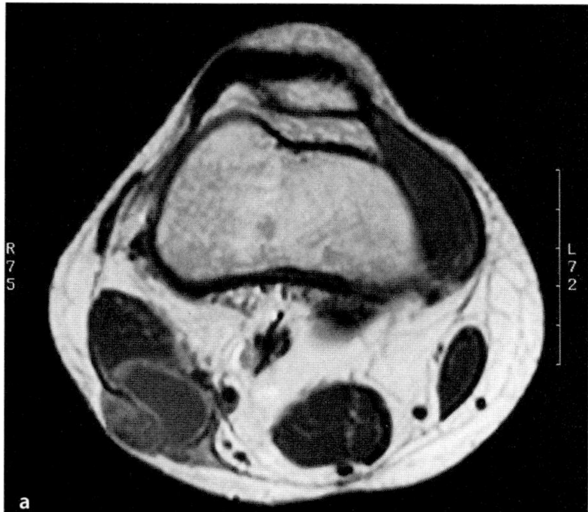
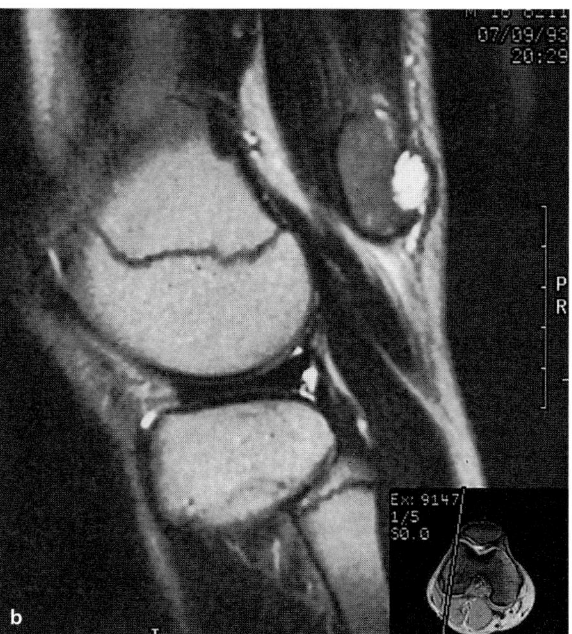

Fig. 22.2a, b. pPNET of the thigh in a 16-year-old boy. **a** Axial spin echo T1-weighted MR image after gadolinium contrast injection. **b** Sagittal turbo spin echo T2-weighted MR image. Mass lesion originating peripherally in the biceps femoris muscle, infiltrating the dorsal fascia. There are two distinctive tumor components. A first one, located at the periphery, shows intermediate signal intensity on T1-weighted image after contrast injection. A second part is located more deeply, and presents as a homogeneous low signal intensity component with a faint peripheral enhancing rim (**a**). On the T2-weighted image the first component shows extremely high signal intensity while the second exhibits low signal intensity and a very low signal intensity peripheral rim (**b**). The first component proved to be the pPNET with characteristic signal intensities, while the second part shows signal intensity-characteristics of chronic hemorrhage

On T1-weighted MR image after intravenous administration of contrast, the tumor shows rapid enhancement [39] (Fig. 22.1). On T2-weighted MR images these neoplasms tend to show a bright, frequently heterogeneous appearance [22, 39] (Figs. 22.1, 22.2). Similar radiologic features are seen in extraskeletal Ewing's sarcoma, Ewing's sarcoma, and other small round (blue) cell tumors [22].

Rib destruction, invasion of the pleura by the tumor and pleural effusion are other common features of Askin tumors [5, 17, 39].

MRI is superior to CT in revealing involvement of surrounding anatomic structures, in particular vascular elements and bone marrow [22, 39].

Differential diagnosis should be made with Ewing's sarcoma of bone and extraskeletal Ewing's sarcoma of the chest wall [27]. Neuroblastoma should be considered when the tumor has a mediastinal or paraspinal localization [18]. Rhabdomyosarcoma and malignant lymphoma must also be taken into consideration. Most important, however, is that the differential diagnosis considers the possibility of an Askin tumor when a chest wall mass in a child or a young adult is being assessed (Fig. 22.6).

22.2 Extraskeletal Ewing's Sarcoma

22.2.1 Definition

Extraskeletal Ewing's sarcoma is a rare soft tissue tumor, histologically indistinguishable from the osseous form. The major differences are in the age group of prevalence and the site of predilection. These tumors are commonly deeply located and have diameters ranging from 5 to 10 cm. On pathology, the tumor is multilobulated, richly vascular, and often contains large areas of necrosis, cyst formation, or hemorrhage [15].

22.2.2 Incidence and Clinical Behavior

In contrast to the osseous form, extraskeletal Ewing's sarcoma occurs in somewhat older persons, with a median age of about 20 years (more than 75 % of the patients are between 10 and 30 years of age). This tumor is slightly more common in men and occurs chiefly in the paravertebral and intercostal regions. Soft tissues of the lower extremities and very rarely of the pelvic an hip regions, retroperitoneum, and upper extremities also may be involved [1]. Patients usually present with a rapidly growing mass, which is painful in about one-third of cases. Sensory or motor disturbances are observed if the tumor involves the spinal cord or peripheral nerves. Metastatic spread – most commonly to lungs or skeleton – and recurrence are common and observed in nearly 65 % of cases [15, 27].

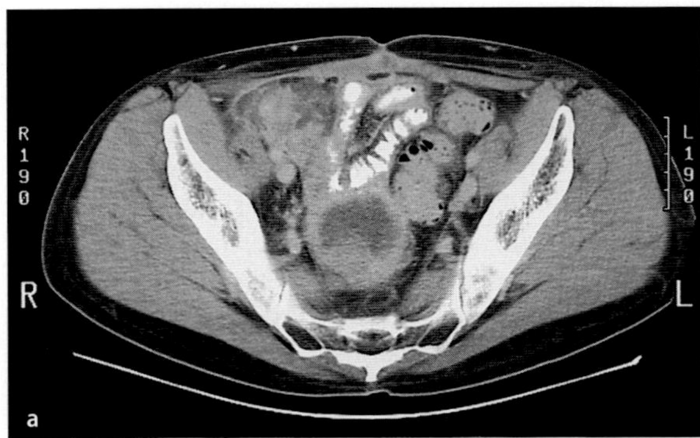

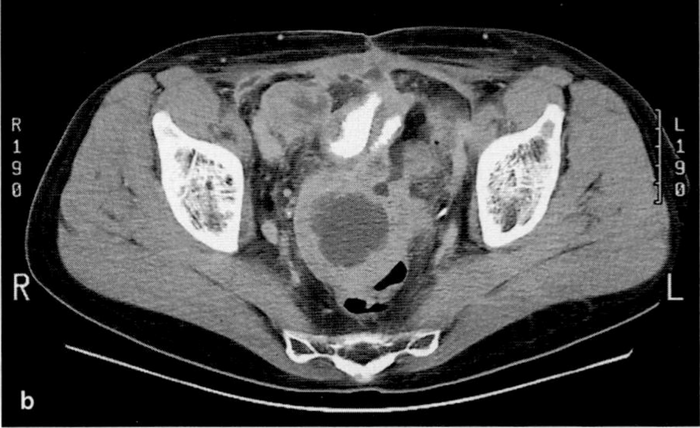

Fig. 22.3 a, b. Extraskeletal Ewing's sarcoma of the pelvis in a 36-year-old man. **a** CT after iodinated contrast injection. **b** Section at a lower level than in a. Hourglass-shaped soft tissue tumor in the pelvis, with major tumor component in a right anterolateral position to the rectum and smaller component anteriorly in the right iliac fossa. Ill-defined, hypodense area without enhancement within the major tumor component, suggesting a necrotic center of the tumor (**a**). Necrotic areas within both tumor components are more clearly seen at the caudal section (**b**). Sequel from previous laparotomy and thickening of bowel walls following radiotherapy are observed at both levels

22.2.3 Imaging Characteristics

22.2.3.1 Imaging Studies Other than MRI

Plain radiographs reveal only a nonspecific soft tissue mass of widely variable size. Small areas of amorphous calcifications are not observed in untreated tumors but may develop during chemotherapy [27]. On ultrasound, these tumors are mostly well circumscribed. Ultrasound features are mostly those of a hypoechoic or partly anechoic mass, although a mixed echo pattern may also be recognized [27]. Unenhanced CT scans show either low attenuation throughout the tumor or only focal areas of hypodensity. Enhancement on postcontrast scans is moderate but variable and reflects the different vascularization pattern [27] (Fig. 22.3).

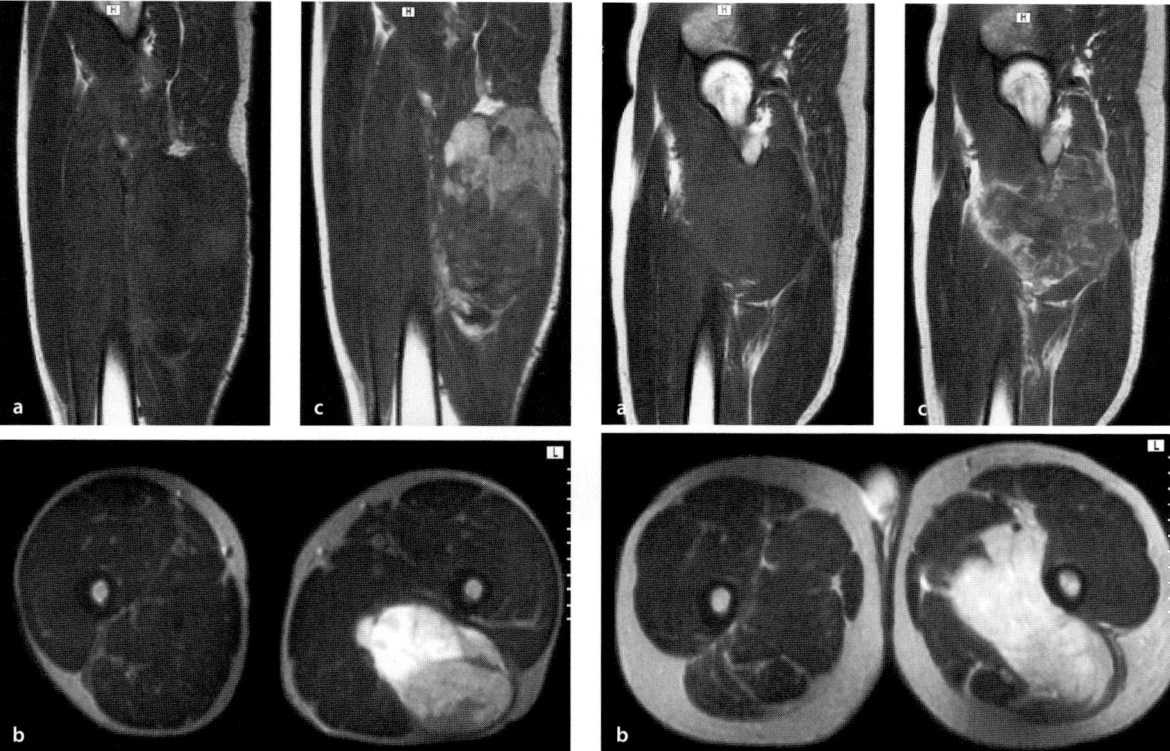

Fig. 22.4a–c. Extraskeletal Ewing's sarcoma of the left thigh in a 29-year-old man. **a** Sagittal spin echo T1-weighted MR image. **b** Axial spin echo T2-weighted MR image. **c** Sagittal spin echo T1-weighted MR image after gadolinium contrast injection. A large polylobular mass at the posterior aspect of the femur is seen. On the T1-weighted image, the lesion appears inhomogeneous, and signal intensity is nearly equal to that of surrounding muscle. Ill-defined, slightly hyperintense area posteriorly in the lesion suggests intratumoral hemorrhage. On the T2-weighted image the polylobular shape of the lesion is confirmed by presence of several lobules with different appearance. Some lobules are very bright and contain low intensity septations, while others have intermediate signal intensity, equal to that of fat. Demarcation from surrounding muscle and subcutaneous fat is sharp (**b**). Highly variable degree of enhancement is observed at the various tumor constituents. Pronounced, but inhomogeneous enhancement is observed at the cranial parts of the tumor. A mottled, only slightly enhancing pattern is observed at the lower pole of the tumor (**c**)

Fig. 22.5a–c. Extraskeletal Ewing's sarcoma at the infratrochanteric region of the left thigh in a 32-year-old man. **a** Sagittal spin echo T1-weighted MR image. **b** Axial spin echo T2-weighted MR image. **c** Sagittal spin echo T1-weighted MR image after gadolinium contrast injection. Presence of a polylobular low-intensity mass medial to the proximal third of the left femur. The mass is homogeneous and slightly hyperintense to muscle on the T1-weighted image (**a**). On the T2-weighted image the lesion has an inhomogeneous appearance. Signal intensity surpasses that of subcutaneous fat (**b**). After contrast medium injection, inhomogeneous pattern of enhancement is observed at the tumor. Central unenhancing areas are likely to represent intratumoral necrosis (**c**). Notice the absence of bony erosion and cortical involvement despite the intimate contact over a long distance

22.2.3.2 MRI

On MRI extraskeletal Ewing's sarcoma presents as a well-circumscribed mass within the involved muscle (Figs. 22.4, 22.5). Intermediate signal intensity is observed on T1-weighted images. T2-weighted images demonstrate a heterogeneous, mottled appearance of the mass containing areas of high signal intensity. Heterogeneous enhancement is observed after administration of gadolinium chelates [1] (Fig. 22.6).

22.2.3.3 Imaging Strategy

None of the findings of the various imaging modalities are characteristic for extraskeletal Ewing's sarcoma. The role of imaging consists mainly of establishing local tumor extent. Despite the nonspecific findings extraskeletal Ewing's sarcoma should be included in the differential diagnosis when a noncalcified soft tissue mass is observed in the paravertebral region of the chest or in an extremity, especially in the appropriate age group.

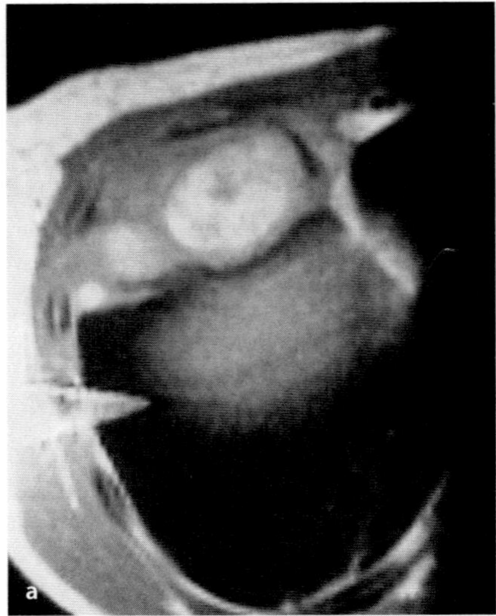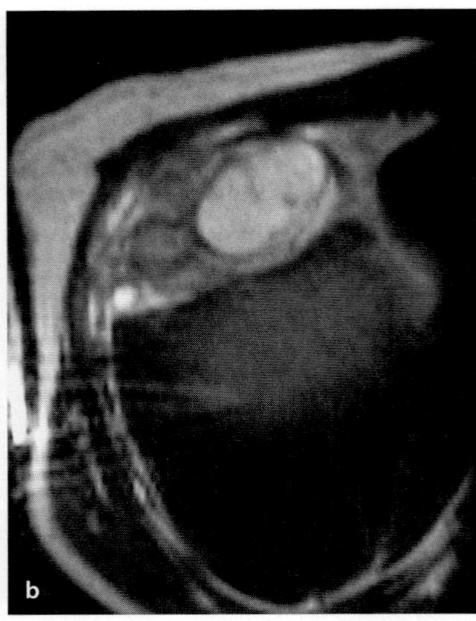

Fig. 22.6 a, b. Askin tumor (pNET) in a 19-year-old man presenting with a mass lesion at the anterior thoracic wall. **a** Axial spin echo T1-weighted MR image after gadolinium contrast injection. **b** Axial spin echo T2-weighted MR image. Presence of a multinodular, enhancing mass lesion at the arterior aspect of the thoracic wall (a). On T2-weighted images the nodules present with different signal intensities (b). Age, localization, morphology and signal intensity charcteristics are in favor of a pNET of the chest wall, also called Askin tumor

Things to remember:

1. Peripheral primitive neuroectodermal tumors and extraskeletal Ewing's sarcoma are small blue cell tumors, sharing phenotypical and genotypical characteristics.
2. They are aggressive and poorly differentiated neoplasms, occurring mainly in children and young adults.
3. Askin tumor is a pPNET with preferential location at the thoracopulmonary region.
4. Imaging features of both pPNET and Ewing's sarcoma are hardly to differentiate from other malignant soft tissue tumors, they frequently contain areas of cystic degeneration, necrosis and hemorrhage.

References

1. Allam K, Sze G (1994) MR of primary extraosseous Ewing sarcoma. Am J Neuroradiol 15:305–307
2. Alobid I, Bernal-Sprekelsen M, Alos L, Benitez P, Traserra J, Mullol J (2003) Peripheral primitiveneuroectodermal tumor of the left maxillary sinus. J Acta Otolaryngol 123(6):776–778
3. Ambros IM, Ambros PF, Strehl S, KOvar H, Gadner H, Salzer-Kuntschik M (1991) MIC2 is a specific marker for Ewing's sarcoma and peripheral primitive neuroectodermal tumors. Evidence for a common histogenesis of Ewing's sarcoma and peripheral primitive neuroectodermal tumors from MIC2 expression and specific chromosome aberration. Cancer 67(7):1886–1893
4. Angervall L, Enzinger FM (1975) Extraskeletal neoplasm resembling Ewing's sarcoma. Cancer 36: 240–251
5. Askin FB, Rosai J, Sibley RK, Dehner LP, McAllister M (1979) Malignant small cell tumor of the thoracopulmonary region in childhood: a distinctive clinicopathologic entity of uncertain histogenesis. Cancer 43:2438–2451
6. Aurias A, Rimbaut C, Buffe D (1983) Chromosomal translocations in Ewing's sarcoma. N Engl J Med 309:496–497
7. Brinkhuis M, Wijnaendts LC, van der Linden LC, van Unnik AJ, Voute PA, Baak JP, Meijer CJ (1995) Peripheral primitive neuroectodermal tumor and extra-osseous Ewing's sarcoma: a histological, immunohistochemical and DNA flow cytometric study. Virchows Arch A Pathol Anat Histopathol 425(6):611–616
8. Burge H, Novotny D, Schiebler M, Delamy D, McCartney W (1990) MRI of Askin's tumor. Case report at 1.5 T. Chest 97:1252–1254
9. Contesso G, Llombart-Bosch A, Terrier P, Peydro-Olaya A, Henry-Amar M, Oberlin O, Habrand J-L, Dubousset J, Tursz T, Spielmann M, Genin J, Sarrazin D (1992) Does malignant small round cell tumor of the thoracopulmonary region (Askin tumor) constitute a clinicopathologic entity? Cancer 69:1012–1020
10. Cuvelier A, L,Her P, Schill H, Jancovici R, Bassoulet J, Vauterin G, Allard P (1990) Sarcomes d'Ewing et tumeurs neuroectodermiques peripheriques. A propos d'un cas de localisation latero-thoracique. Rev Pneumol Clin 46(3):116–122
11. Czekalla R, Fuchs M, Stolze A, Nerlich A, Poremba C, Schaefer KL, Weirich G, Hofler H, Schneller F, Peschel C, Siewert JR, Schepp W (2004) Peripheral primitive neuroectodermal tumor of the stomach in a 14-year-old boy: a case report. Eur J Gastroenterol Hepatol 16(12):1391–1400
12. Dehner LP (1986) Peripheral and central primitive neuroectodermal tumors. A nosologic concept seeking a concensus. Arch Pathol Lab Med 110: 997–1005
13. Dehner LP (1993) Primitive neuroectodermal tumor and Ewing's sarcoma. Am J Surg Pathol 17(1):1–13
14. El Hayek M, Trad O, Islam S (2004) Congenital peripheral primitive neuroectodermal tumor refractory to treatment. J Pediatr Hematol Oncol 26(11):770–772
15. Enzinger FM, Weiss SW (1995) Primitive neuroectodermal tumors and related lesions. In: Enzinger FM, Weiss SW (eds) Soft tissue tumors. Mosby, St. Louis, pp 929–964
16. Faubert C, Inniger R (1991) MRI and pathological findings in two cases of Askin tumors. Neuroradiology 33:277–281
17. Fink IJ, Kurtz DW, Cazenave L, Lieber MR, Miser JS, Chandra R, Triche TJ (1985) Malignant thoracopulmonary small-cell ('Askin') tumour. Am J Radiol 145:517–520
18. Franken Jr EA, Smith JA, Smith WL (1977) Tumours of the chest wall in infants and children. Pediatric Radiology 6:13–18

19. Fujii Y, Hongo T, Nakagawa Y (1989) Cell culture of small round cell tumor originating in the thoracopulmonary region: evidence for derivation from a primitive pluripotent cell. Cancer 64:43–51

20. Gonzalez-Crussi F, Wolfson SL, Misugi K, Nakajima T (1984) Peripheral neuroectodermal tumors of the chest wall in childhood. Cancer 54:2519–2527

21. Horiguchi Y, Nakashima J, Ishii T, Hata J, Tazaki H (1994) Primitive neuroectodermal tumor of the retroperitoneal cavity. Urology 44(1):127–129

22. Ibarburen C, Haberman JJ, Zerhouni EA (1996) Peripheral neuroectodermal tumors. CT and MRI evaluation. Eur J Radiol 21:225–232

23. Indrees M, Gandhi C, Betchen S, Strauchen J, King W, Wolfe D (2005) Intracranial peripheral primitive neuroectodermal tumors of the cavernous sinus: a diagnostic peculiarity. Arch Pathol Lab Med 129(1):e11–e15

24. Kransdorf MJ (1995) Malignant soft-tissue tumors in a large referral population: distribution of diagnosis by age, sex and location. Am J Roentgenol 164:129–134

25. Kurashima K, Muramoto S, Ohta Y, Fujimura M, Matsuda T (1994) Peripheral neuroectodermal tumor presenting pleural effusion. Intern Med 33(12):783–785

26. Nelson RS, Perlman EJ. Askin FB (1995) Is esthesioneuroblastoma a peripheral neuroectodermal tumor? Hum Pathol 26(6):639–641

27. O'Keefe F, Lorigan JG, Wallace S (1990) Radiological features of extraskeletal Ewing's sarcoma. Br J Radiol 63:456–460

28. Peres E, Mattoo TK, Poulik J, Warrier I (2004) Primitive neuroectodermal tumor (PNET) of the uterus in a renal allograft patient: a case report. Pediatr Blood Cancer 44(3)283–285

29. Ravaux S, Bousquet JC, Vancina S (1990) Tumeur d'Askin chez un homme de 67 ans, presentant un cancer de la prostate. Aspects tomodensitometriques. J Radiol 71(3):233–236

30. Saifuddin A, Robertson RJH, Smith SEW (1991) The radiology of Askin tumors. Clin Radiol 43:19–23

31. Schmidt D, Herrmann C, Jurgens H, Harms D (1991) Malignant peripheral neuroectodermal tumor and its necessary distinction from Ewing's sarcoma. A report from the Kiel Pediatric Tumor Registry. Cancer 68(10):2251–2259

32. Scotta MS, De Giacomo C, Maggiore G, Corbella F, Coci A, Costello A (1984) Malignant small cell tumour of the thoracopulmonary region in childhood: a case report. Am J Ped Haemat Oncol 6(4):459–462

33. Shamberger RC, Tarbell NJ, Perez-Atayde AR, Grier HE (1994) Malignant small round cell tumor (Ewing's-PNET) of the chest wall in children. J Pediatr Surg 29(2):179–184

34. Stefanko J, Turnbull AD, Helson L, Lieberman P, Martini N (1988) Primitive neuroectodermal tumours of the chest wall. J Surg Oncol 37:33–37

35. Tanida S, Tanioka F, Inukai M, Yoshioka N, Saida Y, Imai K, Nakamura T, Kitamura H, Sugimura H (2000) Ewing's sarcoma/peripheral primitive neuroectodermal tumor (pPNET) arising in the omentum as a multilocular cyst with intracystic hemorrhage. J Gastroenterol 35(12):933–940

36. Triche TJ, Askin FB (1983) Neuroblastoma and the differential diagnosis of small round blue cell tumors. Hum Pathol 14:569–596

37. Triche TJ, Askin FB, Kissane JM (1986) Ewing's sarcoma and the differential diagnosis of small round blue cell tumors. In: Finegold (ed) Pathology of neoplasia in children and adolescents. Saunders, Philadelphia: 145–195

38. Von Schlippe M, Whelan JS (1995) Primitive neuroectodermal tumour of the chest wall. Ann Oncol 6(4):395–401

39. Winer-Muram HT, Kauffman WM, Gronemeyer SA, Jennings SG (1993) Primitive neuroectodermal tumors of the chest wall (Askin tumors): CT and MR findings. Am J Roentgenol 161:265–268

40. Yunis EJ (1986) Ewing's sarcoma and related small round cell neoplasms in children. Am J Surg Pathol 10 [Suppl]:54–62

Lesions of Uncertain Differentiation

23

H.R. Degryse, F.M. Vanhoenacker

Contents

23.1 Introduction

As one may expect, the lesions of unknown differentiation constitute a very heterogeneous group of both neoplasms and tumor-like lesions. In the past, these tumors were also labeled as being 'of uncertain origin'. In view of the knowledge that these tumors do not arise from their normal cellular counterparts, the former classification based on 'histiogenetic' concepts, was no longer valuable. The current classification is based on terms of 'differentiation', which depends on patterns of gene expression. For a lot of tumors, discussed in this chapter, the line of differentiation that they are recapitulating is not clear. In contrast, for some other tumors, although the line of differentiation can be identified, the cellular counterpart cannot be identified in normal mesenchymal tissues. Consideration of their local growth pattern and clinical behavior allows further distinction between benign and malignant lesions, as presented below.

23.2 Classification

Tumors and tumor-like lesions of uncertain differentiation are commonly classified using the WHO classification, which has become the gold standard. Therefore, except for some minor changes, the latest version of this classification, is used throughout this chapter.

23.3 Benign Lesions of Uncertain Differentiation

23.3.1 Tumoral Calcinosis

20.3.1.1 Definition

Tumoral calcinosis is a rare disease of unknown origin. In its classic presentation, the condition is characterized by multiple, calcified masses resembling neoplasms located in the soft tissues near large joints. These masses are thought to originate from bursal calcifications, extending with growth to adjacent tissues, but rarely causing bone erosion [42, 54]. Despite their location in the vicinity of the joints, they do not involve the synovium itself [54]. The size of the lesions is variable, but most are between 2 and 10 cm in diameter. However, large lesions with diameters exceeding 20 cm are not uncommon. The mass is considered to be a granulomatous reaction to a foreign body, which may be active or inactive. Activity is suggested on imaging when the mass contains cystic spaces, whereas collagen sclerosis without fluid indicates inactivity. Both metabolic and traumatic etiologies have been proposed [16, 54]. At present the disorder is believed to be caused by an inborn error of phosphorus metabolism and is inherited in an autosomal dominant mode, but has a variable clinical expressivity [41]. Calcified soft tissue, masses are the best known and most common clinical component of tumoral calcinosis, but pathologic calcification may also occur in other tissues, such as bone marrow, teeth, skin, and vessels. All of these components may be variably expressed in affected individuals [41].

23.3.1.2 Incidence and Clinical Behavior

Tumoral calcinosis usually presents as periarticular masses in young adults. Few cases have been reported in young children [20]. About two-thirds of the reported cases involve blacks. One-third to half of the cases affect siblings. There is no apparent sex predominance. The most common presentation of tumoral calcinosis is a large, firm mass that is located along the extensor surfaces of, in order of decreasing frequency, hip, shoulder, and elbow. Location in the knee region is rare, but seems more common in children [20]. These masses tend to grow slowly over a period of years. Nearly two-thirds of the patients have multiple lesions, some of which are bilateral and symmetrical. Most masses are asymptomatic and do not limit the range of motion of adjacent joints unless they become large. Symptoms may result from compression of neural structures or from ulceration of the overlying skin. Following ulceration, superinfection of the masses may lead to formation of fistulas that drain a chalky, milk-like fluid [16, 42].

23.3.1.3 Imaging

■ **Imaging Studies Other than MRI.** Plain radiographs reveal globular, amorphous calcific opacities separated by radiolucent lines in a para-articular distribution. In some cases, fluid–fluid levels are demonstrated on upright radiographs [29, 42] (Fig. 23.1). These features reflect the multinodular composition of the lesions with

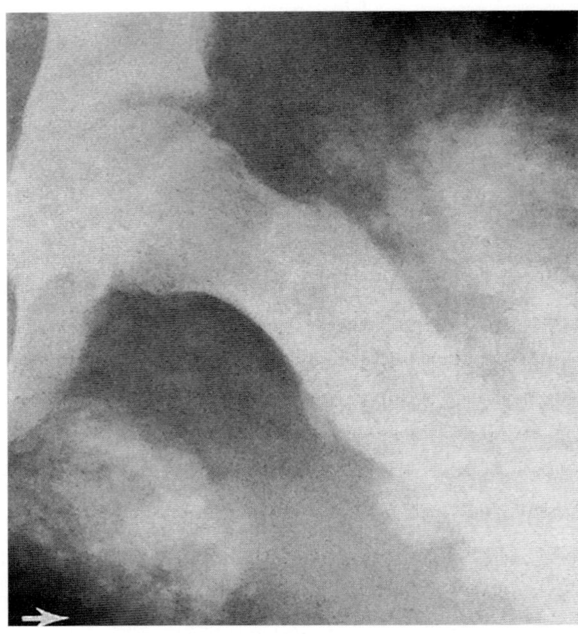

Fig. 23.1. Tumoral calcinosis of the left hip region in a 12-year-old boy. Plain radiographs reveal multinodular, calcified masses in the ischiogluteal and trochanteric regions. Fluid–fluid levels are seen in the ischiogluteal lesion (*arrow*). (Reproduced from [42], with permission)

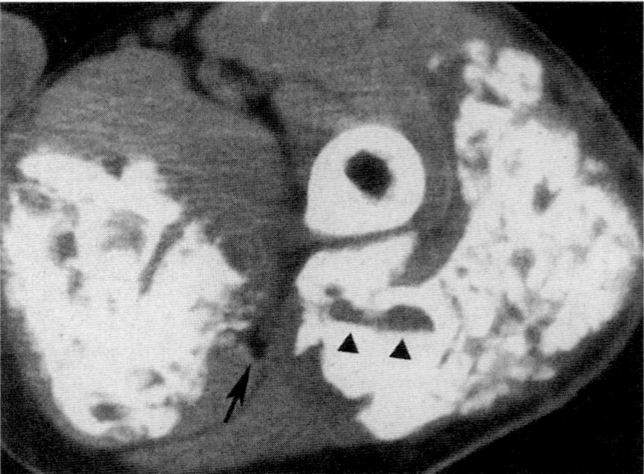

Fig. 23.2. Tumoral calcinosis of the left thigh in a 12-year-old boy. Axial CT of the left thigh obtained at the level just distal to the lesser trochanter demonstrates two calcified masses. The lesions are composed of multiple calcific nodules. Some nodules have thick walls, while others contain fluid–fluid levels (*arrowheads*). (Reproduced from [42], with permission)

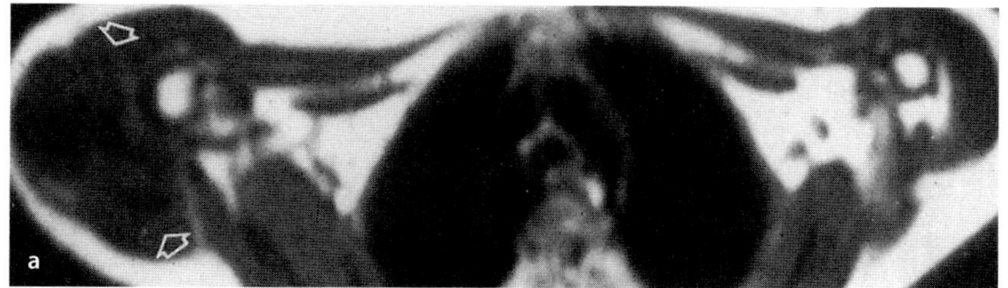
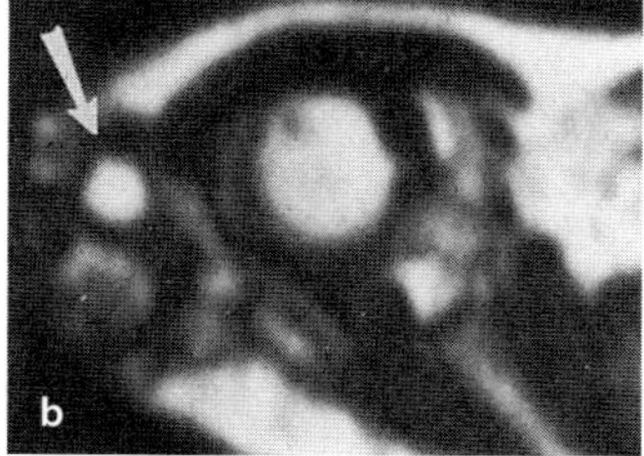

Fig. 23.3 a, b. Tumoral calcinosis of the right shoulder in a 12-year-old boy. **a** Axial spin echo T1-weighted MR image. **b** Axial spin echo T2-weighted MR image. Both sequences show a large rounded mass. The bulk of the mass is formed by a large nodular component with low signal intensity on the T1-weighted image (**a**) and high signal intensity on the T2-weighted image (**b**), and probably represents an inflammatory reaction in the soft tissues. Small nodular areas have low signal intensity on both spin echo sequences and correspond to calcific deposits. (Reproduced from [42], with permission)

radiolucent fibrous septa that separate the cystic components containing the calcareous material. Despite the large size of the lesions, there are no associated bony abnormalities. There is no evidence of skeletal osteoporosis as in patients with renal insufficiency and secondary hyperparathyroidism [16]. Computed tomography (CT) is superior in demonstrating the internal architecture of the lesions. Two distinctive CT appearances are noted [42]. Most commonly the mass is composed of several large cystic components, outlined by thin layers of calcium and high-attenuation septations (Fig. 23.2). The center of most of the cysts has low attenuation. Calcium layering may be seen in the dependent portion of the cysts and is referred to as the "sedimentation sign" Infrequently, CT reveals a mass constituted of multiple small nodules with attenuation of solid rather than of cystic lesions.

■ **MRI Findings.** On magnetic resonance imaging (MRI), as a result of the long T1 – longitudinal relaxation time of the calcific components, tumoral calcinosis appears on T1-weighted images as an inhomogeneous nodular mass lesion of low signal intensity. In contrast, T2-weighted images reveal mostly high signal intensity, despite large calcific deposits (Fig. 23.3). Two distinctive appearances are noticed: a nodular pattern in which areas of very high signal intensity alternate with areas of signal void, or a more diffuse and less bright signal pattern. The latter images, especially when obtained in the axial plane, are the most informative, as the high signal intensity due to long T2 values reflects the inflammatory reaction. This is absent in metabolically stable lesions [42].

■ **Imaging Strategy.** The diagnosis of tumoral calcinosis is mostly apparent when calcified masses are observed along the extensor surface of joints in the most common locations: hips, shoulders, elbows, and feet. Demonstration of the sedimentation sign is important as this reflects activity of the lesion, indicating its potential to grow or shrink in response to therapy [42]. For this purpose, upright conventional radiographs or CT images in the axial plane are recommended. CT furthermore allows the best assessment of the extent of the lesion and evaluation of the cortex of adjacent bone [54]. Despite its low sensitivity in disclosing calcific components, MRI is superior to all other imaging techniques in demonstrating the inflammatory component. This is explained by the long T2 values associated with the granulomatous reaction characteristic of tumoral calcinosis [42].

23.3.2 Intramuscular Myxoma

23.3.2.1 Definition

Intramuscular myxoma is a benign tumor of mesenchymal origin, histologically characterized by the presence of abundant, avascular myxoid stroma in which relatively small numbers of stellate or spindle-shaped cells and reticulum fibers are embedded. The macroscopic appearance is rather stereotypic: most tumors are ovoid or rounded and have a gelatinous consistence. Paucity of vascular structures within the lesion is obvious. On section, the surface has a gray-white or white aspect, depending on the relative amounts of collagen. Occasionally the lesion contains multiple small fluid filled cavities [1, 16, 25]. Size of the lesion mostly ranges between 5 and 10 cm in diameter, although quite large lesions with diameter surpassing 20 cm have been observed (Figs. 23.4 and 23.5). An association exists between multiple intramuscular myxomas and fibrous dysplasia of bone, and is referred to as Mazabraud's syndrome. [1, 19, 25, 57] (Figs. 23.6–23.8). In the vast majority of patients with Mazabraud's syndrome polyostotic fibrous dysplasia is present. Osseous involvement by fibrous dysplasia commonly occurs in the same anatomical region of the myxomas [16, 57]. Malignant transformation of fibrous dysplasia to osteogenic sarcoma in patients with Mazabraud's syndrome has been reported in the literature [38]. Furthermore, the existence of a relationship between myxoma of the soft tissues and McCune-Albright syndrome (fibrous dysplasia, usually polyostotic in type, café-au-lait spots, and endocrinopathy including, but not limited to, precocious puberty, especially in women) has been mentioned [16, 19].

Intramuscular myxomas are considered to be mesenchymal tumors arising from fibroblasts [34] A traumatic factor in the genesis is unlikely, since a history of trauma is only present in less than 25% of cases. Although familial incidence is not increased, the occasional association with fibrous dysplasia raises the possibility of a basic metabolic error of both tissues. Therefore, soft tissue myxoma has been considered by some authors to be "an extraskeletal manifestation of fibrous dysplasia" [57, 62].

23.3.2.2 Incidence and Clinical Behavior

Occurring almost exclusively in individuals between the fifth and seventh decades, intramuscular myxoma is a tumor of adult life. The tumor is rare in young persons and virtually nonexistent in children. Female patients outnumber male patients by a narrow margin [16, 33]. In the majority of cases the only sign is a solitary, painless mass that is firm and often fluctuant on palpation. At the time of diagnosis most lesions measure 5–10 cm in diameter. Pain occurs in less than 25% of cases. The rate of tumor growth is variable, and occasionally there is no apparent growth over a long period of time. There is no close relationship between the size and age of the lesion. The areas most frequently involved are the large muscles of the thigh, shoulder, buttocks, and upper arm. Although the majority of myxomas are solitary lesions, occasionally multiple myxomas are observed. When these occur in the same region of the body, they are nearly always associated with fibrous dysplasia of bone (Figs. 23.6–23.8). The bones involved by fibrous dysplasia are usually in the vicinity of the myxoma [16, 25, 63]. A long interval – sometimes up to 20 or 30 years – is observed between the appearance of the fibrous dysplasia, which is noted during the growth period, and the myxoma. This combination of multiple intramuscular myxomas and fibrous dysplasia has a remarkable predilection for the right limb [62]. Following surgery, recurrence of intramuscular myxoma is rare.

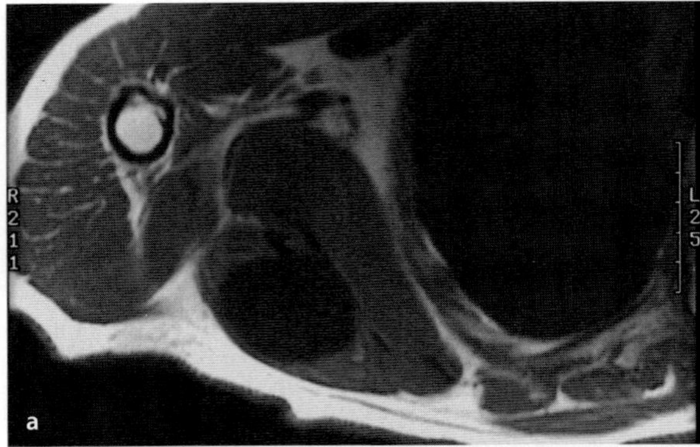
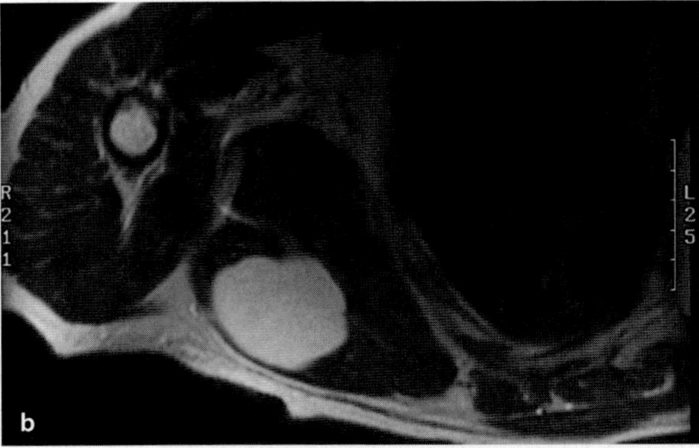
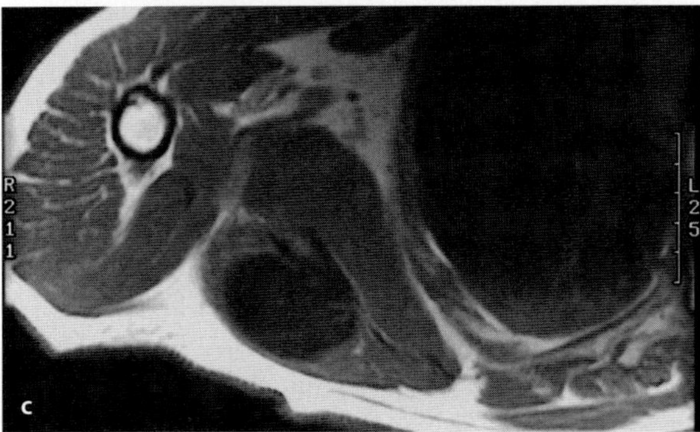

Fig. 23.4a–c. Intramuscular myxoma at the right scapular region in a 68-year-old man. **a** Axial spin echo T1-weighted MR image. **b** Axial spin echo T2-weighted MR image. **c** Axial spin echo T1-weighted MR image after gadolinium contrast injection. Large, rounded, intramuscular lesion at the infraspinate fossa is seen. The mass is well circumscribed and homogeneous on both spin echo sequences, hypointense to muscle on the T1-weighted image and hyperintense to fat on the T2-weighted image (**a, b**). After contrast medium injection, only a few enhancing strands are observed within the lesion. The major parts of the lesion do not enhance. This pattern of enhancement illustrates well the sparse vascularization of the lesion

Fig. 23.5a–f. Intramuscular myxoma of the calf: **a** axial spin echo T1-weighted MR image; **b** axial STIR T2-weighted MR image; **c** sagittal spin echo T1-weighted MR image; **d** sagittal spin echo T1-weighted MR image after gadolinium contrast injection; **e** axial spin echo T1-weighted MR image with fat suppression; **f** axial spin echo T1-weighted MR image with fat suppression after gadolinium contrast injection. Oval-shaped mass within the soleus muscle is observed. The lesion is sharply outlined. On T1-weighted images, the lesion is hypointense to muscle (**a,c,e**). T2-weighted images reveal a homogeneously hyperintense aspect of the tumor, with signal intensity of fluid (**b**). Following injection of contrast medium, no enhancement is observed at the periphery of the lesion, while the central part shows a definite enhancement (**d,f**). The areas of enhancement correspond to regions with high amount of solid myxoid tissue

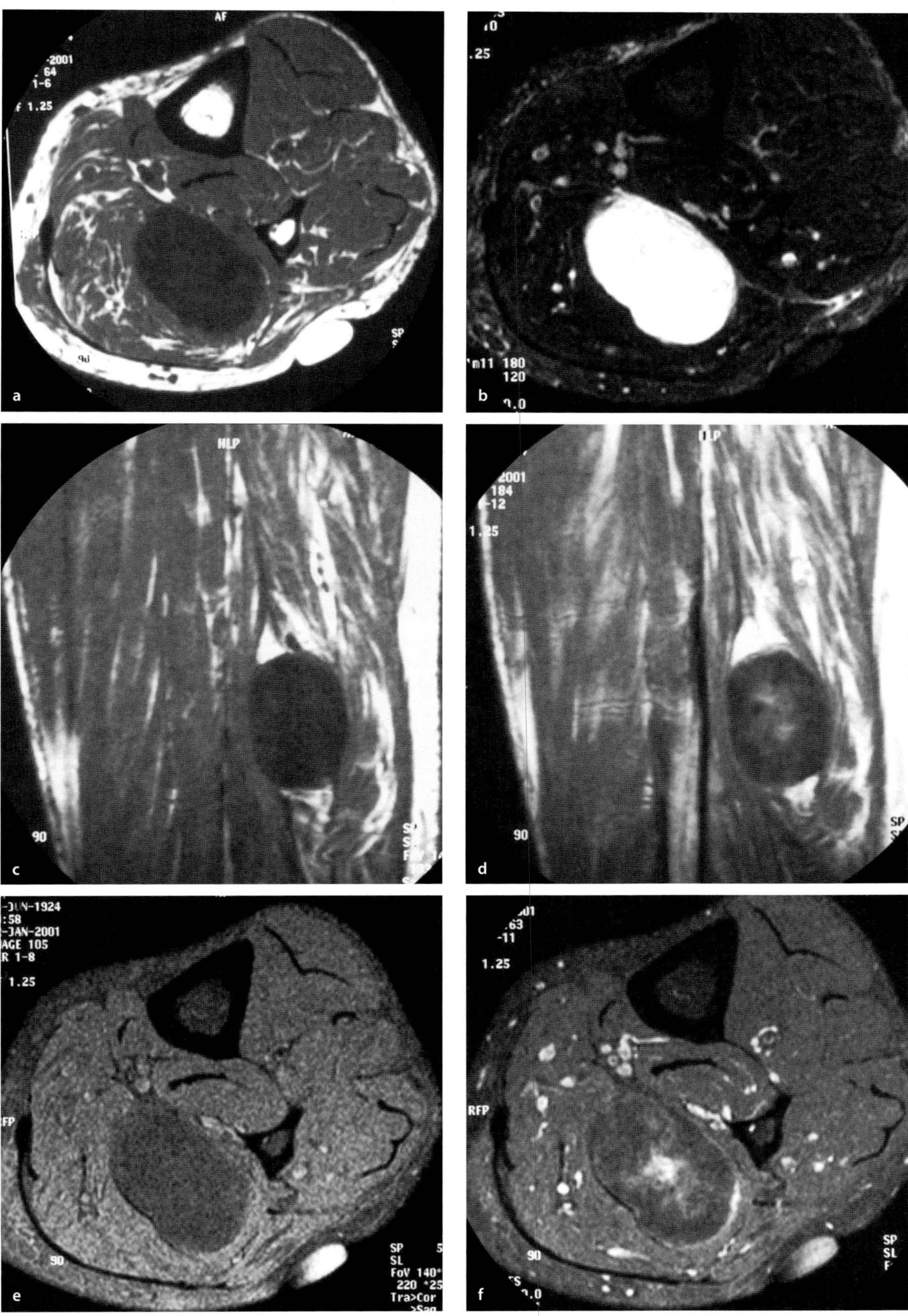

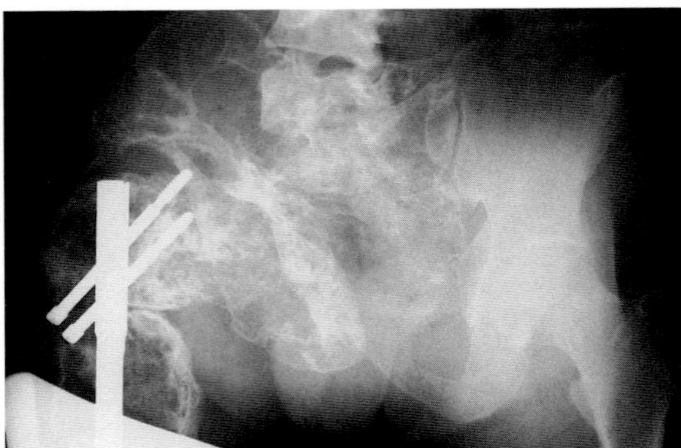

Fig. 23.6. Multiple intramuscular myxomas with polyostotic fibrous dysplasia of bone of lumbar spine, pelvic bones, and femur in a 35-year-old man. Plain radiograph discloses multiple multilocular cystlike lesions with a ground-glass appearance, separated from each other by thin septations within the fifth lumbar vertebra, the right pelvic bones, and right femur, corresponding to fibrous dysplasia. These involved bones are markedly deformed. Endomedullary osteosynthetic material at the femur witnesses previous pathologic fracture. (Courtesy of Trigaux JP, Nisolle SF, Cliniques Universitaires U.C.L. de Mont-Godinne, Belgium)

23.3.2.3 Imaging

■ **Imaging Studies Other than MRI.** As intramuscular myxomas do not contain calcifications, conventional radiographs are of little value in the diagnosis: they may be normal or reveal a nonspecific soft tissue mass. On CT the myxoma presents as a sharply demarcated mass within skeletal muscle. The attenuation of the lesion is intermediate between that of water and muscle, and ranges typically between 10 and 60 Hounsfield units [14, 25, 33, 43] (Fig. 23.7). However, attenuation values close to those of fat have been reported and may be misleading, as they mimic a fat-containing neoplasm [33]. Owing to the paucity of vascular structures within the lesion, the myxoma presents as a poorly vascularized soft tissue mass surrounded by well-vascularized muscle on angiograms.

■ **MRI Findings.** On MRI intramuscular myxoma presents as a well-circumscribed, homogeneous intramuscular mass. Signal intensity is low (less than or equal to that of muscle) on T1-weighted images and very high (brighter than fat) on T2-weighted images, quite similar to the signal characteristics of fluid [1, 25, 33, 48] (Figs. 23.4 and 23.8). In some cases of myxoma the presence of fat has been demonstrated. As a result, the appearance on MRI of these myxomas may be indistinguishable from that of liposarcoma [31, 33, 34]. Following administration of gadolinium chelates, inhomogeneous enhancement is observed. The degree of enhancement seems proportional to the amount of solid myxoid tissue and fibrous septa, which are both variable in degree within the myxoma [25]. The areas of low signal intensity on the contrast enhanced images represent cystic areas on histologic examination [4, 48].

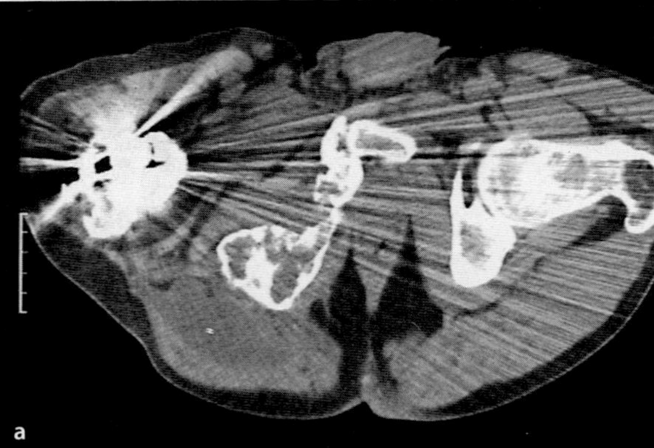

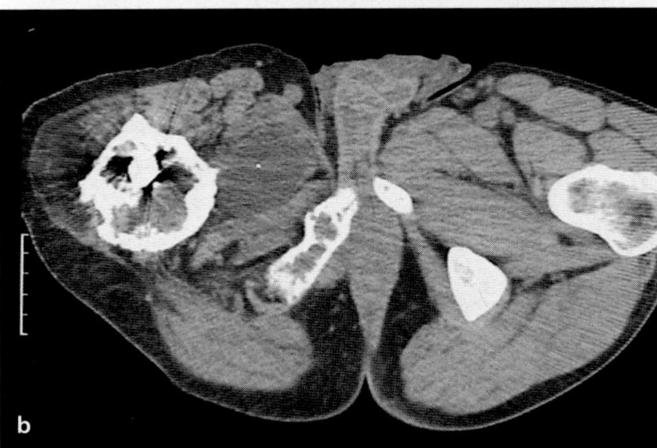

Fig. 20.7a, b. Multiple intramuscular myxomas with polyostotic fibrous dysplasia of bone of lumbar spine, pelvic bones, and femur in a 35-year-old man (same patient as in Fig. 20.5). **a** CT at the level of the hips. **b** CT at the level of right trochanteric region. CT confirms the replacement of medullary fat of the right ischium and femur by fibrous tissue. Expansion and thickening of the overlying cortex. These findings correspond to fibrous dysplasia of bone. In addition, well-delineated, nonenhancing, homogeneously hypodense soft tissue masses are observed within the right gluteal (**a**) and adductor (**b**) muscles, corresponding to intramuscular myxomas. (Courtesy of Trigaux JP, Nisolle SF, Cliniques Universitaires U.C.L. de Mont-Godinne, Belgium)

Fig. 23.8a–h. Multiple intramuscular myxomas with polyostotic fibrous dysplasia of bone of lumbar spine, pelvic bones, and femur in a 35-year-old man (same patient as in Fig.20.5). **a,b** Coronal spin echo T1-weighted MR images at the level of the right femoral diaphysis (**a**) and gluteal muscles (**b**). **c–e** Axial spin echo T1-weighted MR images at the level of the iliac wings (**c**), hips (**d**), and trochanteric regions (**e**). **f–h** axial spin echo T2-weighted MR images at the level of the iliac wings (**f**), hips (**g**), and trochanteric regions (**h**). The intramuscular myxomas appear as homogeneous, very low intensity soft tissue masses within the right adductor (**a, e**) and gluteal (**b, d**) muscles (*arrowheads*). The areas of the right pelvic bones, right femur, and lumbar vertebrae that are involved by fibrous dysplasia (see also Fig.20.5) have a lobular appearance with low signal intensity (*arrows*). On T2-weighted images, both myxomas are very bright, indicating long T2 relaxation times of their myxoid matrix. The gluteal myxoma is composed of several lobules, separated from each other by low intensity septations. The areas involved by fibrous dysplasia of bone are best observed at the level of the right iliac wing. Due to cystic degeneration these areas appear extremely bright on T2-weighted images. Artifacts are observed on all images in the right hip region. These are due to magnetic field inhomogeneity, which is caused by the metallic hip prosthesis. (Courtesy of Trigaux JP, Nisolle SF, Cliniques Universitaires U.C.L. de Mont-Godinne, Belgium).

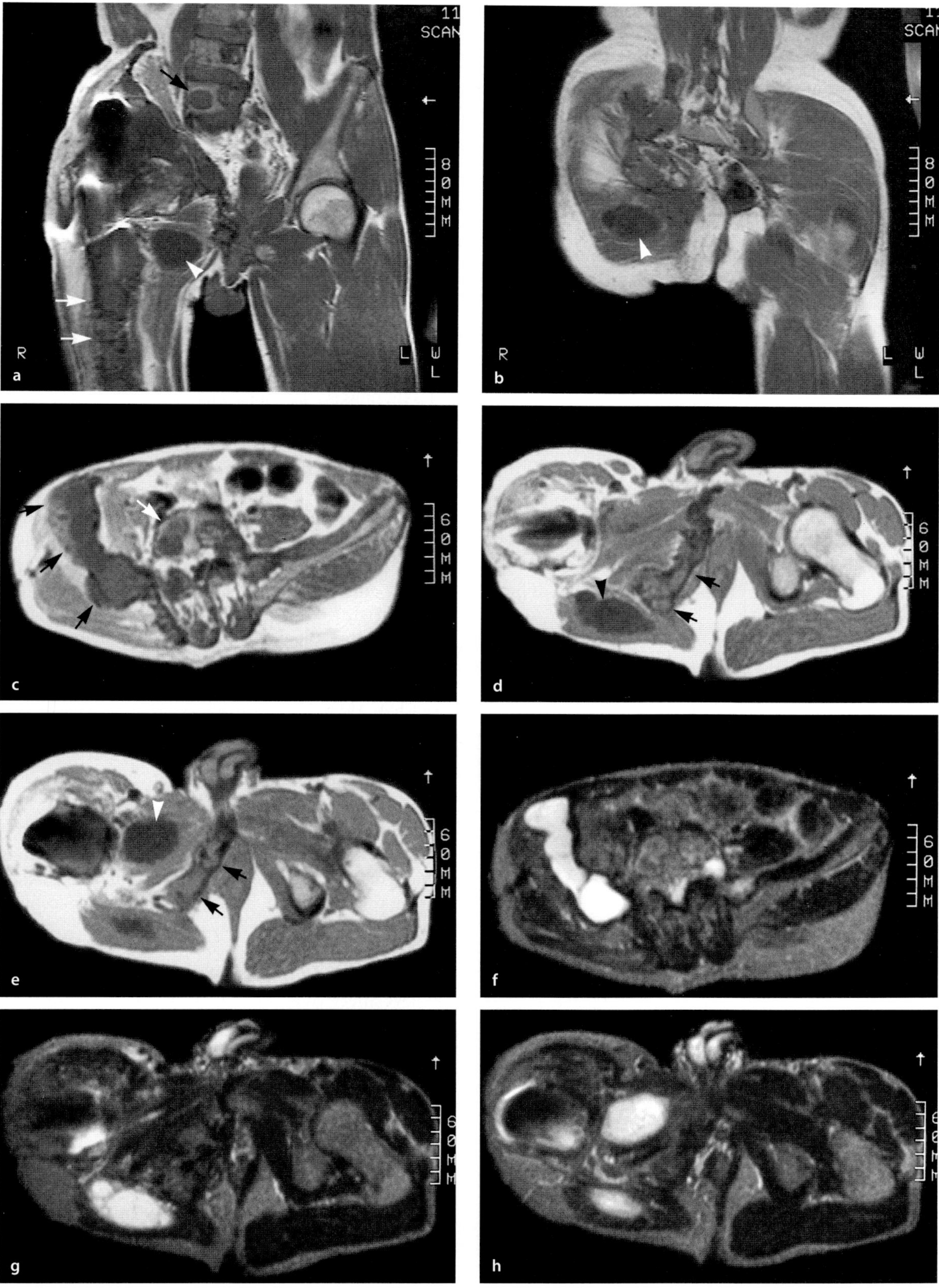

■ **Imaging Strategy.** Conventional radiographs are of little value for the diagnosis of intramuscular myxoma. An exception is made in the case of patients with both multiple myxomas and fibrous dysplasia, but in these cases conventional radiographs are used primarily for investigation of the bony lesions (Fig. 23.6). Mazabraud's syndrome should always be taken into account when fibrous dysplasia occurs with one or more soft tissue masses. CT – like MRI – may reveal misleading findings by demonstrating fat densities within a myxoma that suggest a lipomatous tumor (lipoma or liposarcoma). Sarcomas, particularly with myxoid degeneration, may resemble myxomas both radiologically and histologically. Although MRI is the preferred imaging technique for staging, the MRI findings of intramuscular myxoma are not specific [33, 49].

23.3.3 Miscellaneous Myxoma-like Lesions

Like intramuscular myxomas, this group encompasses other lesions which are all characterized by the presence of abundant myxoid matrix, a small number of cells, and paucity of vascular structures. For most of these lesions, the recurrence rate is greater than that of intramuscular myxoma.

23.3.3.1 Aggressive Angiomyxoma

■ **Definition.** Aggressive angiomyxoma is a rare, slowly growing neoplasm, which predominantly occurs in the pelvic soft tissue in women. The tumor has a gelatinous appearance, and its diameter ranges from a few centimeters to more than 20 cm. Although this tumor has a locally aggressive behavior, distant metastases have not been reported [16, 39].

■ **Incidence and Clinical Behavior.** The majority of angiomyxomas occur in adults, predominantly in women between ages of 25 and 60 years. This tumor has a predilection for the gluteal, perineal, and pelvic regions. Although a slow growth pattern is seen, the tumor is focally infiltrative, often extending into the paravaginal and perirectal regions. Metastatic spread is not observed. Recurrence rate after surgical removal is high [16, 39].

■ **Imaging.** On CT aggressive angiomyxoma has a variable appearance. It has been described either as a predominantly cystic mass containing solid components or as a solid mass containing low-density areas [39, 63]. MRI reveals a high signal intensity mass on T2-weigthed images. The lesion shows a tendency to grow around the pelvic floor muscles, without disrupting them. The tumor only causes displacement of the pelvic organs.

23.3.3.2 Omental-Mesenteric Myxoid Hamartoma

■ **Definition.** Omental-mesenteric myxoid hamartoma is a very rare benign neoplasm occurring in the omentum and mesentery of infants during the first year of life. Macroscopically these tumors appear as a solitary yellow mass or multiple, grapelike nodules within a mucoid and well-vascularized matrix [16].

■ **Incidence and Clinical Behavior.** Few cases have been reported, as this condition is extremely rare. The tumor has a benign behavior and causes abdominal distension and malaise. Its clinical course reflects the benign nature of this disease [16].

■ **Imaging.** A search of the literature reveals no reports on imaging findings.

23.3.3.3 Juxta-articular Myxoma and Meniscal Cyst

■ **Definition.** Meniscal cyst (previously designated as juxta-articular "myxoma") is characterized by depositions of myxoid material in the juxta-articular tissues of the knee and occasionally with myxoid changes within the underlying cartilage. The term "parameniscal cyst" refers to small types of such lesions. Calcification of the myxoid matrix may occur in older lesions [6, 16]. Further discussion is beyond the scope of this chapter (see Chap. 19).

23.3.3.4 Myxoma of the Jaws

■ **Definition.** Although primarily a bone tumor, myxoma of the jaws may manifest as a myxomatous swelling or mass in the soft tissues near the mandible or maxilla. It is characterized by higher cellularity and cellular pleomorphism than other myxomas [16].

■ **Incidence and Clinical Behavior.** Most myxomas of the jaws affect young adults. In its common presentation, the tumor overlies an osteolytic defect in the mandible and/or maxillary bone and may displace or destroy teeth, penetrate into the maxillary sinus, or involve soft tissues of the face [16].

■ **Imaging.** Myxoma of the jaws is seen radiologically as an expansile, well-circumscribed, multilocular radiolucency within the jaw bone. CT is recommended for assessing the extent of the lesion (Fig. 23.9). MRI is superior for demonstrating the extent of soft tissue involvement, but is inferior to CT for evaluating the underlying bony lesion [9] (Figs. 23.9 and 23.10).

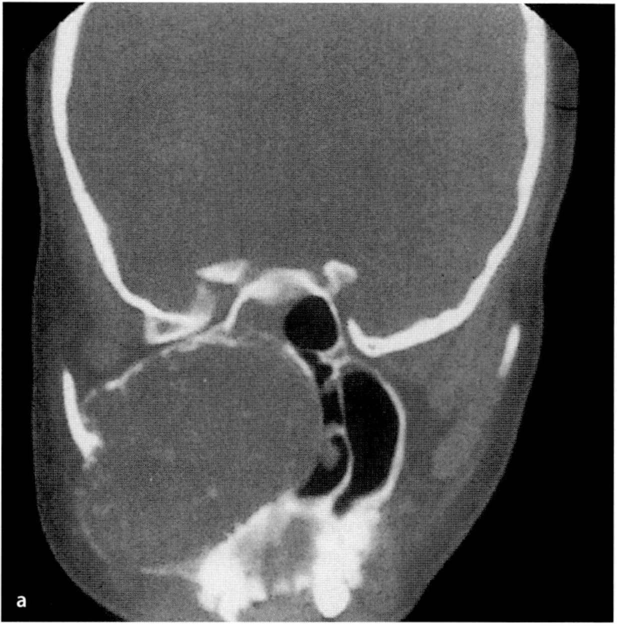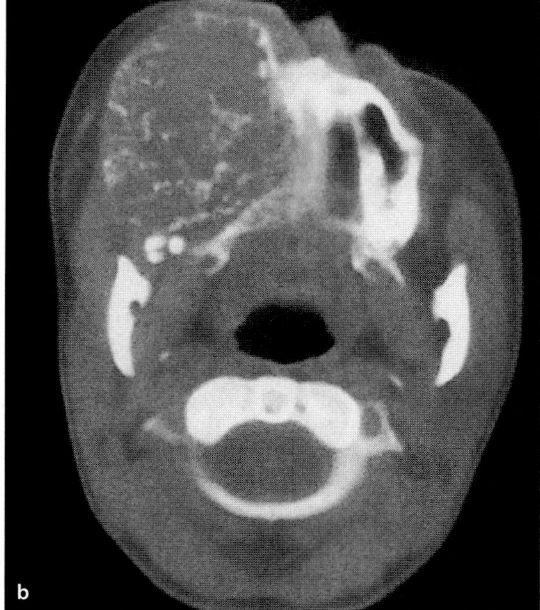

Fig. 23.9 a, b. Myxofibroma of the jaws in an 18-year-old woman. **a** Coronal CT. **b** Axial CT. Presence of an expansive myxofibroma replacing the right maxillary antrum. Expansion, thinning, and destruction of the surrounding bony margins is obvious. Bony trabeculations are well seen within the lesion. (Reproduced from [9], with permission)

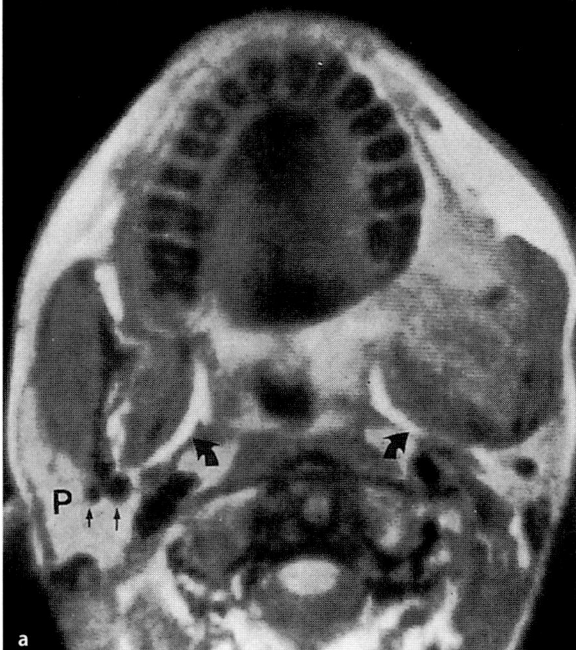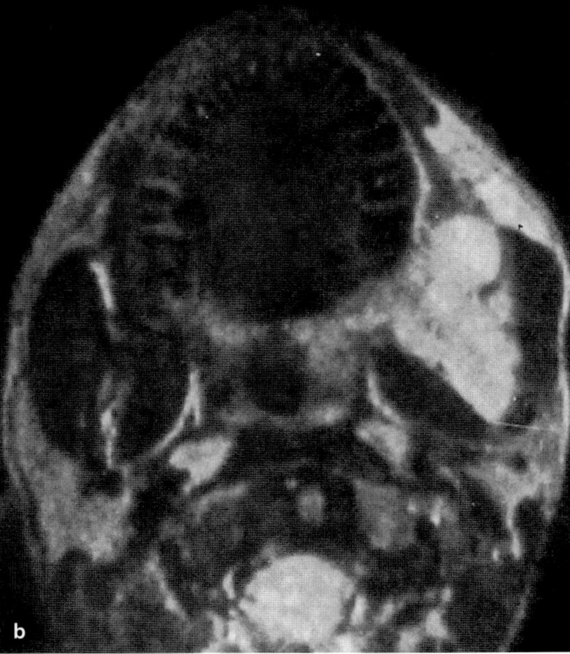

Fig. 23.10 a, b. Myxofibroma of the jaws in a 16-year-old boy. **a** Axial spin echo proton density-weighted MR image. **b** Axial spin echo T2-weighted MR image. Expansive lesion at the left ascending ramus of the mandible is seen. On the proton density-weighted image, the myxofibroma has increased signal intensity compared with the pterygoid and masseter muscles. The T2-weighted image reveals high signal intensity of the tumor, surpassing that of fat. Tumor margins are sharp. Note the bright signal of the parapharyngeal fat (*curved arrows*) and the presence of vascular structures (*straight arrows*) within the parotid gland (*P*). (Reproduced from [9], with permission)

23.3.3.5 Cutaneous and Cardiac Myxomas, Spotty Pigmentation, and Endocrine Overactivity (Carney's Complex)

■ **Definition.** The combination of cutaneous and cardiac myxomas, spotty pigmentation, and endocrine overactivity (Carney's complex) has also been described as "NAME" and "LAMS" syndrome [16]. Cardiac myxomas, as an isolated disorder, are rare benign neoplasms of the heart. The left atrium is the most common location (75%), followed by the right atrium (20%) and finally the ventricles (5%) [18].

■ **Incidence and Clinical Behavior.** The triad of these disorders occurs predominantly in young adults. Men and women are equally affected. Some patients may also have multicentric myxoid fibroadenomas of the breast, adrenocortical hyperplasia, and calcifying Sertoli cell tumors of the testis. Cardiac myxomas not accompanied by any other disorder more frequently affect women. They most commonly affect adults who are 30–60 years of age. This condition has no increased familial incidence [16]. Some atrial myxomas have been reported to cause distal intracranial aneurysms, distant parenchymal masses, and bony metastases [27].

■ **Imaging.** Cardiac myxomas are hypervascular tumors. Echocardiography is actually the preferred imaging technique for diagnosis, but MRI, scintigraphy, angiography, and cine-CT have all proved useful [18].

23.3.3.6 Cutaneous Myxoid Cyst

■ **Definition.** Cutaneous myxoid cyst consists of a small nodule in fingers or toes. The nodule is slow growing and rarely becomes larger than 2 cm. Many of these lesions contain small, fluid-filled cavities [16].

■ **Incidence and Clinical Behavior.** This lesion presents as a soft, dome-shaped nodule of the distal and dorsal portion of the fingers and occasionally the toes. It occurs at any age and has a definite female predominance. Some of these lesions are covered by verrucous skin and are associated with dystrophic changes of the nail [16].

■ **Imaging.** Cutaneous myxoid cysts may be seen on ultrasound of the nodules in fingers or toes. Conventional radiographs occasionally reveal signs of osteoarthritis in the terminal joints [16].

23.3.3.7 Dermal Mucinoses

■ **Definition.** The term "dermal mucinoses" is applied to myxoid changes of the dermis that may occur in rare cases of discoid lupus erythematosus and dermatomyositis [16].

■ **Incidence and Clinical Behavior.** These are a group of changes of the dermis that occur in rare cases of discoid lupus erythematosus or dermatomyositis [16].

■ **Imaging.** Owing to their superficial location, imaging techniques are not recommended for the diagnosis of dermal mucinoses.

23.3.3.8 Ganglion Cyst

For a detailed discussion of ganglion cysts, we refer to Chap. 19 and to [4, 23, 32, 48].

20.3.4 Amyloid Tumor

23.3.4.1 Definition

Amyloid tumors in the soft tissues are rare. The majority of these lesions are secondary types of amyloidosis, which has a well-known association with multiple myeloma, various chronic infections, and inflammatory diseases such as tuberculosis, osteomyelitis, and rheumatoid arthritis. Amyloidosis of the musculoskeletal system more frequently involves bone and/or joints [16, 58]. Primary amyloidosis with deposits in the soft tissues is extremely rare. Amyloid tumors are slowgrowing nodules or masses. They are lobulated and have a whitish or pinkish yellow waxy surface. Cartilage formation and ossification may occur in some amyloids [16].

23.3.4.2 Incidence and Clinical Behavior

These are rare and most commonly observed as a manifestation of secondary amyloidosis, which develops frequently in association with plasmacytoma or a variety of chronic infections or inflammatory diseases. Primary amyloidosis is very rare, appears usually late in life and affects male more often than female patients [58]. These tumor-like lesions are located in the region of the groin, abdominal wall, breast, neck, and orbit. Small nodules have also been observed in the eyelids and the skin [16].

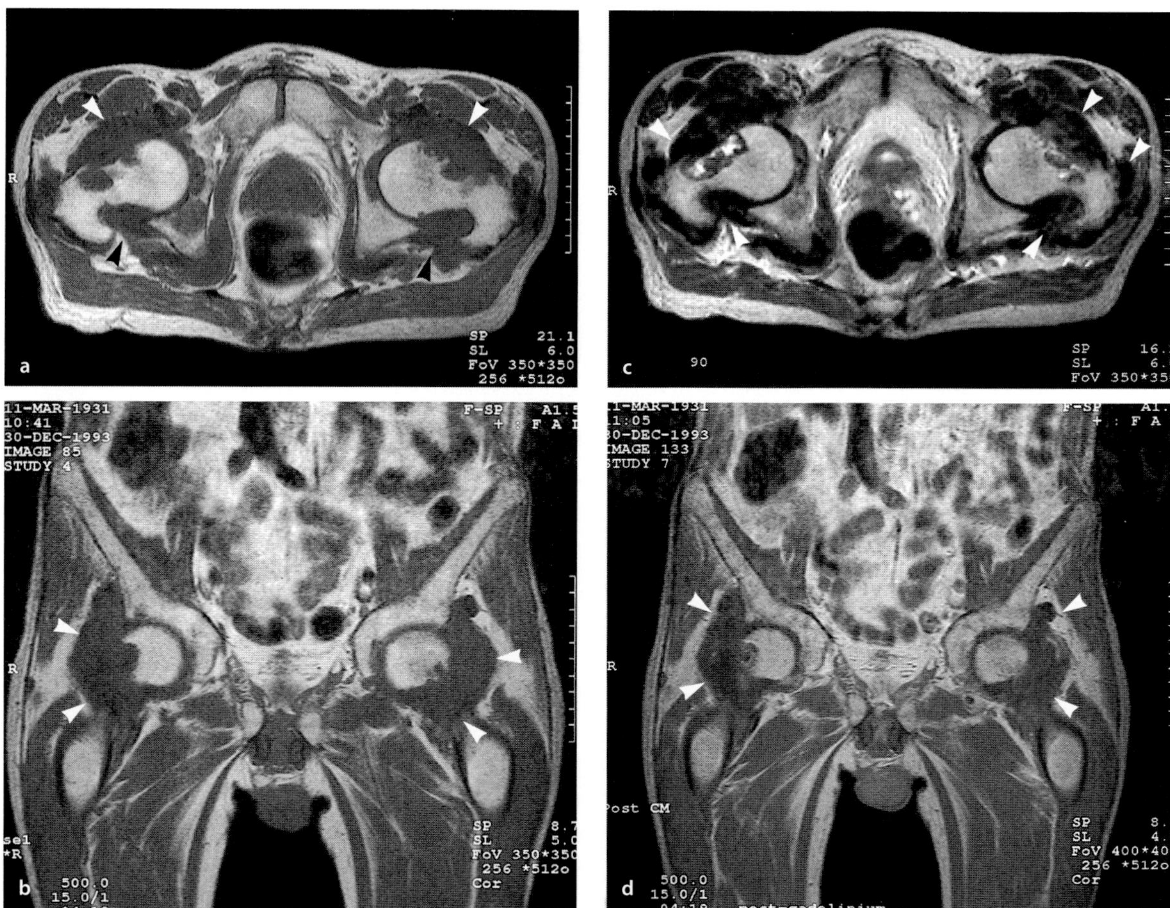

Fig. 23.11 a–d. Secondary amyloidosis involving the hip joints in a 62-year-old man. **a** Axial spin echo T1-weighted MR image. **b** Coronal spin echo T1-weighted MR image. **c** Axial turbo spin echo T2-weighted MR image. **d** Coronal spin echo T1-weighted MR image after gadolinium contrast injection. MR images disclose extensive depositions within both hip joints (*arrowheads*) which are homogeneous with low signal intensity on T1-weighted images and with signal voids on T2-weighted images. Multiple rounded to ovoid lesions in the femoral neck bilaterally. On T2-weighted images, these intraosseous lesions are markedly hyperintense at the center and sharply outlined by a low intensity rim, while on T1-weighted images, the intraosseous depositions have the same MR characteristics as the intra-articular amyloid depositions (**a–c**). No enhancement is observed at the intra-articular amyloid depositions (*arrowheads*). Intermediate enhancement occurs at the intraosseous components (**d**)

23.3.4.3 Imaging

Amyloid tumors present as nonspecific soft tissue masses on plain radiographs and CT. On MRI, they have low to intermediate signal intensity on T1- and T2-weighted images, with signal intensities between those of fibrocartilage and muscle [57]. No enhancement is observed following administration of gadolinium chelates. The appearance of amyloid on MRI is shown in two cases of secondary amyloidosis. In the first case amyloidosis involved the hip joints (Fig. 23.11), whereas in the second case amyloid tumors were seen in the submandibular region in a patient with multiple myeloma (Fig. 23.12).

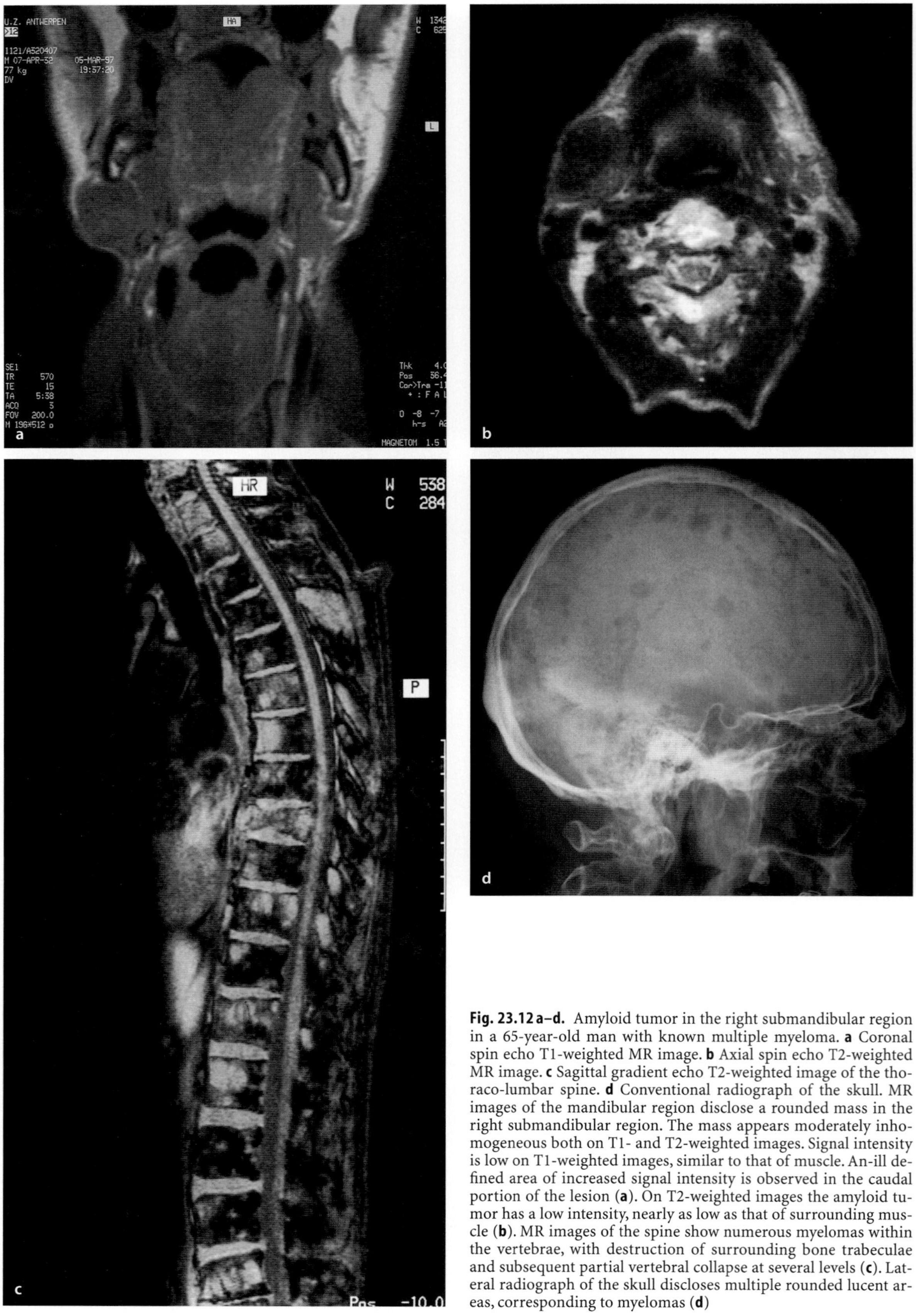

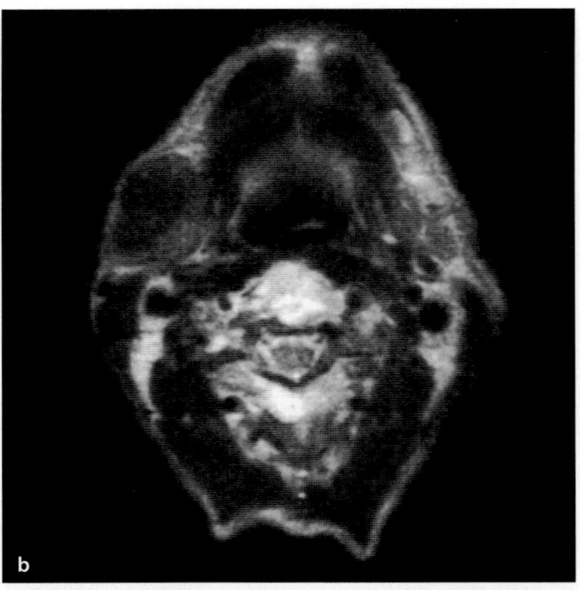

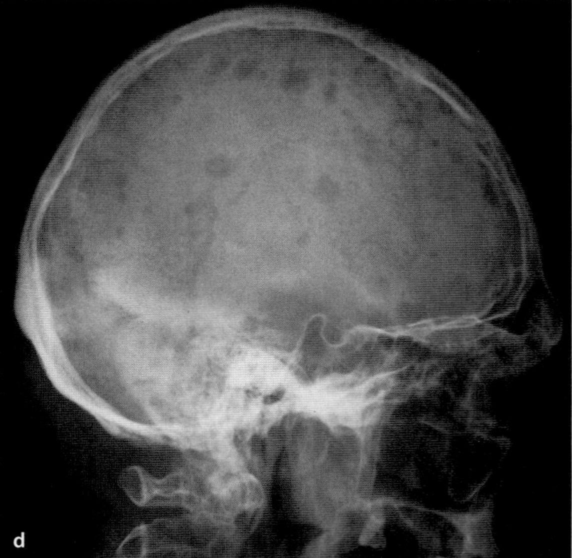

Fig. 23.12 a–d. Amyloid tumor in the right submandibular region in a 65-year-old man with known multiple myeloma. **a** Coronal spin echo T1-weighted MR image. **b** Axial spin echo T2-weighted MR image. **c** Sagittal gradient echo T2-weighted image of the thoraco-lumbar spine. **d** Conventional radiograph of the skull. MR images of the mandibular region disclose a rounded mass in the right submandibular region. The mass appears moderately inhomogeneous both on T1- and T2-weighted images. Signal intensity is low on T1-weighted images, similar to that of muscle. An-ill defined area of increased signal intensity is observed in the caudal portion of the lesion (**a**). On T2-weighted images the amyloid tumor has a low intensity, nearly as low as that of surrounding muscle (**b**). MR images of the spine show numerous myelomas within the vertebrae, with destruction of surrounding bone trabeculae and subsequent partial vertebral collapse at several levels (**c**). Lateral radiograph of the skull discloses multiple rounded lucent areas, corresponding to myelomas (**d**)

23.3.5 Parachordoma

23.3.5.1 Definition

The term "parachordoma" has been applied to a rare tumor of uncertain histogenesis but with a characteristic histologic appearance. The tumor forms a lobulated mass with diameter averaging 3.5 cm. Usually it involves the soft tissues of the extremities adjacent to tendons, synovium, or bones [10, 16].

23.3.5.2 Incidence and Clinical Behavior

Parachordoma is a rare tumor, which affects both adolescents and adults. The lesion predominates in the extremities or peripheral parts of the body where it is deeply seated near tendons, synovium, and osseous structures [10]. Although recurrence has been observed following excision, parachordoma is considered a benign lesion.

23.3.5.3 Imaging

A search of the literature reveals no reports of imaging findings.

23.4 Malignant Lesions of Uncertain Differentiation

23.4.1 Synovial Sarcoma

Although synovial sarcoma is a misnomer, as it is not derived from true synovial cells, we will not go into the details of this nosological discussion.

23.4.1.1 Definition

Synovial sarcoma is a clinically and morphologically well-defined entity. It occurs primarily in the para-articular region, usually in close relationship with tendon sheaths, bursae and joint capsules. It is, however, uncommon in joint cavities. On rare occasions, but widely reported in the radiological literature, it is also encountered in areas without any apparent relationship to synovial structures, such as in the pharynx, the larynx, the tongue, the maxillofacial region, the middle ear, precoccygeal and paravertebral regions, the mediastinum, the thoracic and abdominal wall, the heart or even in intravascular and intraneural locations [7, 45, 46, 50, 55, 56]. Only synovial sarcoma associated with the locomotor system is discussed in this chapter.

23.4.1.2 Incidence and Clinical Behavior

■ **Epidemiology.** Synovial sarcoma is the fifth most commonly reported soft tissue malignancy, accounting for approximately 5–10 % of all malignant mesenchymal neoplasms [15, 30, 45]. It is most prevalent in adolescents and young adults between 15 and 40 years of age [30] (Table 23.1). Men are more susceptible than women with an average ratio of 2:1. There is no predilection for any particular race.

■ **Clinical Behavior and Gross Findings.** The most typical presentation is that of a palpable deep-seated soft-tissue mass. It is usually associated with pain or tenderness and may cause functional impairment of the adjacent joint. Severe functional disturbances or weight loss are infrequent. Although uncommon, involvement of nearby nerves may cause pain, numbness or paresthesia.

It is still uncertain whether trauma contributes to the development of synovial sarcoma or not. Although in many patients there is a definite history of trauma, the majority has no such antecedents. When reported, the interval between the episode of trauma and the detection of synovial sarcoma ranges from a few weeks to as much as 40 years. However there are also reports of patients who sustain injuries after the presence of a mass had been noted, which suggests that, at least in some cases, the relationship between both is purely coincidental.

As mentioned before, synovial sarcoma occurs predominantly in the extremities (80–90 %), mostly near large joints, especially the knee joint (30 %) [15] (Table 23.2). These tumors are intimately related to tendons, tendon sheaths, and bursal structures, usually beyond the confines of the joint capsule. In less than 5 % of all cases, synovial sarcoma arises in the joint space itself.

■ **Pathology.** The name of the lesion is derived from the microscopic resemblance of synovial sarcoma to normal synovium, although its origin is probably from undifferentiated mesenchymal tissue [45]. Unlike most other types of sarcomas, the tumor is composed of two morphologically different types of cells that form a characteristic biphasic pattern: epithelial cells, which resemble those of carcinoma, and fibrosarcoma-like spindle cells. There are transitions between both types of cells, suggesting a close generic relationship. Depending on the relative presence of these types of cells and on their differentiation, synovial sarcomas can be classified into four different types.

The *first type* is the biphasic synovial sarcoma that is characterized by the coexistence of morphologically different but histogenetically related epithelial and spindle cells. Calcification with or without ossification is

Table 23.1. Age distribution of 345 cases of synovial sarcoma according to Enzinger et al. [15]

Age range	No. of cases	Percentage
0–10 years	12	3%
10–20 years	94	27%
20–30 years	85	25%
30–40 years	57	17%
40–50 years	52	15%
50–60 years	25	7%
60–70 years	11	3%
70–80 years	6	2%
80–90 years	3	1%
Total	345	100%

Table 23.2. Localization of synovial sarcoma modified from Enzinger et al. [15]

Head-neck	31		9%
Neck		12	3%
Pharynx		7	2%
Larynx		7	2%
Other		5	1%
Trunk	28		8%
Chest		10	3%
Abdominal wall		9	2.5%
Other		9	2.5%
Upper extremities	80		23%
Shoulder		22	6%
Elbow/upper arm		20	6%
Forearm/wrist		24	7%
Hand		14	4%
Lower extremities	206		60%
Hip-groin		22	6%
Thigh/knee		102	30%
Lower leg/ankle		33	10%
Foot		45	13%
Other		4	1%
Total	345	345	100%

present in about 30% of tumors. The degree of vascularity varies from a few scattered vascular structures to numerous dilated vascular spaces. In less well differentiated tumors hemorrhage may be prominent.

The *second type* is the monophasic fibrous synovial sarcoma with a predominant or even exclusive spindle cell pattern. This type is relatively common. Its clinical presentation is identical to the biphasic type.

The *third type* of synovial sarcoma is the monophasic epithelial form. This is a rarely recognized neoplasm with a predominant or exclusive epithelial cell pattern.

It is difficult to render the diagnosis of this tumor with certainty since it closely resembles other more frequently occurring epithelial and mesenchymal tumors, such as metastatic and adnexal carcinoma, malignant melanoma, malignant epitheloid schwannoma and epitheloid sarcoma.

The *final type* of synovial sarcoma that is histologically recognized is the poorly differentiated type. Its incidence is estimated at 20%. It behaves more aggressively and metastasizes in a greater percentage of cases. Microscopically this tumor is composed of small oval or spindle-shaped cells, intermediate in appearance between epithelial and spindle cells. It has a rich vascular pattern with dilated vascular spaces.

Multicystic formation is a common occurrence in synovial sarcoma. The cyst wall is thickened and composed of fibrous septa. Within the cyst, there are often several internal septa, consisting of tumor cells proliferating over the dense collagenous fibrous tissue without a lining pattern. Tumor cells may become detached from the septa in the internal lumen. Furthermore, dilated hemangiopericytomatous vasculatures can be prominent within those septa.

Chromosomal rearrangements have been reported in association with synovial sarcoma, consisting of t(X;18)(p11–2;q11–2) translocation [13].

23.4.1.3 Imaging

The majority of synovial sarcomas present on *radiographs* as round or oval, lobulated masses. They are usually located close to a large joint, particularly the knee joint. In 5–30% of cases there is periosteal reaction, bone erosion (related to pressure from the adjacent tumor) or even bone invasion [45]. The most characteristic finding is the presence of multiple small densities caused by focal calcifications or ossifications. This feature is seen in about 20–30% of cases [45]. It may range from very fine stippling to marked calcifications or even bone formation, typically in the periphery of the lesion [45]. When present, these opacities differentiate synovial sarcoma from liposarcomas and myxoid chondrosarcomas. The irregular shape of the calcifications helps to make the differentiation from hemangioma. In some cases, extensive ossification is present, resembling osseous or cartilaginous lesions such as soft tissue chondroma, extra-articular synovial chondromatosis, ossifying myositis, tumoral calcinosis, or osteosarcoma, both parosteal and extraskeletal. Cases with extensive calcification have been reported to have a better prognosis, with higher survival rates [45, 52].

Angiography usually reveals a prominent vascularity, not only of the primary tumor, but also of the metastases. This is especially true for the monophasic and poorly differentiated type of tumor [37]. There is exten-

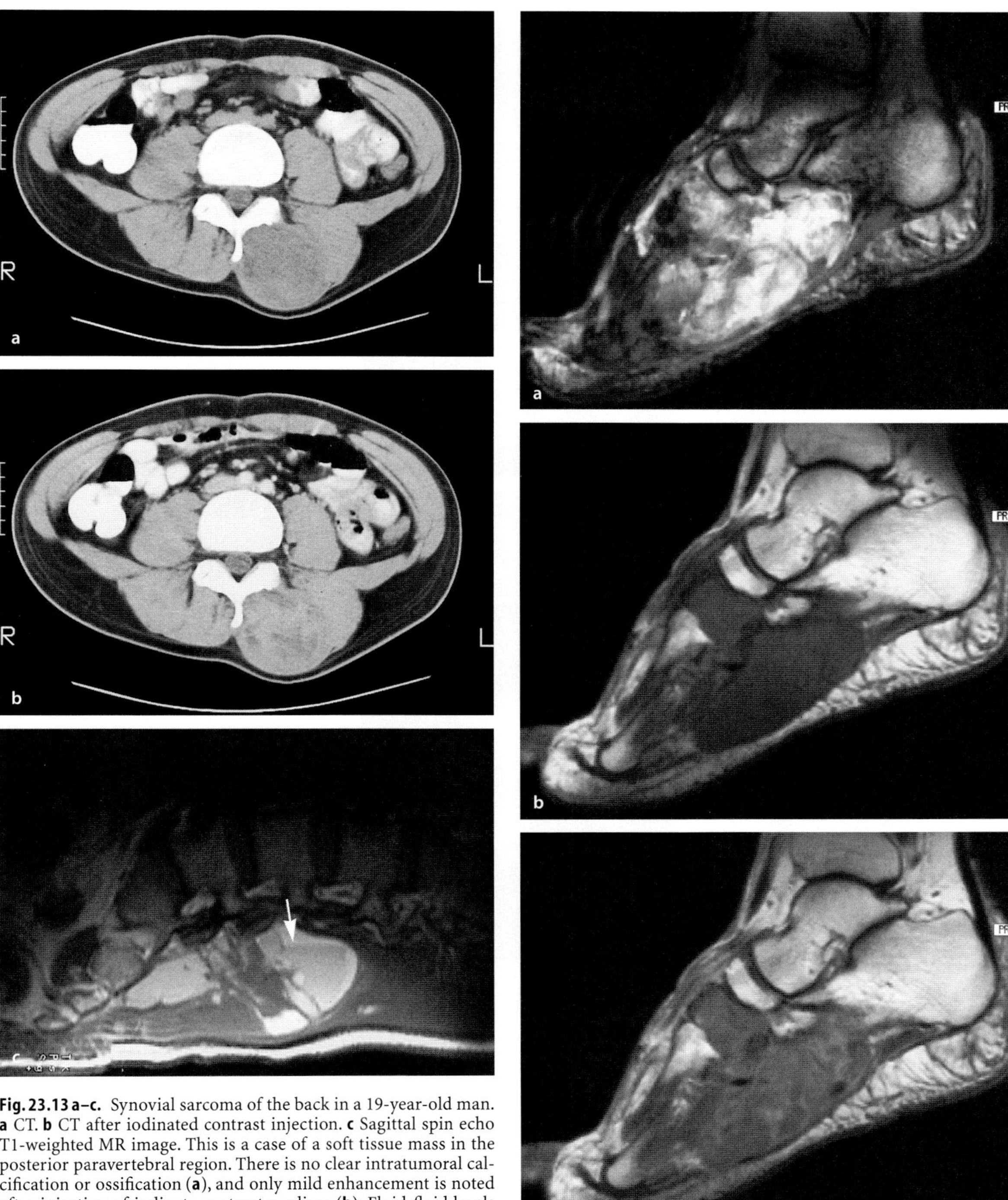

Fig. 23.13 a–c. Synovial sarcoma of the back in a 19-year-old man. **a** CT. **b** CT after iodinated contrast injection. **c** Sagittal spin echo T1-weighted MR image. This is a case of a soft tissue mass in the posterior paravertebral region. There is no clear intratumoral calcification or ossification (**a**), and only mild enhancement is noted after injection of iodinate contrast medium (**b**). Fluid-fluid levels can sometimes be seen on the T1-weighted image (**c**), but are a rare and nonspecific sign (*arrow*)

Fig. 23.14 a–c. Synovial sarcoma of the foot in a 37-year-old man. **a** Sagittal gradient-recalled echo T2*-weighted MR image. **b** Sagittal spin echo T1-weighted MR image. **c** Sagittal spin echo T1-weighted MR image after gadolinium contrast injection. Synovial sarcoma is generally hypointense on a T1-weighted image (**b**) and hyperintense on a T2-weighted image (**a**). Large lesions such as this one are usually heterogeneous and may show internal septation (**a**). Marked enhancement is correlated to the extensive vascular supply of these tumors (**c**). Bone invasion is less frequent (5–30%), but can be quite important (**c**). The sole of the foot is a common localization of synovial sarcoma in young adults

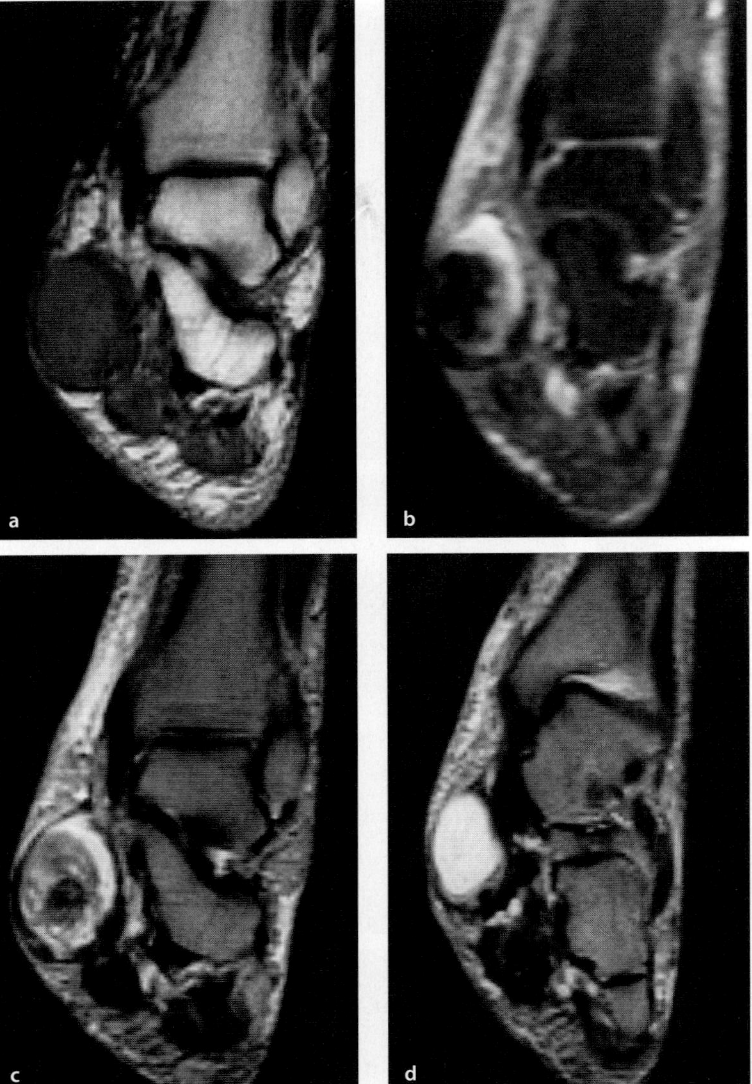

Fig. 23.15 a–d. Synovial sarcoma at the medial side of the ankle. **a** Coronal T1-weighted MR image. **b** Contrast-enhanced coronal fat-suppressed T1-weighted MR image. **c, d** Coronal fat-suppressed T2-weighted MR images. Oval mass, medially at the ankle joint, with inhomogeneous low signal intensity (**a**). Strong contrast uptake is seen at the periphery of the lesion (**b**). A triple signal pattern is seen within the lesion with signal intensities similar to fluid, intermediate and low signal intensities (**c, d**)

sive neovascularity and nonhomogeneous staining. Occasionally the lesion is hypovascular.

Ultrasound characteristics are those of a well-defined, solid vascular tumor with prominent arterial and venous components. There may be internal cystic components due to internal hemorrhage [47]. Internal calcifications are noted in 20–30%. Ultrasound appears useful as a detection method of local recurrence, in the guiding of fine needle biopsy and in the examination of children [24]. In the early postoperative period (less than six months after surgery) inhomogeneous hypoechogenic lesions cannot be differentiated with certainty as recurrent tumor, hemorrhage, edema, granulation tissue, abscess formation or any combination of these. Performed with high-frequency transducers a lesion is considered to be a recurrent tumor when a discrete nodular hypoechogenic mass is present. Areas of diffuse abnormal echogenicity without evidence of a discrete nodule can be classified as non-tumoral.

CT shows a soft tissue mass, which may infiltrate adjacent structures, having a slightly higher density than muscle [45] (Fig. 23.13). Joint invasion is present when the soft tissue mass projects into the expected confines of a joint capsule or when an intraarticular ligament or tendon is involved. Although bony involvement can be identified on both MR imaging and CT, cortical bone erosion or invasion is better depicted on CT. Intratumoral calcification or ossification is also more easily seen on CT than on MR imaging. Because of its extensive vascular supply, synovial sarcoma enhances markedly after injection of contrast medium.

On *MR imaging* most synovial sarcomas (>90%) are hypointense relative to fat, and nearly isointense relative to muscle on T1-weighted MR images [45]. In rare cases

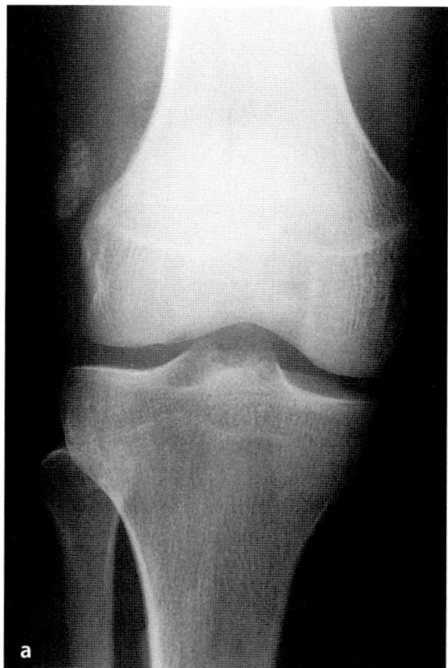

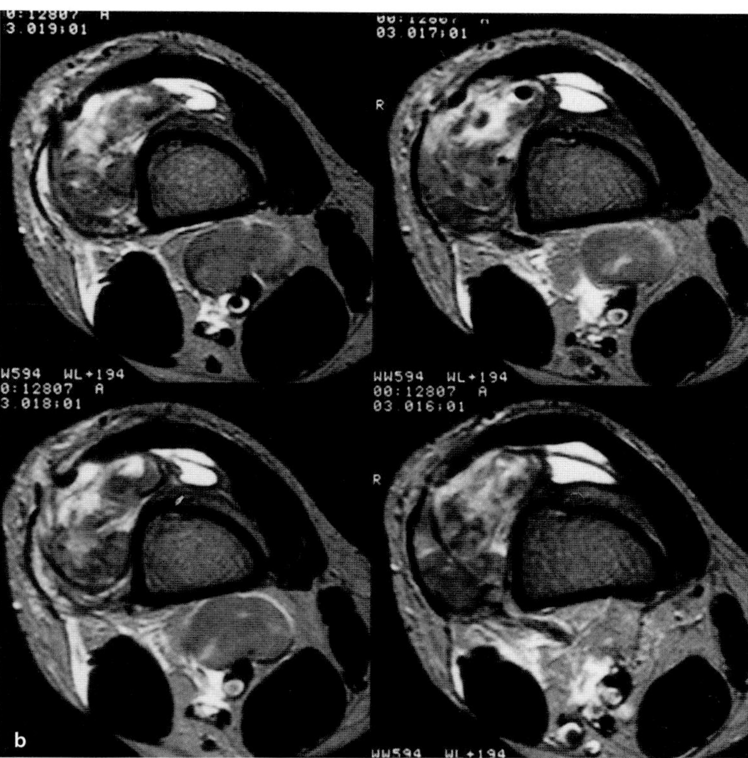

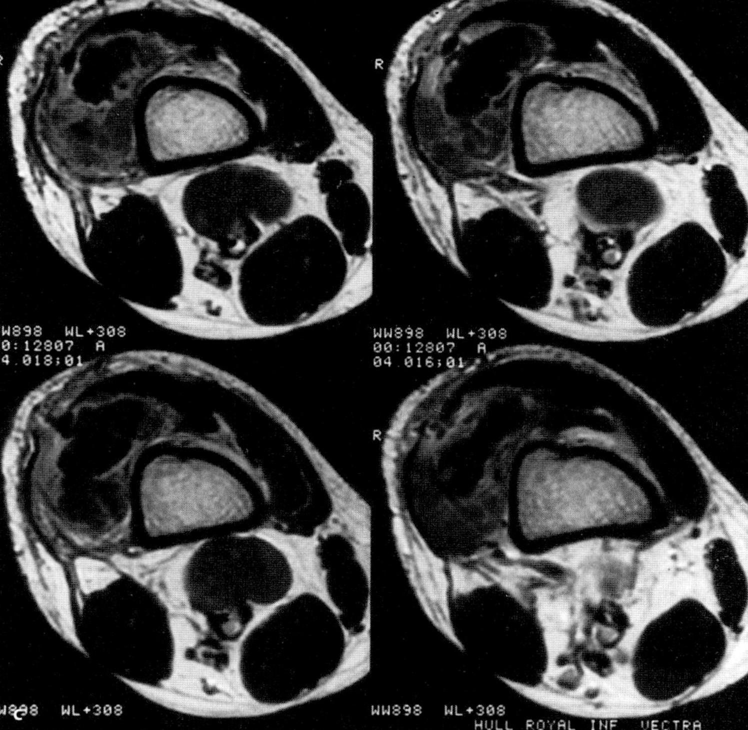

Fig. 23.16 a–c. Synovial sarcoma of the knee. **a** Anteroposterior radiograph of the right knee. **b** Axial T2-weighted MR image at the distal femur. **c** Axial T1-weighted MR image after intravenous gadolinium administration. A crumbly calcification is seen within a palpable soft tissue mass at the lateral side of the knee. Calcifications are seen in up to 30% of synovial sarcomas (**a**). The tumor is of mixed signal intensity with hypointense and hyperintense areas, as well as components of intermediate signal intensity ('triple signal'); the tumor looks to be arising outside the joint, but extends down the lateral patellar retinaculum into the superolateral aspect of the knee joint (**b**). There is marked peripheral contrast enhancement within the mass, with a central irregularly delineated area of non enhancement. There are enlarged lymph nodes around the neurovascular bundle in the popliteal fossa (**c**). (Case courtesy of Dr. A. M. Davies, Birmingham)

the tumor may be mostly hyperintense due to extensive intratumoral hemorrhage. Small areas of high signal on T1-weighted images are more often encountered (45%) [26, 45]). They probably correspond with small foci of hemorrhage, since these areas are of high signal on T2-weighted images too. Fluid-fluid levels, although not very frequent (15–25%) and not specific, can be a striking finding. Areas of previous hemorrhage with fluid-fluid levels or high signal intensity on all pulse sequences, may be associated with a worse prognosis [45] (Figs. 23.13–23.17). On T2-weighted images marked inhomogeneity is the rule, and various degrees of internal septation may be noted [44] (Figs. 23.14 and 23.17). This is especially true for lesions more than 5 cm in diameter which show this heterogeneous signal pattern in more than 85% of cases, vs 60% for smaller lesions [26]. A triple signal pattern on T2-weighted images is described in one third of all synovial sarcomas [26, 52]. It consists of high signal similar to fluid, intermediate signal intensity equal to or slightly hyperintense relative to fat, and low signal intensity closer to that of fibrous tissue. This triple signal pattern on T2-weighted images together with the small high signal foci on T1-weighted images is suggestive for synovial sarcoma (Figs. 23.15 and 23.16). More than half of all lesions are intimately related to bone. There seems to be no notable difference between the MR imaging characteristics of the mono- and biphasic pathologic subtypes.

Heterogeneous enhancement after injection of contrast material is generally seen. Hypervascular areas are strongly enhancing, whereas necrotic and cystic areas remain hypointense. Hypervascularity may be quantified by a dynamic contrast enhanced MR examination. Enhancement of tumor within 7 s after arterial enhancement is a reliable sign, occurring consistently in synovial sarcoma. Other previously described so-called malignant dynamic contrast-enhanced MR imaging features, such as early plateau or washout phase and peripheral enhancement are not always found in synovial sarcoma [60].

Well-defined or reasonably well-defined margins are seen in some cases of synovial sarcoma. This finding has been described as a probable sign of benignity [50, 52]. This may be one of the reasons why synovial sarcoma is the malignant tumor most frequently misdiagnosed as benign [5, 52]. Neurovascular involvement may be suspected in cases where the tumor margin abuts and displaces the neurovascular bundle. In one study this was confirmed at operation in two out of five cases [44]. MR often fails to demonstrate small calcifications seen on plain films or CT. Therefore the MR images of soft tissue and bone tumors should be interpreted with corresponding CT images and plain films.

The differential diagnosis on MR imaging of an inhomogeneous septate mass with infiltrative margins and located in close proximity to a joint, a tendon or a bursa is very limited. Without the history of trauma or signs of

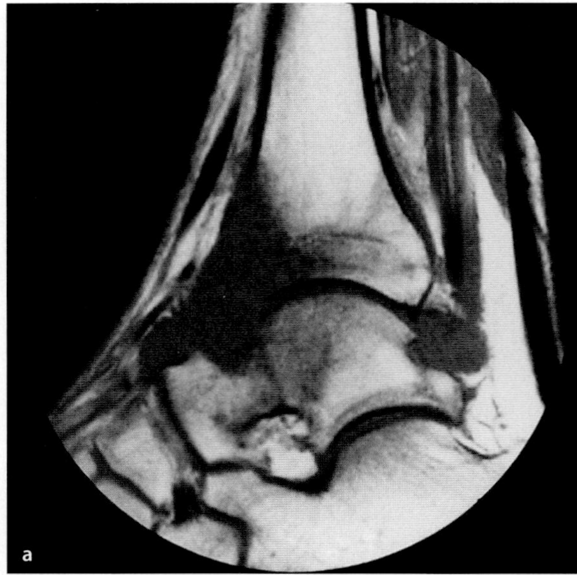

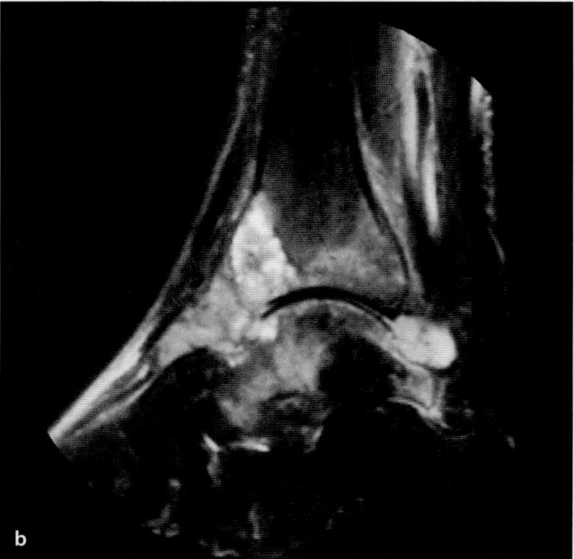

Fig. 23.17 a, b. Synovial sarcoma developing within the ankle joint. **a** Sagittal T1-weighted MR image. **b** Sagittal STIR image. A low signal intensity mass is present within the anterior and posterior recess of the ankle joint. There is associated erosion of the talar neck. The anterior cortex of the distal tibia is destroyed. Bone marrow edema is seen within the distal tibia and in the talus (**a**). The tumor is of high signal intensity on T2-weighted images, with some internal low signal intensity septa. The adjacent bone invasion and bone marrow edema is better appreciated than on the T1-weighted images (**b**). (Case courtesy of Dr. A.M. Davies, Birmingham)

infection, a malignant neoplasm is the most likely consideration. Especially in combination with soft tissue calcifications, the diagnosis of a synovial sarcoma should be preferred. However a septate configuration can also be seen in two types of benign soft tissue masses: hemangioma and synovial or ganglion cysts [61]. Typically these benign tumors are sharply marginated

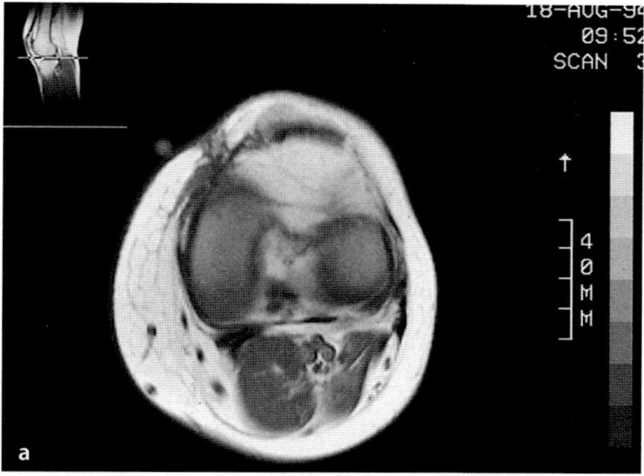

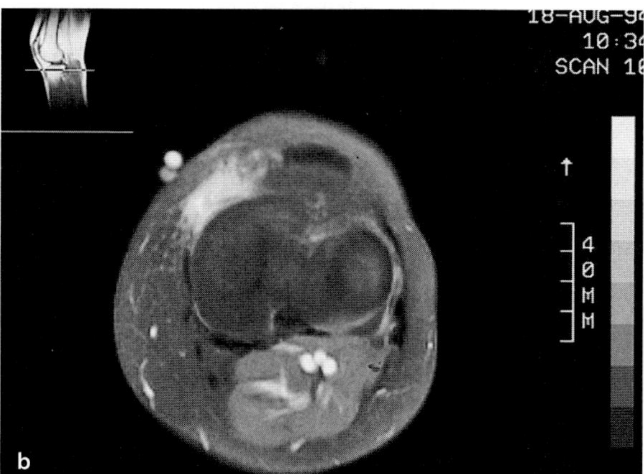

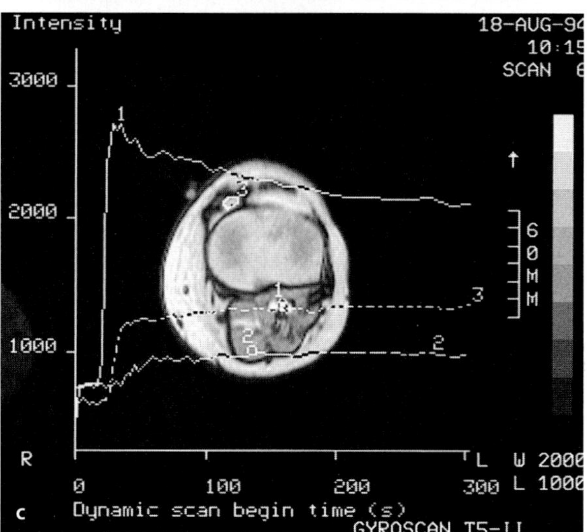

Fig. 23.18 a–c. Recurrent synovial sarcoma. **a** Axial spin echo T1-weighted MR image. **b** Axial, fat-suppressed, spin echo T1-weighted MR image after gadolinium contrast injection. **c** Signal intensity-versus-time curve calculated on a gradient-recalled echo T1-weighted MR image during gadolinium contrast injection. Synovial sarcoma quite frequently recurs after surgical excision. In this case a small hypointense lesion located deep in the scar tissue can be noted on the T1-weighted image (**a**). After gadolinium injection clear enhancement of this region can be noted on the fat-suppressed images (**b**). Dynamic imaging during bolus contrast injection (**c**) demonstrates the higher and more rapid uptake of contrast medium by this tissue (3) than by normal muscle (2). Repeat surgery disclosed recurrent tumor

and have a homogeneous hyperintense signal that is much brighter than that of the subcutaneous fat on T2-weighted images. The pattern of contrast enhancement may be helpful as well in the differential diagnosis.

■ **Treatment, Prognosis and Detection of Tumor Recurrence.** Treatment of synovial sarcoma consists of wide local excision or limb amputation, usually in combination with chemotherapy and/or radiation therapy. Despite this aggressive therapy, metastatic disease or local recurrence is found in approximately 80% of patients. Metastases most frequently affect the lung (59–94% of distant tumor spread). Additional sites of metastatic disease include lymph nodes (4–18%) and bone (8–11%). Soft tissue metastases are rare. Local recurrence occurs in 20–26% of patients, and presents usually within two years after initial diagnosis. The five-years survival rate is approximately 27–55%. Favorable prognostic factors with synovial sarcoma include extensive calcification, younger patient age, lesions less than 5 cm in diameter, and neoplasms located in the extremities [45]. According to Tateishi, other prognostic MRI parameters include the presence of hemorrhage, cysts or the presence of a triple signal. Together with proximal tumor distribution, large tumor size and the absence of calcification, these parameters are associated with high tumor grade and a less favorable prognosis [59.

The value of MRI in the early detection of tumor recurrence will be discussed in detail in Chap. 28, dealing with imaging posttreatment (Fig. 23.18).

23.4.2 Alveolar Soft Part Sarcoma

23.4.2.1 Definition

Constituting less than 1% of all soft tissue sarcomas, alveolar soft tissue sarcoma is one of the least common malignant soft tissue tumors [17]. The term refers to the pseudoalveolar pattern formed by aggregates of large granular cells surrounded by vascular channels mimicking the alveolar pattern of the respiratory alveoli. These tumors are highly hypervascular and frequently surrounded by thick, tortuous blood vessels. This is responsible for the considerable hemorrhage which often occurs during surgical removal [3]. On section they consist of yellow-white to gray-red tissue, often with large necrotic or hemorrhagic areas [17]. Despite a relatively benign appearance – mitoses and pleomorphism are rare – alveolar soft part sarcoma is one of the most malignant soft tissue tumors. Metastatic spread develops early in the course of the disease, is common, and is observed in 40–70% of patients [8, 11, 22, 36]. Preferential sites of metastases are the lungs, followed by the brain and skeleton. Tumor recurrence is high and is noted in 20–30% of cases [36].

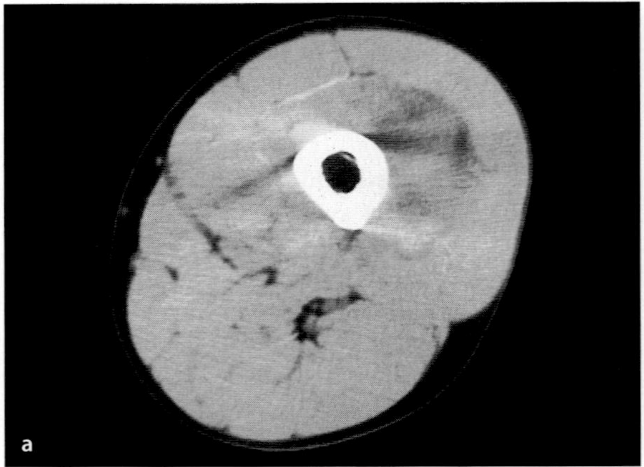
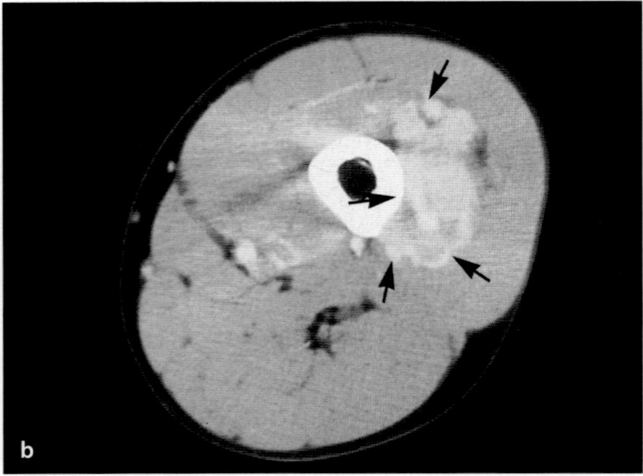

Fig. 23.19 a, b. Alveolar soft part sarcoma of the left thigh in a 26-year-old man. **a** Plain CT. **b** CT after iodinated contrast injection. Presence of a soft tissue mass at the lateral aspect of the femur with unsharp delineation from adjacent vastus intermedius and lateralis muscles. On native CT, the lesion is slightly hypodense relative to muscle. After contrast medium injection, pronounced enhancement of the lesion is seen. Thick, strongly enhancing structures are observed and correspond with enlarged vessels within the tumor (*arrows*) (**b**)

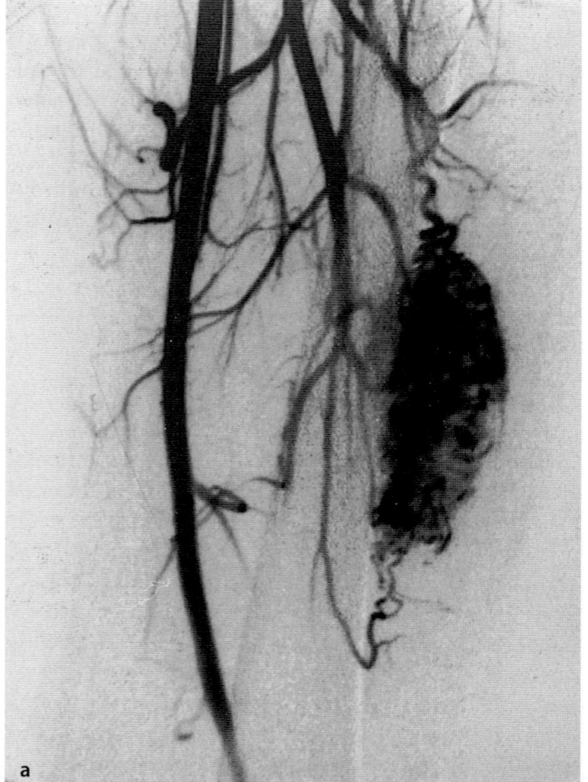
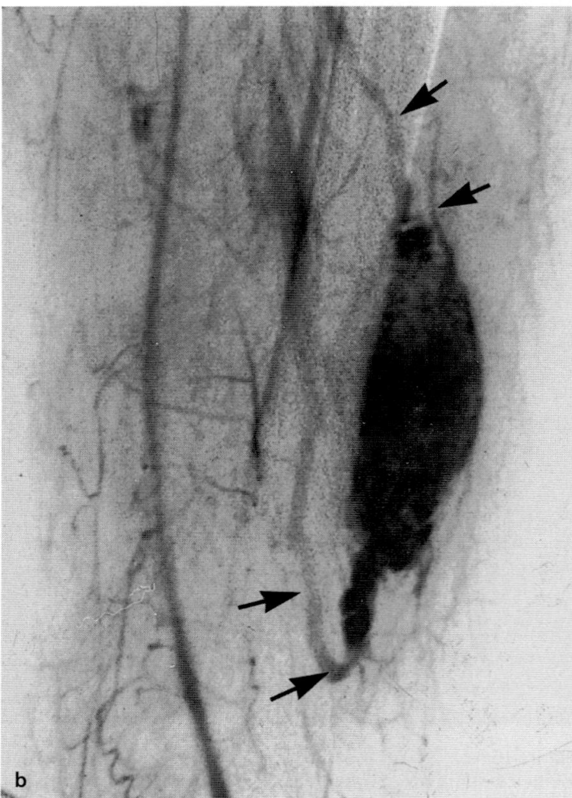

Fig. 23.20 a, b. Alveolar soft part sarcoma of the left thigh in a 26-year-old man (same patient as in Fig. 23.19). **a** Arteriography of the left femoral artery, early phase. **b** Arteriography of the left femoral artery, late parenchymatous – early venous phase. During early arteriographic phase a highly vascularized mass lateral to the femoral shaft is observed. Thick, tortuous arteries are seen all over the lesion (**a**). A few moments later, during staining with contrast medium at the lesion, early venous drainage is observed at the upper and lower pole of the lesion (*arrows*)

23.4.2.2 Incidence and Clinical Behavior

Alveolar soft part sarcoma can be seen at any age, but occurs predominantly in older children, adolescents, and young adults, between 11 and 35 years of age. A female predominance is observed in most series [8, 17]. At least 60% of these tumors occur in the muscles or fascial planes of the lower limb, with the anterior portion of the thigh being most commonly affected. In decreasing order of incidence, head and neck, upper extremity, and the trunk are the other most frequently involved areas [8, 17, 36]. In children and infants head and neck region, particularly the orbit and tongue, are the most common sites of origin. Alveolar soft part sarcoma usually presents as a slowly growing, painless mass. Occasionally pulsations may be observed on palpation. These are explained by the very rich vascularization of the tumor. At the time of diagnosis, the diameter of most tumors surpasses 5 cm.

The large majority of lesions are asymptomatic. Therefore, metastases in the lung or brain may be the first manifestation of the disease [17]. Metastatic spread is present in more than one third of the cases at the time of initial diagnosis [3, 36].

23.4.2.3 Imaging

■ **Imaging Studies Other than MRI.** On conventional radiographs, alveolar soft part sarcoma presents as a nonspecific mass which may occasionally show punctate calcifications [22, 40]. The tumor can erode the adjacent bone. Chest radiographs may reveal pulmonary metastases. Ultrasound may also disclose the tumor and shows a variable echo pattern within it. Doppler ultrasound may emphasize the marked vascularity of the lesion [11]. CT discloses the delineation of the tumor better. On nonenhanced scans, the tumor is slightly hypodense or even isodense compared with surrounding muscle. Contrast-enhanced scans show a very pronounced enhancement and may also demonstrate numerous dilated vessels within the tumor [8, 11, 22, 49] (Fig. 23.19). Angiography shows a hypervascular mass, with arteriovenous shunting and early draining veins [11,22] (Fig. 23.20).

■ **MRI Findings.** Alveolar soft part sarcomas appear bright both on T1- and T2-weighted images (Fig. 23.21). This is probably due to slowly flowing blood in some tumor vessels [11, 22, 40]. On all sequences, multiple areas of signal void are observed within the lesion, suggesting small calcifications or rapid flow within distended vessels [8, 11, 22]. On T1-weighted images most lesions appear homogeneous, whereas on T2-weighted images the pattern becomes inhomogeneous. This sign is important for indicating the malignant nature of the lesion, as it is observed in 72% of malig-

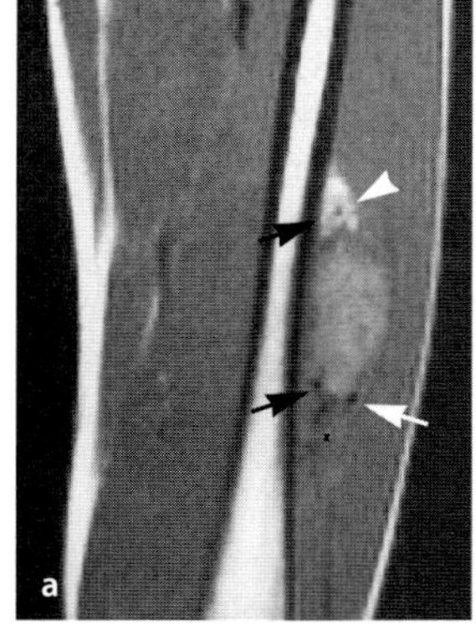
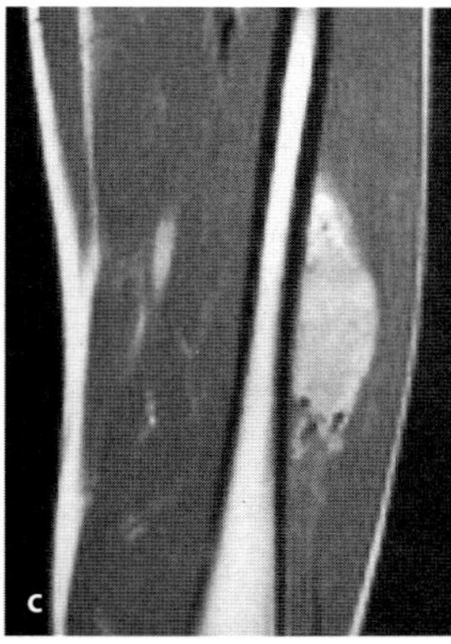
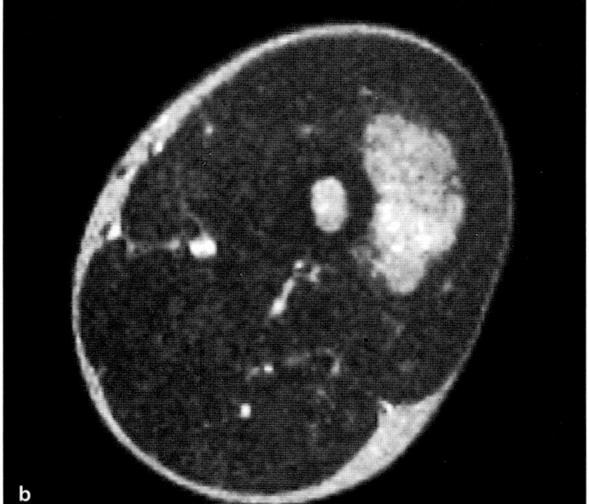

Fig. 23.21 a–c. Alveolar soft part sarcoma of the left thigh in a 26-year-old man (same patient as in Fig. 23.19). **a** Coronal spin echo T1-weighted MR image. **b** Axial spin echo T2-weighted MR image. **c** Coronal spin echo T1-weighted MR image after gadolinium contrast injection. A well-delineated, ovoid, nearly homogeneous mass lesion lateral to the femur is seen. On T1-weighted images, signal intensity is higher than that of muscle, but lower than that of fat. Triangular region with fat signal intensity at the upper pole of the lesion (*arrowhead*). Punctate to tortuous zones with signal void both at the upper and lower poles of the lesion corresponding to rapidly flowing blood within dilated blood vessels (*arrows*) (**a**). T2-weighted images disclose a mottled aspect of the lesion. Signal intensity equals that of fatty tissue. After contrast medium injection, intense enhancement is seen within the lesion. Notice the sharp peripheral demarcation of the lesion and the intact aspect of underlying bones

nant lesions and only in 12.5% of benign lesions [23]. Following administration of gadolinium chelates intense, but inhomogeneous, enhancement is noted [4, 8].

■ **Imaging Strategy.** Plain radiographs are of little value in the diagnosis of alveolar soft part sarcoma as they reveal only nonspecific findings. Conventional chest radiographs are indicated for the detection of pulmonary metastases, although for this purpose, CT of the thorax is more sensitive and should be recommended during initial staging and in surveillance following therapy. Contrast-enhanced CT allows better delineation of the tumor by showing muscle infiltration. Doppler ultrasound, CT, MRI, and angiography all emphasize the hypervascular nature of this tumor. The presence of low intensity septations on T2-weighted images only and the change from an homogeneous pattern on T1-weighted images to inhomogeneous on T2-weighted images are useful criteria for indicating the malignancy of the mass [23]. Together with the bright appearance of these tumors on both T1- and T2-weighted images, the radiologic findings may be helpful in characterizing these lesions [3, 11, 22, 23, 40].

23.4.3 Epithelioid Sarcoma

23.4.3.1 Definition

The term "epithelioid sarcoma" was applied by Enzinger in 1970 to refer to a distinctive neoplasm that commonly involves the soft tissues of the extremities, most frequently of the hand. This tumor presents as a solitary or irregular multinodular mass located in the dermis or deep-seated and attached to tendons or fascia. The size of the lesion is variable and ranges from several millimeters to more than 15 cm in diameter. Central degeneration and necrosis are common features. Lesions located in the dermis often ulcerate through the skin. The tumor may spread along the neurovascular bundles, may invade the vessels, and, hence, metastasize. In general, tumors located in the proximal extremity reveal a more aggressive course than those arising in the distal extremities [21]. The cause, histogenesis, and nature of this neoplasm remain unknown [17].

23.4.3.2 Incidence and Clinical Behavior

Epithelioid sarcoma represents the most common soft tissue sarcoma of the hand. Although it may occur at any age, the tumor is found most commonly in adolescents and young adults between 10 and 35 years of age. Children and older persons are only rarely affected. This tumor is twice as common in men as in women. The principal sites of involvement are the distal upper extremity, involved in 58% of cases, particularly the hands and forearms. This main site of involvement is followed by the distal and proximal extremity, at 15 and 12% respectively. Trunk, head and neck region, with the exception of the scalp, are seldom involved [21]. Lesions may be located in the subcutis or are deep-seated, usually attached to tendons, tendon sheaths, or fascial structures. Epithelioid sarcoma presents as a firm, hard nodule that may be solitary or multiple. These nodules are slowly growing and painless. Ulceration through the skin is common in intradermal lesions. Metastases, pre-dominantly to the regional lymph nodes and lung, are observed in less than half of the cases. These develop mostly within the first year after diagnosis, but may be late and become apparent many years after excision of the primary tumor. Recurrences, often multiple, are common and have been reported in 77% of cases [17].

23.4.3.3 Imaging

■ **Imaging Studies Other than MRI.** Radiographs, CT, and ultrasound usually reveal a soft tissue mass. In 20–30% of cases, ossification or a speckled pattern of calcification is observed within the nodule. In rare cases the tumor causes cortical thinning or erosion of underlying bone [17, 21].

■ **MRI Findings.** No characteristic MRI features of epithelioid sarcoma exist [21]. Hence, MRI does not enable a specific diagnosis of this tumor. On T1-weighted images the tumor appears mostly homogeneous, and is isointense with muscle (Fig. 23.22). Occasionally lesions may be heterogeneous, with either areas of increased signal, due to foci of hemorrhagic necrosis, or with relative central hypointensity, corresponding to extensive intratumoral necrosis. In contrast, on T2-weighted images, the tumor is hyperintense to muscle, hypo-, iso- or hyperintense to fatty tissue. A majority of lesions is homogeneous on these T2-weighted sequences. Peritumoral edema affecting the surrounding muscles is observed in nearly 70% of cases. It typically appears as a high signal intensity area on T2-weighted or STIR images, with variable shape: or it may present as a feathery, radial pattern of increased signal intensity, extending for a maximum of 2 cm into the adjacent muscle, or as an extensive area of abnormal signal, involving completely at least one muscle [21]. Other common findings include tumor encasement of the adjacent neurovascular bundle and enlarged regional lymph nodes. The latter often show the same increased signal intensity on T2-weighted images as the primary tumor. Inhomogeneous but strong enhancement is observed following administration of gadolinium chelates, except at the areas of central necrosis [21].

■ **Imaging Strategy.** As a result of the location of these lesions, the diagnosis is mainly based on the clinical aspect, findings on palpation, and results of biopsy. In spite of the variable appearance of the lesion, suspicion for epithelioid sarcoma should arise in all patients with multiple soft tissue nodules or persistent punched out-ulcers involving the skin and subcutaneous tissues, with enlarged draining lymph nodes, particularly when the mass is located in the distal portion of an extremity [21]. As for all soft tissue tumors, MRI seems to be superior to all other imaging techniques for assessing the extent of the tumor.

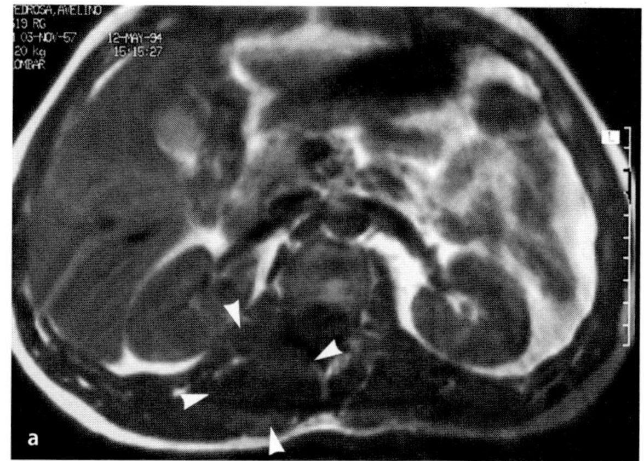

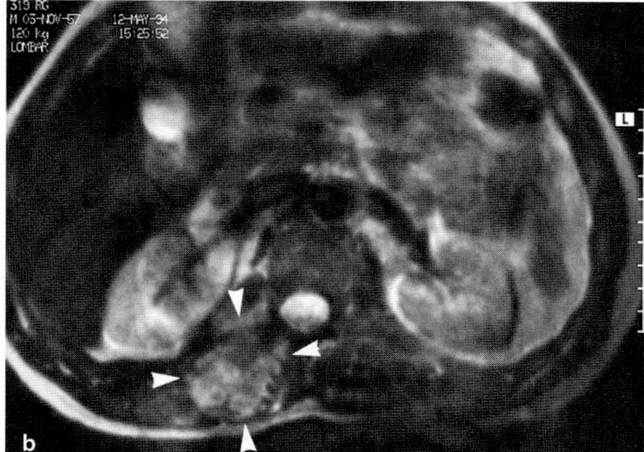

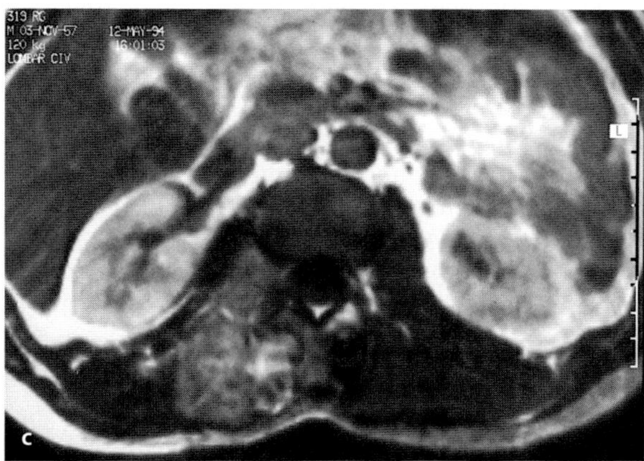

Fig. 23.22 a–c. Epithelioid sarcoma in the lumbar paraspinal region in a 37-year-old man. **a** Axial spin echo T1-weighted MR image. **b** Axial spin echo T2-weighted MR image. **c** Axial spin echo T1-weighted MR image after gadolinium contrast injection. On the T1-weighted image the tumor in the right paraspinal region appears nearly isointense with adjacent muscle and is only visible because of a moderate mass effect that causes asymmetry and distortion of the intermuscular fat planes (*arrowheads*) (**a**). On the T2-weighted image, the signal intensity of the nodular components within the irregularly outlined lesion is high but intermediate between that of muscle and subcutaneous fat (*arrowheads*) (**b**). After contrast medium injection, strong but inhomogeneous enhancement is observed within the tumor

23.4.4 Clear Cell Sarcoma

23.4.4.1 Definition

Clear cell sarcoma (malignant melanoma of the soft parts) is an extremely rare, slow-growing malignant tumor, the cells of which are capable of producing melanin. In contrast to malignant melanoma of the skin, clear cell sarcomas are more deeply located and mostly arise in the soft tissues of the limbs, in the vicinity of tendons, aponeuroses, and fascial structures. Tumor size ranges from 1 cm to more than 10 cm. Since the lesion is mostly well delineated, and lacks perilesional edema, bone invasion, satellite nodules, or intratumoral necrosis, it may be misinterpreted as a non-aggressive mass [16]. Besides its histological appearance, current diagnosis relies to a large degree on the immunohistochemical analysis, since the presence of the melanocytic marker S-100 protein and the melanoma-specific HMB-45 monoclonal antibody is considered very sensitive for the diagnosis of clear cell sarcoma [53].

23.4.4.2 Incidence and Clinical Behavior

Clear cell sarcomas are rare, accounting for only 0.8–1% of all malignancies of the musculoskeletal system [17]. Young adults between the ages of 20 and 40 years are most frequently affected. However, clear cell sarcoma has also been reported in both very young and very old persons. The tumor predominates in females. The extremities are the most commonly involved areas. Lesions located in the lower limb (foot and ankle, knee, thigh) outnumber those in the upper limb. The head and neck region and the trunk are seldom affected. The tumor presents as a slowly growing mass, which cases pain or tenderness in nearly half of the cases. The skin overlying the lesion remains uninvolved, except in bulky lesions ulcerating to the epidermis. Despite the tumor's slow growth and prolonged clinical course, the prognosis is poor as the recurrence rate is high and the development of metastases common [17].

23.4.4.3 Imaging

■ **Imaging Studies Other than MRI.** Radiographs do not contribute substantially to the diagnosis and may only show the presence of a nonspecific, non calcified soft tissue mass. Involvement of the underlying bone is uncommon, but if present an important finding [12, 51]. Angiography reveals variable vascularization of the sarcoma, and may show either hypervascular or poorly vascularized lesions [17].

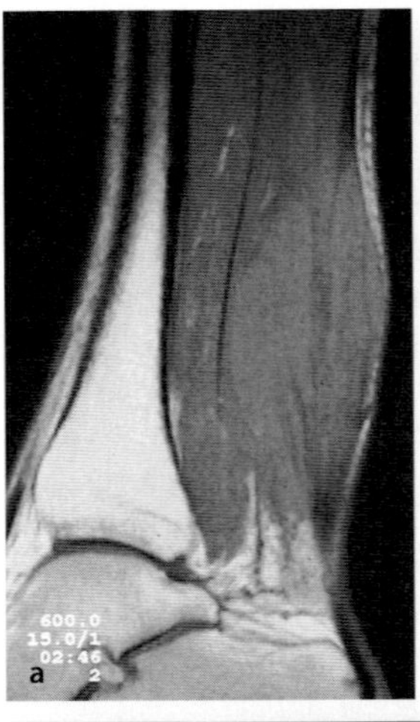
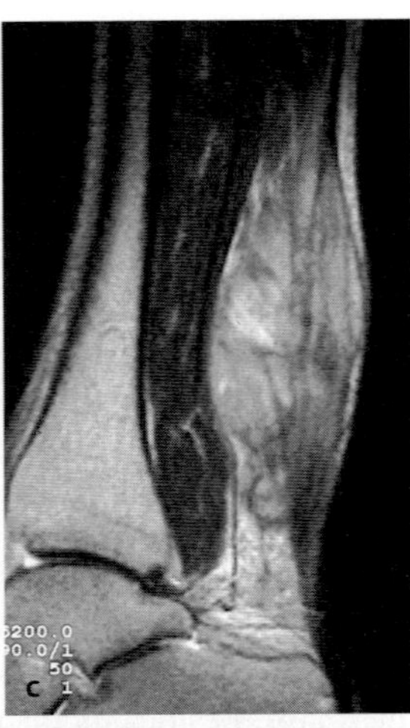
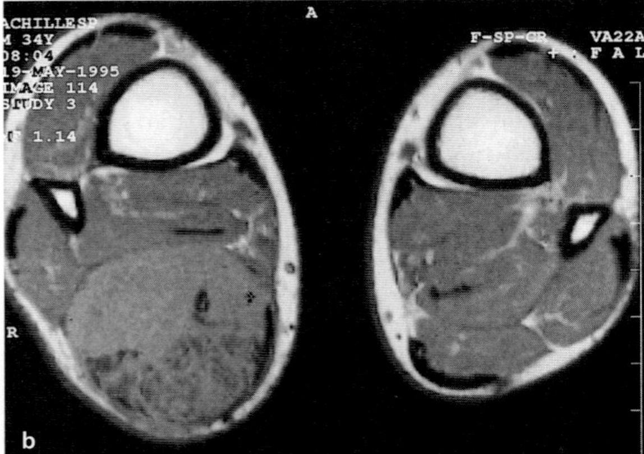
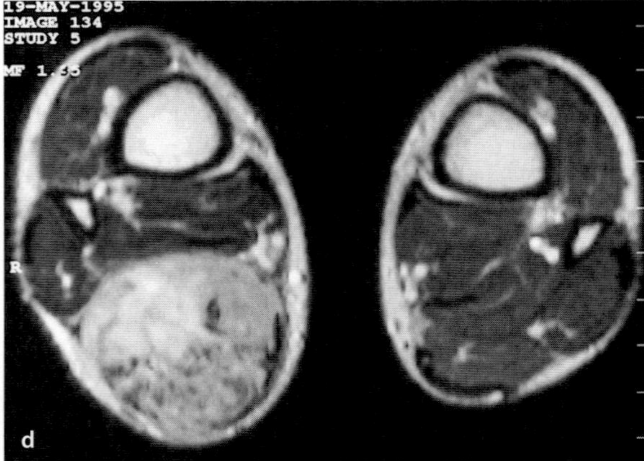

Fig. 23.23 a–d. Clear cell sarcoma of the left calf in a 34-year-old man. **a, b** Sagittal and axial spin echo T1-weighted MR images. **c, d** Sagittal and axial turbo spin echo T2-weighted images. Presence of a large, fusiform mass extending along the Achilles tendon. On the sagittal T1-weighted image the lesion appears homogeneous. On the axial view, numerous hypointense, curvilinear dashes are observed within the posterior portion of the mass. The bulk of the mass is nearly homogeneous and is slightly hyperintense to muscle on the T1-weighted images. Fat planes between tumor and adjacent muscles are partially obliterated (**a, b**). On the T2-weighted images, fine, low intensity septations are observed between the markedly hyperintense components of the lesion (**c, d**). The curvilinear dashes of signal voids, as described on T1-weighted images, persist on these T2-weighted images. In view of their posterior location they may represent dense fibrous tissue in remnants of the invaded Achilles tendon (**d**)

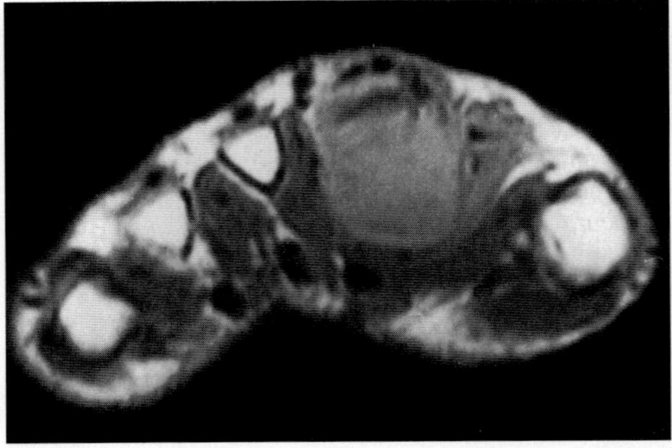

Fig. 23.24. Clear cell sarcoma of the left hand in a 41-year-old man. Axial spin echo T1-weighted MR image. Demonstration of a rounded mass in the second digit. The mass appears hyperintense and homogeneous on this image. Destruction of the metacapal bone is noted and confirms the aggressive behavior of the tumor. (Reprinted from [12])

■ **MRI Findings.** On MRI, clear cell sarcomas present as elliptical, smoothly outlined masses (Fig. 20.23). A large majority of lesions are homogeneous both on T1- and T2-weighted images. Bone destruction and intratumoral necrosis are rare, and were observed in 10 and 5% respectively in a series of 21 cases (Fig. 23.24) [12, 17]. On T1-weighted images, most clear cell sarcomas have a slightly increased signal intensity, compared with muscle (Figs. 23.23–23.25). This results from shortening of the T1 relaxation time, which is due to the paramagnetic effect of intralesional melanin. Since hyperintensity on T1-weighted images is rarely seen in soft tissue tumors, this observation is a quite characteristic sign, which allows narrowing the list of differential diagnoses [12, 17]. Nearly 85% of clear sarcomas are hyperintense to muscle on T2-weighted images (Figs. 23.23 and 23.25). At first sight, this may be surprisingly, as shortening of the T2 time- and hence hypointensity on T2-weighted images might be expected because of the paramagnetic effect of melanin. However, since signal intensity on T2-weighted images also depends on intra- and extracellular water content, it has been suggested that hyperintensity of clear cell sarcomas on T2-weighted images could be caused by a low nucleo-cytoplasmic index, by abundance of loose connective tissue between the cellular nests, or by high amount of myxoid stroma, found in these hyperintense lesions [12, 17]. Following administration of gadolinium, strong enhancement is observed in the majority of cases.

■ **Imaging Strategy.** Various imaging techniques do not provide characteristic features of clear cell sarcoma. MRI is the imaging technique of choice for demonstrating the extent of the tumor, yet it also lacks specificity. Of interest, however, is the fact that high signal intensity

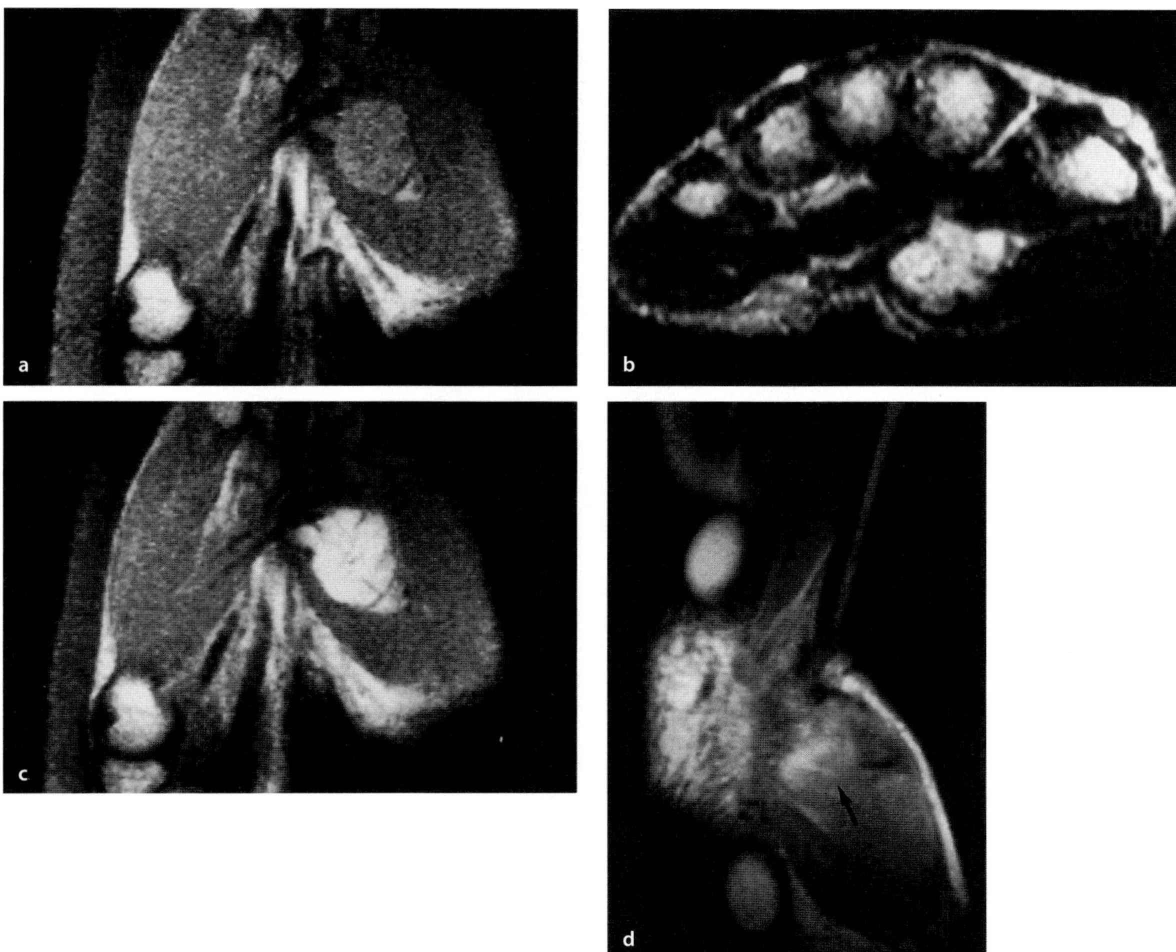

Fig. 23.25 a–d. Clear cell sarcoma of the right hand in a 25-year-old woman. **a** Coronal spin echo T1-weighted MR image. **b** Axial fast spin echo T2-weighted MR image. **c** Coronal spin echo T1-weighted MR image after gadolinium contrast injection. **d** Coronal spin echo T1-weighted MR image after gadolinium contrast injection, performed 6 weeks after initial surgery. Presence of a well circumscribed mass within the thenar muscle. The mass is slightly hyperintense relative to muscle on native T1-weighted images (**a**). On T2-weighted images signal intensity is high. There is no peritumoral edema (**b**). Following gadolinium contrast injection, strong homogeneous enhancement is seen (**c**). Since the images did not display aggressive characteristics, the surgeon decided to perform an excisional biopsy. Pathological examination, however, revealed clear cell sarcoma. Section margins were borderline. On the MR examination, performed 6 weeks after initial surgery, an indeterminate enhancing area was observed on the T1-weighted images after gadolinium contrast injection (**d**). Subsequently, the thenar muscle was widely excised. Pathological examination disclosed small nests of malignant cells. Since then a transradial-ulnar amputation has been performed. At 19 months after initial therapy no metastatic disease has been demonstrated. (Reprinted from [12])

on T1-weighted images, which most commonly reflects the presence of fat or methemoglobin within a tumor, may also be caused by the presence of melanin and may hence point to the nature of the lesion. Furthermore, it should be stressed that clear cell sarcoma often has a benign appearance on MRI studies, but nevertheless behaves as a relentless, highly malignant soft tissue sarcoma. Therefore, when a well-defined, homogeneous, strongly enhancing mass with slightly higher signal intensity than that of muscle on native T1-weighted images is encountered, the differential diagnosis should include clear cell sarcoma.

23.4.5 Malignant Mesenchymoma

23.4.5.1 Definition

The term "malignant mesenchymoma" refers to a group of malignant soft tissue tumors that are characterized by the presence of two or more different tissue components in the same neoplasm. This group is further subdivided into two subcategories. The first category is the smallest one and comprises those tumors that are characterized by coexisting rhabdomyosarcomatous and

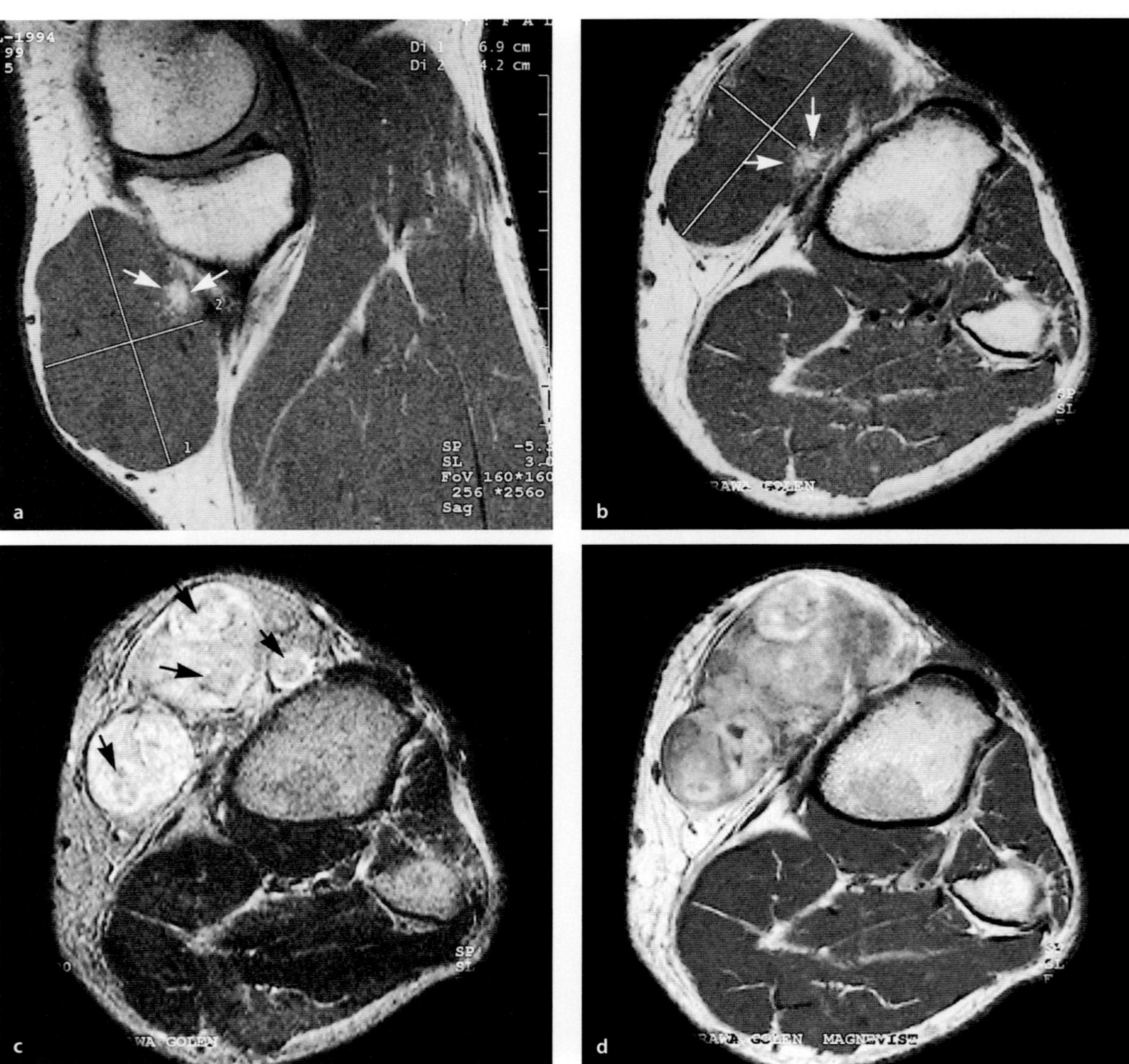

Fig. 23.26a–d. Mesenchymoma of the proximal third of the left leg in a 44-year-old woman. **a, b** Sagittal and axial spin echo T1-weighted MR images. **c** Axial spin echo T2-weighted MR image. **d** Axial spin echo T1-weighted MR image after gadolinium contrast injection. Presence of an ovoid soft tissue mass within the subcutaneous fat layer, just anterior to the tibia. The mass is sharply outlined. On the T1-weighted images, a nearly homogeneous appearance with low signal intensity in the major portions of the tumor is seen. A high signal intensity nodule is observed in the posterior aspect of the tumor, indicating the presence of fat within the tumor (*arrows*) (**a, b**). On the T2-weighted image multiple rounded to ovoid, very hyperintense nodules are shown. Irregular low intensity areas are seen within these nodules (*arrows*). Likewise, the tissue between the nodules presents with low signal intensity (**c**). The gross appearance of the tumor is much more inhomogeneous on T2- than on T1-weighted images. Likewise, the pattern of enhancement is inhomogeneous. The strongest enhancement is observed at the periphery of the nodular components of the tumor in the same areas that are very bright on T2-weighted images (**c, d**)

liposarcomatous elements in the same neoplasm. The second category is much larger and consists of neoplasms containing a specific type of sarcoma together with more or less prominent foci of malignant cartilaginous or osseous tissue [17]. The origin of these tumors remains unclear. Many authors now assume that these tumors arise from primitive mesenchymal cells that have differentiated along multiple cell lines [17].

23.4.5.2 Incidence and Clinical Behavior

As may be expected from the heterogeneity of this group of tumors, clinical presentation is widely variable. However, most of these tumors affect older persons, nearly always older than 55 years.

Occurrence in children and young adults is only rarely seen. The retroperitoneum and thigh are frequently involved. The prognosis is depending from the prevalent mesenchymal component [17].

23.4.5.3 Imaging

■ **Imaging Studies Other than MRI.** Although no reports of imaging findings have been published, the radiographic appearance of these tumors is expected to be related to the prevalent tissue component.

■ **MRI Findings.** The MRI findings in the case presented in Fig. 23.26 include a nearly homogeneous mass on T1-weighted images. On T2-weighted images, the tumor seemed to be composed of multiple hyperintense nodules with a hypointense center. Gadolinium-enhanced T1 -weighted images disclosed strong enhancement of the tumor parts that were very bright on unenhanced T2-weighted images.

Things to remember:
1. Tumoral calcinosis is characterized by multiple calcified masses along the extensor surface of the joints.
   A "sedimentation sign" may be seen on upright radiographs or CT images in the axial planes.
   High signal intensity areas on T2-weighted images may reflect an inflammatory component.
2. When multiple intramuscular myxomas are encountered, one should look for associated fibrous dysplasia to exclude Mazabraud's syndrome.
3. An amyloid tumor has a low signal intensity on all pulse sequences.
4. Synovial sarcoma is a misnomer, as it is not derived from true synovial cells.
   The presence of a triple signal on T2-weighted images, together with high signal intensity areas on T1-weighted images and calcifications on CT-scan or radiographs are suggestive for a synovial sarcoma.
5. A clear cell sarcoma should be considered in the differential diagnosis, when a well-defined extremity lesion with a relatively high signal intensity on T1-weighted images and strong enhancement pattern is seen in a young patient.

References

1. Abdelwahab IF, Kenan S, Hermann G, Klein MJ, Lewis MM (1993) Case report: intramuscular myxoma of the left forearm. Bull Hosp Joint Dis 53:15–17
2. Armstrong SJ, Wakeley CJ, Goddard PR, Watt I (1992) Review of the use of MRI in soft tissue lesions. Clin Radiol 46:311–317
3. Asvall J, Hoeg K, Kleppe K, Prydz PE (1969) Alveolar soft part sarcoma. Clin Radiol 20:426–432
4. Benedikt RA, Jelinek JS, Kransdorf MJ, Moser RP, Berrey BH (1994) MR Imaging of soft-tissue masses: role of Gadopentetate dimeglumine. J Magn Reson Imaging 4:485–490
5. Blacksin MF, Siegel JR, Benevenia J, Aisner SC (1997) Synovial sarcoma: frequency of nonaggressive MR characteristics. J Comput Assist Tomogr 21:785–789
6. Burk DL, Dalinka MK, Karal E et al. (1988) Meniscal and ganglion cysts of the knee: MR evaluation. Am J Roentgenol 150:331–336
7. Carrillo R, el-Naggar AK, Rodriguez-Peralto JL, Batsakis JG (1992) Synovial sarcoma of the tongue: case report and review of the literature. J Oral Maxillofac Surg 50:904–906
8. Castillo M, Lee YY, Yamasaki S (1992) Infratemporal alveolar soft part sarcoma: CT, MRI and angiographic findings. Neuroradiology 34:367–369
9. Cohen MA, Mendelsohn DB (1990) CT and MR imaging of myxofibroma of the jaws. J Comput Assist Tomogr 14:281–285
10. Dabska M (1977) Parachordoma: a new clinico-pathologic entity. Cancer 40:1586
11. Daly BD, Cheung H, Gaines PA, Bradley MJ, Metreweli C (1992) Imaging of alveolar soft part sarcoma. Clin Radiol 46:253–256
12. De Beuckeleer LH, De Schepper AM, Vandevenne JE et al. (2000) MR imaging of clear cell sarcoma (malignant melanoma of the soft parts): a multicenter correlative MRI-pathology study of 21 cases and literature review. Skeletal Radiol 29:187–195
13. Diard F, Hauger O, Kind M, Moinard M, Bonnefoy O (2004) Les synovialosarcomes. In: Laredo JD, Tomeni B, Malghem J et al. (eds) Conduite à tenir devant une image osseuse ou des parties molles d'allure tumorale. Sauramps Médical, Montpellier, pp 429–442
14. Ekelund L, Herrlin K, Rydholm A (1981) Intramuscular myxoma. Skeletal Radiol 7:15–19
15. Enzinger FM, Weiss SW (1995) Synovial sarcoma. In: Enzinger FM, Weiss SW (eds) Soft tissue tumors, 3rd edn. St Louis, Mosby, pp 735–786
16. Enzinger FM, Weiss SW (1995) Benign soft tissue tumors of uncertain type. In: Enzinger FM, Weiss SW (eds) Soft tissue tumors, 3rd edn. Mosby, St Louis, pp 1039–1066
17. Enzinger FM, Weiss SW (1995) Malignant soft tissue tumors of uncertain type. In: Enzinger FM, Weiss SW (eds) Soft tissue tumors, 3rd edn. Mosby, St Louis, pp 1067–1093
18. Fueredi GA, Knechtges TE, Czarnecki DJ (1989) Coronary angiography in atrial myxoma: findings in nine cases. Am J Roentgenol 152:737–738
19. Glass-Royal MC, Nelson MC, Albert F, Lack EE, Bogumill GP (1989) Case report 557. Skeletal Radiol 18:392–398
20. Greenberg SB (1990) Tumoral calcinosis in an infant. Pediatr Radiol 20:206–207
21. Hanna SL, Kaste S, Jenkins JJ, Hewan-Lowe K, Spence JV, Gupta M, Monson D, Fletcher BD (2002) Epitheloid sarcoma: clinical, MR imaging and pathologic findings. Skeletal Radiol 31:400–412
22. Hermann G, Abdelwahab IF, Klein MJ, Kenan S, Lewis MM (1993) Case report 796. Skeletal Radiol 22:386–389
23. Hermann G, Abdelwahab IF, Miller TT, Klein MJ, Lewis MM (1992) Tumour and tumour-like conditions of the soft tissue: magnetic resonance imaging features differentiating benign from malignant masses. Br J Radiol 65:14–20
24. Hodler J, Yu JS, Steinert HC, Resnick D (1995) MR Imaging versus alternative imaging techniques. Magn Reson Imaging Clin N Am 3:591–608
25. Iwasko N, Steinbach LS, Disler D, Pathria M, Hottya GA, Kattapuram S, Varma DGK, Kumar R (2002) Imaging findings in Mazabraud's syndrome: seven new cases. Skeletal Radiol 31:81–87
26. Jones BC, Sundaram M, Kransdorf MJ (1993) Synovial sarcoma: MR imaging findings in 34 patients. Am J Roentgenol 161:827–830
27. Jungreis CA, Sekhar LN, Martinez AJ, Hirsch BE (1989) Cardiac myxoma metastatic to the temporal lobe. Radiology 170:244
28. Kaplan PA, Williams SM (1987) Mucocutaneous and peripheral soft-tissue hemangiomas: MR imaging. Radiology 163:163–166
29. Kolawole TM, Bohrer SP (1974) Tumoral calcinosis with "fluid levels" in the tumoral masses. Am J Roentgenol 120:461–464

30. Kransdorf MJ (1995) Malignant soft-tissue tumors in a large referral population: distribution of diagnosis by age, sex and location. Am J Roentgenol 164:129–134
31. Kransdorf MJ, Jelinek JS, Moser RP, Utz JA, Brower AC, Hudson TM, Berrey BH (1989) Soft-tissue masses: diagnosis using MR imaging. Am J Roentgenol 153:541–547
32. Kransdorf MJ, Jelinek JS, Moser RP (1993) Imaging of soft tissue tumors. Radiol Clin North Am 31:359–372
33. Kransdorf MJ, Moser RP, Jelinek JS, Weiss SW, Buetow PC, Berrey BH (1989) Intramuscular myxoma: MR features. J Comput Assist Tomogr 13:836–839
34. Kransdorf MJ, Moser RP, Meis JM, Meyer CA (1991) From the archives of the AFIP. Fat-containing soft-tissue masses of the extremities. Radiographics 11:81–106
35. Kransdorf MJ, Murphey MD (1999) Case 12: Mazabraud syndrome. Radiology 212:129–132
36. Liebermann PH, Brennan MF, Kimmel M, Erlandson RA, Garin-Chesa P, Flehinger BY (1989) Alveolar soft part sarcoma. A clinico-pathologic study of half a century. Cancer 63:1–13
37. Lois JF, Fischer HJ, Mirra JM, Gomes AS (1986) Angiography of histopathologic variants of synovial sarcoma. Acta Radiol Diagn 27:449–454
38. Lopez-Ben R, Pitt M, Jaffe KA, Siegal GP (1999) Osteosarcoma in a patient with McCune-Albright syndrome and Mazabraud's syndrome. Skeletal Radiol 28:522–526
39. Llauger J, Pérez C, Coscojuela P, Palmer J, Puig J (1990) Aggressive angiomyxoma of pelvic soft tissue: CT appearance. Urol Radiol 12:25–26
40. Lorigan JG, O'Keefe FN, Evans HL, Wallace S (1989) The radiologic manifestations of alveolar soft part sarcoma. Am J Roentgenol 153:335–339
41. Lyles KW, Burkes EJ, Ellis GJ et al. (1985) Genetic transmission of tumoral calcinosis: autosomal dominant with variable clinical expressivity. J Clin Endocrinol Metab 60:1093–1096
42. Martinez S, Vogler JB, Harrelson JM, Lyles KW (1990) Imaging of tumoral calcinosis: new observations. Radiology 174:215–222
43. McCook TA, Martinez S, Korobkin M et al. (1981) Intramuscular myxoma. Skeletal Radiol 7:15–19
44. Morton MJ, Berquist TH, McLeod RA, Unni KK, Sim FH (1991) MR imaging of synovial sarcoma. Am J Roentgenol 156:337–340
45. Murphey MD, Kransdorf MJ, Smith SE (1999) Imaging of soft tissue neoplasms in the adult: malignant tumors. Semin Musculoskeletal Radiol 1:39–58
46. O'Keeffe LJ, Ramsden RT, Birzgalis AR (1993) Primary synovial sarcoma of the middle ear. J Laryngol Otol 107:1070–1072
47. Petasznik R (1999) Ultrasound in acute and chronic knee injury. Radiol Clin North Am 37:797–830
48. Peterson KK, Renfrew DL, Feddersen RM, Buckwalter JA, El-Khoury GY (1991) Magnetic resonance imaging of myxoid containing tumors. Skeletal Radiol 20:245–250
49. Radin DR, Ralls PW, Boswell WD, Lundell C, Halls JM (1984) Alveolar soft part sarcoma: CT findings. J Comput Assist Tomogr 8:344–345
50. Rangheard AS, Vanel D, Viala J, Schwaab G, Casiraghi O, Sigal R (2001) Synovial sarcomas of the head and neck: CT and MR imaging findings of eight patients. Am J Neuroradiol 22:851–857
51. Raynor AC, Vargas-Crotes F, Alexander RW et al. (1979) Clear cell sarcoma with melanin-pigment: a possible soft-tissue variant of malignant melanoma. Case report. J Bone Joint Surg Am 61A:276
52. Sanchez Reyes JM, Alcaraz Mexia M, Quinones Tapia D, Aramburu JA (1997) Extensively calcified synovial sarcoma. Skeletal Radiol 26:671–673
53. Schnarkowski P, Peterfy CG, Johnston JO, Weidner N (1996) Clear cell sarcoma mimicking peripheral nerve sheath tumor. Skeletal Radiol 25:197–200
54. Seeger LL, Butler DL, Eckardt JJ, Layfield L, Adams JS (1990) Tumoral calcinosis-like lesion of the proximal linea aspera. Skeletal Radiol 19:579–583
55. Shaw GR, Lais CJ (1993) Fatal intravascular synovial sarcoma in a 31-year-old woman. Hum Pathol 24:809–810
56. Spielmann A, Janzen DL, O'Connell JX, Munk PL (1997) Intraneural synovial sarcoma. Skeletal Radiol 26:677–681
57. Sundaram M, McDonald D, Merenda G (1989) Intramuscular myxoma: a rare but important association with fibrous dysplasia of bone. Am J Roentgenol 153:107–108
58. Tagliabue JR, Stull MA, Lack EE, Lloyd RJ, Nelson MC (1990) Case report 610. Skeletal Radiol 19:448–452
59. Tateishi U, Hasegawa T, Beppu Y, Satake M, Moriyama N (2004) Synovial sarcoma of the soft tissues. Prognostic significance of imaging features. J Comput Assist Tomogr 28:140–148
60. van Rijswijk CS, Hogendooren PC, Taminiau AH, Bloem JL (2001) Synovial sarcoma: dynamic contrast-enhanced MR imaging features. Skeletal Radiol 30:25–30
61. Wang SC, Chhem RK, Cardinal E, Cho KH (1999) Joint sonography. Radiol Clin North Am 37:653–668
62. Wirth WA, Leavitt D, Enzinger FM (1971) Multiple intramuscular myxomas: another extraskeletal manifestation of fibrous dysplasia. Cancer 27:1167–1173
63. Yaghoobian J, Zinn D, Ramanathan K, Pinck RL, Hilfer K (1987) Ultrasound and computed tomographic findings in aggressive angiomyxoma of the uterine cervix. J Ultrasound Med 6:209–212

Pseudotumoral Lesions

R. Salgado, J. Alexiou, J.-L. Engelholm

24

Contents

24.1 Introduction

Tumor-like soft tissue lesions are a common clinical problem. Their etiology is very broad ranging from pure anatomic variants over post-traumatic events, to metabolic conditions and many other origins. A common feature of many of these lesions is the fact that they are mostly reactive in nature. Several of these conditions are self-limiting, or do not require significant intervention.

Although it is possible to estimate the incidence of true soft tissue tumors, it is more difficult to estimate the incidence of pseudotumors, and this for several reasons. First, many patients often do not seek medical advice for benign lesions (e.g. hematoma) or for normal anatomic variants (e.g. accessory soleus muscle). Moreover, many radiologists are not familiar with the spectrum of non-tumoral masses, as such adding to the confusion between these pseudotumoral processes and a 'true' tumoral process. As a consequence, in a significant number of instances these pseudotumoral masses require a biopsy for a definite diagnosis.

In this chapter, we will discuss infectious and inflammatory pseudotumoral lesions, hemorrhage (hematomas) and gout, as well as normal variants and vascular lesions which may simulate tumoral disease. Other pseudotumoral pathology such as nodular fasciitis and elastofibroma, ganglion and synovial cysts, pigmented villonodular synovitis and arteriovenous malformations will be discussed in specific chapters.

24.2 Clinical Behavior and Imaging

24.2.1 Normal Anatomy Variations and Muscular Anomalies

On occasion, a variation on normal anatomy can simulate a soft tissue tumor, causing unnecessary surgery [114]. Muscular anomalies or variants reported in the upper limbs include accessory palmaris longus muscle (Fig. 24.1), duplication of the hypothenar muscle, anomalous extensor indicis and extensor digitorum brevis muscles, and Langer's axillary arch [114].

In the lower extremities, anatomic variants occur almost exclusively in the soleus muscle [31]. Though present from birth, an accessory soleus muscle usually manifests in the late adolescent age because of muscle hypertrophy secondary to increased physical activity, especially in athletes [92]. It arises either from the anterior surface of the soleus muscle or from the soleal line of the tibia and fibula, and appears as a soft tissue mass between the medial malleolus and the Achilles tendon [31, 92]. Up to 25% of patients may present with an asymptomatic soft-tissue swelling medial to the calcaneum [92] (Fig. 24.2). Symptoms, when present, have been attributed to closed compartment ischemia and are accentuated by exercise [31].

Herniation of muscle through fascial planes can also mimic a tumor. It can be found in athletes, soldiers or other professions requiring great strains on the legs. Most of the herniations have a constitutional origin, where muscle strain or –hypertrophy leads to rupture of fascia on specific constitutional weaker locations [81]. The anterior tibial compartment is a common location for muscle herniations, where the herniation is palpable as a soft tissue mass [53]. Herniation of the m. extensor digitorum longus, m. peroneus longus and brevis, and m. gastrocnemius is also possible [81]. This can be asymptomatic, but also more prominent after exercise [81]. Herniations can be multiple and bilateral [11] (Fig. 24.3).

The diagnosis of a muscular anomaly is mainly based on knowledge of the most common locations, and the aspect of the lesion on ultrasound and MR imaging. Both anatomy variations and muscle herniations can be depicted with ultrasound, where the suspicious mass is identified as having the same echographic characteristics as normal muscular tissue. The ability of dynamic evaluation further increases the diagnostic accuracy. As expected, the signal characteristics on MR imaging of these lesions are identical to skeletal muscle on all pulse sequences, as long as there is no adjacent edema or contusion. When in doubt, a dynamic MR examination with forced dorsiflexion and plantar flexion of the ankle allows a better evaluation of the changes in shape and size of a muscle herniation [11, 81]. MR imaging of the fascial defect is possible but difficult.

Other anomalies such as an accessory breast or nipple may mimic a soft tissue tumor (Fig. 24.4). It is usually present along the primitive milk line above or below the normal breast location, and is the most frequently encountered congenital anomaly of the breast [71]. Other more rare locations include the axilla, scapula, thigh and labia majora [70], since the primitive milk line ex-

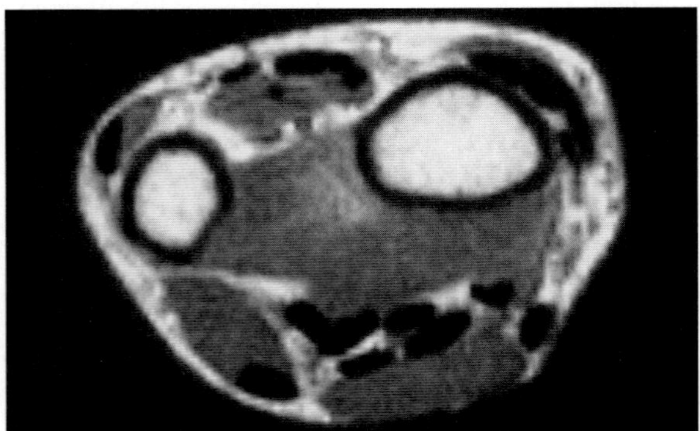

Fig. 24.1. Accessory palmaris longus muscle in a 15-year-old boy. Axial T1-weighted MR image after gadolinium contrast injection. The MR image reveals an additional mass, located superficially of the flexor digitorum tendons, with similar MR characteristics as normal skeletal muscle

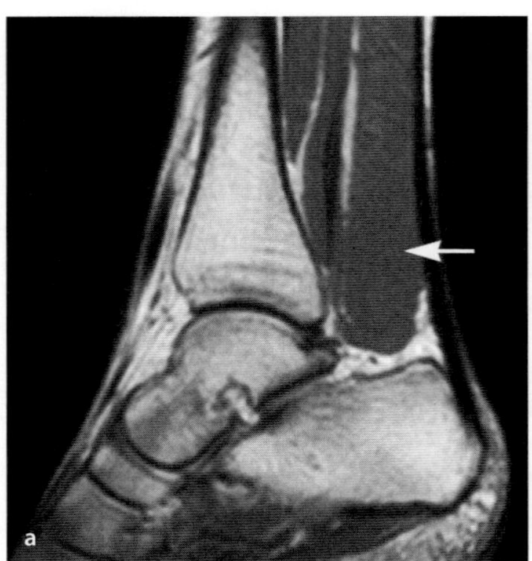
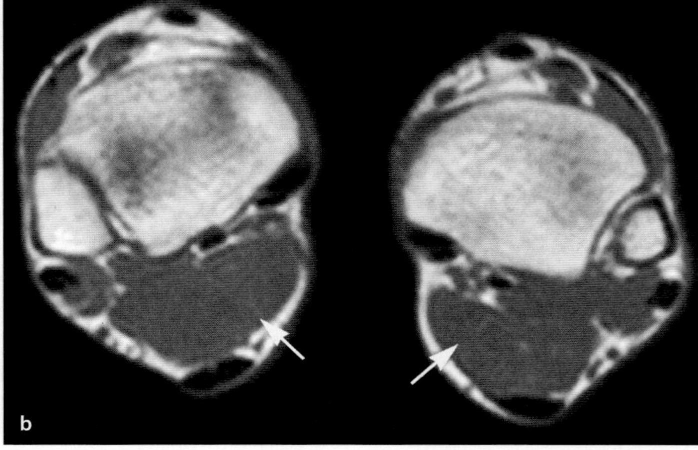

Fig. 24.2 a, b. Accessory soleus muscle in an adult man: **a** sagittal spin echo T1-weighted MR image; **b** axial spin echo T1-weighted MR image. There is a muscle belly within Kagher's fat triangle, anterior to the Achilles tendon (*arrows*). Signal intensity and bilateral presentation of abnormality are in favor of accessory soleus muscle

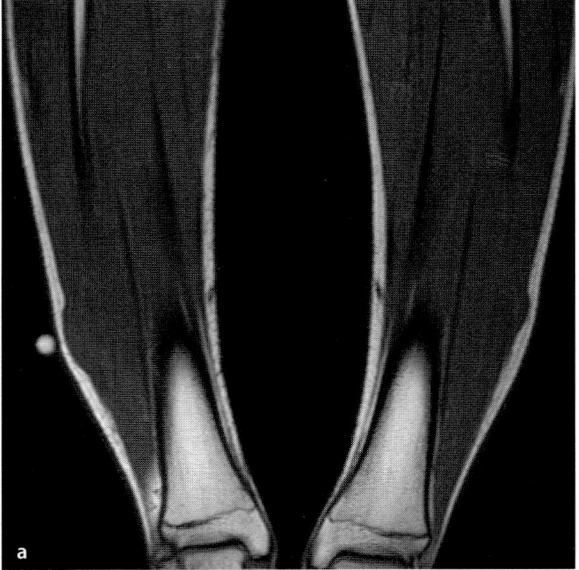

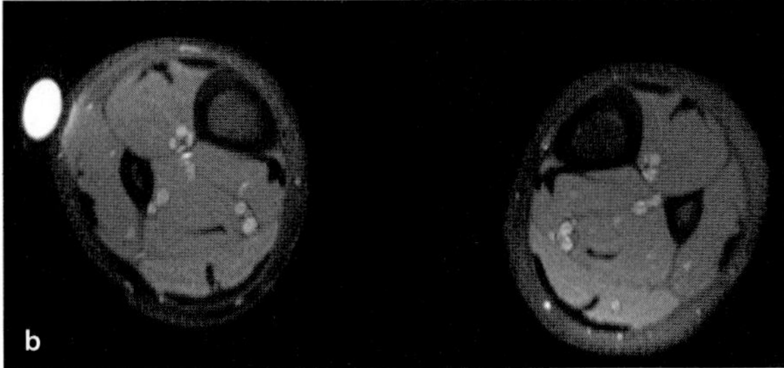

Fig. 24.3 a, b. Long standing bilateral muscle herniation in a 15-year-old male: **a** coronal spin echo T1-weighted MR image; **b** axial turbo spin echo T2-weighted MR image with fat suppression. A focal bulging of the peroneus muscle compartment is seen, more pronounced on the right side. As expected, this protruding mass has the same signal characteristics of normal muscle tissue

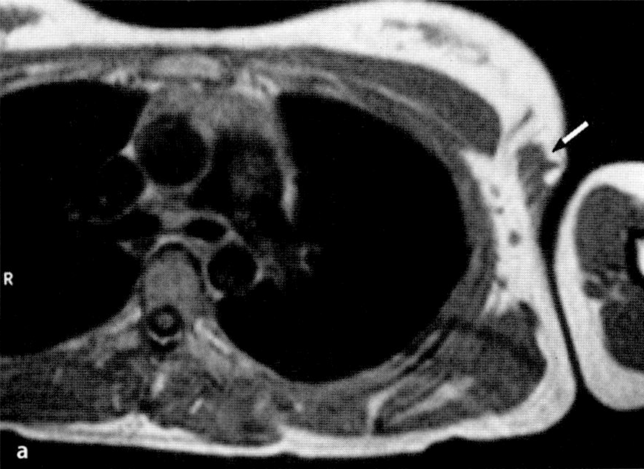

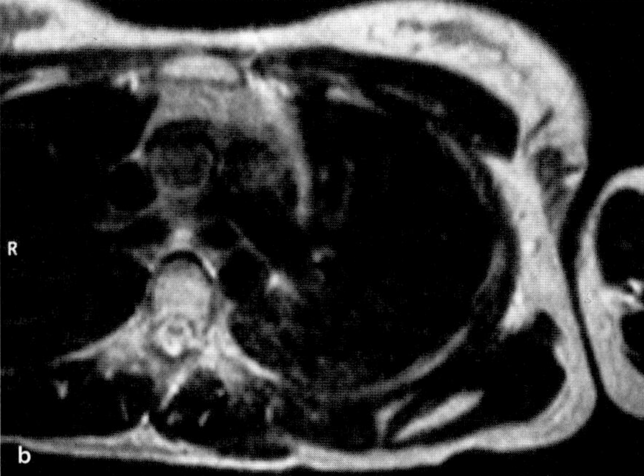

Fig. 24.4 a, b. Accessory breast in a 17-year-old girl: **a** axial spin echo T1-weighted MR image; **b** axial turbo spin echo T2-weighted MR image. Presence of a small soft tissue mass ventrolateral to the left pectoralis muscle on both spin echo sequences, with signal intensities comparable to the signal intensity of normal adjacent breast (*arrows*)

tends from the axilla to the groin. Accessory breasts are subject to the same physiological and pathological changes as proper breast tissue. This means that although they are often dismissed as cosmetic curiosities, they have nevertheless potential for pathologic degeneration [40] and may be associated with significant congenital abnormalities [71].

24.2.2 Inflammatory and Infectious Lesions

24.2.2.1 Cellulitis

Acute infectious cellulitis is an infection of the subcutaneous fat not extending beyond the superficial fascial planes (Figs. 24.5 and 24.6). It is usually associated with a hemolytic group A Streptococcus infection. Cellulitis will only on rare occasions present as a soft tissue mass [112]. An association with abscesses, ascending lym-phangitis, regional lymphadenitis, osteomyelitis and pyoarthrosis is possible [49]. Lymphedema may mimic infectious cellulitis; but the latter is more localized than lymphedema, which tends to affect the entire extremity.

CT shows diffuse infiltration of the subcutaneous fat and thickening of the skin. On MRI, cellulitis appears as an ill-defined area, hypointense on T1-weighted sequences and hyperintense on T2-weighted sequences [100]. Cellulitis may be diagnosed when T2-weighted images reveal subcutaneous thickening with fluid collections, and when subcutaneous tissue, superficial fascia or both show contrast enhancement [106]. The depth of soft-tissue involvement of the infection can be best evaluated on T2-weighted images [100]. However, as the sensitivity of magnetic resonance imaging exceeds the specificity, the extent of the deep fascial involvement can be overestimated [106], leading to the wrong diagnosis of necrotizing fasciitis.

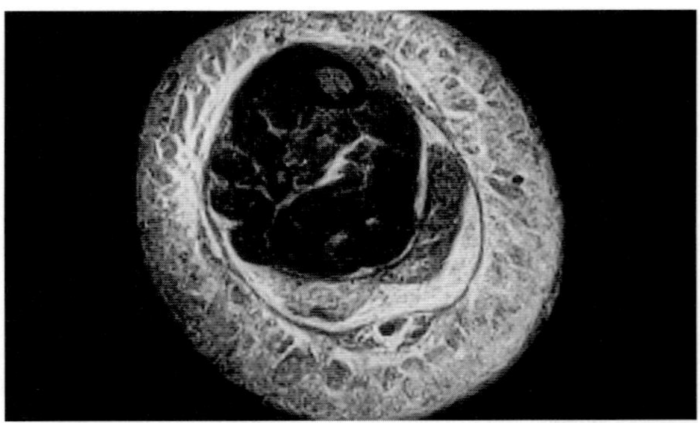

Fig. 24.5. A 24-year-old woman with an infection of the lower leg. Axial turbo spin echo T2-weighted MR image. Thickening of the skin and subcutaneous fat, with multiple septations of high signal intensity, corresponding to edema/cellulitis. The gastrocnemius muscle also has an abnormal signal intensity, and appears atrophic

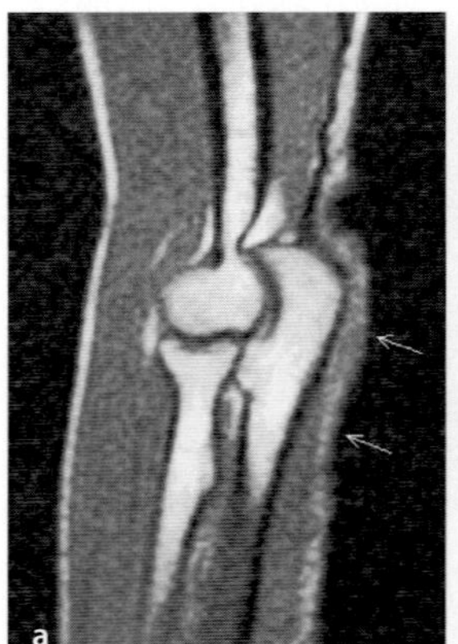
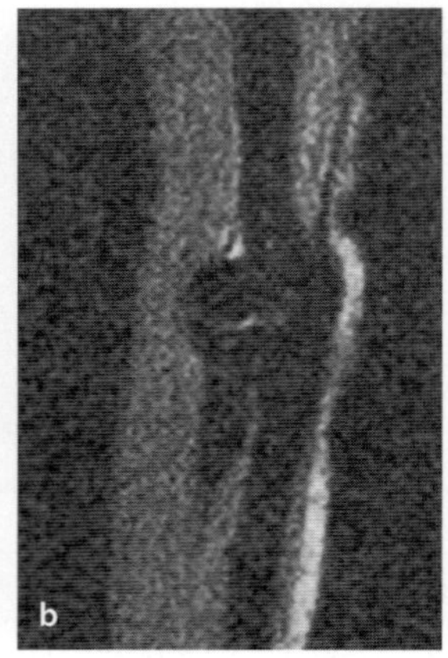

Fig. 24.6 a, b. Erysipelas of the elbow and forearm in a 21-year-old man: **a** sagittal spin echo T1-weighted MR image; **b** sagittal, fat suppressed T2-weighted MR image. Edema of the subcutaneous tissue having characteristic low signal intensity on T1-weighted images (**a**) and high signal intensity on fat suppressed T2-weighted images (**b**). Although erysipelas is a clinical diagnosis, MR imaging nicely documents the subcutaneous infiltration and excludes deeper-seated lesions

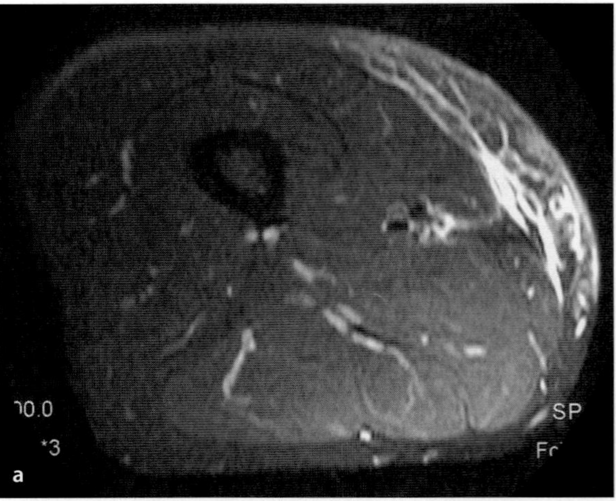
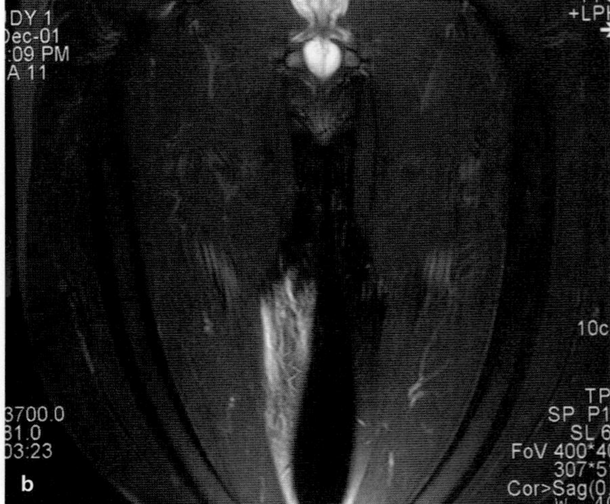

Fig. 24.7 a, b. A 36-year-old previously healthy male with a rapidly spreading reddish skin discoloration and swelling of the right upper leg: **a** axial turbo spin echo T2-weighted MR image with fat suppression; **b** coronal turbo spin echo T2-weighted MR image with fat suppression. The images reveal subcutaneous thickening and reticular infiltration, extending to a thickened superficial adductor fascia. The adductor muscles are normal. The acute presentation, the extension up to the superficial muscle fascia, and the lack of intramuscular signal changes were highly suggestive for this surgically proven necrotizing fasciitis

24.2.2.2 Necrotizing Fasciitis

Necrotizing fasciitis is a rare soft tissue infection, involving deep fascial planes. It has a predilection for older patients, especially for those with malignancy, poor nutrition, alcohol- or drug abuse. It can also be found after trauma, or around foreign bodies in surgical wounds. However, it is important to remember that it can also appear in otherwise healthy subjects with no known risk factors (Fig. 24.7). Early recognition is critical, since this entity is a surgical emergency. The clinical course can be fulminant and the mortality rate can be as high as 73% [100]. The causative organisms are mostly group A hemolytic streptococcus and *Staphylococcus aureus*, on occasion acting in synergy. Other both aerobic and anaerobic pathogens may also be involved.

Necrotizing fasciitis has similar signal behavior on MR as cellulitis, except for a deeper extension. A hyperintense signal on T2-weighted images in deep fasciae with fluid collections, thickening, and peripheral enhancement after intravenous contrast medium injection, suggest necrotizing fasciitis [106]. However, this is not typical for necrotizing soft-tissue infection, as other non-necrotizing conditions can have similar MR signal characteristics [74]. When no deep fascial involvement is revealed with MR imaging, necrotizing fasciitis can be excluded [106].

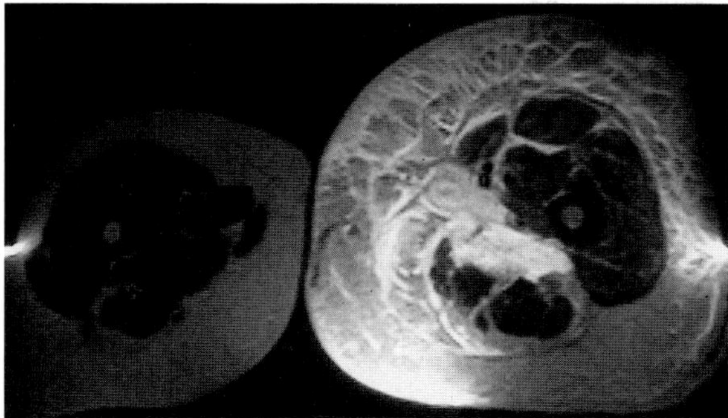

Fig. 24.8. Lymphedema of the left upper leg in a 48 year-old woman, with a history of vulval carcinoma treated with surgery, radio- and chemotherapy. Axial turbo spin echo T2-weighted MR image. There is an important thickening of the subcutaneous fat secondary to lymphedema, probably as a consequence of the intrapelvic surgery. Note the important increase in volume of the left thigh compared with the contralateral leg. An inflammation of the left adductor muscles can also be seen

24.2.2.3 Lymphedema and Lymphangitis

Lymphedema is classified as primary or secondary lymphedema. The primary form is more common in children and is associated with a variety of hereditary or genetic syndromes [125]. Secondary lymphedema has no age preference. Local causes include trauma, surgery, infection, chronic inflammation and radiotherapy (Fig. 24.8). It can also be associated with systemic disease, with a more generalized edema. Secondary lymphedema is usually a clinical diagnosis.

Imaging has a role in the evaluation of primary lymphedema, where magnetic resonance can help in the detection and differentiation of a mass without evident cause [112].

MRI of chronic lymphedema reveals deformity of lymphatics at different tissue levels [73]. In the subcutaneous tissue it shows a diffuse edema or a honeycomb pattern consistent with reticular lymphangiectasia and "lakes" with increased signal intensity on T2-weighted images [73].

Lymphography and lymphoscintigraphy can give additional information on lymphatic morphology and function [125].

24.2.2.4 Abscess

A soft tissue abscess is a well-delineated fluid collection surrounded by a well vascularized fibrous pseudocapsule. It can present as a soft tissue mass without a suggestive history or symptoms [53], and the radiologist must therefore always consider a possible infectious origin of a mass with undetermined characteristics [67]. In one-third of cases, abscesses are multiple [53] (Fig. 24.11). Associated inflammation is possible, dis-

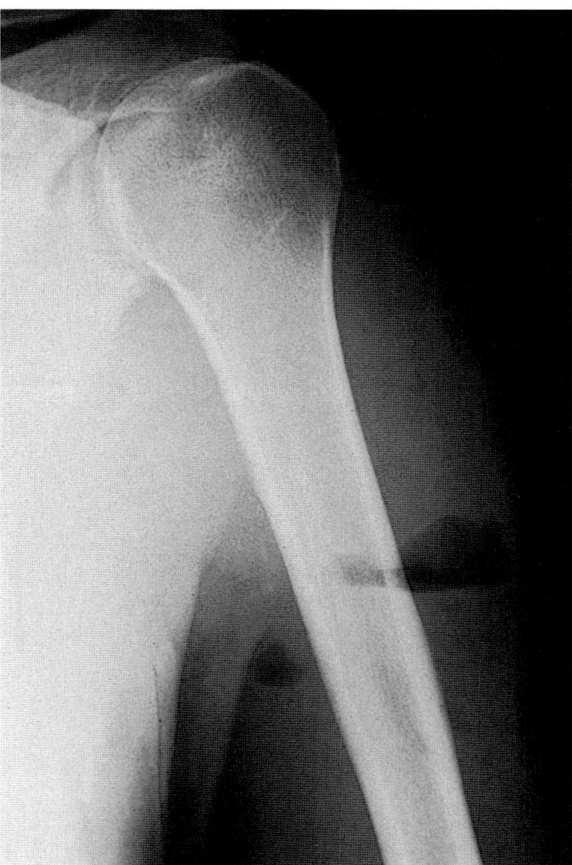

Fig. 24.9. Gas gangrene of the upper arm in a young man. Plain radiograph. Presence of a soft tissue swelling with intralesional air collection and fluid-fluid level, indicating soft tissue abscess

torting normal muscle anatomy and fascial planes [5]. Depending on the causal organism and degree of inflammation, the margins of an abscess can be well-defined or infiltrating [59].

Conventional radiography has little value, unless there is gas development within the abscess (Fig. 24.9). Ultrasound shows an elongated or lobulated fluid collection. It is also useful in guiding an aspiration biopsy or percutaneous catheter drainage. MR is superior to CT in the detection and delineation of the abscess and better demonstrates the characteristic collar-button shape of some abscesses [123]. Even ultra-low field MR is a useful method for detecting soft tissue infections [51].

On MR imaging, an abscess is hypointense to isointense relative to muscle tissue on T1-weighted images. On T2-weighted images, the central portion of the abscess is usually hyperintense, but the capsule may display an isointense or hypointense signal intensity relative to subcutaneous fat [53]. On T1-weighted images the pseudocapsule can have a variable signal intensity compared to skeletal muscle. After intravenous contrast medium injection, a peripheral rim of enhancement is

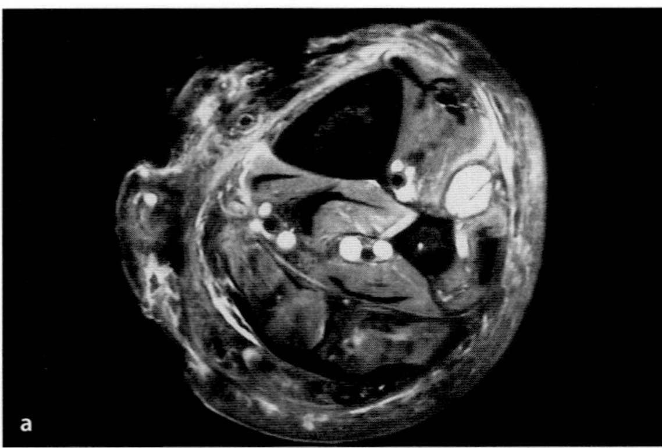

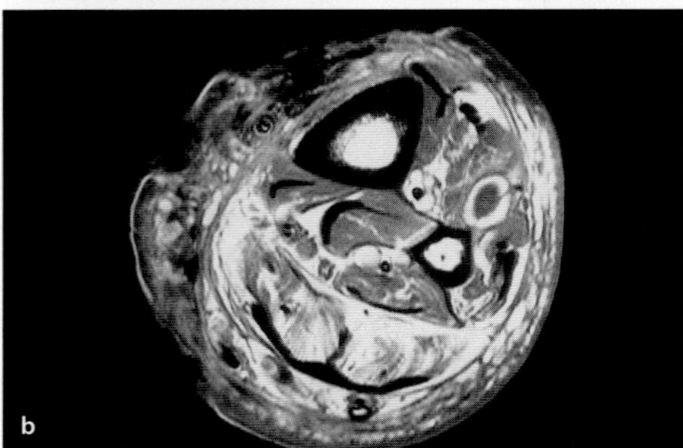

Fig. 24.10 a, b. A 65-year-old man with untreated diabetes mellitus: **a** axial proton-density weighted MR image with fat suppression; **b** axial spin echo T1-weighted MR image after gadolinium contrast administration. Besides a diffuse cellulitis and lymphedema, the images also reveal a fluid collection, located in the lower leg between the extensor digitorum and tibialis anterior muscles, with spontaneous high signal intensity on the proton-density images (**a**). After contrast administration a peripheral enhancement can be seen, corresponding to granulation tissue at the periphery of a soft tissue abscess (**b**)

seen, corresponding to the inflammatory and cellular component of the abscess [107] (Fig. 24.10).

A variable degree of peripheral edema in muscle and subcutaneous tissue can be seen, displaying a hyperintense signal intensity on T2-weighted images. Inhomogeneity on T2-weighted sequences may be a consequence of intralesional gas bubbles and/or necrotic material [123].

The described signal characteristics can be different in an immunocompromised host [53]. The peripheral edema usually seen on T2-weighted images is sometimes absent. Similarly, T1-weighted images will not always show the pseudocapsule. The infected fluid in the center of the abscess can have an inhomogeneous signal intensity [9]. If the content is sufficiently viscous, it can even show mild increased signal intensity on T1-weighted images [9]. Enhancement after intravenous contrast medium injection can also be absent [53].

In the proximity of bone, a soft tissue abscess is often associated with osteomyelitis or a periosteal reaction.

24.2.2.5 Pyomyositis

Pyomyositis, also called bacterial myositis, is a rare cause of single or multiple abscesses of skeletal muscle of unknown etiology. It was initially mainly found in tropical regions where lack of footwear, insect bites, and minor trauma, if untreated, may lead to pyomyositis. Diabetes, HIV-infection and malignancy can, as immune-compromising conditions, however, also predispose to pyomyositis [96, 98], as such contributing to an increased incidence of this disease in industrialized regions with a more temperate climate. It is considered one of the most common musculoskeletal complications of AIDS [104]. In 70–90% of cases the infection is caused by *Staphylococcus aureus* [96, 98]. Other pathogens such as *Streptococcus pyogenes, Mycobacterium tuberculosis, Mycobacterium avium-intracellulare, Nocardia asteroides, Cryptococcus neoformans,* and *Toxoplasma, Salmonella,* and *Microsporidia* species have also been reported [68, 126].

In general, normal skeletal muscle has a high intrinsic resistance to bacterial infection and abscess formation. Therefore, some authors suggest that underlying muscle damage may facilitate the onset of pyomyositis. This is supported by the presence of previous trauma to the affected muscles in 20–50% of cases [18, 24].

The clinical course can be divided into three stages. Pyomyositis initially presents as localized pain in one muscle group with induration of the overlying skin. Signs of systemic inflammation as low-grade fever and mild elevation of the white blood cell count may also be present. In a second stage there is increasing pain, fever, and edema of the affected muscle. Aspiration of the lesion at this time reveals pus. In the third stage, a clear abscess may be noted with necrosis of the muscle. Blood cultures are positive in only 5% of cases, and in 1.8% the outcome is fatal due to sepsis and shock [75, 126].

However, symptoms may be absent when the lesion is deep-seated or due to a superimposed transient bacteriemia [10].

The muscles of the thigh and gluteus region are most often affected (Figs. 24.11 and 24.12). Pyomyositis has also been described in the obturator, serratus anterior, deltoideus, triceps, biceps, iliopsoas, gastrocnemius, abdominal and paraspinal muscles [18, 56, 98]. In AIDS patients pyomyositis may be multifocal (43% of cases in the study of Fleckenstein et al. [34]). Multiplicity of lesions in AIDS patients is not specific for pyomyositis, and may be found in other pathologic conditions such as polymyositis, Kaposi sarcoma, and lymphoma [34].

On T1-weighed images the abscess collection has a low signal intensity compared with surrounding muscle tissue. On occasion, a high intensity peripheral rim is noted, probably representing blood breakdown products [75]. Pus in the abscess can have an intermediate to high signal on T1-weighed images depending on the

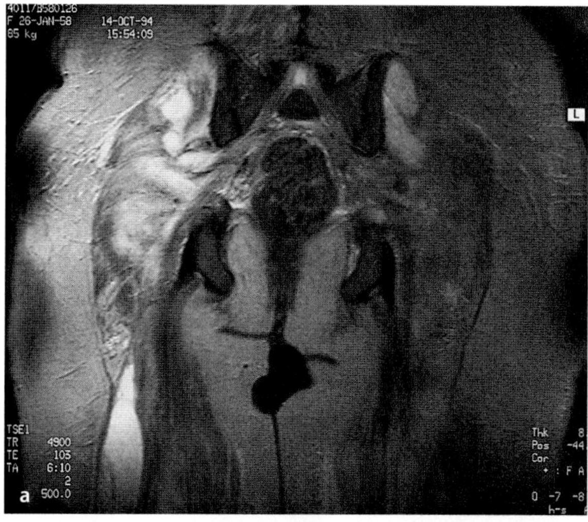

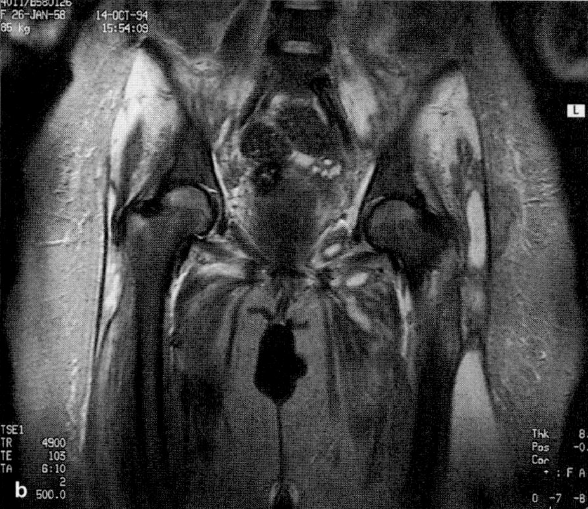

Fig. 24.11 a,b. Multiple abscesses in a 36-year-old woman: **a** coronal turbo spin echo T2-weighted MR image; **b** coronal turbo spin echo T2-weighted MR image at a more ventral level. There is a polylobulate mass in the right gluteal region and a fusiform one at the right thigh (**a**). More ventrally there are multiple oval lesions in both gluteal areas, at the left thigh and at the left pelvic floor (**b**). All lesions have the same high signal intensity on turbo spin echo T2-weighted images. Clinical and laboratory findings together with a characteristic appearance on MR imaging are indicative for pyomyositis with multiple soft tissue abscesses. Smaller abscesses (**b**) were not visible on other imaging modalities

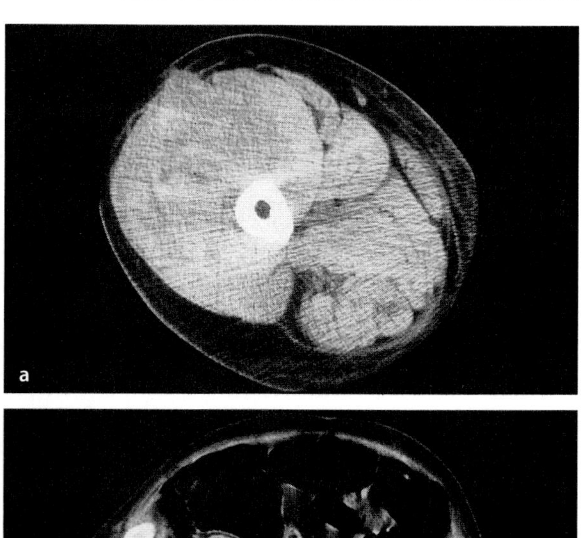

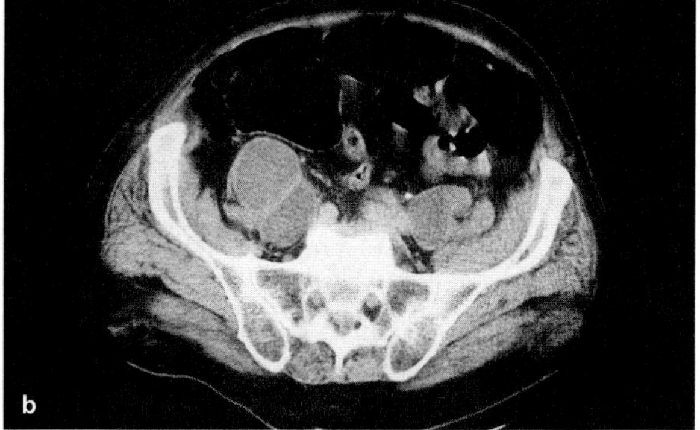

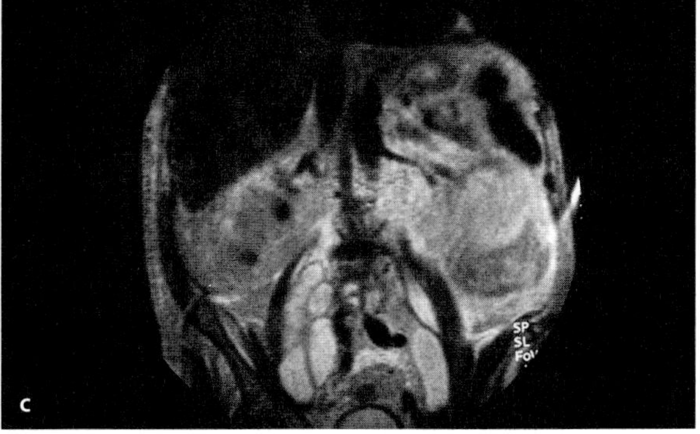

Fig. 24.12 a–c. Pyomyositis in: **a** a 48-year-old man; **b,c** a 72-year-old man, both after minor trauma during travel in tropical regions. CT scan (**a,b**), coronal T2-weighted MR image (**c**). In the first patient, CT scan shows a distinctive increase in size of the vastus medialis, intermedius and lateralis muscles of the right leg, with multiple ill-defined low-density areas (**a**). Similar findings can be seen in the second patient, with an ill-defined collection located between the L4-L5 intervertebral disc and the right psoas muscle (**b**). This is better illustrated on the coronal MR-image, which shows bilateral descending soft tissue abscesses between the spine and the psoas muscles (**c**). These two cases demonstrate the typical history, location and imaging characteristics of pyomyositis

protein content. T2-weighed images reveal a hyperintense collection in the affected muscle, with increased signal in the surrounding muscle tissue representing edema, organized phlegmonous collections or hyperemia [104, 118]. Intravenous administration of contrast material can further discriminate between viable and necrotic muscle tissue, the latter lacking enhancement.

On occasion the imaging presentation of pyomyositis can be confused with a sarcomatous lesion, especially when further clinical and biochemical information is inconclusive. Key elements in the differential diagnosis

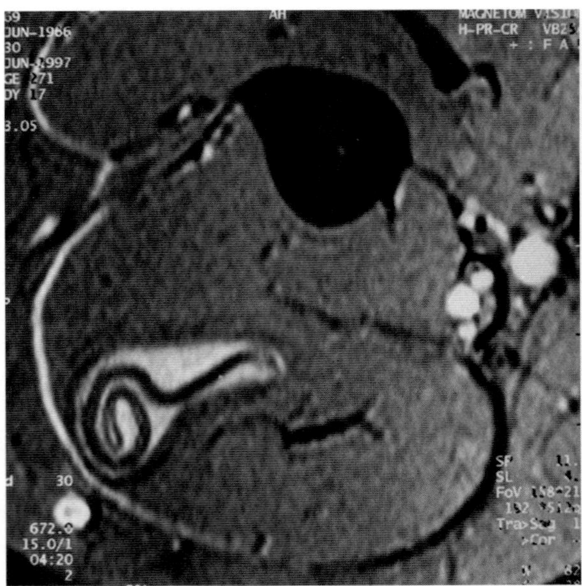

Fig. 24.13. A 31-year-old woman with a hydatid cyst in the biceps brachii muscle. Transverse fluid-attenuated inversion recovery MR image. This unusual MR image demonstrates the presence of a tapeworm in the brachialis muscle, surrounded by high signal intensity fluid and a capsule. After excision of the cyst, the tapeworm was identified as *Echinococcus granulosus*. Reproduced with permission from: Tacal et al. (2000) Coexistence of intramuscular hydatid cyst and tapeworm. Am J Roentgenol 174:575–576

favoring an infectious origin are the extend of the perilesional inflammatory reaction and the possible association of cellulitis (in the absence of previous surgery or local radiotherapy) [67].

Gallium scintigraphy is very sensitive for detection [128]. Since no anatomical detail is obtained, it must be reserved for those cases where in spite of very suggestive clinical findings CT or MRI give no additional relevant information [98]. Scintigraphy can also detect additional abscesses on a distance of the primary lesion [98].

24.2.2.6 Hydatid Cystic Disease

Hydatid cystic disease is a parasitic disease, usually caused by the *Echinoccoccus granulosus* tapeworm parasite (Fig. 24.13). Infection by *Echinococcus multilocularis* is more rare, but has a more invasive nature sometimes mimicking a malignant lesion [97]. Hydatid cystic disease is a rare finding in Western countries. It is more common in parts of South America, the Middle East, Africa, Australia and Mediterranean areas with sheep rearing, where the parasite is endemic. Ingestion of contaminated water or food and contact with dogs are known causes of infection. Liver and lungs are the organs most frequently involved, although it may affect any organ [97]. Other locations contribute for only 10–15% of the cases. Soft tissue involvement is unusual

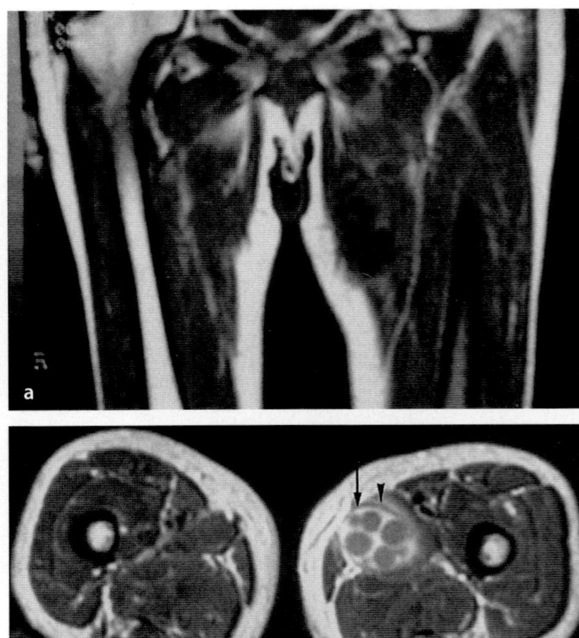

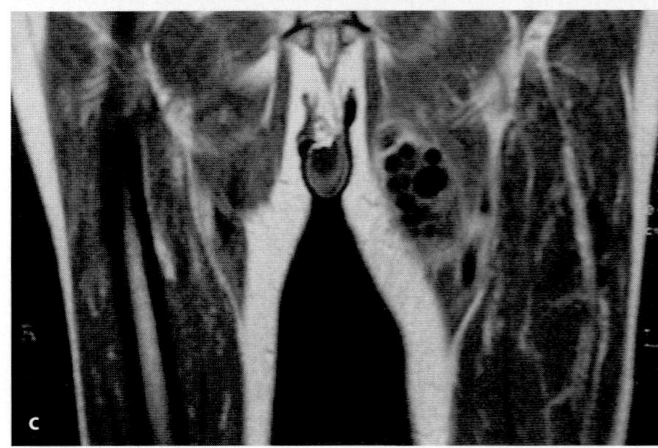

Fig. 24.14a–c. Muscular hydatid cyst on the medial aspect of the left thigh: **a** coronal T1-weighted MR image; **b** axial proton density-weighted MR image; **c** coronal T1-weighted MR image after gadolinium contrast injection. The T1-weighted image shows multiple daughter cysts within the intermediate signal mother cyst. These daughter cysts contain low-density fluid on proton-density images, compared with the high intensity of the mother cyst fluid (**b**). A low intensity rim "pericyst" (*arrow*) and peripheral high intensity soft tissue inflammatory infiltration (*arrowhead*) are observed. Because of vascularization of the pericyst, peripheral enhancement can be seen after gadolinium contrast injection (**c**). Scolices were not observed in the microscopic study. Reproduced with permission from: García-Díez AI et al. (2000) MRI evaluation of soft tissue hydatid disease. Eur Radiol 10:462–466

(1.75–2.42%), since intramuscular growth of a cyst is countered by muscle contractility and lactic acid [1, 14, 97]. Soft tissue hydatid cysts are nevertheless usually intramuscular, most frequently found in the head, neck, trunk and the root of the extremities [37]. A subcutaneous localization is also possible [20].

The imaging characteristics of soft tissue involvement resemble those of hydatid cysts found in the liver [78], showing a multiseptate or multicystic mass surrounded by a rim. Typically, the lesion consists of a mother cyst, containing multiple daughter cysts (Fig. 24.14). On T1-weighted images these daughter cysts are seen as hypointense cysts within the intermediate signal of the mother cyst. The signal intensity of the daughter cysts on T2-weighted images can be high or low, some authors suggesting a relation with the presence and absence, respectively, of viable scolices [37]. Still, the value of MRI in determining the vitality of the cysts remains controversial [37].

A rim of low [37] and/or high signal intensity [82] on T2-weighted images, surrounds the lesion. This rim is composed of three layers: an endocyst, ectocyst and pericyst. The pericyst develops as a reaction following compression and inflammation of surrounding tissue. It is well vascularised, enhancing after intravenous contrast injection [37, 82].

MR has proven superior over ultrasound in detecting this multivesicular structure [78]. More solid appearances are also possible, making it sometimes difficult to differentiate it with other soft tissue tumors [78, 115]. Even in these cases, MR can often reveal the vesicular nature of the lesion, which if frequently still focally preserved.

24.2.2.7 Other Inflammatory Myopathies

Inflammatory myopathies include focal myositis, nodular myositis, proliferative myositis and diabetic muscle infarction. Clinically, inflammatory myopathies often present as a diffuse swelling of the thigh or calf, with or without tenderness. Only on rare occasions they present as a solitary soft tissue mass. These different entities are only distinguishable by their histologic appearances [53], often requiring a biopsy for correct diagnosis.

On MR imaging studies, myopathies are characterized by non-focal hypointense areas on T1-weighted images and hyperintense signal on T2-weighted images [53] (Fig. 24.15). These diffuse signal changes are even better seen when a T2-weighted fat suppression sequence is used [45]. The infiltration crosses the fascial planes.

Differential diagnosis includes infectious myositis, trauma, muscular denervation, muscular dystrophy (such as Duchenne's [72] or Becker's muscular dystrophy), rhabdomyolysis, polymyositis, dermatomyositis [46] and soft tissue malignancy. In most of these cases, clinical and laboratory tests will permit to make the correct diagnosis.

■ **Focal Myositis.** Focal myositis is a relative rare usually self-limiting soft tissue pseudotumor. It is usually found in the lower extremities, 50% of the cases being

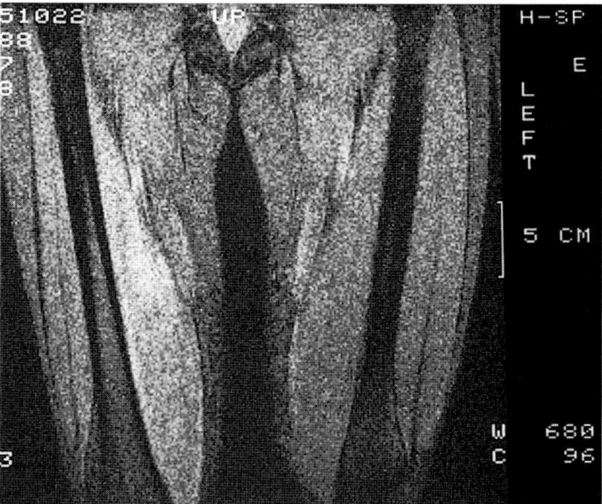

Fig. 24.15. Diabetic myositis of the thigh in a 23-year-old woman. Coronal gradient echo T2*-weighted MR image. Diffuse hyperintensity of the right vastus medialis muscle on T2*-weighted images caused by muscle inflammation in diabetes

located in the thigh and 25% in the lower leg [44]. Other more rare locations include the neck, tongue, perioral region, forearm, hand, abdomen, eyelids, and paraspinal muscles [61]. There is no sex or age predilection [61].

Typically, focal myositis presents as a local intramuscular soft tissue mass, which can rapidly grow in a few weeks (Fig. 24.16). In more than 50% of the cases pain is the main symptom [44]. Usually the process is limited to one muscle, but involvement of multiple muscles has been reported [33, 44]. Previous studies noted that about one third of the patients with focal myositis evolve to polymyositis or a polymyositis-like syndrome [33], suggesting that focal myositis is a localized form of polymyositis. Kransdorf et al. also reported a case that evolved to a myositis ossificans-like lesion [61]. A S-1 radiculopathy has also been described as a cause of unilateral calf enlargement and focal myositis [113], although this swelling can also occur without inflammatory signs (Fig. 24.17) [27].

MR-characteristics are described as a heterogeneous signal pattern, with increased signal intensity on T2-weighted images, in one or more muscle groups [61]. An extensive surrounding edema may be seen. A focal mass, when visualized, may enhance less than the surrounding edema [61].

■ **Diabetic Muscle Infarction.** Diabetic muscle infarction is a rare complication of diabetes mellitus. Patients with poorly controlled type 1 insulin-dependent diabetes mellitus and severe end-organ damage are most frequently affected, although it may occur in a well-controlled patient without known diabetic complications [55]. Although the pathogenesis is still to be completely clarified, the most likely hypothesis is that the muscle

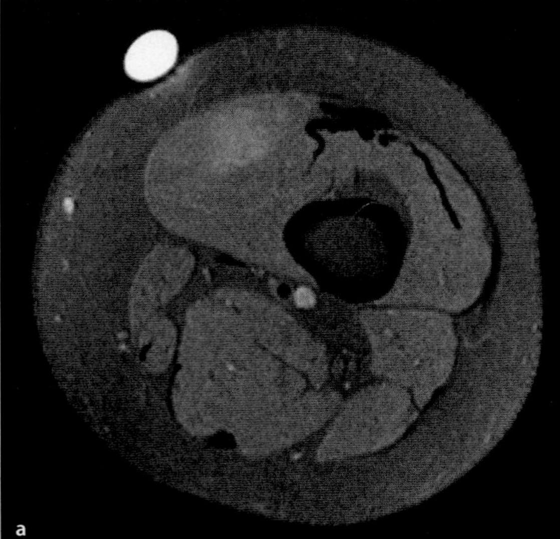

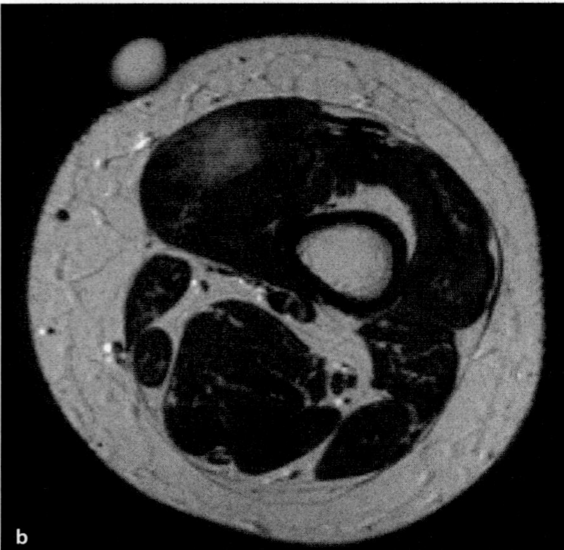

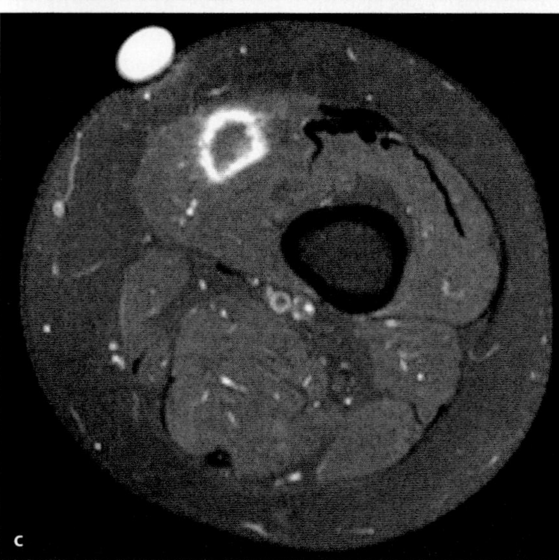

Fig. 24.16a–c. A 39-year-old woman with pain in the left upper leg: **a** axial spin echo T1-weighted MR image with fat suppression; **b** axial turbo spin echo T2-weighted MR image; **c** axial spin echo T1-weighted MR image with fat suppression after intravenous contrast administration. A focal mass with increased signal intensity compared to muscle on both T1- and T2-weighted images is seen (**a,b**). After contrast administration a clear peripheral enhancement is seen (**c**)

infarction is secondary to vascular disease such as arteriosclerosis and diabetic microangiopathy [108, 117], while some authors suggest an alteration in the coagulation-fibrinolysis system [93].

Diabetic muscle infarction typically presents as a sudden onset of severe pain in the thigh (especially in the quadriceps muscle) or calf, with diffuse enlargement of the involved muscle or muscle groups. After subsequent partial resolution a painful palpable mass can be found in up to one third of the cases [117]. Bilateral involvement has been described, with a reported frequency varying from 8% to more than one third of the cases [55, 87, 111, 117].

Clinically, it is frequently misdiagnosed as an abscess, neoplasm or myositis, often requiring a biopsy for further evaluation [17, 29, 55]. Commonly there is elevated erythrocyte sedimentation rate, but no leucocytosis. This can be helpful in the differentiation from pyomyositis [55].

MRI findings in conjunction with clinical information and laboratory studies may reliably give the diagnosis without need of biopsy [17, 54, 55], although this is not universally accepted [29]. As a consequence, the role of a biopsy remains controversial. Histopathologic findings are consistent with edematous and necrotic tissue.

MR images display enlargement of the involved muscles, with uniform increased signal intensity on T2-weighted and inversion recovery images demonstrating the edematous and inflammatory changes (Fig. 24.15) [17, 29, 54, 55]. T1-weighted images show normal or decreased signal intensity in the involved muscles, the swelling being sometimes less appreciated on this sequence [55].

Perifascial and subcutaneous edema are best evaluated on inversion recovery and fat-suppressed T2-weighted images. Additionally, MRI can detect subclinical muscle infarction months before the onset of clinical symptoms [55]. Ultrasound can further complement the MRI findings [29].

Atypical presentations have been reported as a high signal of the affected muscle on T1-weighted images, presumably reflecting intramuscular hemorrhage [109].

Whether intravenous contrast medium injection can be helpful in the differentiation with pyomyositis, muscle abscess or a necrotic tumor, is not clearly established [29].

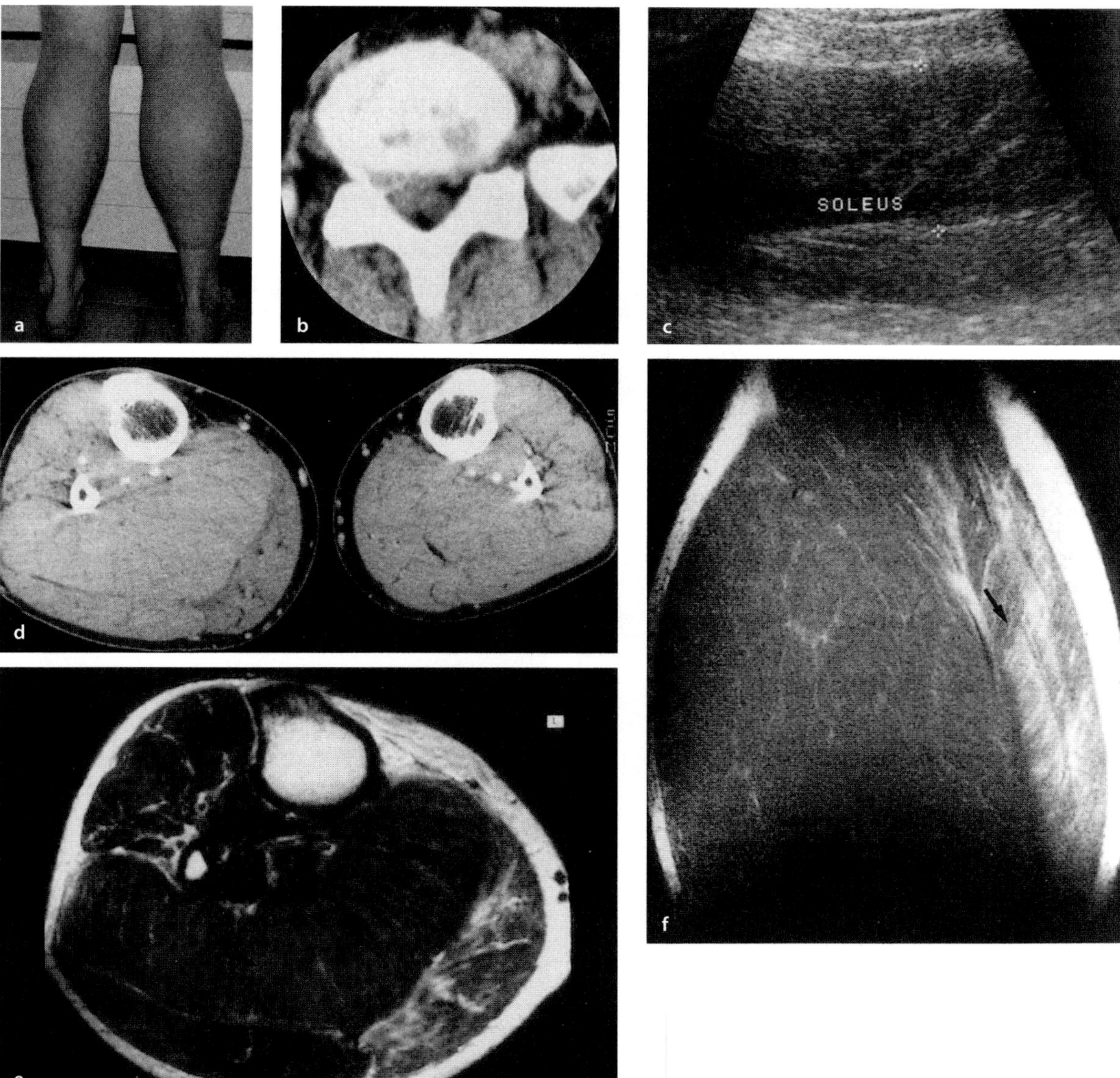

Fig. 24.17 a–f. A 41-year-old man with unilateral right-sided calf enlargement, following chronic ipsilateral S1 radiculopathy: **a** clinical photograph; **b** axial CT scan of the lumbar spine; **c** ultrasonography of the right lower limb; **d** axial CT scan of the lower limbs; **e** axial spin echo T1-weighted MR image; **f** coronal spin echo T1-weighted MR image. The clinical photograph (**a**) demonstrates a clinically painless and progressive enlargment of the right calf. CT images at the level of the lumbar spine reveal a since three years known right-sided disc herniation compressing the S1 nerve root (**b**). In the right lower limb, ultrasound shows reflective linear strands within the muscle belly of the soleus muscle (**c**), while on CT an enlarged circumference of the right lower leg is shown compared with the left leg (**d**). Note the hypertrophy of the soleus muscle and decreased density of the medial head of the gastrocnemius muscle. MR-images (**e, f**) confirm the true muscular hypertrophy of the soleus and gastrocnemius muscles. The muscle fibers are intermingled with fine linear streaks of high signal intensity, corresponding to tiny fatty bands (*arrow*) in pseudohypertrophy

24.2.2.8 Bursitis

Bursae are spaces near joints containing small amounts of fluid, reducing friction between different structures. More than 140 different bursae have been described. The clinical most important are the trochanteric, subdeltoideal, ischiogluteal, pes anserina, iliopsoas, retrocalcaneal and olecranon bursae, because they are the most commonly affected ones [66].

The amount of fluid may increase due to inflammation following overuse, direct trauma or infection, resulting in a soft tissue mass. Non-infectious bursitis is generally produced by repeated movements generating microtrauma in the tendon sheaths, the bursae or the tendons. It may also be a first manifestation of rheumatoid arthritis [110].

Infectious bursitis is a more rare pathology, usually associated with *Staphylococcus aureus* infection. Only a

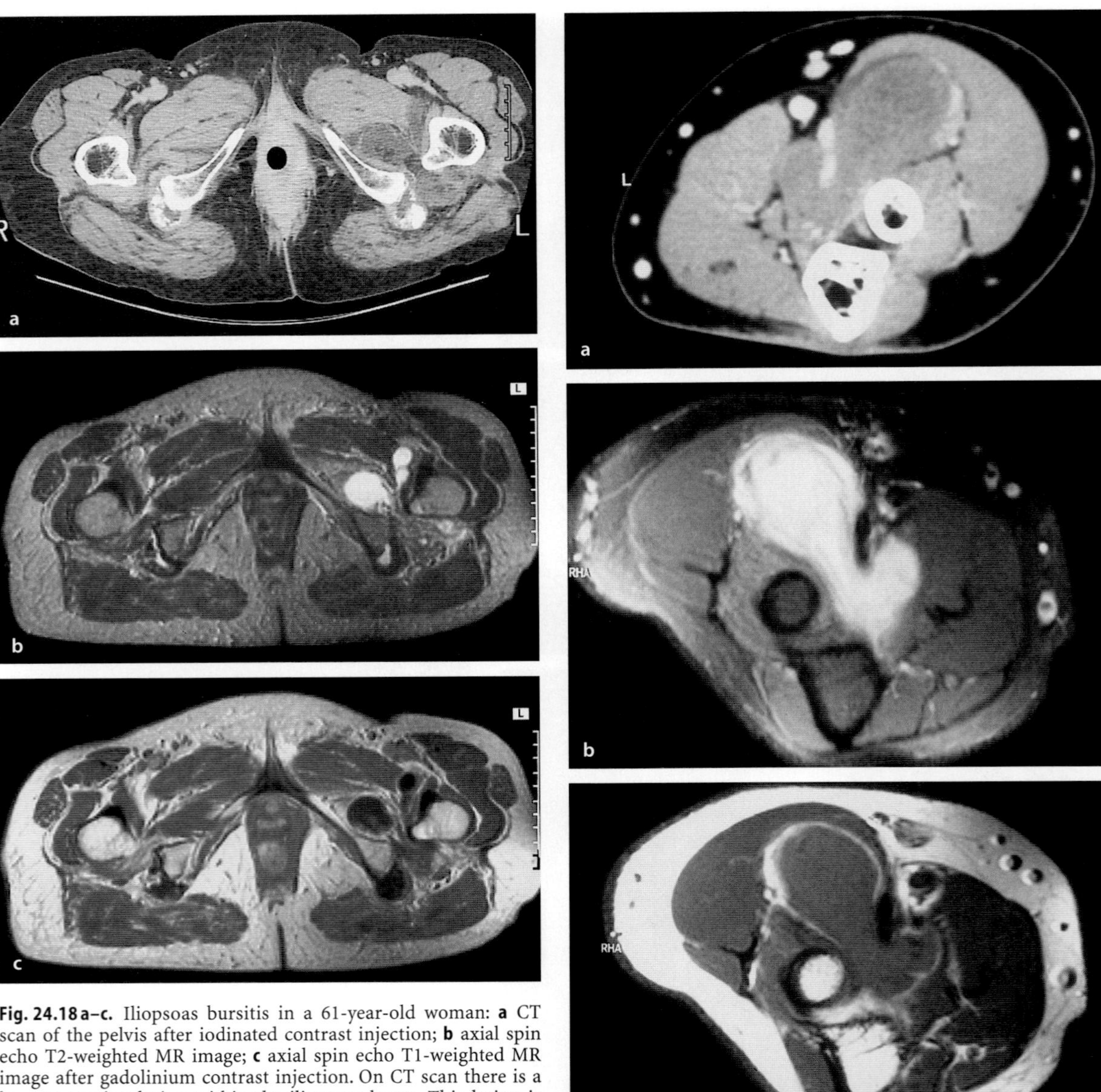

Fig. 24.18 a–c. Iliopsoas bursitis in a 61-year-old woman: **a** CT scan of the pelvis after iodinated contrast injection; **b** axial spin echo T2-weighted MR image; **c** axial spin echo T1-weighted MR image after gadolinium contrast injection. On CT scan there is a low attenuation lesion within the iliopsoas bursa. This lesion is closely related to a collar button mass extending between the ischial tuberosity and lesser trochanter. Compared to the precontrast images, not shown, there is only faint peripheral enhancement (**a**). The lesion is hyperintense on T2-weighted images (**b**) and shows a subtle peripheral enhancement after contrast injection (**c**). There are small intralesional fatty components visible as well on CT scan as on MR imaging. This case shows characteristic localization and MR appearance of an extended iliopsoas bursitis

Fig. 24.19 a–c. A 31-year-old man with a localized swelling in the right elbow: **a** CT scan after iodinated contrast administration; **b** axial turbo spin echo proton-density weighted MR image; **c** axial spin echo T1-weighted MR image after gadolinium contrast administration. A bilobular structure can be seen at the ventral aspect of the elbow, against the proximal radius and ulna, with a low attenuation on CT scan (**a**). The relation with the tendon of the biceps brachii muscle is further illustrated on the MR images, where the lesion has a high signal intensity on the proton-density weighted MR images (**b**), and an intermediate signal intensity on the T1-weighted images (**c**). After gadolinium contrast administration there is peripheral enhancement, more pronounced at the cranial extend of the lesion (**c**). This case nicely demonstrates morphology, location and imaging characteristics illustrative for a bicipito-radialis bursitis

minority of cases is attributed to beta-hemolytic streptococci. The olecranon, pre- and infrapatellar bursa are among the most affected ones, presumably because of their superficial location they are the most prone to trauma and subsequent infection [36, 67]. Nevertheless, a clear history of trauma is not always found.

Due to the increased fluid content, bursitis tends to be hypointense on T1-weighted images and proton density-weighted images, and hyperintense on T2-weighted images. The anatomic location is characteristic (e.g. iliopsoas bursitis) (Figs. 24.18 and 24.19). Enhancement of hypertrophied synovium and surrounding soft tissue edema can be seen after intravenous contrast injection in both infected and non-infected bursitis [6].

No single imaging feature is able to reliably distinguish infectious from non- infectious bursitis [6, 36, 41]. However, the combination of bone erosions with marrow edema is more suggestive for septic bursitis [41]. Other features favoring an infectious origin are marked synovial thickening, synovial edema, soft tissue edema and a complex appearance of the lesion [36, 41].

24.2.3 Granulomatous Myopathies

In tropical regions, a rare granulomatous myositis associated with *Mycobacterium tuberculosis*, atypical mycobacterial infections, sarcoidosis, syphilis, actinomycosis and parasites can be found.

Tuberculous infection of soft tissue without involvement of deeper structures like lymph nodes, bones, or joints is uncommon (Fig. 24.20) [112]. Without proper treatment, it can evolve to a cold abscess. A periosteal reaction in adjacent bone can sometimes be found [112].

24.2.3.1 Sarcoidosis

Sarcoidosis is a systemic granulomatous disorder which can affect multiple organs. Muscle involvement is rare and occurs in 1.4–6% of patients with sarcoidosis [43, 91]. Three main clinical presentations of muscular sarcoidosis can be distinguished: an acute myositic form, a diffuse atrophic form and a nodular form [89, 116]. Clinical symptoms are often absent.

The acute myositis type occurs exclusively in the early stage of sarcoidosis, presenting as myalgia secondary to inflammation. MR imaging is usually negative, presumably because of the sparse distribution and small size of epithelioid cell granulomas [90].

In the diffuse atrophic myopathic form patients can present with myalgia, muscle weakness, and atrophy [89]. The muscles of de proximal portions of the extremities are frequently involved [80]. MR imaging findings are non-specific revealing proximal muscle atrophy

with fatty replacement [85]. Differentiation from a corticoid myopathy is mainly based on clinical and laboratory findings.

The least common form is the nodular presentation, presenting as a single or multiple sarcoid nodules (Fig. 24.21). They may or may not be clinically palpable. These nodules appear elongated, and extend along muscle fibers [89]. On ultrasound examination, sarcoid nodules present with a hyperechoic center and a hypoechoic peripheral zone [89]. They may also present with well-defined borders and an overall hypoechogenic aspect [116].

On MR imaging, the nodules may have a star-shaped hypointense center on all axial pulse sequences ("dark star" sign), which is believed to correspond with fibrous tissue, and does not enhance after intravenous contrast administration [90, 91, 122]. However, this central structure is not present in the acute stage of the disease. It can also be absent in small nodules (<10 mm), presumably because of the short time of granulomatous inflammation in these small structures.

The peripheral area of the nodules is slightly hyperintense compared to muscle on T1-weighted images, with homogeneous high signal intensity on T2-weighted images. There is homogeneous enhancement after intravenous contrast administration, secondary to the high cellularity of granulomas and edema [116].

Coronal and sagittal images may show the "three stripes" sign, consisting of a hypointense inner stripe and hyperintense outer stripes [89]. However, after steroid therapy the sarcoid nodules may disappear [116], or only the inner stripe may be visualized [91].

Gallium-67 scintigraphy shows increased uptake in the nodules [89], but is further nonspecific.

24.2.3.2 Cat Scratch Disease

Cat scratch disease is a benign, self-limiting cause of regional lymphadenitis affecting mostly children and young adults. In more than 90% of the cases there is a history of recent contact with cats, cat scratch or both. In contrast, the site of inoculation is not always found. The Gram-negative bacillus *Rochalimae henselae*, also called *Bartonella henselae*, is the micro-organism most often incriminated. In an otherwise healthy host, the adenitis resolves spontaneously within three weeks to several months, even without antibiotic therapy [30]. Atypical manifestations can mimic neoplastic disease.

Cat scratch disease has a wide spectrum of clinical manifestations, ranging from regional lymphadenitis to disseminated infection. Common locations include the neck, groin and epitrochlear region [38]. A typical case includes skin lesions and an associated enlarged painful reactive adenopathy commonly presenting along a single lymph node chain. Involved glands can have diame-

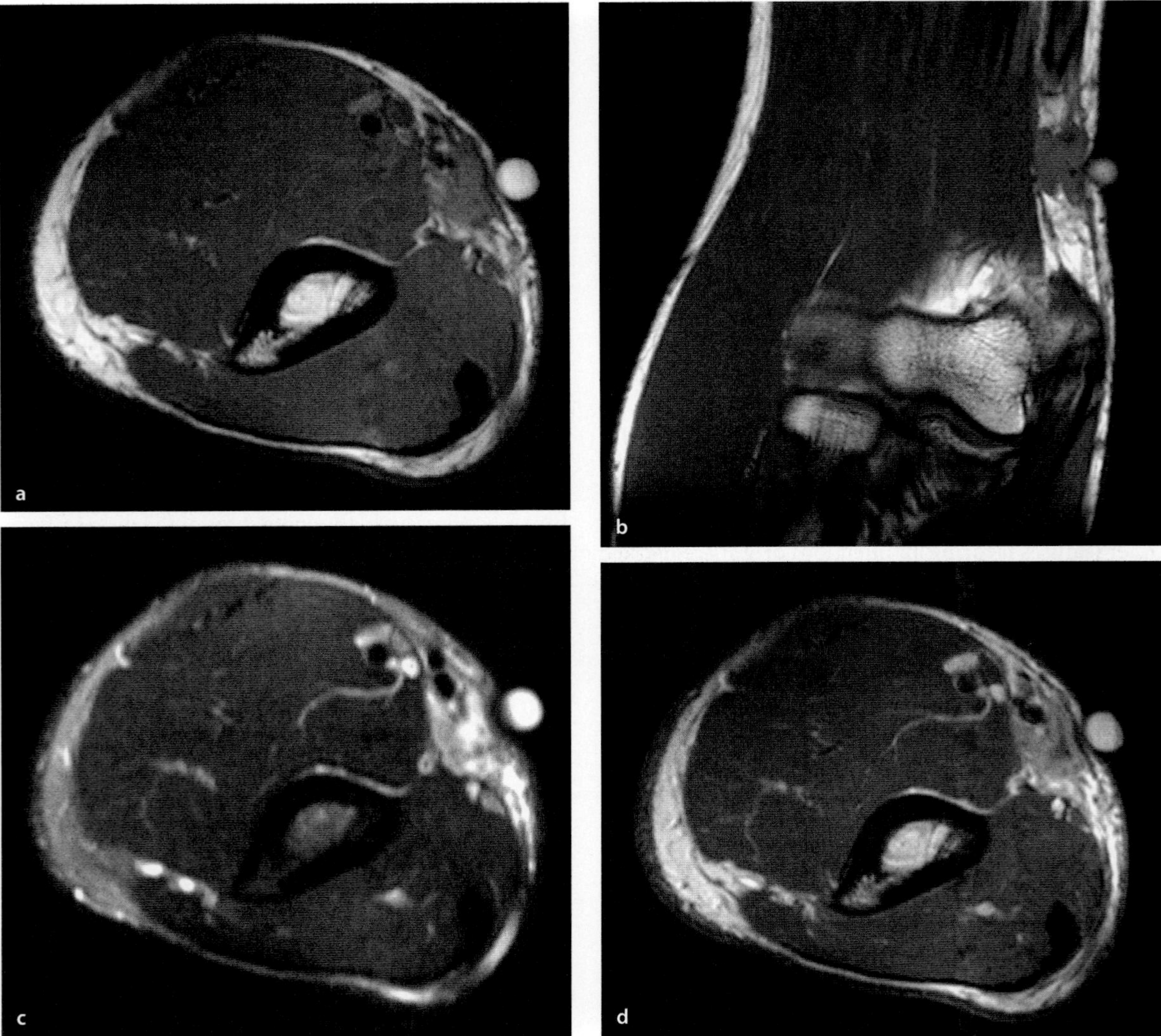

Fig. 24.20 a–d. A 28-year-old man with a swelling at the right elbow since one month: **a** axial spin echo T1-weighted MR image; **b** coronal spin echo T1-weighted MR image; **c** axial turbo spin echo T2-weighted MR image; **d** axial spin echo T1-weighted MR image after intravenous contrast administration. T1-weighted images reveal a small, polynodular mass lesion of intermediate signal intensity at the right elbow region within the subcutaneous fat, adjacent to the medial vascular bundle (**a,b**). There is envelopment of the adjacent vein. The mass is inhomogeneous and of overall high signal intensity on T2-weighted images (**c**). After intravenous contrast administration there is moderate, merely peripheral enhancement (**d**). A biopsy revealed this mass to be a rare soft tissue manifestation of tuberculosis

ters up to 5 cm [76]. Single node involvement is most common, but multiple node involvement at a single site is also possible [59]. Disseminated infection is unusual (5–10%) [76], most frequently seen in immune-compromised patients. Neurological involvement is uncommon [76]. Histologically the soft tissue masses resemble granulomatous disease.

CT shows a soft tissue mass corresponding to involved lymph nodes. Central necrosis can be seen as a low attenuation [30, 59]. MR-images reveal the regional lymphadenopathy as homogeneous or heterogenic masses surrounded by edema [30, 38]. T1-weighted images show an homogeneous isointense signal intensity compared to muscle (Fig. 24.22) [30, 38]. On T2-weighted images the area of the mass and surrounding edema becomes hyperintense. After intravenous contrast injection there may be homogeneous or slight peripheral enhancement of the involved lymph nodes and adjacent soft tissue edema [30, 38].

Bone involvement is rare, usually presenting as lytic lesions [50]. A periosteal reaction and associated sclerosis can be found [50]. A single osteolytic lesion can simulate histiocytosis X [8].

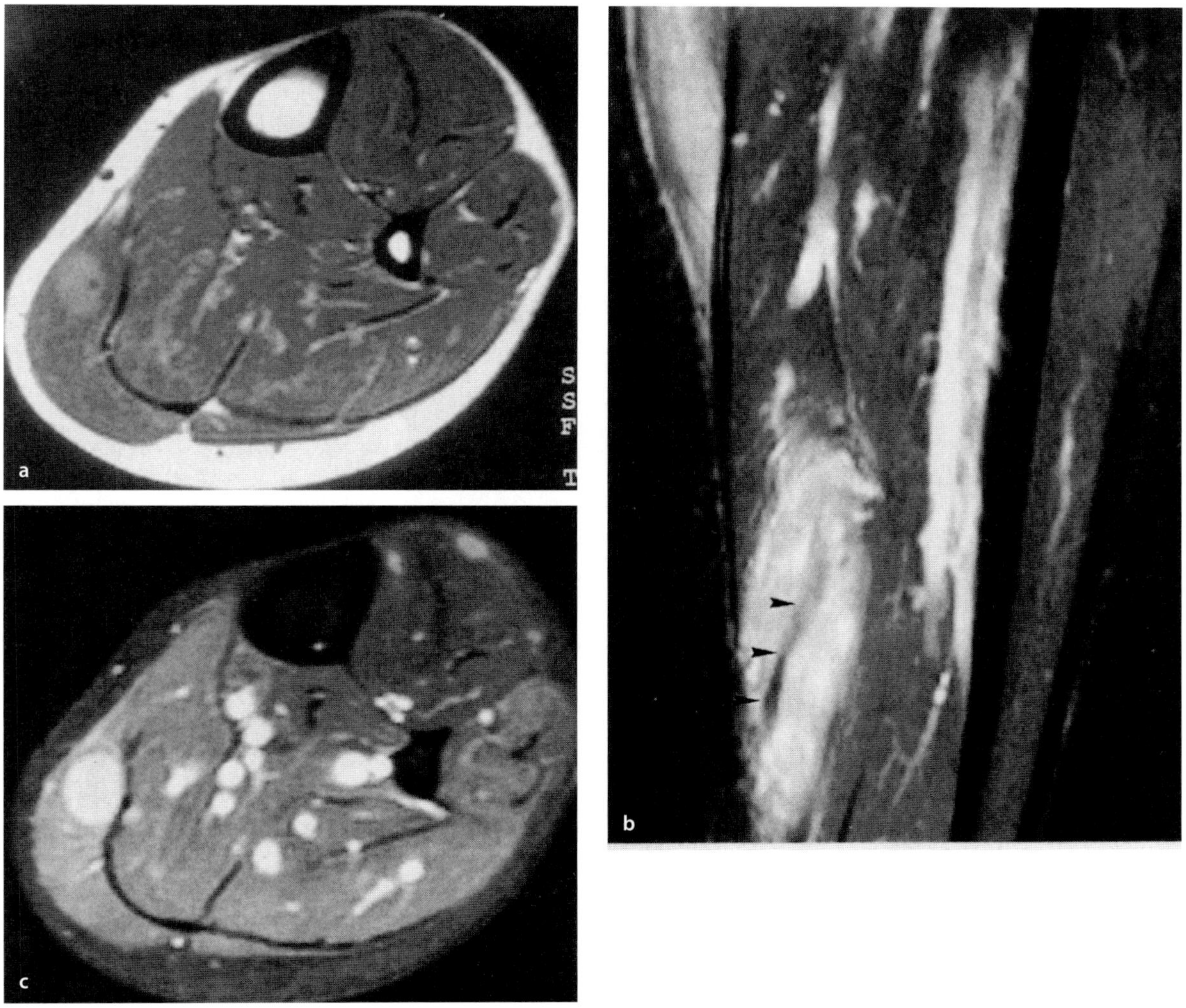

Fig. 24.21 a–c. A 56-year-old woman with a tender palpable mass in the left calf: **a** axial spin echo T1-weighted MR image; **b** sagittal spin echo T1-weighted MR image with fat suppression; **c** axial spin echo T1-weighted MR image with fat suppression after intravenous contrast administration. A nodular lesion, slightly hyperintense compared to muscle, is shown on the axial T1-weighted image (**a**), with a central hypointense center presumably corresponding to fibrous tissue. After intravenous contrast administration, a homogeneous enhancement of this large and other smaller nodules is seen (**c**). The sagittal image (**c**) further demonstrates the three layer composition, with a linear low intensity stripe interposed between two high intensity areas (**b**), longitudinally extending between normal muscle tissue. This case illustrates a rare soft tissue presentation of sarcoidosis

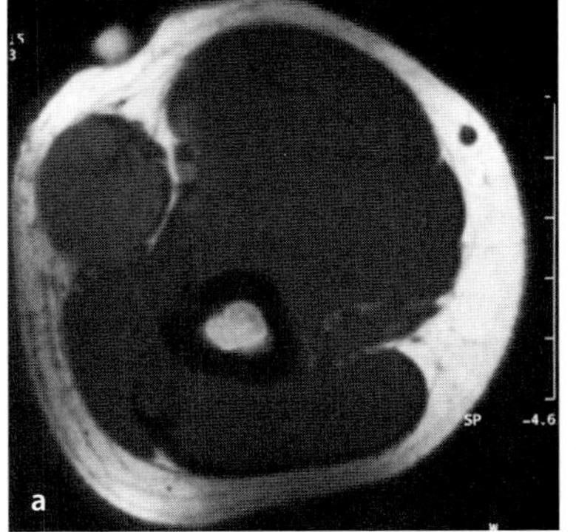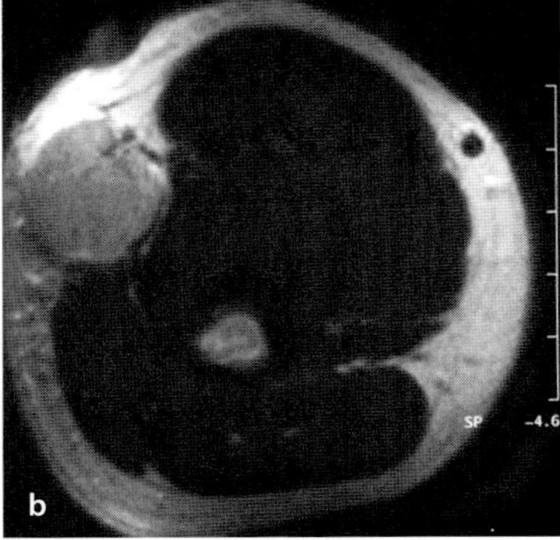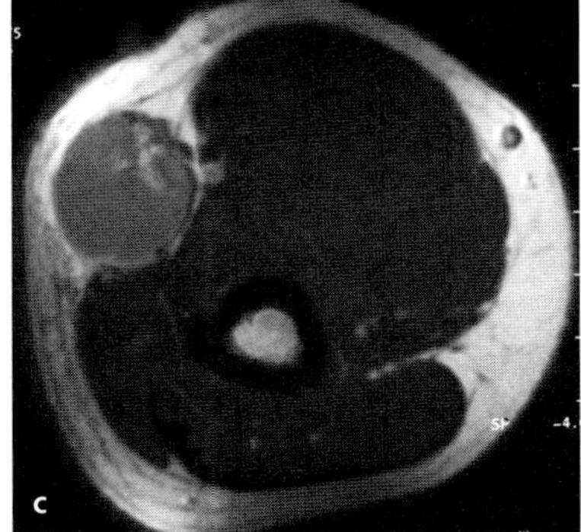

Fig. 24.22 a–c. Cat scratch disease in a 15-year-old boy: **a** axial spin echo T1-weighted MR image; **b** axial turbo spin echo T2-weighted MR image; **c** axial spin echo T1-weighted MR image after intravenous contrast administration. A round, well-defined lesion is located adjacent to the neurovascular bundle at the left elbow. On T1-weighted images (**a**) the lesion has slightly higher and relative homogeneous signal intensity compared to muscle, with a more intermediate signal intensity on T2-weighted images (**b**). After contrast administration there is moderate, mostly homogeneous enhancement of this mass

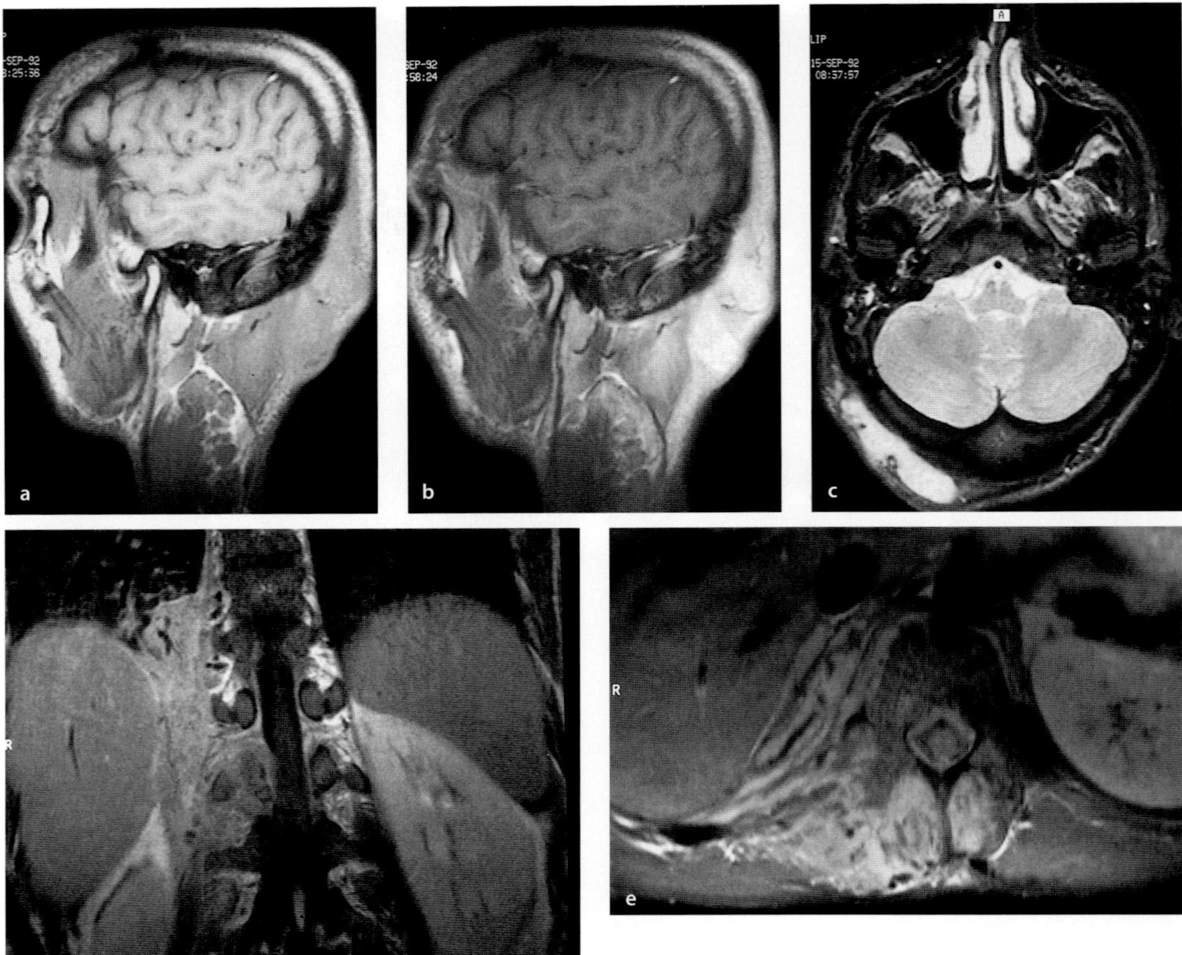

Fig. 24.23 a–e. Actinomycotic abscess in a 21-year-old man (**a–c**) and a 23-year-old man (**d,e**): **a** sagittal spin echo T1-weigted MR image; **b** sagittal T1-weighted MR image after gadolinium contrast injection; **c** axial T2-weighted MR image; **d** coronal spin echo T1-weighted MR image; **e** axial turbo spin echo T2-weighted MR image with fat suppression. In the first patient, there is a collar-button-like mass involving the right splenius and semispinalis muscles which is isointense to muscle on T1-weighted images (**a**) and hyperintense on T2-weighted images (**c**). After contrast injection there is moderate enhancement of the lesion without evidence of necrosis (**b**). After resection of the slowly growing mass the lesion proved to be an actinomycotic abscess. In the second patient, the images show an ill-defined structure of homogeneous intermediate signal intensity on T1-weighted images (**d**) at the level of the paraspinal muscles on a low thoracic level. The lesion extends both cranially and caudally, invading the right psoas muscles and the spine (**d, e**)

24.2.3.3 Injection Granulomas

Injection granulomas are most often encountered in the upper outer quadrant of the buttocks and in the deltoid muscle [103]. The typical location and the absence of muscle distortion are the clues to the diagnosis. On CT they appear as small well-defined nodules, most often containing calcifications. These lesions are hypointense on T1-weighted MR images. On T2-weighted images, injection granulomas can be hyperintense or hypointense, depending on whether the major pattern of the lesion is inflammatory or fibrous. This pattern depends on the time elapsed after injection.

24.2.3.4 Actinomycosis

Actinomycosis is a chronic, suppurative and granulomatous bacterial infection, usually caused by *Actinomycosis israelii*. Clinically a cervicofacial, abdominopelvic or pulmonary form can be distinguished. Soft tissue manifestation often presents as a subacute cellulitis. On clinical examination a wooden hard, palpable mass is often found. It commonly evolves to abscess formation. More unusual presentations can mimic tuberculosis, aspergillosis or a malignant tumor [7, 62].

It can affect the head and neck, thorax, spine, abdomen and cutis [7, 53, 95, 124]. Histologically, the presence of "sulfur granules" containing colonies of *Actinomyces* is considered pathognomonic [12], although their absence does not rule out the infection.

Ultrasound is useful in identifying the abscess formation and guides aspiration for culture of the organism [53]. MR characteristics are not specific, resembling abscess formation or a centrally necrotizing tumor (Fig. 24.23) [7]. It further illustrates the infiltrative nature, showing often a lesion which invades and crosses tissue planes.

24.2.4 Traumatic Lesions

24.2.4.1 Hematoma and Contusion

A contusion is caused by a capillary rupture that provokes bleeding between the tissue muscle fibers, resulting in edema and inflammatory reaction (Fig. 24.24). Contusions are not always painful, may present as a mass and thereby cause clinical confusion. A soft tissue contusion appears on MR images as a diffuse interstitial infiltration due to edema. It is hyperintense on T2-weighted images but without architectural muscle distortion. However, the muscle can increase in volume, owing to inflammation.

The ultrasound appearance of hematomas is variable in time. Acute hematomas are hyperechoic and they become more hypoechoic with aging. They may have well-defined or irregular margins. Dynamic evaluation may be valuable in diagnosing an associated muscle tear (Fig. 24.25). On CT, acute hematoma appears as a hyperdense area (Fig. 24.26). However, MR imaging with its superior sensitivity and specificity has replaced CT in the imaging of hematomas in all circumstances.

The MR imaging appearance of muscular hematomas has many resemblances with that of intracranial hemorrhage [13, 94]. This reflects a similar pathophysiology of forming hemoglobin breakdown products, which are the main constituents of a musculoskeletal hemorrhagic collection. The magnetic properties of these degradation products are mostly related to the oxidation and binding state of iron in the heme unit, closely correlated with the age of the hematoma. Nevertheless, other factors like anatomic location, local partial pressure of oxygen, pH, presence of an underlying lesion and field strength of the MR unit also influence the resulting image.

To understand adequately the evolving signal characteristics of musculoskeletal hemorrhages, a basic knowledge of the underlying pathophysiological changes is necessary.

■ **Pathophysiology of Hemoglobin Degradation.** In intact erythrocytes, hemoglobin freely alternates between oxy- and deoxyhemoglobin. In both forms the iron in

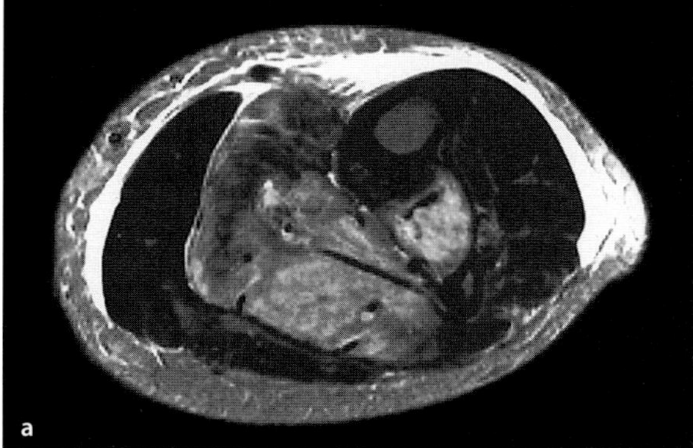
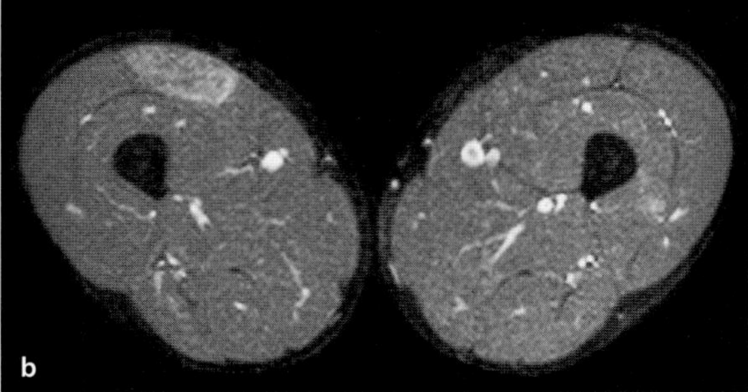

Fig. 24.24 a, b. Muscle contusion of the left calf in a 27-year-old woman, one day after an operation of 8-h duration in lithotomy position (**a**) and of the right thigh in a 29-year-old soccer player: **a** axial turbo spin echo T2-weighted MR image; **b** axial, fat suppressed (STIR) MR image. Increased signal intensity of soleus and posterior tibial muscles with high signal intensity strands and fluid collections within the subcutaneous compartment (**a**). MRI dramatically illustrates muscle contusion and subcutaneous edema due to long standing compression. In the second patient increased signal intensity of the rectus femoris muscle is seen. MR imaging is not able to differentiate muscle contusion from focal myositis

the heme ring is in its reduced or *ferrous* form (+2 oxygenation state), this being necessary for oxygen exchange. The relatively hypoxic environment of an acute hematoma (hours to days) promotes the release of oxygen, thereby disturbing this balance and quickly transforming oxyhemoglobin into deoxyhemoglobin.

In an early subacute hematoma (a few days), the shortage of oxygen as an energy source causes mitochondrial respiration to cease, in that way inactivating antioxidant metabolic pathways. This causes oxidation of deoxyhemoglobin into methemoglobin, which is in the *ferric* form (+3 oxygenation state).

So far, these processes have taken place in intact red blood cells. However, in a late subacute hematoma (seven days to one month) integrity of the cell membrane is lost, allowing methemoglobin to migrate extracellularly.

This extracellular methemoglobin is further transformed into compounds named hemichromes. The final iron-containing degradation product is hemosiderin, formed by lysosomal degradation in macrophages.

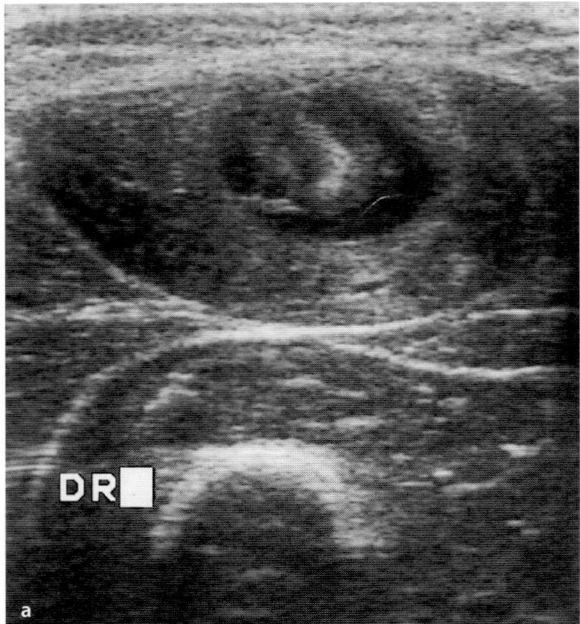

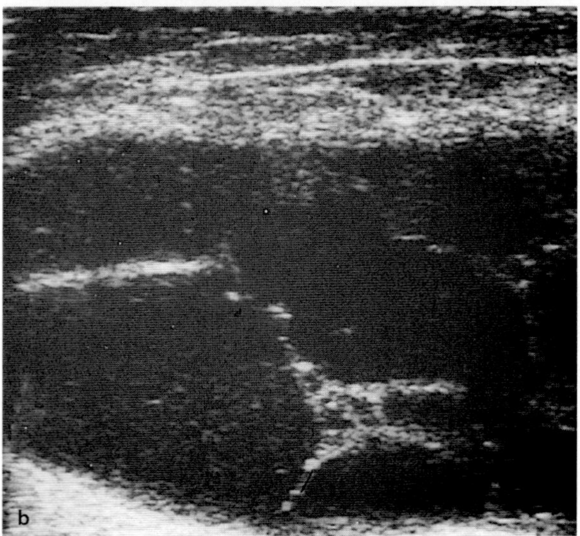

Fig. 24.25 a, b. Hematoma in acute and chronic stage in two adult men **a** axial ultrasound one day after trauma; **b** longitudinal ultrasound 12 days after trauma, in another patient. Hyperechoic center (ruptured muscle) within a heterogeneous hypoechoic mass (hematoma), known as 'clapper-in-the-bell sign' (**a**). Target appearance of a subacute hematoma following muscle rupture of the vastus intermedius muscle. Ultrasound in another patient with hematoma in a chronic stage demonstrates a multilocular anechoic mass with multiple septa formed by fibrin strands (**b**)

■ **Proton-electron Dipole-dipole Relaxation Enhancement.** Proton-electron dipole-dipole (PEDD) relaxation enhancement is the capacity of paramagnetic electrons to enhance the return of the magnetization vector to equilibrium after an RF-pulse, thereby causing T1 shortening. In order for a compound to be paramagnetic, it must have unbound electrons. This is the case for deoxyhemoglobin and methemoglobin. Oxyhemoglobin has no free electrons, and is as such diamagnetic.

PEDD relaxation enhancement only occurs if there is interaction between water protons and the paramagnetic heme iron atom. This is only the case in intra- and extracellular methemoglobin. High signal intensity on T1-weighted images in a hematoma indicates therefore a subacute stage of the collection.

■ **MR Signal Characteristics.** A *hyperacute* hematoma (a few hours old) is seldom investigated with MRI. Since the transition from oxyhemoglobin into deoxyhemoglobin happens very fast, imaging of oxyhemoglobin as the main compound only occurs in rare instances, like, e.g., in an aneurysm. This translates in a high signal on T2-weighted images reflecting high water content of the collection.

In an *acute* hematoma the signal characteristics are dominated by intracellular deoxyhemoglobin. Since there is no PEDD interaction, the hematoma is iso- or slightly hypointense on T1-weighted images compared with muscle. Susceptibility effects also lead to low signal on T2-weighted images, but only well seen on high field strength systems[13].

A hematoma in the *early subacute* stage is characterized by the presence of intracellular methemoglobin, which has PEDD interaction. This produces a high signal intensity on T1-weighted images, often visualized as a high-intensity peripheral rim (Fig. 24.27a). This high-intensity rim is a useful sign, as it may be the only clue that the mass is a hematoma. Susceptibility effects persists on T2-weighted images.

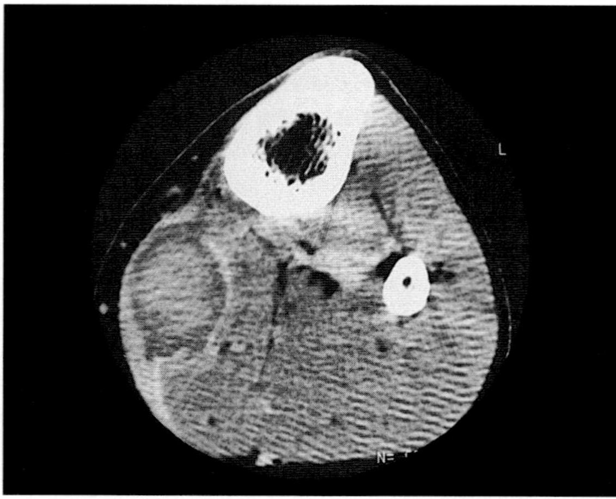

Fig. 24.26. Hematoma of the calf in a 30-year-old man. CT scan. At the medial side of the flexor compartment, there is a rounded area of decreased attenuation with a central zone of hyperdensity. This case is illustrative for a subacute hematoma with serous fluid at the periphery and cloth formation at the center of the lesion

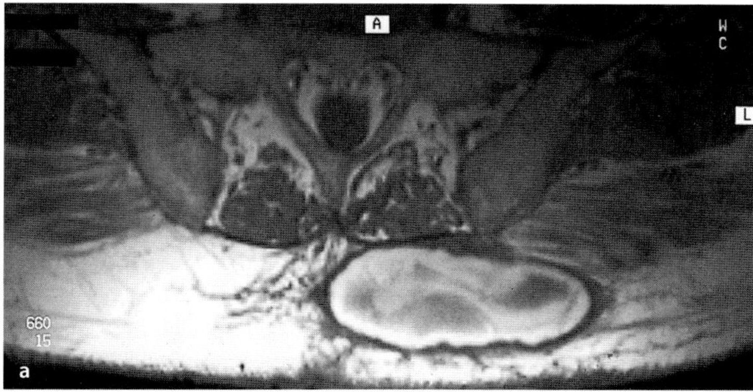

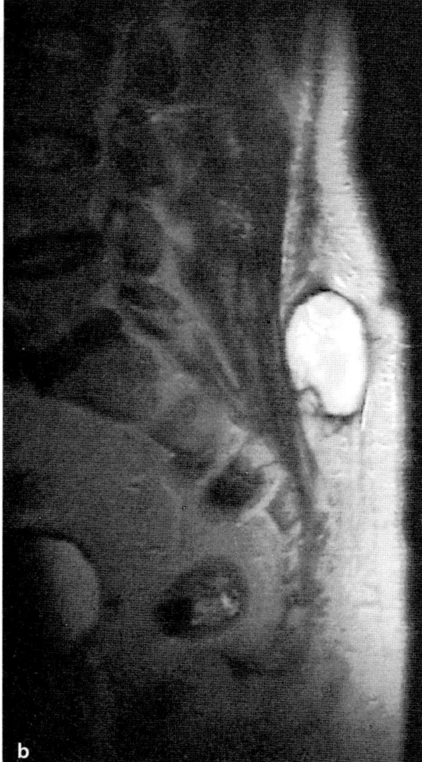

Fig. 24.27 a, b. Subacute hematoma of the low back in a 45-year-old man: **a** axial spin echo T1-weighted MR image; **b** sagittal turbo spin echo T2-weighted MR image. There is an oval mass within the subcutaneous tissue on the left side of the low back. Intermediate signal intensity of the center, high signal intensity of the periphery and low signal intensity of a small peripheral rim on T1-weighted images are a consequence of the presence of respectively intra- and extracellular methaemoglobin and hemosiderin (**a**). On T2-weighted images, overall signal intensity is very high, exception made for a low signal intensity peripheral rim caused by hemosiderin (**b**). Signal intensities are characteristic for a subacute hematoma

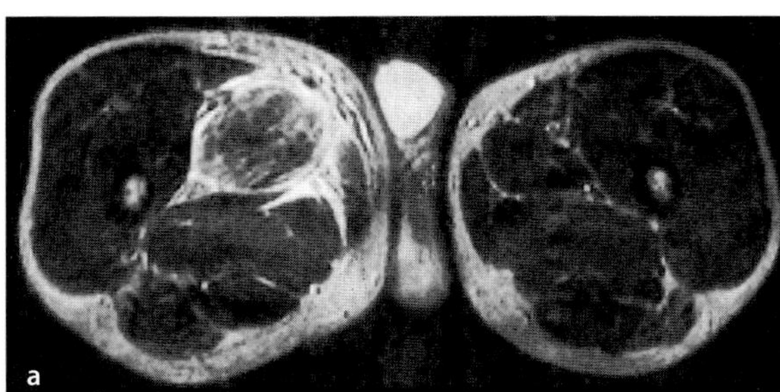

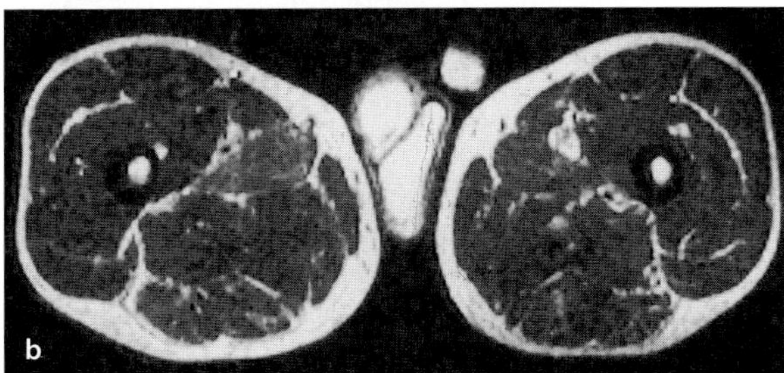

Fig. 24.28 a, b. Hematoma of the right thigh in a 70-year-old man: **a** axial SE T2-weighted MR image; **b** axial spin echo T2-weighted MR image four weeks later. There is a mass at the medial aspect of the right thigh. Signal intensity on T2-weighted images is heterogeneous and mostly low (**a**). On a control MR examination four weeks later, the volume of the lesion has decreased considerably. Signal intensity remains low (**b**). Low signal intensity on T2-weighted images is seldom seen in malignant soft tissue tumors and in this case due to the presence of hemosiderin. Follow-up examinations are useful for diagnosis of hematoma

When loss of cell compartmentalization occurs in *late subacute* hematomas, extracellular methemoglobin is present. PEDD interaction is still at hand, giving T1 shortening. However, T2-weighted images now reveal a high signal intensity (Fig. 24.27b). Diffuse edema is also present within the muscle in acute and subacute hematomas. Therefore, on T2-weighted images, the hematoma may be outlined by an area of high signal intensity.

Finally, hemosiderin in a *chronic* hematoma has no PEDD effect, and also produces susceptibility effects on T2-weighted images. This results in low signal intensity on T1-weighted images, and particularly on T2-weighted images. Furthermore, this phenomenon is accelerated at the periphery of the collection, resulting in a peripheral hypointense rim whereas the central portion of the hematoma may remain hyperintense (Fig. 24.29) [13].

It is important to differentiate hematoma from hemorrhagic tumor, because hemorrhage may obscure tumor tissue. T1-weighted images with fat suppression can aid in the differentiation, further discrimination methemoglobin from fatty tissue [39]. The best features suggesting hematoma are the progressive decrease in size of the lesion, the presence of fluid-fluid levels and the time-dependent signal intensity changes (Figs. 24.27 and 24.28). Conversely, the presence of enhancing nodules after contrast medium administration may suggest the presence of tumor [53]. Nevertheless, organized hematomas can show some enhancement.

When in doubt a biopsy should be performed to establish a firm diagnosis, especially if there is an increase in size of the hemorrhagic mass.

A chronic expanding hematoma is an entity characterized by its persistence and increasing size for more than one month after the initial hemorrhage [101]. MR reveals a heterogeneous signal intensity on both T1- and T2-weighted images, with a peripheral rim of low signal intensity [4].

24.2.4.2 Foreign Body Reactions

Foreign bodies such as plastic, wood, glass, and silica may penetrate the soft tissues and produce an inflammatory reaction. Clinically, a foreign body reaction first appears as a painful soft tissue swelling, and after a quiescent period of weeks or months the symptoms may reappear [114]. If not removed immediately, a foreign body can become encapsulated with fibrous tissue and form a granuloma. The presence of histiocytes and giant cells with a surrounding inflammatory reaction is useful in establishing the diagnosis.

Different imaging methods have each their advantages and limitations in the evaluation of foreign bodies. Radio-opaque bodies can be demonstrated on conventional radiographs. When the lesion is in or near bone, radiographs can show osteolytic and/or osteoblastic bone lesions [64, 105]. Since a positive history of penetrating trauma is not always obvious, and some lesions can be radiolucent, a foreign body reaction can be mistaken for a neoplasm [64, 105].

Ultrasound is a primary imaging tool when conventional radiographs fail in detecting the foreign object. Its use in the detection and guided retrieval of a suspected foreign body has been well established [15]. Ultrasound shows large differences in acoustic impedance between hyperechoic foreign bodies and hypoechoic surrounding inflammatory tissue (Fig. 24.30).

On MR imaging studies the foreign body itself is usually low, due to the presence of few mobile protons in the commonly found foreign materials (glass, wood, metal, ...) [53, 64, 84]. However, dispersed oil droplets

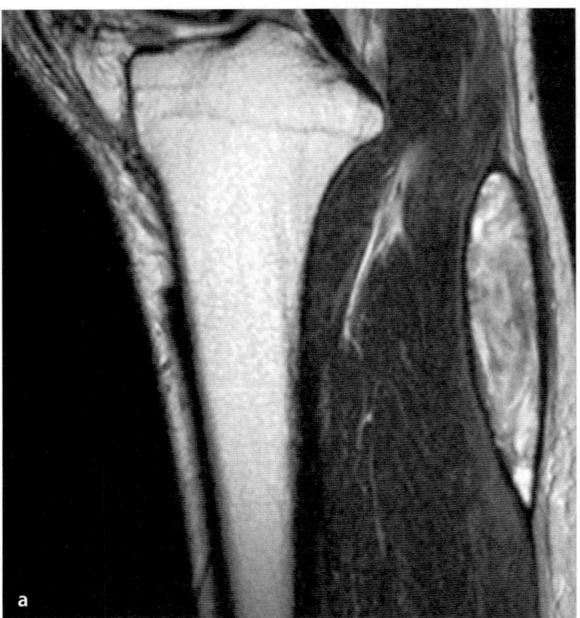

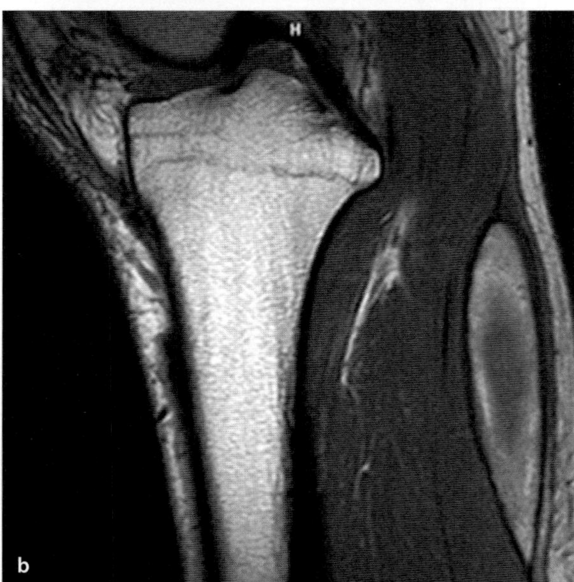

Fig. 24.29 a, b. Long standing swelling posterior in the lower leg in a 30-year-old man: **a** sagittal spin echo T1-weighted MR image; **b** sagittal turbo spin echo T2-weighted MR image. On T1-weighted image different strands of high signal intensity are seen, corresponding with extracellular methemoglobin (**a**). The central lower signal intensity on T2-weighted image is caused by susceptibility effects (**b**). A clear low signal intensity hemosiderin ring is clearly demonstrated on both images. These signal characteristics correspond with a chronic hematoma

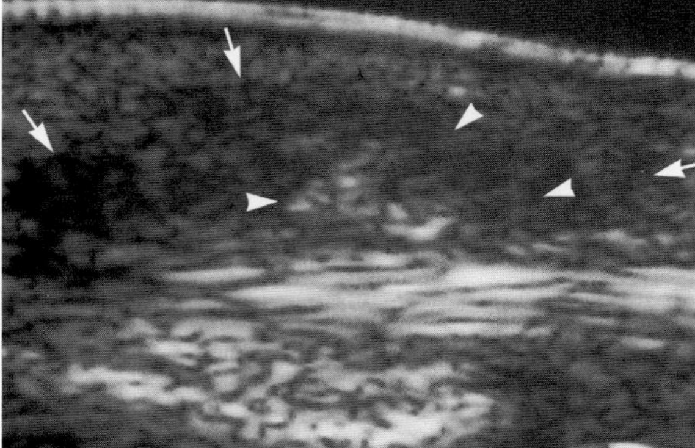

Fig. 24.30. Epidermoid inclusion cyst on foreign body (thorn) in a 40-year-old rose-grower. Ultrasound of the index finger, longitudinal scan. There is a triangular hyperechoic structure (*arrowheads*) within a zone of decreased reflectivity (*arrows*) at the ventral aspect of the finger. The thorn is visible by the surrounding edema and cyst formation

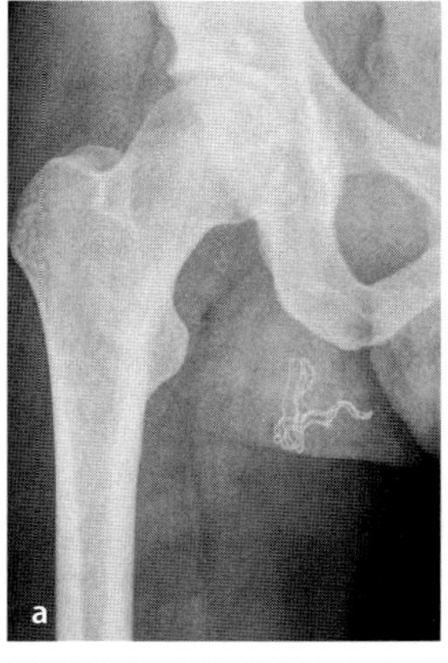
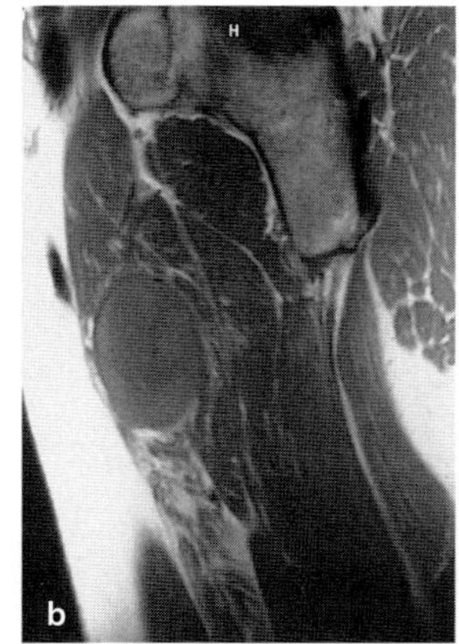
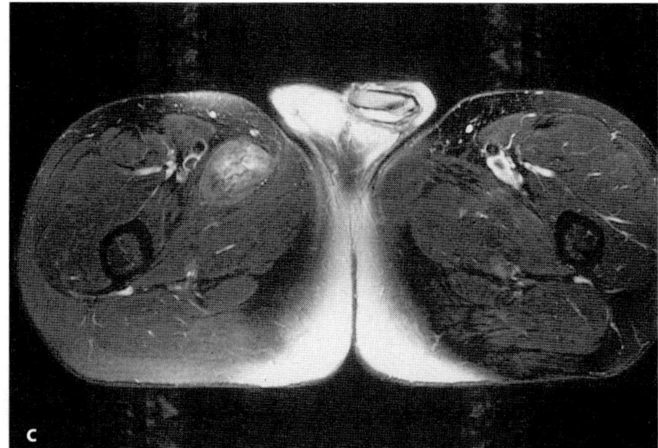
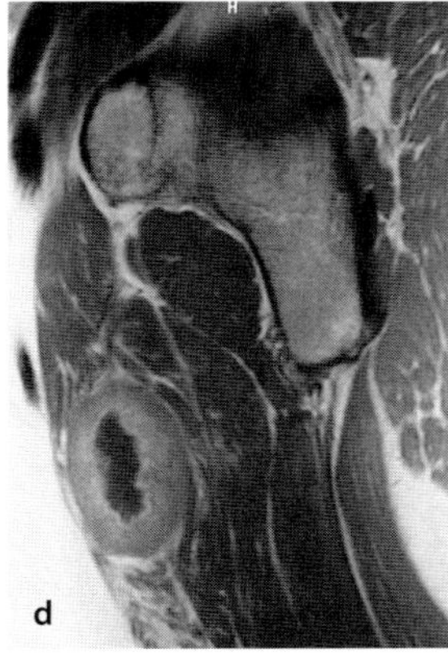

Fig. 24.31 a–d. Foreign body in a 31-year-old man with a textiloma (gossypiboma) three years after orthopedic surgery: **a** plain radiograph of the right proximal thigh; **b** sagittal spin echo T1-weighted MR image; **c** axial fat saturated turbo spin echo T2-weighted MR image; **d** Sagittal spin echo T1-weighted MR image after gadolinium contrast administration. Presence of a foreign body, corresponding with a retained surgical sponge (**a**). A well-circumscribed nodular lesion is seen at the anteromedial aspect of the right thigh, with a slight hypointense center on T1-weighted MR images (**b**). On T2-weighted MR images, the lesion is inhomogeneous and has a predominantly intermediate signal intensity (**c**). No sign of necrosis is observed. After gadolinium contrast administration, there is strong enhancement of the periphery of the lesion (**d**)

can induce a granulomatous reaction and present as subcutaneous soft tissue masses with high signal on T1-weighed images [69].

The foreign body reaction appears isointense to muscle on T1-weighted images and hyperintense compared to subcutaneous fat on T2-weighted images. It is usually seen as an elongated mass without well-defined margins and surrounded by edema, best seen on T2-weighted images. The foreign body itself is hypointense both on T1-weighted images and T2-weighted images [53, 64] (Fig. 24.31).

24.2.4.3 Calcific Myonecrosis

Calcific myonecrosis is an uncommon and late sequela of trauma, occurring with a reported delay ranging from 10 to 64 years after an initial traumatic event [48, 119]. The average age at the time of diagnosis is 56 years [48]. A fusiform soft tissue mass develops in the traumatized compartment, often mimicking a neoplastic process [65, 88, 129]. It is almost exclusively found in the lower extremities, especially in the anterior and lateral compartments of the leg. Other reported more unusual locations include the foot [48] and upper extremities [65].

The exact pathogenesis is still unknown. It usually occurs after trauma of the femur or tibia, with subsequent development of compartment syndrome, although it also can take place after neurovascular injury without compartment syndrome [65]. One hypothesis states that the occurrence of compartment syndrome leads to decreased regional circulation with necrosis and fibrosis [88]. The end result is cystic degeneration of the involved muscle, with plate-like calcification of a rind of fibrous tissue around the central liquefaction zone or hematoma. The expansive character of the lesion is believed to be secondary to intralesional hemorrhage [88]. Some investigators believe that pathologic processes like post-traumatic cysts of soft tissue, chronic expanding hematoma and calcific myonecrosis share a common pathophysiological mechanism [48]. Mentzel proposes the unifying term of 'ancient hematoma' to describe these entities [83].

Plain radiographs show a fusiform mass with plate- or plaque-like peripheral calcifications, which may precipitate in the cystic area of the lesion (Fig. 24.32a). Concomitant smooth bone erosions in adjacent bone may be present, usually with no or minimal periosteal reaction. However, erosions can be extensive thereby mimicking a soft tissue sarcoma. A liquid center can be seen on CT.

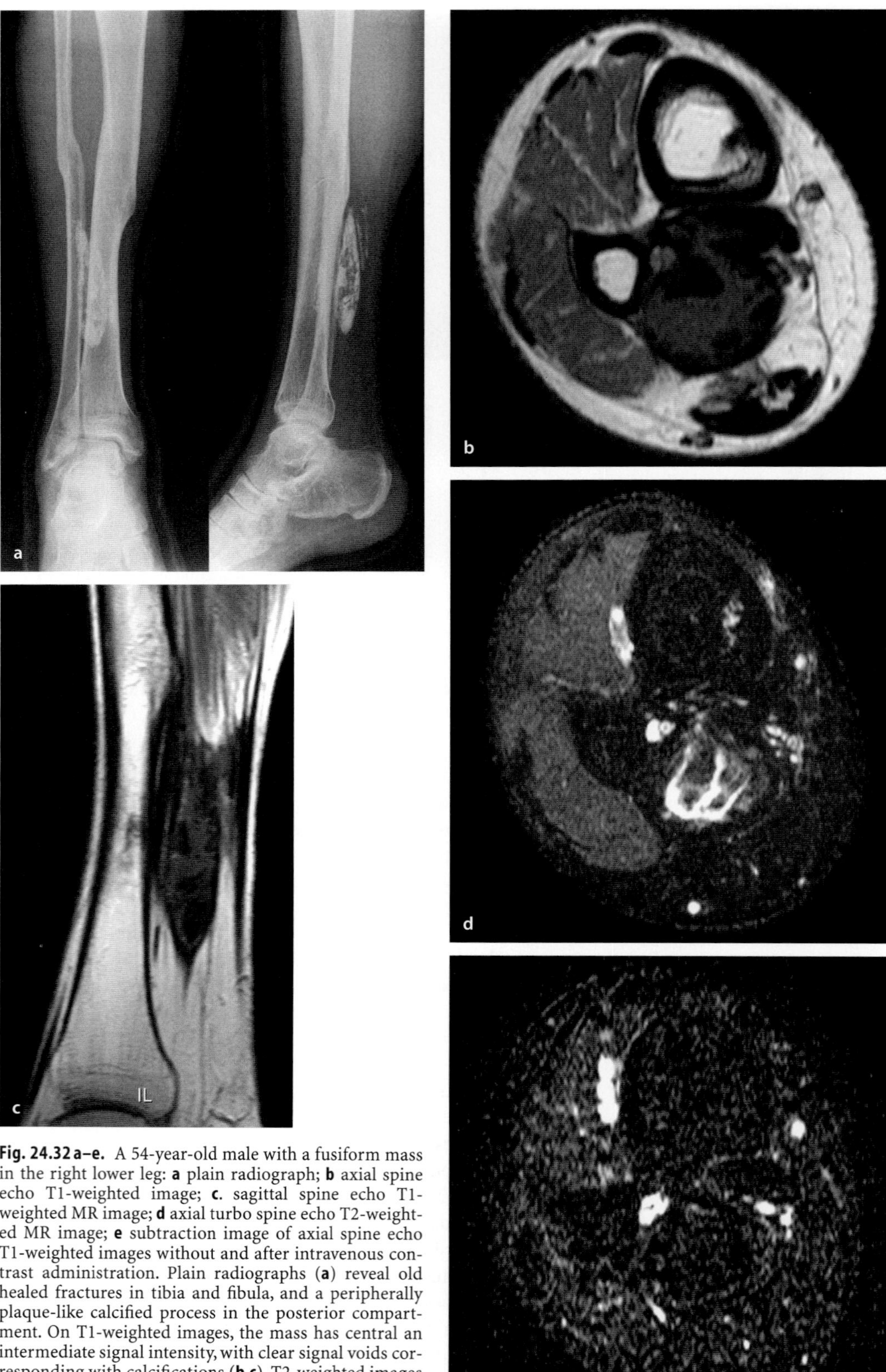

Fig. 24.32 a–e. A 54-year-old male with a fusiform mass in the right lower leg: **a** plain radiograph; **b** axial spine echo T1-weighted image; **c**. sagittal spine echo T1-weighted MR image; **d** axial turbo spine echo T2-weighted MR image; **e** subtraction image of axial spine echo T1-weighted images without and after intravenous contrast administration. Plain radiographs (**a**) reveal old healed fractures in tibia and fibula, and a peripherally plaque-like calcified process in the posterior compartment. On T1-weighted images, the mass has central an intermediate signal intensity, with clear signal voids corresponding with calcifications (**b,c**). T2-weighted images further demonstrate focal areas of bright signal, equivalent with fluid (**d**). No enhancement is noted after intravenous contrast administration (**e**)

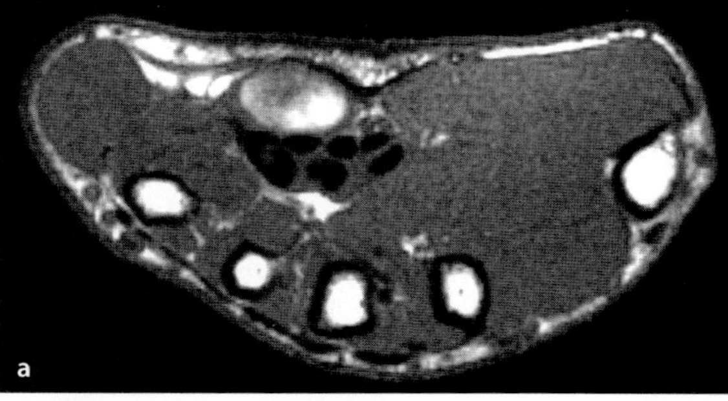
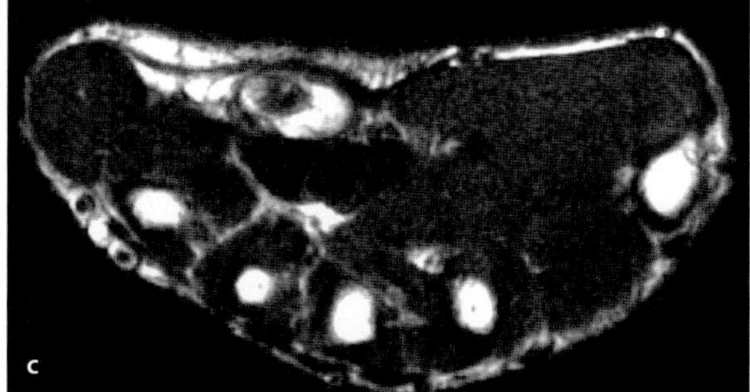
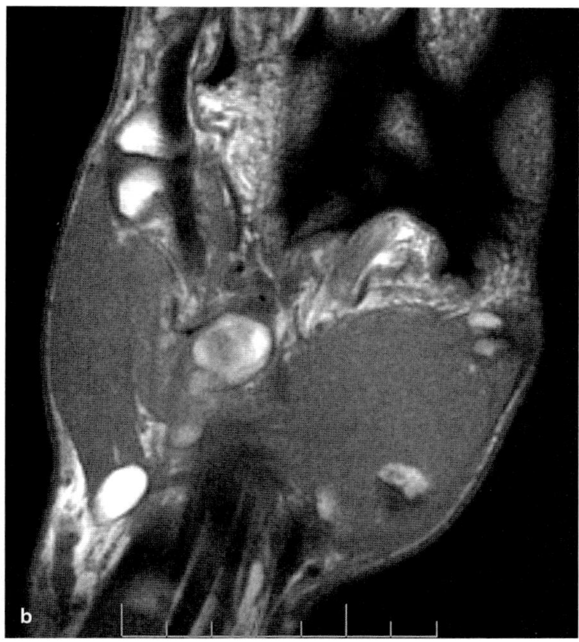

Fig. 24.33 a–c. A 40-year-old man with a painless pulsatile soft tissue swelling at the palmar side of the right hand: **a** axial spin echo T1-weighted MR image; **b** coronal spin echo T1-weighted MR image; **c** axial turbo spin echo T2-weighted MR image. The images reveal a mass in Guyon's canal, anteriorly to the retinaculum flexorum and posteriorly to the transverse ligament. The mass has two components; one which is of high signal intensity on both T1- and T2-weighted images, and another which is low on T2-weighted images and of intermediate signal intensity on T1-weighted images. The location of the lesion, the clinical presentation and history point to a pseudoaneurysm of the ulnar artery as seen in the hypothenar hammer syndrome

MR signal characteristics range from a homo- to heterogeneous soft tissue mass on T1- and T2-weighted images (Fig. 24.32b–e) [48, 65, 112, 119]. T1-weighed images reveal a fusiform mass with commonly intermediate signal intensity in the central fluid region. The mass appears rather heterogeneous on T2-weighted images, with focal bright areas of high signal consistent with fluid while the rest of the lesion demonstrates an intermediate signal intensity. Hypointense peripheral areas can be seen corresponding to signal void by the calcified outer layer. There is typically no enhancement after intravenous contrast administration.

Infection of the mass without recent surgical interventions is very rare but has been reported [48].

24.2.4.4 Hypothenar Hammer Syndrome

The hypothenar hammer syndrome is a rare clinical entity, with a typical presentation of unilateral digital ischemia due to embolic digital artery occlusion from a thrombosed palmar ulnar artery. It was initially described by Guttani (1772) and Von Rosen (1934), while the term was more recently first coined by Conn [25, 26]. It is commonly found in males around the age of 40 who usually in an occupational context repeatedly strike an object with the heel of the palm of the dominant hand. This causes damage to the superficial division of the distal ulnar artery as it passes over the hamate bone in the hypothenar region (Fig. 24.33).

While most cases are unilateral, Ferris found in a large series a striking incidence of similar changes in the asymptomatic and less traumatized hand [32]. Based on the findings in this series, he hypothesized that this syndrome occurs in persons with preexisting fibrodysplasia of the palmar ulnar artery, which are therefore more prone to develop artery damage when subjected to repetitive local trauma.

The diagnosis is mainly based clinical history and physical findings of unilateral digital ischemia. Angiography shows either segmental ulnar artery occlusion in the affected palm or 'corkscrew' elongation with alternating stenoses and ectasia [32]. Multiple digital artery occlusions are further demonstrated.

Treatment is mostly conservative, with surgery only used in rare instances.

24.2.5 Skin Lesions

24.2.5.1 Pilomatricoma

Pilomatricoma, formerly known as calcifying epithelioma of Malherbe, is a benign slow-growing superficial tumor of the hair follicle, most commonly seen in children and young adults [63]. The term "pilomatrixoma" was also previously used, better indicating its histological origin from hair matrix cells. The lesion is typically found (in decreasing order of prevalence) in the head, neck, upper extremities, trunk and lower extremities, presenting as a solitary subcutaneous calcified mass. Non-calcified pilomatricomas are also possible [79]. Most lesions are small, usually less than 3 cm, but larger masses have been reported [52]. A rare association of multiple pilomatricomas with myotonic dystrophy, Steinert disease, Turner syndrome, sarcoidosis and Gardner syndrome has been described [42, 63, 99].

MR images reveal a well-defined subcutaneous tumor, with intermediate signal intensity on T1-weighted images and low-to-intermediate signal intensity on gradient echo and T2-weighted images (Fig. 24.34) [28]. T2-weighted fat-suppressed images may show bands of hyperintense signal radiating away from a lower signal intensity center towards the periphery [47]. On gadolinium-enhanced T1-weighted images, enhancement is possible but not necessary [28, 47, 52, 79]. A possible inhomogeneous appearance is due to the amorphous calcification of the tumor.

A pilomatrix carcinoma is an uncommon aggressive form, representing up to 9% of benign pilomatricomas at any age [77]. Local invasion is possible, but distant metastasis is rare.

24.2.5.2 Granuloma Annulare

Granuloma annulare is a benign inflammatory dermatosis of unknown cause, characterized by formation of dermal papules that tend to form rings. It typically presents as a rapidly growing, solitary, painless, subcutaneous nodule without calcification in children less than five years old. In that population it is according to Kransdorf the most biopsied benign soft tissue mass in the lower extremity [58].

Clinically four forms can be distinguished: three cutaneous forms (erythematous, perforating and generalized) and the subcutaneous form. It is this latter form that can present as a soft tissue mass and requires local staging by imaging modalities.

Radiographs generally display a soft tissue mass of increased density in the subcutaneous compartment, without evidence of bone involvement or mineralization [60, 124]. Ultrasound reveals an ill-defined solid

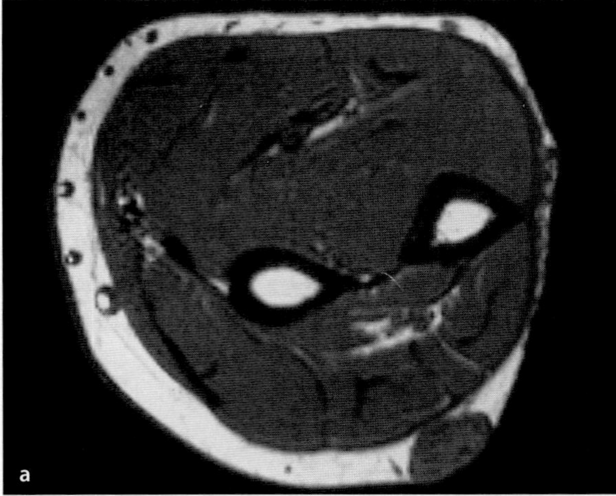

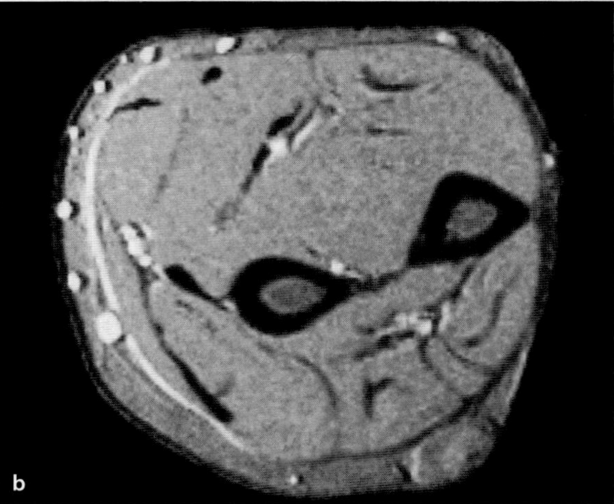

Fig. 24.34 a, b. A 60-year-old man with a subcutaneous lesion in the left lower arm: **a** axial spin echo T1-weighted MR image; **b** axial gradient echo T2-weighted MR image. The images reveal a well-defined nodular mass in the subcutaneous fat, with no specific signal characteristics (**a,b**). A biopsy confirmed the diagnosis of a pilomatricoma

mass that is hypoechoic to surrounding fat [124]. It excludes a vascular or cystic lesion [2].

The MR characteristics of subcutaneous granuloma annulare have been described by several authors [23, 60, 124]. T1-weighted images show an ill-defined subcutaneous mass, isointense to muscle, with a slightly hypointense signal intensity compared to fat on T2-weighted images (Fig. 24.35) [124]. These findings are conform the study of Kransdorf, who reported findings of relative decreased signal intensity on all pulse sequences [60]. Nevertheless, T2-weighted images may show a heterogeneous hyperintense lesion [23].

After intravenous contrast injection a diffuse enhancement can be seen.

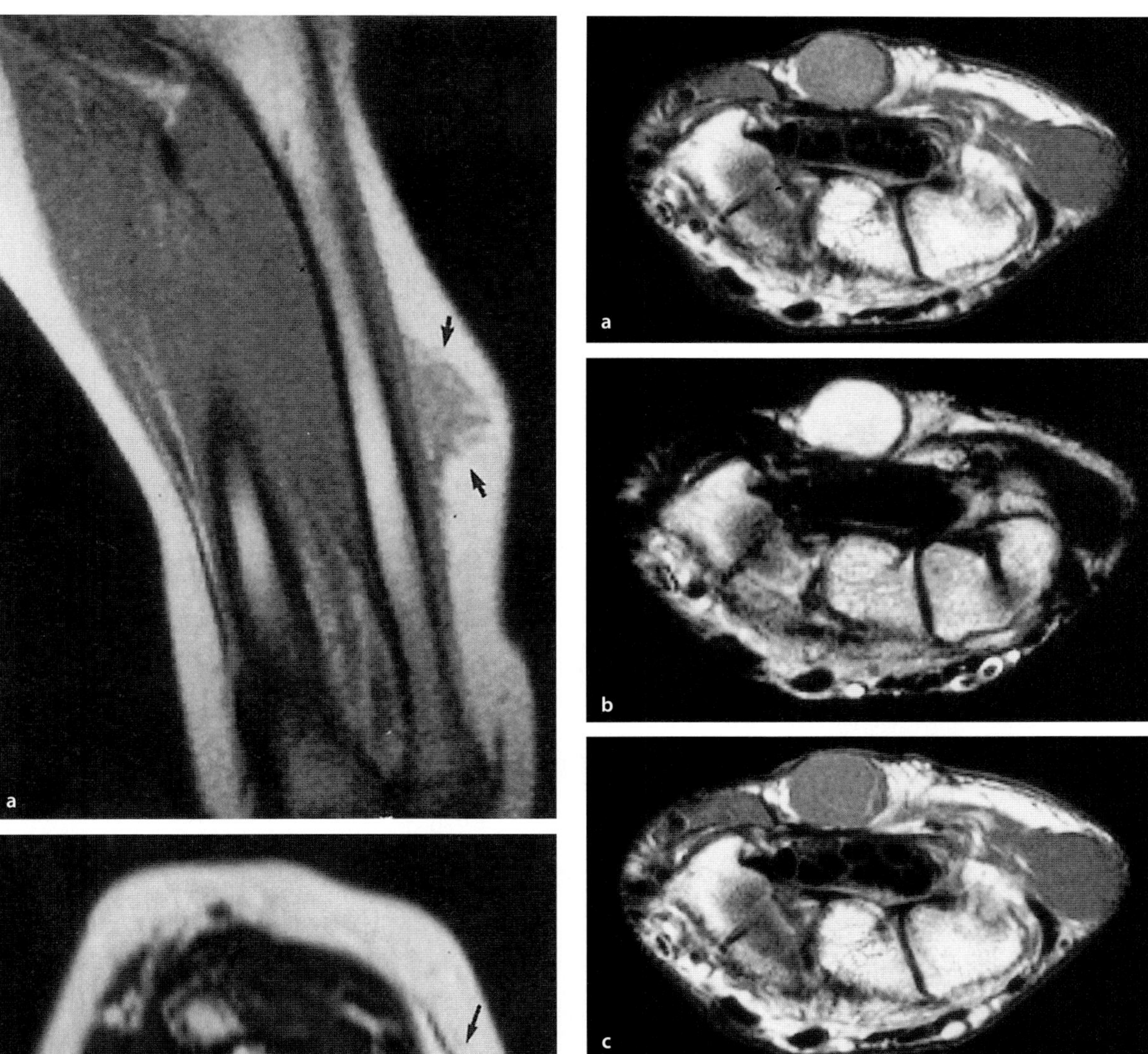

Fig. 24.36 a–c. A 35-year-old man with an epidermal inclusion cyst at the palmar aspect of the left wrist: **a** axial spin echo T1-weighted MR image; **b** axial turbo spin echo T2-weighted MR image; **c** axial spin echo T1-weighted MR image after gadolinium contrast administration. A well-circumscribed nodular lesion with low signal intensity on T1-weighted MR images (**a**), and high signal intensity on T2-weighted MR images (**b**) is seen. There is only slight peripheral enhancement after gadolinium contrast administration (**c**)

Fig. 24.35 a, b. A four-year-old girl with a small but rapidly growing nodule on the extensor aspect of the left forearm: **a** sagittal spin echo T1-weighted MR image; **b** axial spin echo T2-weighted MR image. The lesion appears isointense to muscle on T1-weighted images (**a**), with a small hyperintense peripheral rim on T2-weighted images (**b**). The peripheral high signal rim on T2-weighted images is suggestive for a small zone of perilesional edema. These findings are compatible with a subcutaneous Granuloma annulare in a child

24.2.5.3 Epidermal Inclusion Cyst (Infundibular Cyst)

Epidermal inclusion cysts are benign subcutaneous cysts formed by the cystic enclosure of epithelium within the dermis. They are filled with a mixture of keratin and lipid-rich debris [112]. Commonly they are iatrogenic [102], resulting from mechanical obstruction, scarring or inflammation [59]. Lesions can occur anywhere, but are mostly found in the head, neck and trunk. Less than 10% occur in the extremities [112].

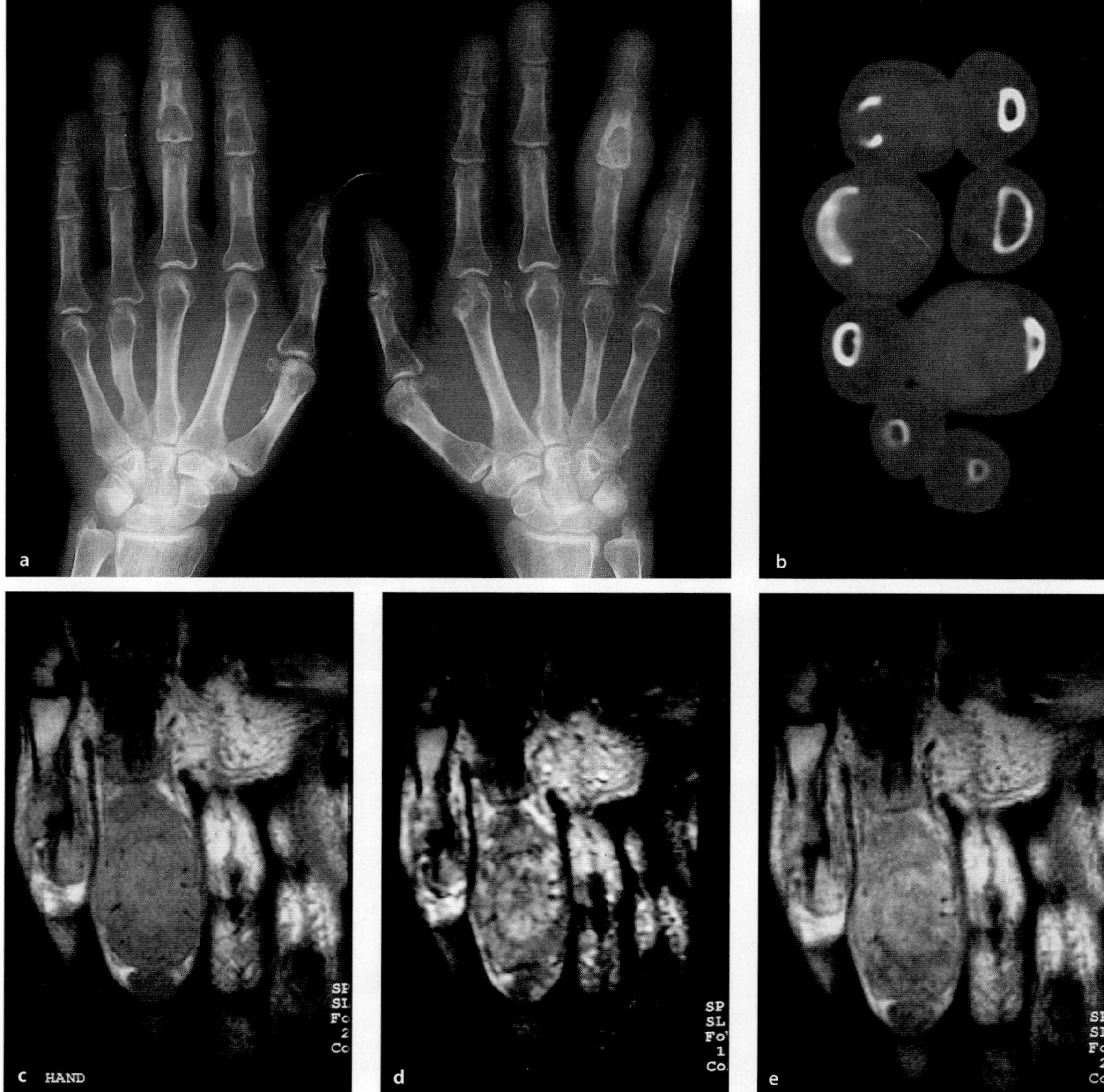

Fig. 24.37 a–e. Gout of both hands in a 65-year-old man: **a** plain radiograph; **b** CT scan; **c** coronal T1-weighted MR image; **d** coronal T2-weighted MR image; **e** coronal T1-weighted MR image after gadolinium contrast administration. Presence of soft tissue masses, multiple erosive lesions and ectopic calcifications on both hands (**a**). CT scan confirms the bone erosions and concomitant soft tissue masses (**b**). On MR imaging the tophi have an intermediate signal intensity on both T1- and T2-weighted MR images (**c, d**), showing enhancement after gadolinium contrast administration (**e**). Imaging characteristics of gouty tophi in a patient with clinical and biochemical evidence of gout

The MR findings resemble that of a simple cyst, with signal characteristics varying with the protein content of the cyst. High protein content can appear hyperintense to muscle on T1-weighted images. Cysts may rupture, provoking a foreign body reaction, granulomatous reaction or abscess formation (Fig. 24.36) [59]. On occasion, they may be multiloculated.

24.2.6 Crystal Depositions

24.2.6.1 Gout and Pseudogout

Gout is a metabolic disorder characterized by hyperuricemia and deposits of monosodium urate monohydrate crystals in periarticular soft tissues. In pseudogout, depositions consist of calcium pyrophosphate dihydrate crystals (CPPD). The disorders most frequently

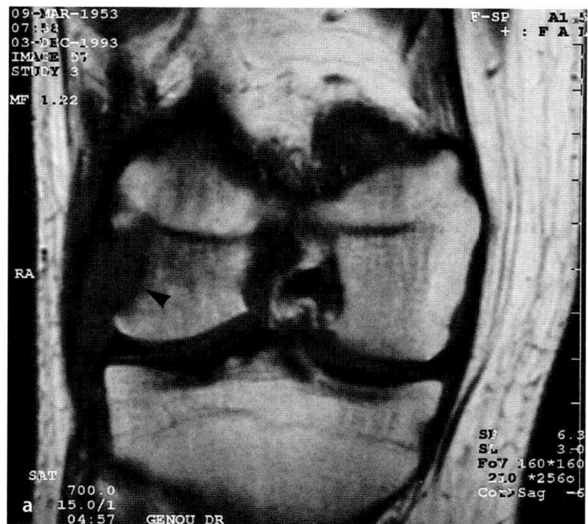

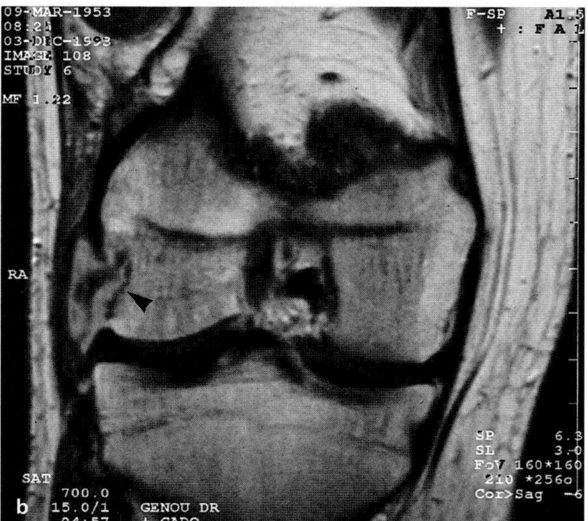

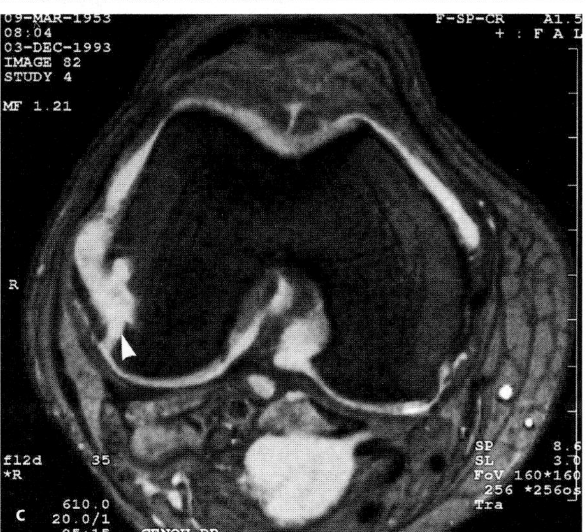

Fig. 24.38 a–c. Tophaceous gout of the knee in a 40-year-old man: **a** coronal spin echo T1-weighted MR image; **b** coronal spin echo T1-weighted MR image after gadolinium contrast injection; **c** axial gradient echo T2-weighted MR image. Presence of a mass lesion eroding the lateral femoral condyle. The lesion is of intermediate signal intensity on T1-weighted images and enhances markedly after contrast injection. The erosive character of the lesion and concomitant joint effusion are better appreciated on T2-weighted images. Presence of a Baker's cyst is a consequence of increased intraarticular pressure. This case is illustrative for a gouty arthritis with important synovial hypertrophy

affect the first metatarsophalangeal joint, followed by the ankle, knee, wrist, fingers and elbow. Clinical and radiographic findings are usually diagnostic (Figs. 24.37–24.39). On occasion, these conditions may present as s soft tissue mass [16]. Calcification of the mass is possible, more frequently seen in pseudogout.

The MR imaging features of gouty arthritis include synovial thickening and joint effusion [120]. Both conditions display a low to intermediate signal intensity on T1-weighted images [59, 120]. T2-weighted images characteristics vary from a heterogeneously hypointense to hyperintense mass on T2-weighted images [16, 59, 112], depending on the degree of inflammation. Diffuse enhancement after intravenous contrast injection may be seen [19] (Figs. 24.37–24.39).

24.2.6.2 Calcific Tendinosis

Calcific tendinosis, also known as calcific tendonitis or calcium hydroxyapatite disease, is a self-limiting inflammatory disorder, characterized by the deposition of hydroxyapatite crystals in tendons and periarticular soft tissue. It mostly seen in the shoulder, but other locations as hip, hand and wrist are also possible [59].

In an initial phase calcium deposits are contained within the tendons, producing no significant clinical symptoms [86]. As the deposits increases in size, the resultant increased tension in the tendon leads to pain. At this time a bursitis (e.g. in the shoulder) can also develop secondary to mass effect. This stage clinically often presents as an acute event, mimicking recent trauma. An adhesive periarthritis can subsequently develop.

Radiography has an important role, revealing amorphous calcification or a radio-opaque dense mass at the suspected site. Bone erosion of the adjacent cortical bone is not common but has been reported [22, 35], presumably secondary to inflammation at the tendon insertion or mass effect. This can lead to the wrong diagnosis of an aggressive neoplasm, especially when previous imaging studies are not available. While periarticular calcifications are typically encountered at the tendon attachment sites, they can occur in and around ligamentous structures with concomitant inflammation [3].

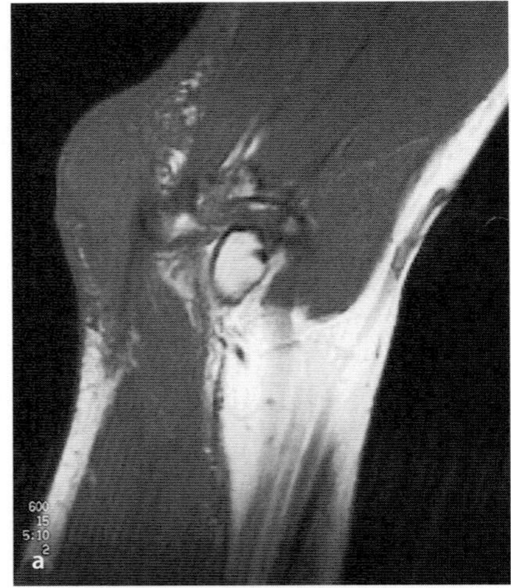

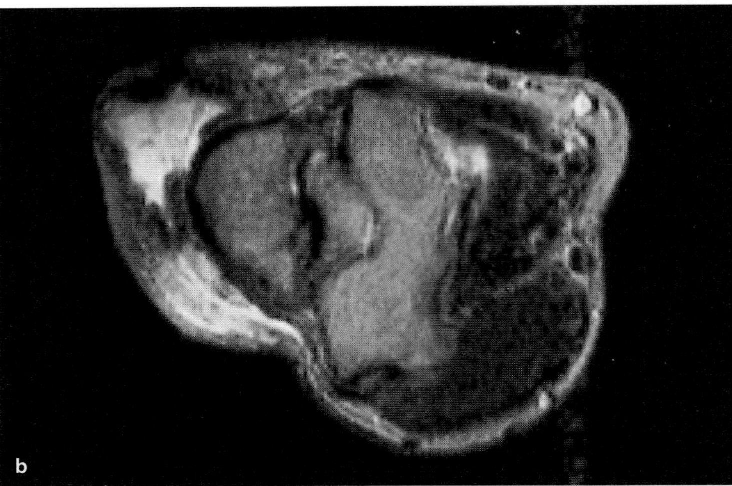

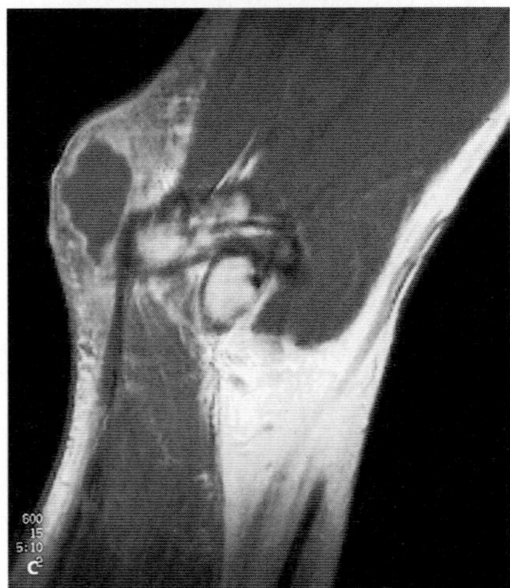

Fig. 24.39 a–c. Gouty bursitis of the elbow in a 60-year-old man: **a** sagittal spin echo T1-weighted MR image; **b** axial spin echo T2-weighted MR image; **c** sagittal spin echo T1-weighted MR image after gadolinium contrast injection. In the subcutis overlying the olecranon, there is a mass with intermediate signal intensity on T1-weighted images, high signal intensity at the center on T2-weighted images and with peripheral enhancement after contrast injection. MR images demonstrate increased amount of fluid and thickened vascularized wall in a case of gouty bursitis. Low signal intensity of the peripheral wall on T2-weighted images might be a consequence of hemosiderin and/or urate crystals

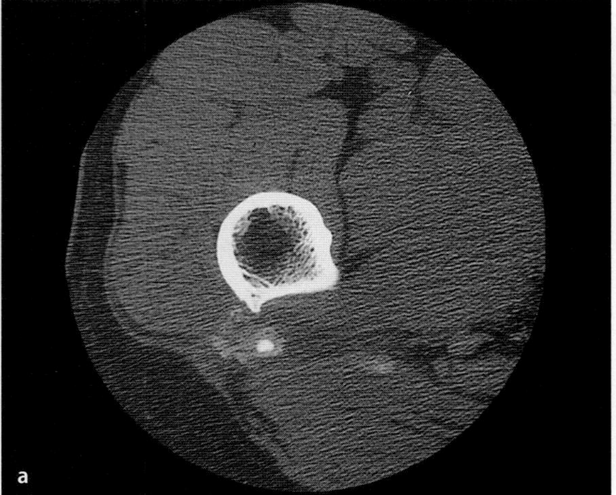

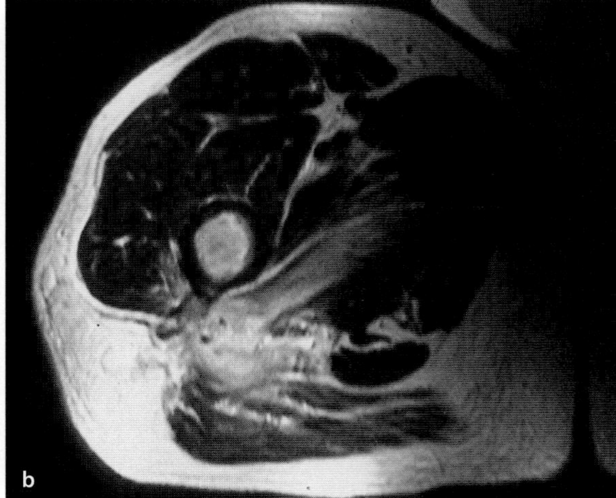

Fig. 24.40 a, b. A 47-year-old man with a painful right thigh, but no history of trauma: **a** CT scan; **b** axial turbo spin echo T2-weighted MR image. Multiple calcifications located posteriorly of the femur are present on CT scan (**a**). MR imaging reveals an ill-defined process of increased signal intensity at the gluteus mus-cles, with edema extending in the gluteus maximus, adductor magnus and vastus lateralis muscles. Multiple small soft tissue calcifications posterior form the linea aspera can be seen. These imaging findings are characteristic of calcific tendonitis of multiple muscles, mainly the right gluteus maximus muscle

Both T1- and T2-weighted images demonstrate a signal void in the area of calcification (Fig. 24.40). A high signal intensity in surrounding muscles related to edema can be seen on T2-weighted images [59, 112]. Bone marrow edema can also incidentally be found [22], on occasion mimicking an osseous metastasis [57, 127].

24.2.7 Vascular Lesions

Adventitial cystic disease of the popliteal artery is an unusual condition of uncertain etiology in which a mucin-containing cyst forms within the adventitia of the popliteal artery, narrowing the arterial lumen and causing symptoms of intermittent lower extremity claudication. Arteriography shows a focal, smoothly tapered stenosis of the popliteal artery at the level of the femoral condyles. Contrast-enhanced CT scan may show a non-enhancing cyst-like mass causing extrinsic compression of an enhancing arterial lumen, with rim enhancement after intravenous contrast administration [59, 112]. MR imaging may reveal cyst-like structures closely invested in a compressed artery, with no specific signal intensity (Fig. 24.41). Today, MR angiography is a valuable non-invasive imaging modality in the evaluation of these lesions.

The presence of a pulsatile mass with bruit in close proximity to an artery in a patient with a history of trauma suggests the diagnosis of aneurysm. Likewise, when a soft tissue tumor entirely surrounds and obliterates a major artery, an aneurysm or a pseudoaneurysm should be considered. Peripheral arterial aneurysms are most commonly found in the popliteal artery, often in association with widespread atherosclerotic disease.

An aneurysm or pseudoaneurysm is recognized on MR by the following features: signal void in regions of flowing blood, hyperintensity on T1- and T2-weighted images due to subacute hemorrhage, and hypointense areas caused by hemosiderin deposits [59]. Moreover, MR imaging demonstrates a characteristic flow-related artifact in the direction of the phase encoding gradient [114]. A major vein engulfed by or adjacent to a mass should evoke a lesion of venous origin [114].

Congenital arteriovenous malformations are characterized by dilated, tortuous blood vessels, infiltrating muscles. Posttraumatic acquired arteriovenous malformations have also been reported [24]. On MR imaging, the appearance of an arteriovenous malformation is similar on T1- and T2-weighted images and is characterized by hypointense, serpiginous blood vessels of low signal intensity due to flow-void effects [24].

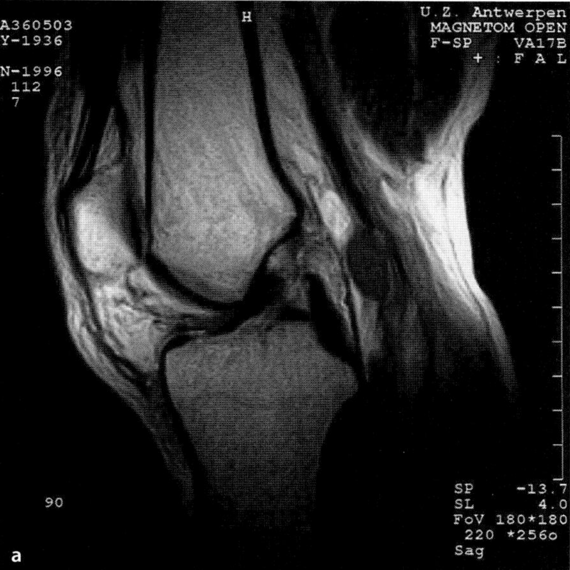

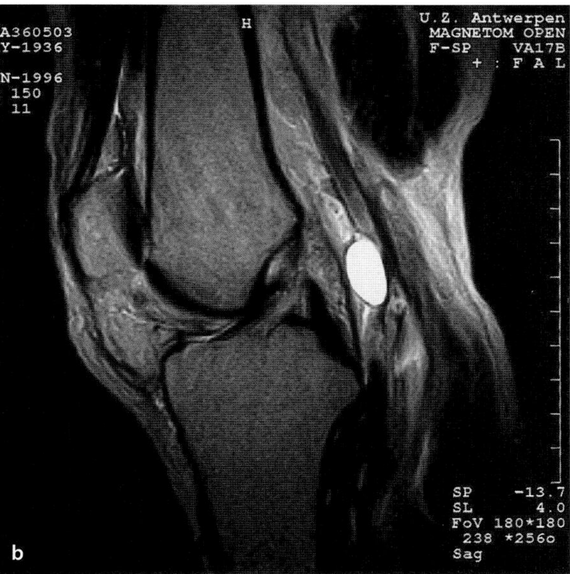

Fig. 24.41 a, b. A 46-year-old man with claudicatio intermittens: **a** axial spin echo T1-weighted MR image; **b** axial turbo spin echo T2-weighted MR image. MR imaging reveals a well-defined cystic process around the popliteal artery, hypointense on T1-weighted images (**a**), and hyperintense on T2-weighted images (**b**). These findings are suggestive for an adventitial cyst around the popliteal artery

Things to remember:

1. As demonstrated, soft tissue pseudotumors encompass a vast range of pathologies varying from normal anatomic variants, inflammatory and infectious lesions, posttraumatic masses and other. Knowledge of the common presentation of these entities in combination with relevant clinical findings can direct the clinician to the correct diagnosis, thereby limiting the need for invasive procedures in these often reactive benign lesions. The radiological approach of soft tissue pseudotumors thereby is no different than for their 'true' tumoral counterparts.

2. Finally, when confronted with a mass with undetermined imaging characteristics, an infectious or inflammatory origin has always to be included in the differential diagnosis.

References

1. Abi F, el Fares F, Khaiz D, Bouzidi A (1989) Unusual localizations of hydatid cysts. Apropos of 40 cases. J Chir (Paris) 5:307–312
2. AbiEzzi SS, Miller LS (1995) The use of ultrasound for the diagnosis of soft-tissue masses in children. J Pediatr Orthop 5:566–573
3. Anderson SE, Bosshard C, Steinbach LS, Ballmer FT (2003) MR imaging of calcification of the lateral collateral ligament of the knee: a rare abnormality and a cause of lateral knee pain. Am J Roentgenol 1:199–202
4. Aoki T, Nakata H, Watanabe H, Maeda H, Toyonaga T, Hashimoto H, Nakamura T (1999) The radiological findings in chronic expanding hematoma. Skeletal Radiol 7:396–401
5. Beauchamp NJ Jr, Scott WW Jr, Gottlieb LM, Fishman EK (1995) CT evaluation of soft tissue and muscle infection and inflammation: a systematic compartmental approach. Skeletal Radiol 5:317–324
6. Beltran J (1995) MR imaging of soft-tissue infection. Magn Reson Imaging Clin North Am 4:743–751
7. Berchtenbreiter C, Bruning R, Auernhammer A, Reiser M (1999) Misleading diagnosis of retroperitoneal actinomycosis. Eur Radiol 9:1869–1872
8. Berg LC, Norelle A, Morgan WA, Washa DM (1998) Cat-scratch disease simulating Histiocytosis X. Hum Pathol 6:649–651
9. Berquist TH, Ehman RL, King BF, Hodgman CG, Ilstrup DM (1990) Value of MR imaging in differentiating benign from malignant soft-tissue masses: study of 95 lesions. Am J Roentgenol 6:1251–1255
10. Boothroyd AE, Carty H (1995) The painless soft tissue mass in childhood – tumour or not? Postgrad Med J 831:10–16
11. Braunstein JT, Crues JV III (1995) Magnetic resonance imaging of hereditary hernias of the peroneus longus muscle. Skeletal Radiol 8:601–604
12. Brown JR (1973) Human actinomycosis. A study of 181 subjects. Hum Pathol 3:319–330
13. Bush CH (2000) The magnetic resonance imaging of musculoskeletal hemorrhage. Skeletal Radiol 1:1–9
14. Cangiotti L, Muiesan P, Begni A, de Cesare V, Pouche A, Giulini SM, Tiberio G (1994) Unusual localizations of hydatid disease: an 18 year experience. G Chir 3:83–86
15. Cardinal E, Chhem RK, Beauregard CG (1998) Ultrasound-guided interventional procedures in the musculoskeletal system. Radiol Clin North Am 3:597–604
16. Chaoui A, Garcia J, Kurt AM (1997) Gouty tophus simulating soft tissue tumor in a heart transplant recipient. Skeletal Radiol 10:626–628
17. Chason DP, Fleckenstein JL, Burns DK, Rojas G (1996) Diabetic muscle infarction: radiologic evaluation. Skeletal Radiol 2:127–132
18. Chauhan S, Jain S, Varma S, Chauhan SS (2004) Tropical pyomyositis (myositis tropicans): current perspective. Postgrad Med J 943:267–270
19. Chen CK, Yeh LR, Pan HB, Yang CF, Lu YC, Wang JS, Resnick D (1999) Intra-articular gouty tophi of the knee: CT and MR imaging in 12 patients. Skeletal Radiol 2:75–80
20. Chevalier X, Rhamouni A, Bretagne S, Martigny J, Larget-Piet B (1994) Hydatid cyst of the subcutaneous tissue without other involvement: MR imaging features. Am J Roentgenol 3:645–646
24. Christin L, Sarosi GA (1992) Pyomyositis in North America: case reports and review. Clin Infect Dis 4:668–677
22. Chung CB, Gentili A, Chew FS (2004) Calcific tendinosis and periarthritis: classic magnetic resonance imaging appearance and associated findings. J Comput Assist Tomogr 3:390–396
23. Chung S, Frush DP, Prose NS, Shea CR, Laor T, Bisset GS (1999) Subcutaneous granuloma annulare: MR imaging features in six children and literature review. Radiology 3:845–849
24. Cohen JM, Weinreb JC, Redman HC (1986) Arteriovenous malformations of the extremities: MR imaging. Radiology 2:475–479
25. Conn J Jr, Bergan JJ, Bell JL (1970) Hand ischemia: hypothenar hammer syndrome. Proc Inst Med Chic 2:83
26. Conn J Jr, Bergan JJ, Bell JL (1970) Hypothenar hammer syndrome: posttraumatic digital ischemia. Surgery 6:1122–1128
27. De Beuckeleer L, Vanhoenacker F, De Schepper A Jr, Seynaeve P, De Schepper A (1999) Hypertrophy and pseudohypertrophy of the lower leg following chronic radiculopathy and neuropathy: imaging findings in two patients. Skeletal Radiol 4:229–232
28. De Beuckeleer LH, De Schepper AM, Neetens I (1996) Magnetic resonance imaging of pilomatricoma. Eur Radiol 1:72–75
29. Delaney-Sathy LO, Fessell DP, Jacobson JA, Hayes CW (2000) Sonography of diabetic muscle infarction with MR imaging, CT, and pathologic correlation. Am J Roentgenol 1:165–169
30. Dong PR, Seeger LL, Yao L, Panosian CB, Johnson BL Jr, Eckardt JJ (1995) Uncomplicated cat-scratch disease: findings at CT, MR imaging, and radiography. Radiology 3:837–839
31. Ekstrom JE, Shuman WP, Mack LA (1990) MR imaging of accessory soleus muscle. J Comput Assist Tomogr 2:239–242
32. Ferris BL, Taylor LM Jr, Oyama K, McLafferty RB, Edwards JM, Moneta GL, Porter JM (2000) Hypothenar hammer syndrome: proposed etiology. J Vasc Surg 1(1):104–113
33. Flaisler F, Blin D, Asencio G, Lopez FM, Combe B (1993) Focal myositis: a localized form of polymyositis? J Rheumatol 8:1414–1416
34. Fleckenstein JL, Burns DK, Murphy FK, Jayson HT, Bonte FJ (1991) Differential diagnosis of bacterial myositis in AIDS: evaluation with MR imaging. Radiology 3:653–658
35. Flemming DJ, Murphey MD, Shekitka KM, Temple HT, Jelinek JJ, Kransdorf MJ (2003) Osseous involvement in calcific tendinitis: a retrospective review of 50 cases. Am J Roentgenol 4:965–972
36. Floemer F, Morrison WB, Bongartz G, Ledermann HP (2004) MRI characteristics of olecranon bursitis. Am J Roentgenol 1:29–34
37. Garcia-Diez AI, Ros Mendoza LH, Villacampa VM, Cozar M, Fuertes MI (2000) MRI evaluation of soft tissue hydatid disease. Eur Radiol 3:462–466
38. Gielen J, Wang XL, Vanhoenacker F, De Schepper H, De Beuckeleer L, Vandevenne J, De Schepper A (2003) Lymphadenopathy at the medial epitrochlear region in cat-scratch disease. Eur Radiol 6:1363–1369
39. Gielen JL, De Schepper AM, Parizel PM, Wang XL, Vanhoenacker F (2003) Additional value of magnetic resonance with spin echo T1-weighted imaging with fat suppression in characterization of soft tissue tumors. J Comput Assist Tomogr 3:434–441

40. Giron GL, Friedman I, Feldman S (2004) Lobular carcinoma in ectopic axillary breast tissue. Am Surg 4:312–315
41. Graif M, Schweitzer ME, Deely D, Matteucci T (1999) The septic versus nonseptic inflamed joint: MRI characteristics. Skeletal Radiol 11:616–620
42. Harper PS (1972) Calcifying epithelioma of Malherbe. Association with myotonic muscular dystrophy. Arch Dermatol 1:41–44
43. Heckmann JG, Stefan H, Heuss D, Hopp P, Neundorfer B (2001) Isolated muscular sarcoidosis. Eur J Neurol 4:365–366
44. Heffner RR Jr, Armbrustmacher VW, Earle KM (1977) Focal myositis. Cancer 1:301–306
45. Hernandez RJ, Keim DR, Chenevert TL, Sullivan DB, Aisen AM (1992) Fat-suppressed MR imaging of myositis. Radiology 1:247–249
46. Hernandez RJ, Sullivan DB, Chenevert TL, Keim DR (1993) MR imaging in children with dermatomyositis: musculoskeletal findings and correlation with clinical and laboratory findings. Am J Roentgenol 2:359–366
47. Hoffmann V, Roeren T, Moller P, Heuschen G (1998) MR imaging of a pilomatrixoma. Pediatr Radiol 4:272
48. Holobinko JN, Damron TA, Scerpella PR, Hojnowski L (2003) Calcific myonecrosis: keys to early recognition. Skeletal Radiol 1:35–40
49. Hopkins KL, Li KC, Bergman G (1995) Gadolinium-DTPA-enhanced magnetic resonance imaging of musculoskeletal infectious processes. Skeletal Radiol 5:325–330
50. Hopkins KL, Simoneaux SF, Patrick LE, Wyly JB, Dalton MJ, Snitzer JA (1996) Imaging manifestations of cat-scratch disease. Am J Roentgenol 2:435–438
51. Hovi I, Hekali P, Korhola O, Valtonen M, Valtonen V, Taavitsainen M, Kivisaari A, Hopfner-Hallikainen D, Raininko R, Porkka L et al. (1989) Detection of soft-tissue and skeletal infections with ultra low-field (0.02 T) MR imaging. Acta Radiol 5:495–499
52. Ichikawa T, Nakajima Y, Fujimoto H, Koyama A, Honma M, Yatsuzuka M, Ohtomo K, Uchiyama G, Ushigome S, Ohba S (1997) Giant calcifying epithelioma of Malherbe (pilomatrixoma): imaging features. Skeletal Radiol 10:602–605
53. Jelinek J, Kransdorf MJ (1995) MR imaging of soft-tissue masses. Mass-like lesions that simulate neoplasms. Magn Reson Imaging Clin North Am 4:727–741
54. Jelinek JS, Murphey MD, Aboulafia AJ, Dussault RG, Kaplan PA, Snearly WN (1999) Muscle infarction in patients with diabetes mellitus: MR imaging findings. Radiology 1:241–247
55. Khoury NJ, el-Khoury GY, Kathol MH (1997) MRI diagnosis of diabetic muscle infarction: report of two cases. Skeletal Radiol 2:122–127
56. King RJ, Laugharne D, Kerslake RW, Holdsworth BJ (2003) Primary obturator pyomyositis: a diagnostic challenge. J Bone Joint Surg Br 6:895–898
57. Kraemer EJ, El-Khoury GY (2000) Atypical calcific tendinitis with cortical erosions. Skeletal Radiol 12:690–696
58. Kransdorf MJ (1995) Benign soft-tissue tumors in a large referral population: distribution of specific diagnoses by age, sex, and location. Am J Roentgenol 2:395–402
59. Kransdorf MJ (1997) Imaging of soft tissue tumors:masses that may mimic soft tissue tumors. In: Kransdorf MJ (ed) Imaging of soft tissue tumors, 1st edn. Saunders, Philadeplhia
60. Kransdorf MJ, Murphey MD, Temple HT (1998) Subcutaneous granuloma annulare: radiologic appearance. Skeletal Radiol 5:266–270
61. Kransdorf MJ, Temple HT, Sweet DE (1998) Focal myositis. Skeletal Radiol 5:283–287
62. Kumar A, Detrisac DA, Krecke CF, Jimenez MC (1991) Actinomycosis of the thigh presenting as a soft-tissue neoplasm. J Infect 2:187–190
63. Lan MY, Lan MC, Ho CY, Li WY, Lin CZ (2003) Pilomatricoma of the head and neck: a retrospective review of 179 cases. Arch Otolaryngol Head Neck Surg 12:1327–1330
64. Laor T, Barnewolt CE (1999) Nonradiopaque penetrating foreign body: "a sticky situation". Pediatr Radiol 9:702–704
65. Larson RC, Sierra RJ, Sundaram M, Inwards C, Scully SP (2004) Calcific myonecrosis: a unique presentation in the upper extremity. Skeletal Radiol 5:306–309
66. Larsson LG, Baum J (1986) The syndromes of bursitis. Bull Rheum Dis 1:1–8
67. Lebon C, Malghem J, Lecouvet F, Vande Berg B, Maldague B (2003) Pseudotumeurs des parties molles. In: Encycl Méd Chir, Editions Scientifices et Médicales. Elsevier SAS, Paris
68. Lee DJ, Sartoris DJ (1994) Musculoskeletal manifestations of human immunodeficiency virus infection: review of imaging characteristics. Radiol Clin North Am 2:399–411
69. Lee SY, Lee NH, Chung MJ, Chung GH (2004) Foreign-body granuloma caused by dispersed oil droplets simulating subcutaneous fat tissue on MR images. AJR Am J Roentgenol 4:1090–1091
70. Lesavoy MA, Gomez-Garcia A, Nejdl R, Yospur G, Syiau TJ, Chang P (1995) Axillary breast tissue: clinical presentation and surgical treatment. Ann Plast Surg 4:356–360
71. Lewis EJ, Crutchfield CE III, Ebertz MJ, Prawer SE (1998) Report of a nipple nevus and an overview of accessory mammary tissue. Cutis 5:243–246
72. Liu GC, Jong YJ, Chiang CH, Jaw TS (1993) Duchenne muscular dystrophy: MR grading system with functional correlation. Radiology 2:475–480
73. Liu NF, Wang CG (1998) The role of magnetic resonance imaging in diagnosis of peripheral lymphatic disorders. Lymphology 3:119–127
74. Loh NN, Ch'en IY, Cheung LP, Li KC (1997) Deep fascial hyperintensity in soft-tissue abnormalities as revealed by T2-weighted MR imaging. Am J Roentgenol 5:1301–1304
75. Major NM, Tehranzadeh J (1997) Musculoskeletal manifestations of AIDS. Radiol Clin North Am 5:1167–1189
76. Margileth AM (1993) Cat scratch disease. Adv Pediatr Infect Dis 1–24
77. Marrogi AJ, Wick MR, Dehner LP (1992) Pilomatrical neoplasms in children and young adults. Am J Dermatopathol 2:87–94
78. Martin J, Marco V, Zidan A, Marco C (1993) Hydatid disease of the soft tissues of the lower limb: findings in three cases. Skeletal Radiol 7:511–514
79. Masih S, Sorenson SM, Gentili A, Seeger LL (2000) Atypical adult non-calcified pilomatricoma. Skeletal Radiol 1:54–56
80. Matsuo M, Ehara S, Tamakawa Y, Chida E, Nishida J, Sugai T (1995) Muscular sarcoidosis. Skeletal Radiol 7:535–537
81. Mellado JM, Perez del Palomar L (1999) Muscle hernias of the lower leg: MRI findings. Skeletal Radiol 8:465–469
82. Memis A, Arkun R, Bilgen I, Ustun EE (1999) Primary soft tissue hydatid disease: report of two cases with MRI characteristics. Eur Radiol 6:1101–1103
83. Mentzel T, Goodlad JR, Smith MA, Fletcher CD (1997) Ancient hematoma: a unifying concept for a post-traumatic lesion mimicking an aggressive soft tissue neoplasm. Mod Pathol 4:334–340
84. Monu JU, McManus CM, Ward WG, Haygood TM, Pope TL Jr, Bohrer SP (1995) Soft-tissue masses caused by long-standing foreign bodies in the extremities: MR imaging findings. Am J Roentgenol 2:395–397
85. Moore SL, Teirstein AE (2003) Musculoskeletal sarcoidosis: spectrum of appearances at MR imaging. Radiographics 6:1389–1399
86. Moseley HF (1963) The natural history and clinical syndromes produced by calcified deposits in the rotator cuff. Surg Clin North Am 1489–1493
87. Nguyen B, Brandser E, Rubin DA (2000) Pains, strains, and fasciculations: lower extremity muscle disorders. Magn Reson Imaging Clin North Am 2:391–408
88. O'Keefe RJ, O'Connell JX, Temple HT, Scully SP, Kattapuram SV, Springfield DS, Rosenberg AE, Mankin HJ (1995) Calcific myonecrosis. A late sequela to compartment syndrome of the leg. Clin Orthop 318:205–243
89. Otake S (1994) Sarcoidosis involving skeletal muscle: imaging findings and relative value of imaging procedures. Am J Roentgenol 2:369–375
90. Otake S, Banno T, Ohba S, Noda M, Yamamoto M (1990) Muscular sarcoidosis: findings at MR imaging. Radiology 1:145–148

91. Otake S, Imagumbai N, Suzuki M, Ohba S (1998) MR imaging of muscular sarcoidosis after steroid therapy. Eur Radiol 9:1651–1653

92. Palaniappan M, Rajesh A, Rickett A, Kershaw CJ (1999) Accessory soleus muscle: a case report and review of the literature. Pediatr Radiol 8:610–612

93. Palmer GW, Greco TP (2001) Diabetic thigh muscle infarction in association with antiphospholipid antibodies. Semin Arthritis Rheum 4:272–280

94. Parizel PM, Makkat S, Van Miert E, Van Goethem JW, van den Hauwe L, De Schepper AM (2001) Intracranial hemorrhage: principles of CT and MRI interpretation. Eur Radiol 9:1770–1783

95. Park JK, Lee HK, Ha HK, Choi HY, Choi CG (2003) Cervicofacial actinomycosis: CT and MR imaging findings in seven patients. Am J Neuroradiol 3:331–335

96. Patel SR, Olenginski TP, Perruquet JL, Harrington TM (1997) Pyomyositis: clinical features and predisposing conditions. J Rheumatol 9:1734–1738

97. Polat P, Kantarci M, Alper F, Suma S, Koruyucu MB, Okur A (2003) Hydatid disease from head to toe. Radiographics 2:475–494; quiz 536–477

98. Pretorius ES, Hruban RH, Fishman EK (1996) Tropical pyomyositis: imaging findings and a review of the literature. Skeletal Radiol 6:576–579

99. Pujol RM, Casanova JM, Egido R, Pujol J, de Moragas JM (1995) Multiple familial pilomatricomas: a cutaneous marker for Gardner syndrome? Pediatr Dermatol 4:331–335

100. Rahmouni A, Chosidow O, Mathieu D, Gueorguieva E, Jazaerli N, Radier C, Faivre JM, Roujeau JC, Vasile N (1994) MR imaging in acute infectious cellulitis. Radiology 2:493–496

101. Reid JD, Kommareddi S, Lankerani M, Park MC (1980) Chronic expanding hematomas. A clinicopathologic entity. J Am Med Accoc 24:2441–2442

102. Reinherz RP (1993) Epidermal inclusion cysts. J Foot Ankle Surg 3:247

103. Resendes M, Helms CA, Fritz RC, Genant H (1992) MR appearance of intramuscular injections. Am J Roentgenol 6:1293–1294

104. Restrepo CS, Lemos DF, Gordillo H, Odero R, Varghese T, Tiemann W, Rivas FF, Moncada R, Gimenez CR (2004) Imaging findings in musculoskeletal complications of AIDS. Radiographics 4:1029–1049

105. Sakayama K, Fujibuchi T, Sugawara Y, Kidani T, Miyawaki J, Yamamoto H (2004) A 40-year-old gossypiboma (foreign body granuloma) mimicking a malignant femoral surface tumor. Skeletal Radiol (Sep 8 - Epub ahead of print)

106. Schmid MR, Kossmann T, Duewell S (1998) Differentiation of necrotizing fasciitis and cellulitis using MR imaging. Am J Roentgenol 3:615–620

107. Schoenberg NY, Beltran J (1994) Contrast enhancement in musculoskeletal imaging. Current status. Radiol Clin North Am 2:337–352

108. Scully RE, Mark EJ, McNeely WF, Ebeling SH, Phillips LD (1997) Case records of the Massachusetts General Hospital. Weekly clinicopathological exercises. Case 20-1997. A 74-year-old man with progressive cough, dyspnea, and pleural thickening. N Engl J Med 26:1895–1903

109. Sharma P, Mangwana S, Kapoor RK (2000) Diabetic muscle infarction: atypical MR appearance. Skeletal Radiol 8:477–480

110. Smith JW (1995) Infectious arthritis. In: Mandell GL BJ, Dolin R (eds) Mandell, Douglas and Bennett's principles and practice of infectious diseases, 4th edn. Churchill Livingstone, New York

111. Spengos K, Wohrle JC, Binder J, Schwartz A, Hennerici M (2000) Bilateral diabetic infarction of the anterior tibial muscle. Diabetes Care 5:699–701

112. Stoker DJ, Saifuddin A (1999) The radiologic features of nonneoplastic tumors of soft tissue. Semin Musculoskelet Radiol 1:81–96

113. Streichenberger N, Meyronet D, Fiere V, Pellissier JF, Petiot P (2004) Focal myositis associated with S-1 radiculopathy: report of two cases. Muscle Nerve 3:443–446

114. Sundaram M, Sharafuddin MJ (1995) MR imaging of benign soft-tissue masses. Magn Reson Imaging Clin North Am 4:609–627

115. Tacal T, Altinok D, Yildiz YT, Altinok G (2000) Coexistence of intramuscular hydatid cyst and tapeworm. Am J Roentgenol 2:575–576

116. Tohme-Noun C, Le Breton C, Sobotka A, Boumenir Z, Milleron B, Carette M, Khalil A (2004) Imaging findings in three cases of the nodular type of muscular sarcoidosis. Am J Roentgenol 995–999

117. Trujillo-Santos AJ (2003) Diabetic muscle infarction: an underdiagnosed complication of long-standing diabetes. Diabetes Care 1:241–245

118. Trusen A, Beissert M, Schultz G, Chittka B, Darge K (2003) Ultrasound and MRI features of pyomyositis in children. Eur Radiol 5:1050–1055

119. Tuncay IC, Demirors H, Isiklar ZU, Agildere M, Demirhan B, Tandogan RN (1999) Calcific myonecrosis. Int Orthop 1:68–70

120. Van Slyke MA, Moser RP Jr, Madewell JE (1995) MR imaging of periarticular soft-tissue lesions. Magn Reson Imaging Clin North Am 4:651–667

124. Vandevenne JE, Colpaert CG, De Schepper AM (1998) Subcutaneous granuloma annulare: MR imaging and literature review. Eur Radiol 8:1363–1365

122. Vanhoenacker P, Brijs S, Geusens E, De Man R, Dujardin P, Tanghe W (1994) MR imaging of primary muscular sarcoidosis. Case report. Rofo 6:570–571

123. Wall SD, Fisher MR, Amparo EG, Hricak H, Higgins CB (1985) Magnetic resonance imaging in the evaluation of abscesses. Am J Roentgenol 6:1247–1224

124. Wee SH, Chang SN, Shim JY, Chun SI, Park WH (2000) A case of primary cutaneous actinomycosis. J Dermatol 10:651–654

125. Wright NB, Carty HM (1994) The swollen leg and primary lymphoedema. Arch Dis Child 1:44–49

126. Wu CM, Davis F, Fishman EK (1998) Musculoskeletal complications of the patient with acquired immunodeficiency syndrome (AIDS): CT evaluation. Semin Ultrasound CT MR 2:200–208

127. Yang I, Hayes CW, Biermann JS (2002) Calcific tendinitis of the gluteus medius tendon with bone marrow edema mimicking metastatic disease. Skeletal Radiol 6:359–361

128. Yousefzadeh DK, Schumann EM, Mulligan GM, Bosworth DE, Young CS, Pringle KC (1982) The role of imaging modalities in diagnosis and management of pyomyositis. Skeletal Radiol 4:285–289

129. Zohman GL, Pierce J, Chapman MW, Greenspan A, Gandour-Edwards R (1998) Calcific myonecrosis mimicking an invasive soft-tissue neoplasm. A case report and review of the literature. J Bone Joint Surg Am 8:1193–1197

Soft Tissue Metastasis

A. De Schepper, S. Khan, J. Alexiou, L. De Beuckeleer

25

Contents

25.1 Introduction

The spread and growth of metastases are the most dramatic manifestations of malignancy in cancer. According to Liotta and Stetler-Stevenson, 30 % of patients with newly diagnosed solid tumors (except skin neoplasms other than melanoma) have detectable secondary lesions, and 60 % have microscopic or macroscopic metastases as early as the time of primary tumor treatment [30]. Although soft tissues, and in particular skeletal muscles, represent about 40 % of the total body weight, they are infrequently affected by primary tumors and even more rarely by metastatic lesions. Rates of 1 % of all neoplasms, but 6 % in patients under the age of 25, are reported [7, 8, 64]. The low incidence of these primary and secondary tumors is probably responsible for the poor understanding of their natural evolution [64].

Since radiologists are infrequently involved in diagnostic work-up of skin lesions, except for melanoma, cutaneous metastases are discussed only briefly in this chapter.

25.2 Metastatic Process and Distribution

The metastasizing process consists of a series of sequential steps in which malignant cells are released from the primary tumor and disseminate in other organs where they create new tumor foci [30, 44]. Common routes of spread are hematogenous and/or lymphatic; spread along anatomical structures such as fascial planes or nerve sheaths is rather rare. The pattern of metastatic spread depends on properties of the tumor cell itself, on biologic differences in the organs, and on a variety of immunologic and nonimmunologic mechanisms in the tumor-bearing host [15, 20, 23, 37]. A number of studies have been undertaken to determine why metastases develop in parts remote from the primary tumor.

The reasons for the rarity of metastases in skeletal muscle may be related to blood flow, tissue pressure, and metabolism. Skeletal muscles are well vascularized and have a variable flow, in contrast to organs such as liver, brain, and lungs, where the blood flow is relatively constant. During exercise the flow in skeletal muscle may be increased by up to 800 times. Blood turbulences may be responsible for the destruction of tumor cells. Metabolites such as lactic acid may create an environment which is hostile to carcinogenesis [51, 31]. Enzyme inhibitors or some proteases may increase the relative resistance of muscle tissue against metastatic deposits [54, 56]. As a corollary to the reported increased growth of some tumors by hypoxia in vitro, it can be expected that hyperoxia and an increase in reactive metabolites, namely products of cellular oxidation reduction (superoxide dismutase), protect against tumor invasion [33, 55]. According to Weiss, experimentally denervated muscle showed greater cancer cell survival than electrically stimulated muscle [66]. Humoral and cellular immunity together with cell surface properties contribute to the organ-specific mechanism of tumor spread [15, 30, 37].

It has been demonstrated that trauma may favor development of metastases [2, 11, 16]. This can be a consequence of increased adherence of tumor cells to vessels

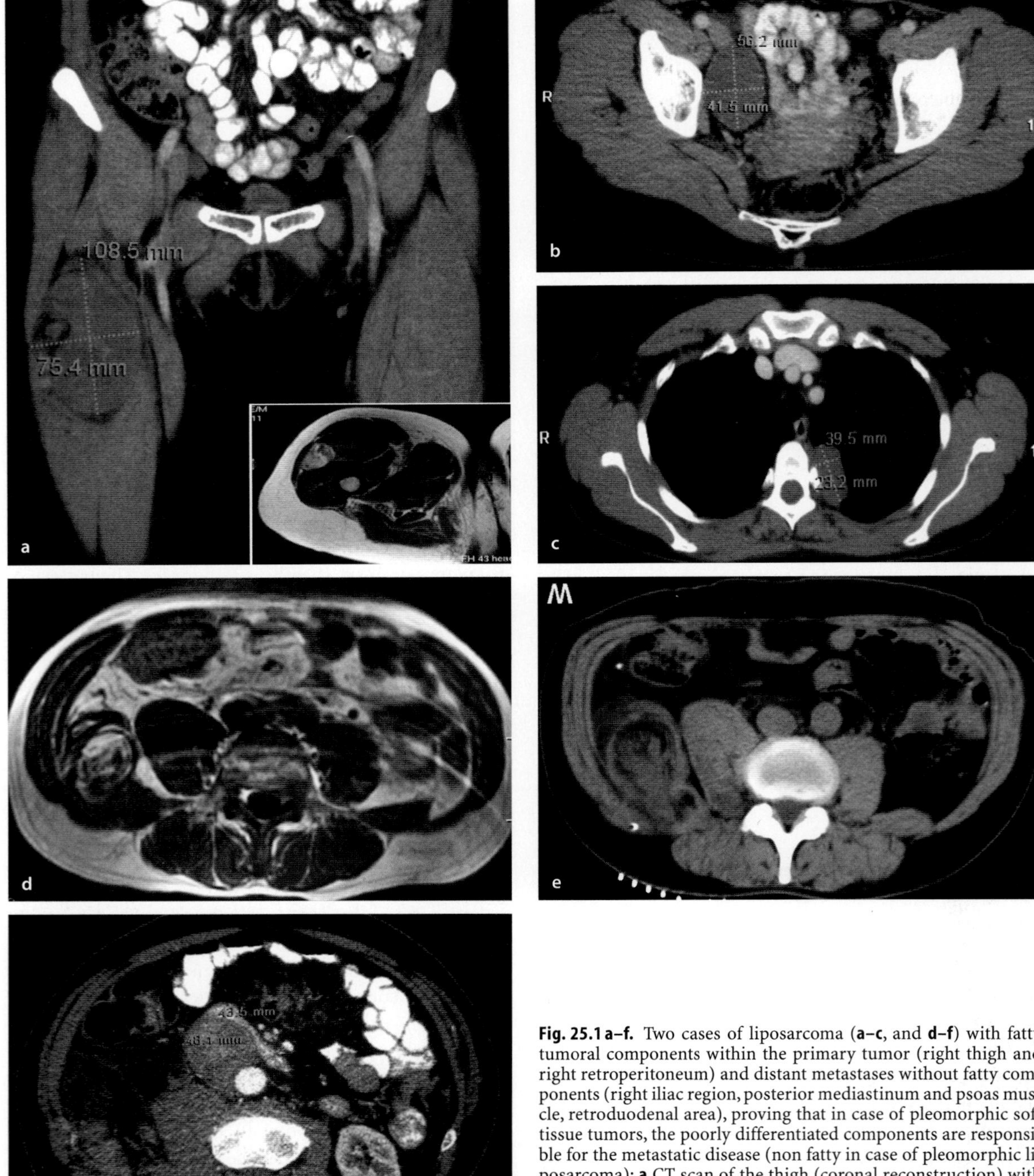

Fig. 25.1 a–f. Two cases of liposarcoma (**a–c**, and **d–f**) with fatty tumoral components within the primary tumor (right thigh and right retroperitoneum) and distant metastases without fatty components (right iliac region, posterior mediastinum and psoas muscle, retroduodenal area), proving that in case of pleomorphic soft tissue tumors, the poorly differentiated components are responsible for the metastatic disease (non fatty in case of pleomorphic liposarcoma): **a** CT scan of the thigh (coronal reconstruction) with in detail a T1-weighted MR image of the upper pole of the tumor; **b** CT scan of the pelvis; **c** CT scan of the chest, mediastinal window; **d** axial SE T1-weighted MR image of the retroperitoneum; **e** CT scan of the same region; **f** CT scan of the upper abdomen

resulting from endothelial damage and to alteration in the coagulation mechanism and peripheral flow [1, 2, 16]. Nevertheless, the effect of the coagulation mechanism remains controversial [16]. The effect of a local tumor growth-promoting factor produced by dead or dying cells was reported by Fisher et al. [16, 56]. Enzyme activity from leukocytes generating tumor cell chemotactic factors from C5 (fifth component of complement) may contribute to the possible role of injury and/or inflammation in the metastatic process [38].

In case of multiple tumoral components of different differentiation, poorly differentiated components are responsible for metastatic disease, e.g. non-fatty, cellular components metastasize in cases of pleomorphic liposarcoma while fatty components do not (Fig. 25.1)

25.3 Incidence

In comparison to primary malignant tumors, metastases to the soft tissues are sparsely reported. In various series of autopsies the proportion of metastases to soft tissues varies considerably, ranging from 0.8 % in the study of Willis to 16 % in that by Pearson and 52 % in the Buerger study [9, 68]. The varying incidences reported in these articles may be explained, firstly, by the fact that Willis probably sampled only one or two muscles instead of nine as in Pearson's study and 12 as in the Buerger study. Secondly, Pearson and Buerger included microscopic metastatic foci in their results. Another reason for the higher frequency described by Buerger is that their study only concerned patients affected by leukemia or lymphoma, which commonly metastasize [32, 59] (Fig. 25.1).

Statistics are biased by the fact that limbs are usually not studied in necropsies (except when a mass is apparent), and even when they are it is virtually impossible to examine the entire soft tissue compartment. In addition, clinical evidence of metastases to soft tissues is rarely reported. Sudo et al. reported on four cases of metastasis in a 15-year period during which 147 primary soft tissue sarcomas were treated [58]. During a 16-year period, Herring et al. observed only 15 patient with metastasis to muscle, in contrast to 54,000 new carcinomas in the same institution [24]. Petasnick et al. in their study of 35 soft tissue masses reported 3 metastases out of 12 malignant lesions. Weekes et al. in a study of 84 soft tissue tumors listed 41 primary neoplasms and 9 secondary lesions.

In our experience, out of 53 patients with secondary tumoral lesions in muscles examined over the past 7 years, 26 had melanomas as primary tumor, 4 had breast cancer, 3 colonic carcinoma, and 3 soft tissue sarcoma. Differences in the population obviously influence study results.

According to Willis, the majority of muscle metastases occur in the abdominal wall and the pectoral, deltoid, psoas, erector spinal, and thigh muscles. All metastases reported by Shridhar et al. originated from lung cancer and were located in proximal skeletal muscles [56, 61]. Schultz et al. showed secondary involvement in the muscles of the chest wall, thigh, calf, quadratus lumborum, and, more often, in the iliopsoas and the gluteal muscles [49]. Sudo et al. report that metastases develop commonly in the muscles neighboring the trunk such as paravertebral, gluteal, and thigh muscles [58]. Anecdotal cases demonstrate the predominance of the metastases in the proximal muscles. These metastases

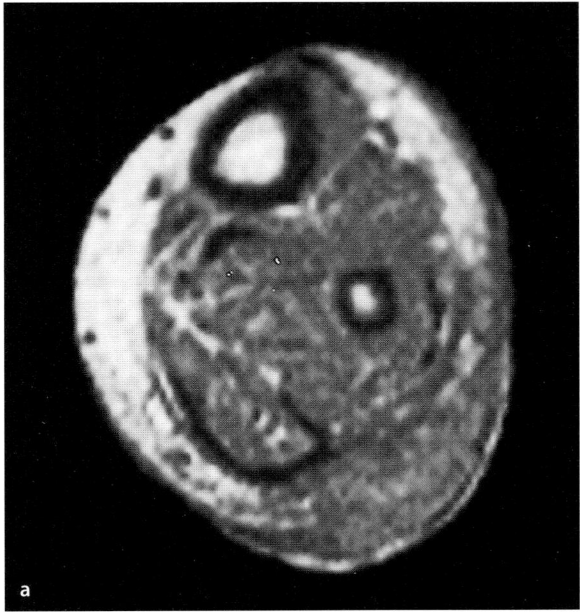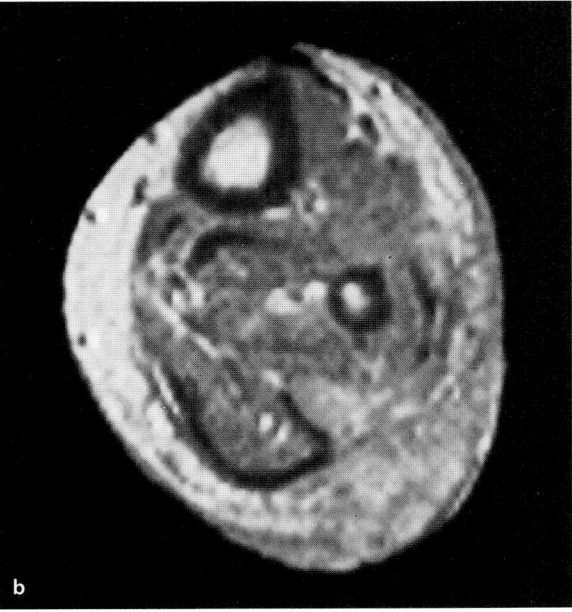

Fig. 25.2 a, b. Acute leukemia in a 61-year-old man. **a** Axial spin echo T1-weighted MR image. **b** Axial spin echo T1-weighted MR image after gadolinium contrast injection. Diffuse infiltration of the skin and the subcutis of the calf. Infiltration is isointense compared to muscle on the T1-weighted image (**a**), and mostly hyperintense to fat on a T2-weighted image (not shown). There is slight enhancement after contrast injection (**b**). Myeloblastic infiltration of the soft tissues with nonspecific MRI features, in a patient with acute leukemia

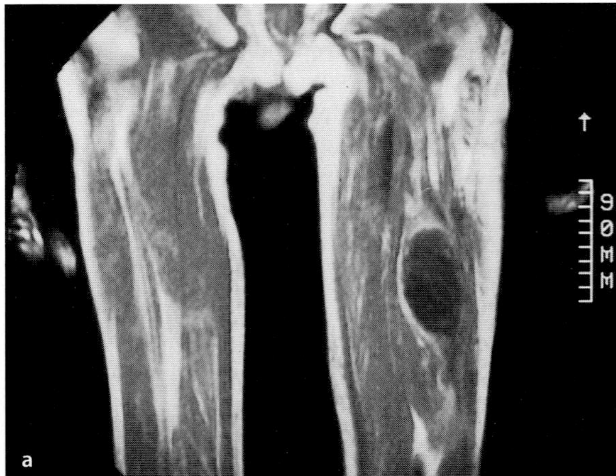

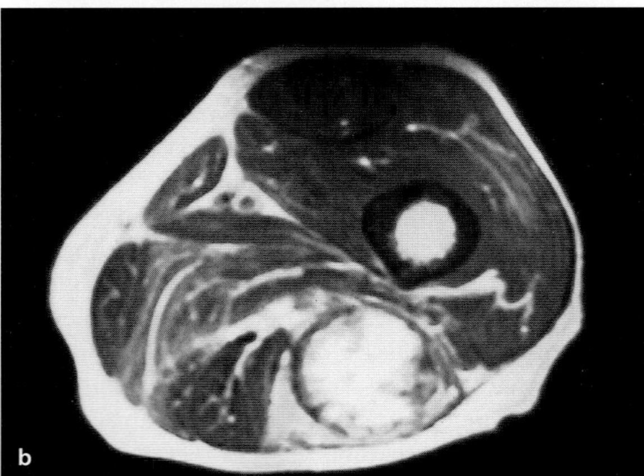

Fig. 25.3 a, b. Metastasis of a Pancoast's tumor in a 46-year-old man. **a** Coronal spin echo T1-weighted MR image. **b** Axial turbo spin echo T2-weighted MR image. Well-defined, oval mass at the dorsal aspect of the left thigh. The lesion is of low signal intensity on the T1-weighted image (**a**), of extremely high signal intensity on the T2-weighted image (**b**), and inhomogeneous on both sequences

generally originate from tumors of the pancreas, colon, kidney, lung, uterus, stomach, hypopharynx, thyroid, and prostate [28, 35, 41, 42, 46, 53, 56, 57, 58, 65]. Metastases distal to the knee and elbow are extremely rare [21, 29]. The primary tumors responsible for these distal lesions are bronchial carcinomas and breast, kidney, or testicle cancers [29].

Overall, the most common cause of soft tissue metastases are lung, renal and colon primaries [3, 5]. A significant number of cases are due to unknown primary carcinoma and the histopathological features are of undifferentiated tumor. Histological diagnosis most commonly seen is adenocarcinoma predominantly from lung and gastrointestinal tract [61]. Squamous cell carcinomas and renal clear cell carcinomas are other frequent cause of metastases [12]. Sarcomas are uncommon cause of metastases to the soft tissues.

Bone-forming muscle metastases have been linked to gastric adenocarcinoma or to breast, ovary, thyroid, colon, bladder, skin, and prostate cancers or to osteogenic sarcomas [24, 36, 40, 49].

Skin metastases are easier to detect and are discovered in 0.2–9 % of autopsies in cancer patients [47].

The incidence of metastases from soft tissue sarcomas to the skin and subcutaneous tissue is about 10 %, leiomyosarcoma being the most frequently reported primary tumor [64]. Cutaneous lesions are also described in lymphoma, leukemia, and melanoma [8, 32, 39]. Cutaneous metastases generally arise in a late stage of cancer and have a poor prognosis [24, 46].

In women the most frequent cancer responsible for secondary cutaneous lesions arises from breast (69 %), colon (9 %), skin (5 %; melanoma), lung (4 %), and ovaries (4 %). In men metastases originate from lung cancer (24 %; Fig. 25.2), colonic carcinoma (19 %; Fig. 25.3), melanoma (13 %), squamous cell carcinoma of the oral cavity (12 %), kidney, and stomach cancer (6 % each) [49].

25.4 Clinical Behavior

An intramuscular mass is first suspected to be a primary tumor rather than a metastasis. Oncologic patients with pain in large muscles and negative radiographic or radionuclide evaluation for osseous metastases are suspected of having soft tissue metastases [56]. Skeletal muscle metastases often present as a firm and tender mass deeply rooted within the muscle and with a diameter of more than 5 cm. Presentation with pain is commonly seen in skeletal muscle metastases while primary sarcomas tend to be painless [12, 18, 29, 42, 49, 56]. Small lesions are often asymptomatic and are discovered as incidental findings on CT or MR [45].

Cutaneous and subcutaneous metastases tend to be painless and are better felt when underlying muscles are actively contracted [21, 56]. They are generally 0.5–2 cm in diameter when discovered [39]. Subcutaneous metastases are firm and freely movable [21].

Mostly primary tumors are discovered before metastases, but in a minority metastases may be the first sign of malignancy [28, 35, 42, 49, 58]. The incidence of soft tissue metastasis without a known primary is about 0.8% [12]. In some cases they have been observed before lung or liver metastases or appeared as the first sign of recurrence [21, 35, 53, 57]. In rare instances, however, no primary tumor is found [14]. In our series a soft tissue metastasis was the first symptom of malignancy in 2 out of 53 patients.

Malignant subcutaneous lesions must be differentiated from benign nodules (such as sebaceous cysts, lipomas or injection granulomas) and blood vessels [39].

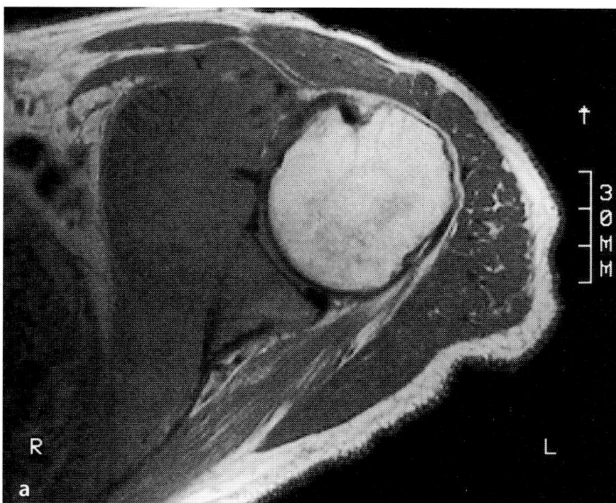

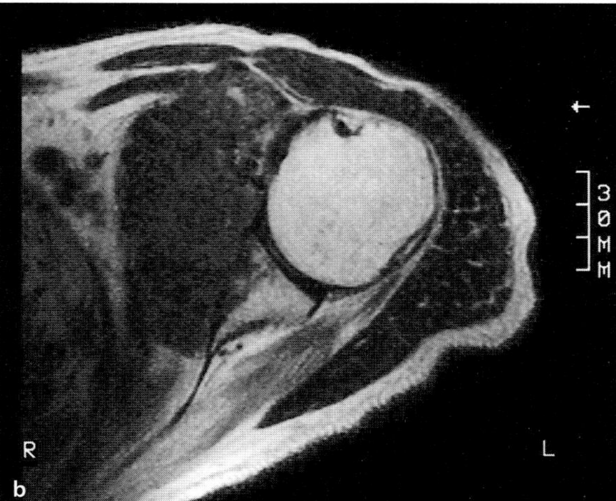

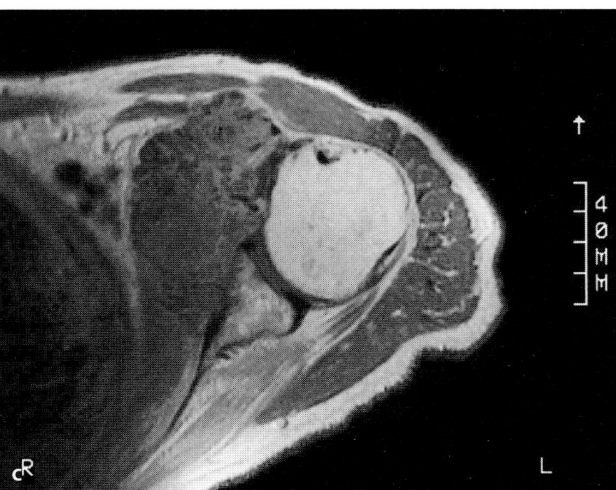

Fig. 25.4a–c. Metastasis of colon carcinoma in a 60-year-old man. **a** Axial spin echo T1-weighted MR image. **b** Axial turbo spin echo T2-weighted MR image. **c** Axial spin echo T1-weighted MR image after gadolinium contrast injection. There is a heterogeneous, ill-defined mass at the ventral aspect of the left shoulder with involvement of the scapula (**b**). Involvement of the scapula is better demonstrated on the T1-weighted image (**a**) while tumoral invasion of the joint is suspected on the postcontrast image (**c**). The lesion is of rather low signal intensity on both sequences. There is slight enhancement after contrast injection. This case demonstrates the staging properties (bone and joint involvement) of MRI

Multiple masses may be seen in metastases, neurofibromatosis, fibromatosis, lipomas, and myxomas (see Table 11.10).

The prognosis of secondary intramuscular lesions is not well known, but they are often considered as a sign of generalized tumor spread, and most patients die within a few months despite various treatments [56, 58]. The number and location of lesions affect the clinical outcome [6]. Therefore it is mandatory to perform a complete physical examination, chest radiograph, liver ultrasound, and bone scintigraphy whenever a secondary lesion is discovered.

The optimal treatment in muscle metastases is not well known. There are only a few reports on surgical or radiation therapy [28, 29, 41, 56]. Wide excision of a solitary metastasis of soft tissue sarcoma may sometimes render a patient disease free [25]. Surgery may be attempted to palliate pain refractory to radiotherapy [24, 56]. Chemotherapy is instituted for metastases of certain types of tumor such as melanoma and can be administered by local intra-arterial perfusion.

25.5 Imaging

25.5.1 Imaging Modalities other than MRI

The imaging investigation of a suspected soft tissue mass begins with a plain radiograph to exclude a bone deformity (such as an exuberant osseous callus due to a previous trauma) and a bone lesion (such as osseous metastases invading soft tissues) which may simulate a soft tissue tumor. Plain radiographs may also detect calcifications or ossifications narrowing the differential diagnosis, including hemangioma (phleboliths), osteochondromatosis (rice bodies) and myositis ossificans (peripheral calcification) [50]. They may demonstrate local bone involvement such as periosteal reaction, scalloped areas near the soft tissue mass, or concomitant osseous lesions not contiguous to the mass itself.

Plain radiographs should be obtained with low kilovoltage that enhances differences in radiographic density between soft tissues such as fat and muscle.

Although some authors originally maintained that CT was superior to MRI in detecting cortical bone destruction, more recent studies have confirmed these two modalities to be comparable [60].

Metastatic infiltration of skeletal muscle generally appears on CT as an area of decreased attenuation with a varying degree of definition [24, 43, 49]. Sometimes detection is more difficult, and a lesion may be suspected only from a slight asymmetry of soft tissues when comparing with the opposite side.

The use of contrast medium helps in detection and definition of extent of the lesions. Muscle metastases often present with rim enhancement and central hypo-

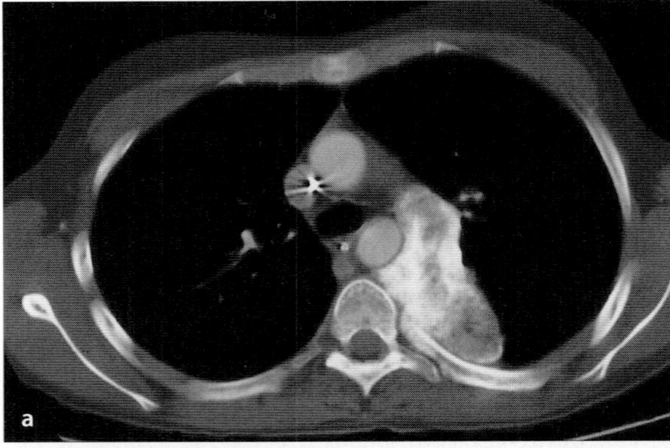

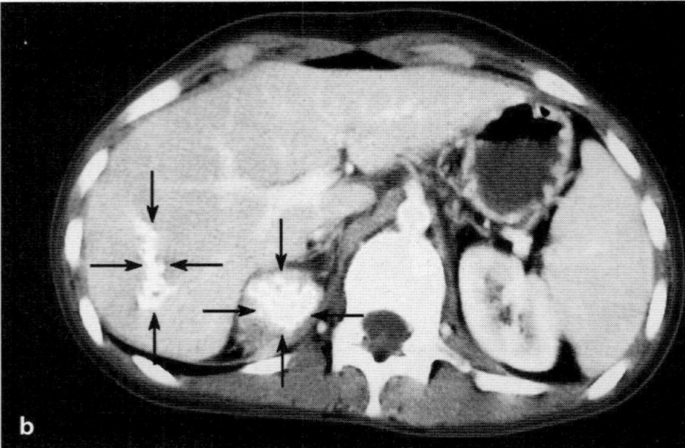

Fig. 25.4. Calcified/ossified metastases of an osteosarcoma of the left femur in 17-year-old boy. **a** CT scan of the chest. **b** CT scan of the upper abdomen. A well-delineated calcified/ossified mass is seen at the posteromedial aspect of the left hemithorax, invading the posterior mediastinum. A similar lesion is noted at the right liver (segment 6) and in the right adrenal region (*arrows*)

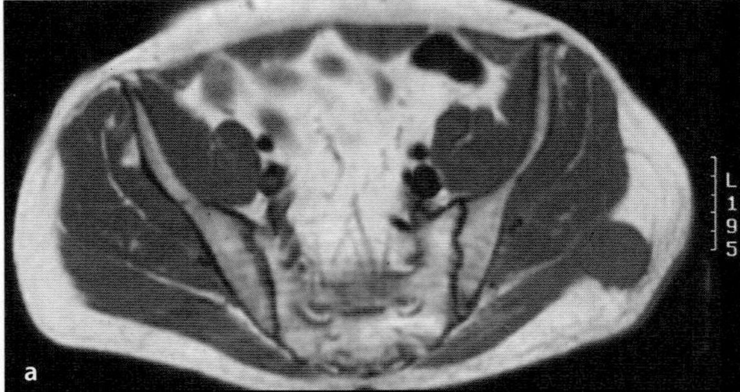

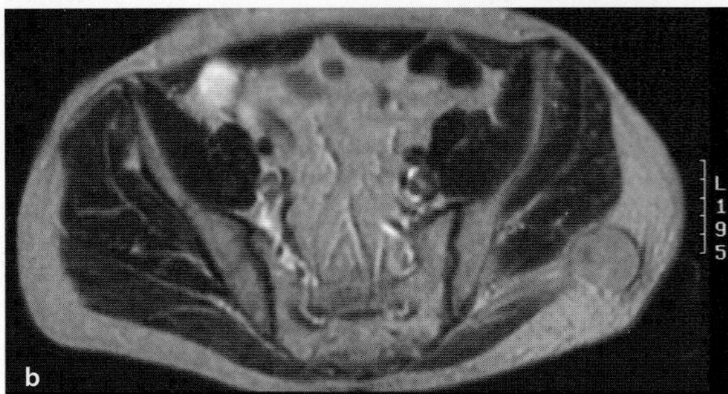

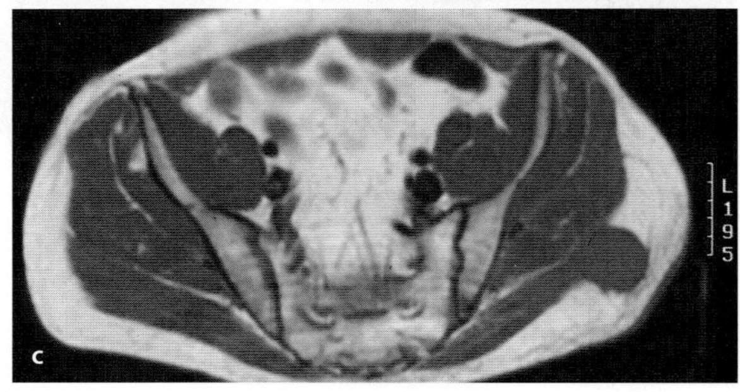

Fig. 25.6 a–c. Metastasis in the left gluteal region in a 55-year-old man with primary neuroendocrine malignancy. **a** Axial spin echo T1-weighted MR image. **b** Axial spin echo T2-weighted MR image. **c** Axial spin echo T1-weighted MR image after gadolinium contrast injection. A well-defined nodule is visualized in the subcutaneous fat of the left buttock. The lesion appears isointense compared to muscle on the T1-weighted image (**a**), isointense to fat on the T2-weighted image (**b**), and is slightly enhanced after contrast injection (**c**). Atypical presentation of a metastasis at the left buttock

attenuation [24, 42]. CT, however, cannot differentiate metastases from primary tumors. CT is currently replaced by MRI in evaluating soft tissue masses, because CT information is generally superfluous rather than being complementary.

Diagnosis of calcified metastases and differential diagnosis with myositis ossificans is easier on CT than on MRI (Fig. 25.5).

CT is not able to differentiate between benign and malignant subcutaneous nodules, except for subcutaneous lipomas, injection granulomas, and sebaceous cysts.

Since the introduction of CT and MRI, indications for angiography are limited to the differentiation of arteriovenous malformations from other soft tissue masses.

Ultrasound is a sensitive, noninvasive, and inexpensive imaging technique but is poor in terms of specificity. It may help in detection and further evaluation of soft tissue masses. Differentiating between diffuse and well-delineated lesions, solid, mixed, and cystic lesions and guiding percutaneous biopsies are well-known advantages of this method.

When associated with color Doppler, the degree of intratumoral blood flow in solid lesions can be assessed, and the response to nonsurgical therapy can be monitored.

Scintigraphy is of less value in evaluating soft tissue metastases, except for the detection of metastases of osteogenic sarcoma [17]. 99 mTc-Labeled methylene diphosphonate bone scan may show areas of increased activity in soft tissues, corresponding to metastatic locations, but the uptake of the radionuclide tracer may occur both in calcified and in noncalcified secondary soft tissue lesions [17, 22, 36, 40]. A case of metastasis detected by Ga-67 scintigraphy has also been reported. The use of monoclonal antibodies labeled with isotopic components may refine the method [70].

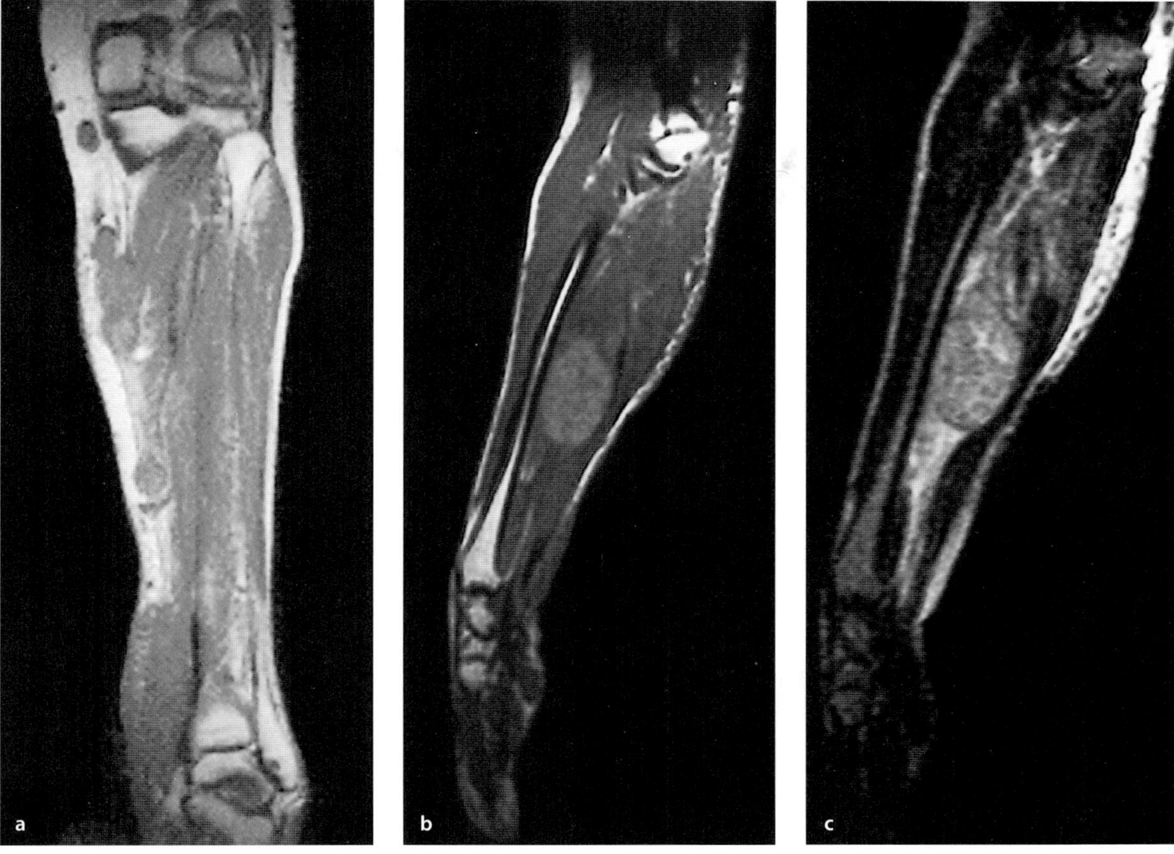

Fig. 25.7 a–c. Metastasis of malignant melanoma of the lower leg in a 64-year-old woman (**a**) and of the forearm in a 48-year-old man (**b, c**). **a** Coronal spin echo T1-weighted MR image. **b** Sagittal spin echo T1-weighted MR image. **c** Sagittal spine echo T2-weight-ed MR image. The paramagnetic property of the free radicals in melanin is responsible for the high signal intensity of metastasis of malignant melanoma on T1-weighted images

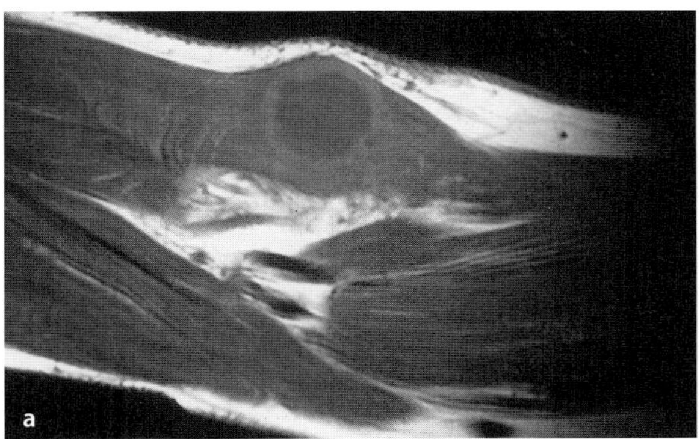

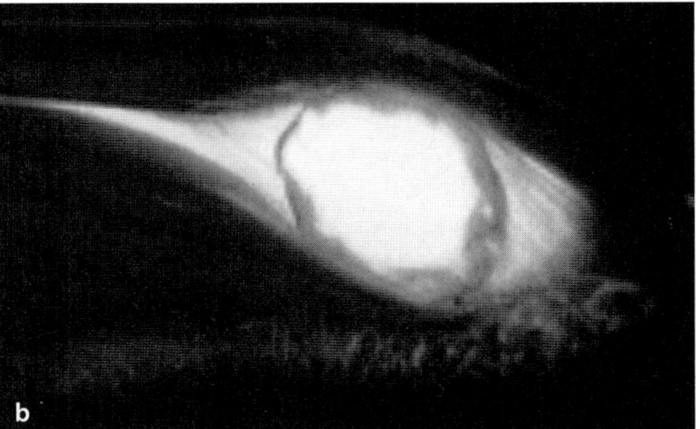

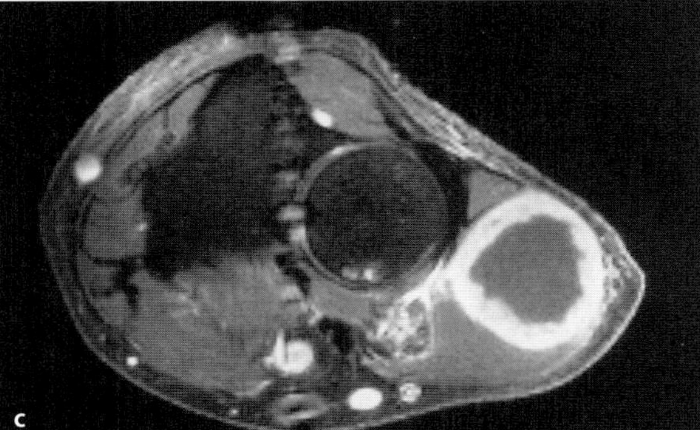

Fig. 25.8 a–c. Metastasis of a spinocelluar carcinoma of the lung in a 76-year-old man. **a** Coronal spin echo T1-weighted MR images. **b** Coronal fat-suppressed turbo spin echo T2-weighted image. **c** Axial spin echo T1-weighted MR image after gadolinium contrast injection. Lateral to the head of the radius there is a fusiform mass with a hypo-intense center and a hyperintense peripheral zone compared with the signal intensity of normal muscle (**a**). On T2-weighted images, the center of the lesion is hyperintense while the peripheral zone is of lower signal intensity (**b**). After contrast injection, the peripheral zone exhibits an early and intense enhancement (**c**). This "inverted target sign" is highly suggestive for high-grade malignancy

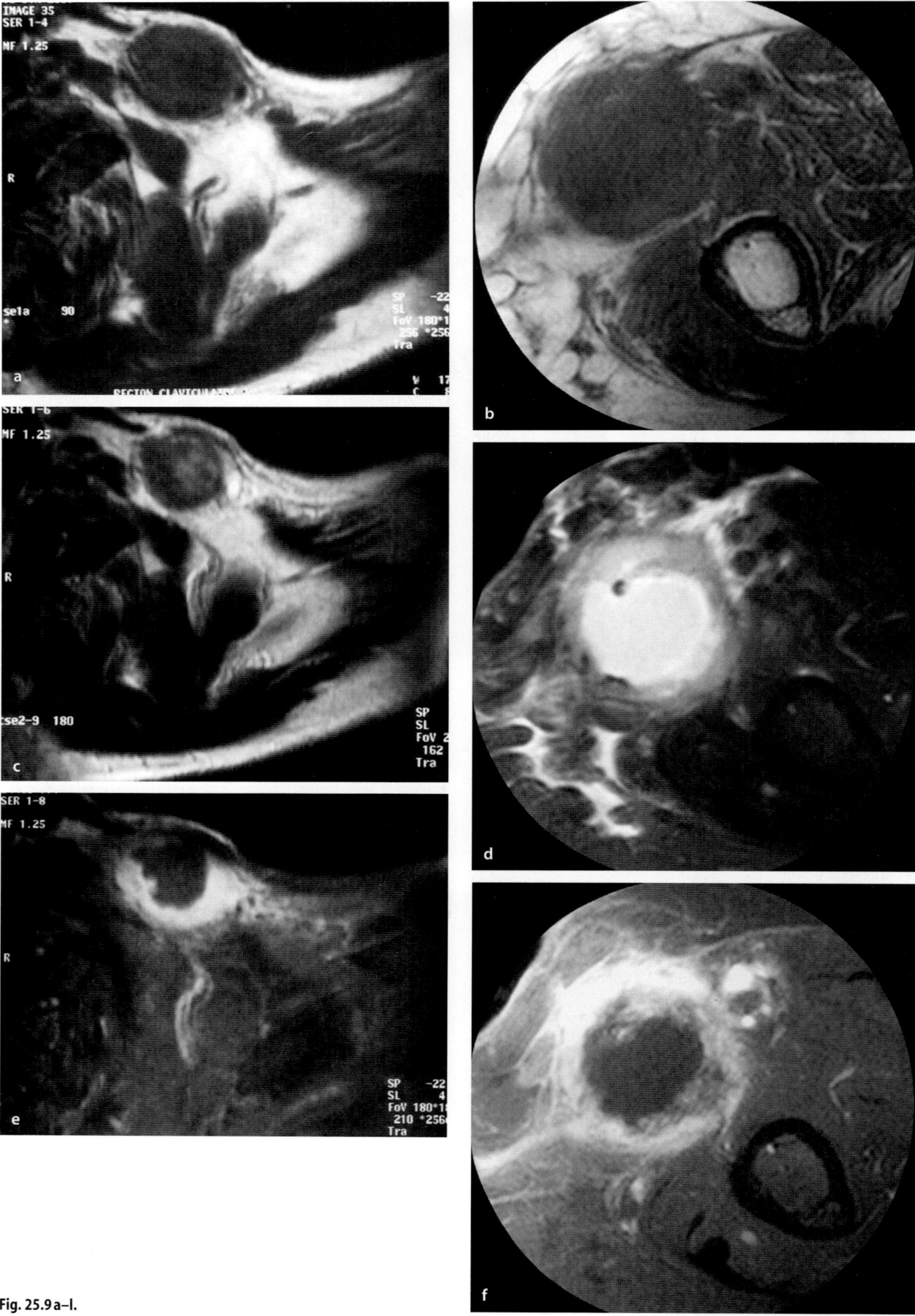

Fig. 25.9 a–l.

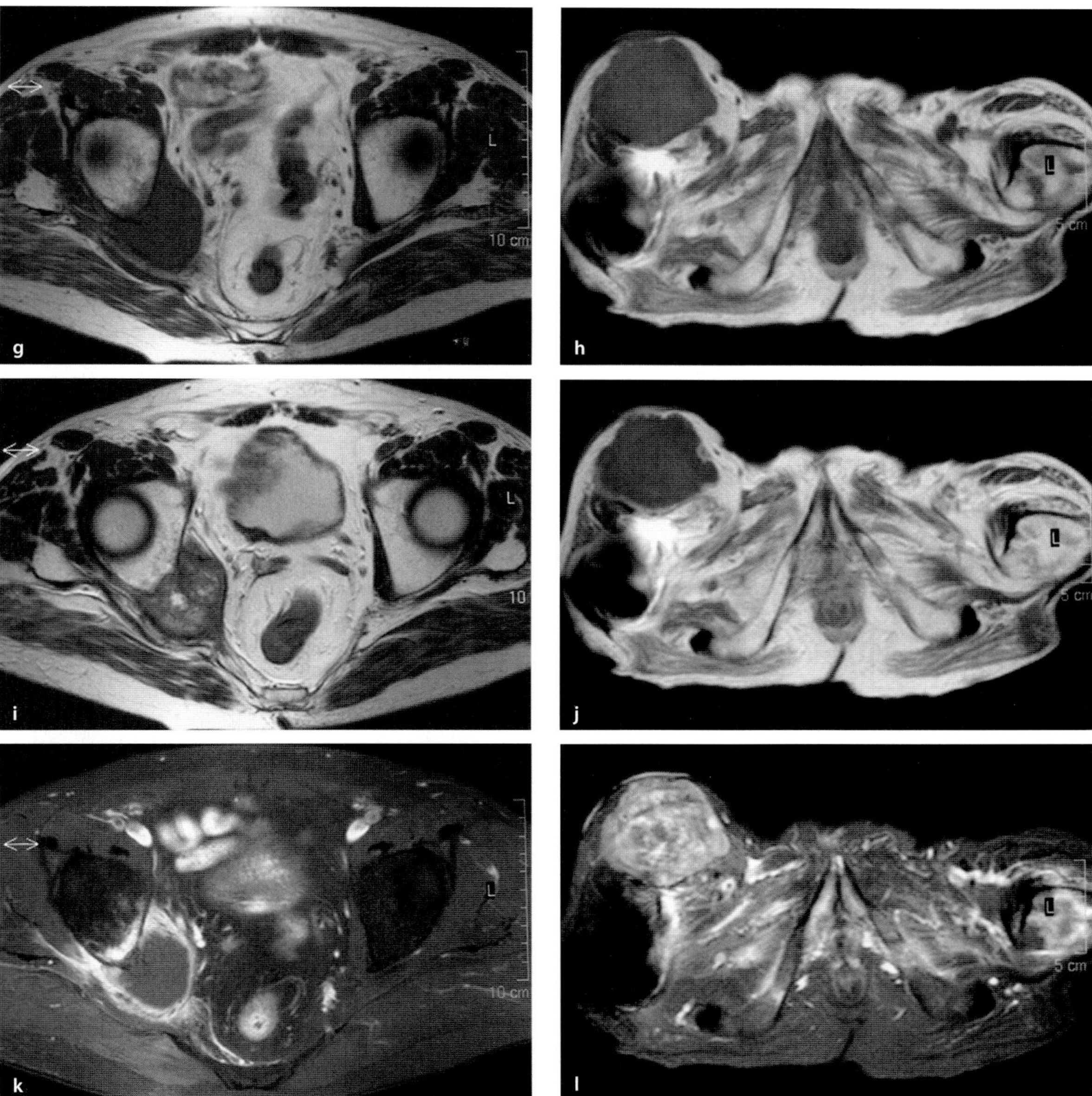

Fig. 25.9 a–l. Four cases of soft tissue metastasis from respectively: **a–c** a papillary renal carcinoma; **d–f** a squamous cell carcinoma; **g–i** an undifferentiated adenocarcinoma; **j–l** a lung carcinoma (**j, k, l**). All four patients show with the most common presentation of soft tissue metastasis, i.e. low to intermediate signal intensity and non homogeneity on T1-weighted MR images, intermediate to high signal intensity with or without peripheral, hypointense rim ("inverted target" sign) on T2- weighted MR images and with only peripheral enhancement after gadolinium contrast administration. Figures **a, d, g**, and **j** are axial SE T1- weighted MR images; **b, e, h**, and **k** are axial SE T2- weighted MR images; and **c, f, i**, and **l** are axial SE T1-weighted MR images after gadolinium contrast injection

Generally considered non-specific. However, peritumoral edema with central necrosis was the feature most commonly seen on MRI. In our own series metastases mostly present as non-homogeneous lesions with low signal intensity on T1- and high signal intensity on T2-weighted MR images, with peripheral enhancement after Gadolinium contrast administration, central necrosis and perilesional edema (Fig. 25.8, 25.9).

25.5.2 Magnetic Resonance Imaging

MRI offers much better soft tissue contrast resolution than all other techniques previously reported, and it has multiplanar imaging capability useful in tumor assessment and preoperative planning [10, 13]. MRI of soft tissue metastases is described in only a small number of cases. In these cases the lesions had lower signal intensity than fat and were isointense to muscle on T1-weighted images; they were hyper- or isointense relative to fat, and always presented with a higher signal intensity than muscle on T2-weighted images [24, 42, 58]. These features are generally considered nonspecific (Fig. 25.6).

In certain cases, for example in metastases of mucinous adenocarcinoma of the colon or pancreas, marked hypointensity is seen on T2-weighted images as a consequence of the high ratio between nuclei and cytoplasm and the limited extracellular space (Figs. 25.4 (11, 12)).

Metastases from melanoma have a higher signal intensity than muscle and a lower signal intensity than fat on T1-weighted images (Fig. 25.7); on T2-weighted images they have intermediate signal intensity. These signal intensity characteristics are the consequence of the paramagnetic stable free radicals in melanin, although some authors suggest an influence of iron associated with hemorrhage or chelated metal ions [4, 69]. Comparable MRI features have also been described in cases of pleomorphic liposarcoma and intratumoral hemorrhage [60].

Secondary tumoral lesions may present either as a regular or an irregular, well-marginated mass or as an ill-defined mass [39]. It may show a homogeneous or heterogeneous signal intensity on both T1- and T2-weighted images and a moderate to strong enhancement after intravenous injection of paramagnetic contrast. In some of our cases, a hypointense rim was seen on T2-weighted images, creating an "inverted target" sign (Figs. 25.8, 25.9). Small masses tend to be homogeneous and large ones more heterogeneous.

As shown by Kransdorf, the probability of malignancy of a mass increases with its size and heterogeneity. This is a consequence of the outgrowth of their vascular supply, which can provoke subsequent infarction and necrosis. Intratumoral bleeding can also be seen in metastases [40] (Fig. 25.10) (see also Chap. 11).

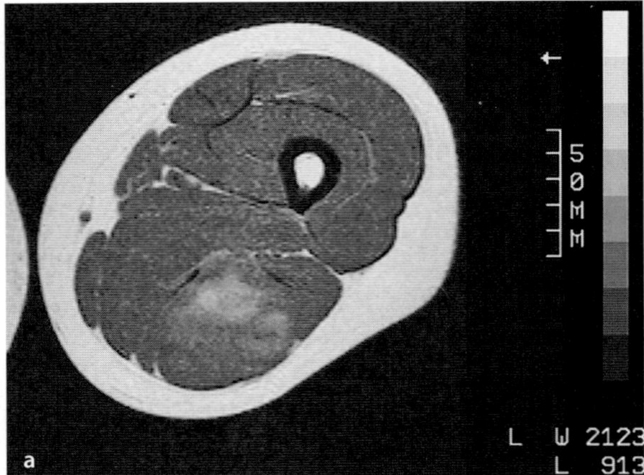

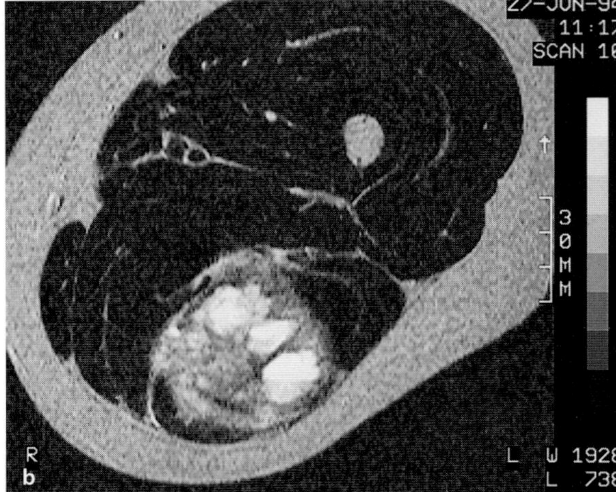

Fig. 25.10 a, b. Metastasis of an osteosarcoma in a 23-year-old man. **a** Axial spin echo T1-weighted MR image. **b** Axial turbo spin echo T2-weighted MR image. Ill-defined mass within the hamstrings with intralesional areas of high signal intensity on the T1-weighted image (**a**), presence of fluid-fluid levels on the T2-weighted image with low signal intensity (hemosiderin) of the dependent portion (**b**). Both MRI features suggest intralesional bleeding, a parameter with low specificity in prediction of malignancy

Although many authors state that MRI cannot reliably distinguish between benign and malignant soft tissue tumors, the use of criteria such as signal intensity, homogeneity, margins, neurovascular invasion, growth rate, septation in the tumor, extension beyond one compartment, bone destruction, and signal changes in adjacent tissues, together with clinical findings often affords better distinction between benign and malignant lesions [10, 34].

The use of gadolinium chelates may facilitate distinction between tumor, muscle, and edematous tissue and provides information on tumor vascularity and necrosis [48] (Figs. 25.4, 25.8, 25.9 and 25.11).

The use of color Doppler imaging, blood pool scintigraphy, and dynamic MRI contrast studies (see Chaps. 2,

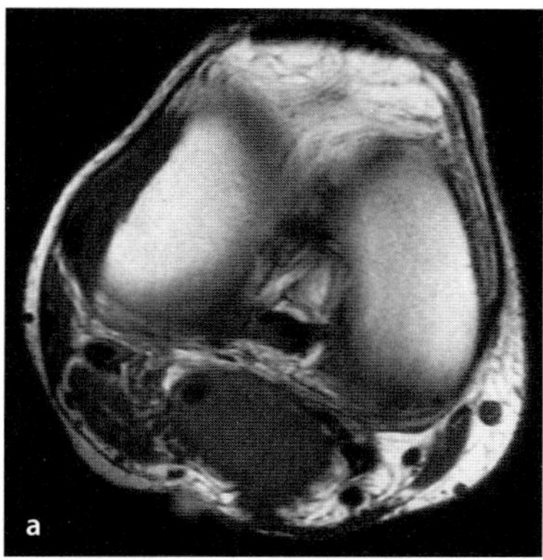 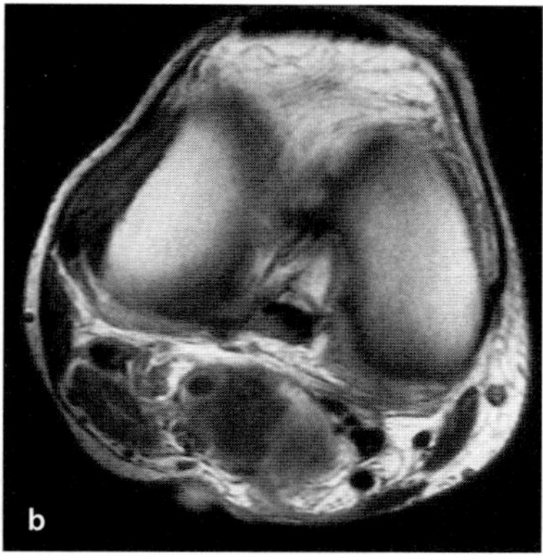 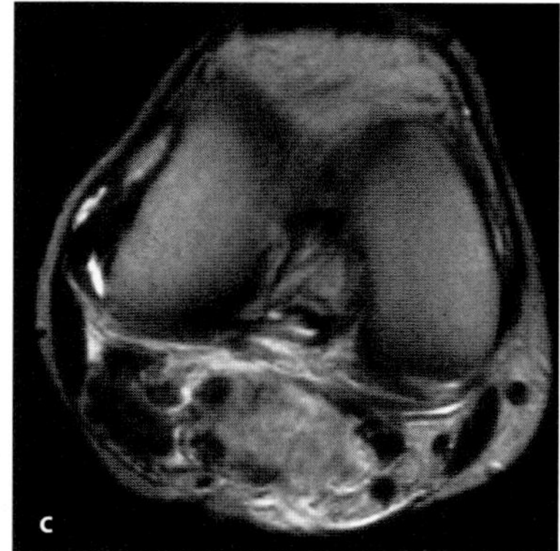

Fig. 25.11a–c. Metastasis of a clear cell sarcoma in a 35-year-old man. **a** Axial spin echo T1-weighted MR image. **b** Axial spin echo T1-weighted MR image after gadolinium contrast injection. **c** Axial turbo spin echo T2-weighted image. Rounded, well-delineated mass in the popliteal fossa surrounding and encasing the popliteal artery. The lesion is of intermediate signal intensity on both T1- and T2-weighted images and shows a large area of non-enhancement on T1-weighted images after gadolinium contrast injection

4, 6) may be useful in monitoring results of chemotherapy [62, 63]. A decrease in vascularity and perfusion is correlated with good response and vice versa.

25.6 Imaging and Diagnostic Strategy

The presence of metastases means progressive disease, which changes the therapeutic strategy.

Cutaneous nodules are easily detected by clinical examination and do not require imaging except if extension to deeper tissues is suspected. Surgical excision of skin lesions is often performed without preoperative radiological investigation.

Because imaging of subcutaneous metastases is non-specific, and because nontumoral lesions such as lymphocele, hematoma, abscess, and reactive lymphadenopathy are frequent in cancer patients, other investigators advocate biopsy as a first-choice investigation [24, 43, 56, 58, 67].

A third possible strategy consists in full imaging to determine the appropriate technique of management, i. e., fine needle, trocar, open biopsy, or "en bloc" excision [52].

In the evaluation of a deeper seated nodule in a patient with known primary cancer and without known metastatic disease, the general imaging strategy (as for primary soft tissue tumors) must be followed (see Chap. 12).

If a patient with known primary cancer and known metastatic disease presents with a deeper seated nodule, imaging procedures must be restricted to guidance of some therapeutic acts, i. e., palliative therapy in the case of intractable pain caused by metastases or drainage of paraneoplastic abscesses. One must be aware of paraneoplastic coagulopathy, which is often seen in patients with lymphoma or leukemia and represents a contraindication for biopsy.

25.7 Prognosis and Management

The majority of patients diagnosed with soft tissue metastasis have poor prognosis with very shortened life span, dying in less than nine months [61, 12]. The number and location of lesions affect the clinical outcome. Therefore, it is mandatory to perform a complete physical examination, chest radiograph, liver ultrasound and bone scintigraphy whenever a secondary lesion is discovered.

Treatment options are limited and tend to be palliative. Surgical excision is rarely carried out due to increased morbidity and poor prognosis.

On the contrary, attempts at surgical excision may result in rapid recurrence and widespread metastasis and rapidly shorten the life span. This has been noted in cases of lung and colon skeletal metastases [58, 3, 28]. Hence, any surgical excision requires good understanding of the primary cancer and thorough preoperative planning. However, there are sporadic reports of increased life span in cases of renal and lung metastases. Chondroblastoma metastasis excision have better result even in the presence of multiple metastases provided there is no lung metastasis [26]. Surgery may be used with improvement in prognosis in patients with metastasis from chondroblastoma, chondrosarcoma and osteosarcoma.

Generally, radiotherapy or chemotherapy is used in controlling the disease process mainly with the aim of palliation.

25.8 Conclusion

Soft tissue metastasis should be considered in the diagnosis of soft tissue mass, particularly when it is painful. Good history with judicious use of various radiological imaging modalities should narrow down the differential and may pinpoint the diagnosis. But more likely the findings are non-specific and biopsy would shed light on the diagnosis.

Things to remember:

1. Skeletal muscle metastases are rare which can be explained by vascular, metabolic and traumatic etiopathogenetic circumstances.
2. Primary tumors responsible for soft tissue metastases are adenocarcinomas and squamous cell carcinomas, mostly originating from lung, kidney and gastro-intestinal tract.
3. Soft tissue metastases are frequently painful lesions, in contradistinction with primary soft tissue tumors, which are mostly painless.
4. Multiplicity of lesions and known primary tumor may help in diagnosing soft tissue metastases.
5. Most metastases have nonspecific features on imaging except for metastases of osteosarcoma (intralesional ossification), and melanosarcoma (increased SI on T1-weighted MR images).
6. MR-findings of low SI on T2-weighted MR images, due to hypercellularity and increased nucleo-cytoplasmatic index and especially the "Inverted Target Sign" (high SI on T2-weighted MR images with low SI peripheral rim and inversion of SI's after Gd contrast admininistration, i.e. peripheral enhancement and lack of central enhancement, due to central necrosis) are more specific features seen in soft tissue metastases.
7. Diagnosis of soft tissue metastases will change diagnostic and therapeutic strategies. Surgical excision is seldomly curative.

References

1. Agostino D, Cliffton EE (1965) Trauma as a cause of localization of blood-borne metastases: preventive effect of heparin and fibrinolysin. Ann Surg 161(1):97–102
2. Alexander JW, Altemeier WA (1964) Susceptibility of injured tissue to hematogenous metastases: an experimental study. Ann Surg 159(6):933–943
3. Araki K, Kobayashi M, Ogata T, Takuma K (1994) Colorectal carcinoma metastatic to skeletal muscle. Hepatogastroenterology 41:405–408
4. Atlas SW, Braffman BH, LoBrutto R, Elder DE, Herlyn D (1990) Human malignant melanomas with varying degrees of melanin content in nude mice: MR imaging, histopathology, and electron paramagnetic resonance. J Comput Assist Tomogr 14(4):547–554
5. Avery GR (1988) Metastatic adenocarcinoma masquerading as a psoas abscess. Clin Radiol 39:319–320
6. Berdeaux DH, Moon TE, Meyskens FL Jr (1985) Clinical-biologic patterns of metastatic melanoma and their effect on treatment. Cancer Treat Rep 69(4):397–401
7. Bongartz GM, Vestring T (1991) Soft tissue tumours. MR State of the art ECR 91; CC 811:193–198
8. Boothroyd AE, Carty H (1995) The painless soft tissue mass in childhood – tumor or not? Postgrad Med 71:10–16
9. Buerger LF, Monteleone PN (1966) Leukemic-lymphomatous infiltration of skeletal muscle. Cancer 19:1416–1422
10. Chang AE, Matory YL, Dwyer AJ, Hill SC, Girton ME, Steinberg SM, Knop RH, Frank JA, Hyams D, Doppman JL, Rosenberg SA (1987) Magnetic resonance imaging versus computed tomography in the evaluation of soft tissue tumors of the extremities. Ann Surg 205:340–348
11. Cohen HJ, Laszlo J (1972) Influence of trauma on the unusual distribution of metastases from carcinoma of the larynx. Cancer 29:466–471
12. Damron TA, Heiner J (2000) Distant soft tissue metastases: a series of 30 new patients and 91 cases from the literature. Ann Surg Oncol 7:526–534
13. Demas BE, Heelan RT, Lane J, Marcove R, Hajdu S, Brennan MF (1988) Soft-tissue sarcomas of the extremities: comparison of MR and CT in determining the extent of disease. AJR Am J Roentgenol 150: 615–620
14. Didolkar MS, Fanous N, Elias EG, Moore RH (1977) Metastatic carcinomas from occult primary tumors. Ann Surg 186:625–630
15. Fidler IJ, Hart IR (1981) The origin of metastatic heterogeneity in tumors. Eur J Cancer 17:487–494
16. Fisher B, Fisher ER, Feduska N (1967) Trauma and localization of tumor cells. Cancer 20:23–30
17. Flowers WM Jr (1974) 99 mTc-polyphosphate uptake within pulmonary and soft-tissue metastases from osteosarcoma. Radiology 112:377–378
18. Fornage BD (1991) Tumeurs musculaires. In: Fornage BD (ed) Echographie des membres. Vigot, Paris, pp 47–86
19. Glockner JF, White LM, Sundaram M, McDonald DJ (2000) Unsuspected metastases presenting as solitary soft tissue lesions: a fourteen-year review. Skeletal Radiol 29:270–274
20. Gorelik E, Fogel M, De Batselier P, Katzav S, Feldman M, Segal S (1982) Immunobiological diversity of metastatic cells. In: Liotta LA, Hart IR (eds) Tumor invasion and metastasis. Nijhoff, Hague, pp 133–146
21. Gottlieb JA, Schermer DR (1970) Cutaneous metastases from carcinoma of the colon. JAMA 213:2083
22. Hain SF, Cooper RA, Aroney RS, King S, Roach PJ (1999) Soft-tissue uptake of colonic metastases. Clin Nucl Med 24:358–359
23. Hart IR, Talmadge JE, Fidler IJ (1981) Metastatic behavior of a murine reticulum cell sarcoma exhibiting organ-specific growth. Cancer Res 41:1281–1287
24. Herring CL Jr, Harrelson JM, Scully SP (1998) Metastasic carcinoma to skeletal muscle. A report of 15 patients. Clin Orthop Relat Res 355:272–281
25. Huth JF, Eilber FR (1988) Patterns of metastatic spread following resection of extremity soft-tissue sarcomas and strategies for treatment. Semin Surg Oncol 4:20–26
26. Khalili K, White LM, Kandel RA, Wunder JS (1997) Chondroblastoma with multiple distant soft tissue metastases. Skeletal Radiol 26:493–496
27. Kline TA, Neal HS, Holroyde CP (1976) Needle aspiration biopsy. Diagnosis of subcutaneous nodules and lymph nodes. JAMA 235:2848–2850
28. Laurence AE, Murray AJ (1970) Metastasis in skeletal muscle secondary to carcinoma of the colon-presentation of two cases. Br J Surg 57:529–530
29. Letanche G, Dumontet C, Euvrard P, Souquet PJ, Bernard JP (1990) Metastases distales des cancers bronchiques. Métastase osseuse et métastase des tissus mous. Bull Cancer 77:1025–1030
30. Liotta LA, Stetler-Stevenson WG (1993) Principles of molecular cell biology of cancer: cancer metastasis. In: De Vita VL Jr, Hellman S, Rosenberg SA (eds) Cancer: principles and practice of oncology, 4th edn. Lippincott, Philadelphia, pp 134–149
31. Magee T, Rosenthal H (2002) Skeletal muscle metastases at sites of documented trauma. Am J Roentgenol 178:985–988
32. Malloy PC, Fishman EK, Magid D (1992) Lymphoma of bone, muscle, and skin: CT findings. AJR Am J Roentgenol 159:805–809

33. Marklund SL, Westman NG, Lundgren E, Roos G (1982) Copper- and zinc-containing superoxide dismutase, manganese-containing superoxide dismutase, catalase, and glutathione peroxidase in normal and neoplastic human cell lines and normal human tissues. Cancer Res 42:1955–1961

34. Moulton JS, Blebea JS, Dunco DM, Braley SE, Bisset III GS, Emery KH (1995) MR imaging of soft-tissue masses: diagnostic efficacy and value of distinguishing between benign and malignant lesions. AJR Am J Roentgenol 164:1191–1199

35. Mulsow FW (1942) Metastatic carcinoma of skeletal muscles. Am J Surg 55:112–114

36. Narvaez JA, Narvaez J, Clavaguera MT, Juanola X, Valls C, Fiter J (1998) Bone and skeletal muscle metastases from gastric adenocarcinoma: unusual radiographic, CT and scintigraphic features. Eur Radiol 8:1366–1369

37. Nicolson GL, Winkelhake JL (1975) Organ specificity of bloodborne tumour metastasis determined by cell adhesion? Nature 255:231–233

38. Orr FW, Varani J, Kreutzer DL, Senior RM, Ward PA (1979) Digestion of the fifth component of complement by leukocyte enzymes. Am J Pathol 94:75–83

39. Patten RM, Shuman WP, Teefey S (1989) Subcutaneous metastases from malignant melanoma: prevalence and findings on CT. AJR Am J Roentgenol 162:1009–1012

40. Peh WCG, Shek TWH, Wang S-C, Wong JWK, Chien EP (1999) Osteogenic sarcoma with skeletal muscle metastases. Skeletal Radiol 28:298–304

41. Pellegrini AE (1979) Carcinoma of the lung occurring as a skeletal muscle mass. Arch Surg 114:550

42. Perrin AE, Goichot B, Greget M, Lioure B, Dufour P, Marcellin L, Imler M (1997) Metastases musculaires révélatrices d'un adenocarcinome. Rev Med Interne 18:328–331

43. Pollen JJ, Schmidt JD (1979) Diagnostic fine needle aspiration of soft tissue metastases from cancer of the prostate. J Urol 121:59–60

44. Poste G, Fidler IJ (1980) The pathogenesis of cancer metastasis. Nature 283:139–145

45. Pretorius ES, Fishman EK (2000) Helical CT of skeletal muscle metastases from primary carcinomas. AJR Am J Roentgenol 174:401–404

46. Rao UNM, Hanan SH, Lotze MT, Karakousis CP (1998) Distant skin and soft tissue metastases from sarcomas. J Surg Oncol 69:94–98

47. Safai B (1993) Cancers of the skin: tumors metastatic to skin. In: De Vita VL Jr, Hellman S, Rosenberg SA (eds) Cancer: principles and practice of oncology, 4th edn. Lippincott, Philadelphia p 1692

48. Schoenberg NY, Beltran J (1994) Contrast enhancement in musculoskeletal imaging. Radiol Clin North Am 32:337–352

49. Schultz SR, Bree RL, Schwab RE, Raiss G (1986) CT detection of skeletal muscle metastases. J Comput Assist Tomogr 10:81–83

50. Schütte HE, van der Heul RO (1990) Pseudomalignant, non-neoplastic osseous soft-tissue tumors of the hand and foot. Radiology 176:149–153

51. Seely S (1980) Possible reasons for the high resistance of muscle to cancer. Med Hypoth 6:133–137

52. Shives TC (1993) Biopsy of soft-tissue tumors. Clin Orthop Rel Res 289:32–35

53. Sidhu PS, Lewis M, Nicholson DA (1994) Soft tissue metastasis from a renal cell carcinoma. Br J Urol 74:799–801

54. Sorgente N, Kuettner KE, Soble LW, Eisenstein R (1975) The resistance of certain tissues to invasion. II. Evidence for extractable factors in cartilage which inhibit invasion by vascularized mesenchym. Lab Invest 32:217–222

55. Sridhar KS, Plasse TF, Holland JF, Shapiro M, Ohnuma T (1983) Effects of physiological oxygen concentration on human tumor colony growth in soft agar. Cancer Res 43:4629–4631

56. Sridhar KS, Rao RK, Kunhardt B (1987) Skeletal muscle metastases from lung cancer. Cancer 59:1530–1534

57. Stulc JP, Petrelli NJ, Herrera L, Lopez CL, Mittelman A (1985) Isolated metachronous metastases to soft tissue of the buttock from a colonic adenocarcinoma. Dis Colon Rectum 28:117–121

58. Sudo A, Ogihara Y, Shiokawa Y, Fujinami S, Sekiguchi S (1993) Intramuscular metastasis of carcinoma. Clin Orthop Rel Res 296:213–217

59. Suenaga M, Sanada I, Tsukamoto A, Sato M, Kawana F, Shido T, Miura K, Tominaga R (1993) Trisomy 4 in a case of acute myelogenous leukemia accompanied by subcutaneous soft tissue tumors. Cancer Genet Cytogenet 71:71–75

60. Sundaram M, McGuire MH, Herbold DR, Beshany SE, Fletcher JW (1987) High signal intensity soft tissue masses on T1-weighted pulsing sequences. Skelet Radiol 16:30–36

61. Tuoheti Y, Okada K, Osanai T, Nishida T, Ehara S, Hashimoto M et al. (2004) Skeletal muscle metastases of carcinoma: a clinicopathological study of 12 cases. Jpn J Clin Oncol 34:210–214

62. Verstraete KL (1995) Categorical course: introductory and advanced MRI: techniques with clinical applications. Presented at the joint meeting of the Society of MR and the Society for MR in Medicine and Biology. Nice, August 25

63. Verstraete KL, De Deene Y, Roels H, Dierick A, Uyttendaele D, Kunnen M (1994) Benign and malignant musculoskeletal lesions: dynamic contrast-enhanced MR imaging parametric "first-pass" images depict tissue vascularization and perfusion. Radiology 192:835–843

64. Vezeridis MP, Moore R, Karakousis CP (1983) Metastatic patterns in soft-tissue sarcomas. Arch Surg 118:915–918

65. Ward AJ, Bourke JB (1984) Skeletal muscle metastasis from prostatic carcinoma. J Urol 131:769

66. Weiss L (1989) Biomechanical destruction of cancer cells in skeletal muscle: a rate-regulator for hematogenous metastasis. Clin Exp Metastasis 7:483–491

67. Williams JB, Youngberg RA, Bui-Mansfield LT, Pitcher JD (1997) MR imaging of skeletal metastases. AJR Am J Roentgenol 168:555–557

68. Willis RA (1952) The spread of tumours in the human body. Butterworths, London, pp 284–285

69. Woodruff WW Jr, Djang WT, McLendon RE, Heinz ER, Voorhees DR (1987) Intracerebral malignant melanoma: high-field-strength MR imaging. Radiology 165:209–213

70. Zartman GM, Thomas MR, Robinson WA (1987) Metastatic disease in patients with newly diagnosed malignant melanoma. J Surg Oncol 35:163–164

Soft Tissue Lymphoma

26

P. Bracke, F.M. Vanhoenacker, J. Gielen,
A.M. De Schepper

Contents

26.1 Introduction

Lymphoma can involve any part of the musculoskeletal system. Primary lymphoma has initially been described involving the skin, subcutaneous tissues (mycosis fungoides), muscles, synovium, nerve roots and bone. Secondary lymphomatous involvement of the musculoskeletal system is common, while primary malignant soft tissue lymphoma is rare and accounts for only 0.1–2% of soft tissue tumors [20, 29]. An increased incidence has been noted in recent years, possibly related to an increase in the number of immunocompromised patients [23]. Classification of malignant lymphoma continues to evolve from increased understanding of normal lymphoid cell differentiation as well as from observations on behavior and response to therapy within lymphoma subtypes. Therefore comparing studies and data should be made with precaution, respecting the fact that lymphomas have been classified by several systems over the past 30 years.

The purpose of further classifying non-Hodgkin's lymphomas into specific categories is to describe the individual behavior and to develop appropriate treatment strategies for each type of lymphoma.

The most common classification system used in the 1980s-1990s was the International Working Formula-tion (IWF). The IWF divided non-Hodgkin's lymphomas into three grades based on the microscopic appearance. This type of histological grading into low-grade, intermediate-grade and high-grade lymphoma is found throughout case reports and in the literature [26, 29].

Since the utilization of the IWF, additional work is done that further classifies non-Hodgkin's lymphomas into individual cancers, each with specific features and behavior. This newer system is called the Revised European American Lymphoma (REAL) classification (1994). This REAL classification was so far updated in 1999 with the WHO modification [11] which recognizes three major categories of lymphoid malignancies based on morphology and cell lineage: B-cell neoplasms, T-cell/natural killer (NK)-cell neoplasms, and Hodgkin's lymphoma.

Almost all cases described in the literature and reflected in our series are non-Hodgkin's lymphomas, the majority of the B-cell type.

Histological and immunophenotypic studies show a range of small lymphocytic, follicular, mixed, small noncleaved and large cell (anaplastic, immunoblastic and centroblastic) lymphoma. Only a minority of T- cell lymphoma of the soft tissues is reported in the literature [1, 6, 16, 18, 26].

A distinctive subtype of soft tissue lymphomas has been reported by Isaacson and Wright [13] in 1983 and named MALTomas, where "MALT" stands for *mucosal associated lymphoid tissue*. These are the extra-nodal equivalent of monocytoid (marginal zone) B-cell lymphomas occurring in lymphoid organs such as the lymph node. Although MALT lymphomas occur most frequently in the stomach, they have also been described in various nongastrointestinal sites, such as salivary gland, conjunctiva, thyroid, orbit, lung, breast, kidney, skin, liver, and prostate, as well as the central nervous system. Most of these organ systems lack native lymphoid tissue but acquire MALT in close association with chronic inflammation or autoimmune processes. MALT lymphomas appear to have similar clinical, pathological and molecular features regardless of the organ of origin.

In the revised REAL-WHO classification, the MALT lymphomas were definitively classified among the marginal zone B-cell lymphomas.

26.2 Epidemiology

The disease mainly affects patients in their sixth to seventh decades. There is no sex predilection. As far as race is described in literature, there have been no black patients with primary soft tissue lymphoma. Ninety-five percent of lymphomas occur in the extremities, with 75% in the lower extremities [19]. Earlier studies also report a minor predilection for the gluteus and psoas muscles [3]. Primary soft tissue lymphoma is rather rare, the reported frequency depending on the strictness of definition. Lymphomas originating at soft tissue account for 0.11–2% of primary lymphomas.

Although extranodal lymphomas are common in HIV-1-positive disease in general, there are only a few reports of primary soft tissue non-Hodgkin's lymphoma in the literature [28].

MALToma represents about 8% of all non-Hodgkin's lymphomas [13]. Nongastrointestinal locations represent about 30–40% of all low-grade mucosa-associated lymphoid tissue (MALT) lymphomas.

26.3 Pathogenesis

Little is known about the etiology and pathogenesis of soft tissue lymphoma. An association has been described between B-cell lymphoma and rheumatoid arthritis [9]. Chronic local immune stimulation may have a significant role in the pathogenesis of these lymphomas, unlike the frequently reversible and EBV-positive lymphomas that occur in rheumatoid patients undergoing immunosuppressive therapy.

An increased incidence of soft tissue lymphomas has been described in patients who have previously undergone orthopedic surgery using metallic implants and after joint replacement, in acquired immune deficiency syndrome, and after organ transplantation with immunosuppressive treatment [4, 16, 25]. Some studies also suggest a possible correlation between dioxin pollution, the use of chlorinated drinking water, the exposure to chlorophenols or phenoxy herbicides and the presence of soft tissue sarcoma and non-Hodgkin's lymphoma.

26.4 Clinical Manifestations

The clinical presentation is non-specific. Lymphomas are relatively large tumors at presentation, varying from 2 cm to more than 15 cm. The soft tissue mass is often the only clinical finding. Pain and tenderness may be present and are more often found in case of lymphoma than in soft tissue sarcoma. In some cases increased serum levels of lactate dehydrogenase are found [5]. The general signs associated with the nodal type of lymphoma are only found in less than 2% of reported cases.

In rare cases, a nephrotic syndrome can be the initial presentation of soft tissue lymphoma [8, 18]. Locations such as stomach, intestine, skin, endocrine and salivary glands, as well as central nervous system, can present with atypical, nonspecific signs and symptoms related tot the site of origin. Neurological and skin involvements usually dominate the clinical presentation of intravascular lymphomatosis (IL) and mycosis fungoides. IL is a rare entity, only recently included in the lymphoma classification, whose main characteristics result from tumoral infiltration of the blood vessels, presenting with skin rash or neurological symptoms due to necrotic or demyelinating disorders.

26.5 Radiological Imaging

Plain radiographs are usually of little help in the assessment of soft tissue lymphoma, as they rarely show associated bone abnormalities.

On ultrasound, lesions are relatively heterogeneous, hyporeflective or isoreflective in comparison with adjacent muscles. The infiltrative pattern of the lesions can be appreciated by their rather irregular borders towards the adjacent muscle groups. Ultrasound can easily depict the infiltration of the subcutaneous fat by the tumor. In some cases, apparent coarsening of fibroadipose septa and swelling of muscle bundles may occur [2]. As with other soft tissue tumors, ultrasound has a very low specificity but can be used for monitoring therapy and biopsy guiding. Ultrasound can especially be used in the follow up of skin involvement.

Computed tomography shows lesions with an attenuation similar to that of muscle [17, 24]. As a consequence the lesion often cannot be distinguished from adjacent muscle fibers and presents as a diffuse soft tissue swelling. In the same way, a clinically apparent mass lesion in non-Hodgkin's lymphoma should not be neglected on the basis of an apparently unremarkable CT scan. After intravenous administration of iodinated contrast material enhancement of soft tissue lymphomas is mostly poor, though diffuse [8].

Angiography is of little or no value; lymphomas mostly present as hypovascular mass lesions [3].

On magnetic resonance imaging lymphomas merely present as large masses with signal intensities comparable to or slightly lower than adjacent muscles on T1-weighted images. In our own series of non-Hodgkin's soft tissue lymphoma, however, we found areas of mild hyperintensity on T1-weighted images in 10 out of 14

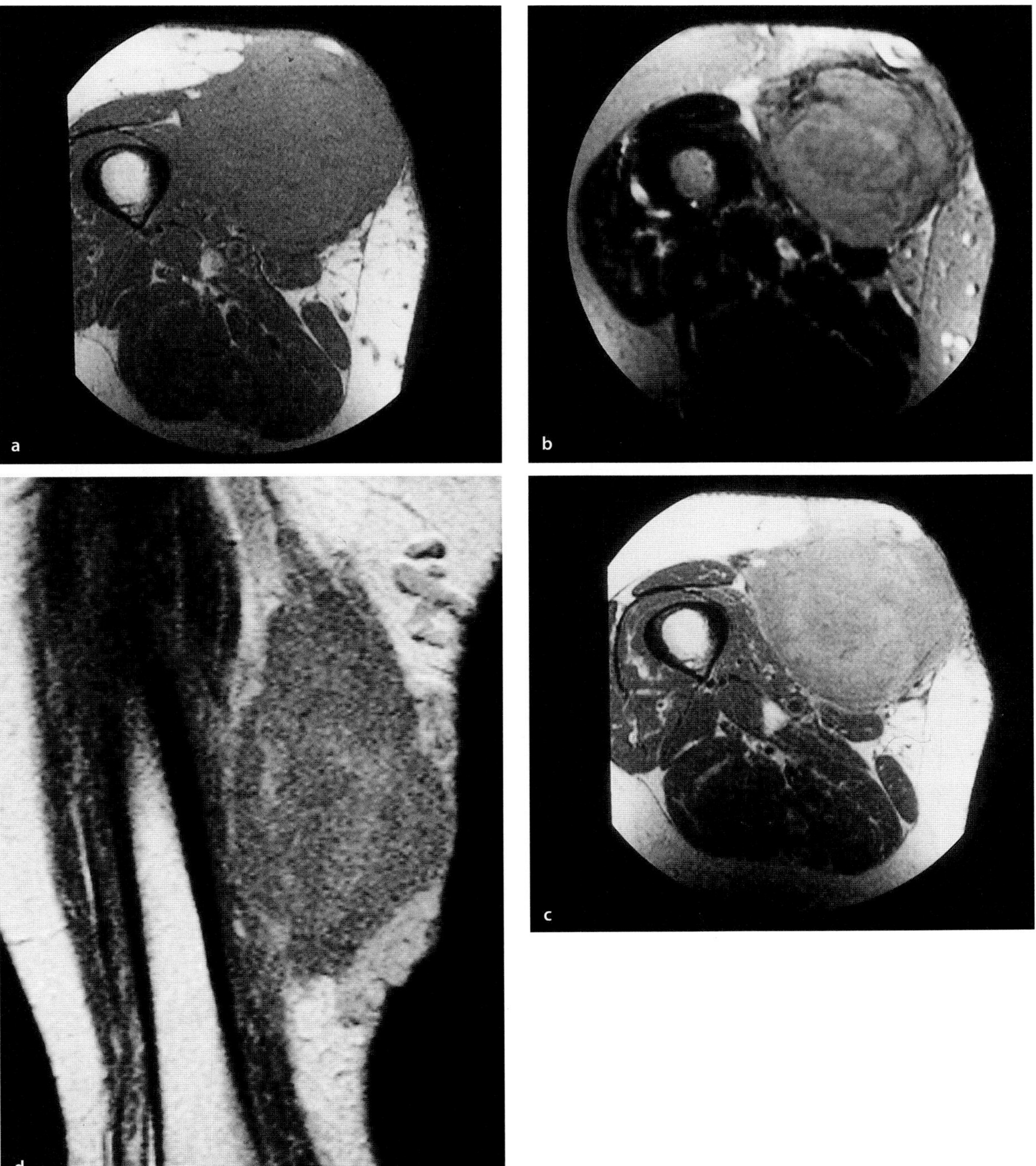

Fig. 26.1 a–d. Biopsy-proven non-Hodgkin's lymphoma of the quadriceps muscle in a 64-year-old woman: **a** axial spin-echo T1-weighted MR image; **b** axial spin-echo T2-weighted MR image; **c, d** axial and coronal spin-echo T1-weighted MR images after gadolinium contrast injection. On a T1-weighted image the lesion presents as a nodular mass, infiltrating the fascia and superficial fibers of the rectus femoris, vastus intermedius and adductor longus muscles. The lesion has a slightly higher signal intensity than adjacent muscle. There is extensive tumoral spread into the subcutis and cutis resulting in venous obstruction and superficial varices (**a**). After contrast injection there is a diffuse, moderately heterogeneous contrast enhancement providing a good differentiation between muscle fibers and tumor on T1-weighted images (**c,d**). On a T2-weighted image the extent of the lesion can be depicted better owing to the hyperintense appearance relative to the low signal intensity of muscle (**b**)

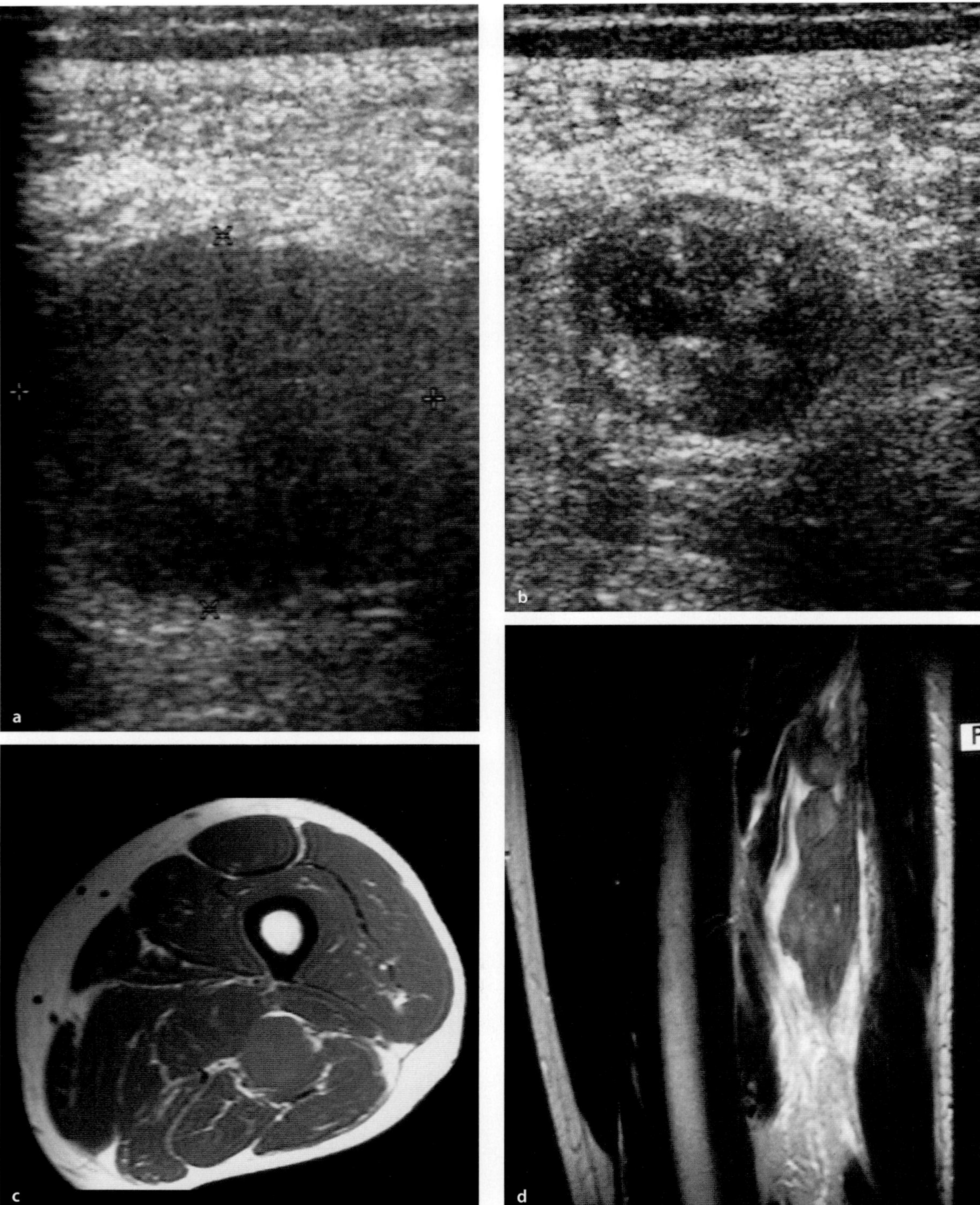

Fig. 26.2 a–e. A 66-year-old man with left sciatica presenting with a type-B non-Hodgkin's lymphoma in and around the sciatic nerve: **a, b** ultrasound; **c** axial spin-echo T1-weighted MR image; **d** sagittal spin-echo T2-weighted MR image. A nodular type of lesion is found on ultrasound between the hamstring muscles. The lesion is sharply demarcated and presents with similar, but more heterogeneous echogenicity to that of the hamstring muscles (**a**). In the caudal border of the lesion, hyper-echogenicity is due to in-filtration of the tumor in the surrounding fat (**b**). On T1-weighted images there is a nodular lesion in the center of the hamstrings along the neurovascular bundle. The lesion has a mildly hyperintense to iso-intense appearance, making differentiation with adjacent muscle groups relatively difficult (**c**). On T2-weighted images a mildly hyperintense, bead-like lesion extending along the nerve root with irregular fat planes towards the biceps femoris (caput longum) muscle is seen

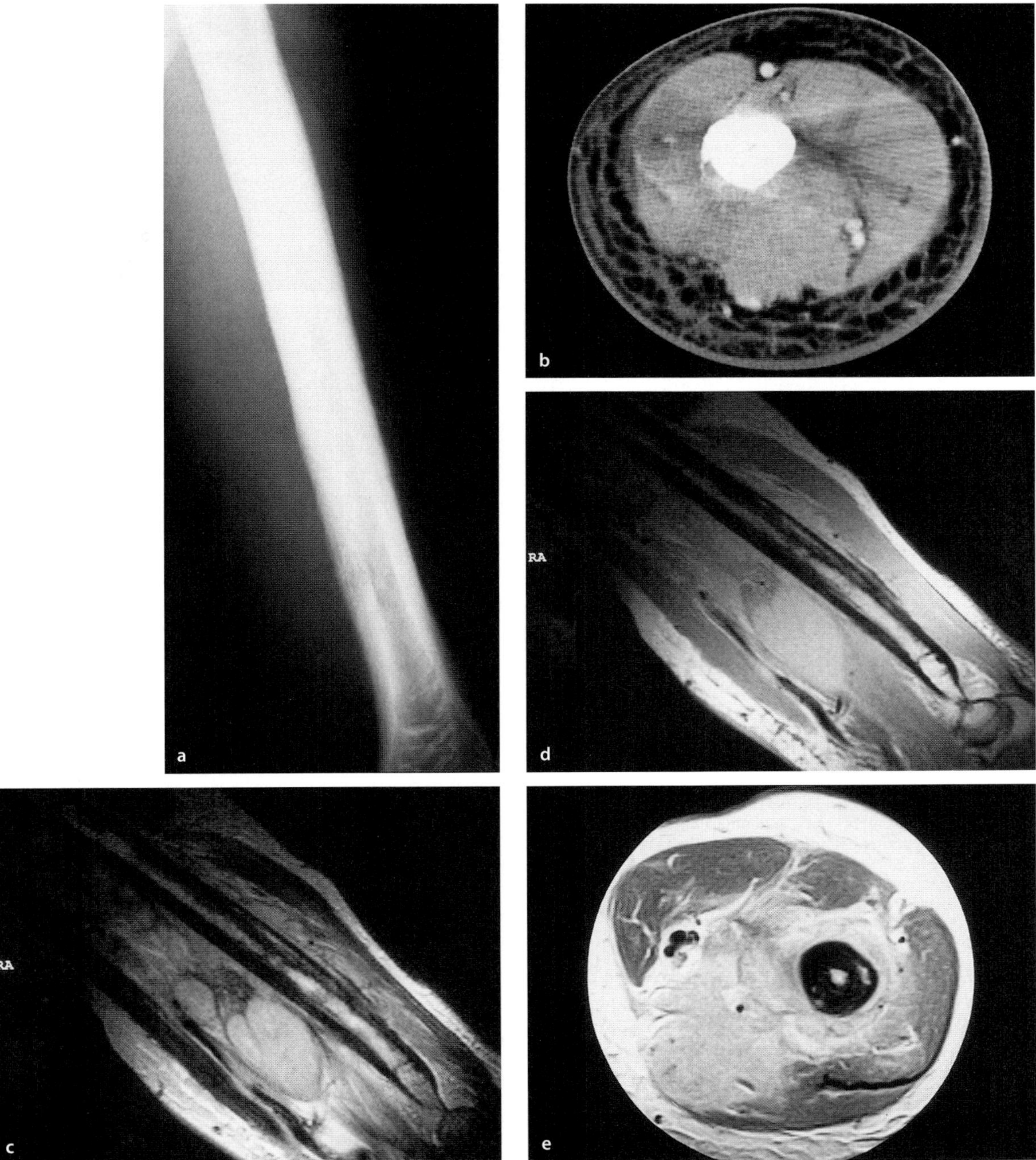

Fig. 26.3 a–d. A 64-year-old man with a palpable soft tissue mass at the left upper arm (non-Hodgkin's lymphoma): **a** radiography of the left humerus; **b** CT scan after iodinated contrast injection; **c,d** sagittal spin echo T1-and T2- weighted MR images; **e** axial spin echo T1-weighted MR image after gadolinium contrast administration. The initial radiographic examination reveals a permeated aspect of the cortex of the left humerus of a lengthy area with linear and irregular periosteal abnormalities (**a**). Contrast-enhanced CT-scan shows a diffuse iso-attenuating infiltrating mass, whereas the borders of the lesion cannot be distinguished from the adjacent muscle fibers. The density of the bone marrow is abnormal (**b**). The higher signal intensity of the tumor on corresponding T1- and T2-weighted images (**c,d**) is indicative of a diffuse infiltrating mass extending along the humeral shaft and infiltrating the brachioradial and triceps compartments. The bony 'wrap-around' sign of the tumor resulting in periosteal reaction at the humeral diaphysis and in bone marrow involvement is considered highly suggestive of soft tissue lymphoma. T1-weighted images after gadolinium contrast administration allow evaluation of tumor extension into different compartments and exclusion of invasion of the neurovascular bundle (**e**)

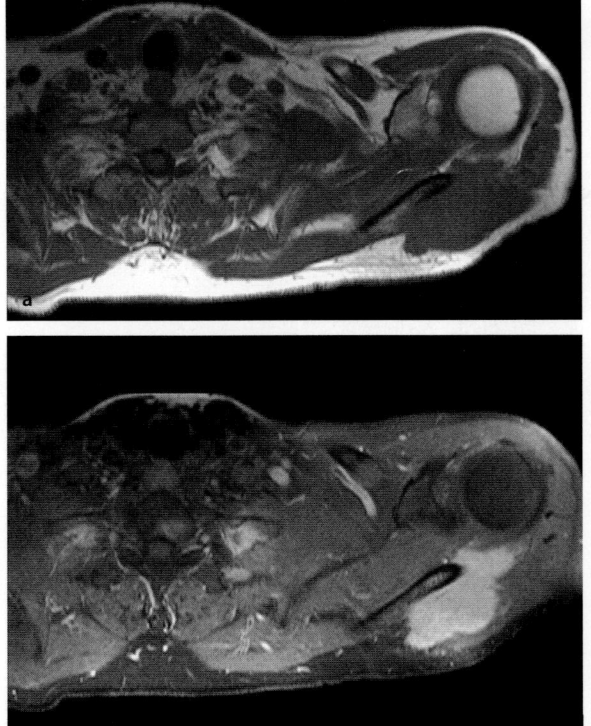

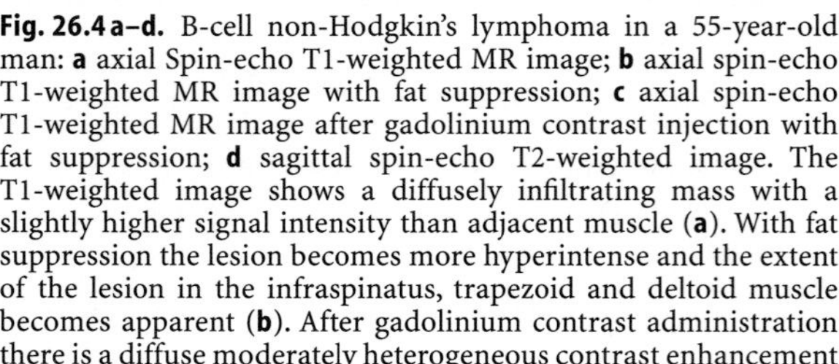

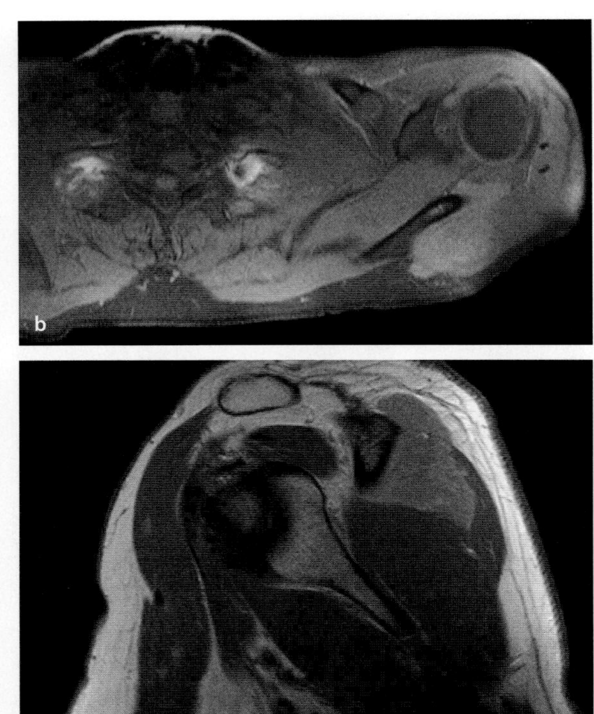

Fig. 26.4a–d. B-cell non-Hodgkin's lymphoma in a 55-year-old man: **a** axial Spin-echo T1-weighted MR image; **b** axial spin-echo T1-weighted MR image with fat suppression; **c** axial spin-echo T1-weighted MR image after gadolinium contrast injection with fat suppression; **d** sagittal spin-echo T2-weighted image. The T1-weighted image shows a diffusely infiltrating mass with a slightly higher signal intensity than adjacent muscle (**a**). With fat suppression the lesion becomes more hyperintense and the extent of the lesion in the infraspinatus, trapezoid and deltoid muscle becomes apparent (**b**). After gadolinium contrast administration there is a diffuse moderately heterogeneous contrast enhancement providing a good differentiation between muscle fibers and tumor on the T1-weighted image (**c**). On the T2-weighted image, the lesion is better depicted owing to the hyperintense appearance relative tot the low signal intensity of muscle, illustrating the extent of tumoral involvement with a sharp transition zone to the surrounding trapezoid muscle (**d**). The T2-weighted image and the T1-FS-weighted image after gadolinium demonstrate an intact aspect of the cortical bone of the scapula with a sharp demarcation between the relative hyperintense tumor and the cortical bone of the scapula (**c,d**).

cases. T1-weighted images with fat suppression demonstrate a hyperintense aspect of the infiltrating lesion in comparison to the surrounding muscle tissue. Lesions tend to be hyperintense on T2-weighted images. Only one report describes a relative low to isointense signal of lymphoma on T2-weighted images with a hyperintense signal on STIR images [21]. In our studies we have two similar patients presenting with a low SI on T2-weighted images. After intravenous administration of gadolinium-DTPA there is a mild to moderate, diffuse enhancement. There are in general no signs of necrosis or hemorrhage before treatment (Figs. 26.1–26.5).

Two different morphological patterns are encountered: a more polynodular, which is usually more superficial and a deeper, diffuse infiltrative pattern. In both cases lesions behave aggressively, often infiltrating multiple muscle groups, with no respect for compartment boundaries. The transition of the tumor is irregular without cleavage planes towards adjacent muscle fibers (Figs. 26.1 and 26.2). Infiltration along the neurovascu-

lar bundle and extension through subcutaneous strands is often present (5 out of 11 cases in our series). The strands are hypointense on TI-weighted images and mildly hyperintense on T2-weighted images. The strands show little or no gadolinium-DTPA enhancement. Often there is encasement of major vascular structures.

MR is the imaging technique of choice for demonstrating neurovascular encasement and defining the extent of cortical bone and marrow involvement. Lymphoma can infiltrate and/or surround the cortical bone with changes in the signal intensity of the adjacent marrow. In these cases, differentiation between secondary soft tissue lymphoma by extracortical spread of primary bone lymphoma and primary soft tissue lymphoma with secondary bone involvement is often not possible. The first possibility is supported by findings of Hicks, the second by findings of Moulopoulos [12, 22].

Moulopoulos [22] reviewed a series of 13 stage IV lymphomas with bone involvement. If tumor was pre-

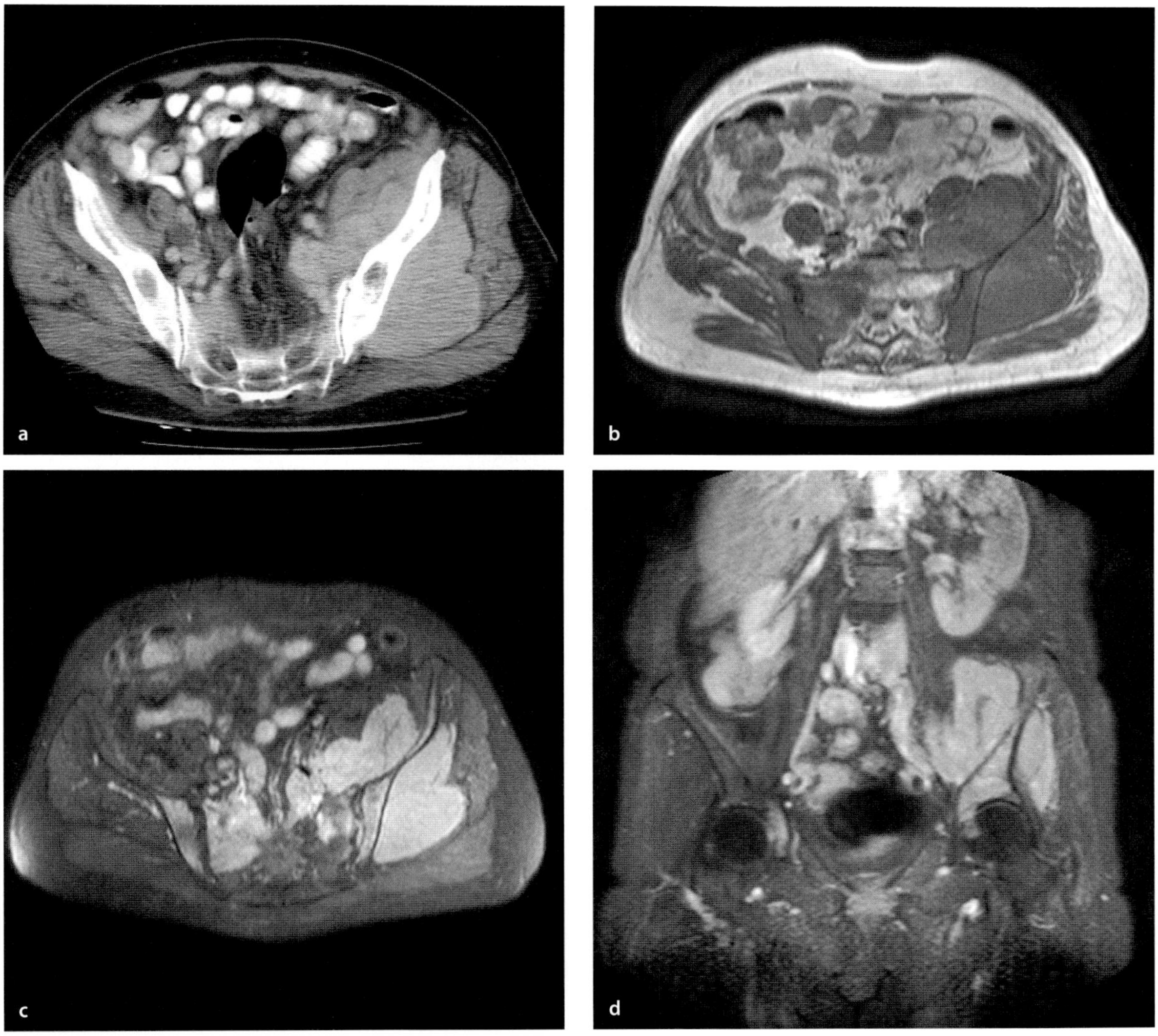

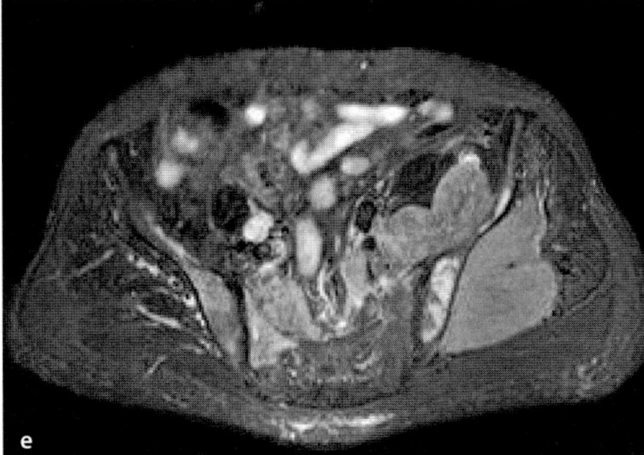

Fig. 26.5 a–e. Giant B-cell lymphoma in a 68-year-old woman: **a** axial CT image after IV contrast injection; **b** axial spin-echo T1-weighted MR image; **c** axial spin-echo T1-weighted MR image after gadolinium contrast injection with fat suppression; **d** coronal spin-echo T1-weighted MR image after gadolinium contrast injection with fat suppression; **e** axial spin-echo STIR-weighted image. CT image after contrast shows a butterfly-shaped lesion consisting of a soft tissue mass enveloping the cortical bone of the iliac crest. The lesion shows a homogeneous contrast enhancement making the lesion mildly hyperdense in comparison to the gluteal and iliac muscles (**a**). The T1-weighted image shows no apparent destruction of the iliac wing. The lesion is rather homogeneous presenting with a signal intensity similar to the surrounding muscle structures (**b**). Both T1- and T2-weighted images with fat suppression illustrate focal areas of abnormal bone marrow due to permeative bone infiltration characteristic of lymphoma without apparent bone destruction. The presentation is typical for the "wrap-around" sign seen in bone and soft tissue lymphoma (**c–e**). The hyperintensity of the lesion after fat suppression allows better evaluation of the tumor extent and better delineate the transition of tumoral tissue to normal gluteal and iliac muscle fibers. The tumor enhances homogeneously showing minor internal septation (**c,d**)

sent on either side of the bony cortex but the contour of the affected bone was preserved, it was described as 'wrapped-around' (Fig. 26.5). This wrap-around sign is indicative of a primary soft tissue lymphoma and is not found in patients with myeloma or metastases.

Hicks et al. [12] recently showed that the absence of cortical destruction in the case of a soft tissue mass adjacent to a bone lymphoma does not exclude the possibility of an extension of the primary bone disease into adjacent soft tissues. In their study of primary bone lymphoma, they showed the presence of intracortical channels which are filled with tumoral material.

In those studies, however, the intraosseous component preceded the development of a soft tissue mass or was very extensive in proportion to the soft tissue mass itself. In our series the soft tissue component of the tumors was accompanied by only a mild endomedullary component in four cases. The soft tissue component was obviously more extensive than the bone marrow abnormalities. Intracortical channels were not shown either before or after intravenous gadolinium-DTPA administration. Consequently these lesions are considered primary soft tissue lymphoma with secondary bony involvement.

26.6 Nuclear Medicine

Similar to systemic lymphoma, gallium and positron emission tomography show a marked accumulation of radionuclide and are therefore used in the follow-up and therapy of soft tissue lymphoma. A diffuse, widespread accumulation of radioisotope in the affected muscle can also be seen in rhabdomyolysis [18]. Rhabdomyolysis can be a sequel of lymphoma, as a result of the tendency of malignant lymphoma to increase the amount of muscle damage. Muscle damage may be caused by diffuse infiltration into muscles, by affection of multiple neighboring muscle compartments and metastasizing into other soft tissues, as well as a sequel of cytotoxic actions. This can account for the number of patients reported with renal dysfunction associated with muscle lymphomas.

The different imaging modalities are complementary rather than competitive in the evaluation of malignant lymphoma. The imaging characteristics are not specific for lymphoma subtypes.

26.7 Staging

In addition to characterization, imaging techniques are mandatory to determine the stage or local and distant cancer spread. All new treatment information is categorized and evaluated by the stage of the disease. AJCC Manual for Staging Cancer is used to stage lymphoma

Table 26.1. Staging of lymphoma

Stage I Involvement of a single lymph node region (I) or of a single extra-lymphatic organ or site (IE)
Stage II Involvement of two or more lymph node regions on the same side of the diaphragm (II) or localized involvement of extra-lymphatic organ or site and of one or more lymph node regions on the same side of the diaphragm (IIE)
Stage III Involvement of lymph node regions on both sides of the diaphragm (III) which may also be accompanied by localized involvement of extralymphatic organ or site (IIIE) or by involvement of the spleen (IIIS) or both (IIISE)
Stage IV Diffuse or disseminated involvement of one or more extra-lymphatic organs or tissues with or without associated lymph node enlargement

(Table 26.1). It was originally developed for Hodgkin's disease, and later expanded to include non-Hodgkin's lymphoma.

Determining the local extent of the cancer requires MRI, distant spread may be studied by CT of the abdomen and thorax, MRI of the brain and skeletal scintigraphy and/or PET-scan and blood tests. Although an extranodal presentation of lymphoma means stage IV disease (involves one or more organs outside the lymph system or a single organ and a distant lymph node site) imaging will be used to exclude involvement of other nodal or organ involvement.

26.8 Differential Diagnosis

Lymphoma in an extranodal site can be confused with a wide variety of both inflammatory as well as neoplastic conditions.

Fine-needle aspiration biopsy (FNAB), core biopsy or open biopsy is mandatory for a definite diagnosis. In the majority of cases, it is possible to obtain a specific diagnosis and subtype of soft tissue lymphoma using FNAB [30]. Reliable differentiation of lymphoma from other small round cell tumors, such as rhabdomyosarcoma or Ewing's sarcoma and from metastatic carcinoma is necessary for therapeutic purposes. Light microscopy is usually sufficient for diagnosis. However, myxofibrosarcoma (formerly known as malignant fibrous histiocytoma) may be difficult to distinguish from Hodgkin's disease. This resemblance occurs more often in the presence of tumors in which histiocyte-like cells are intermingled with chronic inflammatory cells [7]. In these cases immunohistochemical examination is mandatory. Leu-M1 is a marker for Reed-Sternberg cells, which are not found in myxofibrosarcoma. Anaplastic, sarcomatoid lymphoma appearing primarily in the soft tissues without peripheral lymphadenopathy can create considerable diagnostic difficulties even for the pathologist, as it may be mistaken for sarcoma [1]. An accurate histological diagnosis is essential, because treatment of a muscle mass based on histological diagnosis of an undifferentiated neoplasm may lead to unnecessary radical surgery [27].

Diagnosing non-Hodgkin's lymphoma requires a great deal of skill, and an expert pathologist. The use of Fluorescence In Situ Hybridization (FISH), DNA microarray technology and the use of CD Markers are just some of the tests and technologies that may be used to achieve a correct diagnosis.

Moreover, a correct diagnosis of primary lymphoma is essential because the long-term prognosis is usually good if the tumor is properly managed. Collaboration between the radiologist and pathologist is a prerequisite for a correct diagnosis. In this regard, the presence of adenopathies and the infiltrative pattern of lymphomas in contrast to sarcomas can help pathologists in orienting the tissue diagnosis. Tumor size is not a prognostic tool in predicting survival [10]. Staging for systemic disease is done by thoracic and abdominal CT and/or MR.

Things to remember:
1. Whenever a soft tissue mass is encountered, which is iso- to slightly hyperintense on T1-weighted images and hyperintense on T2-weighted images with a diffuse infiltrative pattern extending into different muscle groups, lymphoma should be included in the differential diagnosis.
2. A soft tissue mass wrapped around bone is especially suspect for extranodal primary soft tissue lymphoma.

References

1. Axiotis CA, Fuks J, Jennings TA, Kadish AS (1988) Peripheral T-cell lymphoma presenting as a soft tissue mass of the extremity. Arch Pathol Lab Med 112:850–851
2. Beggs I (1997) Primary muscle lymphoma. Clin Radiol 52:203–212
3. Bruneton JN, Drouillard J, Balu-Maestro C et al. (1990) Imaging of malignant lymphoma of muscular sites. J Radiol 71:185–189
4. Chevalier X, Amoura Z, Viard JP, Souissi B, Sobel A, Gherardi R (1993) Skeletal muscle lymphoma in patients with the acquired immunodeficiency syndrome: a diagnostic challenge. Arthritis Rheum 36:426–427
5. Damron TA, Le MH, Rooney MT, Vermont A, Poiesz BJ (1999) Lymphoma presenting as a soft tissue mass: a soft tissue sarcoma simulator. Clin Orthop 360:221–230
6. Ellstein J, Xeller C, Fromowitz F, Elias JM, Saletan S, Hurst LC (1984) Soft tissue T-cell lymphoma of the forearm: a case report. J Hand Surg Am 9:346–350
7. Enzinger F, Weiss SW (1995) In: Enzinger FM, Weiss SW (eds) Soft tissue tumors, 3rd edn. Mosby, St Louis, p 367
8. Girad T, Nochy D, Montravers F (2004) Intravascular large B-cell lymphoma revealed by a nephritic syndrome: a one year remission induced by a high frequency CHOP and rituximab. Leuk Lymphoma 45(8):1703–1705
9. Goodlad JR, Hollowood K, Smith MA, Chan JK, Fletcher CD (1999) Primary juxtaarticular soft tissue lymphoma arising in the vicinity of inflamed joints in patients with rheumatoid arthritis. Histopathology 34:199–204
10. Grunshaw ND, Chalmers AG (1992) Skeletal muscle lymphoma. Clin Radiol 45:399–400
11. Harris NL, Jaffe ES, Kiebold J, Flandrin G, Muller-Hermelink HK, Vardiman J (2000) Lymphoma classification-from controversy to consensus: the REAL and WHO Classification of lymphoid neoplasms. Ann Oncol 11(suppl 1):3–10
12. Hicks DG, Gokan T, O'Keefe RJ et al. (1995) Primary lymphoma of bone: correlation of MR imaging features with cytokine production by tumor cells. Cancer 75:973–980
13. Isaacson P, Wright DH (1983) Malignant lymphoma of mucosa associated lymphoid tissue: a distinctive type of B-cell lymphoma. Cancer 52:1410–1416
14. Lanham GR, Weiss SW, Enzinger FM (1989) Malignant lymphoma. A study of 75 cases presenting in soft tissue. Am J Surg Pathol 13:1–10
15. Lee VS, Martinez S, Coleman RE (1997) Primary muscle lymphoma: clinical and imaging findings. Radiology 203:237–244
16. Lum GH, Cosgriff TM, Byrne R, Reddy V (1993) Primary T-cell lymphoma of muscle in a patient infected with human immunodeficiency virus. Am J Med 95:545–546
17. Malloy PC, Fishman EK, Magid D (1992) Lymphoma of bone, muscle and skin: CT findings. Am J Roentgenol 159:805–809
18. Masaoka S, Fu T (2002) Malignant lymphoma in skeletal muscle with rhabdomyolysis: a report of two cases. J Orthop Sci 7(6):688–693
19. Maurer R, Tanner A, Honegger HP, Schmid U, Schmid L (1988) Primary non-Hodgkin lymphoma of the muscles. Schweiz Med Wochenschr 18:354–357
20. Meister HP (1992) Malignant lymphomes of soft tissues. Verh Dtsch Ges Pathol 76:140–145
21. Metzler JP, Fleckenstein JL, Vuitch F, Frenkel EP (1992) Skeletal muscle lymphoma: MRI evaluation. Magn Reson Imaging 10:491–494
22. Moulopoulos LA, Dimopoulos MA, Vourtsi A, Gouliamos A, Vlahos L (1999) Bone lesions with soft tissue mass: magnetic resonance imaging diagnosis of lymphomatous involvement of the bone marrow versus multiple myeloma and bone metastases. Leuk Lymphoma 34:179–184
23. Murphey MD, Kransdorf MJ, Smith SE (1999) Imaging of soft tissue neoplasms in the adult: malignant tumors. Semin Musculoskeletal Radiol 3:39–58
24. Panicek DM, Lautin JL, Schwartz LH, Castellino RA (1997) Non-Hodgkin lymphoma in skeletal muscle manifesting as homogeneous masses with CT attenuation similar to muscle. Skeletal Radiol 26:633–635
25. Radhi JM, Ibrahiem K, al-Tweigeri T (1998) Soft tissue malignant lymphoma at sites of previous surgery. J Clin Pathol 51:629–632
26. Salamao DR, Nascimento AG, Lloyd RV, Chen MG, Habermann TM, Strickler JG (1996) Lymphoma in soft tissue: a clinicopathologic study of 19 cases. Hum Pathol 27:253–257
27. Schwalke MA, Rodil JV, Vezeridis MP (1990) Primary lymphoma arising in skeletal muscle. Eur J Surg Oncol 16:70–73
28. Sipsas NV, Kontos A, Panayiotakopoulos GD (2002) Extranodal non-Hodgkin lymphoma presenting as a soft tissue mass in the proximal femur in a HIV+ patient. Leuk Lymphoma 43(12):2405–2407
29. Travis WD, Banks PM, Reiman HM (1987) Primary soft tissue lymphoma of the extremities. Am J Surg Pathol 11:359–366
30. Wakely P, Frable WJ, Kneisl JS (2001) Soft tissue aspiration cryopathology of malignant lymhoma and leukemia. Cancer 93(1):35–39

Imaging of Soft Tissue Tumors in The Pediatric Patient

27

A.M. De Schepper, L.H. De Beuckeleer,
J.E. Vandevenne

Contents

27.1 Introduction

Tumors of the musculoskeletal system are rare in childhood and, when discovered, are worrisome to both parents and physicians.

In Kransdorf's series from the Armed Forces Institute of Pathology (AFIP), only 1,330 (5%) of 26,854 soft tissue tumors arose in utero and in young children (0–5 years) and only 7% in children between 6 and 15 years old [2, 5]. In our series of 982 histologically proven soft tissue tumors, 4% were found in children of 0–5 years and 9% in those of 6–15 years [6].

Fortunately, most soft tissue tumors arising in children are benign. In a study performed in Denmark, only 14% of 76 neonates with a congenital malignancy had a soft tissue sarcoma [8]. In the United States, evidence exists that malignancies among children younger than 15 years are increasing in incidence, except for Wilms' tumor and soft tissue and bone sarcoma [9]. In a series of the AFIP, 79% of soft tissue tumors in children between 0 to 5 years old are benign, as are 70% in those from 6 to 15 years [2, 5]. In our pediatric series of soft tissue tumors, 90% of the tumors were benign. In contrast, only 60% of soft tissue tumors in adults are benign. The difference in incidences between these two centers could be explained by the referral nature of the AFIP series, with a higher incidence of malignant tumors accumulated during a ten-year period, whereas

our series included patients referred to our large community university hospital primarily to undergo diagnostic imaging procedures, especially magnetic resonance (MR) imaging of a soft tissue mass.

Some tumors are more frequently encountered in the pediatric age group (Table 27.1) [10–32]. Most common malignant tumors in children between 0 and 5 years are fibrosarcoma (36% of all malignant soft tissue tumors in this age group), rhabdomyosarcoma (21%), giant cell fibroblastoma (7%), dermatofibrosarcoma protuberans (6%), angiomatoid malignant fibrous histiocytoma (5%) and malignant peripheral nerve sheath tumor (5%). In children between 6 and 15 years, the most common malignant tumors are angiomatoid "malignant" fibrous histiocytoma (16%), synovial sarcoma (13%), rhabdomyosarcoma (11%), fibrosarcoma (8%), and malignant fibrous histiocytoma (7%). Traditionally, pediatric oncologists have arbitrarily divided soft tissue sarcomas into two groups: rhabdomyosarcoma (RMS), the most common soft tissue sarcoma of childhood, and non-RMS soft tissue sarcomas (NRSTS), a biologically and clinically heterogeneous assortment of tumors. The most common NRSTS in childhood are synovial sarcoma, malignant fibrous histiocytoma, malignant peripheral nerve sheath tumor, and fibrosarcoma. RMS is more common in children less than 10 years of age, whereas the NRSTS predominate in the older age groups [40]. On the contrary, in the files of the Kiel Pediatric Tumor Registry (n=4272 soft tissue malignancies) rhabdomyosarcomas are by far the most frequent sarcomas (44.6% of the cases), followed in decreasing order of frequency by the family of Ewing tumors (peripheral primitive neuroectodermal tumors and extraosseous Ewing's sarcomas; altogether 22.3%), malignant peripheral nerve sheath tumors (8.1%), synovial sarcomas (5.0%), leiomyosarcomas (3.2%), fibrosarcomas (2.4%), extrarenal malignant rhabdoid tumors (2%), and alveolar soft tissue sarcomas (1.1%). A further group (11.3%) includes rare tumors, intermediate fibrohistiocytic tumors, and unclassified sarcomas. Embryonal rhabdomyosarcomas are 2.5 times more frequent than the alveolar rhabdomyosarcomas, which are prognostically unfavorable and located predominantly in the extremities

Table 27.1. Common soft tissue (pseudo) tumors in childhood

Tumor subtype	Preferential age	Location, clinical information	Important histological features
Fibroblastic/myofibroblastic tumors			
Fibromatosis colli	Newborn	Neck region Lower portion of the sternocleido-mastoid muscle Unilateral, fusiform Spontaneous regression	Fibroblastic proliferation
Fibrous hamartoma	0–2 years	Upper portion of the extremities (axillary and inguinal region) Subcutaneous tissue	Fibrocollagenous, myxoid and mature adipose components
Infantile digital fibromatosis	0–1 years	Dorsolateral aspect of the fingers and toes (II-V) Single or multiple	Presence of intracytoplasmatic inclusion bodies
Myofibromatosis	0–2 years	Nodules in head and neck region Visceral nodules Osteolytic lesions Single or multiple Spontaneous regression of the bone and soft tissue lesions when no visceral involvement exists	Abundance of myofibroblasts Highly vascular central area Central fibrosis and calcifications
Infantile hemangio-pericytoma (same spectrum as myo-fibroma(tosis)	0–1 year	Head and neck, retroperitoneum, (lower) extremities	Branching vascular spaces lined by normal endothelium, with pericytes in between
Juvenile hyaline fibromatosis	2 months to 4 years	Multiple (sub)cutaneous nodules in head and neck region, foot, thigh Gingival hyperplasia Mental retardation Flexion contractures Osteolytic lesions (systemic disease)	Homogeneous eosinophilic ground substance in which a few spindle cells are embedded
Infantile fibromatosis	0–5 years	Head and neck region, limb girdles, proximal extremities Infiltrating soft tissues	Immature type: primitive mesenchymal cells and fibroblasts Mature type: mature fibroblasts and collagen
Inflammatory myo-fibroblastic tumor	Children and young adults	Lung, mesentery and omentum Rare in soft tissues Mass, fever, weight loss and pain	Spindled myofibroblasts, fibroblasts and inflammatory cells
Calcifying aponeu-rotic fibroma	<12 years M/F = 2/1	Rare tumor Hands and feet Deep palmar fasciae	Fibroblast-like cells with blunt nuclei and abundant cytoplasm in a parallel (cord-like) orientation Nodular deposits of calcification
Low and High grade Myofibrosarcoma		Low grade: infiltrative Deep soft tissues (head-neck) No metastases High grade: may metastasize	Myofibroblasts Nuclear pleomorphism Resemble MFH
Infantile (congenital) fibrosarcoma	0–1 years (20% at birth)	Hands>feet Large, infiltrating lesion Better prognosis than adult form, metastases rare	Primitive fibroblasts, highly cellular, prominent mitotic activity, interlacing fascicles sometimes in a herringbone pattern
Fibrohistiocytic tumors			
Juvenile xantho-granuloma	0–6 months	Skin or deep seated Single or multiple Macronodular form associated with multiple organ involvement	Uniform histiocytes, xanthomatous cytoplasm, and eosinophils
Lipomatous (pseudo) tumors			
Lipoblastoma-lipoblastomatosis	0–4 years M/F=2/1	Extremities, subcutis, chest Invasive growth pattern with extension into preformed spaces. (intercostal space, neuroforamina)	Immature lipoblasts, myxoid matrix, lobular architecture, fibrous septa
Fibrolipohamartoma of nerve (neural fibrolipoma)	<20 years	Distal upper extremities (median nerve) Sausage-like, spaghetti-like, fusiform	Proliferation of fatty and fibrous components surrounding the nerve

Table 27.1. *(continued)*

Tumor subtype	Preferential age	Location, clinical information	Important histological features
Muscular tumors			
Fetal rhabdomyoma	0–3 years M>F	Head and neck Superficial Single	Bland primitive spindled cells, fetal myotubules, myxoid stroma
Embryonal rhabdomyosarcoma	0–15 years	19% of all childhood soft tissue sarcomas Head and neck (40%), Extremities (more in adults) Early metastatic potential	Small cells with round hyper-chromatic nuclei, rhabdomyoblasts (eosino- philic cytoplasm)
Vascular tumors			
Juvenile (infantile) capillary hemangioma	0–1 year F>M	1/200 births, involutes by age of 7 years in 75–90% of cases Biphasic growth curve: initial proliferation, spontaneous involution Head and neck (periparotid) Skin, subcutaneous tissues Association with Klippel-Trenaunay-Weber syndrome	Small vessels lined by flattened endothelial cells
Cavernous hemangioma	0–5 years F>M	Upper portion of the body Deep seated, intramuscular No spontaneous involution Association with Kasabach-Merritt and Maffucci's syndromes	Dilated spaces filled with blood, serpentine channels Flattened endothelium Dystrophic calcification, ossification (phleboliths) (30–50%)
Intramuscular hemangioma	15–30 years F=M	Thigh, deep intramuscular location	Reactive, fatty overgrowth
Arteriovenous hemangioma (malformation)	Young children	Superficial or deep location	
Synovial hemangioma	Adolescents	Pain, swelling, decreased range of motion Monoarticular (knee, elbow) Repetitive episodes of intra-articular bleeding	50%: Cavernous type of hemangioma 25%: Capillary type of hemangioma
Angiomatosis	10–20 years	Limbs, viscera Soft tissue, bone, visceral involvement	Mixture of capillary, cavernous and arterio-venous lesions Mature adipose tissue
Lymphangioma	0–2 years	Head and neck (75%), axilla (20%) Capillary, cavernous and cystic (cystic hygroma) types Soft fluctuant mass	Noncommunicating lymphoid tissue lined by lymphatic endothelium
Neurogenic tumors			
Neurofibroma	Rare in children 20–30 years F=M	Superficial, subcutis Neck, limbs (Neurofibromatosis I)	Originates in the nerve Consists of Schwann cells and fibroblasts Zonal distinction
Schwannoma	Rare in children 20–70 years F=M	Head and neck, limbs	Eccentric location on a nerve Schwann cells in a collagenous matrix, Antoni A and B cells
Primitive neuroectodermal tumors			
Extraskeletal Ewing's sarcoma PNET Askin tumor (PNET of chest wall)	10–30 years	Trunk (paravertebral region and chest wall), extremities Rapidly growing	Small, round blue cells Rich in collagen Highly vascularized Areas of hemorrhage, necrosis
Tumors of uncertain differentiation			
Fibrous Histiocytoma Angiomatoid	Children Young adults	Extremities Rare metastases Noninvasive	Multinodular proliferation of eosino- philic, histiocytoid or myoid cells Pseudoangiomatoid spaces Thick fibrous pseudo-capsule Pericapsular lymphoplasmacytic infiltrate

Table 27.1. *(continued)*

Tumor subtype	Preferential age	Location, clinical information	Important histological features
Pseudotumors			
Myositis ossificans	9–40 years M>F	Extremities (lower>upper) Related to trauma Intramuscular Solitary Self-limiting	"Zoning" phenomenon (centripetal maturation)
Fibroplasia ossificans progressiva	0–6 years	Calcification – ossification of ligaments, muscles, tendons and fat Thumb and great toe malformation	Early stage: edema, proliferation of fibroblasts Advanced stage: deposition of abundant collagen Late stage: ossification – calcification at the center of the lesion
Subcutaneous granuloma annulare	4–15 years	Subcutaneous nodule(s) Dorsal aspect of the hands, feet, forearms, arms, legs, thighs	Fibrinoid degeneration of collagen surrounded by palisading fibroblasts and histiocytes

and the trunk. With regard to clinical findings, histology, molecular biology and prognosis, embryonal and alveolar rhabdomyosarcomas have to be considered as two different tumor types. The family of Ewing tumors includes extraosseous Ewing's sarcoma and peripheral primitive neuroectodermal tumors (synonym: malignant peripheral neuroectodermal tumors), the former tumors without and the latter with neural differentiation. Many cases of infantile malignant peripheral nerve sheath tumors and infantile fibrosarcomas are low-grade malignancies and are prognostically more favorable than their "adult" counterparts [26]. The most common benign masses in young children between birth and 5 years are hemangioma (15% of all benign tumors in this age group), fibromatosis (11%), granuloma annulare (10%), infantile myofibromatosis (8%), and lipoblastoma (8%). The most frequent benign tumors in older children (6 to 15 years) are fibrous histiocytoma (17%), nodular fasciitis (16%), hemangioma (13%), and fibromatosis (5%) [2, 5].

The location of soft tissue masses in children varies. In children younger than 6 years of age, almost 60% of benign and malignant lesions occur within the head and neck region, the lower extremity, or the trunk. In children of 6 to 15 years old, benign tumors most often occur in the hand or wrist, the head and neck region, and the lower extremities [2, 5], whereas malignant soft tissue tumors in this age group are more common in the lower or upper extremity or the trunk. Rhabdomyosarcomas in the pediatric age group have a different anatomic distribution when compared with non-rhabdomyosarcoma tumors in children and soft tissue tumors in adults [34]. Many of the primary sites of childhood rhabdomyosarcoma, such as the orbit, bladder, prostate, and paratesticular region are virtually never primary sites of the non-rhabdomyosarcoma tumors in children and of other soft tissue sarcomas in adults [34].

Pediatric soft tissue sarcoma may occur as a second malignant neoplasm due to treatment of a prior primary childhood malignancy and/or genetic susceptibility. In a series of 25 patients treated for different primary tumors second malignant neoplasms occurred after a median of 8 years and included rhabdomyosarcoma, malignant peripheral nerve sheath tumor, extraosseous Ewing family tumor, leiomyosarcoma, fibrosarcoma and synovial cell sarcoma [4]

27.2 The Role of Imaging

Not all masses require imaging evaluation. Most cutaneous or subcutaneous masses are very small and are often excised without imaging studies. Other benign masses (capillary hemangioma) may be recognized by experienced dermatologists, pediatricians, or surgeons and are not evaluated with imaging because of characteristic clinical presentation.

Because the young patient frequently has nonspecific symptoms, and complaints are often initially neglected, diagnosis may be delayed. Indeed, children often have injuries related to play, and pain and soft tissue masses may thus be attributed to former trauma. Unfortunately, when dealing with malignant soft tissue tumors, therapeutic options and long-term survival are strongly related to the disease stage at the time of diagnosis. Therefore, when symptoms persist, an adequate physical examination and dedicated imaging studies (plain film and/or CT, ultrasonography, MR imaging) should be performed [35].

To achieve the best outcome, patients with soft tissue sarcomas should be sent to specialized oncologic centers to receive optimal diagnostic and therapeutic management [36]. In our center, the cases of all patients are presented to an Advisory Board on Bone and Soft Tissue Tumors. Diagnostic problems are discussed, appropri-

Table 27.2. Imaging findings in soft tissue (pseudo) tumors in childhood (*WI* weighted image/s)

Tumor subtype	Plain film/CT	Ultrasonography	MR imaging
Fibrous (pseudo) tumors			
Fibromatosis colli	None	Homogeneous Reflectivity depends on age of the lesion	T1-WI: intermediate SI T2-WI: intermediate SI

Fibrous hamartoma	None	Homogeneous (?)
		
		Increased reflectivity
			T1-WI: inhomogeneous,
			  intermediate SI
			T2 WI: inhomogeneous,
			  low to intermediate SI

Infantile digital fibromatosis	None	Not reported	T1-WI: intermediate SI

Myofibromatosis	Intralesional "cornflake"
	  calcifications
	Osteolytic lesions of long bones
	  (metaphyseal, eccentric),
	  spine, ribs
	Hypodense, inhomogeneous
	  mass with intralesional
	  calcifications (CT)
	Slightly, patchy, or marked
	  enhancement (CT)
		Hyperreflective intralesional
		  dots (calcifications)
			T1-WI: homogeneous,
			  low to intermediate SI
			T2-WI: inhomogeneous,
			  intermediate to high SI

Infantile hemangio-pericytoma	Marked enhancement (CT)	Not specific	Vascular channels T2-WI: low SI (high flow) T2-WI: high SI (slow flow)
Juvenile hyaline fibromatosis	Osteolytic lesions (long bones, epiphyseal), acro-osteolysis	Not reported	T2-WI: high SI

Infantile fibromatosis	Homogeneous, iso-to hyperdense
	  to muscle, enhancing after
	  contrast injection (CT)
		Hyporeflective, ill defined	T1-WI: low to intermediate
			T2-WI: low, intermediate to high SI
			Infiltrative margins (57%)
			Marked enhancement (72%)

Calcifying aponeurotic fibroma	Stippled calcifications	Not reported	T1-WI: intermediate SI T2-WI: intermediate SI
Infantile (congenital) fibrosarcoma	Associated bone involvement	Not reported	Nonspecific
Fibrohistiocytic tumors			
Juvenile xantho-granuloma		Not reported	Not reported
Lipomatous (pseudo) tumors			

Lipoblastoma	Hypodense, inhomogeneous mass
	  (Fatty components)
		Hyperreflective,
		  homogeneous lesion (CT)
			T1-WI: inhomogeneous,
			  low to intermediate SI
			T2-WI: high SI

Fibrolipohamartoma of nerve (neural fibrolipoma)	Associated macrodactyly	Increased reflectivity
		  of enlarged neural bundles
			Inhomogeneous, fascicular sign
			  (axial images)
			Neural components:
			  low SI on T1- and T2- WI
			Fatty components: increased SI
			  on T1- and T2-WI

Muscular tumors			
Fetal rhabdomyoma	Not reported	Not reported	Non-specific
Embryonal rhabdo-myosarcoma	Associated bone involvement Bony metastasis	Intratumoral calcifications and necrosis	Non-specific T1-WI: intermediate SI T2-WI: high SI
Vascular tumors			
Juvenile capillary hemangioma	Non-specific enhancing mass (CT)	Non-specific	T1-WI: low SI (areas with high SI: fat) T2-WI: high SI Marked enhancement

Cavernous hemangioma	Phleboliths (30%)
	Mass with serpentine vascular
	  components (CT)
		Nonspecific, complex mass
		Phleboliths
		  (acoustic shadowing)
			Vascular spaces: fluid-fluid levels
			Phleboliths: signal voids
			T2-WI: heterogeneous mass,
			  high SI (circular, linear, serpentine)
			Marked enhancement

Table 27.2. *(continued)*

Tumor subtype	Plain film/CT	Ultrasonography	MR imaging
Vascular tumors			
Intramuscular hemangioma	Phleboliths (rare) Serpentine enhancement (CT) Reactive periosteal reaction (rare)	Complex reflectivity Phleboliths Doppler: low vascular resistance	T1-WI: low to intermediate SI with high SI areas (fatty components) T2-WI: very high SI (vascular components) Intermediate SI (non-vascular fatty components) Marked enhancement
Arteriovenous hemangioma (malformation)			Prominent serpentine vessels Fast flow (low SI on T1- andT2- WI)
Synovial hemangioma	Bone erosions (resembling PVNS or hemophilic arthropathy) Joint effusion (hemarthrosis)	Not specific	T1-WI: Low-to-intermediate SI with high SI areas (fatty components) T2-WI: very high SI (vascular components) Marked enhancement
Angiomatosis Lymphangioma	Lytic, multifocal lesions Multilocular mass, with fibrous septations (CT) Water density (CT) Calcifications (rare)	Not reported Polylobular Solid and cystic components intervening septa	See hemangiomas T1-WI: low SI T2-WI: high SI Heterogeneous enhancement Septal enhancement Fluid-fluid levels(bleeding)
Neurogenic tumors			
Neurofibroma	Bone erosions Hypodense mass (CT) Little or no enhancement (CT)	Hypoechoic, ovoid mass	T1-WI: low SI (almost identical to SI of muscle) T2-WI: high SI Variable enhancement Target appearance
Schwannoma	Bone erosions Hypo- to iso-dense mass (CT) Strong enhancement (CT) Central cystic changes (CT)	Hypoechoic, solid mass Posterior signal reinforcement (50%)	T1-WI: low SI (almost identical to SI of muscle) T2-WI: high SI Strong enhancement (heterogeneous in large lesions)
Primitive neuroectodermal tumors			
Extraskeletal Ewing's sarcoma	Well-circumscribed mass (CT)	Mixed reflectivity (hyporeflective)	Non-specific
PNET-Askin tumor	Heterogeneous mass with low attenuation (CT) Variable enhancement (CT)	Hyporeflective cystic components	T1-WI: heterogeneous, low to intermediate SI T2-WI: heterogeneous, high SI Marked heterogeneous enhancement Intratumoral hemorrhage and necrosis
Tumors of uncertain differentiation			
Fibrous histiocytoma Angiomatoid	Children Young adults	Extremities Rarely metastases Non-invasive	Multinodular proliferation of eosinophilic, histiocytoid or myoid cells Pseudoangiomatoid spaces Thick fibrous pseudocapsule Pericapsular lymphoplasmacytic infiltrate
Pseudotumors **Myositis ossificans** Early stage	No abnormalities	Well-defined, elongated hyporeflective mass Moderate distal acoustic enhancement	T1-WI: intermediate SI T2-WI: high SI (seldom rim of low SI) Edema around the lesion
Subacute stage	Non-ossified center with peripheral rim of mature bone		T1-WI: intermediate or slightly increased SI T2-WI: high SI (rim of low SI) Edema around the lesion Foci of low SI (ossification) Seldom fluid-fluid levels (hemorrhage)

Table 27.2. *(continued)*

Tumor subtype	Plain film/CT	Ultrasonography	MR imaging
Chronic stage	Considerable ossification	Well-defined hyperreflective peripheral rim (calcifications) with acoustic shadowing	T1-WI: low SI surrounding core of fatty marrow T2-WI: low SI surrounding core of fatty marrow No edema around the lesion Foci of low SI (ossification)
Fibroplasia ossificans progressive	Bony bridges ectopic calcification Short thumbs and fifth fingers	Not reported	Nonspecific
Subcutaneous granuloma annulare	Nonspecific subcutaneous nodule(s) Poorly defined mass with variable attenuation and enhancement (CT)	Hypoechoic, relatively poorly defined lesion	T1-WI: low SI T2-WI: low to intermediate SI T1-WI+Gd: strong enhancement

Table 27.3. **Table 27.3.** Diseases concomitant with soft tissue masses

Mass	Concomitant disease(s)
Angiomatosis	Concomitant osseous involvement
Infantile myofibromatosis	Concomitant osseous involvement+nodular soft tissue tumors
Infantile fibromatosis	
Juvenile hyaline fibromatosis	Concomitant osseous involvement+nodular soft tissue tumors+ hypertrophic gingiva+flexion contractures+acro-osteolysis
Cavernous hemangioma(s)	Maffucci's disease
Schwannoma(s)	Neurofibromatosis
Neurofibroma(s)	
Fibrolipohamartoma of the median nerve	Macrodystrophia lipomatosa of the digits
Lymphangioma	Turner syndrome Noonan syndrome Fetal alcohol syndrome Down syndrome Familial pterygium colli

ate therapeutic approaches are formulated, and the follow-up of previously presented patients is noted. The importance of constant data communication is stressed by M. Lawrence, who has stated that clinical trials will continue to be vital to the refinement of clinical management of all sarcomas in both children and adults [34].

In this regard we organized the "Belgian Soft Tissue Neoplasm Registry", which is a multi-institutional databank containing actually more than 1500 histologically proven soft tissue tumors.

The diagnostic gain reached in the last decade, together with new developments in therapeutic regimens for soft tissue tumors, enables the surgeon to use reconstructive and limb salvage procedures instead of radical or wide amputation or even mutilating disarticulation. Newer methods of diagnosis (dynamic contrast-enhanced MR imaging, PET scan, molecular biology, immunology, and cytogenetics) may give us additional insight into the biology of tumors and may help us in tailoring therapeutic strategies according to these biologic and imaging characteristics [37–42].

The following discussion provides an overview of imaging techniques applicable to soft tissue tumors in the pediatric patients. Because of the number of soft tissue masses found in the pediatric patient, this review presents the findings in tabular format. The clinical, histologic, and imaging features of benign, malignant, and pseudotumoral soft tissue masses most frequently encountered in children and concomitant diseases are presented in Tables 27.1–27.3 [10–32]. As a guideline for the reader, other tables present the most common locations for tumors (Table 27.4), multiplicity (Table 27.5), different shapes associated with specific soft tissue tumors (Table 27.6), and specific MR features, including presence of signal voids (Table 27.7), fluid-fluid levels (Table 27.8), and signal intensities on spin echo MR sequences (Table 27.9).

Neuroblastoma and ganglioneuroma are two tumors that often affect young children. However, because they

Table 27.4. Preferential location of soft tissue tumors

Location	Tumor
Neck	Cystic hygroma – lymphangioma
Sternocleidomastoid	Capillary hemangioma
muscle	Fibromatosis colli
Trunk	Askin (PNET) tumor
Axilla	Cystic hygroma-lymphangioma
Upper limb	
Wrist	Ganglion cyst
Wrist, volar aspect	Fibrolipohamartoma of median nerve
Hand, volar aspect	Fibrolipohamartoma of median nerve
Finger, dorsal aspect	Digital fibroma
Lower limb	
Thigh	Fibrohamartoma of infancy
Knee	Synovial hemangioma
Knee, tibiofibular joint	Ganglion cyst
Ankle	Ganglion cyst
Foot, extensor aspect	Ganglion cyst
Upper and lower limbs	Myositis ossificans
Hand and feet	Calcifying aponeurotic fibroma
Joints, periarticular	Synovial hemangioma
Cutis, subcutis	Dermatofibrosarcoma protuberans

Table 27.6. Shape

Fusiform (ovoid)	Neurofibroma Lipoma
Dumbbell	Neurofibroma
Moniliform	Neurofibroma
Round	Cyst Schwannoma
Serpiginous	Hemangioma Lymphangioma

Table 27.7. Intratumoral signal void

Flow	Hemangioma (capillary) Arteriovenous malformation
Calcification	Hemangioma (phlebolith) Lipoma (well-differentiated and dedifferentiated) Myositis ossificans (marginal) Myofibromatosis

Table 27.5. Multiplicity

Venous malformation
Lipoma (5–8%)
Neurofibroma
Dermatofibrosarcoma protuberans
Desmoid

Table 27.8. Fluid- fluid levels

Hemangioma
Cystic lymphangioma
Synoviosarcoma
Hematoma

Table 27.9. Signal intensities on spin echo sequences

High SI on T1-WI+intermediate SI on T2-weighted images	Lipoma Lipoblastoma Fibrolipohamartoma
High SI on T1+high SI on T2-weighted images	Hemangioma Lymphangioma Subacute hematoma Low-flow a-v malformation
Low SI on T1+high SI on T2-weighted images	Cyst
Intermediate SI on T1+high SI on T2-weighted images	Neurogenic tumors
Low to intermediate SI on T1-weighted+low SI on T2-weighted images	Fibrolipohamartoma Acute hematoma (few days) Old hematoma High-flow a-v malformation Mineralized mass Scar tissue Subcutaneous granuloma annulare High-grade malignancies

do not arise in the peripheral musculoskeletal system, they are beyond the scope of this chapter and are not included. Some other tumors that are not characteristic for the pediatric age group but seldom arise in children (e.g. elastofibroma, giant cell tumor of the tendon sheath, non-rhabdomyosarcomas, ...) are also not included in the list.

27.3 Imaging Modalities

27.3.1 Ultrasonography

When a child has been referred for diagnostic work-up of a suspected soft tissue mass, ultrasonography must be the first imaging modality, because it can readily demonstrate the presence of a mass without intravenous contrast medium, requires only minimal cooperation of the child and no sedation, does not expose the child to radiation, and is reproducible and inexpensive. When masses are located in the subcutaneous region, standoff pads are often useful. Dynamic US examination of a soft tissue mass (e.g. flexion or extension maneuvers) often allow the sonographer to evaluate the relationship of the lesion to the underlying fascia, muscles or tendons.

The shape, volume, borders and compressibility of small masses are readily recognizable, as are the relationships to adjacent structures. Deeper seated or larger tumors are more difficult to examine adequately because anatomic landmarks are lacking and depth penetration is limited. To achieve deeper penetration and a wider field of view in an anatomic compartment, transducers with lower frequency (5 MHz) are necessary, but they lower the spatial resolution of the method.

Ultrasonography makes it possible to differentiate between solid and cystic tumors. The specificity of this method is very low however, mostly resulting in the inability of the sonographer to give an accurate tissue-related diagnosis. Since there are no pathognomonic ultrasound criteria for grading soft tissue tumors, ultrasonography often does not allow to differentiate between benign and malignant soft tissue masses.

Some soft tissue masses, with a characteristic shape, echogenicity, or both, are neurogenic tumors (oval, hyporeflective masses with posterior acoustic enhancement in more than 50 % of our tumors studied), lipomas (oval, mostly well-circumscribed, homogeneous masses with iso-, hypo- or hyperreflective presentation), ganglion cysts (anechoic and rounded masses), hemangiomas (irregular, circumscribed, or infiltrating, hypo- or slightly hyperreflective lesions, often containing phleboliths characterized by echogenic foci with posterior acoustic shadowing), and lymphangiomas (polylobular, poorly defined masses with cystic and solid components, separated by intervening septa) [43, 44].

Color Doppler ultrasound examination and spectral analysis help quantify the degree of vascularization and analysis of flow patterns and are useful in diagnosing tumor vascularity (such as occurs in hemangiomas), evaluating response to local or systemic chemotherapy, and in guiding biopsy procedures [43, 45]. When non-palpable recurrences are detected by means of ultrasonography, CT or MR imaging, intraoperative ultrasound-guided localization may be necessary. Despite the excellent application of Color Doppler ultrasound in the evaluation of the response of soft tissue sarcoma to chemotherapy, we disagree with Menke and Solbiati [44, 46] that ultrasonography is useful in early detection of recurrent or residual disease. We have often found the results of ultrasonography as the first-line examination to be inconclusive for recurrence, whereas those provided by MR imaging, especially with the newer dynamic techniques [38], have been more accurate and we now regard MRI as mandatory for the preoperative work-up when a recurrent mass has been noted.

Ultrasonography may also be useful in detecting retained foreign bodies in patients with a pseudotumoral inflammatory mass, and in diagnosing a ganglion cyst, bursitis, or abscess.

However, where ultrasonography fails, MR imaging is an accurate problem-solver for evaluating tumor-like conditions (e.g. abscess, hematoma, myositis, accessory muscle).

The overall value of ultrasonography has to be relativated. In a recent study by Brouns et al. [7] about delay in diagnosis of soft tissue sarcoma, wrong diagnosis on ultrasound was cited as the most frequent reason for this delay.

27.3.2 Plain Film/CT

Plain films are of only limited value in diagnostic work-up of a child with a soft tissue mass. Involvement of adjacent osseous structures may be detected (e.g. in myofibromatosis, juvenile hyaline fibromatosis, infantile fibrosarcoma, and angiomatosis). Associated bone alterations may be detected (e.g. macrodactyly in fibrolipohamartoma) and the presence and morphology of intralesional calcifications (e.g. hemangiomas, myofibromatosis) or ossifications may be evaluated and lead to a correct (differential) diagnosis. Plain films may also contribute to the differential diagnosis against pseudotumoral lesions (e.g. myositis ossificans).

CT examination allows confirmation of the presence of a clinically suspected mass. The ability to perform imaging in axial plane and the presence of the contralateral part of the body within the field of view allows the detection of deep-seated tumors even when they are small. Involvement of the adjacent bony structures is much more accurately appreciated than on plain films, and intralesional calcifications, fat, fluid, vessels, blood, and gas may be adequately recognized on CT. However current indications for CT are few in number, because MR imaging is the accepted primary technique for evaluating soft tissue tumors.

27.3.3 MR Imaging

MR imaging is a powerful diagnostic tool in the work-up of soft tissue tumors in children. However, motion artifacts may be a major problem in MR imaging. A number of simple measures can be taken to obtain high-quality images. It is of the utmost importance to immobilize the patient adequately and comfortably on the scanner table. Tape, sponges, Velcro straps, and vacuum cushions may be used to immobilize the limbs of the child. In children older than 6 years of age sedation is not needed. Younger children (especially those under 3 years of age), require sedation if adequate images are to be achieved. In our institution, chloral hydrate (0.5 ml/kg body weight) is administered p.o., following a standardized protocol. Peripheral saturation is monitored by way of pulse oximetry.

Dedicated surface coils should be used as much as possible to improve the signal-to-noise ratio and spatial resolution. The imaging protocol for work-up of soft tissue tumors consists of T1- and T2-weighted images and is similar to those of the adult [47]. Spin echo T2-weighted images are frequently replaced by fast spin echo or turbo spin echo weighted sequences because acquisition times are shorter. A major disadvantage of fast SE T2-weighed imaging is the high SI of fat. Gradient echo sequences have less value in work-up of soft tissue tumors, but may be used to demonstrate susceptibility artifacts when one suspects the presence of hemosiderin.

STIR sequences and fat-saturated T1- and T2-weighted sequences are now frequently used because they have a higher sensitivity in lesion detection.

Gadolinium-enhanced T1-weighted images are performed to define the local tumor extent, to demonstrate intratumoral necrosis and to follow-up tumors [38]. MR features of pediatric soft tissue tumors are presented in Tables 27.6–27.9.

When CT, MR imaging, or both do not allow a specific diagnosis of a benign condition, an open or percutaneous biopsy must be performed. Because more than 70 % of all soft tissue masses in children are benign, it is important not to perform a biopsy on 'do-not-touch' lesions and to restrict biopsies only to tumors that show signs of malignancy or aggressiveness [48]. To avoid areas of necrosis or hemorrhage, accurate percutaneous biopsies can be performed under guidance of ultrasonography or CT scan [49]. Fluid collections can be aspirated using fine needles, and solid tumors be biopsied using large-core needles. For performance of MR-guided percutaneous biopsies, an open or 'dough-nut' magnet configuration is more attractive as this makes the child more accessible.

27.3.4 Angiography

The role of angiography in the diagnostic work-up of soft tissue masses is currently restricted to preoperative vascular mapping or therapeutic embolization of highly vascularized tumors.

It does not allow accurate differentiation of benign from malignant tumors and only rarely provides a precise tissue-related diagnosis.

It requires catheterization, iodinated contrast media, ionizing radiation, all of which should be avoided, whenever possible, in the pediatric patient with a soft tissue tumor. If knowledge of tumor vascularity is mandatory for accurate therapeutic planning, MR angiography of affected body areas may become an alternative method.

27.4 Role of Imaging in Staging and Tissue Characterization

Soft tissue tumors, like all tumors, grow in a centrifugal fashion until resistance is met. In soft tissue, the barriers consist of major fibrous septa, and the origins and insertions of muscles. As the natural barriers are encountered, growth tends to occur in the plane of least resistance, which in the case of soft tissue tumors means in a longitudinal fashion, i.e. in the compartment of origin. As the tumor grows, the host responds by creating a reactive fibrovascular tissue which forms a true limiting capsule in the case of benign lesions. Aggressive lesions compress the host reactive tissue into a "pseudocapsule" containing fingerlike or nodular tumoral foci called "satellite lesions". In highly aggressive lesions tumoral foci are found beyond the reactive zone within the compartment of origin. They are called "skip metastases".

The *staging* system of the Musculoskeletal Tumor Society (Enneking system) and of the American Joint Committee on Cancer Staging for tumors of mesenchymal origin are based on the interrelationship of significant variables such as the grade (low, medium, high), the site (compartment), and the presence or absence of metastases [50, 51]. Although the Musculoskeletal Tumor Society system is the system predominantly used for the grading of soft tissue sarcomas in adults and of non-rhabdomyosarcomas in children, the American Joint Committee on Cancer system, based on the tumor-lymph node-metastases (TNM) classification supplemented by histological grade, is also used for these tumors [52].

Rhabdomyosarcoma poses a particular problem because this tumor presents in a wide variety of clinical settings and histological types, with different mechanisms of spread and with different prognoses. Because all rhabdomyosarcomas are highly malignant, anatomical sites and TNM data are more important than microscopic grading. The current systems for staging rhabdomyosarcoma are the more widely used TNM system of the American Joint Committee and the revised system of the Intergroup Rhabdomyosarcoma Study [53, 54], which are based on the TNM classification and on the status of the patient at presentation. Anatomical site is an important prognostic variable and is used as a major grouping [53, 54]. Most children with cancer are treated in specialized centers and are entered on clinical research protocols; thus, most of the common pediatric neoplasms are effectively staged and imaging studies have an important role [54]. Radiography, CT and MR imaging can demonstrate bone involvement, which will change the surgical stage of a soft tissue tumor. Bone scintigraphy is used for screening for bone metastases, and CT scan of the chest is the preferred method for detection of pulmonary metastases. Local staging is best achieved by MR imaging. The multiplanar capabilities and the unique soft tissue resolution of the method allow exact definition of location, extent, and relationship with surrounding muscular, fascial, neurovascular, subcutaneous and osseous structures. Coronal or sagittal images demonstrate the full extent of the involved compartment. Recently, fluorodeoxyglucose (F-18) PET was found to have the potential for grading soft tissue sarcomas because of its ability to show different metabolic rates among different tumor grades, although there is some overlap [39].

Characterization of a tumor consists of both grading and the tissue-specific diagnosis [41].

Although histology is the gold standard for diagnosing soft tissue tumors, prediction of a specific histological diagnosis remains one of the ultimate goals of each new imaging technique. If imaging studies could provide a specific diagnosis or a limited differential diagnosis, decisions on biopsy and treatment could be simplified. Furthermore, if a definite diagnosis could be made, most soft tissue masses arising in children would not need an aggressive work-up and biopsy could be avoided.

Because of high intrinsic contrast resolution, it was anticipated that MR imaging would be useful in characterizing tissues and in providing tissue-specific diagnosis of soft tissue tumors. Unfortunately, MR tissue characterization may be limited for two reasons. First of all, MR images only provide indirect information about tumor histology by showing signal intensities related to some physicochemical properties of tumor components (e.g. fat, blood, water, collagen) and, consequently, reflect gross morphology of the lesion rather than underlying histology. Soft tissue tumors belonging to the same histologic group may have a different composition or different proportions of tumor components resulting in different MR signals; this feature is well exemplified by the group of lipomatous tumors. Only lipomas and well-differentiated liposarcomas are predominantly fatty, while lipoblastomas have less than 25% fat.

The second difficulty in obtaining a tissue-specific diagnosis on soft tissue tumors on MR imaging is related to the time-dependent changes that occur during natural evolution or as a consequence of therapy. Young fibrous tumors are highly cellular, with a high water content that results in high SI on T2-WI. Over time, they become more collagenous and less cellular, which results in a decrease in SI that is more characteristic of fibrous tissue. Another example of time-related changes is the signal intensity of large malignant tumors, which undergoes changes as a consequence of intratumoral necrosis, bleeding, or both.

The highest confidence in characterization occurs with the benign masses (lipomas, hemangiomas, benign neurogenic tumors, periarticular cysts, hematomas, and abscesses) seen in the pediatric patient [47, 55]. For example, Laor and Burrows reported on the ability of MR imaging to differentiate between different subtypes of hemangiomas [56]. Lesions characterized by high flow on the GRE images, were further examined with SE sequences. When a mass lesion is noted on T1- or T2-weighted SE MR images with high flow, it is reasonable to conclude that it corresponds to an infantile capillary hemangioma, whereas a high flow pattern without obvious mass represents an arteriovenous hemangioma. A mass lesion with slow flow on GRE sequences, corresponds to a venous hemangioma or a lymphangioma. Vascular lesions that exhibit slow flow on gradient echo sequences are differentiated by means of their enhancement pattern. Diffusely enhancing lesions correspond to venous hemangiomas, whereas septal enhancement is seen in lymphangiomas [56].

The imaging parameters for predicting the malignancy of soft tissue tumors in adults and children have been discussed by several groups [57, 60] and include size, shape, margin, homogeneity of signal intensity on different sequences, contrast enhancement on both static and dynamic studies, peritumoral edema, hemorrhage/necrosis, growth rate, and extent (intra- or extra-compartmental, bone involvement and neurovascular displacement/encasement). Few studies have been published on differentiation between benign and malignant soft tissue tumors in children. One must always approach an apparently benign, small, well-circumscribed tumor carefully, and masses should be considered to be indeterminate unless the tissue-specific diagnosis can be given with reference to the child's age, signal features, and location [47].

Things to remember:

1. Soft tissue tumors are rare in childhood and adolescence. They are mostly benign. Hemangiomas are the most common benign, rhabdomyosarcomas the most common malignant soft tissue tumors.

2. Notwithstanding the limitations of ultrasound, it remains the first choice diagnostic modality in children suspect of having a soft tissue tumor.

3. Plain radiography and CT scan are best suited for demonstration of calcified lesions or intralesional calcifications.

4. MR imaging is also in children the main modality of grading, staging and characterizing (definition of a tissue specific diagnosis) soft tissue tumors.

5. Because long term survival of children with malignant soft tissue tumors in strongly related to disease stage at the time of diagnosis, early detection is mandatory.

6. Rhabdomyosarcomas have a staging system apart where TNM, anatomical site and clinical status at presentation are major variables.

7. Tissue specific diagnosis by imaging is achievable in a lot of benign tumors but difficult in the malignant group.

8. Children with a soft tissue tumor should be treated in specialized centers as well for diagnosis as for treatment and follow-up.

References

1. Ahn JM, Yoon HK, Suh YL et al. (2000) Infantile fibromatosis in childhood: findings on MR imaging and pathologic correlation. Clin Radiol 55(1):19–24
2. Berquist T, Ehman R, King B, et al. (1990) Value of MR imaging in differentiating benign from malignant soft tissue masses: study of 95 lesions. AJR Am J Roentgenol 155:1251–1255
3. Billings SD, Giblen G, Fanburg-Smith JC (2005) Superficial low-grade fibromyxoid sarcoma (Evans tumor): a clinicopathologic analysis of 19 cases with a unique observation in the pediatric population. Am J Surg Pathol 29(2):204–210
4. Bisogno G, Sotti G, Nowicki Y et al. (2004) Soft tissue sarcoma as a second malignant neoplasm in the pediatric age group. Cancer 100(8):1758–1765
5. Bleyer WA (1993) What can be learned about childhood cancer from *"Cancer statistics review 1973-1988"*?. Cancer 15:3229–3236
6. Borch K, Jacobsen T, Olsen JH, et al (1994) Neonatal cancer in Denmark 1943–1985. Ugeskr Laeger 156:176–179
7. Brouns F, Stas M, De Wever I (2003) Delay in diagnosis of soft tissue sarcomas. Eur J Surg Oncol 29(5):440–445
8. Clasby R, Tilling K, Smith MA, Fletcher CD (1997) Variable management of soft tissue sarcoma: regional audit with implications for specialist care. Br J Surg 84:1692–1696
9. Colon F, Upton J (1995) Pediatric hand tumors. Hand Clin 11:223–243
10. Conrad EU, Bradford L, Chansky HA (1996) Pediatric soft-tissue sarcomas. Orthop Clin North Am 27:655–664
11. Crim J, Seeger L, Yao L, et al (1992) Diagnosis of soft tissue masses with MR imaging: can benign masses be differentiated from malignant ones? Radiology 185:581–586
12. De Maeseneer M, Vande Walle H, Lenchik L, et al. (1998) Subcutaneous granuloma annulare: MR imaging findings. Skeletal Radiol 27:215–217
13. De Schepper A, Ramon F, Degryse H (1992) Statistical analysis of MRI parameters predicting malignancy in 141 soft tissue masses. Rofo Fortschr Geb Rontgenstr Neuen Bildgeb Verfahr 156:587–591
14. De Schepper AMA, Parizel PM, Ramon F, De Beuckeleer L, Vandevenne J (1997) Imaging of soft tissue tumors, 1st edn. Springer, Berlin Heidelberg New York
15. Eary JE, Conrad EU (1999) Positron emission tomography in grading soft tissue sarcomas. Semin Musculoskeletal Radiol 3:135–138
16. Enzinger FM, Weiss SW (1995) Soft tissue tumors, 3rd edn. Mosby, St Louis
17. Fanburg-Smith J (1999) Immunohistochemistry in the evaluation of soft tissue tumors. Semin Musculoskeletal Radiol 3:145–172
18. Fleming ID (1992) Staging of pediatric cancers. Semin Surg Oncol 8:94–97
19. Fletcher BD, Hanna SL (1996) Pediatric musculoskeletal lesions simulating neoplasms. Magn Reson Imaging Clin N Am 4:721–747
20. Fornage B (1999) Soft tissue masses: the underutilization of sonography. Semin Musculoskeletal Radiol 3:115–134
21. Fornage BD, Eftekari F (1989) Sonographic diagnosis of myositis ossificans. J Ultrasound Med 8:463–46
22. Gallego MS, Millan JM, Gil-Martin R, et al. (1987) Juvenile hyalin fibromatosis: radiographic and pathologic findings of a new case. J Med Imaging 1:251–257
23. Garcia-Pena P, Mariscal A, Abellan C, et al. (1999) Juvenile xanthogranuloma with extracutaneous lesions. Pediatr Radiol 22:377–378
24. Ha TV, Kleinman PK, Fraire A, et al. (1994) MR imaging of benign fatty tumors in children: report of four cases and review of the literature. Skeletal Radiol 23:361–367
25. Harms D (1995) New entities, concepts, and questions in childhood tumor pathology. Gen Diagn Pathol 141:1–14
26. Harms D (2004) Soft tissue malignancies in childhood and adolescence. Pathological and clinical relevance based on data from the kiel pediatric tumor registry. Handchir Mikrochir Plast Chir 36(5):268–274
27. Ibarburen C, Haberman JJ, Zerhouni EA (1996) Peripheral primitive neuroectodermal tumors. CT and MRI evaluation. Eur J Radiol 21:225–232
28. Janssens de Varebeke S, De Schepper A, Hauben E, et al. (1996) Subcutaneous diffuse neurofibroma of the neck: a case report. J Laryngol Otol 110:182–184
29. Johnson GL, Baisden BL, Fishman EK (1997) Infantile myofibromatosis. Skeletal Radiol 26:611–614
30. Karabocuoglu M, Baraser N, Aydogan U, et al. (1992) Development of Kasabach-Merritt syndrome following needle aspiration of a hemangioma. Pediatr Emerg Care 8:218–220
31. Khong PL, Chan GC, Shek TW et al. (2002) Imaging of peripheral PNET: common and uncommon locations. Clin Radiol 57(4):272–277
32. Kransdorf M (1995) Malignant soft tissue tumors in a large referral population: distribution of specific diagnoses by age, sex and location. Am J Roentgenol 1995;164:129–134
33. Kransdorf M (1995) Benign soft tissue tumors in a large referral population: distribution of specific diagnoses by age, sex and location. AJR Am J Roentgenol 164:395–402
34. Kransdorf MJ, Murphey MD, Temple HT (1998) Subcutaneous granuloma annulare: radiologic appearance. Skeletal Radiol 27:266–270
35. Laor T, Burrows PE (1998) Congenital anomalies and vascular birthmarks of the lower extremities. Magn Reson Imaging Clin N Am 6:497–519
36. Lawrence W Jr (1994) Soft tissue sarcomas in adults and children: a comparison. CA Cancer J Clin 44:197–199
37. Letson GD, Greenfield GB, Heinrich SD (1996) Evaluation of the child with a bone or soft tissue neoplasm. Orthop Clin North Am 27:431–451

38. Mende U, Ewerbeck V, Krempien B, et al. (1992) Die Sonographie in der therapieorientierten Diagnostik und Nachsorge von primären Knochen- und Weichteiltumoren. Bildgebung 59:4–14
39. Merton DA, Needleman L, Alexander AA, et al. (1992) Lipoblastoma: diagnosis with computed tomography, ultrasonography, and color Doppler imaging. J Ultrasound Med 11:549–552
40. Meyer William H, Spunt Sheri L (2003) Soft tissue sarcomas of childhood. Cancer Treatment Reviews 30(3):269–280
41. Moulton J, Blebea J, Dunco D, et al. (1995) MR imaging of soft tissue masses: diagnostic efficacy and value of distinguishing between benign and malignant lesions. AJR Am J Roentgenol 164:1191–1199
42. Murphey MD, Fairbairn KJ, Parman LM, et al. (1995) From the archives of the AFIP. Musculoskeletal angiomatous lesions: radiologic-pathologic correlation. Radiographics 15:893–917
43. O'Keeffe F, Lorigan JF, Wallace S (1990) Radiological features of extraskeletal Ewing sarcoma. Br J Radiol 63:456–460
44. Ozbek SS, Arkun R, Killi R, et al. (1995) Image-directed color Doppler ultrasonography in the evaluation of superficial solid tumors. J Clin Ultrasound 23:233–238
45. Peabody TD, Simon MA (1996) Making the diagnosis. Keys to a successful biopsy in children with bone and soft-tissue tumors. Orthop Clin North Am 27:453–459
46. Peck RJ, Metreweli C (1988) Early myositis ossificans. Clin Radiol 39:586–588
47. Rubin BP, Fletcher JA, Fletcher MD (1999) Basic concepts in molecular cytogenetics of soft tissue tumors for the clinician. Semin Musculoskeletal Radiol 3:173–182
48. Schankwiler RA, Athey PA, Lamki N (1989) Aggressive infantile fibromatosis. Pulmonary metastases documented by plain film and computed tomography. Clin Imaging 13:127–129
49. Schultz E, Rosenblatt R, Mitsudo S, Weinberg G (1993) Detection of a deep lipoblastoma by MRI and ultrasound. Pediatr Radiol 23:409–410
50. Shapeero LG, Vanel D, Verstraete K, Bloem JL (1999) Dynamic contrast-enhanced MR imaging for soft tissue sarcomas. Semin Musculoskeletal Radiol 3:101–114
51. Solbiati L, Rizzatto G (1995) Ultrasound of superficial structures. High frequencies, Doppler and interventional procedures, 1st edn. Churchill Livingstone, Edinburgh
52. Springfield DS (1994) Staging systems for musculoskeletal neoplasia. Instr Course Lect 43:537–542
53. Stocker JT, Mosijczuk AD (1998) Handling the pediatric tumor. Am J Clin Pathol 109 [(4) Suppl 1]:S1–S3
54. Sundaram M (1999) MR imaging of soft tissue tumors: an overview. Semin Musculoskeletal Radiol 3:15–20
55. Temple HT (1999) Clinical evaluation and treatment of soft tissue tumors. Semin Musculoskeletal Radiol 3:5–14
56. Upton J, Coombs C (1995) Vascular tumors in children. Hand Clin 11:307–337
57. van der Woude HJ, Verstraete KL, Hogendoorn PC, et al. 1998) Musculoskeletal tumors: does fast dynamic contrast-enhanced subtraction MR imaging contribute to the characterization? Radiology 208:821–828
58. Vazquez E, Enriquez G, Castellote A, et al. (1995) US, CT, and MR imaging of neck lesions in children. Radiographics 15:105–122
59. Wolf RE, Enneking WF (1996) The staging and surgery of musculoskeletal neoplasms. Orthop Clin North Am 27:473–481
60. Yang WT, Ahuja A, Metreweli C (1997) Sonographic features of head and neck hemangiomas and vascular malformations: review of 23 patients. J Ultrasound Med 16:39–44

Part 4
Imaging After Treatment

Follow-Up Imaging of Soft Tissue Tumors

28

C.S.P. Van Rijswijk

Contents

28.1 Introduction

Soft tissue sarcomas are a rare and heterogeneous group of sarcomas with variable biology and pattern of recurrence (local and distant). Prognosis of soft tissue sarcoma is dominated by local recurrence and distant metastasis [1]. Approximately one-third of all patients with soft tissue sarcomas will develop local recurrence or distant metastatic disease, with the highest risk in the first few years after treatment; however late recurrences after 5 years do occur [2–4]. The overall survival mainly depends on the development of metastatic disease.

The patterns of recurrence vary with the anatomic site of the primary tumor [5]. Patients with extremity and superficial trunk primaries have a higher predilection for metastases and a lower probability of loco-regional recurrences. In contrast, patients with retroperitoneal or head and neck tumors have a higher tendency towards loco-regional recurrences compared to metastases.

28.2 Loco-regional Recurrence

The benefit of early detection of local recurrence depends on the availability of therapeutic options that can prolong survival. Radical compartmental resection with or without adjuvant radiotherapy and/or chemotherapy may provide long-term salvage in patients with a local recurrence of soft tissue sarcoma [6]. The tendency for local recurrence depends on tumor site, size, grade and adequacy of surgical margins. Although about 2–20 % of all resections will have positive margins and this is a

well-known important risk factor for local recurrence, its impact on overall survival remains controversial [1, 4, 7].

Several guidelines have been recommended for the follow-up of soft tissue sarcoma consisting of a combination of clinical history, physical examination, blood tests, chest radiographs, computed tomography (CT) and magnetic resonance (MR) imaging [8–13]. Most institutions rely on consensus-based guidelines due to the absence of evidence-based guidelines. Surveillance strategies that, through early detection and treatment, improve survival and quality of life while minimizing costs have yet to be identified in randomized clinical trials. Only few studies have been reported on the efficacy of surveillance strategies for the follow-up of soft tissue sarcoma [8, 9, 14]. According to Whooley et al. clinical assessment and physical examination are the most useful tools for evaluating loco-regional recurrence whereas routine MR imaging of the primary tumor site and laboratory blood tests appear ineffective strategies. In a retrospective review of 141 patients they detected by routine surveillance imaging (imaging of primary tumor site was performed on an annual basis) only one

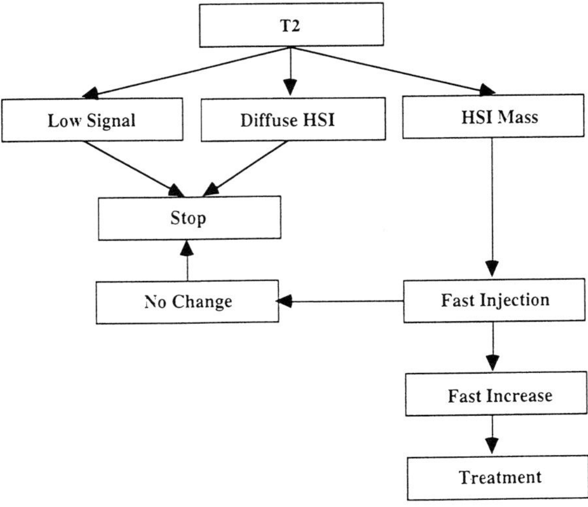

Fig. 28.1. Flowchart of MR imaging in the follow-up of aggressive soft tissue tumors

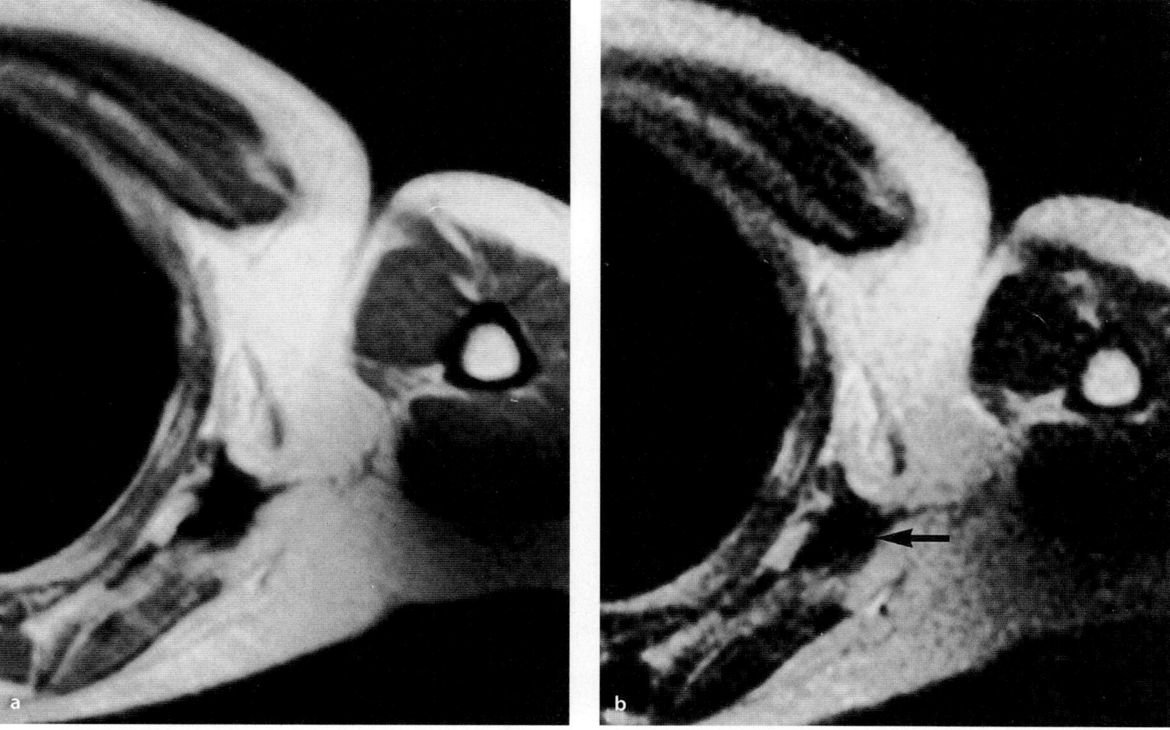

Fig. 28.2 a, b. Malignant soft tissue tumor studied after surgery and radiotherapy in a 30-year-old male: **a** axial T2-weighted MR image shows low signal intensity (*arrow*) indicative of no recurrence; **b** the scar also has low signal on T1-weighted MR image

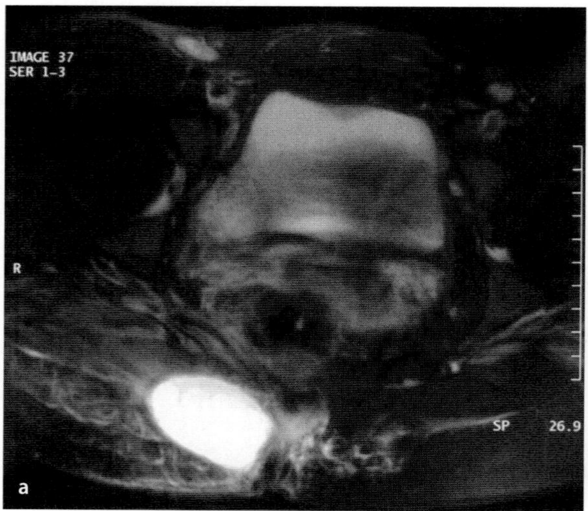

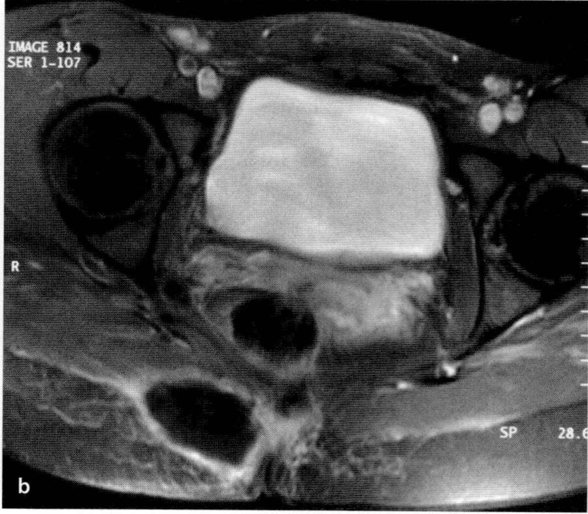

Fig. 28.3 a, b. Three months after resection of desmoid-type fibromatosis of the pelvis in a 26-year-old female: **a** axial T2-weighted MR image shows a well-defined mass with homogeneous high signal intensity; **b** on axial fat suppressed T1-weighted MR image after intravenous administration of gadolinium chelate is only a small rim of enhancement seen consistent with a postoperative seroma that resolved spontaneously

asymptomatic local recurrence; all others were found on physical examination of the primary site [8, 14]. However, MR imaging has shown to be useful in patients in whom physical examination is hampered due to radiotherapy changes.

When indicated, MR imaging is the most useful technique for identifying suspected local recurrence or residual disease after incomplete resection [15]. A T2-weighted MR sequence with fat saturation or short tau inversion recovery (STIR) sequence is considered to be

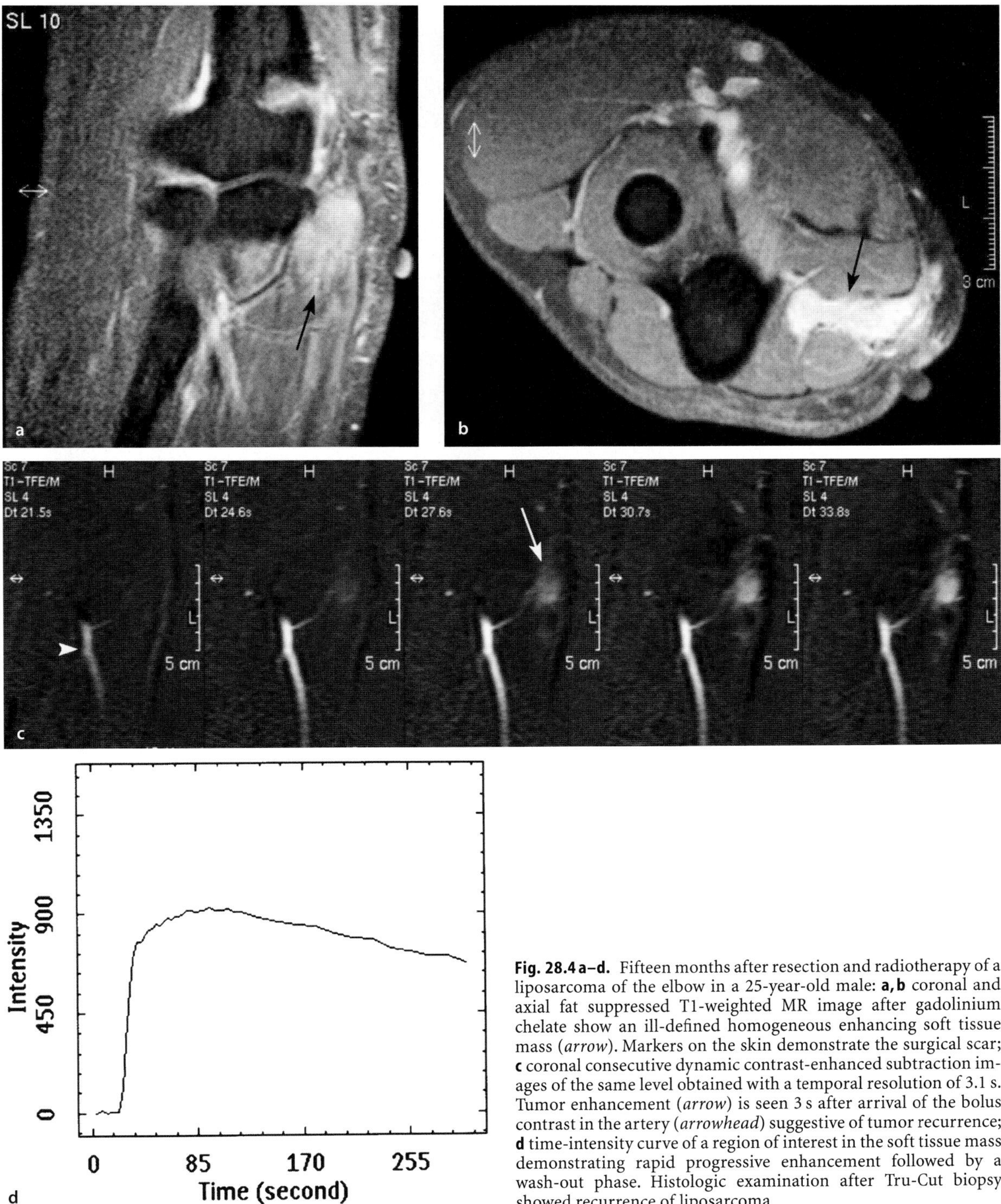

Fig. 28.4 a–d. Fifteen months after resection and radiotherapy of a liposarcoma of the elbow in a 25-year-old male: **a, b** coronal and axial fat suppressed T1-weighted MR image after gadolinium chelate show an ill-defined homogeneous enhancing soft tissue mass (*arrow*). Markers on the skin demonstrate the surgical scar; **c** coronal consecutive dynamic contrast-enhanced subtraction images of the same level obtained with a temporal resolution of 3.1 s. Tumor enhancement (*arrow*) is seen 3 s after arrival of the bolus contrast in the artery (*arrowhead*) suggestive of tumor recurrence; **d** time-intensity curve of a region of interest in the soft tissue mass demonstrating rapid progressive enhancement followed by a wash-out phase. Histologic examination after Tru-Cut biopsy showed recurrence of liposarcoma

the most useful first step for detecting recurrent tumor (Fig. 28.1). The morphology of the lesion and the signal intensity contribute to the definition of its character. Low signal intensity on T2-weighted images or diffuse high signal intensity on T2-weighted images excludes tumor recurrence in 99 % of patients. Mature scar tissue usually exhibits low signal intensity (Fig. 28.2) because of its fibrous tissue content, as described in previous studies. Diffuse high signal intensity with a feather-like appearance, without mass-effect, generally represents post-therapy change or inflammation. High signal intensity mass-like lesions on T2-weighted images require further examination with intravenous gadolinium chelates [16].

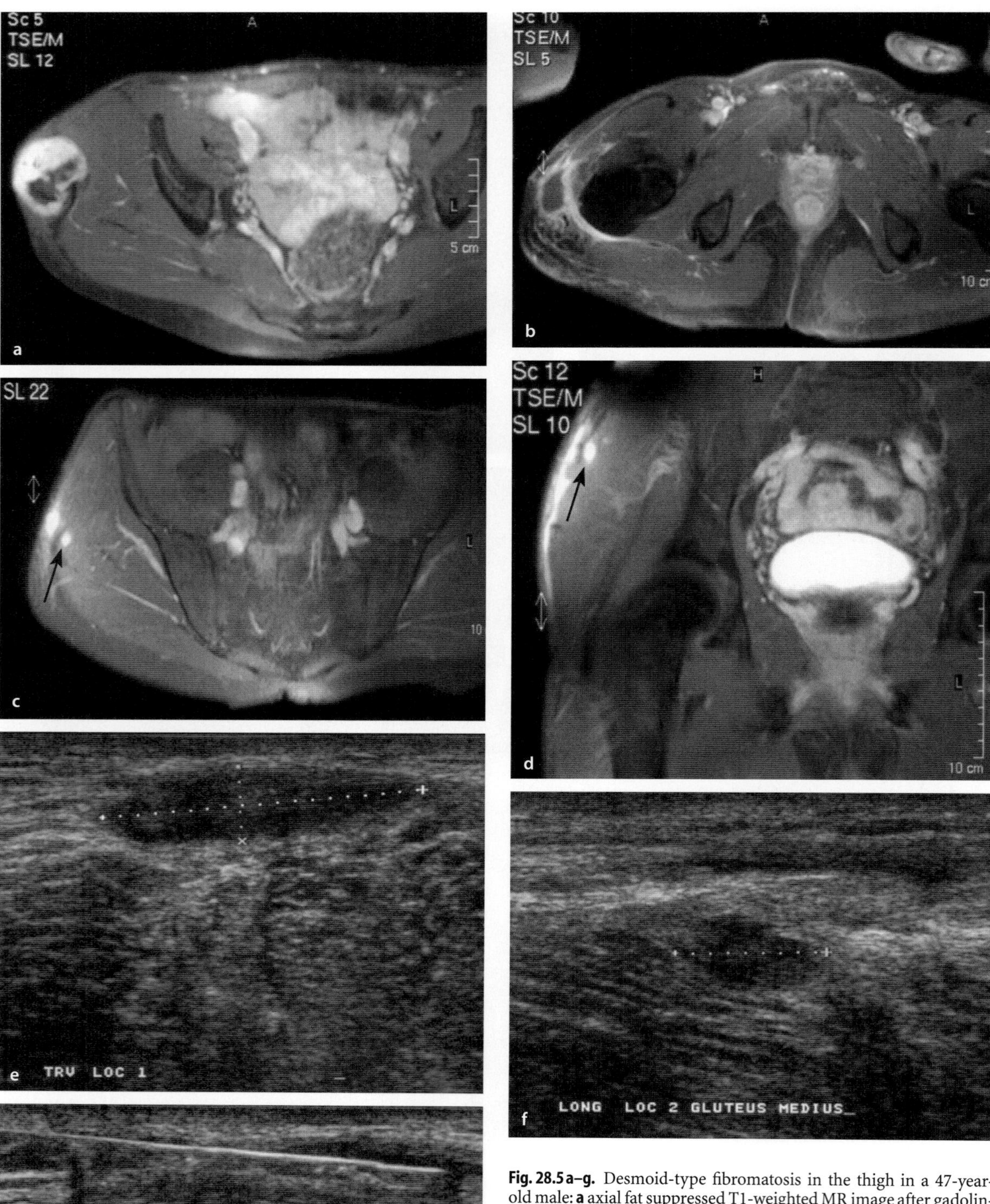

Fig. 28.5 a–g. Desmoid-type fibromatosis in the thigh in a 47-year-old male: **a** axial fat suppressed T1-weighted MR image after gadolinium chelate. The relatively well-defined soft tissue mass shows inhomogeneous enhancement. The non-enhancing area demonstrated low signal intensity on all pulse sequences; **b** three months after resection, axial fat suppressed T1-weighted MR image after gadolinium chelate reveals a postoperative seroma; **c,d** twelve months after resection, axial and coronal fat suppressed T1-weighted MR image after gadolinium chelate. Spontaneous regression of the postoperative seroma but appearance of new small intramuscular enhancing nodules suggestive of multifocal recurrence (*arrow*); **e,f** the nodules were identified on ultrasound as hypoechoic soft tissue masses; **g** ultrasound guided histological Tru-Cut biopsy was performed and recurrence of desmoid-type fibromatosis was confirmed

Standard T1-weighted spin echo sequences after contrast medium injection (gadolinium chelates) can be used to distinguish non-enhancing post-therapy hygroma, seroma or hematoma from enhancing tumor recurrence, post-therapy fibrosis, granulation tissue or inflammatory masses (Fig. 28.3). Absence of contrast enhancement indicates no recurrent tumor. On these standard contrast-enhanced images, the differentiation between recurrent viable tumor and post-therapy fibrosis or inflammatory pseudomasses may remain difficult. However, in these cases dynamic contrast-enhanced MR imaging may prove helpful. Dynamic contrast-enhanced MR imaging allows differentiation between inflammation and recurrent or residual tumor. After a rapid bolus injection of contrast, viable tumor exhibits rapid progressive increase of signal intensity followed by wash out or plateau phase whereas the signal from inflammatory changes will also increase but later [17] (Fig. 28.4).

Each case of a suspicious (recurrent) mass should be treated as if it is a new sarcoma. Confirmation should be obtained by cytological sampling or core-needle (Tru-Cut or Jamshidi) biopsy after loco-regional re-staging by MR imaging. Histological biopsy should always be performed after MR imaging because reactive changes hemorrhage and edema secondary to biopsy may hamper interpretation of MR images and therefore interfere with staging.

Preliminary studies of positron emission tomography (PET) demonstrate the potential of PET with FDG as an additional tool for detecting local recurrence of soft tissue sarcoma. Moreover, PET seems particularly useful in patients with extensive histories of surgery and radiation therapy; in the setting in which MR imaging interpretation can be difficult [18, 19].

Desmoid-type fibromatoses are benign fibroblastic proliferations that arise in the deep soft tissues and are characterized by infiltrative growth in the surrounding soft tissue structures and the absence of a pseudocapsule. Local recurrence is frequent and often related to the adequacy of surgical resections. Routine follow-up MR imaging of patients with desmoid-type fibromatosis seems justified not only to detect (often asymptomatic) local recurrence but also to evaluate the natural behavior of these lesions [20] (Fig. 28.5).

28.3 Metastases

Early detection of pulmonary metastases is an important component of surveillance because the overall survival of sarcoma patients mainly depends on the development of distant metastases (Fig. 28.6). Metastatic spread is found predominantly in the lungs, and about 70% of all patients who develop metastases will have distant disease confined to the lungs [21]. Pulmonary metastasectomy is considered a standard practice since there is indeed a small population that can be cured. Whooley et al. studied the cost-effectiveness of chest radiograph surveillance in primary soft tissue sarcomas in a retrospective analysis. They proved the utility of chest radiograph surveillance on the basis of a review of 74 patients with first recurrence confined to the lungs (79% of all first recurrences). Although chest CT is recommended as part of the staging evaluation for all patients with high-grade soft tissue sarcomas due to higher sensitivity than chest radiographs, the role of CT in the surveillance of metastatic disease has not been invested yet. However, extrapolations of results of chest CT at time of initial staging didn't demonstrate cost-effectiveness of routine use of surveillance chest CT over chest radiographs when the risk of pulmonary metastatic disease was low (thus in low-grade tumors) [9, 22].

Things to remember:
1. Although only few studies have been reported on post-treatment surveillance, intensive observation by clinical history, physical examination and chest radiographs (and cross-sectional MR imaging and chest CT when indicated) seems to be an effective follow-up approach in patients with soft tissue sarcoma. A rational and practical surveillance algorithm should include routine office visits (with clinical assessment and chest radiograph) every four months for two years, every six months for three years, and then annually. Additional MR imaging should be performed based upon the reliability of physical examination and suspicion for deep-seated recurrence in perspective of patient risk stratification. Subsequently, patients with retroperitoneal and head or neck soft tissue sarcoma may require MR imaging for routine follow-up.
2. The use of MR imaging as a surveillance method for early detecting loco-regional recurrences before clinical symptoms requires further prospective studies. When indicated MR imaging is the method of choice for re-staging loco-regional recurrence. The evaluation of soft tissue sarcoma or aggressive soft tissue tumors in the follow up should begin with a T2-weighted sequence. If there is a mass with high signal intensity on T2-weighted MR images additional contrast-enhanced MR sequences should be used to differentiate recurrent tumor from postoperative granulation tissue.

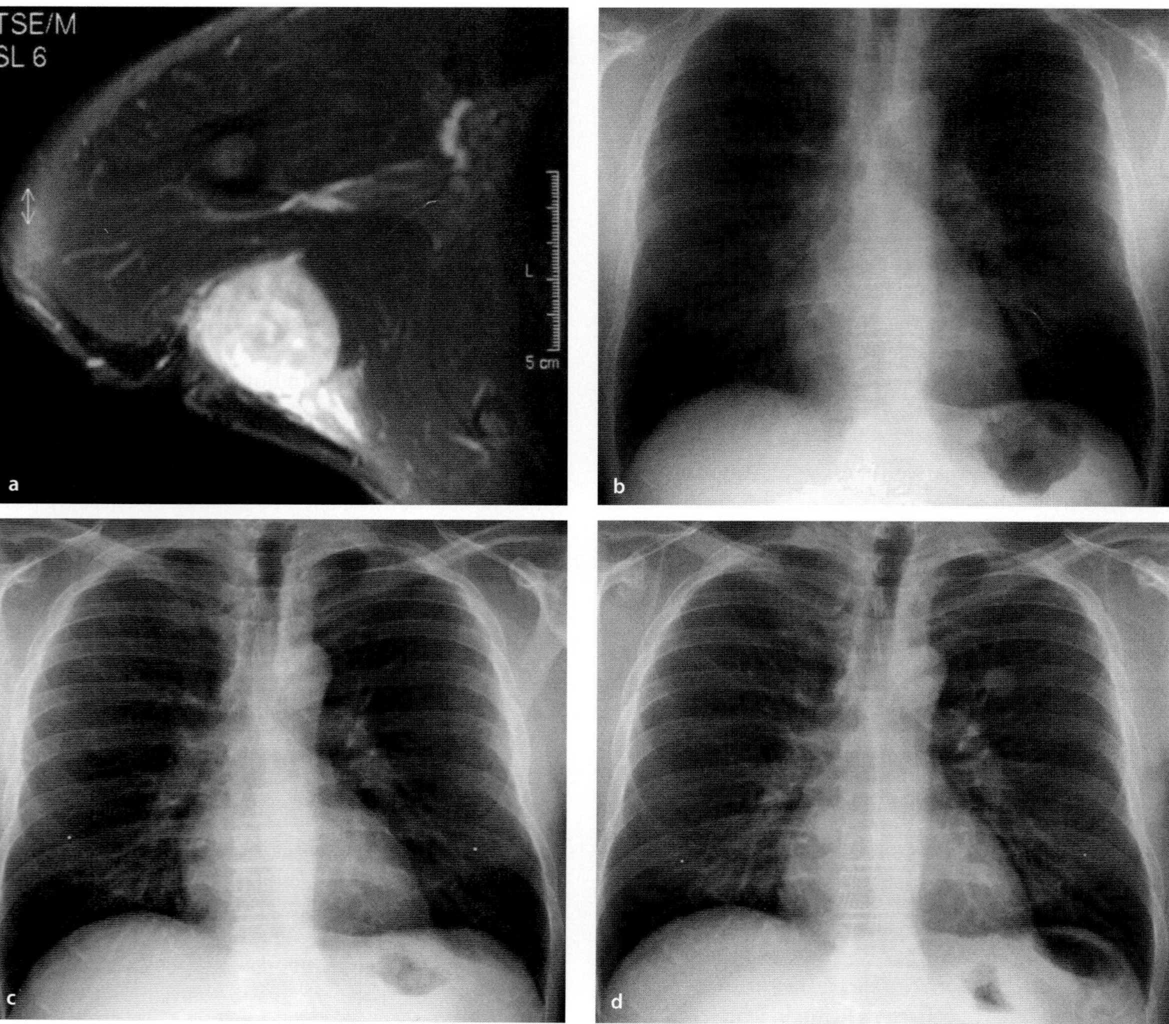

Fig. 28.6a–d. Myxofibrosarcoma of the axilla in a 42-year-old man: **a** fat suppressed axial T2-weighted MR image of the axilla. Staging chest CT at time of diagnosis demonstrated no lung metastases; **b** three weeks after resection, normal chest radi-ograph; **c** three months after resection, normal chest radiograph; **d** six months after resection, a new solitary lung nodule in the left upper lobe is demonstrated. Metastasectomy was performed

References

1. Zagars GK, Ballo MT, Pisters PW et al. (2003) Prognostic factors for patients with localized soft-tissue sarcoma treated with conservation surgery and radiation therapy: an analysis of 225 patients. Cancer 97(10):2530–2543
2. Huth JF, Eilber FR (1988) Patterns of metastatic spread following resection of extremity soft-tissue sarcomas and strategies for treatment. Semin Surg Oncol 4(1):20–26
3. Gibbs JF, Lee RJ, Driscoll DL, McGrath BE, Mindell ER, Kraybill WG (2000) Clinical importance of late recurrence in soft-tissue sarcomas. J Surg Oncol 73(2):81–86
4. Lewis JJ, Leung D, Casper ES, Woodruff J, Hajdu SI, Brennan MF (1999) Multifactorial analysis of long-term follow-up (more than 5 years) of primary extremity sarcoma. Arch Surg 134(2):190–194
5. Gerrand CH, Bell RS, Wunder JS et al. (2003) The influence of anatomic location on outcome in patients with soft tissue sarcoma of the extremity. Cancer 97(2):485–492
6. Singer S, Antman K, Corson JM, Eberlein TJ (1992) Long-term salvageability for patients with locally recurrent soft-tissue sarcomas. Arch Surg 127(5):548–553
7. Trovik CS, Bauer HC, Alvegard TA et al. (2000) Surgical margins, local recurrence and metastasis in soft tissue sarcomas: 559 surgically-treated patients from the Scandinavian Sarcoma Group Register. Eur J Cancer 36(6):710–716
8. Whooley BP, Gibbs JF, Mooney MM, McGrath BE, Kraybill WG (2000) Primary extremity sarcoma: what is the appropriate follow-up? Ann Surg Oncol 7(1):9–14
9. Kane JM III (2004) Surveillance strategies for patients following surgical resection of soft tissue sarcomas. Curr Opin Oncol 16(4):328–332
10. Patel SR, Zagars GK, Pisters PW (2003) The follow-up of adult soft-tissue sarcomas. Semin Oncol 30(3):413–416
11. Beitler AL, Virgo KS, Johnson FE, Gibbs JF, Kraybill WG (2000) Current follow-up strategies after potentially curative resection of extremity sarcomas: results of a survey of the members of the society of surgical oncology. Cancer 88(4):777–785
12. Davies AM, Vanel D (1998) Follow-up of musculoskeletal tumors. I. Local recurrence. Eur Radiol 8(5):791–799

13. Goel A, Christy ME, Virgo KS, Kraybill WG, Johnson FE (2004) Costs of follow-up after potentially curative treatment for extremity soft-tissue sarcoma. Int J Oncol 25(2):429–435
14. Whooley BP, Mooney MM, Gibbs JF, Kraybill WG (1999) Effective follow-up strategies in soft tissue sarcoma. Semin Surg Oncol 17(1):83–87
15. Vanel D, Lacombe MJ, Couanet D, Kalifa C, Spielmann M, Genin J (1987) Musculoskeletal tumors: follow-up with MR imaging after treatment with surgery and radiation therapy. Radiology 164(1):243–245
16. Panicek DM, Schwartz LH, Heelan RT, Caravelli JF (1995) Non-neoplastic causes of high signal intensity at T2-weighted MR imaging after treatment for musculoskeletal neoplasm. Skeletal Radiol 24(3):185–190
17. Vanel D, Shapeero LG, Tardivon A, Western A, Guinebretiere JM (1998) Dynamic contrast-enhanced MRI with subtraction of aggressive soft tissue tumors after resection. Skeletal Radiol 27(9):505–510
18. Kole AC, Nieweg OE, van Ginkel RJ et al. (1997) Detection of local recurrence of soft-tissue sarcoma with positron emission tomography using [18F]fluorodeoxyglucose. Ann Surg Oncol 4(1):57–63
19. Johnson GR, Zhuang H, Khan J, Chiang SB, Alavi A (2003) Role of positron emission tomography with fluorine-18-deoxyglucose in the detection of local recurrent and distant metastatic sarcoma. Clin Nucl Med 28(10):815–820
20. Vandevenne JE, De Schepper AM, De Beuckeleer L et al. (1997) New concepts in understanding evolution of desmoid tumors: MR imaging of 30 lesions. Eur Radiol 7(7):1013–1019
21. Billingsley KG, Lewis JJ, Leung DH, Casper ES, Woodruff JM, Brennan MF (1999) Multifactorial analysis of the survival of patients with distant metastasis arising from primary extremity sarcoma. Cancer 85(2):389–395
22. Fleming JB, Cantor SB, Varma DG et al. (2001) Utility of chest computed tomography for staging in patients with T1 extremity soft tissue sarcomas. Cancer 92(4):863–868

Subject Index